ATLAS OF PEDIATRIC EMERGENCY MEDICINE

ATLAS OF PEDIATRIC EMERGENCY MEDICINE

Binita R. Shah, MD, FAAP

Professor of Emergency Medicine
Professor of Pediatrics
Departments of Emergency Medicine and Pediatrics
SUNY Downstate Medical Center
Brooklyn, New York

Director
Pediatric Emergency Medicine
Department of Emergency Medicine
Kings County Hospital Center
Brooklyn, New York

Michael Lucchesi, MD, FACEP

Associate Professor of Emergency Medicine
Department of Emergency Medicine
SUNY Downstate Medical Center
Brooklyn, New York

Chairman
Department of Emergency Medicine
SUNY Downstate Medical Center
University Hospital of Brooklyn
Kings County Hospital Center
Brooklyn, New York

The McGraw-Hill Companies
MEDICAL PUBLISHING DIVISION

New York Chicago San Francisco Lisbon London Madrid Mexico City
Milan New Delhi San Juan Seoul Singapore Sydney Toronto

The McGraw·Hill Companies

ATLAS OF PEDIATRIC EMERGENCY MEDICINE

1 2 3 4 5 6 7 8 9 0 CTP/CTP 0 9 8 7 6

ISBN: 0-07-138713-7

This book was set in Times Roman by TechBooks.
The editors were Andrea Seils, Karen Edmonson, and Regina Y. Brown.
The production supervisor was Catherine Saggese.
The cover designer was Pehrsson Design.
China Translation & Printing Services Ltd. was printer and binder.

DEDICATION

To my children

Ronak Shah, MD and **Toral Shah, BS, PA-C**

For bringing me the unparalleled joy of motherhood and for carrying the "torch" of serving humanity through the practice of medicine.

and

To my husband

Rajni P. Shah, MD

For his unconditional love, unflinching encouragement, and serving as my backbone in pursuit of my professional career.

and

To my mother

Chanchalben

It is because of her perseverance and intense desire that I became a physician.

Binita R. Shah, MD

To my parents

Ann and **John**

Who have always believed in me more than I have ever believed in myself.

and

To my children

Michael, Jessica and **John**

For being the reason why I drag myself out of bed each morning and the reason why I rush home each night.

and

To my wife

Kim

Who has stood by me with faith, love and encouragement throughout my entire career.

Michael Lucchesi, MD

CONTENTS

CHILD MALTREATMENT
Chapter 1

Binita R. Shah

CONDITIONS MISTAKEN FOR CHILD ABUSE AND SEXUAL ABUSE
Chapter 2

Binita R. Shah

INFECTIOUS DISEASES
Chapter 3

Binita R. Shah

CONTRIBUTING AUTHORS

M. Douglas Baker, MD
Professor of Pediatrics
Yale University School of Medicine
Chief, Pediatric Emergency Medicine
Yale-New Haven Children's Hospital
New Haven, Connecticut
Chapter 18

Bonny Baron, MD
Associate Professor of Emergency Medicine
Department of Emergency Medicine
SUNY Downstate Medical Center
Kings County Hospital Center
Brooklyn, New York
Chapter 20

Geetha Chari, MD
Assistant Professor of Neurology
Division of Pediatric Neurology and Clinical Neurophysiology
Department of Neurology
SUNY Downstate Medical Center
Kings County Hospital Center
Brooklyn, New York
Chapter 13
Figure 13-21

Ayman Chritah, DDS, MD
Oral and Maxillofacial Surgeon
Jacobi Medical Center
Bronx, New York
Chapter 20

Mert Erogul, MD
Director, Essential of Clinical Medicine I
SUNY Downstate College of Medicine
Assistant Professor of Emergency Medicine
Department of Emergency Medicine
SUNY Downstate Medical Center
Kings County Hospital Center
Brooklyn, New York
Chapter 8

Kumarie Etwaru, MD
Director, Division of Pediatric Emergency Medicine
Beth Israel Medical Center
New York, New York
Chapter 17

Irma Fiordalisi, MD
Professor of Pediatrics
Head, Section of Pediatric Critical Care
Brody School of Medicine, East Carolina University
Director, Pediatric Intensive Care Unit and Sedation Services
Children's Hospital, University Health Systems of Eastern North Carolina
Greenville, North Carolina
Chapter 14
Figure 14-1
Figure 17-11, 17-13 A and B

Radha Giridharan, MD
Assistant Professor of Neurology
Division of Pediatric Neurology
SUNY Downstate Medical Center
Kings County Hospital Center
Brooklyn, New York
Chapter 13

Glenn D. Harris, MD
Professor of Pediatrics
Director of Pediatric Diabetology
Section of Endocrinology
Brody School of Medicine, East Carolina University
Greenville, North Carolina
Chapter 14
Figure 14-1

Robert J. Hoffman, MD
Director of Research
Department of Emergency Medicine
Beth Israel Medical Center
New York, New York
Chapter 17
Figures 17-5, 17-6 A and B, 17-22 A and B, 17-23 A and B 17-24 A and B

Lewis Kohl, DO
Chairman, Department of Emergency Medicine
Long Island College Hospital
Assistant Professor of Emergency Medicine
SUNY Downstate Medical Center
Brooklyn, New York
Chapter 18
Figure 18-19 to Figure 18-26
Figure 18-30 to Figure 18-37
Figure 18-39 and Figure 18-40

David Listman, MD
Attending, Pediatric Emergency Medicine
Department of Pediatrics
Saint Barnabas Hospital
Bronx, New York
Chapter 20

Kevin J. McSherry, MD
Assistant Professor of Pediatrics
Department of Emergency Medicine
Mount Sinai School of Medicine
New York, NY
Chapter 20

Scott Miller, MD
Director, Pediatric In-patient Services
Department of Pediatrics
Professor of Clinical Pediatrics
SUNY Downstate Medical Center
Brooklyn, New York
Chapter 11

Peter Peacock, MD
Assistant Professor of Emergency Medicine
Department of Emergency Medicine
SUNY Downstate Medical Center
Kings County Hospital Center
Informatics Director, Emergency Medicine Physicians of Brooklyn
Brooklyn, New York
Chapter 9

Eileen C. Quintana, MD, MPH
Assistant Professor of Pediatrics and Emergency Medicine
Drexel University College of Medicine
Hahnemann University Hospital
St. Christopher Hospital for Children
Philadelphia, PA
Chapter 20

Sreedhar P. Rao, MD
Director, Pediatric Hematology and Oncology
Department of Pediatrics
Professor of Clinical Pediatrics
Department of Pediatrics
SUNY Downstate Medical Center
Brooklyn, New York
Chapter 11
Figures 8-16 A and B

Sudha M. Rao, MD
Director, Pediatric Cardiology
Kings County Hospital Center, Brooklyn, New York
Clinical Associate Professor of Pediatrics
New York University School of Medicine
New York, New York
Editor, Chapter 5
Figures 5-6, 5-8 B, 5-22, 12-1 and 12-11

Sarah Rawstron, MD
Director, Pediatric Residency Program
The Brooklyn Hospital Center
Adjunct Assistant Professor of Pediatrics and Medicine
SUNY Downstate Medical Center
Brooklyn, New York
Chapter 4

Karen A. Santucci, MD
Associate Professor of Pediatrics
Yale University School of Medicine
Medical Director, Pediatric Emergency Medicine
Yale-New Haven Children's Hospital
New Haven, Connecticut
Chapters 18 and 20

Ronak R. Shah, MD
Assistant Professor of Emergency Medicine
Staten Island University Hospital
SUNY Downstate Medical Center
Brooklyn, New York
Chapters 17 and 18
Figures 2-13 A, B and Figure 9-3

Anup Singh, MD
Associate Professor of Pediatrics
Drexel University College of Medicine
Chief, Division of Pediatric Nephrology
The Children's Hospital
St. Peter's University Hospital
New Brunswick, NJ
Chapter 16

Mark Spektor, DO
Director, Emergency Services, Brooklyn VA Hospital
Assistant Professor of Emergency Medicine
Department of Emergency Medicine
SUNY Downstate Medical Center
Brooklyn, New York
Chapter 9
Figure 8-18

Karen L. Stavile, MD
Assistant Director, Adult Emergency Services
Kings County Hospital Center
Assistant Professor of Emergency Medicine
Department of Emergency Medicine
SUNY Downstate Medical Center
Brooklyn, New York
Chapter 20

Amy Suss, MD
Director, Division of Adolescent Medicine
Associate Director, Pediatric Residency Program
Associate Professor of Clinical Pediatrics
Department of Pediatrics
SUNY Downstate Medical Center
Brooklyn, New York
Chapter 4

Mark Su, MD
Director of Toxicology and Assistant Residency Director
Department of Emergency Medicine
Assistant Professor of Emergency Medicine
SUNY Downstate Medical Center
Kings County Hospital Center
Brooklyn, New York
Chapter 17
Figures 17-8, 17-9, 17-10, 17-30 A and B, 17-31 A and B

Joseph A. Sykes, MD, FAAP
Pediatric Critical Care Attending
Newark Beth Israel Medical Center
Newark, New Jersey
Chapter 13

David Tran, MD
Assistant Professor of Emergency Medicine
Department of Emergency Medicine
SUNY Downstate Medical Center
Kings County Hospital Center
Brooklyn, New York
Chapter 15

PHOTOGRAPHY AND RADIOGRAPHY CREDITS

Angela Anderson, MD
Associate Professor of Emergency Medicine and Pediatrics
Department of Emergency Medicine
Brown University
Attending Physician
Hasbro Children's Hospital
Providence, Rhode Island
Figure 17-18

Mona Baidwan, MD
Attending Physician
Baidwan Medical Clinic
Winnipeg, Manitoba, Canada
Figure 7-2

Daniel Cooperman, MD
Professor of Orthopaedic Surgery
Department of Orthopaedic Surgery
Case Western Reserve University
University Hospitals of Cleveland
Cleveland, Ohio
Figure 1-10

Pamela Diamantis, MD
Clinical Instructor of Pediatrics
Jacobi Medical Center
Bronx, New York
Figure 2-9

Eugene Dinkevich, MD
Assistant Professor of Pediatrics
SUNY Downstate Medical Center
Brooklyn, New York
Figures 8-14 A and B

Ingrid Dodard, MD
Pediatrician; Mid Hudson Medical Group
Poughkeepsie and Fishkill
New York
Figure 3-50

Mario Eddy Dumas, MD MS FCCP
Assistant Professor of Pediatrics
Division of Pediatric Pulmonary Medicine
University of Sherbrooke School of Medicine
Sherbrooke, Quebec, Canada
Figures 6-4 B and C

Christine Eskenazi, RN
Kings County Hospital Center
Brooklyn, New York
Figure 19-4

Rachael George, MD
Assistant Professor of Emergency Medicine
SUNY Downstate Medical Center
Kings County Hospital Center
Brooklyn, New York
Figure 8-11

Howard Greller, MD
Fellow, Medical Toxicology
New York University / Bellevue Hospital Center
New York City Poison Control Center
New York, New York
Figure 17-26 A and B

Barry Hahn, MD
Assistant Professor of Emergency Medicine
Staten Island University Hospital
SUNY Downstate Medical Center
Brooklyn, New York
Figure 5-8 A and Figure 19-48

Alexander, Imas MD
Pain Management and Rehab Assoc.
Farmington Hills, Michigan
Figure 1-7 A and Figure 1-8 A

Ernesto Jose Jule, MD
Assistant Professor of Emergency Medicine
SUNY Downstate Medical Center
Kings County Hospital Center
Brooklyn, New York
Figure 2-23 and Figure 5-12

Raffi S. Kapitanyan, MD
Emergency Medicine Resident
Department of Emergency Medicine
SUNY Downstate Medical Center
Brooklyn, New York
Figure 19-63 A

Pascale Kersaint, MD
Clinical Assistant Instructor
Department of Pediatrics
SUNY Downstate Medical Center
Brooklyn, New York
Figure 12-9

James G. Linakis, MD
Associate Professor of Emergency Medicine & Pediatrics
Departments of Emergency Medicine and Pediatrics
Brown Medical School
Rhode Island Hospital/Hasbro Children's Hospital
Figure 17-7

Yulianna Kandalina
Ultrasound Technician
Department of Radiology
Staten Island University Hospital
Staten Island, New York
Figure 4-23

Ambreen Khan, MD
Assistant Professor of Emergency Medicine
SUNY Downstate Medical Center
Kings County Hospital Center
Brooklyn, New York
Figure 6-20

Smita Kumar, MD, MPH
Resident, Preventive Medicine
SUNY Stony Brook University Medical Center
New York
Figure 1-4 B

Teresita A. Laude, M.D.
Retired pediatrician and Dermatologist
Staten Island, NY
Figures 7-3, 7-23, 7-38 A, 7-50, 7-54, 7-57, 7-59 and 7-62
Figures 12-12 A and B

Cedma Mark
Pre-hospital Training Coordinator
Department of Emergency Medicine
Kings County Hospital Center
Brooklyn, New York
Figure 17-19

Swati Mehta, M.D.
Clinical Assistant Professor of Pediatrics
Department of Pediatrics
SUNY Downstate Medical Center
Kings County Hospital Center
Brooklyn, New York
Figure 2-25 and Figure 14-5

Andrew Miller, MD
Clinical Assistant Instructor
Department of Emergency Medicine
SUNY at Buffalo School of Medicine
Buffalo, NY
Figures 19-69 A and B

Hiren Muzumdar, MD
Assistant Professor of Pediatrics
Department of Pediatrics
SUNY Downstate Medical Center
Brooklyn, New York
Figures 6-13 A and B

Patricia A. O'Neill, MD
Associate Professor of Surgery
Co-Chief, Division of Trauma and Surgical Critical Care
SUNY Downstate Medical Center
Kings County Hospital Center
Brooklyn, New York
Figure 20-36 and Figure 20-37

Chandrakant Rao, MD
Clinical Associate Professor
Department of Pathology
SUNY Downstate Medical Center
Kings County Hospital Center
Brooklyn, New York
Figure 13-4 and Figure 13-5

Dilip Sen, MD
Assistant Professor of Emergency Medicine
SUNY Downstate Medical Center
Kings County Hospital Center
Brooklyn, New York
Figure 15-10 B

Itchak Schwarzbard, MD
Senior Resident
Department of Orthopedic Surgery
SUNY Downstate Medical Center
Kings County Hospital Center
Brooklyn, New York
Figures 19-67 B and C

Kunal R. Shah, MD
Senior Resident
Department of Pediatrics
UMDNJ-Robert Wood Johnson
Bristol Myers Squibb Children's Hospital
New Brunswick, New Jersey
Figure 11-8

Vikas S. Shah, MD
Pediatric Critical Care Fellow
New York-Presbyterian
Weill Cornell Medical Center
New York, New York
Figure 13-17 and Figure 17-32

Haseeb A. Siddiqi, Ph.D.
Director, Diagnostic Immunology and Clinical Parasitology Laboratories
Kings County Hospital Center
Associate Professor
Departments of Medicine, Pathology, Microbiology and Immunology
SUNY Downstate Medical Center
Brooklyn, New York
Figures 3-68 A and B

Phillip Steiner, MD
Professor Emeritus
Department of Pediatrics
SUNY Downstate Medical Center
Brooklyn, New York
Figures 6-17, 6-18 and 6-19 A, B , C

Michael Stracher, MD
Assistant Professor of Orthopedic Surgery
Department of Orthopedic Surgery
SUNY Downstate Medical Center
Brooklyn, New York
Figure 2-16, Figure 10-23 and Figure 18-8

SPECIAL RADIOGRAPHY CREDITS

(For Contributing Radiographs and Writing Legends):

Sudha Chala, MD
Staten Island University Hospital
Assistant Professor of Radiology
SUNY Downstate Medical Center
Brooklyn, New York
Figures 1-9 A, B and C
All the radiography legends in chapters Child Maltreatment, Cardiology, Respiratory Disorders and Gastrointestinal disorders

Zinn Daniel, MD
Assistant Professor of Radiology
SUNY Downstate Medical Center
Kings County Hospital Center
Brooklyn, New York
Figures 10-16, 10-18 B and C and accompanying legends

William Fischer, MD
Visiting Clinical Associate Professor of Radiology
Department of Diagnostic Radiology
SUNY Downstate Medical Center
Brooklyn, New York
Figures 10-1, 10-2, 10-5 and 10-6 and accompanying legends

Kedar Jambhekar, MD
Intructor in Radiology
University of Arkansas for Medical Sciences
Little Rock, Arkansas
Figures 10-8 A and B, 12-6 B, 13-19, 13-22 D to F and accompanying legends
All the radiography legends in chapters Sexual Abuse, Gynecology and Sexually Transmitted Diseases, Ophthalmology, Otolaryngology, Hematology, Rheumatology, Neurology and Toxicology

PREFACE

The advantage of working in an environment with a plethora of clinical pathology is that one's ability at visual diagnosis becomes finely tuned. Armed with a digital camera and a consent form, an enthusiastic clinician can quickly build a library of educational material in the form of clinical pictures, radiographic images and fascinating stories.

The demands of increasing productivity, decreasing reimbursement from the third party payers and increasing numbers of patients, have led to the training of a generation of physicians who spend their time deciding what tests to order instead of observing and examining their patients. The art of visual diagnosis is an endangered species. The luxury of pondering over a diagnosis with exciting anticipation of the outcome no longer exists. Where once the bedside experience was the highlight of our clinical day, the "art" has been replaced by mechanics. Our trainees are being schooled in processing flow and survival mode ideation.

Sir William Osler once wrote: "Avoid the common and fatal facility of reaching conclusions from superficial observations and being constantly misled by the ease with which our minds fall into the ruts of one or two experiences." The more patients one sees and examines the better one becomes at forming a concise differential diagnosis prior to ordering an expensive, time consuming and often invasive work up. The student of visual diagnosis is not only more likely to make the right diagnosis, but is also more likely to avoid the costly error. We urge our fellow physicians to hold on to the art. By perfecting the tools we were born with and supplementing them with those which we developed, we will continue to have pride in what we do, love our patients and enjoy our careers.

We have made an attempt to write this *Atlas* in the simplest, most understandable and most user friendly manner for the clinicians. Unlike the other books of this type, this *Atlas* features a *consistent format*. The images are presented in the medical sections with a *Definition followed by Etiology, Associated Clinical Features including* appropriate l*aboratory* work-up and *Consultation*. The typical *Clinical Features and Differential Diagnosis* are presented in a box format to provide at -a-glance review of essential diagnostic information. The *Emergency Department Treatment and Disposition* are then emphasized. Each entity ends with *Clinical Pearls* highlighting all the most important "need-to-know" take home clinical information. *Epidemiology, pathophysiology, pharmacokinetics* and toxicity are discussed as indicated. The orthopedic and trauma sections begin with *Mechanism of Injury* followed by *Associated Clinical Features, Consultation, Complications, Emergency Department Treatment and Disposition*. Once again a box format is used for the ease of reference and a quick review highlighting *Clinical Features, Differential Diagnosis or Clinical Pearls*.

This *Atlas* is intended to assist the busy clinician in diagnosis, work-up and disposition. It was written for anyone who steps foot into a Pediatric Emergency Department and has the privilege of taking care of children. It is also the hope of the authors that the experiences we have had and the images we have captured will stimulate the clinicians who are starting their careers to never stop asking questions, always strive to improve the art of visual diagnosis, work on eliminating any fear of patient contact and never stop learning from your patients.

Ars longa vita brevis (Translation: Art is long while life is short). With this quote, Hippocrates reminds us how much there is to learn in a short period and thereby (hopefully) inspire us to be humble, scholarly and better doctors.

Michael Lucchesi, MD

Binita R. Shah, MD

SPECIAL ACKNOWLEDGEMENT

Michael H. Siegel, MD
Clinical Assistant Professor
Department of Diagnostic Radiology
SUNY Downstate Medical Center
Kings County Hospital Center
Brooklyn, New York

Figures 19-55 A and B, 20-15 B to E, 20-16 A and B, 20-17, 20-18 A and B, 20-19 A and B, 20-20 B, 20-25 A to F, 20-26, 20-27, 20-29 A and B, 20-32, 20-33, 20-34

We would like to extend our special thanks to Dr. Siegel. This Atlas could not have been possible without his help. This incredible physician has spent his career at Kings County Hospital, one of the busiest emergency departments in the country. His library of images and teaching files are second to none. This is not what makes him the best emergency radiologist on the face of the planet. What makes this physician unique is his relationship with his emergency medicine colleagues and his frequency and enthusiasm to come to the bedside and see the patient himself. He is a wealth of knowledge, a priceless resource, a respected colleague and a friend. Thank you Mike.

Mark Silverberg, MD, FACEP
Director, Fourth Year Medical Student's Emergency Medicine Rotation
SUNY Downstate College of Medicine
Assistant Professor of Emergency Medicine
Assistant Residency Director
Department of Emergency Medicine
SUNY Downstate Medical Center
Kings County Hospital Center
Brooklyn, New York

Figure 3-1, 3-67, Figures 19-26 A, 19-50 C, 19-62 A, 19-64 A and B
Figures 20-1, 20-3 B, 20-3 D, 20-5, 20-6, 20-29 C, 20-30, 20-31, 20-38, 20-39, 20-41 A, B and C

We would like to thank Dr. Silverberg for contributing multiple images to this Atlas. As a member of our faculty, Mark is often seen dashing through the ED with a consent form and a camera in the hand. This physician is more than a student of a visual diagnosis; he is a master of it.

Charles A. Catanese, MD
Medical Examiner, New York City, New York
Clinical Assistant Professor of Pathology
Department of Pathology
SUNY Downstate Medical Center
Kings County Hospital Center
Brooklyn, New York

Figures 1-2, 1-5 A and B, 1-12, 1-15, 1-16 A, 1-19 A and B, 1-25 B and C, 1-26 A and B and 6-1 B

We would also like to extend our sincere gratitude to Dr. Catanese for contributing his teaching file cases, writing all the accompanying legends and constantly offering his enthusiastic support for this book.

Binita R. Shah, MD

Michael Lucchesi, MD

ACKNOWLEDGEMENTS

We are grateful to all the residents and medical students who rotate through the emergency department, and to our colleagues and nursing staff of the emergency department. They constantly stimulate us by challenging us. Learning from each other as we work together has been a privilege. We thank you all.

We express our sincere gratitude to Ms. Andrea Seils for her countless hours in helping us conceive and organize the initial stages of this book. Without her hard work and constant encouragement, this book would not come to fruition. We also extend our sincere appreciation to Ms. Regina Brown for her editorial diligence, patience, and wonderful guidance, Ms. Karen Edmonson for her sage advice and Ms. Catherine Saggese for her expertise as a production supervisor for this book.

Most importantly, we are indebted to our patients and their families. In spite of their sufferings, they gave us permission to take their photographs without any reservations. *They are the unsung heroes of this book*. We salute them for giving us the privilege of taking care of them and for their kindness in allowing us to learn from them and teach others. We trust that with this book we are in some way repaying the great debt we owe to our patients.

Lastly I would like to convey my special thanks to my computer consultant Mr. Jay Patel. He tirelessly answered every S.O.S. phone call to fix many computer "emergencies" during the preparation of this book including retrieving the manuscripts that I accidentally erased on many occasions or lost them when my lap top "crashed" by "worms". Thank you Jay – you have been a "life-saver" (BRS).

Binita R. Shah, MD

Michael Lucchesi, MD

CHAPTER 1

CHILD MALTREATMENT

Binita R. Shah

DIAGNOSIS — CHILD ABUSE

SYNONYMS

"Battered child syndrome"
Child victimization

Definition

The Child Abuse Prevention and Treatment Act which was passed in 1974 defines child abuse as: "The physical or mental injury, sexual abuse, negligent treatment, or maltreatment of a child under the age of 18 by a person who is responsible for the child's welfare under circumstances which indicate that the child's health and welfare is harmed or threatened thereby." The key aspect of child abuse is maltreatment of a child by parents, guardians, or caregivers. The maltreatment may be in the form of direct physical or sexual abuse, denial of nutrition or medical care, or failure to provide a safe, nurturing environment.

Associated Clinical Features

1. Over 3 million cases of child abuse and neglect are reported annually with an annual mortality of greater than 4000 children.
2. Mechanisms of inflicted injuries range from direct impact (e.g., punching, slapping, or hitting with an object), shaken impact syndrome, penetrating injuries, and injuries related to asphyxiation.
3. Some characteristics of victims of abuse include premature birth, congenital defects, mental retardation, and multiple births.
4. Some characteristics of abusive families include a history of substance abuse, single parent household, young parental age, lack of education, previous incidents of domestic violence, socioeconomic constraints (e.g., poverty and unemployment), and mental health problems.
5. Presenting signs and symptoms range from asymptomatic presentations (e.g., bruising) to seizures, coma, or death, and may involve:
   a. Bruises and contusions (Fig. 1-1; most common injuries of child abuse)
   b. Abusive head trauma (Fig. 1-2; most common cause of death from child abuse)
   c. Blunt abdominal trauma (this carries the second highest mortality rate related to abusive injuries). Inflicted abdominal injuries include ruptured liver or spleen, intestinal perforation, duodenal hematoma, pancreatic injury, and kidney trauma.
   d. Skeletal injuries (see Figs. 1-7 to 1-9)
   e. Burns (see Figs. 1-22 and 1-24)
   f. Poisoning (e.g., poisoning by table salt with water restriction [presenting with hypernatremia], over-the-counter and prescription drugs, laxatives, ipecac, pepper, carbon monoxide, or illicit drugs).
   g. Munchausen syndrome by proxy (a serious disorder of parenting in which illness in a child is either produced or simulated by a parent)
6. Physical examination should include growth parameters (height and weight [failure to thrive] and head circumference [rapidly increasing head size indicative of head injury]).
7. As indicated, evaluation of child abuse includes complete blood count (screening for anemia and platelet count, base line hemoglobin and hematocrit), liver function tests (elevation of transaminase seen with liver injury), and coagulation profile (exclude bleeding disorders).
8. Radiographic skeletal survey
   a. A skeletal survey screening for occult fractures
      1) Mandatory for all patients <2 years of age with evidence of physical abuse
      2) Indicated in infants <1 year of age with evidence of significant neglect and deprivation
      3) The yield from the skeletal survey decreases with increasing age, as the frequency of occult fractures decreases in older children (those between 2 and 5 years of age).

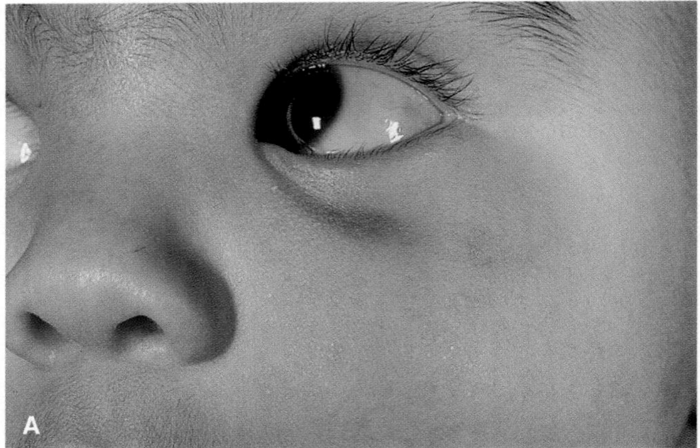

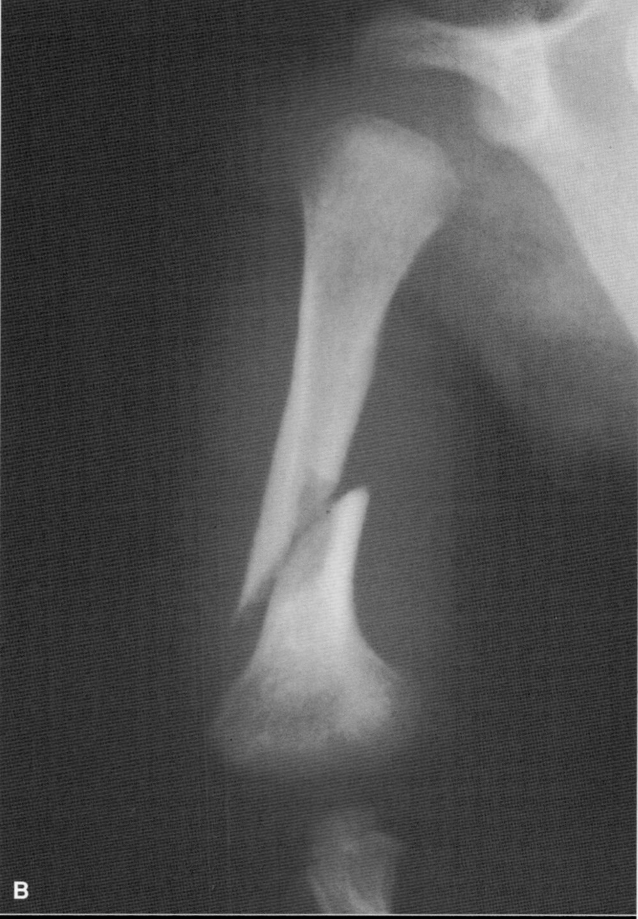

Figure 1-1. Child Abuse

A. Bruise. Bruises are the most common injuries of child abuse. External evidence of inflicted injuries may be very subtle at times as seen in this 3-month-old infant who presented with inconsolable crying. She had a very small bruise in the periorbital region. A skeletal survey revealed a humerus fracture. *B*. Fractured humerus. An oblique fracture at the junction of middle and distal third of the humerus is seen. The humerus and femur are among the most frequently fractured long bones in abusive injuries. The most common type of abusive fractures are spiral (oblique) or transverse. A humerus fracture in a child <3 years of age should raise a strong suspicion of child abuse.

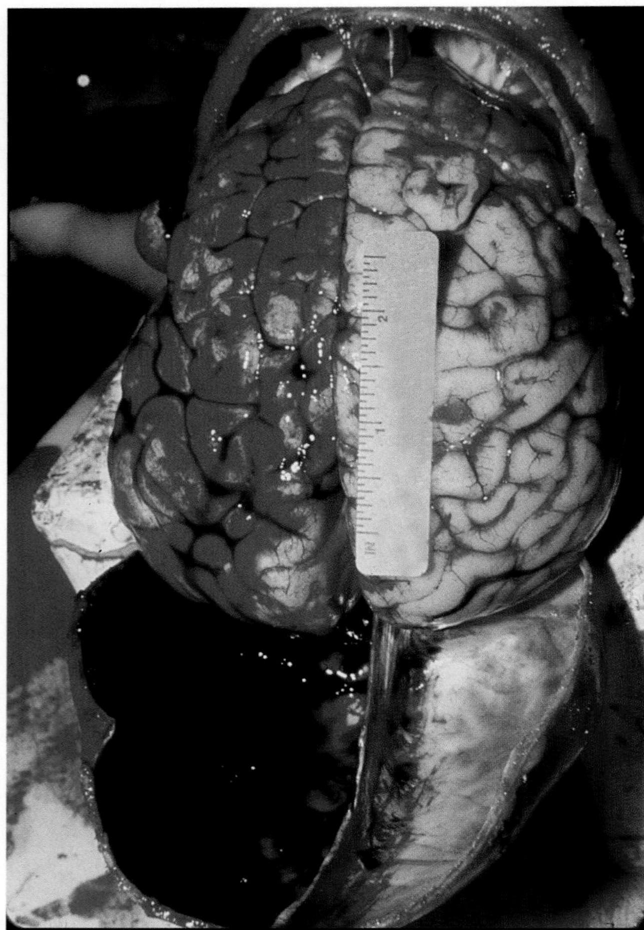

Figure 1-2. Subarachnoid Hemorrhage (SAH) and Subdural Hemorrhage (SDH); Shaken impact Syndrome

An autopsy photograph taken just prior to brain removal shows a SAH on the upper right hand side, SDH in the lower right hand side, and brain swelling with flattened gyral configuration. This 8-month-old infant was seen 4 weeks earlier because of bleeding from the ear, and was sent home with a diagnosis of otitis externa. Subsequently he was seen for facial palsy on the same side as the bloody otorrhea. He was treated with antibiotics with a clinical diagnosis of otitis media with facial palsy. A few days later, he was brought to the ED in cardiopulmonary arrest. He was also found to have skull and multiple rib fractures (otorrhea and facial palsy were found to be due to a basal skull fracture). *Remember: Otitis externa is an exceedingly uncommon diagnosis in infancy, and bloody ear discharge is neither seen in otitis media nor otitis externa.*

    4) Instead of a skeletal survey, appropriate radiographs can be ordered based on the complaints of pain and/or the physical examination in older children.

b. A skeletal survey is usually *not* indicated for:
    1) Children >5 years of age, because acute occult fractures are rarely present in this age group
    2) Siblings of an abused victim without clinical evidence of physical abuse
    3) Victims of isolated sexual abuse

9. Radionuclide bone scans
   a. Bone scans can identify most fractures within the first 48 hours after an injury.
   b. They are helpful in infants and young children with suspected abusive injuries with a negative skeletal survey.
   c. They are helpful in detecting fractures in locations that are difficult to see radiographically (e.g., hands, feet, or ribs).
   d. They are helpful for detecting recent fractures (<7- to 10-day-old rib fractures or subtle diaphyseal fractures).
   e. They serve as a complementary test to radiography, when additional evidence of abusive injuries is required to establish the diagnosis of child abuse.
   f. If a bone scan is used as an initial study, all positive areas must be evaluated further with radiography.
   g. *Injuries cannot be dated on bone scans.*
   h. They are insensitive for detecting cranial injuries.

10. All patients with suspected intracranial injury must undergo cranial CT or MRI or both. Strongly consider doing cranial CT scans in infants <1 year of age with abusive skeletal injuries.

11. Photographs are an important form of documentation. They are usually admissible in legal proceedings as long as they are authenticated (label each photograph on the back with the name and medical record number of the child, the signature of the person taking the picture, and the date and time). A front view of the face (in order to confirm the identity of the child) must be included in addition to photos of the injuries (e.g., bruises).

12. An interview should be conducted in a closed environment with a child old enough to describe the mechanism of injury. These questions should be developmentally appropriate and open-ended (e.g., "Can you tell me what happened to your arm?"), rather than asking leading questions (e.g., "Did your mommy hit you?"). Document the child's and caregiver's *exact* statements about the child's injuries, verbatim.

Consultations

A multidisciplinary team effort should be used (as indicated depending on the injuries), with consultations from a pediatrician, a child abuse consultant, and a social worker, as well as a specialist in pediatric radiology, neurosurgery, surgery, and ophthalmology.

Emergency Department Evaluation and Disposition (General Guidelines)

1. For management of specific injuries and hospitalization, please refer to the sections on the individual entities.

2. All 50 states have child-protection ordinances mandating that professionals who come into contact with children report cases of suspected abuse to the local child protective services agency.

3. Legal issues regarding reporting child abuse:
   a. The law requires reporting all cases of *suspected (but not necessarily proven) as well as known cases of child abuse or child sexual abuse.*
   b. Report to child protective and law enforcement agencies as indicated by local law.
   c. *Mandated reporters* are those individuals who are routinely responsible for a child's health or well-being, and may include medical personnel, teachers, day care workers, and law enforcement professionals.
   d. Mandated reporters who report their suspicions in good faith are protected from lawsuits.
   e. A mandated reporter may be prosecuted for failing to report abuse, and civil malpractice litigation may be brought against a physician or other health care practitioner for failure to recognize or diagnose child abuse or child sexual abuse.
   f. In cases in which a false report is filed, statutes generally provide immunity as long as the report is done in good faith.

4. Documentation in the medical record should be made with great care with a very clear, concise, and legible history, physical examination, and laboratory and radiological findings, because such records may become evidence in a criminal prosecution.

5. Once a diagnosis of abuse is considered likely, the ED physician, in consultation with child protective service workers, must make a decision about the safe disposition of the child and the possibility of further harm if the child returns to the custody of the caregiver in question. Options include immediate placement in foster care (either with a relative or designated foster parent), or temporary hospitalization while awaiting arrangements for transport to a safe environment.

6. Referral to mental health professionals should be made for both the victim and their innocent relatives or caregivers to help them to cope with the emotional trauma of abuse.

7. Once a diagnosis of child abuse or child sexual abuse is made, all other siblings or other minors should be evaluated, if they were also in contact with the alleged perpetrator.

Clinical Pearls: Child Abuse

1. *Any injury to a minor who presents to a clinician may be the result of child abuse.*

2. Openness to a diagnosis of child abuse and/or neglect is *paramount* when examining a child who is potentially injured or abused.

3. It is important to undress the child completely so that a thorough examination may be carried out to evaluate for integumentary or other occult injuries.

4. Remember that many children who are physically abused may also be sexually abused. Exclude sexual abuse by taking a thorough history and performing a thorough physical examination, and order laboratory studies as indicated.

5. Red flags for child abuse include inconsistent, unexplained, and implausible history; delays in seeking treatment; and a history of repeated accidents.

BOX 1-1. A FULL SKELETAL SURVEY

Anteroposterior (AP), posteroanterior (PA), lateral, or oblique views:

AP and lateral views of axial skeleton:

- AP and lateral skull
- Lateral cervical spine
- AP and lateral thorax
- AP pelvis (including mid and lower lumbar spine)
- Lateral lumbar spine

AP views of appendicular skeleton

- AP humeri
- AP forearms
- Oblique PA hands
- AP femurs
- AP lower legs
- AP feet

Important:

- A follow-up skeletal survey about 2 weeks after the initial study increases the diagnostic yield and should be considered when abuse is strongly suspected.
- AP and lateral views of the skull must be taken even when cranial CT has been performed, because skull fractures coursing in the axial plane may be missed with axial CT.
- Oblique views of the thorax increase the yield for detection of rib fractures.
- A "babygram" or full body radiograph (of the entire infant or young child on one or two radiographs) is *NOT acceptable.*
- An abbreviated skeletal survey is *NOT acceptable.*
- At least two views of each fracture should be taken for complete delineation.

BOX 1-2. DATING OF BONE INJURIES

- Dating of the fractures
  (1) Helps in estimating age of injury
  (2) Helps in identifying multiple episodes of trauma, inflicted at different times
  (3) Is based on callus formation, appearance of periosteum, fracture line and soft tissues seen on radiographs

Age of Injury	*Bone Appearance on Radiograph*
0–2 days	Fracture Soft tissue swelling
0–5 days	Visible fragments
<10–14 days	None or minimal periosteal new bone
10–14 days	Immature callus formation Periosteal new bone with calcified periphery and radiolucent center
>21 days	Dense mature callus (uniformly dense and smooth)
>3 months	Only thickened cortex

BOX 1-3. DIFFERENTIAL DIAGNOSIS OF CHILD ABUSE

- Accidental trauma
- Conditions mimicking abusive bruises (see Box 1-5)
- Conditions mimicking abusive burns (see Box 1-18)
- Sudden infant death syndrome or infanticide
- Metabolic conditions with an increased tendency for fractures (see Box 1-8)

Suspect child abuse with any of the following:

- Multiple injuries
- Injuries in different stages of healing
- Delay in seeking medical care
- Inconsistent history
- Injuries inappropriate for child's stage of development
- When the alleged mechanism of injury is not consistent with clinical findings or the child's stage of development
- Frequent episodes of "accidental" poisoning

DIAGNOSIS CUTANEOUS MANIFESTATIONS OF CHILD ABUSE

Definition

1. Cutaneous manifestations of child abuse include bruises, bite marks, and burns.
2. The most common injuries identified in abused children are bruises.
3. A bruise results when blunt force is applied to the skin surface resulting in disruption of capillaries, and with greater force larger blood vessels, leading to extravasation of blood into the dermis or subcutaneous tissues.

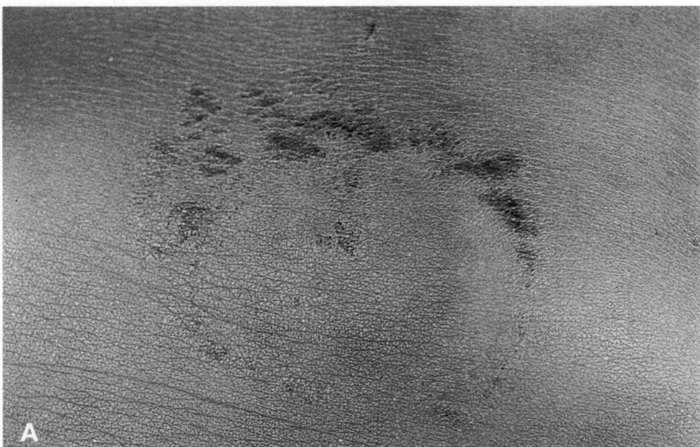

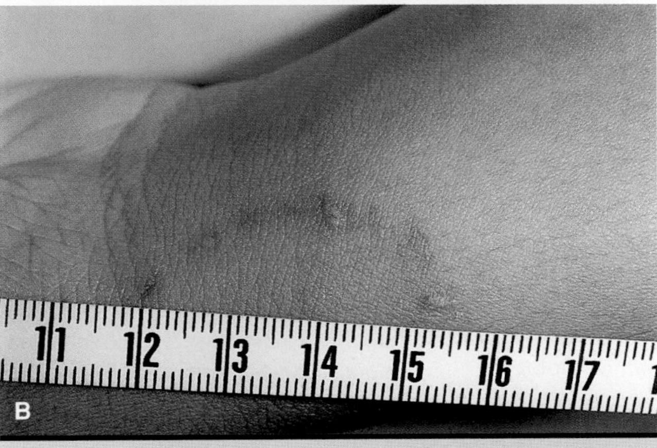

Figure 1-3. Bite Marks

A, B. Bite marks lead to a very distinctive pattern of bruises. They should be suspected when ecchymosis, lacerations, or abrasions are found in an elliptical or oval form (two arched patterns that appear as mirror images of one another if both mandibular and maxillary teeth are used to bite). Canine marks in a bite are the most prominent (or deep) part of the bite. The normal distance between maxillary canine teeth in adult humans is 2.5 to 4 cm, and in a child it is <3 cm. If the intercanine distance is <3 cm, the bite mark may have been inflicted by a child; if it is >3 cm, it was probably inflicted by an adult. As seen here, human bites compress flesh, causing only contusions; animal bites (dogs and other carnivorous animals) tear flesh. Recent bites (and those in a child who has not been bathed) can be swabbed with a saline-soaked cotton swab and sent for DNA analysis, which may help in identifying the perpetrator.

Associated Clinical Features

1. The skin usually is the first place abuse becomes apparent, before visceral, skeletal, and CNS injuries become obvious.
2. When the injury is inflicted by hands, belts, cords, ropes or bites (Fig. 1-3 and 1-4*A*), bruises appear in distinctive patterns. Cords, belts, and ropes can be looped, leading to U-shaped bruises (Fig. 1-4*B*). Linear, rigid objects (e.g., cooking utensils) lead to linear bruises. Sometimes marks are left by the hands of the abuser (Fig. 1-5).

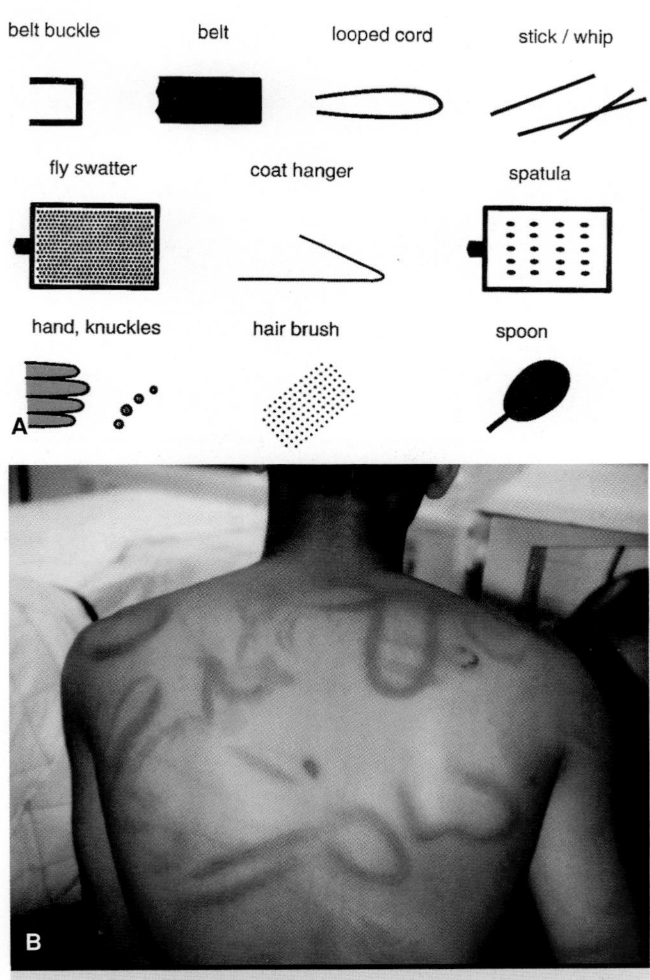

Figure 1-4. Marks Due to Child Abuse

A. Marks from objects. (Reproduced with permission from: Johnson CF: Inflicted injury versus accidental injury. In: *Child Abuse*. Pediatric Clinics of North America. WB Saunders, Philadelphia, Vol. 37, No. 4, August 1990, p. 791). *B*. Loop and linear marks from electrical cord; inflicted injuries.

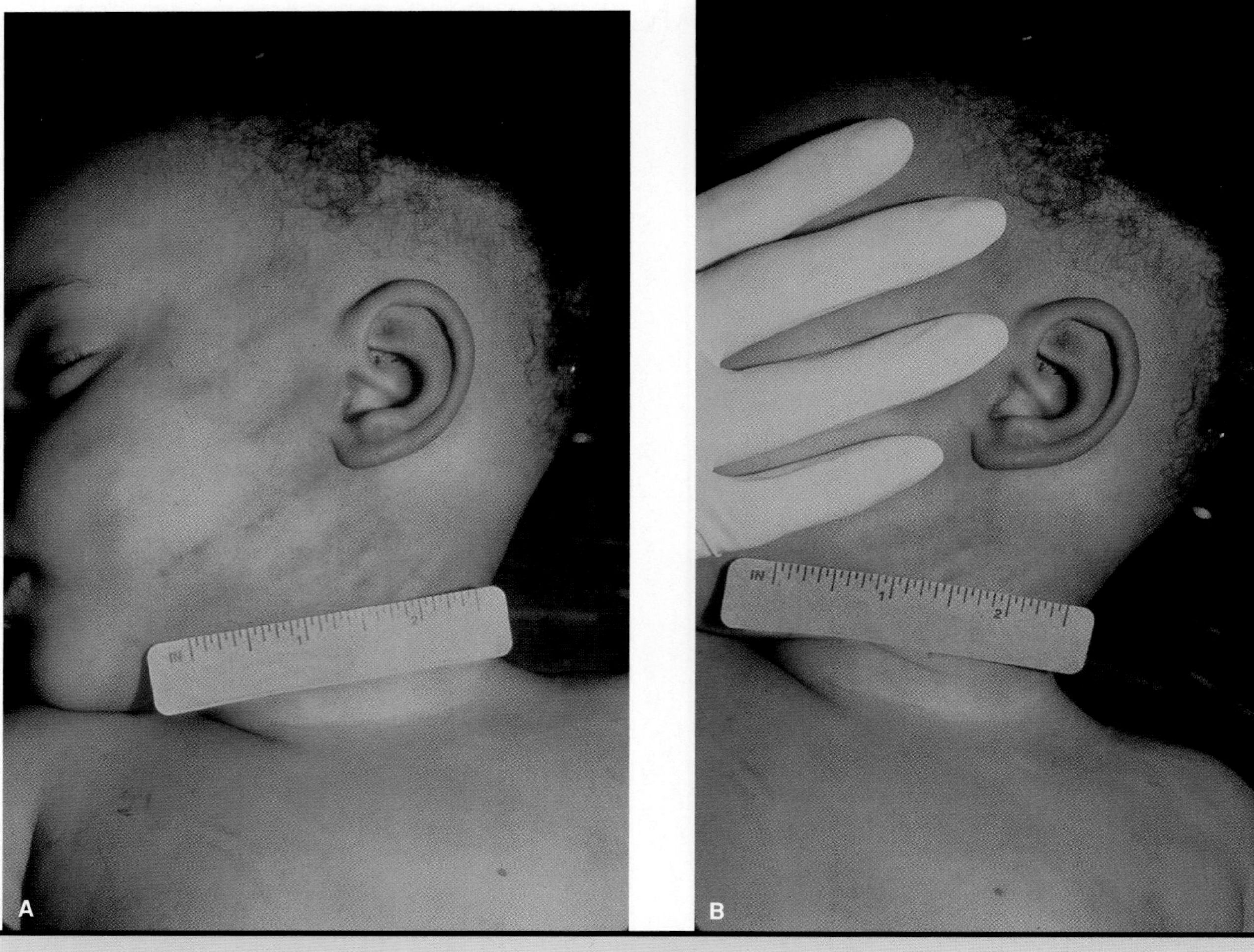

Figure 1-5. Finger Patterns of Child Abuse

A. Finger patterns seen on the face of the same infant shown in Fig. 1-2. *B*. Gloved fingers corresponding to the finger patterns shown in A.

3. For each bruise or contusion document its color, shape, pattern, location, and size (Fig. 1-6).
4. A CBC, platelet count, and coagulation studies (prothrombin time and partial thromboplastin time) may help when a bleeding disorder is suspected. Additional tests like bleeding time and coagulation factors may be indicated in selected cases. Clotting studies may be helpful or lead to confusion at times (e.g., after serious head injury, clotting studies may be abnormal because of consumption of coagulation factors in response to injury). A family history of bleeding disorders will also help (e.g., hemophilia as an X-linked recessive disorder [most commonly seen in males only]).

Consultations

A multidisciplinary team approach should be used (as indicated depending on the injuries) with consultations with a pediatrician, a child abuse consultant, a social worker, and specialists in pediatric radiology, neurosurgery, surgery, and ophthalmology.

Emergency Department Evaluation and Disposition

1. Management of bruises is generally supportive.
2. Assess cardiovascular stability in cases of deep bruises (e.g., thigh).
3. For general guidelines for reporting to child protective agencies, see page 3.

Clinical Pearls: Cutaneous Manifestations of Child Abuse

1. Bruises are the most common injury in physically abused children. Bruises are also a common accidental injury of childhood.

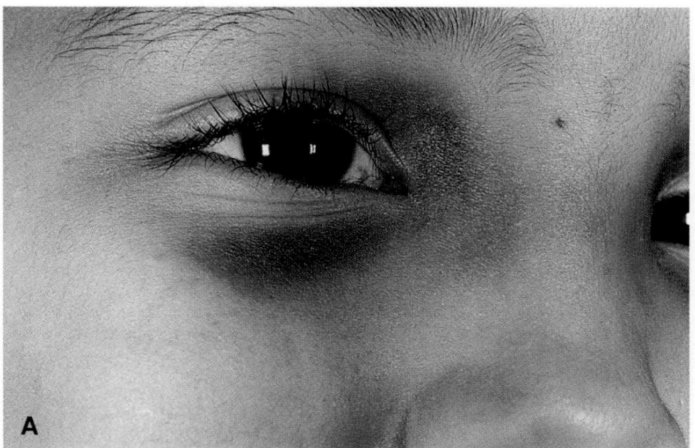

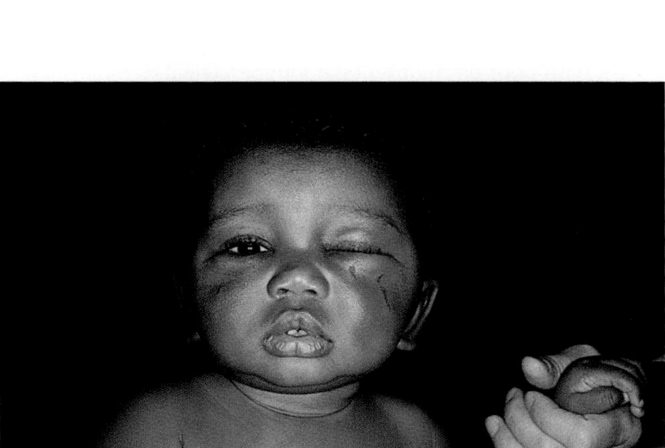

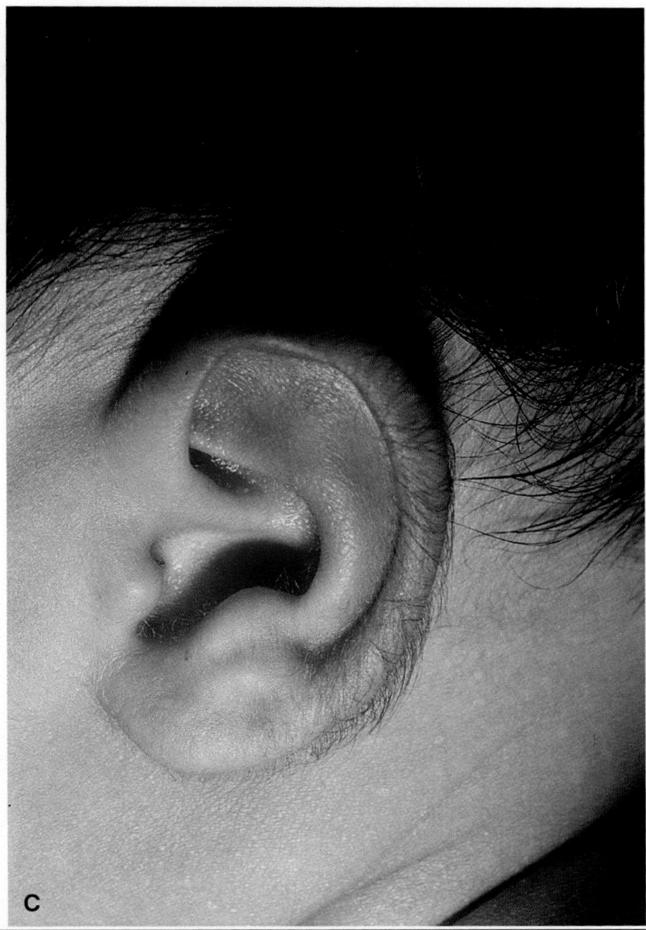

Figure 1-6. Inflicted Bruises

A. Bruises on the relatively well protected areas suggest inflicted injuries. Purple bruise (about 3 to 5 days old) around periorbital region and red bruise (about 1 to 2 days old) on the nasal bridge seen here represent new bruises. *B*. Red bruise (new bruise about 1 to 2 days old) and scratch marks are seen on both cheeks in this infant who was left with his mentally retarded brother. He also had human bite marks on his trunk. *C*. Ears are not frequently injured in childhood accidents. Bruises at these sites are strong indicators of abuse. Ears can be bruised by pulling, pinching, or grabbing them. Inflicted bruises are typically seen on top of the pinna. Pulling the ears can also cause bruises at the junction between the ears and head posteriorly.

2. Dating of bruises is *NOT* absolutely accurate. The color of the bruise depends on its location, depth, and amount of bleeding and circulation in the bruised area.
3. *Remember: Those who can't cruise don't bruise* (meaning that any bruises in young infants who are not yet able to stand or walk should raise concern about abuse, with the exception of infants placed in walkers).

BOX 1-4. BRUISES

Location of bruise or contusion

- Bruises on skin over bony prominences (areas first impacted during a fall) suggest accidental bruises.

Examples:

(1) Anterior tibia (shins)

(2) Knees

(3) Elbows

(4) Forehead

(5) Lower arms and dorsum of hands

- Bruises on relatively well protected areas suggest inflicted injuries.

Examples:

(1) Ears

(2) Cheeks

(3) Frenulum

(4) Neck

(5) Upper arms and trunk

(6) Flanks

(7) Buttocks

(8) Genitalia/groin

(9) Upper anterior and inner thighs

Determination of age of bruise or contusion

- Dating bruises can be difficult due to the variability in their rate of progression.
- Bruises are difficult to see on darkly pigmented skin.
- The color of the bruise may appear different depending on the patient's skin tone.
- The rate of healing of a bruise depends on:
  (1) *Location:* Bruises on the face or genitalia heal faster than bruises on shins due to their excellent blood supply.
  (2) *Depth:* Deep tissue bruises (e.g., thighs or hips) take longer to appear and longer to heal.
  (3) *Amount of bleeding:* Bruises with heavy bleeding take longer to heal.
  (4) *Circulation in the bruised area:* Bruises in areas with poor circulation take longer to heal.

Guidelines for color of bruises:

(1) Red to blue: about 1 to 2 days old

(2) Blue to purple: about 3 to 5 days old

(3) Green: about 6 to 7 days old

(4) Yellow to brown: about 8 to 10 days old

(5) Resolved: at least 13 to 28 days old

(6) It is likely safest to describe bruises as either "new" (red, purple, or blue) or "old" (green, yellow, or brown)

Note: The presence of bruises that have various ages may signify multiple episodes of injury caused by ongoing physical abuse.

BOX 1-5. DIFFERENTIAL DIAGNOSIS OF CONDITIONS MIMICKING ABUSIVE BRUISES

- Accidental trauma
- Raccoon eyes from accidental trauma (see Fig. 2-12)
- Birthmarks
  (1) Mongolian spots (see Fig. 2-1)
  (2) Hemangioma (especially cavernous; see Fig. 7-57)
- Infections
  (1) Systemic bacterial or viral infections associated with petechiae or purpura (see Figs. 3-30 to 3-31)
  (2) Severe infections with disseminated intravascular coagulation (see Figs. 3-28 to 3-29)
- Coagulation defects
  (1) Hemophilia (factor VIII, IX, and X deficiencies)
  (2) Von Willebrand's disease
- Vasculitis
- Henoch-Schönlein purpura (see Fig. 11-8 and Figs. 7-13 to 7-15)
- Platelet dysfunction
- Acute or chronic immune thrombocytopenic purpura (see Fig. 11-7)
- Folk-healing practices (Coining, cupping and moxibustion see Fig. 2-2 to 2-4)
- Dermatological conditions
  (1) Phytophotodermatitis (see Fig. 2-11)
  (2) Cold panniculitis (see Fig. 2-5 and 2-6)
  (3) Subcutaneous fat necrosis
  (4) Erythema nodosum
  (5) Hypersensitivity reactions (e.g., erythema multiforme; see Fig. 7-5)
- Tattooing or dye stains
- Conditions associated with increased skin fragility and bruising
  (1) Osteogenesis imperfecta
  (2) Ehlers-Danlos syndrome

DIAGNOSIS SKELETAL MANIFESTATIONS OF CHILD ABUSE

Associated Clinical Features

1. The reported frequency of fractures associated with child abuse varies from 11 to 55%.
2. Inflicted skeletal injures may involve any part of the axial and appendicular skeleton.
3. Age is the single most important risk factor for abusive skeletal injuries:
   a. Such injuries are seen more frequently in infants and young children than in older children.
   b. About 55 to 70% of all abusive skeletal injuries are seen in infants <1 year of age.
   c. About 80% of abusive fractures are seen in infants <18 months of age.
   d. Only 2% of accidental fractures are seen in infants <18 months of age.
4. Intracranial and visceral injures often coexist with abusive skeletal injuries (Fig. 1-7). About 70% of abuse-related intracranial injuries have associated fractures.
5. Metaphyseal and epiphyseal fractures require forces that are not produced by the usual accidental trauma of infancy, and their presence should raise a strong suspicion for child abuse (Fig. 1-8). Salter-Harris fractures are relatively uncommon in abuse.
6. Radiographic studies that are used for detection of musculoskeletal trauma include a skeletal survey (see Box 1-1), radionuclide scans (see page 3), and MR imaging.

Consultations

A multidisciplinary team approach should be used (as indicated), with consultations with a pediatrician, a child abuse consultant, a social worker, and a specialist in pediatric radiology and orthopedics.

Emergency Department Treatment and Disposition

1. Skeletal fractures related to child abuse are rarely life-threatening; however, recognition of a skeletal injury may be the first indication of child abuse and it serves as an important diagnostic tool. While awaiting completion of the investigation, the patient usually requires hospitalization.

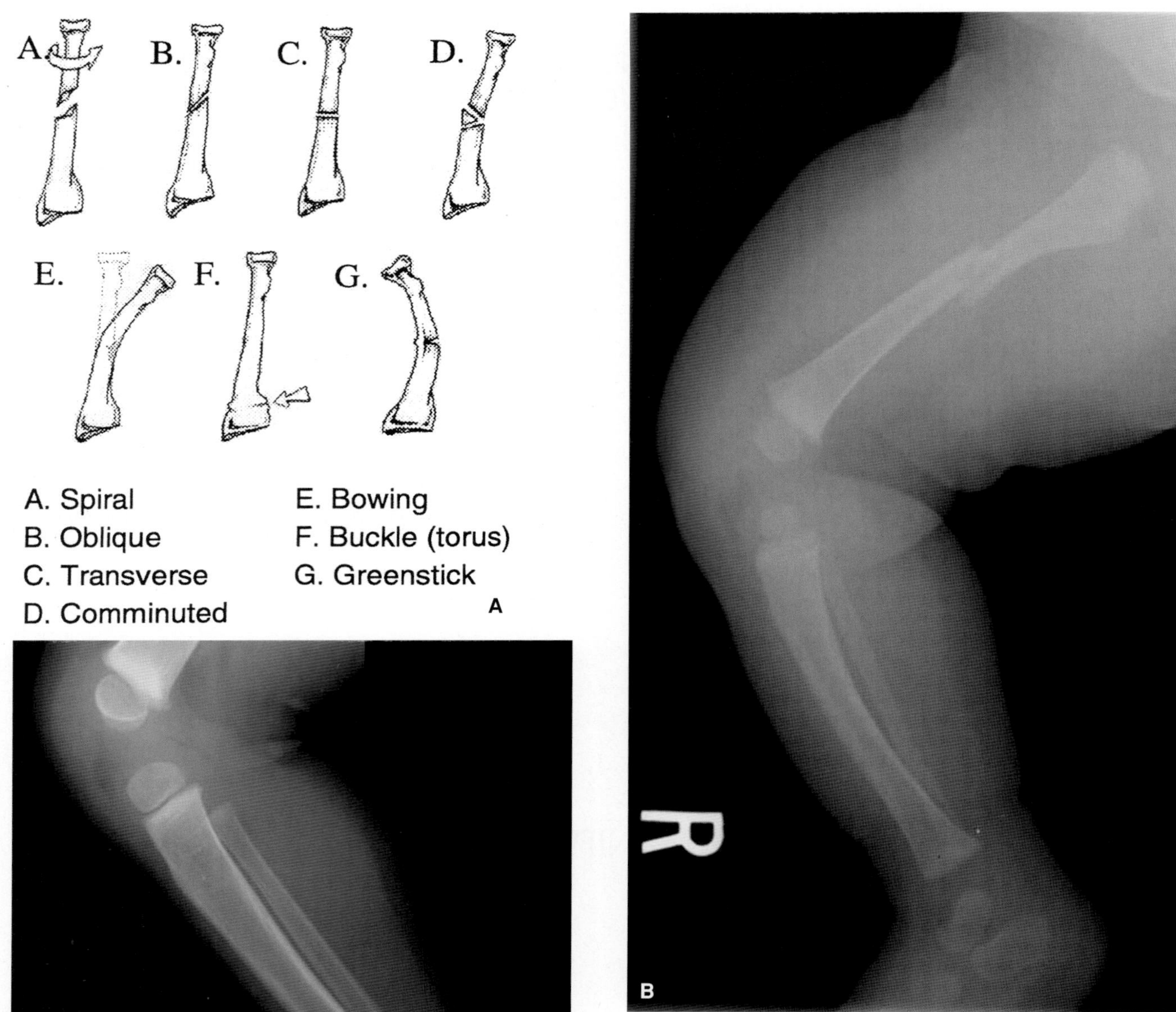

Figure 1-7. Fractures: Inflicted versus Accidental

A. Common fractures in childhood. (Illustrations by Alexander Imas, M.D.) *B*. Femoral shaft fracture; child abuse. An oblique, displaced fracture of the midshaft of the femur in a 4-month-old infant who was brought to the ED with a history of inconsolable crying. Diaphyseal fractures are the most common type of fractures seen in child abuse. The femur is one of the most frequently fractured long bones in abusive injuries. It requires significant force to break the femur; thus a spiral, oblique, or transverse fracture of the femur is highly suspicious of child abuse in an otherwise healthy infant. *C*. Toddler's fracture; accidental injury. A nondisplaced spiral fracture is seen at the distal third of the tibia in a 12-month-old infant. Toddler's fracture is usually seen in the distal third of the tibia in an ambulating or cruising toddler. A skeletal survey was negative and child abuse was excluded by a thorough investigation in this infant.

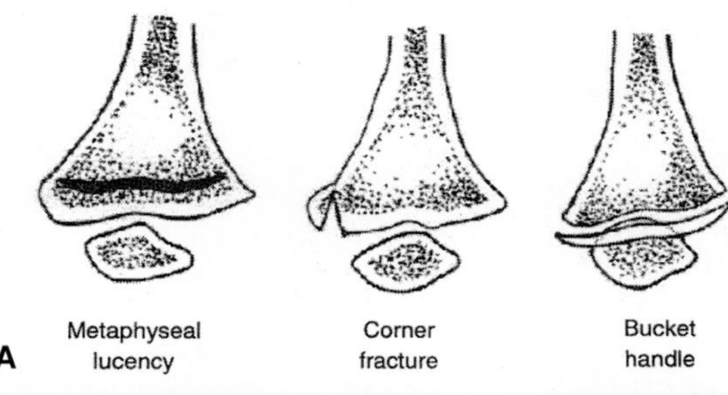

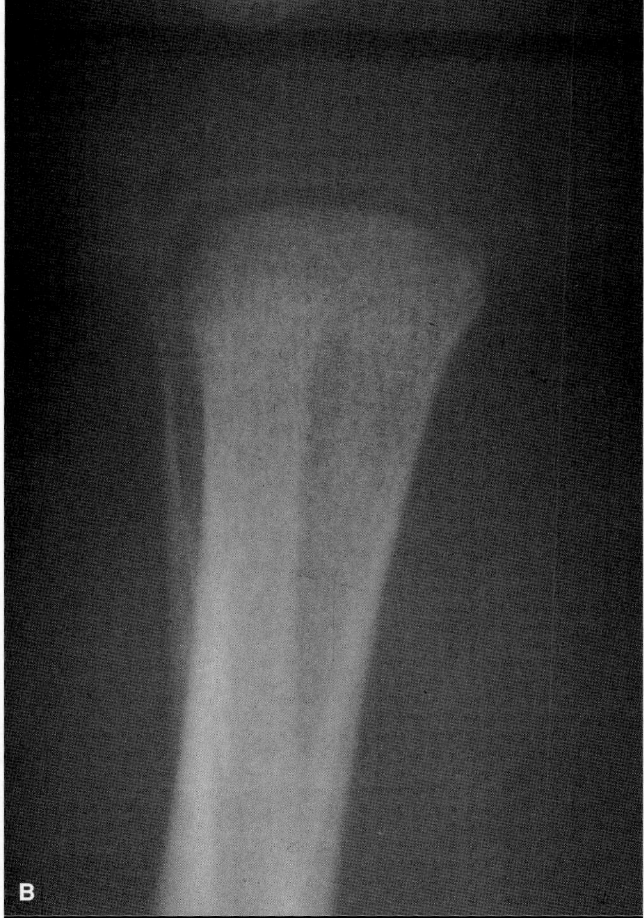

Figure 1-8. Classic Metaphyseal and Epiphyseal Injuries of Child Abuse

A. Metaphyseal-epiphyseal injuries are classic fractures of child abuse and can occur in any long bone adjacent to a growth plate. (Illustrations by Alexander Imas, M.D.) *B*. "Bucket-handle" fracture. Frontal view of distal tibia in a 4-month-old infant. Note the separation of a thin band of metaphysis, representing a "bucket-handle" fracture. (Reproduced with permission from: Shah BR, Laude TL: *Child Abuse and Sexual Abuse. Atlas of Clinical Pediatrics*. WB Saunders, Philadelphia, 2000, p. 36.)

2. For guidelines for reporting cases of suspected abuse to the local child protective services agency, see page ??.
3. Diaphyseal fractures:
   a. Treatment depends on the type, location, and stage of the fracture, and age of the patient.
   b. Immobilization is usually required, with limitation of weight bearing for lower limb fractures.
4. Metaphyseal fractures usually heal without specific treatment and do not need immobilization.

Clinical Pearls: Skeletal Manifestations of Child Abuse

1. Multiple fractures at different stages of healing are pathognomonic for child abuse (Fig. 1-9).
2. Skull fractures, rib fractures and metaphyseal lesions are the predominant type of abusive injuries seen during infancy; long bone fractures are the most common skeletal injury after 1 year of age.
3. Inflicted fractures are more common in infants. Accidental fractures are more common once children become ambulatory. Thus, long bone fractures are more likely the result of accidental trauma after the age of 2 years.
4. Even though diaphyseal fractures are the most common type of fractures seen in child abuse, they are not pathognomonic for abusive injuries, and can also result from accidental injuries.
5. The hallmark finding in fractures caused by nonaccidental trauma is the lack of a plausible explanation.
6. Lack of changes in radiographic findings on a follow-up skeletal survey done approximately 2 weeks after the initial study helps in confirming normal anatomic variants or metabolic bone diseases (e.g., dysplasia) that mimics abusive injuries.
7. The body mass of an infant $<$12 months of age will not ordinarily generate sufficient force to fracture a normal bone in a simple fall from a crib, bed, or couch.
8. Tibial spiral fractures are usually due to accidental trauma unless they occur in nonambulatory young infants.

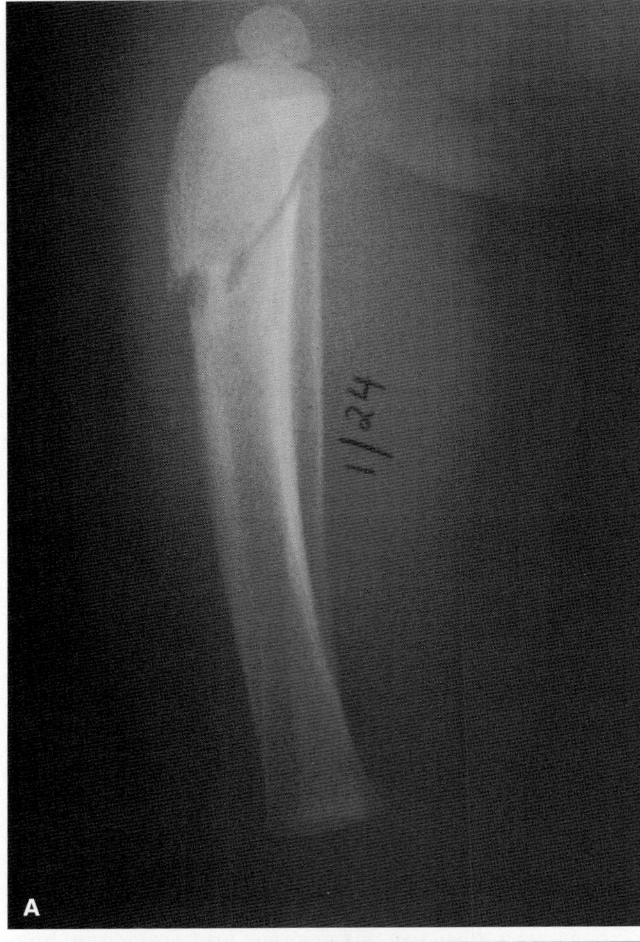

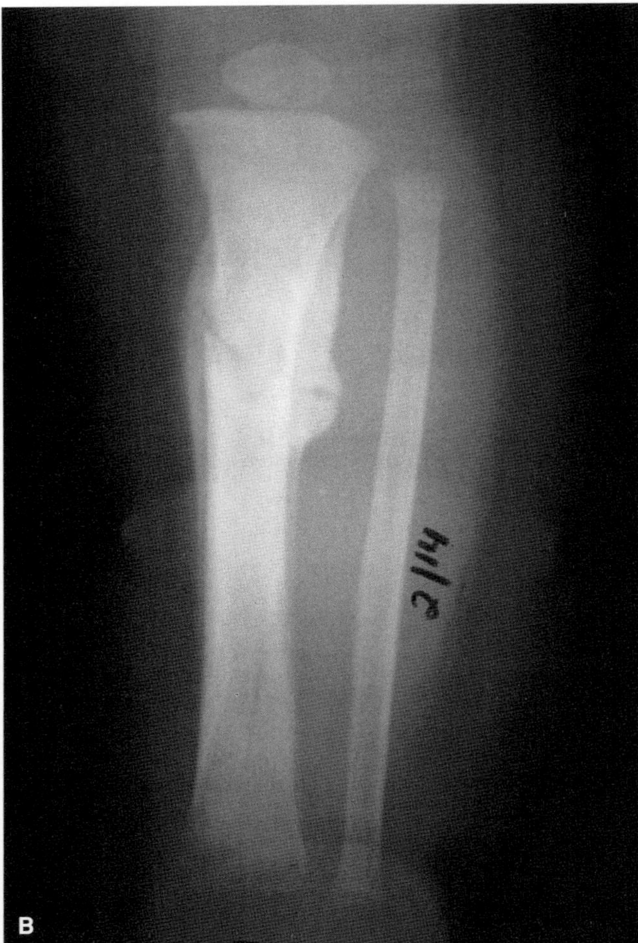

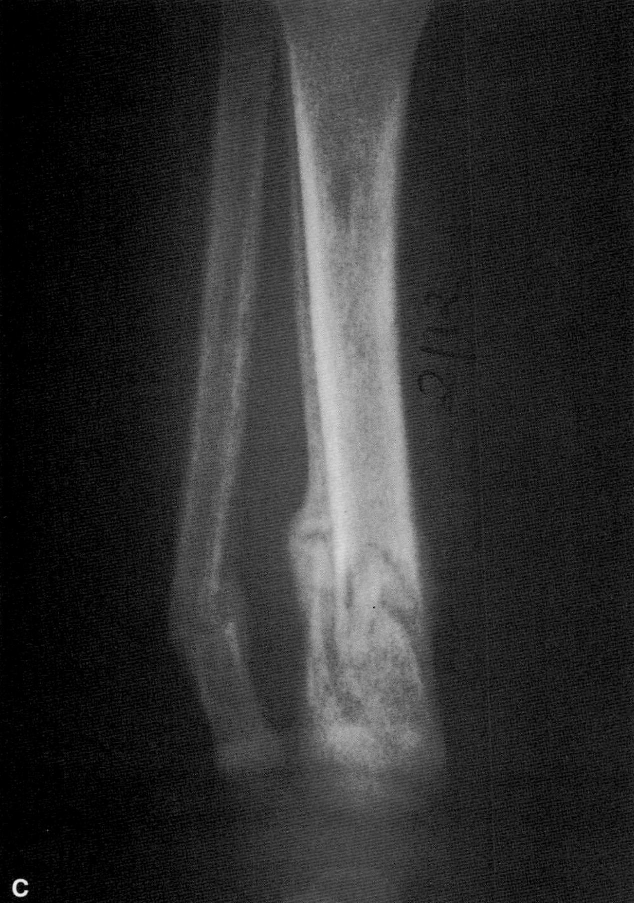

Figure 1-9. Multiple Fractures; Child Abuse

Multiple fractures are seen in a 6-month-old infant at different sites on these radiographs. A spiral fracture of the proximal third of right tibia is seen *A*. A repeat radiograph taken 3 weeks later shows a diffuse periosteal reaction and substantial callus formation *B*. This infant also had a comminuted spiral fracture of the distal third of the left tibia and a transverse fracture of the left fibula (seen on the radiograph with a subperiosteal formation of new bone; *C*). He also had bilateral multiple rib fractures. Toddler or spiral fractures of the tibia in a child who is not walking or cruising is highly suggestive of abuse. The presence of multiple fractures (either injuries of different bones or more than one site of fracture within same bone) and/or fractures in different stages of healing suggests child abuse.

BOX 1-6. CLINICAL FEATURES OF SKELETAL MANIFESTATIONS OF CHILD ABUSE

- Clinical signs and symptoms in a young nonverbal infant:
  (1) Pain manifested by inconsolable crying or irritability
  (2) Crying with movement of affected limb
  (3) Decreased use of a broken extremity (pseudoparalysis)
  (4) Some fractures (e.g. metaphyseal or rib) may not be apparent on examination, and can only be identified by radiographs
  (5) Local swelling and tenderness may be present
  (6) External bruising may or may not be present over the fracture site
- The most common injuries are extremity fractures.
- Common injuries include diaphyseal fractures of the long bones (with femur and humerus fractures being most common), and those of the tibia, ulna, radius, and fibula.
- Common types of fractures include spiral or oblique (due to rotational or torsional forces applied to the limb) and transverse (due to a direct blow or bending force).
- Diaphyseal or metaphyseal fractures are most common.
- Subperiosteal formation of new bone involving the diaphysis indicates abuse (it reflects the presence of a subperiosteal hemorrhage due to traumatic separation of diaphyseal periosteum due to excessive torsional forces).
- Other sites of fractures that are seen in abuse include:
  (1) Fractures about the shoulder girdle (the clavicle, acromion, scapula, and humerus)
  (2) Fractures of the hands and feet
  (3) Spinal fractures
  (4) Craniofacial fractures (mandibular fracture)
  (5) Rib fractures (see Figs. 1-11 and 1-12)
  (6) Skull fracture (see Figs. 1-15 and 1-16)

Note: No diaphyseal fracture by itself is pathognomonic of child abuse.

BOX 1-7. CHILD ABUSE FRACTURES

- *Pathognomonic or "classic" child abuse fractures:*
  a. Classic metaphyseal lesion
  b. Examples: "Bucket-handle" or "corner" fractures or metaphyseal lucency
     (1) Typically found in infants and young children
     (2) Seen with shaken impact syndrome (acceleration-deceleration forces associated with shaking)
     (3) Seen with pulling and twisting of extremities (resulting in excessive tractional and torsional forces)
     (4) Metaphyseal fractures require mechanical forces that are not produced by usual accidental trauma of infancy
     (5) Usually absence of soft tissue swelling or external bruising
     (6) Usually not identified by physical examination
     (7) Most commonly seen in femur, tibia, and humerus
- Fractures *strongly suggestive* of child abuse:
  (1) Multiple fractures (without plausible explanation)
  (2) Multiple fractures, especially bilateral
  (3) Fractures in different stages of healing
  (4) Fractures inconsistent with the history or developmental age of the child
  (5) Fractures with delayed onset of seeking care
  (6) Posterior rib fractures
  (7) Skull fractures (multiple, bilateral, or depressed, crossing suture lines or occipital)
  (8) Sternum fractures
  (9) Spiral fractures in a infant not walking
  (10) Scapular fractures
  (11) Clavicular fractures (not midshaft; sternoclavicular or acromioclavicular)
  (12) Avulsion fractures of the spinous process
  (13) Vertebral body compression and spinous process fractures and subluxations
  (14) Digital fractures (torus fractures of metacarpals and metatarsals, buckle fractures of proximal phalanx)
  (15) Pelvic fracture without history of significant force
- Fractures *less likely* to be abusive:
  (1) Clavicle fractures
  (2) Toddler's fracture of the tibia
  (3) Supracondylar fractures of the humerus
  (4) Torus fractures of long bones
  (5) Pelvic or spiral fractures with a history of significant force

BOX 1-8. DIFFERENTIAL DIAGNOSIS OF CHILD ABUSE FRACTURES

- Accidental trauma
  - (1) Toddler fracture
  - (2) Birth injury (clavicle fracture most common)
- Disorders with increased tendency to fracture
  - (1) Osteogenesis imperfecta (see Fig. 2-20)
  - (2) Rickets (see Figs. 2-17 and 2-19)
  - (3) Metabolic bone disease of prematurity
  - (4) Scurvy
  - (5) Osteoporosis
  - (6) Hypervitaminosis A
  - (7) Coffey's disease
  - (8) Menkes' kinky hair syndrome
- Infection (metaphyseal destructive lesions)
  - (1) Congenital syphilis (see Fig. 4-12)
  - (2) Osteomyelitis (see page 798)
- Sickle cell disease (bony infarction; subperiosteal formation of new bone)
- Malignancy
  - (1) Leukemia
  - (2) Metastatic (e.g., neuroblastoma)
- Normal variants
  - (1) Physiologic periosteal new bone (e.g., seen in long bones of extremities during infancy [usually resolves by 8 months of age], symmetric involvement)
  - (2) Metaphyseal variants like beaks and spurs
  - (3) Ossification center (acromial process)
- Metaphyseal chondrodysplasia, Schmid type
- Congenital indifference to pain

Important: Suspect child abuse if
(skeletal survey is recommended for all infants <2 years of age with any of the following):

- Multiple fractures are present without a plausible explanation
- Fractures are in different stages of healing
- Fractures inconsistent with history or developmental age of the child
- Fractures with delayed onset of seeking care

DIAGNOSIS RIB FRACTURES DUE TO ABUSE

Associated Clinical Features

1. Rib fractures account for up to 29% (range: 5 to 29% in varying reports) of all fractures in children who are victims of physical abuse. A higher incidence of rib fractures is reported in autopsy findings.
2. They are usually seen with violent shaking with anteroposterior thoracic compression in infants (Fig. 1-10) and with direct blows to the chest in older children.
3. Involvement of the posterior arc of a rib is most common; however, fractures can be seen at any rib site in abuse. Posterior rib fractures are due to levering of the posterior neck over the transverse spinous process as the rib cage is vigorously squeezed. There may be associated anterior and costochondral junction fractures.
4. Clinically significant injury to the lungs and heart is uncommon in spite of the high frequency of rib fractures in abused children.
5. Other thoracic injuries that can be seen rarely with rib fractures include pulmonary contusions, pneumothoraces, or pleural effusions.
6. In addition to the initial AP and lateral chest radiographs, right and left posterior oblique views should be obtained to further delineate rib fractures that are seen on the initial radiographs.

Consultations

A multidisciplinary team approach should be used (as indicated), with consultations from a pediatrician, a child abuse consultant, a social worker, and a specialist in pediatric radiology, neurosurgery, and ophthalmology.

Emergency Department Treatment and Disposition

1. For guidelines for reporting cases of suspected abuse to the local child protective services agencies, see page 3.
2. All patients with rib fractures due to child abuse require hospitalization while awaiting additional tests for other injuries (as indicated) and child protective agency investigation.
3. Rib fractures heal rapidly, and do not require any specific therapy.

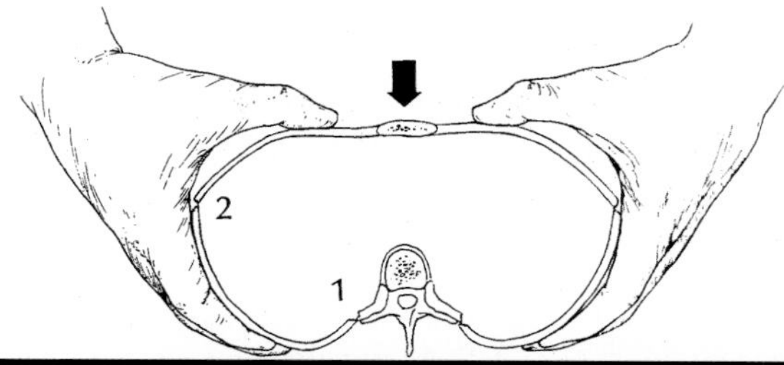

Figure 1-10. Rib Fractures due to Shaking

As the infant is grasped, the assailant's palms are usually situated laterally, with the thumbs positioned anteriorly and the fingers placed posteriorly. With anteroposterior compression of the chest in association with shaking, rib fractures occur initially in the proximal rib over the transverse process of the adjacent vertebra (costovertebral junction; see 1), and subsequently more laterally along the posterior arc of the rib to the midaxillary line (see 2). (Reproduced with permission from: Cooperman DR, Merten DF: Skeletal manifestations of child abuse. In: Reece RM, Ludwig S (eds). *Medical Diagnosis and Management,* 2nd ed. Lippincott Williams & Wilkins, Baltimore, 2001, p. 40.)

Clinical Pearls: Child Abuse Rib Fractures

1. Rib fractures are the most common type of thoracic trauma in physically abused children.
2. Rib fractures are often symmetrically seen at multiple levels and at similar points along arcs of adjacent ribs, and frequently involve middle ribs (Figs. 1-11 and 1-12).

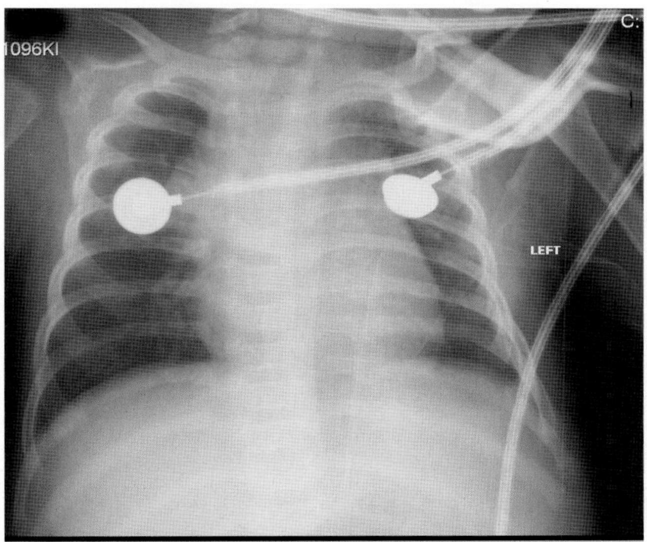

Figure 1-11. Multiple Posterior Rib Fractures

An 8-month-old infant was admitted because of abusive head injury. He did not have any other evidence of external injury. These rib fractures were detected accidentally on skeletal survey. The patient was completely asymptomatic as far as rib fractures were concerned.

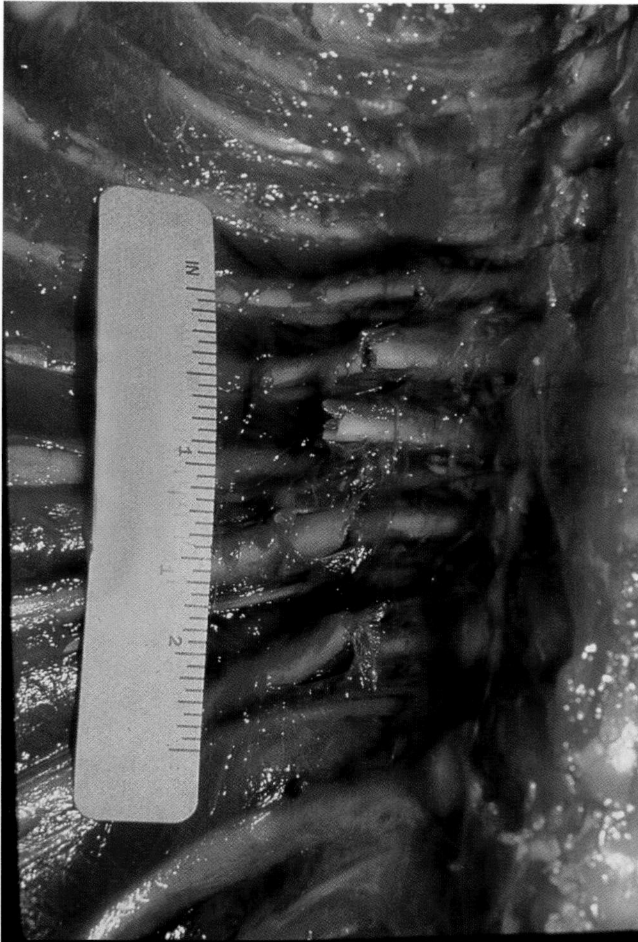

Figure 1-12. Multiple Rib Fractures

Multiple posterior rib fractures (ribs 5 through 11) were seen at autopsy in this 23-month-old infant who died of blunt trauma injuries that included laceration of the lung, liver, and heart.

3. Even though rib fractures are seen in adults following cardiopulmonary resuscitation (CPR), they should *NOT* be considered as a complication of CPR in infants and young children.
4. The presence of rib fractures in the absence of any etiology (e.g., severe motor vehicle accident or metabolic bone disease) should be considered *evidence of child abuse unless and until proved otherwise.* These injuries are quite rare even in the setting of severe accidental trauma in infants.
5. Children with rib fractures from accidental injuries are significantly older than children with rib fractures related to abuse.

BOX 1-9. RIB FRACTURES AND CHILD ABUSE

- Most commonly seen in infants and toddlers
- About 90% are seen in infants <2 years of age
- About 80% are located posteriorly near the costovertebral articulation
- Lateral and anterior fractures are uncommon
- First rib fractures are strongly associated with abuse
- Usually involve multiple ribs
- Usually bilateral symmetrical involvement
- Fractures sometimes occult and not apparent on physical examination
- Fractures do not interfere with breathing in most patients
- Fractures are usually not associated with pulmonary or visceral injuries
- Acute nondisplaced fractures often invisible on plain radiographs
- Fractures are detected radiographically after callus formation and subperiosteal formation of new bone
- Acute fractures (<7 to 10 days postinjury) may be detected by a bone scan or CT scan

BOX 1-10. DIFFERENTIAL DIAGNOSIS OF RIB FRACTURES

- Child abuse unless and until proved otherwise
- Severe vehicular accident or other major accidental trauma (e.g., falls from heights)
- Gunshot wound
- Metabolic bone disease (e.g., osteogenesis imperfecta or osteopenia of prematurity)
- Overenthusiastic physiotherapy (extremely rare; exclude child abuse first)
- Birth trauma (larger newborns; shoulder dystocia)

DIAGNOSIS SKULL FRACTURES DUE TO ABUSE

Associated Clinical Features

1. Child abuse is the most common cause of severe head injury in children younger than 1 year of age.
2. Skull fractures are the second most common form of abusive skeletal injuries and account for 7 to 30% of all fractures seen in abused children.
3. A skull fracture is caused by a forceful blow to the head with a solid object.
4. There is a poor correlation between skull fracture and intracranial injury (in both accidental and abusive trauma), and *the absence of a skull fracture does not exclude the possibility of intracranial injury.*
5. Plain radiographs are the method of choice for identifying fractures. AP and lateral views of the skull must be taken even when cranial CT has been performed, because skull fractures coursing in the axial plane may be missed with axial CT (Fig. 1-13). Bone scans are also not helpful in identifying skull fractures.
6. Cranial CT without contrast should be performed for initial evaluation of all suspected inflicted head injuries (see page 3).
7. Dating of skull fractures is difficult, as they do not heal with evident callus formation like that seen with long bone fractures.

Consultations

A multidisciplinary team approach should be used (as indicated), with consultations from a pediatrician, a child abuse consultant, a social worker, and a specialist in pediatric radiology, neurosurgery, and ophthalmology.

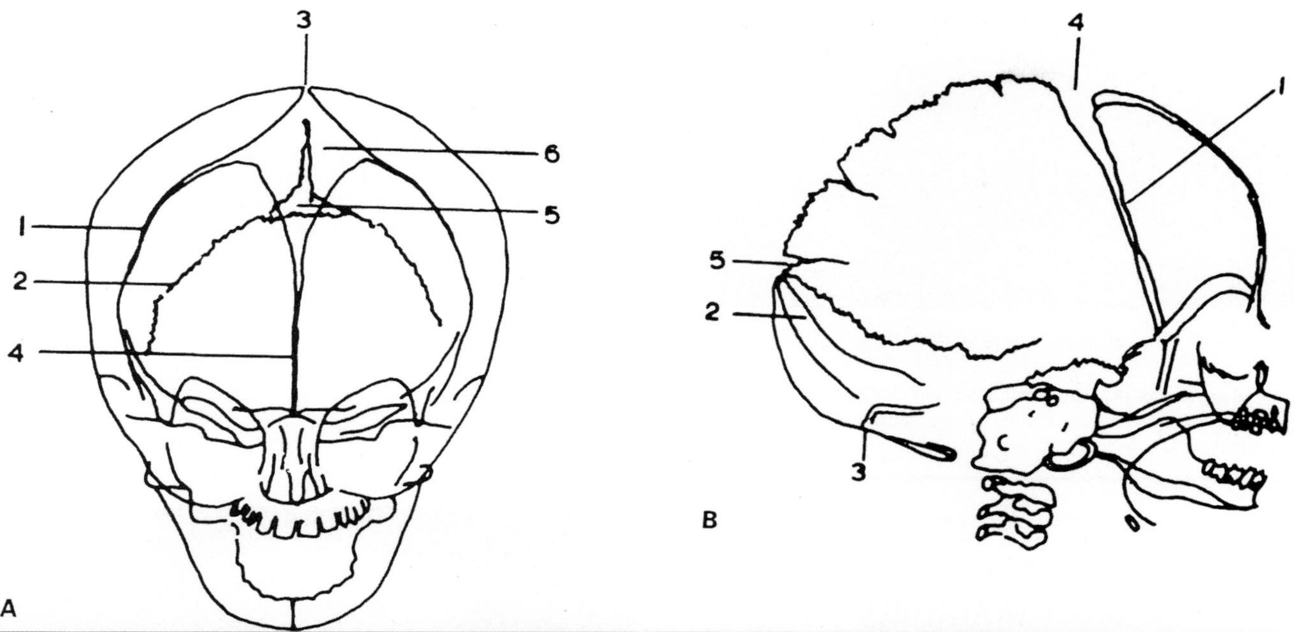

Figure 1-13. Diagrams of the Neonatal Skull

A. Frontal view. 1, coronal suture; 2, lambdoid suture; 3, sagittal suture; 4, metopic suture; 5, anterior fontanelle; 6, posterior fontanelle. *B*. Lateral view. 1, coronal suture; 2, lambdoid suture; 3, mendosal suture; 4, anterior fontanelle; 5, posterior fontanelle. (Reproduced with permission from: Sutton D: The skull. In: Sutton, D (ed). *Textbook of Radiology and Medical Imaging*, Vol. 2, 5th ed. Churchill Livingstone, NY, p. 1377.)

Emergency Department Treatment and Disposition

1. Stabilize the vital signs (if indicated): *A*irway, *b*reathing, *c*irculation, *d*isability, and *e*xposure (*ABCDE*s of the primary survey) in patients presenting with intracranial injuries associated with skull fracture(s).
2. For guidelines for reporting cases of suspected abuse to local child protective services agencies, see page 3.
3. Isolated skull fractures require no specific therapy. They are benign in the majority of cases.
4. Patients need continuing follow-up by their primary care provider for a serious skull fracture or development of a leptomeningeal cyst (seen with a diastatic fracture associated with a dural tear).

Clinical Pearls: Abusive Skull Fractures

1. No pattern of skull fracture is pathognomonic of child abuse; however, skull fractures that are multiple, bilateral, or those that cross suture lines are more likely to be due to abuse than to an accident.
2. Skull fractures that occur in infants after simple accidental falls (e.g., falls <4 feet, such as falling off of a bed or table)

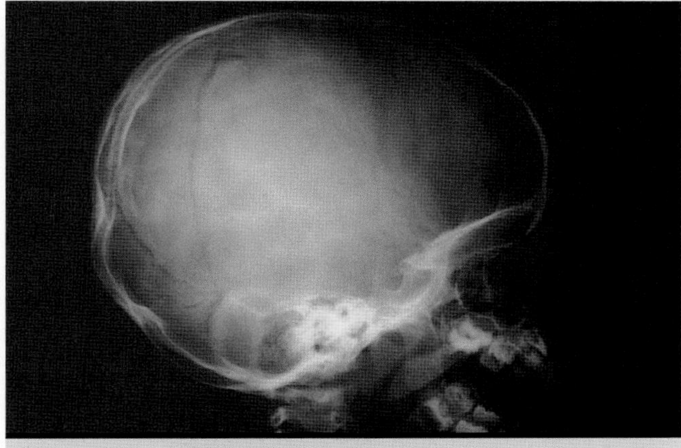

Figure 1-14. Skull Fracture

A 22-month-old infant presented with a history of accidentally tripping and falling down 10 steps onto a concrete floor as he was waking down with the mother. He had a palpable hematoma on the right parietal area; otherwise the examination was normal. A lateral radiograph of the skull reveals a vertical line of lucency involving the parietal bone that is suggestive of a fracture. Neither overlying soft tissue swelling nor suture diastasis is seen. A CT scan was only positive for a fracture in the right parietal bone with overlying soft tissue swelling, without any underlying extra-axial collection or intracranial hemorrhage. The rest of the examination was completely normal and the family had no prior record of abuse with child protective services. This fracture was considered an accidental injury.

are typically single, linear, nondiastatic, and most commonly involve the parietal bone. Fractures associated with simple accidental falls are also not associated with intracranial injury (Fig. 1-14).

3. Suspect abuse in a child presenting with a history of minor trauma with depressed, diastatic, or serious fractures, or complex or multiple fractures, particularly those involving the occipital bone (Figs. 1-15 and 1-16).

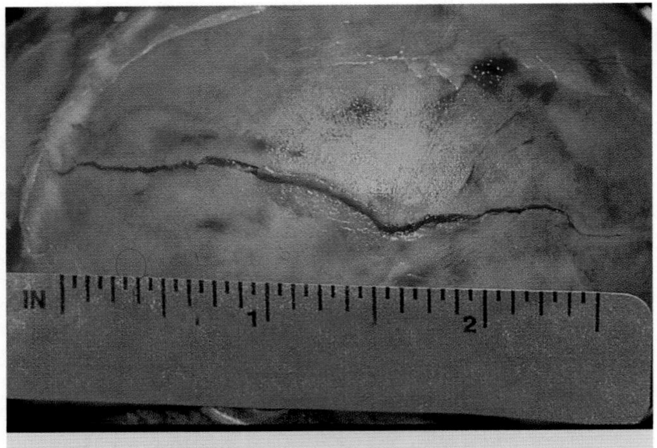

Figure 1-15. Skull Fracture due to Abuse

Intermastoid incision of the scalp in an infant shows a linear skull fracture of the parietal bone. There was brain injury with swelling but no intracranial hemorrhage was noted.

BOX 1-11. COMMON TYPES OF SKULL FRACTURES

Type	Characteristics
• Linear	A single, unbranched line that can be straight, curved, or angulated
• Complex	Comprised of more than one line May be branched or stellate or consist of more than one distinct fracture
• Stellate	A type of complex fracture Fracture lines radiate from a central point
• Comminuted	Complex fracture resulting in separate fragments of bone
• Depressed	Bony fragment is displaced inward toward the brain Often a comminuted fracture May be associated with neurological deficits, usually due to underlying brain involvement
• Diastatic	Fracture margins significantly separated Injuries to sutures can result in diastasis (either in association with a fracture or as an isolated injury)
• Ping-pong	Bone indented but without a distinct fracture
• Basilar	Fracture of base of skull Difficult to identify radiographically CT scan more sensitive than plain films Usually diagnosed by clinical criteria: CSF otorrhea, rhinorrhea, "raccoon" eyes or Battle's sign (see Fig. 2-13)

(Reproduced with permission from: Evaluation of fractures and skeletal injuries. In: Giardino AP, Christian CW, Giardino ER. *A Practical Guide to the Evaluation of Child Physical Abuse and Neglect*. Thousand Oaks, CA, Sage, 1997, p. 112.)

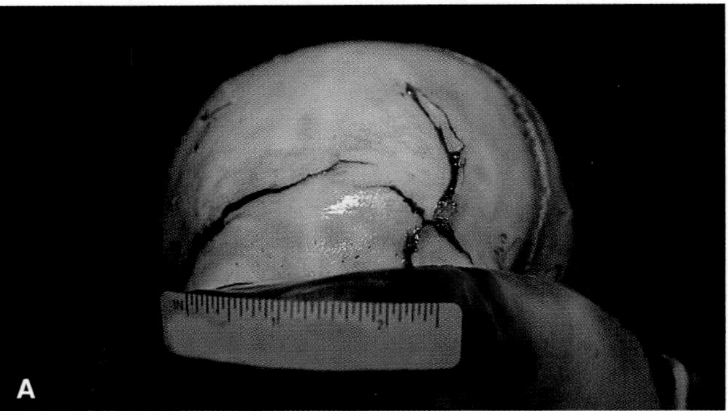

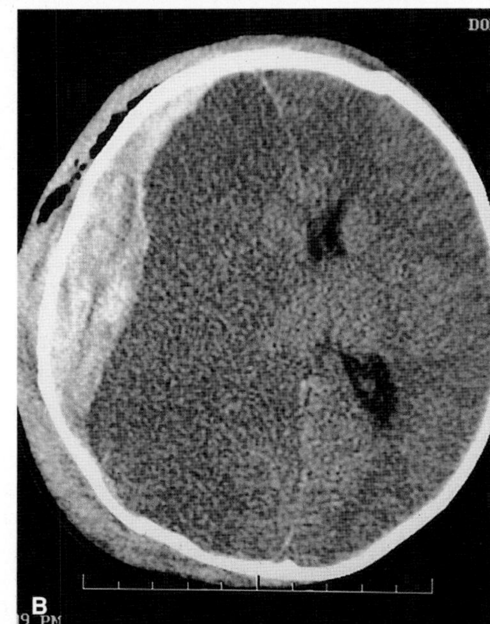

Figure 1-16. Head Injuries due to Abuse

A. Skull fractures. Comminuted skull fractures can be seen radiating from areas subjected to traumatic force in a toddler with an inflicted head injury. This patient's head was slammed against the kitchen counter. He presented in coma with signs of increased intracranial pressure due to an epidural hematoma. (*B*).

BOX 1-12. CLINICAL FEATURES OF SKULL FRACTURES DUE TO CHILD ABUSE

- *Skull fractures due to abuse:*
  (1) Most commonly seen in infants and toddlers
  (2) Soft tissue swelling overlying fracture site may not be seen at the time of presentation, but may become apparent after a few days (when the scalp hematoma liquefies)
  (3) The most common type of fracture in abusive injury and accidental falls is a linear parietal skull fracture
- *Strongly consider abuse if any of the following are present:*
  (1) Involvement of more than one cranial bone (multiple)
  (2) Bilateral fractures
  (3) Complex skull fractures
  (4) Fractures crossing suture lines
  (5) Nonlinear and nonparietal (e.g., occipital fractures)
  (6) Depressed fractures
  (7) Diastatic fractures
  (8) Growing skull fractures

BOX 1-13. DIFFERENTIAL DIAGNOSIS OF SKULL FRACTURES DUE TO ABUSE

- Accidental trauma
- Metabolic bone disease (e.g. osteogenesis imperfecta)

DIAGNOSIS SHAKEN IMPACT SYNDROME

SYNONYMS

Shaken baby syndrome
Whiplash shaken baby syndrome
Whiplash shaken infant syndrome

Associated Clinical Features

1. Abusive head trauma is the most common cause of death from child abuse.
2. About 95% of fatal or life-threatening head injuries in infants during the first year of life are the result of abuse.
3. Abusive head trauma may present with any of the following:
   a. Shaken impact syndrome (SIS)
   b. Intracranial hemorrhages (subdural, subgaleal, or epidural hematoma; Fig. 1-17)
   c. Periorbital ecchymosis
   d. Traction alopecia
4. SIS is the result of violent back-and-forth shaking of an infant, with or without impact, that causes a whiplike action of the unstable infant's head, leading to intracranial, cervical spine, and intraocular injuries. Findings of skull fracture, subgaleal and subperiosteal hemorrhages, and focal cortical contusions suggest that the shaking episode was likely followed by some type of impact (e.g., roughly throwing the infant onto a sofa or into a crib).
5. Findings of SIS may include any of the following:
   a. Subdural hemorrhage
   b. Bilateral chronic subdural hematoma
   c. Intracerebral contusion or hemorrhage; interhemispheric hemorrhage

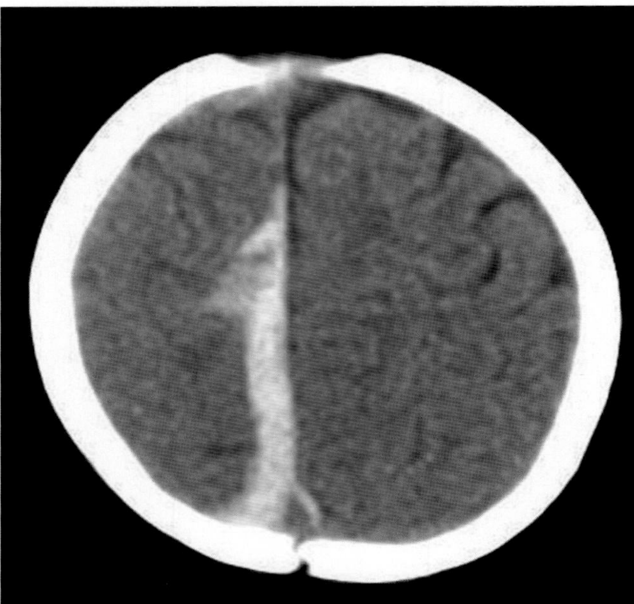

Figure 1-17. Acute Subdural Hematoma

Noncontrast computed tomogram of the brain shows hyperdense area along the right tentorium extending into the posterior interhemispheric fissure, along the falx and over the convexity, suggestive of an acute subdural hematoma. The patient also had a small subdural hematoma in the right frontotemporal region. This 3-month-old infant was brought to the ED with lethargy and signs of Cushing's triad (bradycardia [HR 70 bpm], bradypnea [RR 12/min], and hypertension [BP 114/50 mmHg]); he also had anemia (Hgb 6.97 g/dL). His anterior fontanelle was full; he had no evidence of any external injuries. Subsequently his father confessed to shaking the infant. This patient also had multiple posterior rib fractures involving the seventh through the 10th ribs with callus formation.

d. Subarachnoid hemorrhage
e. Cerebral edema
f. Skull fracture
g. Hematomas of the cervical spinal cord
h. Injuries at the cervicomedullary junction of the spinal cord
i. Retinal hemorrhages (see Box 1-15; Fig. 1-18)
j. Other ocular findings (vitreous hemorrhages, retinal folds, or traumatic retinoschisis) (Fig. 1-19)
k. Tin ear syndrome (a variant of SIS produced by a blow to the side of the head that causes forceful rotational acceleration of the head on the neck); patients present with unilateral bruising of the pinna and ipsilateral cerebral edema, subdural hemorrhage, and retinal hemorrhages.

6. Fundoscopy must be done after the pupils are dilated (if possible, by a pediatric ophthalmologist) in all cases of SIS.

7. Mild to moderate anemia is a typical finding (intracranial blood loss) in SIS. Additional tests should include a coagulation profile (prothrombin time, partial thromboplastin time, fibrinogen, and bleeding time; bleeding diathesis may be seen due to release of cerebral thromboplastin), liver function tests (elevated transaminase levels indicates occult liver injury), and urinalysis (to detect renal injuries)

8. Lumbar puncture (LP) should be performed.
   a. The presence of blood is often mistaken for bloody or traumatic LP.
   b. Centrifuged cerebrospinal fluid (CSF): a xanthochromic supernatant suggests a past cerebral bleed (blood in the CSF for at least 12 to 24 hours).
   c. Chronic subdural bleed: CSF is viscous and yellow.

9. All patients with suspected intracranial injury must undergo CT scan or MRI or both.
   a. CT scan without contrast enhancement
      1) CT is readily available and is performed first (before MRI) as a part of the initial evaluation for suspected head injury.
      2) CT has high sensitivity and specificity for diagnosing acute subdural and epidural hemorrhages that may require emergency surgical intervention.
      3) Subarachnoid and intraparenchymal bleeds are also well demonstrated on CT.
      4) Bone windows may show associated skull and facial fractures.
      5) *CT is better than MRI for evaluation of acute hemorrhage.*
      6) CT allows dating of injuries by documenting changes in the hemoglobin in the affected area.
   b. MRI
      1) Best modality for fully assessing intracranial injury including extra-axial collections, contusions, shear injuries, and brain edema

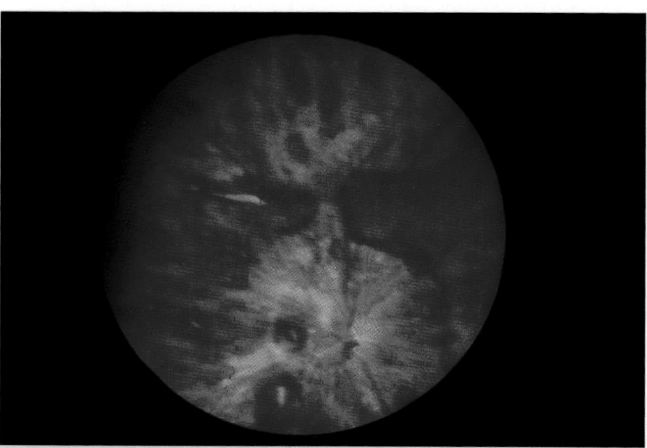

Figure 1-18. Retinal Hemorrhages

Severe, diffuse preretinal and intraretinal blot hemorrhages characteristic of child abuse. Hemorrhages such as these strongly correlate with inflicted injury. (Reproduced with permission from: Christian CW, Lane WG: Ophthalmic involvement in non accidental trauma. In: Hertle RW, Schaffer DB, Foster JA (eds). *Pediatric Eye Disease. Color Atlas and Synopsis.* McGraw-Hill, New York, 2002, p. 106.)

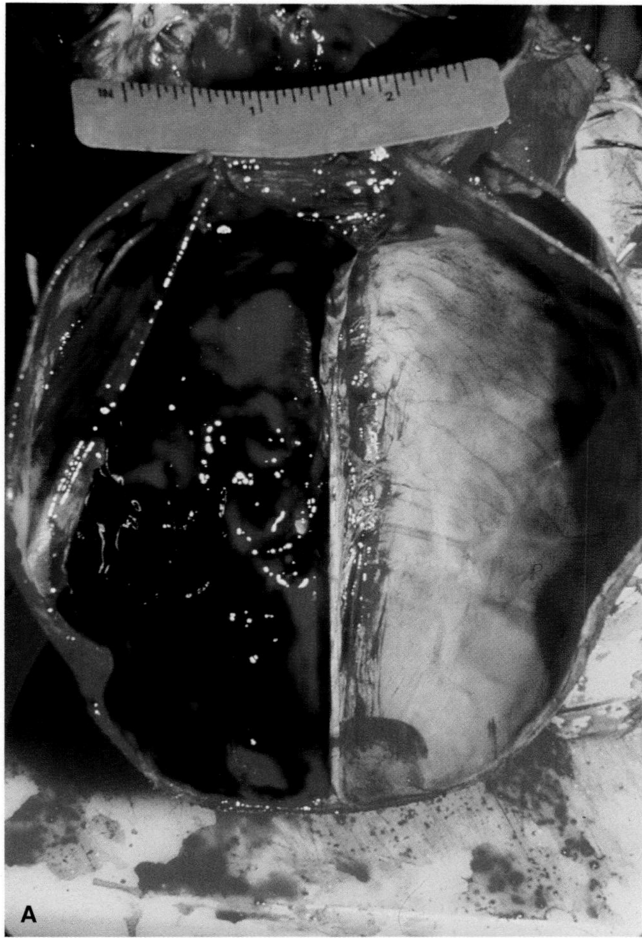

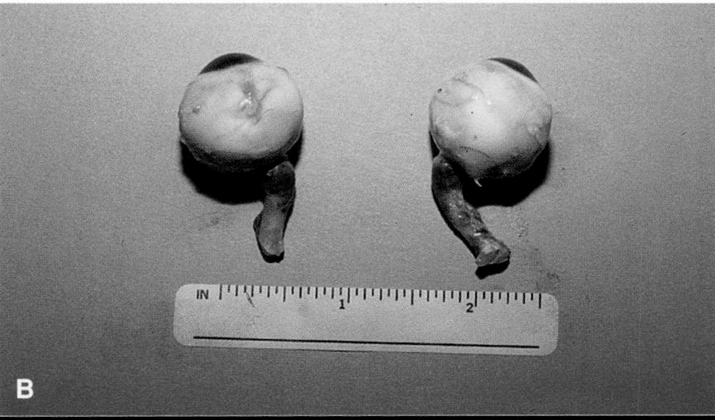

Figure 1-19. Hemorrhages Seen in Shaken Infant Syndrome

A. Acute subdural hematoma. A 6-month-old infant was brought in cardiopulmonary arrest. Per the mother's history he was found in the bed "not breathing." The only findings on examination were Mongolian spots on the buttocks and back of the trunk (these can easily be mistaken for bruises; see Fig. 2-1). Acute subdural hematoma was seen at autopsy. Unlike subdural hemorrhage (SDH), epidural hemorrhage (EDH) may occur with simple and complex skull fractures in association with accidental falls. Thus the presence of EDH alone should not raise the same level of concern for child abuse as that raised by identification of a SDH. *B*. Optic nerve sheath hemorrhages. Eye globes showing hemorrhages. Retinal hemorrhages were also noted on microscopic examination.

2) MRI may not detect acute subarachnoid or subdural hemorrhage; thus MRI should be repeated 5 to 7 days in acutely ill children.
3) MRI offers the highest sensitivity and specificity for diagnosing subacute and chronic injury.

10. Skeletal survey (see Box 1-1)
    a. Mandatory for infants with SIS
    b. A skeletal survey may need to be repeated in 2 weeks to identify new fractures that may not become apparent until they show evidence of healing (usually after 7 to 10 days).
11. Long-term neurological morbidity of SIS may include mental retardation, chronic subdural effusions, hydrocephalus, spastic quadriplegia, seizures, cerebral atrophy, encephalomalacia, or porencephalic cysts.

Consultations

A multidisciplinary team approach should be used, with consultations with a neurosurgeon, a neurologist, an ophthalmologist, a radiologist, a pediatrician, a child abuse consultant, and a social worker.

Emergency Department Treatment and Disposition

1. Assessment of ABCDEs with simultaneous stabilization of vital signs. After stabilization, all patients with intracranial injuries require transfer to the PICU for continuous monitoring. The patient may be brought to the operating room for evacuation of subdural or epidural hematomas.
2. For guidelines for reporting to child protective agency, see page 3.

Clinical Pearls: Shaken Impact Syndrome

1. Cardinal symptoms of SIS include brain injury (subdural hemorrhage and cerebral edema), retinal hemorrhages, and skeletal injuries.
2. SIS is one of the most common causes of intracranial injury in infants <1 year of age.
3. Infants rarely sustain accidental head injury sufficiently severe to result in unconsciousness. Suspect SIS in any infant presenting with altered sensorium, a bulging fontanelle, head circumference $>$90th percentile, or abnormal respiratory patterns despite a normal pulmonary examination.
4. Usually there are *no* external signs of injury in SIS.
5. In a case of a suspected infantile sepsis, examine any bloody spinal fluid for xanthochromia.
6. Perform a dilated retinal exam to look for retinal hemorrhages in any infant presenting with unresponsiveness or cranial soft tissue injuries.

BOX 1-14. CLINICAL FEATURES OF SHAKEN IMPACT SYNDROME

- *Age at presentation:*
  (1) SIS is almost always seen in infants <2 years of age.
  (2) It is most common in infants <1 year of age, and most patients are <6 months of age.
- *Common presenting signs and symptoms:*
  (1) Lethargy or irritability
  (2) Bulging or tense fontanelle
  (3) Apnea or respiratory arrest
  (4) Bradycardia
  (5) Coma
  (6) Poor feeding
  (7) Seizures
  (8) Vomiting
  (9) Usually minimal neurologic deficits
  (10) Head circumference >90th percentile
  (11) Typically there is no external bruising or visible injuries
- *Skeletal injuries strongly suggestive of SIS:*
  (1) Bilateral, multiple, posterior rib fractures
  (2) Metaphyseal fractures of long bones

BOX 1-15. RETINAL HEMORRHAGES AND SHAKEN IMPACT SYNDROME

- Hemorrhages
  (1) Present in 75 to 90% of cases
  (2) Bilateral in 60 to 90% of cases
  (3) Unilateral in 10 to 30% of cases
  (4) Usually last 10 to 14 days; may persist for longer period
  (5) Flame-shaped hemorrhages (superficial retinal nerve fiber layer)
  (6) Dot and blot hemorrhages (intraretinal)
- Mechanism Retinal venous hypertension from significant accelerative or decelerative forces causes rupture of retinal veins.
- *Differential diagnosis of retinal hemorrhages:*
  (1) Birth trauma of vaginal delivery (small flame-shaped hemorrhages rarely persist beyond the first week of life and intraretinal dot or blot hemorrhages disappear by 4 weeks)
  (2) Severe accidental trauma (e.g., motor vehicle accident, blunt eye trauma)
  (3) Nontraumatic (e.g., coagulopathy, carbon monoxide poisoning, sepsis, meningitis, severe hypertension)
  (4) Increased intracranial pressure with papilledema
  (5) Following cardiopulmonary resuscitation (controversial)

Key point: Retinal hemorrhages in infants <2 years of age suggest SIS unless proven otherwise.

(Reproduced with permission from: Shaken impact syndrome. Shah BR, Laude TA: *Atlas of Pediatric Clinical Diagnosis.* WB Saunders, Philadelphia, 2000, p. 30.)

BOX 1-16. DIFFERENTIAL DIAGNOSIS OF SHAKEN IMPACT SYNDROME

- Infections (e.g., sepsis, meningitis)
- Poisoning
- Seizure disorder
- Inborn errors of metabolism
- Altered level of consciousness from other etiologies (see mnemonic COMATOSE PATIENT, Box 13-4)
- Hemorrhagic disease of the newborn (vitamin K deficiency)

DIAGNOSIS INFLICTED BURN INJURIES

Associated Clinical Features

1. About 10 to 25% of pediatric burns are a result of abuse.
2. Burns (both accidental and inflicted) are seen more frequently in children <5 years of age with a peak incidence in infants and toddlers <3 years of age.
3. Classification of burns:
   a. Scalds (due to hot liquids; e.g., tap water, boiling water, tea, coffee, soup, or oil). These are the most common type of burns in both accidental and abusive injuries (Fig. 1-20). In children about 83% of inflicted burn

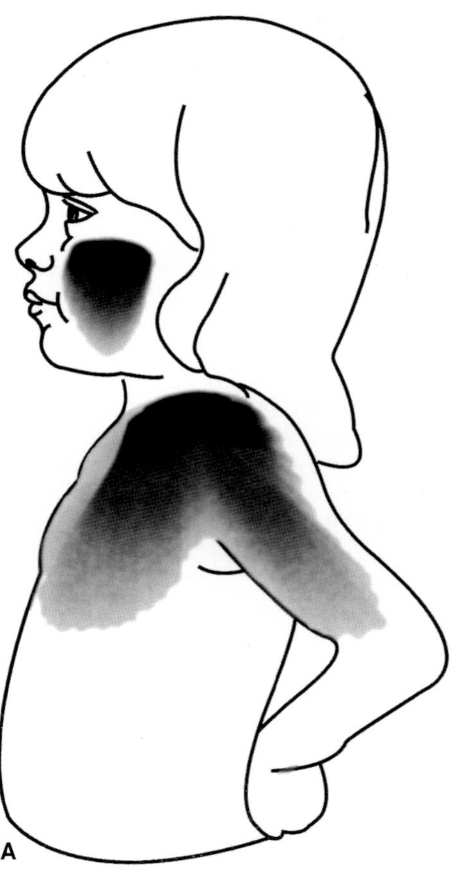

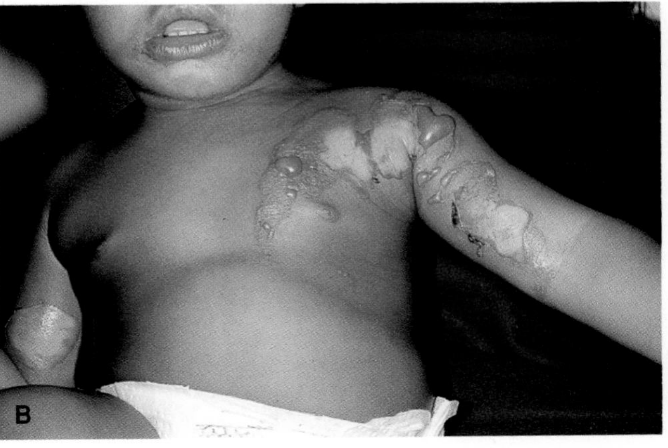

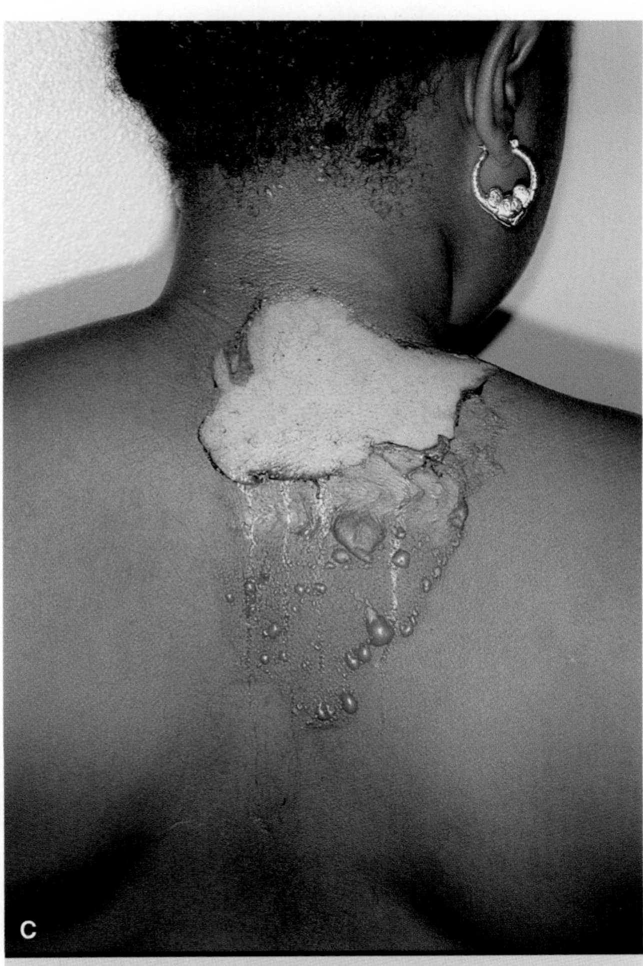

Figure 1-20. Typical Spill Burn Patterns

A. Burn with distribution on anterior trunk. An arrow-shaped configuration occurs due to cooling as the liquid descends. The presence of clothing makes burns more severe by holding hot liquid in close contact with the skin. Accidental spill burns may also show splash marks away from the point of maximal contact. *B*. Accidental spill burn. Accidental first- and second-degree burns to the lower face, shoulder, chest, and hand in this 2-year-old child due to hot tea spilling on him when he reached up and pulled the mug filled with the tea from a table. In a typical spill burn, the hot liquid usually falls onto the child's face and shoulder first (usually the most severe burn is seen at these sites), and as the liquid runs down the body and cools, the burn becomes less severe. *C*. Inflicted splash burn. Hot soup was thrown on the back of this girl as she tried to run away from her father during an argument. Figure 1-20 A is reproduced with permission from: Giardino AP, Christian CW, Giardino ER: *A Practical Guide to the Evaluation of Child Physical Abuse and Neglect* Sage Publications, Thousand Oaks, CA, 1997, p. 79.

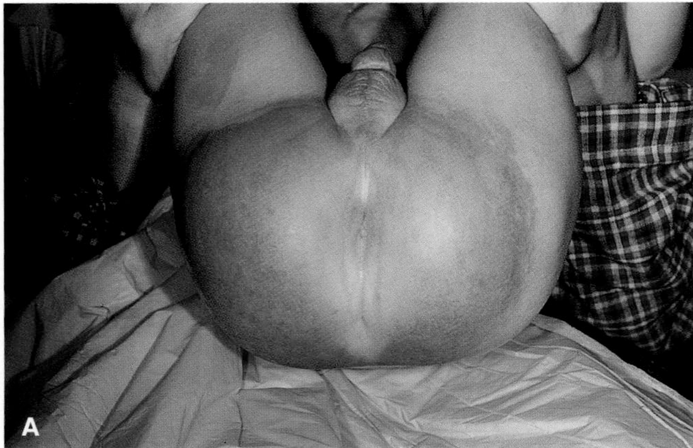

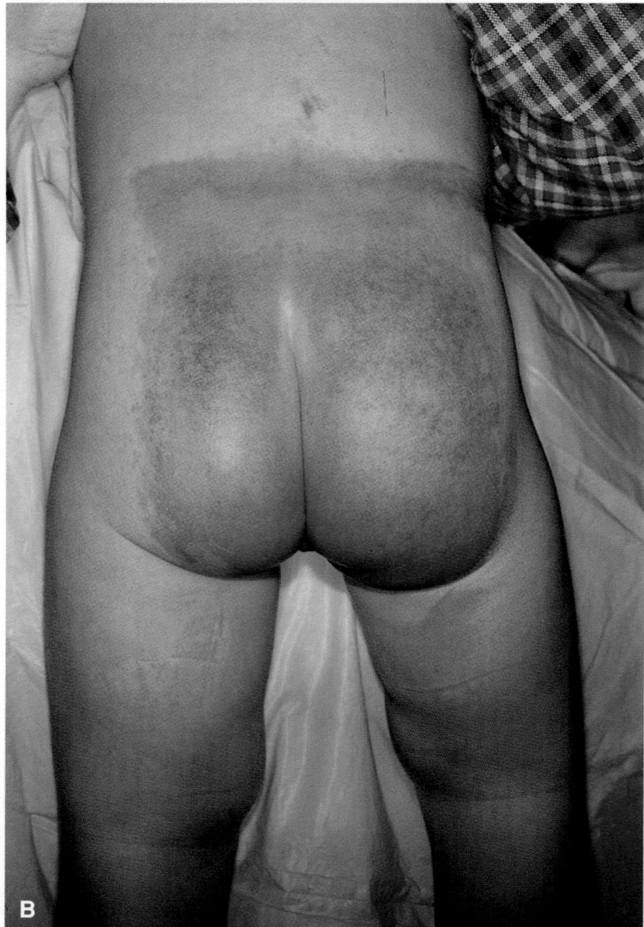

Figure 1-21. Chemical Burn

Burn caused by chlorine bleach that accidentally spilled in this infant's diaper that served as an occlusive dressing. It was difficult to determine if this was an accidental or inflicted injury, and the incident was reported to child protective services. After a thorough investigation, this injury was considered to be accidental.

injuries involve tap water–induced scalds, as opposed to only 15% of accidental scalds.

1) Scalds can be caused by: (a) a spill (hot liquid falls) or splash (hot liquid is thrown); (b) immersion (accidental fall or submersion in hot liquid); or (c) forced immersion (a pattern suggestive of force used to hold the child in the hot liquid is seen).

b. Flame
c. Electrical
d. Chemical (Fig. 1-21)
e. Immersion burns (Fig. 1-22)
   1) Flexion of the hips occurs instinctively as the child's buttocks are held in contact with the hot liquid. Thus the crease between the thigh and abdomen (opposing surfaces of skin) is spared.
   2) "Hole-in-a-doughnut" pattern (Fig. 1-22).
f. Contact burns (hot object is forcibly held against the child's skin; Figs. 1-23 and 1-24)
   1) Second most common type of inflicted burn
   2) Well-circumscribed affected area
   3) Outline of the hot object that was used is seen (e.g., an iron)

Consultations

A multidisciplinary team approach should be used, with consultations from a pediatrician, a child abuse consultant, a social worker, and a surgeon (preferably a specialist in pediatric surgery).

Emergency Department Treatment and Disposition

1. For guidelines to management of burns and indications for hospitalization, please refer to page 689.
2. Sometimes it is very difficult to differentiate between an accidental splash burn and an inflicted splash burn and physical findings may not help to differentiate them. If in doubt, all suspect burns require hospitalization while awaiting further investigation. A thorough history and physical examination to look for other evidence of injury may be helpful (e.g., immunization status, growth parameters, bruises, or poor hygiene).

Clinical Pearls: Inflicted Burn Injuries

1. Stocking-and-glove burn patterns and forced immersion burns are pathognomonic for child abuse.
2. Inflicted immersion burns have a distinct line demarcating the burned and unburned areas and the burn is uniform in depth.
3. Abusive immersion burns are more common in infants and toddlers.
4. Inflicted contact burns frequently are geometric, due to the shape of the object used to inflict the injury. Accidental contact burns occur due to brief contact with a hot object and are less geometric in shape and more superficial.
5. Scalding is the most common mechanism of burn injury for abused children.

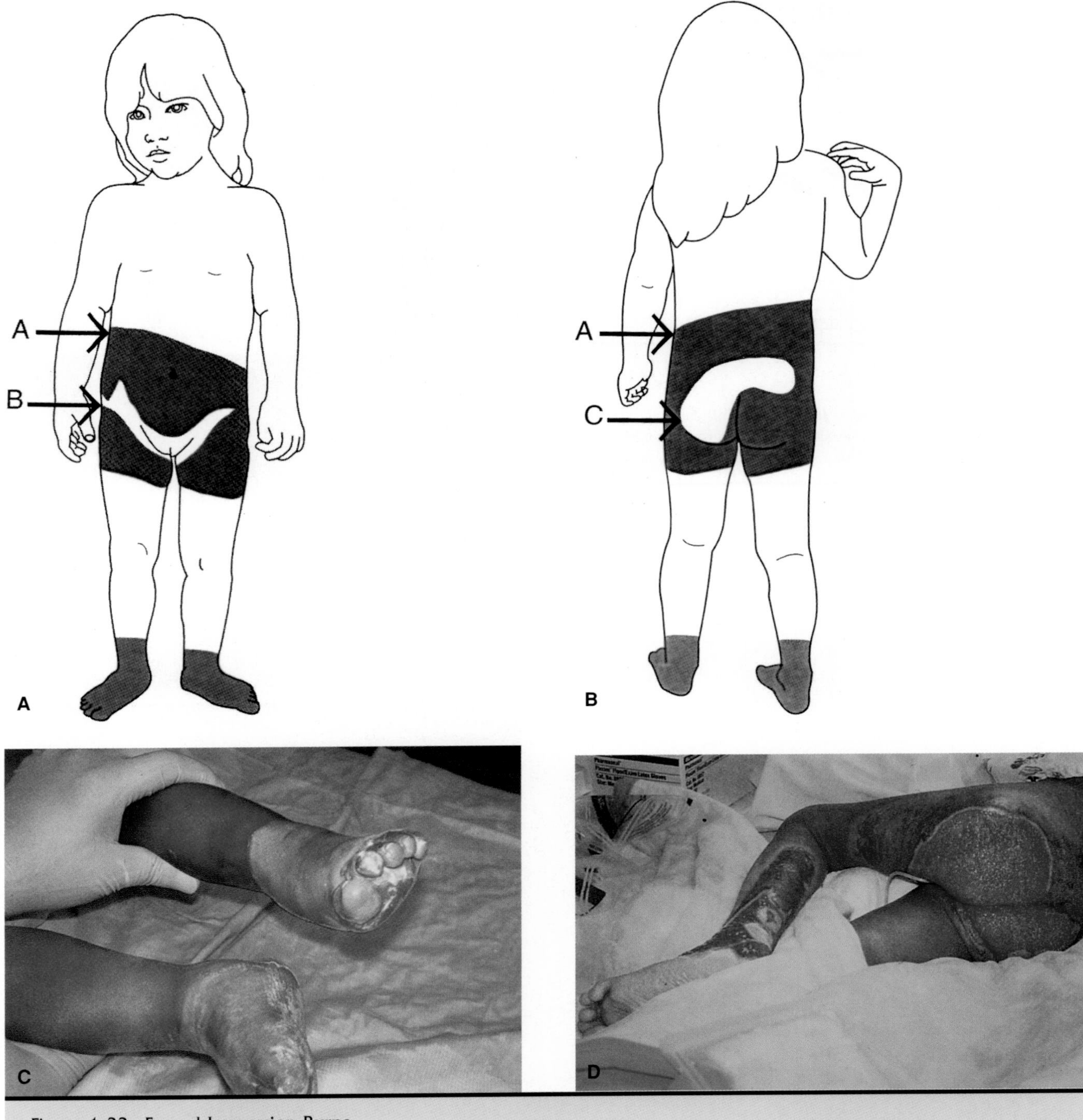

Figure 1-22. Forced Immersion Burns

A. As the child's buttocks are plunged into the hot liquid and held against the porcelain tub, the child instinctively flexes the hips. The burn is well demarcated (A). The crease between the thigh and abdomen is spared (B). *B*. The area of the buttocks that is held against the relatively cooler tub is less severely burned and gives rise to the "hole-in-a-doughnut" pattern (C). The child's heel may come into contact with the hot liquid, and the burn is well demarcated (*A and B*). *C*. Stocking burns. A 20-month-old infant whose feet got dirty and reportedly was left in a basin of hot water. Stocking burns of the feet up to both ankles are due to submersion in scalding water. *D*. A $2^1/_2$-year-old with severe immersion burns to the buttocks and feet. Note evidence of previous healed immersion burns to the same areas. The child was not taken for medical care until she presented with severe brain injury. A skeletal survey revealed a healing supracondylar fracture of the right humerus. (Reproduced with permission from: Giardino AP, Christian CW, Giardino ER: *A Practical Guide to the Evaluation of Child Physical Abuse and Neglect.* Sage Publications, Thousand Oaks, CA, 1997, pages 82-84 and 89.)

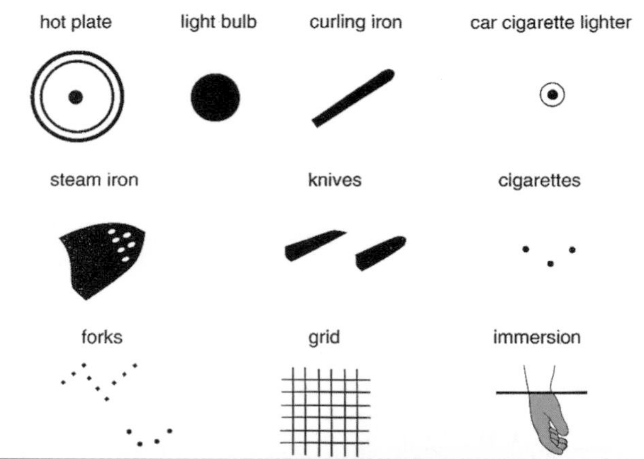

Figure 1-23. Marks from Burns

(Reproduced with permission from: Johnson CF: Inflicted injury versus accidental injury. In: *Child Abuse*, Pediatric Clinics of North America. WB Saunders, Philadelphia, Vol. 37, No. 4, 1990, p. 807).

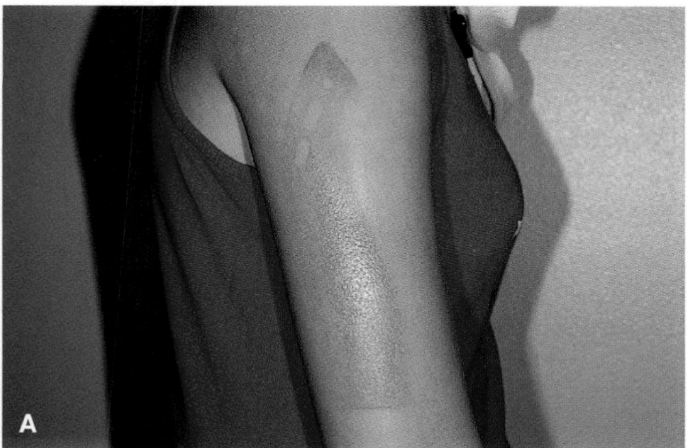

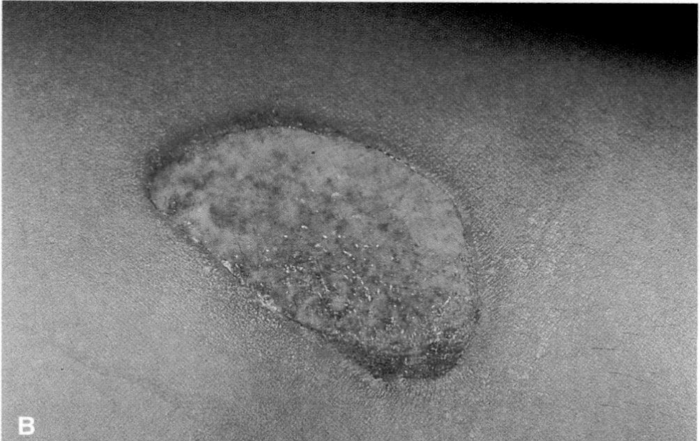

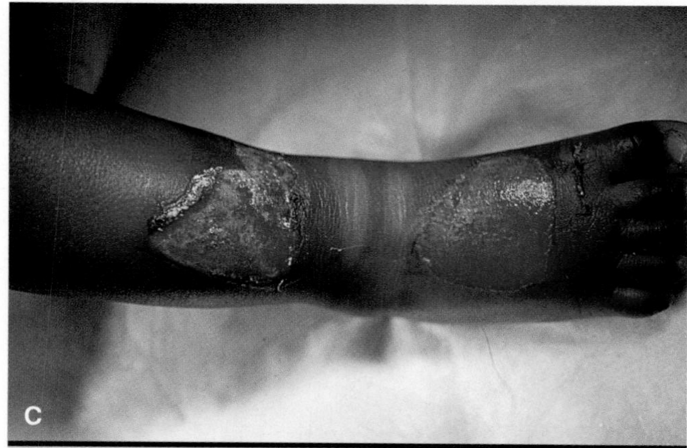

Figure 1-24. Contact Burns

A. Burn from an iron inflicted on this patient by her stepfather during an argument. *B*. A well-defined area of burn inflicted on this child by a heated spoon. *C*. An 8-month-old infant with second- and third-degree burns of the lower extremity inflicted by a hot object because "he was crying too much."

BOX 1-17. CLINICAL FEATURES OF BURNS

Typical accidental spill burn pattern (due to a child reaching up and pulling a container of hot liquid):

- Usually hot liquid falls on the face and shoulder first; the most severe burn is at the point of initial contact; as the liquid runs down the body and cools, the burn becomes narrower and less severe at the perimeter

Forced immersion burn

- Pathognomonic burns of child abuse
- Most common locations are the perineum and extremities
- Well-demarcated burn
- "Hole-in-a-doughnut" pattern (area of buttocks that is held against the relatively cooler tub is less severely burned than the rest of the skin, which is in contact with hot liquid and gives rise to a characteristic pattern)
- Typical glove distribution (from hands being forcibly held in hot liquid)
- Typical stocking burn (from feet being forcibly held in hot liquid)

Cigarette burns

- Round, symmetrical burns, often seen in clusters
- Inner circle of tissue more deeply burned than the periphery
- Average diameter about 8 to 10 mm

BOX 1-18. CONDITIONS MIMICKING INFLICTED BURN INJURIES

- Accidental burns
- Chemical burns
- Infections
  (1) Ecthyma (see Figs. 3-12 and 3-13)
  (2) Blistering distal dactylitis
  (3) Bullous impetigo (see Figs. 3-8 to 3-10)
  (4) Staphylococcal scalded skin syndrome (see Figs. 3-23 to 3-27)
- Folk-healing practices (see Figs. 2-2 to 2-4)
- Arthropod bites (see Fig. 3-11)
- Frostbite (see Figs. 18-6 and 18-7)
- Dermatologic conditions
  (1) Phytophotodermatitis (see Fig. 2-11)
  (2) Severe diaper dermatitis
  (3) Drug eruptions (see Figs. 7-8 to 7-9)
  (4) Epidermolysis bullosa
  (5) Dermatitis herpetiformis

DIAGNOSIS

INFANTICIDE VERSUS SUDDEN INFANT DEATH SYNDROME

SYNONYMS

Crib death or cot death for SIDS

Definitions

1. *Sudden infant death syndrome* (SIDS) is a sudden and unexplained death occurring in a healthy infant younger than 1 year old. SIDS is a diagnosis of exclusion (see Box 1-20).
2. *Infanticide* is an incident of child abuse that is fatal during infancy (Fig. 1-25).

Associated Clinical Features

1. The incidence of SIDS is two to three times higher among African-American and some Native American populations.
2. Contributory factors for SIDS include:
   a. Factors related to sleep (e.g., sleeping in a prone position or sleeping on soft material or a soft surface)
   b. Maternal factors (e.g., young maternal age, maternal smoking during or after pregnancy, lack of prenatal care)

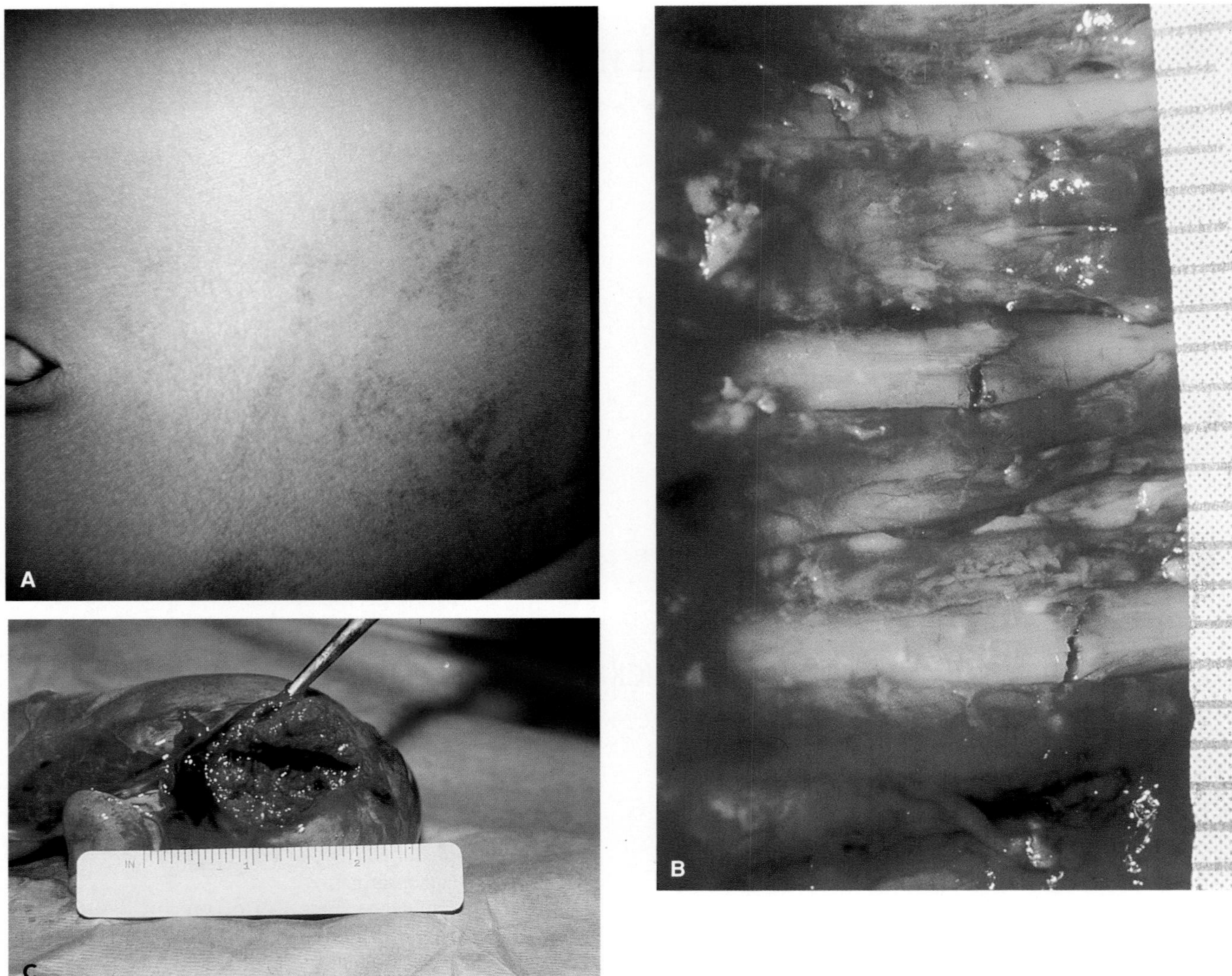

Figure 1-25. Infanticide

A. Abdominal bruise. An infant brought in with cardiopulmonary arrest was found to have this bruise on the abdominal wall. The mother gave a history of finding the baby "not breathing" 4 hours after she had fed the baby. *B*. Rib fractures. Multiple bilateral rib fractures were found at autopsy. *C*. Liver laceration. Liver and mesenteric lacerations were found at autopsy in this infant. Blunt abdominal trauma causes the second highest mortality rate related to abusive injuries. Suspect abusive abdominal trauma in any infant or child with unexplained peritonitis or shock (especially in the presence of bilious vomiting and/or anemia). Inflicted abdominal injuries include ruptured liver or spleen, intestinal perforation, duodenal hematoma, pancreatic injury, and kidney trauma.

   c. Factors related to the infant (e.g., prematurity, low birth weight, male gender)
   d. Environmental factors (e.g., overheating, overwrapping)

3. Estimates of the incidence of infanticide among cases diagnosed as SIDS vary between <1 and 5%.
4. It is impossible to distinguish at autopsy between SIDS and accidental or intentional suffocation with a soft object.
5. Postmortem studies that will be done by the medical examiner include:
   a. Radiographic skeletal survey (before autopsy)
   b. Toxicologic screening (e.g., occult cocaine exposure [a 2.7 to 40% incidence was reported in some postmortem studies])
   c. Metabolic screening for inborn errors of metabolism (analysis of blood or other body fluids such as urine, vitreous humor, CSF, and stomach contents; and tissue

analysis of the brain, liver, kidney, heart, muscle, adrenal glands and pancreas)

Consultations

A medical examiner (ME) or coroner; a child maltreatment specialist or pediatrician with expertise in child maltreatment; consultation with a pediatric pathologist, forensic pathologist, law enforcement officer, social worker, and child protective services agency personnel, as indicated.

Emergency Department Management

1. Once the infant is pronounced dead, approach the family with an empathic, compassionate, supportive, and nonaccusatory manner while attempting to learn more about the

BOX 1-19. NORMAL POSTMORTEM FINDINGS AFTER DEATH

- Evidence of terminal motor activity (e.g., clenched fists)
- Serosanguineous, watery, frothy, or mucoid discharge coming from nose or mouth
- Skin mottling
- Postmortem lividity in dependent portions of the body (Fig. 1-26)
- Postmortem anal dilation

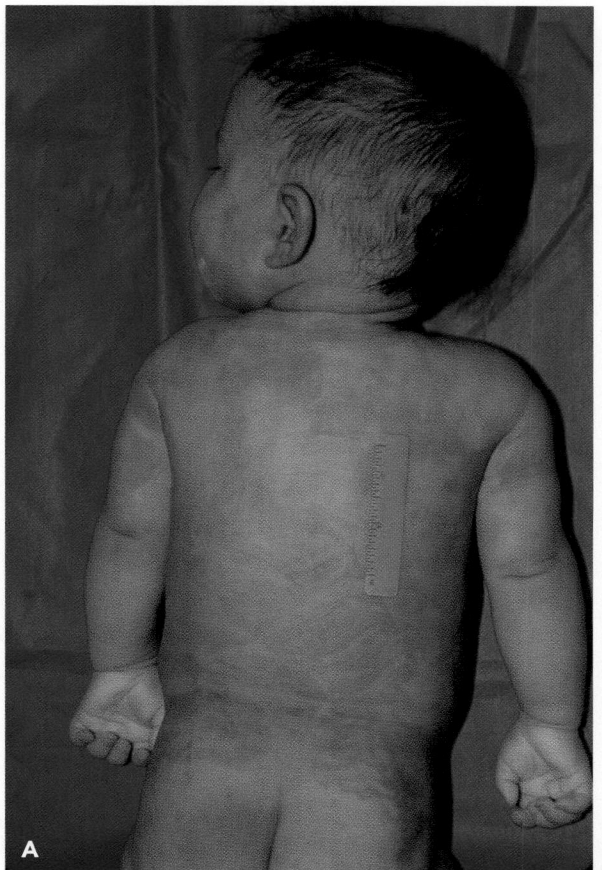

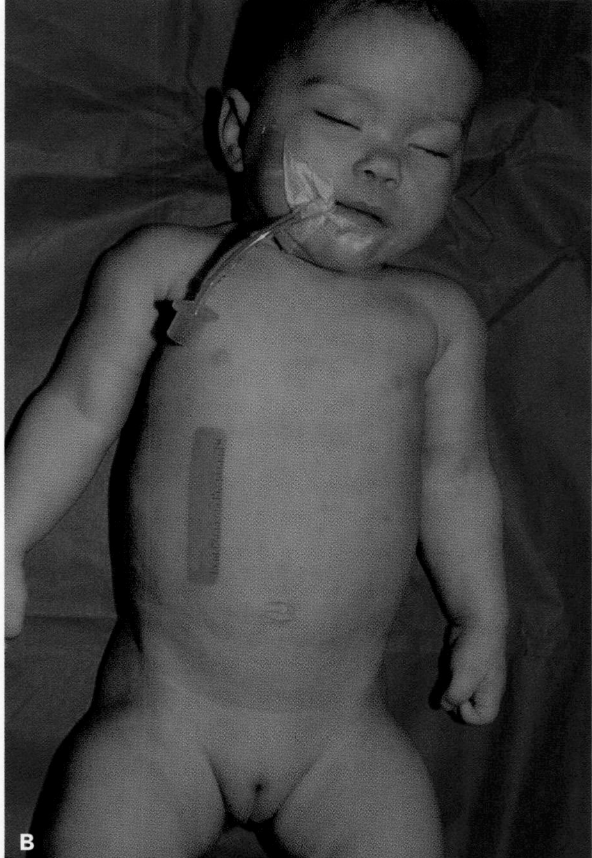

Figure 1-26. Postmortem Lividity (Livor Mortis)

Postmortem lividity is a purplish-blue discoloration due to settling of blood in dependent areas of the body due to gravitational forces. It is usually seen within hours after death on the back if the body was in a supine position, and on the face and front if the body was in a prone position. Within 8 to 12 hours, the skin lesions become nonblanching. This finding can easily be confused with bruises due to child abuse.

BOX 1-20. SUDDEN INFANT DEATH SYNDROME VERSUS INFANTICIDE

SIDS:

- Most common cause of death between 1 and 6 months of age
- Peak incidence between 2 and 4 months of age
- About 90% of SIDS deaths occur before 6 months of age
- A diagnosis of exclusion (if all of the following are unrevealing or normal):
  (1) Complete postmortem exam (including cranium and cranial contents) within 24 hours of death
  (2) Absence of gross or microscopic evidence of trauma or significant disease process
  (3) Thorough death scene investigation findings negative
  (4) Review of clinical history fails to reveal another cause of death
  (5) Normal radiographs (no evidence of trauma on skeletal survey performed before autopsy)
  (6) Other causes of death have been ruled out (e.g., sepsis, meningitis, myocarditis, dehydration, abdominal trauma, congenital lesions, fluid and electrolyte imbalance, inborn errors of metabolism, carbon monoxide asphyxia, drowning, or burns)
  (7) No evidence of current alcohol, drug or toxic exposure (e.g., occult cocaine exposure)

Suspect possible intentional suffocation or infanticide if any of following are present:

- Previous recurrent episodes of cyanosis, apnea, or apparent life-threatening event (ALTE) while under the care of the same person
- Age at death >6 months
- Previous unexplained or unexpected deaths of one or more siblings
- Simultaneous or nearly simultaneous death of twins
- Previous death of infants under the care of the same unrelated person
- Discovery of blood on the infant's nose or mouth in association with ALTEs

circumstances surrounding the infant's death. The reaction of the caregivers or parents should also be noted.

2. Even though a thorough investigation of the death scene will be done by law enforcement officers, try to obtain the details about the observations made by the first-response teams and document in the medical record (e.g., position of the infant; body temperature and rigor; the presence of any marks on the body prior to CPR administration; the type of crib or bed and any defects and the type of mattress [firm versus a water bed]; the presence of a fluffy blanket or comforter, soft stuffed toys or pillows in the crib; the amount of clothing on the baby; the room temperature and type of ventilation and heating). Provide the accurate history to the ME or coroner after carefully interviewing caretaker and family members who were present at the scene.
3. A thorough examination of the dead infant should be done by either a child maltreatment specialist or pediatrician with expertise in child maltreatment. All of the findings must be conveyed to the coroner or ME. In the absence of any external evidence of trauma, a preliminary diagnosis of "probable SIDS" can be given to a previously healthy infant who has died suddenly and without any explainable cause.
4. A definitive diagnosis of SIDS can only be reached after fulfilling the criteria detailed in Box 1-20. Postmortem findings in fatal child abuse most often reveal cranial injuries (e.g., subdural hematoma, intracerebral hemorrhage), intra-abdominal trauma (e.g., liver laceration, hollow viscus perforation, intramural hematoma), burns, and drowning or toxic exposure.

Clinical Pearls: Infanticide versus Sudden Infant Death Syndrome

1. An autopsy must be performed on any infant who dies suddenly and unexpectedly. Infant deaths without postmortem examination should not be attributed to SIDS.
2. Failure to differentiate infanticide from SIDS is costly. By excluding child abuse through a thorough investigation in every sudden and unexplained death, surviving and subsequent siblings can be protected.

Suggested Readings

American Academy of Pediatrics: Child abuse and neglect. *A Guide to References and Resources in Child Abuse and Neglect,* 2nd ed. Elk Grove Village, IL, 1998.

American Academy of Pediatrics: Child abuse and neglect. *A Guide to References and Resources in Child Abuse and Neglect.* Elk Grove Village, IL, 1994.

American Academy of Pediatrics. Committee on Child Abuse and Neglect: Distinguishing sudden infant death syndrome from child abuse fatalities. *Pediatrics* 2001;107:437.

American Academy of Pediatrics. Kellogg N and the Committee on Child Abuse and Neglect: The evaluation of sexual abuse of children: *Pediatrics* 2005;116(2):506.

American Academy of Pediatrics, Committee on Child Abuse and Neglect: Shaken baby syndrome: Inflicted cerebral trauma. *Pediatrics* 1993:92;872.

American Academy of Pediatrics, Section on Radiology: Diagnostic imaging of child abuse. *Pediatrics* 2000;105(6):1345.

Atabaki S, Paradise JE: The medical evaluation of the sexually abused child: Lesions from a decade of research. *Pediatrics* 1999104: 178.

Finkel MA, Giardino AP (eds): *Medical Evaluation of Child Sexual Abuse. A Practical Guide*, 2nd ed. Sage, Thousand Oaks, CA, 2002.

Giardino AP, Christian CW, Giardino ER: *A Practical Guide to the Evaluation of Child Physical Abuse and Neglect.* Sage, Thousand Oaks, CA, 1997.

Jain AM: Domestic violence. Emergency department evaluation of child abuse. *Emerg Med Clin North Am* 1999;17:575.

Kellogg N, American Academy of Pediatrics Committee on Child Abuse and Neglect. The evaluation of sexual abuse in children. Pediatrics. 2005;116(2):506.

Nimkin K, Kleinman PK: Pediatric musculoskeletal radiology. Imaging of child abuse. *Radiol Clin North Am* 2001;39:(4)843.

Reece RM, Ludwig S (eds): Child abuse. *Medical Diagnosis and Management,* 2nd ed. Lippincott Williams & Wilkins, Baltimore, 2001.

CHAPTER 2

CONDITIONS MISTAKEN FOR CHILD ABUSE AND SEXUAL ABUSE

Binita R. Shah

DIAGNOSIS MONGOLIAN SPOTS

Definition

Mongolian spots are benign, grey-blue macular birthmarks characteristically located over the lumbosacral area.

Etiology

1. Mongolian spots are a form of dermal melanocytosis. Melanocytes, in their transit from the neural crest to epidermis during the embryonic period, become arrested in the dermis (migrational arrest). This results in ectopic melanocytes in the dermis.
2. When light strikes the surface of the lesions, all colors of the spectrum are absorbed by the melanin in the dermis except for the blue, which is reflected (Tyndall effect). As time goes by, these melanocytes lose their cell membranes and get processed by macrophages. Clinically this translates into fading of the lesions.

Associated Clinical Features

1. Mongolian spots are seen in >95% of African-American infants, 70 to 80% of Asian infants, 46% of Hispanic newborns, and <10% of Caucasian infants.
2. The diagnosis is made clinically.

Emergency Department Treatment and Disposition

No treatment is required except for reassurance about the benign nature of these lesions.

Clinical Pearls: Mongolian Spot

1. Mongolian spots may be mistaken (especially in a white infant) for ecchymosis resulting from accidental or inflicted injury (bruises due to abuse) (Fig. 2-1).
2. An ecchymotic skin lesion undergoes color changes (see Box 1-4) and resolves within a few days, while mongolian spots *do not undergo this color change* and fade spontaneously over a period of years.

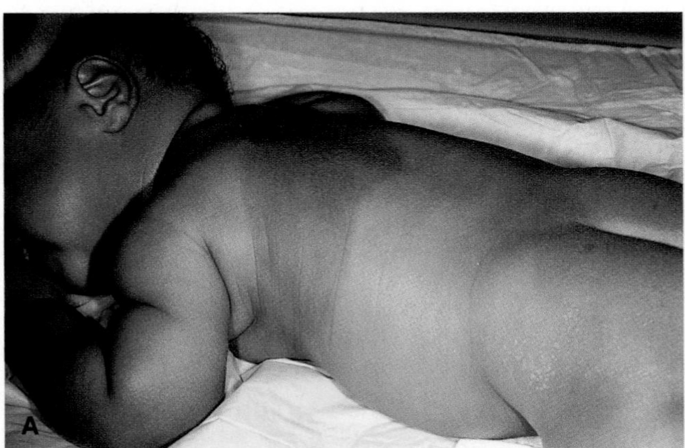

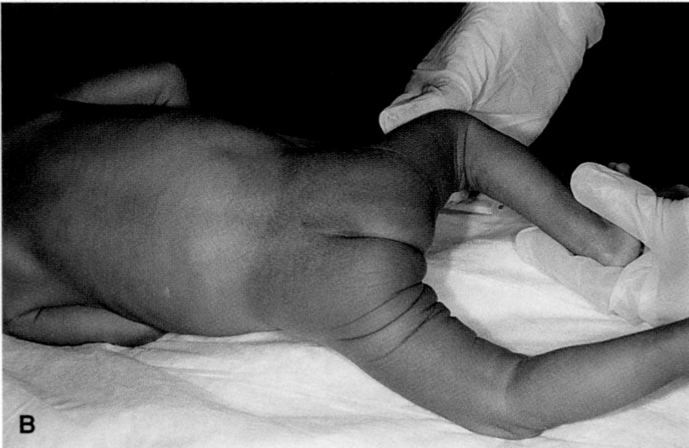

Figure 2-1. Mongolian Spots

A. A bluish-gray, nontender macular lesion is seen on the back of a 5-month-old otherwise healthy African-American infant. This lesion was present since birth. The bluish-gray discoloration is also seen on the sacrogluteal area (the most common site of mongolian spots). The lesion on his back also extends to the anterior chest wall. *B*. This 6-month-old infant was brought to the ED in cardiopulmonary arrest without any vital signs. He had bluish-gray macular lesions on the buttocks and trunk, as well as a small red bruise on his right cheek. There were no apparent causes for his arrest at presentation and his physical examination was otherwise negative. Based on the location and appearance of the lesions, they were thought to be mongolian spots, and this was subsequently confirmed by the absence of any contusions underlying these areas of discoloration. The medical examiner would typically incise areas of skin discoloration to exclude underlying contusions. This infant had a subdural hematoma, retinal hemorrhages, and multiple rib fractures noted at autopsy (shaken infant syndrome; see Fig. 1-19).

BOX 2-1. CLINICAL FEATURES OF MONGOLIAN SPOTS

- Skin lesion
  (1) A flat or macular lesion
  (2) Slate gray or bluish-gray discoloration
  (3) Asymptomatic (*the infant otherwise seems healthy*)
  (4) Nontender (*unlike ecchymosis*)
  (5) Poorly circumscribed lesion
  (6) Usually present since birth
- Number
  (1) Typically single lesion
  (2) May vary from one lesion to several lesions
- Size may vary from a few millimeters to >10 cm
- Location (can be seen anywhere on the body)
  (1) Most common: sacrogluteal area (90% of cases)
  (2) Outside sacrogluteal area (e.g., back, shoulders, flank [10% of cases])
- Natural history
  (1) Lesion may increase in size and intensity until age 2 years
  (2) Lesion generally fades gradually
  (3) Resolves by 5 to 6 years of age in about 96% of cases
  (4) Persists for life in 3 to 4% of cases

BOX 2-2. DIFFERENTIAL DIAGNOSIS: MONGOLIAN SPOT

- Accidental or inflicted injury
- Other forms of dermal melanocytosis
  (1) Examples: blue nevus, nevus of Ito, nevus of Ota (see Fig. 2-7)
  (2) These are permanent lesions (*unlike the majority of mongolian spots*)

DIAGNOSIS FOLK-HEALING PRACTICES

Synonyms

Folk medicine
Pseudo-battering
Coin rubbing (*Cao gio* or scratch the wind or coining)
Spooning (spoon rubbing or *quat sha*)
Cupping (*ventosa* or *ventosos*)

Definition

Folk-healing practices are forms of the folk medicine used by various cultures to treat illness.

Associated Clinical Features

1. Coin rubbing (Figs. 2-2 and 2-3)
   a. Practiced among Southeast Asians (Vietnamese and Cambodians) when a child is sick
   b. Warm oil (e.g., tiger balm or mentholated oil) is applied over the affected region of the body, and then it is vigorously rubbed in with the edge of a coin.
   c. This is done in an attempt to rid the body of "ill wind" or "bad wind" (to reduce fever and chills).
2. Cupping (Fig. 2-4)
   a. Seen in some Eastern European, Latin American, and Russian cultures
   b. Alcohol is applied to the inner rim of the cupping glass and ignited with cotton soaked in alcohol. The cup is applied to the skin after the flame is extinguished. As it cools, a vacuum forms in the cup causing an ecchymotic lesion at the site.
   c. The purpose is to reduce congestion.

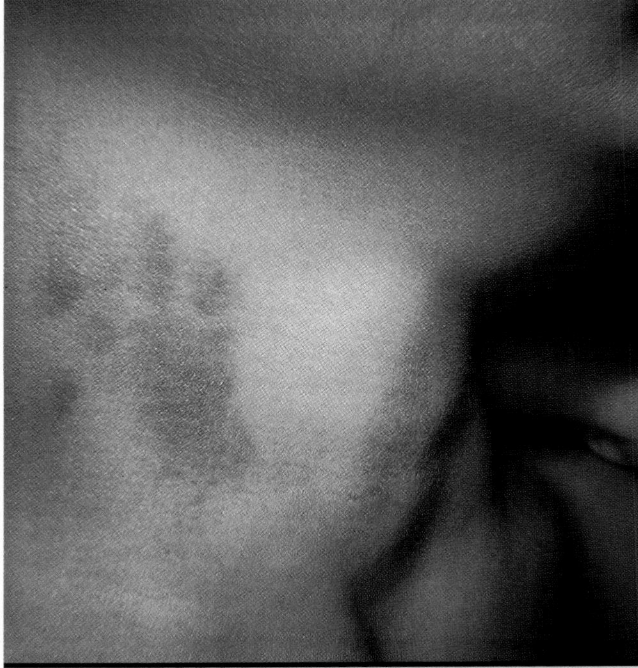

Figure 2-2. Coin Rubbing (*Cao Gio*)

This 6-year-old Cambodian boy was referred to the ED by the school nurse because of suspected child abuse. His mother confessed to inducing this lesion by rubbing his neck with a coin after applying warm mentholated oil. Her intention was to rid the child of fever and cold symptoms.

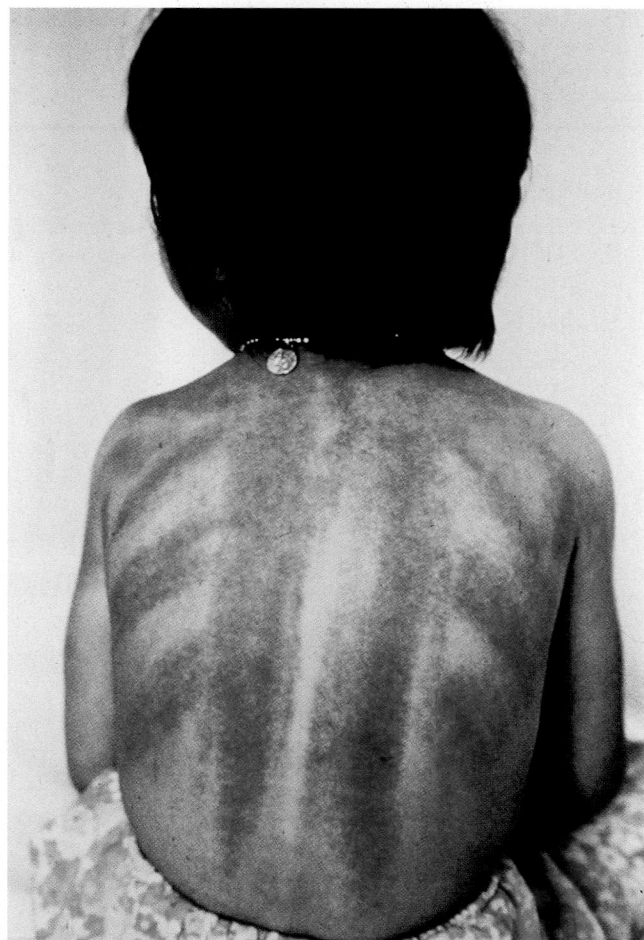

Figure 2-3. Coin Rubbing (*Cao Gio*)

Linear symmetrical lines of purpura in the intercostal spaces in a Cambodian boy produced by rubbing with a hot coin in an effort to cure fever. (Reproduced with permission from: American Academy of Pediatrics: *The Visual Diagnosis of Child Physical Diagnosis*. The C. Henry Kempe National Center on Child Abuse and Neglect. EIK Grove Village, IL, American Academy of Pediatrics 1994, p. 12.)

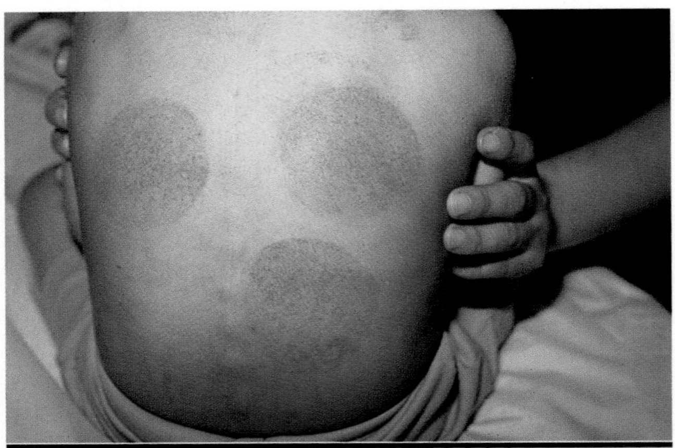

Figure 2-4. Cupping (Ventosa)

A Palestinian boy seen in the ED because of upper respiratory symptoms was found to have three identical round purpura on his back due to cupping. (Reproduced with permission from: Shah BR, Laude TL: *Atlas of Pediatric Clinical Diagnosis*. WB Saunders, Philadelphia, 2000, p. 44.)

3. Spooning
   a. Seen among the Chinese to relieve pain and headache
   b. The skin is scratched with a porcelain spoon until ecchymotic lesions appear.
4. Moxibustion
   a. Practiced among the Chinese
   b. A form of acupuncture
   c. Burning sticks of incense, yarn, cigarettes, or cones of the herb Artemisia are used to make small circular burns on the skin at therapeutic points.
5. *Maquas*
   a. Seen among Arabs, Jews, and Bedouins
   b. Hot metal spits or coals are applied to areas of disease or over a traditional "draining point" to produce burns.
6. *Caida de mollera* (fallen fontanelle)
   a. Seen among Mexicans and Hispanics
   b. An attempt to elevate the fontanelle in children who are dehydrated from vomiting and diarrhea
   c. The child is held upside-down.

Consultation

Consult organizations that sponsor immigrants in order to educate these families about proper medical care and to stop folk healing practices that may be injurious.

Emergency Department Treatment and Disposition

1. These practices are not done to injure the child. They are performed out of ignorance in accordance with well-intentioned cultural beliefs that these practices help the child to heal or recover from illness.
2. Educate parents about the injurious nature of these practices and suggest alternative approaches to treating illness.

Clinical Pearls: Folk-Healing Practices

1. Folk-healing practices may be mistaken for child abuse.
2. These practices are not done by parents to injure the child, and ignorance of these folk-healing practices results in allegations of physical abuse. In misguided attempts to heal

BOX 2-3. CLINICAL FEATURES OF FOLK-HEALING PRACTICES

Coin rubbing (Cao gio)

- A linear pattern of purpura
- Sites (along bony prominences): spine, neck, intercostal spaces
- Usually produces sharp borders of petechiae and purpura
- Often bilateral and symmetric

Cupping

- Round identical purpura
- Circular ecchymotic areas that are often symmetrically distributed
- First- or second-degree burns may be seen
- Sites: back, abdomen, chest

Spooning

- Ecchymotic lesions

Moxibustion

- Small circular incense burns at therapeutic points

Maquas

- Small deep burns at the sites of disease

Caida de mollera (fallen fontanelle)

- Retinal hemorrhages
- Resembles shaken impact syndrome
- Possible closed head injury

their children by using practices that are widely accepted in their culture, these parents may be accused of physically abusing the children, and the trust between the physician and the family may be irrevocably damaged.

3. Physicians should become familiar with folk-healing practices in their community and every effort should be made to prevent their occurrence.

BOX 2-4. DIFFERENTIAL DIAGNOSIS OF COIN RUBBING AND CUPPING

- Purpura or bruises inflicted by child abuse
  (1) Bruises inconsistent with the stated history
  (2) Geometric shapes or patterns to bruises (e.g., cord or loop marks, handprints; see child abuse, Fig. 1-4)
  (3) Multiple bruises in different stages of healing (suggestive of repeated abuse)
  (4) Unusual locations (e.g., genitalia, buttock, cheek)
  (5) Other signs of injury (e.g., skeletal) may be present

DIAGNOSIS COLD PANNICULITIS

SYNONYM

Popsicle panniculitis

Definition and Etiology

1. Cold panniculitis is an inflammation of the subcutaneous fat after prolonged exposure to cold. Popsicle panniculitis is a cold panniculitis specifically caused by sucking on ice (Figs. 2-5 and 2-6).
2. Cold panniculitis is also seen after prolonged application of a cold object to any area of the skin (e.g., ice packs applied to the face of an infant to control supraventricular tachycardia or ice packs applied to the lower extremities after vaccination).
3. Cold panniculitis is believed to occur solely because of the inherent properties of infant body fat, and the degree of fat necrosis is inversely related to the age of the patient. A higher percentage of saturated fatty acids in the subcutaneous fat of neonates and infants (as compared to older children and adults) may explain the increased propensity of baby fat to solidify with prolonged exposure to a cold object.

Associated Clinical Features

1. Popsicle panniculitis is seen especially in infants who suck on popsicles or ice cubes, who do not move them around in the mouth as do adults. As a result, the cold object is in contact with the buccal fat for long periods of time, causing cold injury.
2. Popsicle panniculitis is commonly seen during summertime.
3. A skin biopsy may be performed in doubtful cases. Histologically, nonspecific lobular adipocyte necrosis is observed at the dermal-epidermal junction with a surrounding mixed inflammatory infiltrate.

Consultation

Dermatology (for questionable cases)

Emergency Department Treatment and Disposition

1. Cold panniculitis is a self-limiting condition. There is no specific therapy except reassuring caregivers.
2. Recurrence of panniculitis is common and parents must be educated about the condition.

Clinical Pearls: Cold Panniculitis

1. A diagnosis of cold panniculitis is made by obtaining a history of exposure of the skin to a cold object.
2. Popsicle panniculitis lesions due to sucking on ice are seen adjacent to the corners of the infant's mouth.

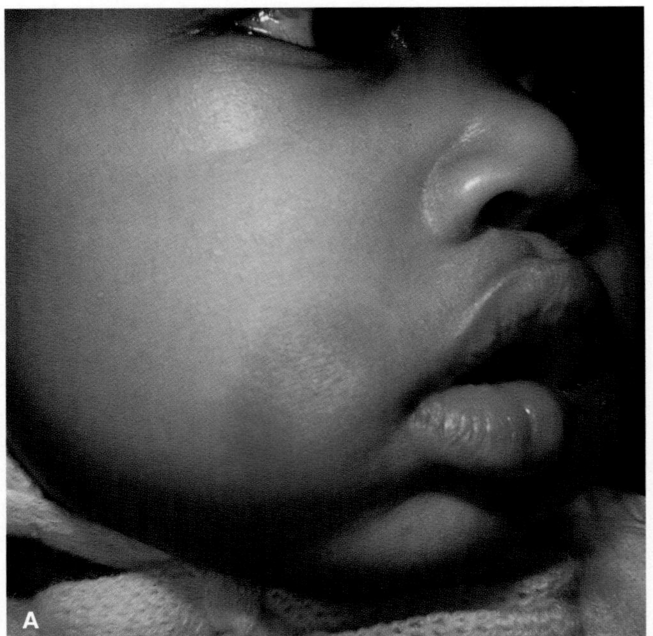
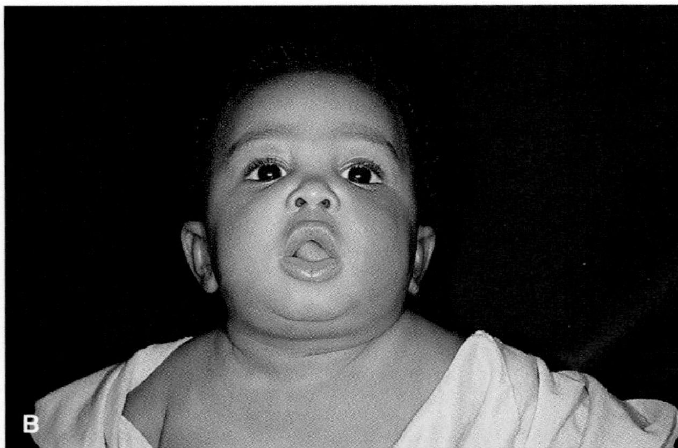

Figure 2-5. Cold Panniculitis

A. A 13-month-old infant was referred for social service clearance and to rule out abuse by a pediatrician when this erythematous and indurated skin lesion near the corner of the mouth was seen during a well baby visit. This lesion was initially interpreted as a red bruise produced by pinching. A history of the infant sucking on an ice cube 2 days prior to appearance of this lesion was subsequently obtained. *B*. A 4-month-old afebrile infant was admitted to differentiate between child abuse and buccal cellulitis in August, during an extreme heat wave. An erythematous, indurated, and mildly tender lesion was present on the cheek. Otherwise this infant was very playful and feeding well. A history of putting ice packs on his cheeks because of the hot weather 2 days prior to appearance of the rash was obtained.

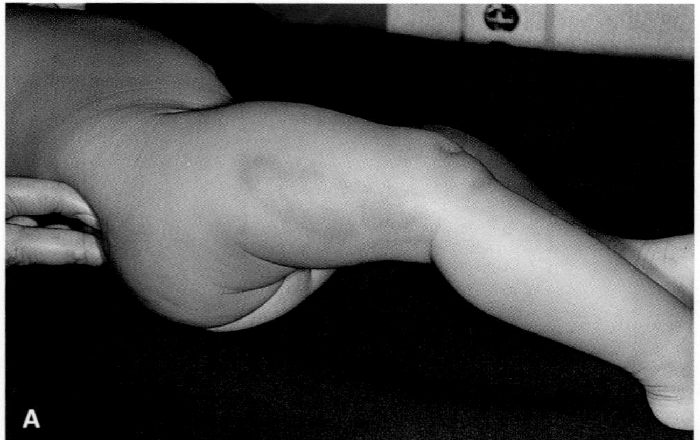
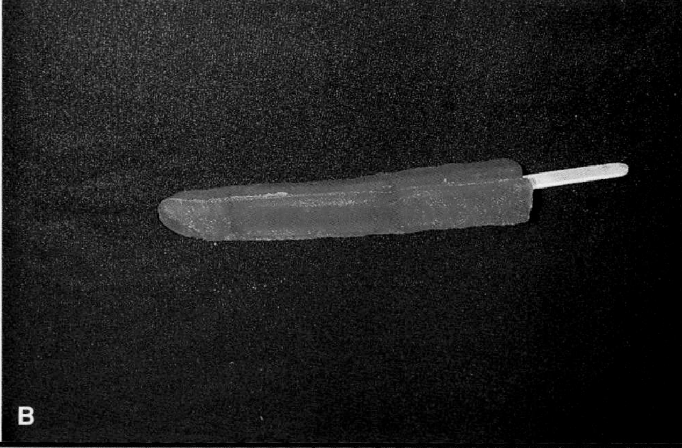

Figure 2-6. Cold Panniculitis

A. A 9-month-old infant presented with an erythematous, indurated, linear "skin rash." This skin lesion was mistaken for a bruise inflicted by a long thin object (e.g., a ruler or belt), and the family was referred to child protective services. The mother said that her 6-year-old son was eating a popsicle (like that shown in Fig. 2-6*B*), and had placed the popsicle on the thigh of the infant. A skin biopsy confirmed the diagnosis of cold panniculitis, and charges were subsequently dropped against the family.

DIAGNOSIS HAIR-TOURNIQUET SYNDROME

SYNONYMS

Hair-thread tourniquet syndrome
External genital tourniquet syndrome (penile tourniquet or clitoral tourniquet syndrome)

Definition and Etiology

Hair-tourniquet syndrome (HTS) involves fibers of hair or thread wrapped around an appendage, producing tissue necrosis.

Associated Clinical Features

1. HTS frequently occurs as an accidental injury.
2. Offending fibers are hair or synthetic fibers from mittens in the cases afflicting fingers.
3. A constricting hair or thread decreases lymphatic drainage. Lymphedema subsequently impedes venous drainage, leading to more edema and eventually preventing arterial flow to the appendage. This obstruction leads to necrosis and tissue loss if not promptly relieved.
4. Hair is thin and has high tensile strength. As the encircling hair dries out it shrinks, cuts through the skin, and becomes enveloped in surrounding edematous tissue, *thus making diagnosis difficult.*
5. Parents usually seek medical attention promptly (before circulatory compromise) due to irritability or inconsolable crying in infants (Fig. 2-14). *Suspect child neglect if there is a delay in seeking medical care;* careful inquiry should be made in such cases.
6. Complications of HTS are variable and depend on the duration of strangulation, but can include amputation of the digit, clitoris, or penis, and partial or complete transection of the urethra.

Emergency Department Treatment and Disposition

1. Prompt removal of the constricting hair or fibers is required to prevent tissue loss.

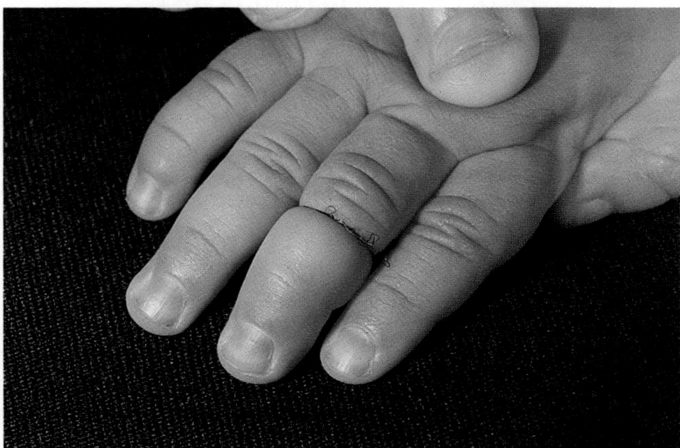

Figure 2-14. Hair-Tourniquet Syndrome

A 4-month-old presenting with inconsolable crying was found to have a hair wrapped around a digit that was erythematous and edematous. One or more hairs may be wrapped around one or more times, so a thorough inspection is required after removal of hair to be sure no strands remain.

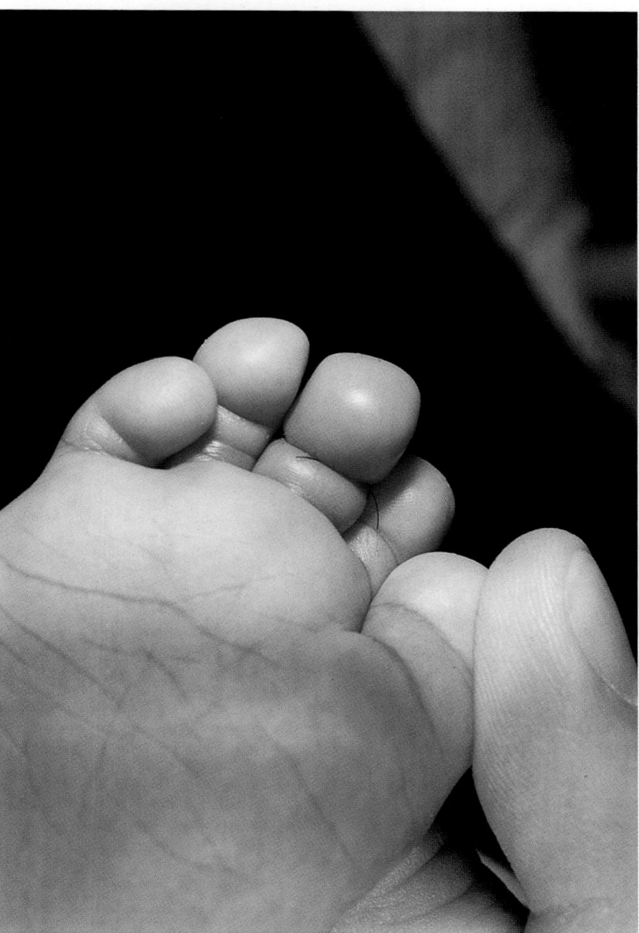

Figure 2-15. Hair-Tourniquet Syndrome

A 2-month-old infant presenting with irritability was found to have a hair wrapped around a toe. This patient underwent a work-up for sepsis before this was discovered. This case illustrates the importance of a thorough physical examination, including all digits and the genitalia, in an infant presenting with irritability or inconsolable crying.

2. Sometimes the end of the hair or fiber is visible and can be used to facilitate removal; otherwise the wound needs exploration to dissect and remove all strands.
3. A meticulous hunt to remove every single stand is required prior to discharging the patient (Fig. 2-15).

Clinical Pearls: Hair-Tourniquet Syndrome

1. Consider the possibility of a tourniquet syndrome in any patient presenting with swelling of an appendage, including the penis or clitoris.
2. Even though most cases of HTS are thought to be unintentional, the possibility of child abuse must be considered when a tourniquet syndrome is diagnosed (e.g., deliberate wrapping of hair around the penis to stop wetting has been reported to be a form of punishment used by some caretakers; Fig. 2-16).
3. A cursory examination of digits or other appendages may fail to identify the problem in an infant presenting with irritability or inconsolable crying. A thorough physical examination of all digits (after removal of socks and mittens) and genitalia is required.

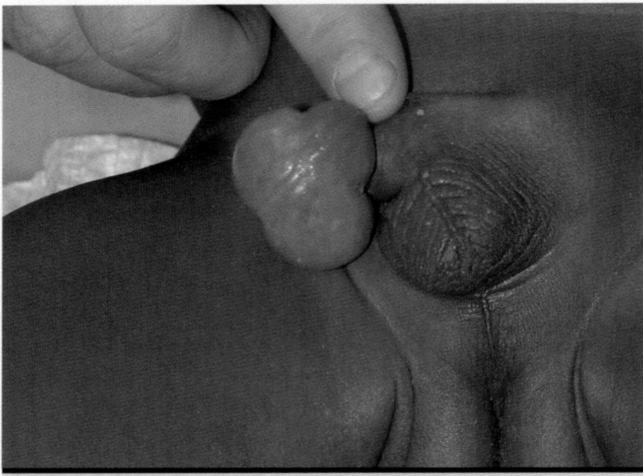

Figure 2-16. Penile-Tourniquet Syndrome

Erythema and edema of the glans penis (paraphimosis) was produced by a hair wrapped around the glans. With extreme swelling of the glans and edema of the coronal sulcus due to venous and arterial occlusion, constricting strands of hair may be difficult to see. In this case, hair was deliberately wrapped around the penis to stop bedwetting, as punishment by his mother.

BOX 2-15. CLINICAL FEATURES OF HAIR-TOURNIQUET SYNDROME

- *Age at presentation:*
  (1) Hair-tourniquet syndrome involving toes or fingers: infants (4 days to 2 years)
  (2) Penile-tourniquet syndrome: infants to 6 years
  (3) Clitoral-tourniquet syndrome: older girls (8 years to adolescence)
- *Symptoms:*
  (1) Inconsolable crying or irritability (young infants)
  (2) Odd gait (older children)
  (3) Genital pain (older children)
- *Signs:*
  (1) Erythema and swelling of involved area (early presentation)
  (2) Gangrene and amputation (late presentation)
- *Common sites:*
  (1) Toes
  (2) Fingers
  (3) Penis
  (4) Clitoris
  (5) Labia

BOX 2-16. DIFFERENTIAL DIAGNOSIS OF HAIR-TOURNIQUET SYNDROME

- Accidental injury
- Child abuse
- Self-inflicted (e.g., older girls with clitoral-tourniquet syndrome)

DIAGNOSIS

NUTRITIONAL RICKETS

SYNONYM

Vitamin D deficiency rickets

Definition

1. Rickets is caused by undermineralization of the cartilaginous epiphyseal growth plate, resulting in excessive accumulation of unmineralized matrix (osteoid).
2. Rickets is seen only in childhood because the growth plate exists only when the skeleton is growing. Failure to calcify osteoid in the adult is called osteomalacia.

Etiology

1. The main function of the vitamin D-parathyroid hormone (PTH)-endocrine axis is to maintain the extracellular fluid concentration of calcium (Ca) and phosphorus (PO_4) at appropriate levels to permit mineralization.
2. The normal product of serum Ca $\times$ PO_4 concentration, with each measured in milligrams per deciliter, is 40; rickets occurs when the Ca $\times$ PO_4 product drops below 30.
3. Nutritional rickets (NR) results from a deficiency of metabolites of vitamin D:
   a. "Sunshine deficiency" (inadequate exposure to sunlight, or factors preventing UV light penetration [e.g., industrial pollution, darkly pigmented skin, abundant clothing])
   b. Dietary vitamin D deficiency (e.g., exclusive breast-feeding without vitamin D supplementation, strict vegan diet)
   c. Fat malabsorption (e.g., celiac disease, extrahepatic biliary atresia)

Associated Clinical Features

1. Laboratory tests suggestive of NR include either low (early) or normal (with secondary hyperparathyroidism) serum Ca level, invariably a low PO_4 level, and an elevated alkaline phosphatase. Liver enzymes, serum albumin, blood urea nitrogen, and creatinine values help in excluding underlying liver or kidney disease as a cause of rickets. Additional tests that help in confirming the diagnosis of NR include an elevated serum PTH and a decreased serum calcidiol (25- hydroxycholecalciferol) value.
2. A single AP view of the knee is obtained in children <3 years of age, to look for rachitic changes at the metaphyses and epiphyses of the femur and tibia (the most rapidly growing bones in infants, which leads to accentuated rachitic changes; Fig. 2-17). In older children, a single AP view of the wrist is obtained. Radiologic changes suggestive of rickets include:
   a. Cupping of metaphyses (concave deformity of the end of the long bone shaft, instead of the normal convex or flat appearance)
   b. Fraying of metaphyses (indistinct, shaggy borders)
   c. Widening of metaphyses
   d. Generalized demineralization (osteopenia) and thinning of the cortex
   e. Pseudofractures
   f. Bowing deformities of long bones
   g. Increased distance (radiolucent zones) between metaphyses and epiphyses

Consultation

Endocrine

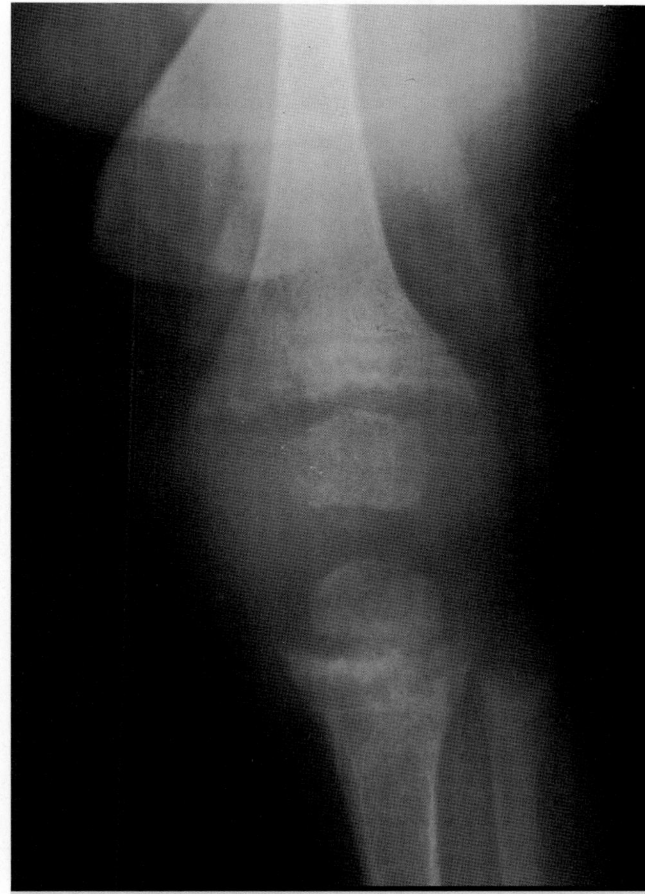

Figure 2-17. Rickets

Frontal view of the knee showing evidence of florid rickets. Note the severe metaphyseal widening, cupping, and fraying of the distal femur and proximal tibia and fibula. Normally the epiphyses should be closer to the metaphyses, and the increased distance seen here between the metaphyses and epiphyses (radiolucent zone) is due to the presence of radiolucent osteoid. Generalized osteopenia can also be seen. This widening of the epiphyseal plates radiographically distinguishes rickets from abuse-related fractures.

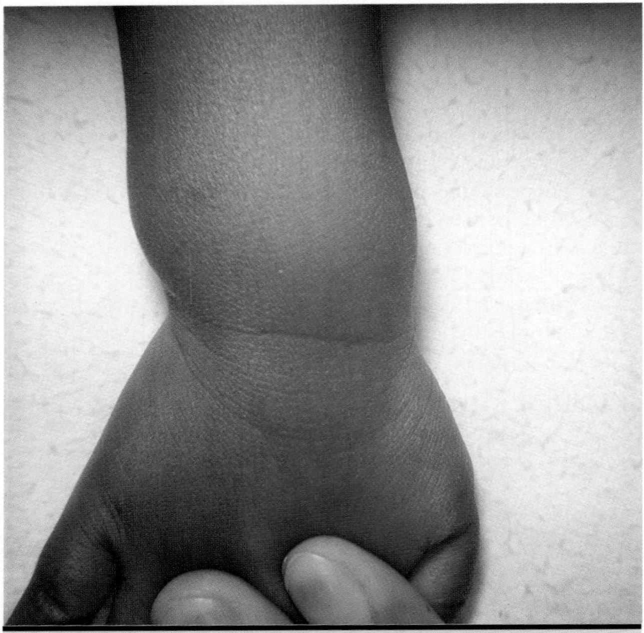

Figure 2-18. Prominent Wrist due to Rickets

Prominent enlargement of the wrist in rickets results from excessive accumulation of osteoid. This finding can be mistaken for abuse (e.g., swelling due to fracture). This African-American infant was exclusively breast-fed without any vitamin D supplementation. He presented with a hypocalcemic seizure (serum Ca 6 mg/dL, PO_4 2.5 mg/dL, and alkaline phosphatase 2500 U/L). In addition to prominent enlargement of the wrists, another manifestation of rickets is bow-legs.

Emergency Department Treatment and Disposition

1. Hospitalize any patient presenting with symptomatic or asymptomatic hypocalcemia associated with NR. These patients need correction of hypocalcemia and initiation of vitamin D therapy.
2. Asymptomatic normocalcemic patients can be referred to a primary care physician or endocrinologist for the treatment of rickets.

Clinical Pearls: Nutritional Rickets

1. Metaphyseal changes of rickets can be mistaken for skeletal injuries of abuse (Fig. 2-19). Rachitic changes seen on the physical examination (and absence of abusive injuries) will help to confirm the diagnosis of rickets.
2. Lucent epiphyseal-metaphyseal junctions seen in rickets may resemble the "bucket-handle" fractures of child abuse. However, widening of the epiphyseal plates distinguishes rickets radiographically from abuse-related fractures.
3. Generalized osteopenia and usually a bilaterally symmetrical pattern of skeletal involvement (rachitic changes) are distinguishing features of rickets.

BOX 2-17. CLINICAL FEATURES OF NUTRITIONAL RICKETS

- *Rachitic deformities:*
  (1) Bow-legs (genu varum; most common see Fig. 14-4)
  (2) Prominent wrists and ankles (excessive accumulation of osteoid; Fig. 2-18)
  (3) Rachitic rosary (enlargement of costochondral junctions)
  (4) Harrison's groove (weakened ribs pulled by muscles, producing flaring over the diaphragm)
  (5) Craniotabes
  (6) Frontal bossing with craniosomatic disproportion
  (7) Knock-knee (genu valgum)
  (8) Kyphoscoliosis (secondary to vertebral softening)
- Generalized muscular hypotonia
- Failure to thrive
- *Hypocalcemia:*
  (1) Asymptomatic
  (2) Seizures (with or without fever)
  (3) Tetany (latent or manifest)

BOX 2-18. CONDITIONS ASSOCIATED WITH METAPHYSEAL CHANGES

- Child abuse
- Rickets due to any of the following etiologies:
  (1) Nutritional rickets (vitamin D-deficiency rickets)
  (2) Familial hypophosphatemic rickets (FHR)
  (3) Vitamin D–dependent rickets, type 1
  (4) Vitamin D–dependent rickets, type 2
  (5) Rickets from other etiologies (e.g., liver disease)
- Metaphyseal dysplasia, Schmidt type
- Congenital syphilis

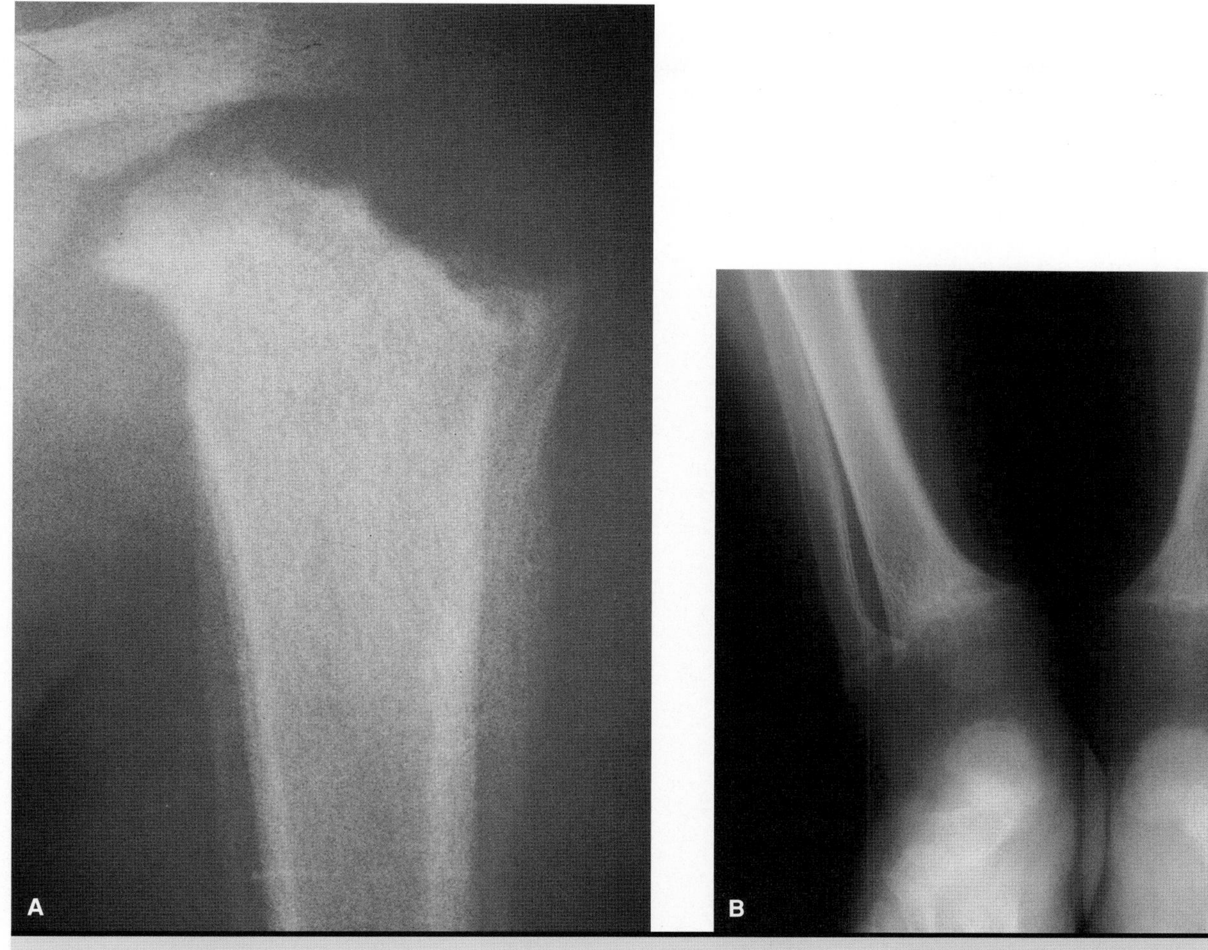

Figure 2-19. Differential of Child Abuse and Rickets

A. Child abuse. Frontal view of the humerus in a 2-year-old child who was physically abused by his stepfather. He had extensive bruises on the skin. Note the extensive periosteal reaction along the shaft, with diffuse metaphyseal irregularity and a corner fracture seen laterally. (Reproduced with permission from: Shah BR, Laude TL: *Atlas of Pediatric Clinical Diagnosis*. WB Saunders, Philadelphia, 2000, p. 35.) *B*. Rickets. Generalized distribution and bilateral, usually symmetrical pattern of skeletal involvement with widening of metaphyses distinguishes rickets radiographically from abuse-related fractures.

DIAGNOSIS OSTEOGENESIS IMPERFECTA

Definition and Etiology

1. Osteogenesis imperfecta (OI) is a genetically inherited disorder of connective tissue resulting from an abnormal quantity or quality of type I collagen. There are four clinical subtypes of OI with variable manifestations that primarily affect the musculoskeletal system. Genetic inheritance varies from autosomal dominant (types I and IV) to autosomal dominant or recessive (types II and III).
2. *Osteopenia* is insufficient bone mass resulting from reduced production of bone, increased breakdown of bone, or both. *Osteoporosis* is a clinical syndrome resulting from osteopenia that can lead to increased bone fragility, susceptibility to fractures, and skeletal deformities. OI is the most common type of osteoporosis syndrome seen in childhood.
3. Clinical classifications of OI include *osteogenesis imperfecta congenita* (extreme bone fragility and fractures with some patients dying in the newborn period) and *osteogenesis imperfecta tarda* (bone fragility manifested later in life with a normal life-span).

Associated Clinical Features

1. OI type I is the most common type, occurring in 1 per 30,000 births.

2. Fractures in OI occur following a slightly traumatic event or spontaneously in an active child.
3. Laboratory tests such as serum calcium, phosphorus, and alkaline phosphatase values are normal, and the coagulation profile is also normal.
4. Radiographic features of OI include osteopenia, thin cortices, bowing, angulation of healed fractures, and normal callus formation at the sites of recent fractures (Fig. 2-20). Most fractures in OI are situated in the diaphysis.
5. When the rare patient with type IV OI presents with a normal physical examination, a negative family history, and no obvious radiographic evidence of OI except recurrent fractures, a punch biopsy of the skin for biochemical analysis of type I collagen in cultured skin fibroblasts may be considered.

Consultations

Orthopedics

Emergency Department Treatment and Disposition

1. Exclude the diagnosis of child abuse.
2. The patient needs a very close follow-up by orthopedics and their primary care physician. Multidisciplinary management with referrals as indicated to a dentist, a geneticist, an endocrinologist, and a social worker for family support are also needed.
3. Goals of therapy include:
    a. Splinting of fractures
    b. Maximizing comfort and function
    c. Management of fractures in patients with only moderate involvement with OI is no different from management of fractures in otherwise normal children.
    d. Orthotics may be needed in children with increased bone fragility, to protect their bones as they move about.
    e. Osteotomies may be needed to straighten bone, and intramedullary rods may be inserted to maintain correct alignment and repair the deformities arising both from fractures and from progressive bowing or bending of the skeleton.
4. Calcitonin therapy may be considered to decrease bone resorption.

Clinical Pearls: Osteogenesis Imperfecta

1. OI is less common than child abuse, and type IV OI (a milder form of OI) often gets misdiagnosed as child abuse. Family history, multiple fractures, angulation of healed bones, wormian bones, osteopenia, and dentinogenesis imperfecta are present in type IV OI. Consultations with a radiologist, a dentist, and a geneticist may be helpful in difficult cases.

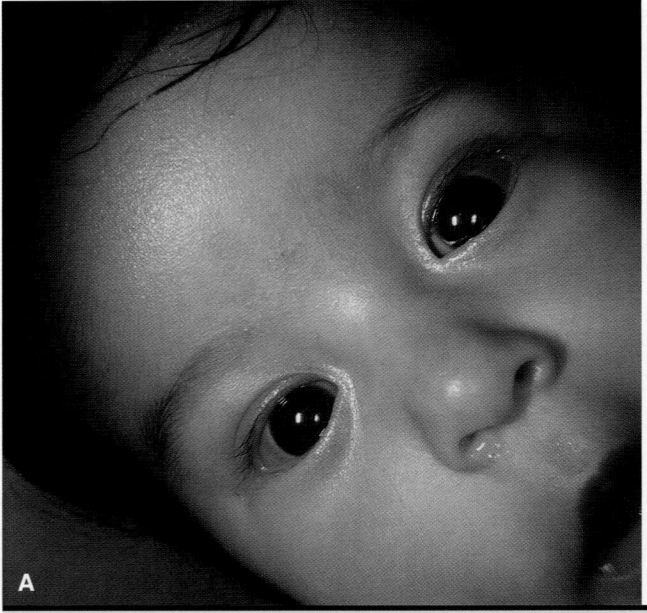
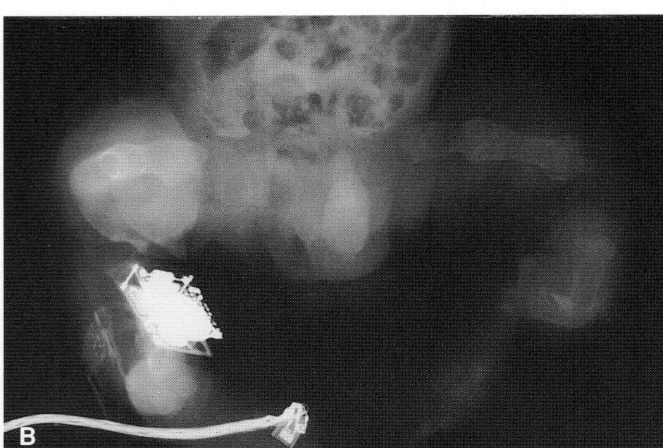

Figure 2-20. Osteogenesis Imperfecta

A. Bilateral blue sclera noted at birth. *B*. Frontal radiograph of the pelvis and lower extremity showing multiple healed fractures with angular deformities of the femur, tibia, and fibula that were noted at birth. This patient also had multiple wormian bones in the skull, multiple fractures with callus formation involving almost all the long bones, multiple rib fractures with callus formation, and generalized osteopenia. Most likely this patient had type II OI. This patient died in early infancy from a respiratory-related complication.

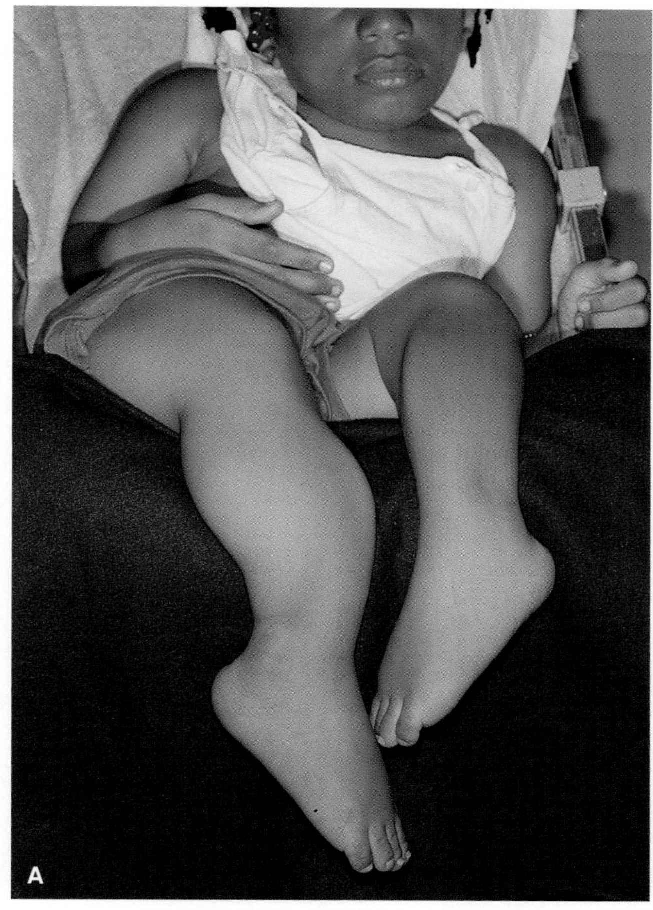

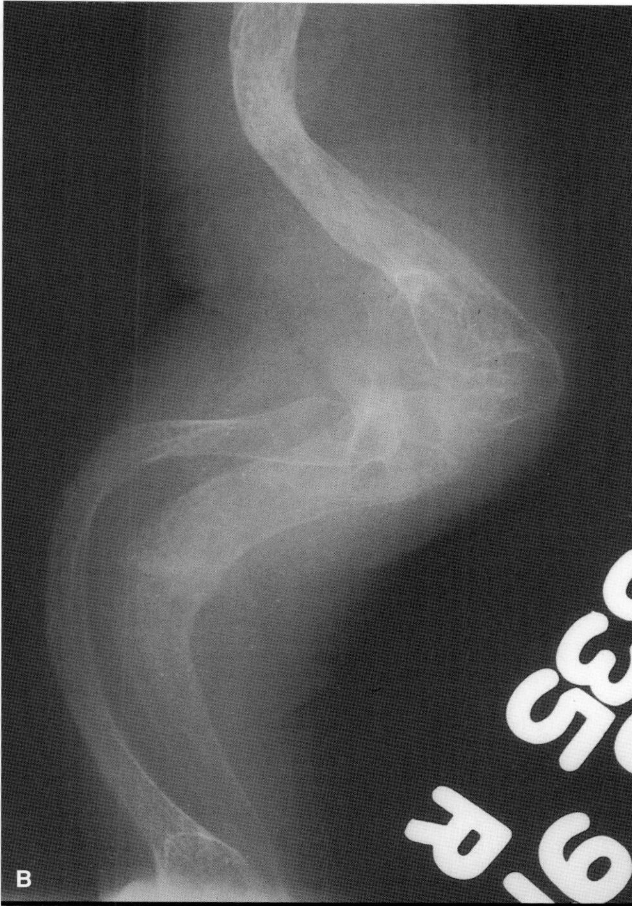

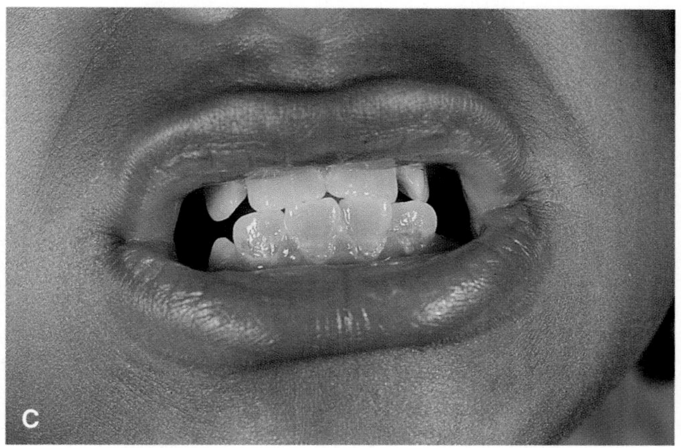

Figure 2-21. Osteogenesis Imperfecta

A. Severe bowing and deformities of both upper and lower extremities are seen in this 8-year-old girl with type III OI. She had normal sclera, triangular facies, and severe bone fragility leading to multiple fractures from early infancy. *B*. Radiograph of the lower extremity showing generalized osteopenia with marked angular deformities of the bones. *C*. Dentinogenesis imperfecta showing transparent yellow, prematurely eroded teeth in the same patient.

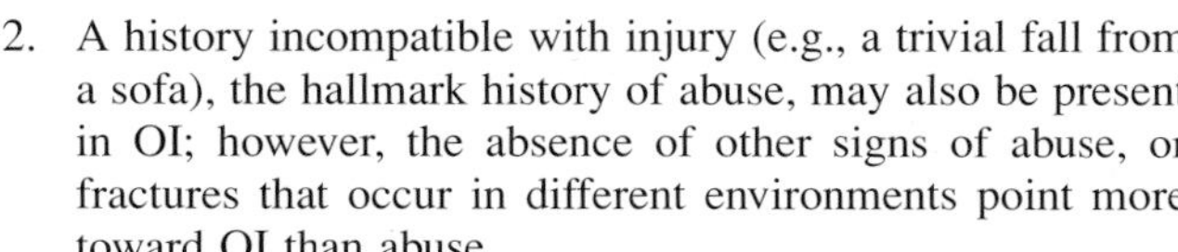

2. A history incompatible with injury (e.g., a trivial fall from a sofa), the hallmark history of abuse, may also be present in OI; however, the absence of other signs of abuse, or fractures that occur in different environments point more toward OI than abuse.
3. Spiral or transverse fractures of long bones are more common in OI than metaphyseal fractures; however, metaphyseal fractures resembling abusive fractures are also seen in OI.

BOX 2-19. CLINICAL FEATURES OF OSTEOGENESIS IMPERFECTA

- Four types of OI (based on phenotype and radiologic features)
  (1) Most common type: type I (~80% of cases)
  (2) Type most commonly mistaken for child abuse: type IV (extremely rare)
  (3) Multiple fractures in utero/perinatal lethal type: type II
  (4) Multiple fractures at birth: types II, III, IV, and less common with type I
  (5) Extreme bone fragility with in utero or early infancy deformities and death: types II and III
- Sclerae
  (1) Blue: types I and II (Fig. 2-20)
  (2) Slightly blue-gray at birth, changing to normal white later: type III
  (3) Normal: type IV
- Repeated fractures (all types)
- Many fractures early and throughout life (type III; Fig. 2-21)
- Variable age of onset of fractures (birth through adulthood): type IV
- Frequency of fractures decreases during puberty: type IV
- Triangular facies with bitemporal bulging: type III
- Wormian skull bones: type IV
- Bowing and multiple angular deformities of the long bones due to fractures
- Spine changes (scoliosis, kyphosis, codfish vertebrae)
- Growth retardation and short stature
- Defective dentinogenesis (teeth transparent, yellow, or gray-blue; prematurely eroded or broken)
- Conductive hearing loss (seen in adolescents and adults)
- Hyperlaxity of ligaments (small joints of hands, feet, knees)
- Easy bruising, fragile skin

BOX 2-20. DIFFERENTIAL DIAGNOSIS OF OSTEOGENESIS IMPERFECTA

- Child abuse
- Achondroplasia
- Congenital hypophosphatasia
- Idiopathic juvenile osteoporosis
- Steroid therapy
- Cystinosis
- Blue sclerae:
  (1) Prematurity (normal secondary to underdeveloped sclerae)
  (2) Ehlers-Danlos syndrome
  (3) Marfan's syndrome
  (4) Trisomy 18 syndrome
  (5) Turner's syndrome

DIAGNOSIS LICHEN SCLEROSUS ET ATROPHICUS

SYNONYMS

Lichen sclerosis
White spot disease
Lichen albus
Guttate scleroderma or circumscribed scleroderma
Balanitis xerotica obliterans (males)

Definition and Etiology

Lichen sclerosus et atrophicus (LSA) is a benign mucocutaneous condition of unknown etiology. It is characterized by white lesions on the genitalia (most common site). When it occurs in males, it is called balanitis xerotica obliterans.

Associated Clinical Features

1. LSA is seen in children between 1 and 13 years of age. It is also seen among adults.
2. It is predominantly seen in girls (F:M ratio 9:1).
3. Most lesions appear spontaneously, but some may be induced by trauma.
4. Intertriginous lesions that involve the groin and perianal area are subject to friction and maceration. The delicate, thin, white, wrinkled, compromised skin breaks down to become hemorrhagic and eroded (thus simulating irritant or *Candida* intertrigo). Bullae may precede erosions.
5. The diagnosis is made clinically. Skin biopsy reveals hyperkeratosis with follicular plugging, hydropic degeneration of basal cells, a bandlike dermal lymphocytic infiltrate, homogenized collagen, and thinned elastic fibers in the upper dermis.
6. Prepubertal LSA usually resolves spontaneously without sequelae in about two-thirds of cases at or just before menarche, leaving a brown hyperpigmented area on skin that had been white and atrophic. Involution is more likely to occur in those in whom the disorder developed at a younger age. About one-third of patients have persistence of LSA into adulthood.
7. Leukoplakia and squamous cell carcinoma have been rarely reported to develop from LSA.

Emergency Department Treatment and Disposition

1. Topical treatments have included estrogen, progesterone, testosterone, antimicrobial and antifungal agents, and petrolatum. In controlled trials many of these agents have been shown to be no more effective than placebo.
2. High-potency topical steroids:
   a. Highly effective in providing relief from the pruritus, and clearing of lesions
   b. Apply bid for 2 weeks
   c. Side effects: vaginal and vulvar candidiasis, atrophy of the vulva from continual application
   d. Discontinue when a favorable response is obtained (usually in 2 weeks or less)
3. Emollients and antipruritic agents may help for symptomatic relief.
4. Topical progesterone 1% and testosterone propionate 2% preparations have also been used for genital lesions; however, one needs to closely monitor girls for signs of virilization.

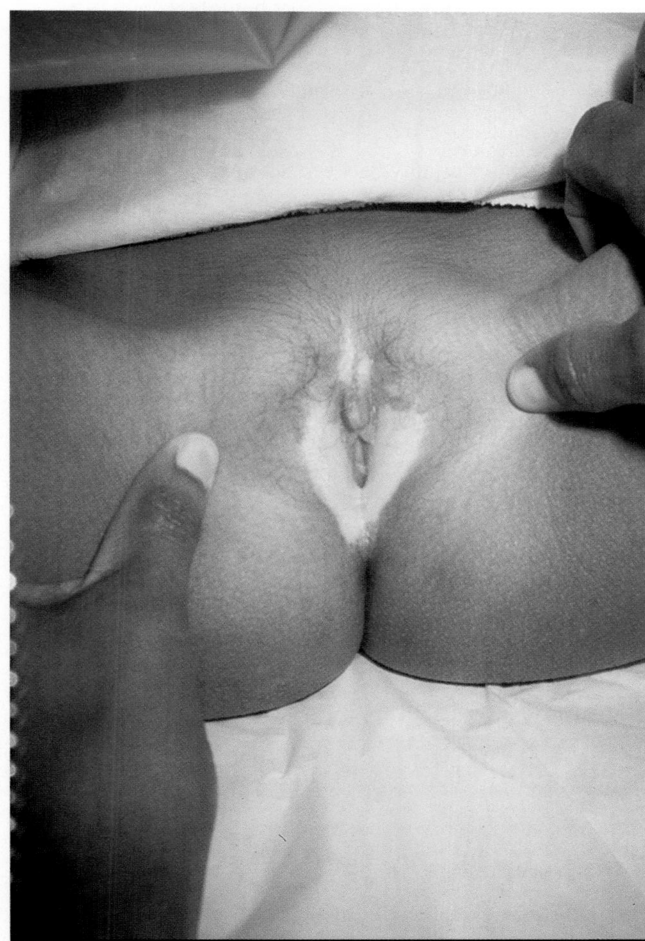

Figure 2-22. Lichen Sclerosus et Atrophicus

An hourglass-shaped porcelain white area of atrophy in the anogenital area in a young girl presenting with pruritus and burning in the vulvar area. This most distinctive pattern is seen in prepubertal females as well as in adults.

BOX 2-21. CLINICAL FEATURES OF LICHEN SCLEROSUS ET ATROPHICUS

Skin lesion

- Starts as ivory-colored shiny, indurated papules that become confluent, then become irregular plaques of variable size
- Plaques may develop hemorrhagic bullae at their margins.
- In later stages, lesions atrophy, and become depressed plaques with a wrinkled surface.

Girls:

(1) Sites: vulvar, perianal, and perineal skin
(2) Purpura of vulva (occasional manifestation)
(3) A porcelain white plaque around the anus and vulva forms a figure-8 or hourglass configuration.
(4) Atrophic plaque may lead to shrinkage of the labia and stenosis of the introitus

Boys:

(1) Onset usually between 4 and 12 years of age
(2) Sites: glans, undersurface of prepuce

Extragenital lesions:

(1) Seen in 42% of cases

(2) Sites: neck, axillae, trunk, periumbilical, flexor surfaces of wrists, around eyes

(3) Appear as atrophic depigmented patches with cigarette paper–like wrinkling of the surface

Signs and symptoms:

- Pruritus, burning, constipation, dysuria, dyspareunia
- Vaginal discharge preceding vulvar lesions (girls)
- Phimosis and recurrent balanitis (boys)

Clinical Pearls: Lichen Sclerosus et Atrophicus

1. LSA is the one of the most common dermatitides mistaken for sexual abuse. Purpura of the vulva, an occasional manifestation of pediatric LSA, mimics sexual abuse and has led to false accusations and unnecessary investigations.
2. LSA lesions are atrophic, depigmented plaques in the anogenital area in the shape of an hourglass in girls (Fig. 2-22).
3. Nearly all affected boys with LSA present with phimosis in a previously retractable foreskin with an atrophic depigmented plaque at the tip of the penis.

BOX 2-22. DIFFERENTIAL DIAGNOSIS OF LICHEN SCLEROSUS ET ATROPHICUS

- Vitiligo in anogenital area (vitiligo has no signs of atrophy)
- Postinflammatory hypopigmentation
- Sexual abuse
- Bacterial vulvovaginitis
- Intertrigo
- Condyloma acuminata
- Pinworm infestation
- Discoid lupus erythematosus
- Morphea (focal scleroderma)
- Lichen planus
- Lichen simplex chronicus
- Leukoplakia

DIAGNOSIS PERIANAL STREPTOCOCCAL DERMATITIS

SYNONYMS

Perianal streptococcal cellulitis
Perianal streptococcal infection or streptococcal perianal disease
Perianal dermatitis

Definition and Etiology

Perianal streptococcal dermatitis (PSD) is a superficial bacterial infection caused by group A beta-hemolytic *Streptococcus* (GABHS) involving the perianal area.

Associated Clinical Features

1. PSD primarily occurs in children between 6 months and 10 years of age.
2. It occurs more commonly in boys (about 70% of cases).
3. Intrafamily spread of this infection has been seen (e.g., due to family members bathing together). Siblings may be either asymptomatic with only GABHS-positive cultures, or they may develop similar dermatitis.

4. The chronic stage of PSD may present *without* any signs of cellulitis; thus, the preferred term to describe this entity is *perianal streptococcal dermatitis*, not cellulitis.
5. PSD is diagnosed by its characteristic distribution and confirmed by a culture obtained from the perianal area.
   a. *A specific request should be made of the laboratory to look for GABHS.*
   b. Culture the index case and family members as indicated.
   c. A moderate to heavy growth of GABHS will confirm the diagnosis (children with asymptomatic perianal colonization have light growth of GABHS).
   d. Direct antigen studies for GABHS may also help (sensitivity about 90%; false-negative results seen early in the course).
   e. A throat culture may also be positive for GABHS.
   f. Acute and convalescent sera for antistreptolysin O or anti-DNAse B are not helpful in making the diagnosis.
   g. Rarely perianal dermatitis may be caused by *Staphylococcus aureus*.
6. Associated other features (e.g., the presence of guttate psoriasis; see page 311) helps in arriving at the correct diagnosis.

Emergency Department Treatment and Disposition

1. PSD should be treated with systemic antibiotic therapy augmented by topical therapy.
2. Drug of choice: penicillin (any of the following):
   a. Penicillin V (dose: 25 to 50 mg/kg per day or 250 mg [400,000 units] for children), given orally bid to tid for 10 days *OR*
   b. A *single dose* of benzathine penicillin G (BPG) given intramuscularly: 600,000 units for children <60 lb and

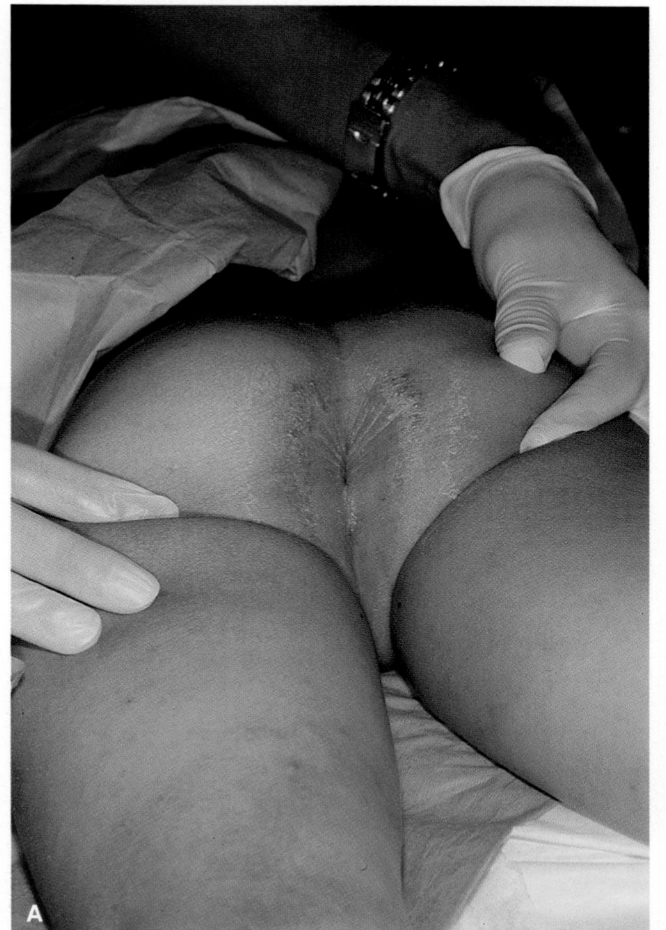

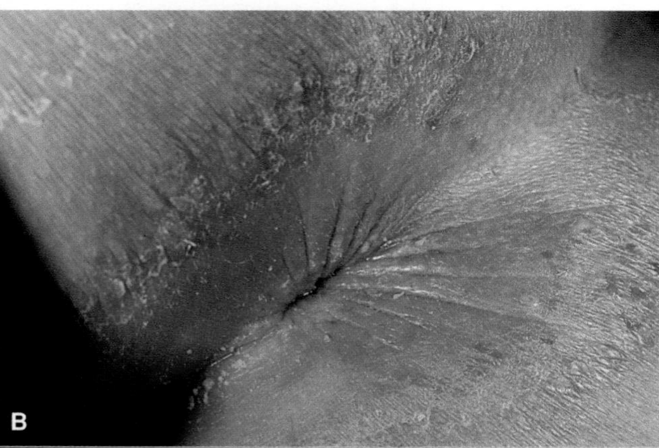

Figure 2-23. Perianal Streptococcal Dermatitis

A. An 8-year-old girl was brought to the ED by a foster mother for evaluation for sexual abuse. This rash, which had been present for several weeks, was treated by different ointments with no response. The patient also had pain on defecation. *B*. A close-up showing perianal erythema, fissuring, and excoriation with crusting at the periphery. A rectal culture was positive for GABHS.

1.2 million units for children >60 lb (to reduce the pain and discomfort, BPG preparations containing procaine may be used).

2. Amoxicillin may be used instead of penicillin (better-tasting preparation).
3. Use erythromycin or clindamycin for patients who are allergic to penicillin. These alternative antibiotic treatments may also be helpful for patients who have not responded to a course of penicillin, or who are infected with *S. aureus*.
4. Topical therapy: mupirocin ointment 2% tid for 10 days
5. The patient needs to be followed by the primary care physician for monitoring of response to therapy, as well as to document bacteriologic cure posttreatment. Recurrences have been seen in about 40% of cases.

BOX 2-23. CLINICAL FEATURES OF PERIANAL STREPTOCOCCAL DERMATITIS

Symptoms:

- Perianal dermatitis (90% of cases)
- Perianal pruritus (80% of cases)
- Painful defecation and rectal pain (50% of cases)
- Perianal pain
- Constipation (fecal-holding behavior)
- Blood-streaked stools (33% of cases)
- Anal discharge
- Usually absence of systemic symptoms (fever or malaise)

Signs around the perianal area may include any of the following:

Acute phase (<6 weeks):

- Bright red erythema confluent from anus outward
- Usually nonindurated
- Moist and tender to the touch
- Lesions have well-demarcated margins.
- Size varies from a few to several centimeters.

Chronic phase:

- Painful perirectal fissures
- Dried mucoid discharge
- Irritation and excoriation
- Proctocolitis
- Bleeding
- Little or no erythema
- Psoriasiform plaques with yellow peripheral crust
- Infection may involve the penis or vulva, leading to vulvovaginitis (commonly mistaken for sexual abuse)

Clinical Pearls: Perianal Streptococcal Dermatitis

1. PSD is a bright-red, sharply demarcated perianal dermatitis caused by GABHS.
2. PSD often gets mistakenly diagnosed as sexual abuse or contact or atopic dermatitis.
3. PSD is often misdiagnosed for long periods, and patients are subjected to treatments for a variety of different diagnoses without success. Failure to respond to prior therapy with topical antifungals or corticosteroids and oral preparations for pinworms are important clues in suspecting PSD.
4. Undiagnosed and inappropriately treated patients with PSD develop perianal fissures, bleeding, pain during defecation, and constipation (Fig. 2-23).

BOX 2-24. DIFFERENTIAL DIAGNOSIS FOR PERIANAL DERMATITIS OR CELLULITIS

- Sexual abuse
- Candidiasis
- Contact dermatitis
- Atopic dermatitis
- Chronic diaper dermatitis
- Seborrheic dermatitis
- Psoriasis
- Pinworm infestation
- Inflammatory bowel disease
- Local trauma (heavy wiping)

DIAGNOSIS

LABIAL ADHESION

SYNONYMS

Labial or vulvar agglutination
Labial fusion
Labial or vulvar synechiae

Definition

Labial adhesion is fusion of the labia minora, usually extending from an area immediately inferior to the clitoris to the fourchette. The extent of the adhesion is variable, and is thickest posteriorly.

Etiology

1. Labial adhesion is an acquired condition.
2. It occurs as a result of labial abrasion that culminates in the labia adhering to one another, following which epithelialization occurs (Fig. 2-24). Fusion of the medial surfaces of the labia minora to each other occurs secondary to local inflammation in the presence of the hypoestrogenic state of a preadolescent child (inflamed or injured epithelium is more likely to agglutinate in a low-estrogen environment).
3. Nonspecific vulvovaginitis, poor perineal hygiene, diaper rash, and use of harsh soaps are some of the most common contributory factors.
4. Other etiologies include conditions such as lichen sclerosus, atopic or seborrheic dermatitis, herpes, and pinworm infections.
5. Trauma and vulvar irritation from sexual abuse may also lead to labial fusion.

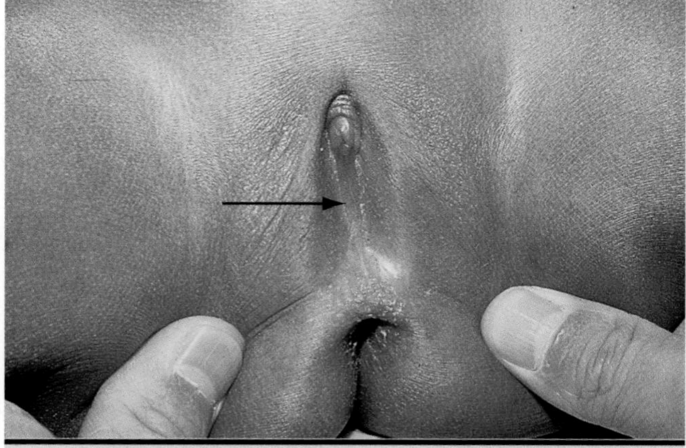

Figure 2-24. Labial Adhesion

A 2-year-old otherwise asymptomatic girl was accidentally found by her parents to have "abnormal looking private parts." With complete adhesions, as seen here, the introitus is not seen, and this is often interpreted by parents as an absence of the vagina. It may also appear that there is no urethral opening through which the child can urinate. A thin line of central raphe (*arrow*) where the labia are fused is seen. Visualization of a midline raphe excludes the diagnosis of imperforate hymen.

Associated Clinical Features

1. The possibility of labial adhesions due to the trauma of sexual abuse should be considered in any girl (especially an older girl) presenting many years after toilet training, as well as in those without any prior history of labial adhesions, those without any predisposing skin condition, or those presenting with thick adhesions that are difficult to treat.
2. Diagnosis of labial adhesions is made clinically by visual inspection of the genitalia.
3. Complications include urinary tract infections (~20 to 40% of cases) related to pooling of urine in the vagina and leading to recurrent vulvovaginitis (due to the constantly moist and irritated vulva) and urethritis.
4. Recurrent labial adhesions may occur.

Emergency Department Treatment and Disposition

1. Generally, no treatment except reassurance is indicated for patients with asymptomatic adhesions. Spontaneous resolution without therapy occurs in the majority of children (>80%) over the course of a year.
2. With endogenous estrogen production and the vaginal pH becoming more acidic at puberty, labial adhesions almost always resolve spontaneously.
3. General measures include:
   a. Reassurance to the family about the presence of normal female genitalia
   b. Improving perineal hygiene (e.g., regular changing of diapers and thorough wiping after each bowel movement, from anterior to posterior)
   c. Removal of irritants (e.g., caustic soaps)
   d. Treatment of diaper dermatitis (e.g., *Candida*)
   e. Loose-fitting cotton underwear
   f. Sitz baths (with either tap water or Burow's solution)
4. For reporting guidelines and management of cases of suspected sexual abuse, see Box 4-4.
5. Estrogen cream (e.g., Premarin)
   a. For patients with nearly complete adhesions with or without urinary symptoms
   b. May be used especially for significant parental anxiety
   c. A small quantity of estrogen cream is applied topically with gentle traction bid for 3 weeks, then at bedtime for 3 weeks (very effective in vast majority of patients).
   d. An additional few weeks of application of an inert ointment (e.g., petroleum jelly) keeps the labia apart while healing is completed.

e. Failure usually results from parents not applying the cream to the correct area.
f. Prolonged use should be discouraged (side effects include breast enlargement and/or tenderness, vulvar pigmentation, and vulvar erythema).

6. Once the adhesions are separated, the patient should be re-examined for any underlying predisposing condition (e.g., the presence of a vaginal septum).
7. The patient should also receive specific therapy for any underlying predisposing condition (e.g., pinworm infection).
8. Agglutinated tissue should *not* be manually forced apart; it is very painful, and the resulting raw surfaces have a greater tendency to reagglutinate. If the patient presents with acute urinary symptoms, a gentle attempt to separate the labia with a Calgiswab can be made (only if adhesions appear to separate easily) after applying 5% lidocaine (Xylocaine ointment) or 2.5% prilocaine (EMLA cream).
9. Surgery is rarely necessary and should be reserved for thick adhesions that have failed medical therapy and manual separation. Sedation or general anesthesia will be required for the procedure, and it can be performed in outpatient surgical suite, either by a gynecologist or a pediatric surgeon. Care after separation is very important; the patient needs topical estrogen therapy for 1 to 2 weeks, followed by 6 to 12 months of daily application of a bland emollient (e.g., petroleum jelly).

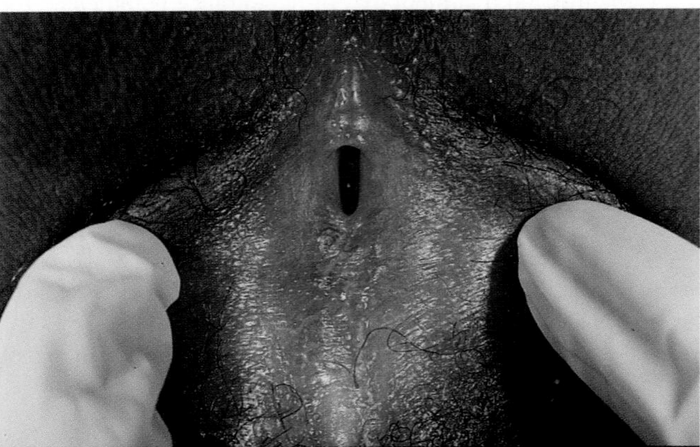

Figure 2-25. Female Circumcision (Infibulation)

This 10-year-old girl underwent excision of her clitoris and labia minora (as ritual female circumcision) during her early childhood in Africa. Scarred tissue and a narrowed introitus as seen here following surgery may mimic labial adhesion or trauma due to sexual abuse. The practice of female circumcision is seen in many countries in Africa, the Middle East, and Muslim populations of Indonesia and Malaysia. This procedure is typically performed on preadolescent children (typically between the ages of 4 and 10 years [range: birth to just before marriage]). The type of mutilation ranges from simple excision of the prepuce of the clitoris to complete excision of all elements of the vulvar region, leaving a very small opening for the passage of urine and menstrual fluid. Female circumcision is illegal in Western countries and is classified as child abuse in some European countries.

Clinical Pearls: Labial Adhesions

1. A thin vertical raphe (line of adherence) over the site of the vaginal orifice in the midline where the labia are adherent is pathognomonic for labial adhesions.
2. Labial adhesions should not be separated manually by force; it leads to adhesion of the raw surfaces, is painful, and causes emotional trauma to the patient.
3. Labial adhesions can also be the result of sexual abuse, but in the absence of other evidence, the presence of adhesions alone is not diagnostic of sexual abuse. In case control studies, no differences are noted in the percentages of abused versus nonabused children with labial adhesions.
4. Scaring following female circumcision may be mistaken for labial adhesions (Fig. 2-25).

BOX 2-25. CLINICAL FEATURES OF LABIAL ADHESIONS

- Most common age at presentation
  (1) Between 3 months and 6 years (peak incidence: 13 to 23 months)
  (2) May be seen at any age
  (3) Rare in newborns (exposure to high levels of maternal estrogens)
  (4) Rare in postpubertal premenopausal women
- Presenting symptoms
  (1) Majority of patients are asymptomatic
  (2) Usually accidentally noted by a parent or by a physician during examination
  (3) Apparent absence of a vaginal opening
  (4) Symptoms of urinary tract infection (dysuria, frequency), urinary retention, or altered urinary stream
- Signs
  (1) A thin vertical raphe in the midline over the site of the vaginal orifice (where labia are adherent)
  (2) Normal female genitalia
  (3) Extent of adhesions varies from child to child
  (4) With complete adhesions:
  Urethra usually not visualized.
  Urine may be seen dribbling at the anterior end (just posterior to the clitoris).
  Hymen and introitus are obscured.
  (5) With partial adhesions:
  A central line of fusion is seen at the posterior fourchette (extending to varying lengths anteriorly).

BOX 2-26. DIFFERENTIAL DIAGNOSIS OF LABIAL ADHESIONS

- Imperforate hymen (see Figs. 10-20 and 10-21)
  (1) Normal urethral orifice should be seen.
  (2) Imperforate hymen seen in the same plane as the urethral orifice on the floor of vestibule.
- Sexual abuse
  (1) *Adhesions may occur due to trauma of sexual abuse.*
  (2) *In the absence of sexual abuse, adhesions may be mistaken for vaginal scars due to hymenal trauma.*
- Ambiguous genitalia
- Congenital absence of the vagina
- Scaring following female circumcision

DIAGNOSIS URETHRAL PROLAPSE

Definition

Urethral prolapse is an eversion of the distal urethral mucosa that protrudes through the urethral meatus. Urethral prolapse may be partial or complete.

Etiology and Associated Clinical Features

1. Predisposing factors include hypoestrogenism (premenarcheal and postmenopausal age groups) resulting in a weak attachment between the inner longitudinal and outer circular-oblique smooth muscle layers of the urethra, allowing separation of these layers during episodes of increased intra-abdominal pressure (e.g., violent coughing, constipation). Preceding trauma (e.g., straddle injury or sexual abuse) may also be contributory.
2. Constriction of the prolapsed mucosa at the urethral meatus may lead to impairment of the venous blood flow with subsequent edema and erythema or purplish appearance of the mucosa. Thrombosis and necrosis of the mucosa results if the process is not corrected.
3. Urethral prolapse is a clinical diagnosis. The prolapse may be large enough that it will conceal the introitus. Retraction of the vulva gently in a downward and lateral direction or placing the child in a knee-chest position may help in appreciating the anatomy clearly with the vaginal introitus seen as a separate structure posterior to the prolapsed urethra (Figs. 2-26 and 2-27).
4. Urinalysis may show red blood cells because of the external irritation of the urethral meatus. Urine culture is usually negative.

Consultation

Urological or surgical consultation for patients with necrotic mucosa or recurrent prolapse

Emergency Department Treatment and Disposition

1. Conservative therapy is used for mild cases without necrotic mucosa. This includes warm sitz baths and emollient cream. If indicated, topical antibacterial therapy or topical estrogen therapy (the distal urethra is estrogen dependent) twice a day for 10 to 14 days can be used.
2. Urethral prolapse usually resolves spontaneously or with the above therapy in 2 to 3 weeks.
3. Indications for surgery (excision and reapproximation of the mucosal edges or CO_2 laser therapy) include prolapse with necrotic mucosa at the time of presentation, persistent prolapse with failed medical therapy, recurrent symptomatic prolapse, or urinary retention.
4. Recurrences may occur weeks to months after the initial resolution following medical therapy. Recurrence is uncommon after surgery.

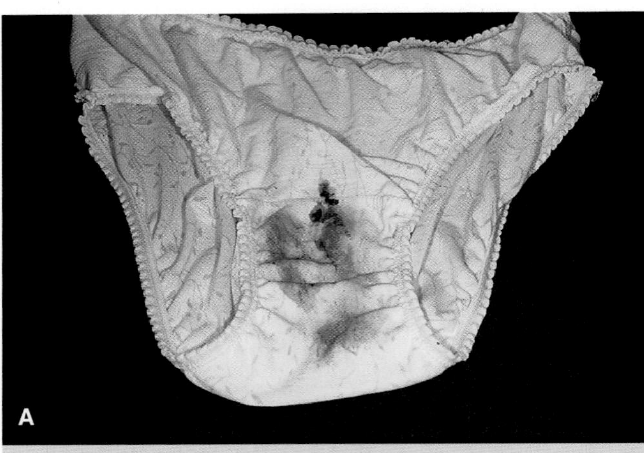

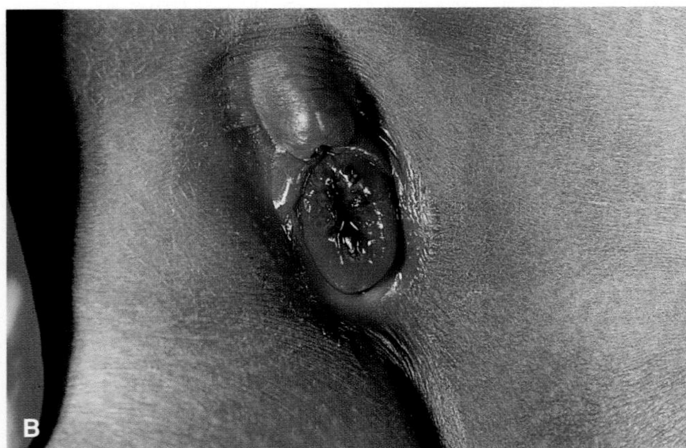

Figure 2-26. Urethral Prolapse

A. Apparent vaginal bleeding. Blood stained underwear from a 5-year-old African-American girl. The mother was very concerned when she noticed bloody spotting on the child's underwear. The patient was cared for by a baby sitter when the mother went to work, and she wanted to rule out sexual abuse. The patient was completely asymptomatic. Painless bleeding or spotting on underwear is the most common symptom of urethral prolapse and frequently gets mistaken for vaginal bleeding by a caretaker. *B*. Urethral prolapse. A doughnut-shaped, hyperemic, edematous mass with a slightly hemorrhagic center is seen. Mucosal prolapse (as seen here) is usually a complete circle forming a doughnut shape and obscuring the vaginal introitus. A dimple in the center indicates the urethral meatus.

Clinical Pearls: Urethral Prolapse

1. Urethral prolapse is the most common cause of apparent vaginal bleeding in premenarcheal girls.
2. Urethral prolapse presents as an interlabial mass. It is the only lesion that has a circular mass of tissue surrounding the urethral meatus. If in doubt, catheterization of the bladder through the central dimple of the mass or observation of the child during voiding will aid in the diagnosis.
3. Clinical findings of urethral prolapse can be mistakenly attributed to sexual abuse, especially when prolapsed mucosa has become hemorrhagic and friable.
4. Urethral prolapse cannot be reduced manually.

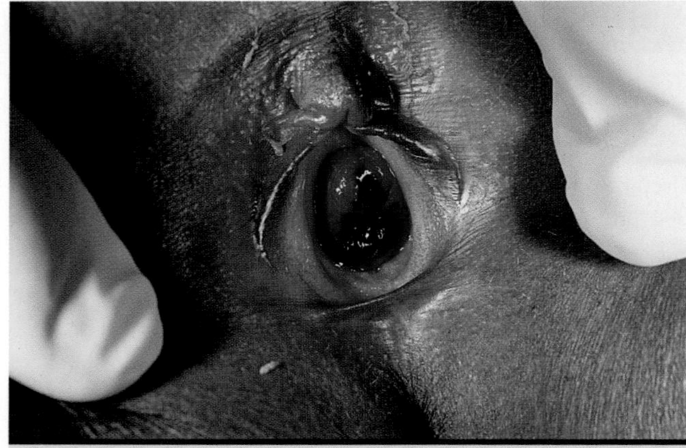

Figure 2-27. Urethral Prolapse

A doughnut-shaped, edematous mass with hemorrhagic mucosa obscuring the vaginal introitus is seen in a 4-year-old African-American girl. This disorder can be mistakenly attributed to trauma caused by sexual abuse.

BOX 2-27. CLINICAL FEATURES OF URETHRAL PROLAPSE

Clinical symptoms (*any of the following*):

- Age at presentation
  (1) Almost exclusively in premenarcheal girls (peak incidence between 4 and 10 years of age)
  (2) Second peak: postmenopausal women
  (3) Rarely reported in newborns and infants
- Racial predilection
  (1) Premenarcheal girls: about 95% of cases occur among African-American girls
  (2) Postmenopausal women: no racial predilection
- Most common symptom (90% of patients): painless bleeding or spotting on underwear
  (1) Bleeding most often mistaken for vaginal bleeding
  (2) Bleeding occasionally mistaken for hematuria or rectal bleeding
- Urinary symptoms
  (1) Dysuria and/or frequency (urethral inflammation)
  (2) Difficult to void
  (3) Urinary retention (depending on the size of the mass, and whether or not it occludes the urethral meatus)
- Perineal discomfort
- Prolapse may be noted on routine examination in a completely asymptomatic patient

Clinical signs of a prolapsed urethra (*any of the following*):

- Cherry-red doughnut or prolapsed cervix-like circular mass at the introitus
- Usually not tender
- May appear as a friable rosette of red or hemorrhagic tissue
- May be ulcerated or gangrenous (necrotic) or infected
- Prolapse may be partial or complete
- Center of the doughnut-shaped mass is the urethral orifice
- A centrally located urethral meatus may not be visible in the presence of severe edema or strangulation

BOX 2-28. DIFFERENTIAL DIAGNOSIS OF URETHRAL PROLAPSE

- Hematoma of hymen
  (1) Trauma from straddle injury
  (2) Nonaccidental trauma (sexual abuse; see Fig. 4-4)
- Hematometrocolpos (see Figs. 10-20 and 10-21)
- Prolapsed ectopic ureterocele
- Prolapse of urethral polyp
- Prolapsed bladder
- Periurethral abscess
- Urethral cysts
- Condylomata acuminata
- Hemangioma
- Sarcoma botryoides

DIAGNOSIS STRADDLE INJURY

Definition

Injuries to the genitalia occur accidentally or intentionally and are either penetrating or nonpenetrating in nature. Straddle injuries are the most common type of accidental injuries to the genitalia and rarely involve penetration.

Associated Clinical Features

1. Straddle injury occurs when soft tissues get crushed between the pubic bone (e.g., pubic symphysis, ischiopubic ramus) and a hard object during impact.
2. Straddle injuries occur when a child accidentally falls on a furniture arm, bed, bicycle crossbar, balance beam, fence, concrete wall, or playground equipment (Figs. 2-28 and 2-29).

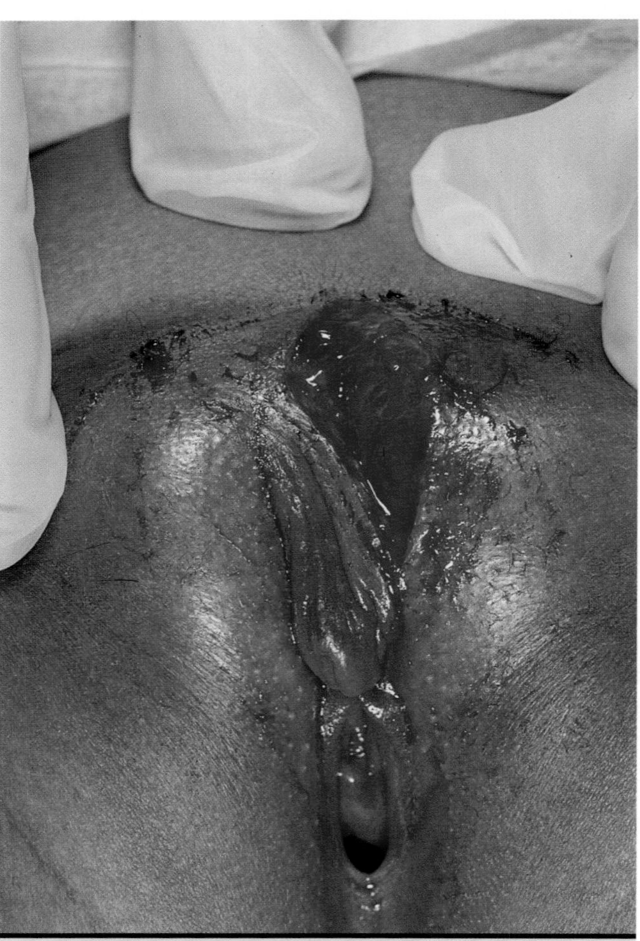

Figure 2-28. Straddle Injury

Laceration of the labia majora extending into periurethral tissue secondary to a fall onto the bar of a bicycle in a 5-year-old girl. Her injury was unilateral and did not involve the urethra, hymen, or vagina.

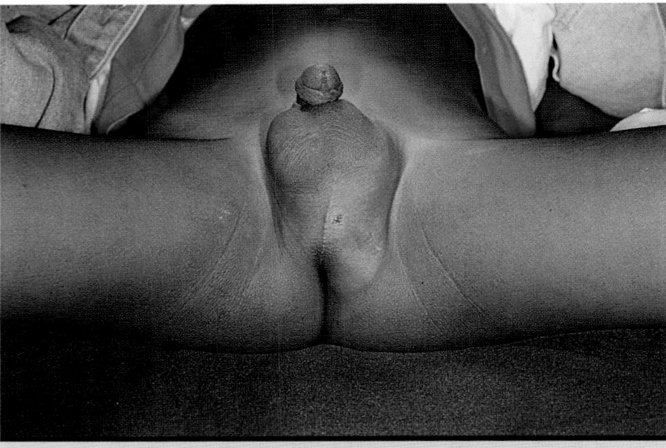

Figure 2-29. Straddle Injury

Unilateral scrotal swelling with bruising and a small abrasion in a 6-year-old boy who fell on a balance beam. Scrotal ultrasound showed a hematoma but the testes were not involved.

BOX 2-29. CLINICAL FEATURES OF STRADDLE INJURY

- Most common type: nonpenetrating injuries
- Findings in girls:

a. Usually unilateral and anterior injury

b. Usual sites and characteristics:
   (1) Typically external genitalia
   (2) Most common: labia majora, labia minora
   (3) Other sites: clitoral hood, clitoris, periurethral tissue, posterior fourchette
   (4) *Usually does not involve the hymen or vagina* (unless accidental penetrating injury)
   (5) Typically linear abrasions, bruising or hematoma of labia majora or minora
   (6) Small posterior fourchette tears
   (7) Swelling and pain
   (8) Bleeding

- Findings in boys:
   (1) Ecchymosis or minor laceration
   (2) Sites: scrotum, penis

BOX 2-30. DIFFERENTIAL DIAGNOSIS OF STRADDLE INJURY

- Sexual abuse (*suspect with any of the following*):
  - (1) Lack of correlation between history and clinical findings
  - (2) Straddle injuries in nonambulatory children
  - (3) Extensive injuries
  - (4) Vaginal, perianal, or hymenal injury without a clear history of penetrating trauma
  - (5) Evidence of other injuries

3. Accidental injury to internal genital structures or the anus is rare (protected by soft tissues of the buttocks and labia and bones of the pelvis).
4. Self-inflicted injuries are exceedingly rare. Normal masturbation in girls is clitoral or labial and does not cause genital injury. Self-inserted foreign bodies also do not cause injuries to the hymen.
5. Other associated injuries (e.g., injury to the urethra) must be excluded.

Consultations

Child abuse consultant or pediatrician and child protective services if the diagnosis is unclear

Emergency Department Treatment and Disposition

1. To minimize discomfort the patient can be advised to take sitz baths.
2. Local application of antibiotics may help in promoting healing.

Clinical Pearls: Straddle Injury

1. Straddle injuries are the most common type of accidental injuries involving the genitalia.
2. Straddle injuries may be difficult to differentiate from injuries due to sexual abuse.
3. A plausible explanation and physical examination that supports the history are important in arriving at the correct diagnosis.

Suggested Readings

American Academy of Pediatrics: Child abuse and neglect. *A Guide to References and Resources in Child Abuse and Neglect,* 2nd ed. Elk Grove Village, IL, 1998.

American Academy of Pediatrics: Child abuse and neglect. *A Guide to References and Resources in Child Abuse and Neglect.* Elk Grove Village, IL, 1994.

American Academy of Pediatrics. Committee on Child Abuse and Neglect: Distinguishing sudden infant death syndrome from child abuse fatalities. *Pediatrics* 2001;107:437.

American Academy of Pediatrics. Committee on Child Abuse and Neglect: Guidelines for the evaluation of sexual abuse of children: Subject review. *Pediatrics* 1999;103(1):186.

American Academy of Pediatrics, Committee on Child Abuse and Neglect: Shaken baby syndrome: Inflicted cerebral trauma. *Pediatrics* 1993:92;872.

American Academy of Pediatrics, Section on Radiology: Diagnostic imaging of child abuse. *Pediatrics* 2000;105(6):1345.

Atabaki S, Paradise JE: The medical evaluation of the sexually abused child: Lesions from a decade of research. *Pediatrics* 1999;104:178.

Bacon JL: Prepubertal labial adhesions: Evaluation of a referral population. *Am J Obstet Gynecol* 2002;187:327.

Finkel MA, Giardino AP (eds): *Medical Evaluation of Child Sexual Abuse. A Practical Guide*, 2nd ed. Sage, Thousand Oaks, CA, 2002.

Giardino AP, Christian CW, Giardino ER: *A Practical Guide to the Evaluation of Child Physical Abuse and Neglect.* Sage, Thousand Oaks, CA, 1997.

Jain AM: Domestic violence. Emergency department evaluation of child abuse. *Emerg Med Clin North Am* 1999;17:575.

Nimkin K, Kleinman PK: Pediatric musculoskeletal radiology. Imaging of child abuse. *Radiol Clin North Am* 2001;39(4):843.

Reece RM, Ludwig S (eds): Child abuse. *Medical Diagnosis and Management,* 2nd ed. Lippincott Williams & Wilkins, Baltimore, 2001.

Rink RC, Kaefer M: Surgical management of intersexuality, cloacal malformation, and other abnormalities of the genitalia in girls. In: Campbell, MF, Walsh PC, Retik AB (eds). *Campbell's Urology,* 8th ed. WB Saunders, Philadelphia, 2002, p. 2428.

Valerie E, Gilchrist BF, Frischer J, et al: Diagnosis and treatment of urethral prolapse in children. *Urology* 1999;54(6):1082.

CHAPTER 3

INFECTIOUS DISEASES

Binita R. Shah

DIAGNOSIS STREPTOCOCCAL PHARYNGITIS

SYNONYM

"Strep throat"

Definition and Etiology

1. "Strep throat" is acute tonsillopharyngitis caused by *Streptococcus pyogenes* or group A beta-hemolytic streptococci (GABHS), which is responsible for the great majority of infections.
2. Strains of other serogroups, especially groups C and G, may occasionally be involved.

Associated Clinical Features

1. Streptococcal pharyngitis is among the most common bacterial infections of childhood (Fig. 3-1).
2. It is seen among schoolchildren between the ages of 5 and 15 years with a peak incidence during the first few years of school.
3. The incubation period is 2 to 4 days.
4. Throat colonization by GABHS varies with geographic location and season, and is seen in 10 to 20% of normal school-aged children. About 30% of children with sore throat have a positive throat culture for GABHS; only half of these have a positive antibody response indicative of active infection rather than colonization. Thus, isolation of GABHS from the pharynx of a child with pharyngeal infection does not necessarily indicate that the infection is caused by GABHS.
5. Clinical judgment alone unfortunately does not predict which children may have GABHS infection as opposed to viral pharyngitis.
6. Diagnostic tests:
   a. Consider doing a throat culture or rapid antigen detection test when a diagnosis of strep throat is strongly suggested (e.g., moderate to severe exudative pharyngitis, petechiae on the palate, tender cervical adenitis [Fig. 3-2], or scarlet fever).
   b. To obtain an adequate sample for a throat culture, vigorous swabbing of the tonsils and posterior pharynx is required.
   c. False-negative cultures occur in up to 10% of symptomatic patients, even with a properly obtained throat swab.
   d. Rapid antigen detection tests that are currently available have a high specificity but vary considerably in sensitivity (between 50 and 90%). Thus, a positive rapid antigen test is diagnostic, but a negative test requires a back-up throat culture.
   e. Serologic tests (e.g., antistreptolysin O titer) confirm recent GABHS infection, but are not helpful in diagnosing acute infection in the ED.
7. Complete blood count, ESR, and C-reactive protein do not help to differentiate between GABHS pharyngitis and pharyngitis from other etiologies. Leukocytosis can be seen in bacterial as well as viral infections. Atypical lymphocytosis and the presence of splenomegaly suggest Epstein-Barr virus infection.

Emergency Department Treatment and Disposition

1. Therapy can be started after a positive rapid antigen detection test.
2. Withholding therapy for 24 to 48 hours while awaiting throat culture results does not increase the risk of acute rheumatic fever (ARF).
3. Antibiotic therapy should be started (before confirmation of test results) with any of the following:
   a. Prior history of ARF
   b. Clinical diagnosis of scarlet fever (see Fig. 3-3)
   c. Suppurative complications (e.g., peritonsillar cellulitis or abscess; see Fig. 9-3)
   d. Lack of availability of follow-up culture results

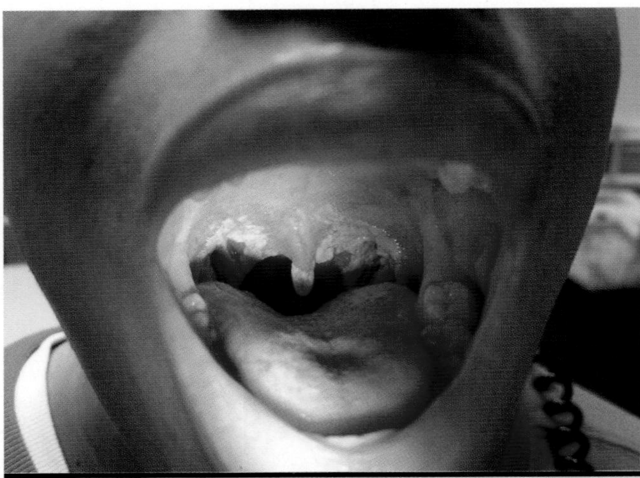

Figure 3-1. Exudative Tonsillopharyngitis

Exudative tonsillopharyngitis in a 9-year-old patient presenting with high fever, sore throat, and tender anterior cervical adenopathy. Her throat culture was positive for GABHS.

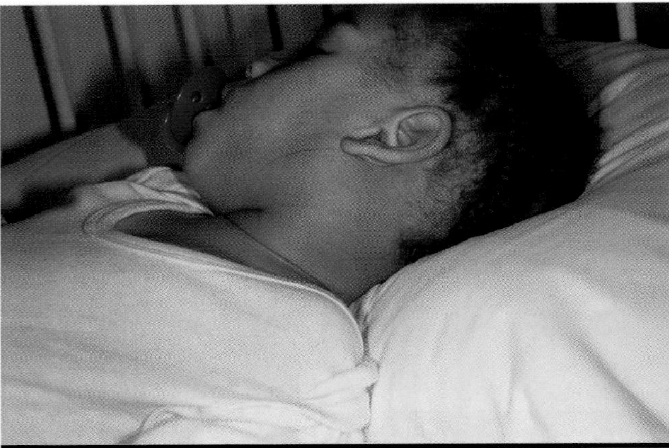

Figure 3-2. Acute Suppurative Cervical Lymphadenitis

Both throat culture and lymph node aspirate culture were positive for GABHS in this 5-year-old girl who presented with erythematous and rapidly enlarging unilateral swelling in the neck (anterior cervical lymphadenitis) associated with high fever and leukocytosis.

4. Drug of choice: penicillin V
   a. Penicillin therapy prevents ARF even when therapy is started as late as 9 days after the onset of acute illness, shortens the clinical course, and decreases toxicity, infectivity, and suppurative complications.
   b. Dose: 250 mg [400,000 units] for children and 500 mg for adolescents and adults, given orally two to three times per day for 10 days *or*
   c. A *single dose* of benzathine penicillin G (BPG) given intramuscularly
      1) 600,000 units for children <60 lb and 1.2 million units for children >60 lb
      2) To reduce pain and discomfort, BPG preparations containing procaine penicillin may be used.
5. For patients allergic to penicillin: erythromycin or clindamycin
6. Amoxicillin (or ampicillin) is often used in place of penicillin V, but these drugs have no microbiologic advantage over penicillin.
7. To prevent ARF, emphasize the importance of completing the *full 10-day course of antibiotic therapy* regardless of the clinical improvement.
8. Children can return to school after 24 hours of antibiotic therapy.
9. Streptococcal pharyngitis is a self-limited disease. Fever abates within 3 to 5 days (in the absence of suppurative complications) and all acute signs and symptoms subside within 1 week. Tonsils (tonsillar hypertrophy) and lymph nodes take several weeks to return to their usual size.
10. Routine post-treatment follow-up culture is not needed unless the patient remains symptomatic or is at particularly high risk of ARF.
11. Repeated courses of antibiotic therapy are also not indicated for asymptomatic patients who remain GABHS-positive after appropriate antibiotic therapy (an exception being patients with a prior history of ARF or those with family members with a history of ARF).

Clinical Pearls: Streptococcal Pharyngitis

1. The most common clinical illness produced by GABHS is acute pharyngotonsillitis.
2. The presence of coryza, cough, conjunctivitis, hoarseness, diarrhea, discrete ulcers, or stomatitis in a child with pharyngitis strongly suggests a viral etiology and not GABHS infection.
3. An abrupt onset of fever, sore throat, headache, abdominal pain, nausea, vomiting, and enlarged tender cervical lymphadenopathy in a school-aged child with exudative pharyngitis strongly suggests GABHS infection.
4. Exudative pharyngitis in children <3 years of age is rarely of streptococcal etiology and diagnostic studies for GABHS are not recommended routinely in this age group.
5. Treat all children with pharyngitis who have either a positive throat culture or a rapid antigen test for GABHS (even though in some cases the presence of GABHS may only represent colonization).

BOX 3-1. CLINICAL FEATURES OF STREPTOCOCCAL PHARYNGITIS

- Age >5 years
- Abrupt onset with high fever
- Sore throat, pain on swallowing, malaise, headache
- Nausea, vomiting, and abdominal pain common
- Tonsillopharyngitis
  (1) Pharynx: beefy red
  (2) Palate and uvula may be edematous, reddened, and covered with petechiae
  (3) Tonsils erythematous, enlarged with patches of a gray-white exudate giving a "strawberry" appearance (intensity of exudates varies from absent in mild cases to formation of a distinct membrane covering entire pharynx in severe cases)
- Tender anterior cervical lymphadenopathy (lymph nodes at the angles of the mandibles)
- Scarlatiniform rash may be present (see scarlet fever, Fig. 3-3)
- With or without history of exposure
- Streptococcosis
  (1) Presentation in toddlers (<2 years of age)
  (2) Signs and symptoms: serous rhinorrhea, variable fever, irritability, anorexia, pharyngitis
  (3) Poor weight gain, suppurative complications, protracted course (4 to 8 weeks)

BOX 3-2. DIFFERENTIAL DIAGNOSIS OF EXUDATIVE TONSILLOPHARYNGITIS

- Other streptococci (groups C and G)
- Adenovirus infection
- Epstein-Barr virus infection
- Herpes simplex virus infection (shallow tonsillar ulcers with gray exudates)
- Diphtheria
- Tularemia
- *Mycoplasma* infections
- *Candida* (immunosuppressed patients; oropharyngeal erythema with white exudates)

BOX 3-3. COMPLICATIONS OF GROUP A BETA-HEMOLYTIC STREPTOCOCCAL INFECTIONS

- Suppurative complications
  (1) Suppurative acute cervical lymphadenitis
  (2) Peritonsillar cellulitis or peritonsillar abscess
  (3) Retropharyngeal abscess
  (4) Acute otitis media
  (5) Acute sinusitis
  (6) Mastoiditis
  (7) Streptococcal pneumonia
  (8) Toxic shock syndrome (*Streptococcus pyogenes*– mediated TSS)
  (9) Intracranial complications (meningitis, brain abscess, thrombosis of venous sinuses [extension through cribriform plate or mastoid bone])
  (10) Bacteremic spread with metastatic infection (septic arthritis, endocarditis, meningitis, brain abscess, osteomyelitis, liver abscess; these complications are extremely rare since the advent of effective therapy)
- Nonsuppurative complications
  (1) Acute rheumatic fever
  (2) Acute glomerulonephritis

DIAGNOSIS — SCARLET FEVER

SYNONYM

Scarlatina

Definition and Etiology

1. Scarlet fever is caused by Group A beta-hemolytic streptococcus (GABHS; *Streptococcus pyogenes*) strains that elaborate streptococcal pyrogenic exotoxins (erythrogenic toxins). The circulating toxin is responsible for the rash and systemic symptoms. The infection occurs in children who lack immunity to the toxin.
2. At least three immunologically distinct erythrogenic toxins are identified. This explains the recurrent episodes of scarlet fever in the same patient.
3. The oropharynx is the portal of entry in the majority of cases. Occasionally a surgical wound may be the portal of entry (*surgical scarlet fever*).

Associated Clinical Features

1. Most cases occur in children between 2 and 8 years of age in winter and early spring.
2. The average incubation period is 2 to 4 days (range: 1 to 7 days).
3. Usual constitutional symptoms are sore throat, headache, malaise, and fever. Vomiting and abdominal pain may occur, and if present before the appearance of the rash, mimic an abdominal surgical condition.
4. Diagnosis is usually made clinically and can be confirmed by a throat culture (for throat culture and additional tests that help in confirming the diagnosis of GABHS, see Streptococcal pharyngitis, on page 67).
5. Scarlet fever is usually a benign condition (see Box 3-3 for suppurative complications).
6. Rarely, severe forms of scarlet fever associated either with local and hematogenous spread of the organism (septic scarlet fever), or with profound toxemia (toxic scarlet fever), present with high fever and marked systemic toxicity. The course may be complicated by arthritis, jaundice, and hydrops of the gallbladder. Such severe forms of the disease are quite infrequent in the antibiotic era.
7. Nonsuppurative late complications include acute rheumatic fever (ARF) and acute poststreptococcal glomerulonephritis.

Emergency Department Treatment and Disposition

1. Treatment is indicated to prevent the suppurative complications and ARF.
2. Drug of choice: penicillin (see Streptococcal pharyngitis, page 68 for details)
3. For patients allergic to penicillin: erythromycin or clindamycin
4. Children can return to school after 24 hours of antibiotic therapy.

Clinical Pearls: Scarlet Fever

1. Scarlet fever occurs most commonly in association with pharyngitis. It rarely occurs with pyoderma or an infected wound.
2. Rash begins as generalized innumerable pinhead-sized papules with a vivid scarlet hue and a sandpaper texture followed by a prominent desquamation of the hands and feet (Fig. 3-3).
3. Pharyngeal and tonsillar involvement are absent in surgical scarlet fever.
4. Skin tenderness is absent in scarlet fever, as opposed to the prominent skin tenderness of staphylococcal scarlatina (staphylococcal scarlet fever).

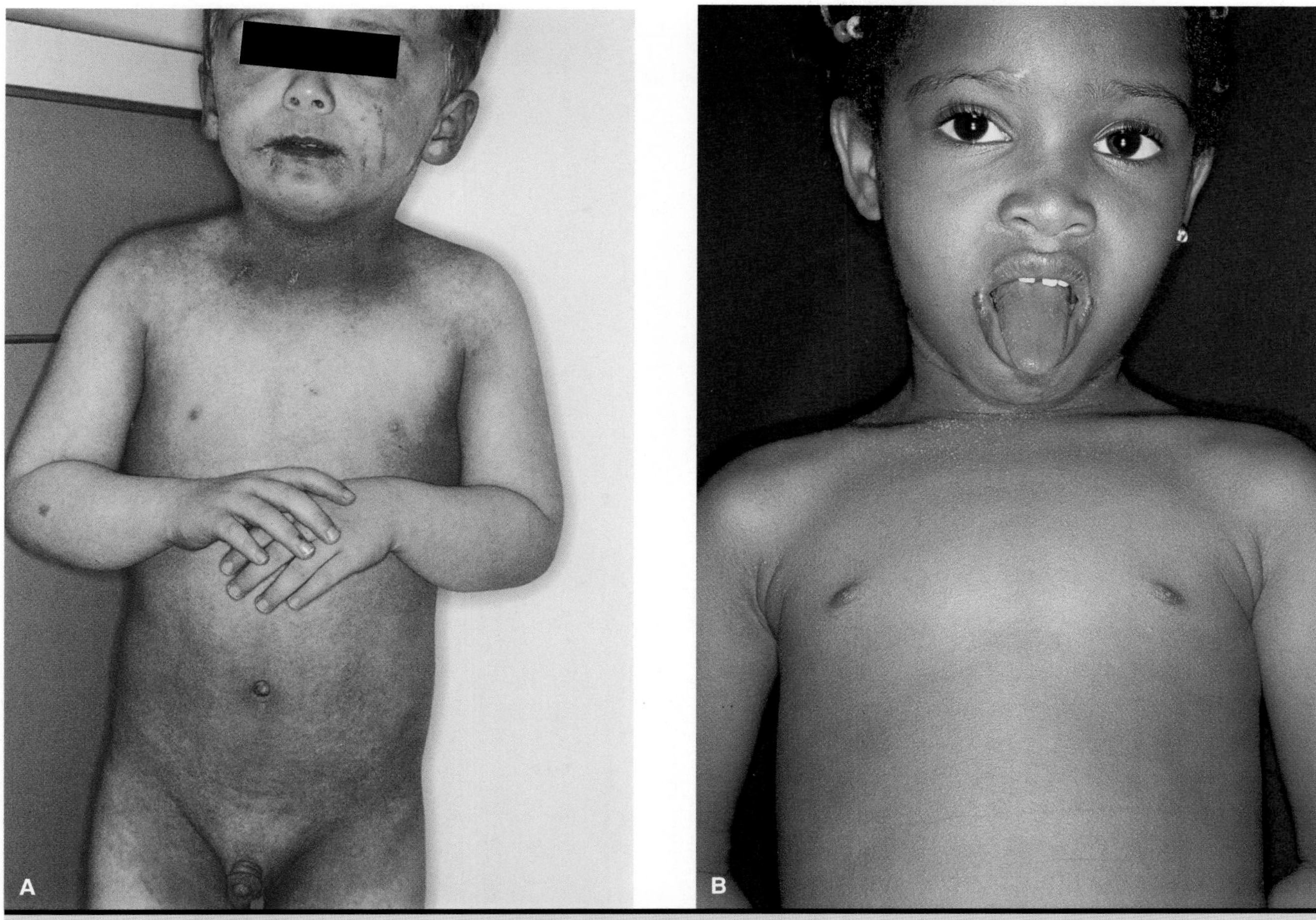

Figure 3-3. Scarlet Fever

A. Erythematous pinhead-size papular rash on the second day of illness. Note the prominence of the rash in the neck, axillas, and groin (all pressure sites). *B*. In dark-skinned patients, the rash of scarlet fever may be palpated more easily than seen. Always feel the texture and you will make the diagnosis in such cases. Note the accentuation of the rash in the neck area. Also note the absence of conjunctival injection and red lips (characteristic features of Kawasaki disease, which can also present with scarlatiniform rash).

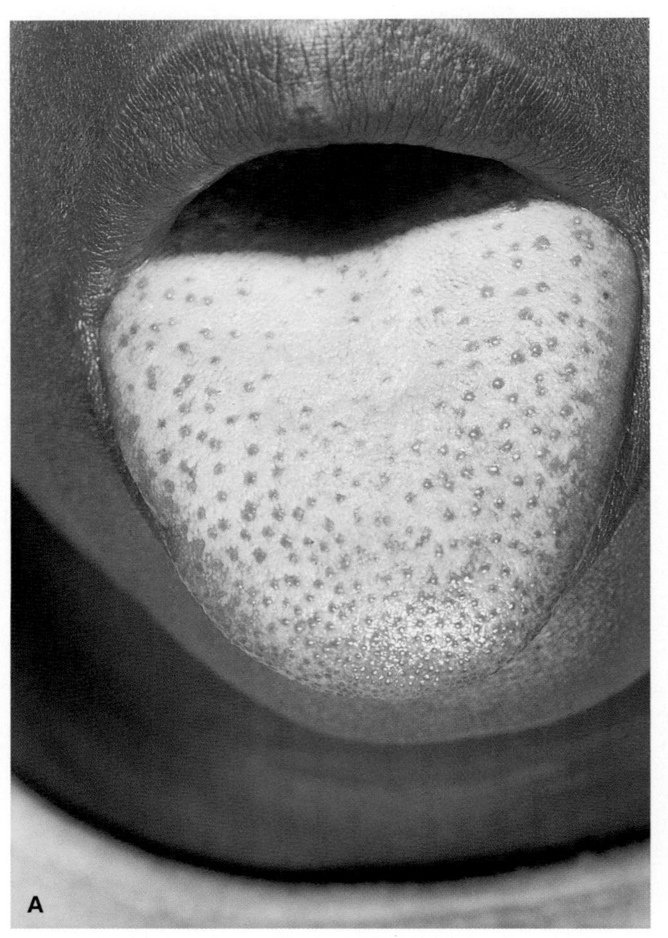

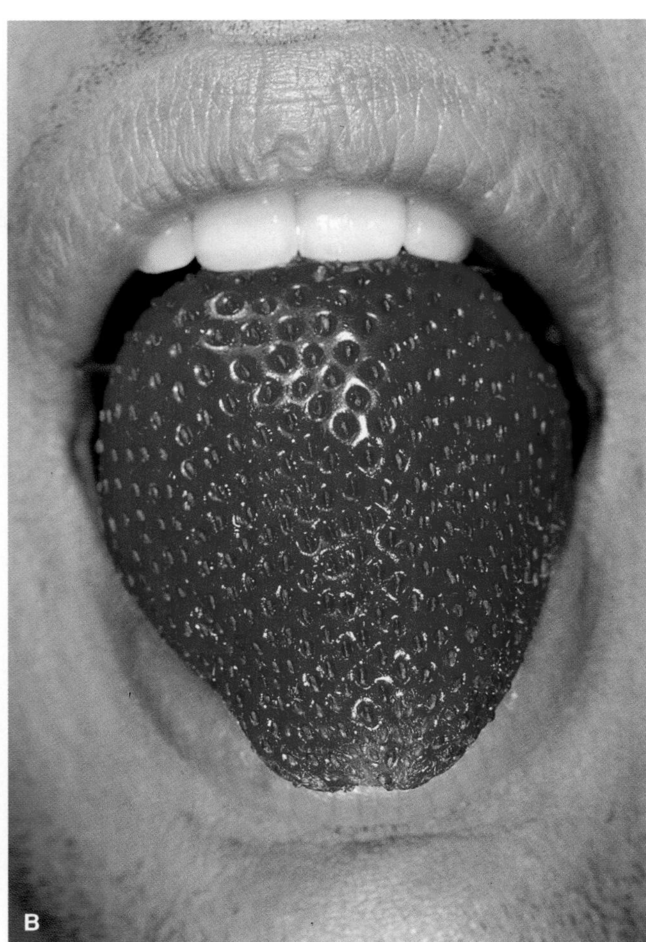

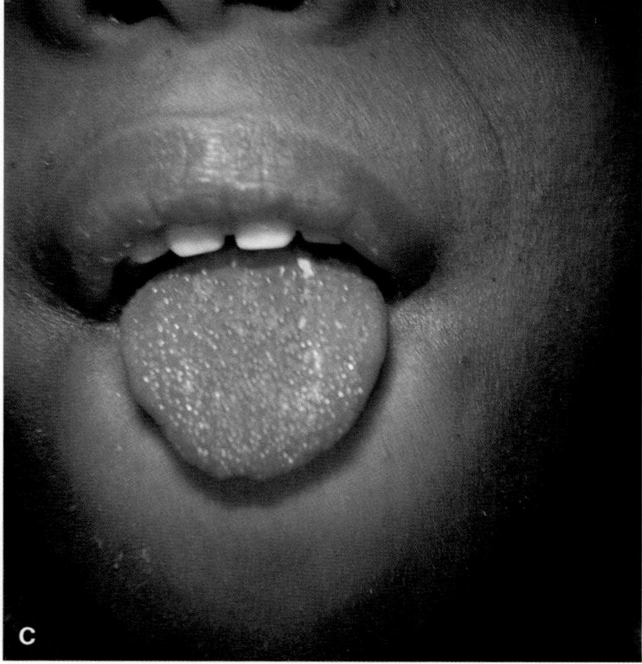

Figure 3-4. "Strawberry Tongue" of Scarlet Fever

A. White strawberry tongue (edematous red papillae projecting through white coated tongue; seen on the second day of illness in a child with scarlet fever). *B*. Red strawberry tongue? (Have you ever seen a "red strawberry tongue" like this?). *C*. Red strawberry tongue (as white coating disappears, red tongue studded with prominent papillae appears; seen on the third day of illness in a child with scarlet fever).

BOX 3-4. CLINICAL FEATURES OF SCARLET FEVER

- Patients usually febrile for 12 to 24 hours followed by appearance of rash
- Circumoral pallor (forehead and cheeks flushed with area around mouth pale)
- Rash
  (1) Initially begins in axilla, groin, and neck; becomes generalized within 24 hours
  (2) A vivid scarlet hue with innumerable pinhead-size papules with the texture of sandpaper or gooseflesh ("sunburn with goose pimples")
  (3) Rash may be palpated more readily than seen in dark-skinned patients
  (4) Blanches prominently when pressure is applied
  (5) Rash more prominent in axillas, groin, and at pressure sites
  (6) Palms, soles, and usually face are spared
  (7) Small vesicular lesions (miliary sudamina) may appear over the abdomen, hands, and feet in severe disease
- Strawberry tongue
  (1) White strawberry tongue (Fig. 3-4): edematous red papillae projecting through the white coated tongue) in the first 2 days *followed by*
  (2) Red strawberry tongue or raspberry tongue (as white coating disappears, red tongue studded with prominent papillae that stand out)
- Tonsillopharyngitis
  (1) Pharynx: beefy red
  (2) Palate and uvula may be edematous, reddened, and covered with petechiae
  (3) Tonsils erythematous and enlarged with patches of a gray-white exudate, giving a strawberry appearance (intensity of exudates varies from absent in mild cases to formation of a membrane covering the entire pharynx in severe cases)
- Pastia's sign: accentuation of rash in the skin folds (antecubital fossa, inguinal area, axillae) with a fine line of petechiae
- Desquamation (Figs. 3-5 and 3-6)
  (1) One of the most characteristic features
  (2) Seen at the end of the first week (between 7 and 10 days)
  (3) Desquamation complete in most cases in 2 to 3 weeks (may continue for as long as 6 to 8 weeks)
  (4) Begins on the face in fine flakes, then precedes over the trunk, hands, and feet
  (5) Extent and duration of desquamation directly related to the intensity of the rash
  (6) Appears as large areas of skin peeling off giving rise to a perforated appearance
  (7) Large sheaths of epidermis may be shed from the palms and soles in a glovelike pattern, exposing new and often tender epidermis beneath

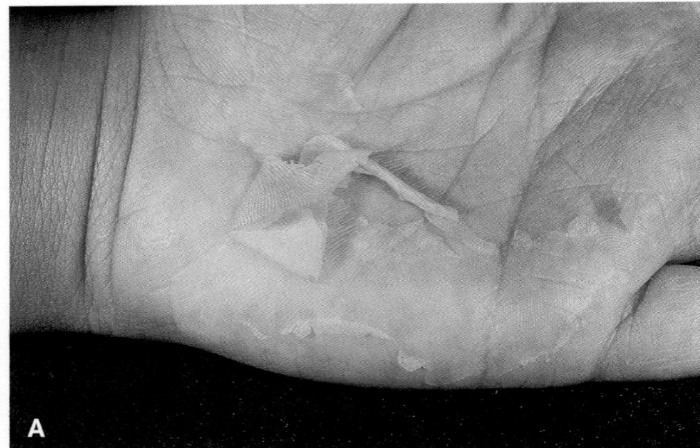

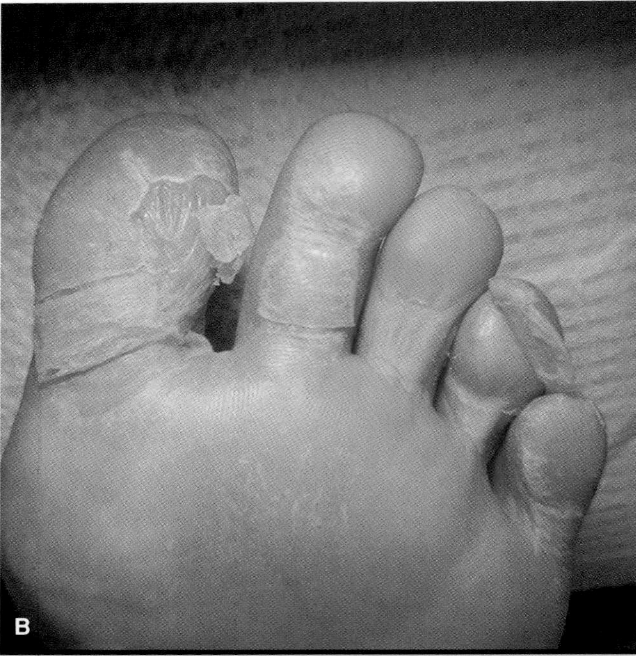

Figure 3-5. Close-Up Photos of Desquamation of the Hand and Foot in Scarlet Fever

A. and *B.* Photographs taken on the eighth day of illness in a child with scarlet fever.

BOX 3-5. DIFFERENTIAL DIAGNOSIS OF STRAWBERRY TONGUE

- Scarlet fever
- Kawasaki disease
- Toxic shock syndrome
  (1) Staphylococcal TSS
  (2) Streptococcal TSS

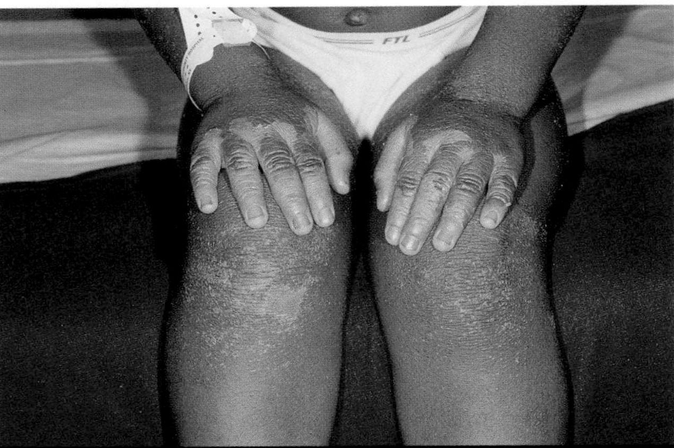

Figure 3-6. Desquamation as Presenting Sign of Scarlet Fever.

This 4 year-old child was brought in because of this prominent (and frightening to the parents) desquamation seen in both hands and lower extremities. He had a sore throat and low-grade fever with "goose bumps" 9 days prior to this finding. Desquamation on the hands and feet may be a presenting sign of scarlet fever (if the initial acute phase is mild and overlooked), necessitating making the diagnosis retrospectively.

BOX 3-6. DIFFERENTIAL DIAGNOSIS OF SCARLET FEVER

- Kawasaki disease
- Staphylococcal scarlatina
- Staphylococcal scalded skin syndrome
- Viral exanthems
  (1) Infectious mononucleosis
  (2) Measles
  (3) Hepatitis B virus
  (4) Coxsackie virus
  (5) Rubella
  (6) Roseola
- Toxic shock syndrome
  (1) Staphylococcal TSS
  (2) Streptococcal TSS
- Drug hypersensitivity reaction
- Severe sunburn
- Mycoplasma pneumoniae infection
- Arcanobacterium haemolyticum infection
  (1) Tonsillopharyngitis with scarlatiniform rash
  (2) Seen in adolescents and young adults
  (3) Absence of strawberry tongue

DIAGNOSIS

IMPETIGO

Synonyms

Impetigo contagiosa
Streptococcal impetigo
Streptococcal pyoderma
Nonbullous impetigo
Impetigo vulgaris

Definition and Etiology

1. Impetigo is a contagious superficial skin infection caused by group A beta-hemolytic streptococcus (GABHS or *Streptococcus pyogenes*) either alone or in combination with *Staphylococcus aureus*.
2. Strains of GABHS that produce impetigo have different M serotypes (e.g., 2, 49, 52) than the M serotypes (e.g., 1, 2, 4,6) found in the strains producing pharyngitis.
3. Impetigo was once thought to be primarily a streptococcal disease, but staphylococci are isolated either alone or in combination with GABHS as the predominant agents from the majority of lesions in recently documented reports.

Associated Clinical Features

1. Most commonly seen in children between 2 and 5 years of age.
2. A diagnosis of impetigo is made clinically and usually no laboratory tests are performed. A gram-stained smear of vesicopustular lesions shows gram-positive cocci in chains with or without gram-positive cocci in clusters. Culture of the exudate (beneath an unroofed crust) reveals GABHS, *S. aureus*, or a mixture of both.
3. Antistreptolysin O titer (ASLO) elevation after streptococcal impetigo is minimal or absent; however, titers of anti-DNAase B and antihyaluronidase increase significantly.
4. Acute poststreptococcal glomerulonephritis (APGN) may develop following impetigo, and treatment of impetigo does not alter the risk of APGN. Acute rheumatic fever has not been reported as a complication of impetigo (for complications of bacterial impetigo, see Box 3-11).
5. Unlike ecthyma caused by GABHS (see page 80), lesions of impetigo remain superficial, do not ulcerate or infiltrate the dermis, and heal without scarring.

Emergency Department Treatment and Disposition

1. Impetigo is self-limiting; however, untreated infection may last for weeks or months.
2. General measures include washing the affected area with antibacterial soap (e.g., Betadine) once or twice a day, and removal of the crusts (facilitated by softening the crusts by soaking with a wet cloth compress) before applying the topical therapy.
3. Topical mupirocin ointment therapy
   a. Effective for solitary lesions
   b. Applied three times per day until all lesions have cleared
   c. As effective as oral antibiotics for most patients
   d. Usually useful for limiting person-to-person spread of GABHS impetigo and for eradicating localized disease
4. Systemic antibiotic therapy is used for:
   a. Multiple site or extensive involvement
   b. Impetigo in multiple family members, child care groups, or athletic teams
   c. Penicillin was the drug of choice in the past for impetigo; however, to cover the mixed pathogens (GABHS and *S. aureus*), now penicillinase-resistant antibiotics (e.g., dicloxacillin) or cephalexin is commonly used.
   d. Antibiotic therapy is usually given orally for 7 to 10 days.
5. Rarely erythromycin-resistant *S. aureus* has been seen, but for most patients erythromycin is still a cheaper alternative therapy (especially in patients with penicillin allergy).

Clinical Pearls: Impetigo

1. Vesiculopustular lesions with yellow or honey-colored firmly adherent crusts are characteristic features.
2. Impetigo is a highly contagious infection. Spread among families, particularly among preschool children, is facilitated by poor hygiene.
3. The second most common clinical illness caused by GABHS is skin infection (pharyngitis being the most common).

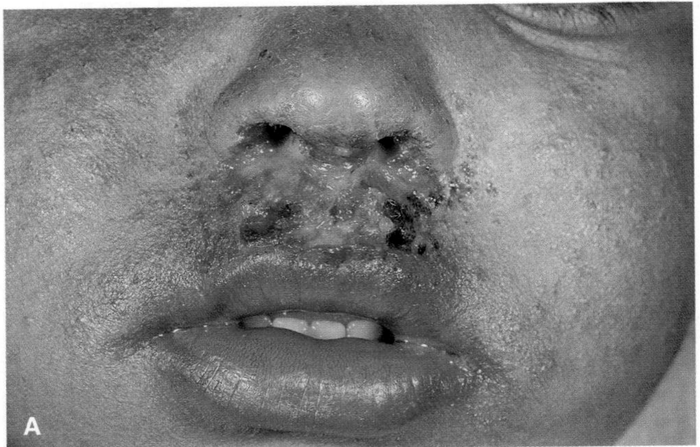

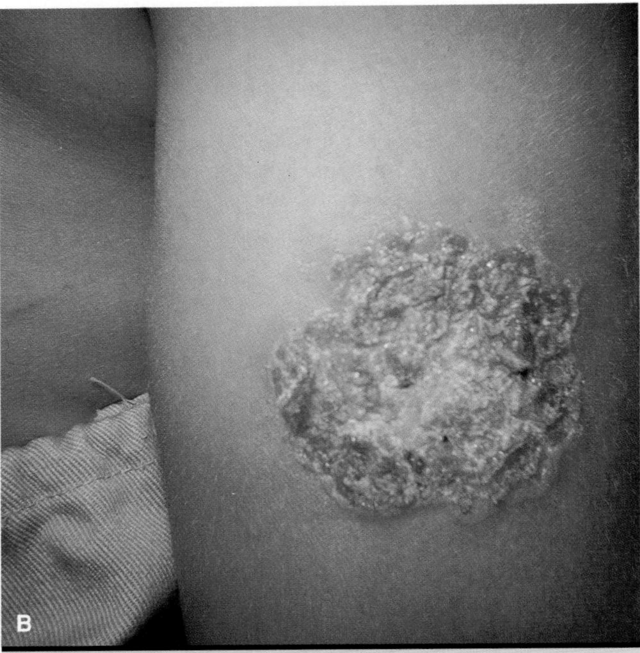

Figure 3-7 Impetigo

A. Exposed body surfaces such as the face (around the nose and mouth) are the most common sites. *B*. Lesion with a honey-colored crust on the upper extremity. Removal of the crust reveals bright red, shiny erosions.

BOX 3-7. CLINICAL FEATURES OF IMPETIGO

- Lesions begin as small vesicles that rapidly become pustules.
- Lesions extend radially and satellite lesions appear beyond the periphery.
- Vesiculopustular lesions rupture, exposing a red, moist base and purulent discharge.
- Purulent discharge dries and forms the thick, yellow or honey-colored firmly adherent crust.
- Lesions have little surrounding erythema.
- Lesions are usually painless and asymptomatic.
- Most common sites
  (1) Exposed body surfaces such as the face (nose and mouth) or extremities (*unlike bullous impetigo*)
  (2) Palms and soles not affected
- Lesions tend to occur on traumatized skin (e.g., insect bite, abrasion) *unlike bullous impetigo*.
- More common in hot, muggy summer months (*unlike bullous impetigo*)
- Pruritus common; scratching lesions helps in their spread (autoinoculation)
- Regional lymphadenopathy common (*unlike bullous impetigo*)
- Absent or minimal constitutional symptoms

BOX 3-8. DIFFERENTIAL DIAGNOSIS OF IMPETIGO

- Staphylococcal impetigo (bullous impetigo)
- Herpes simplex virus infection
- Varicella
- Tinea corporis
- Localized acute pustular psoriasis

DIAGNOSIS

BULLOUS IMPETIGO

Synonyms

Staphylococcal impetigo
Impetigo bullosa

Definition and Etiology

1. Bullous impetigo is a superficial skin infection caused by *Staphylococcus aureus* (most commonly phage group 2, type 71 or 52) that produces exfoliative (epidermolytic) toxin.
2. Bullous impetigo is *not* secondarily infected by *Streptococcus pyogenes* (unlike impetigo due to GABHS, which is usually co-infected by *S. aureus*). *S. aureus* is now known to be the primary pathogen in both forms of impetigo.

Associated Clinical Features

1. Most commonly seen in newborns, infants, and young children aged 2 to 5 years
2. The reservoir for staphylococci is the upper respiratory tract (e.g., nose and conjunctiva) of an asymptomatic person. These asymptomatic carriers spread the pathogen to the skin of infants and young children probably during handling.
3. Infection is initiated by exfoliating toxin produced at the site of infection. The toxin causes intraepidermal cleavage below or within the stratum granulosum.
4. The diagnosis is usually made clinically and can be confirmed by the culture of the aspirate from the lesion. Gram-stained smear will show gram-positive cocci in clusters.
5. Rarely serious secondary infections (e.g., osteomyelitis or septic arthritis) may follow seemingly innocuous superficial impetigo in infants.
6. Patients with recurrent impetigo should be evaluated for nasal carriage of *S. aureus*.

Emergency Department Treatment and Disposition

1. Topical mupirocin ointment is effective for solitary lesions.
2. For multiple and extensive involvement, a penicillinase-resistant antibiotic (e.g., dicloxacillin) or cephalexin is given orally for 7 to 10 days.
3. Rarely, erythromycin-resistant *S. aureus* has been seen, but for most patients erythromycin is still a cheaper alternative therapy (especially in patients with penicillin allergy).
4. Patients with nasal carriage of *S. aureus* leading to recurrent impetigo should be treated with intranasal application of mupirocin for 5 days.

Clinical Pearls: Bullous Impetigo

1. A pathognomonic finding of bullous impetigo is a ring of scale at the periphery of an eroded lesion with a varnished surface.
2. Staphylococci are isolated from the skin lesions of bullous impetigo, as opposed to negative culture results from skin lesions of staphylococcal scalded skin syndrome.

BOX 3-9. CLINICAL FEATURES OF BULLOUS IMPETIGO

- Begins as vesicles that rapidly enlarge to flaccid bullae
- Contents of bullae turn clear to cloudy (pus).
- Lesions may be few and localized to one area or numerous and widely scattered.
- Lesions have little or no surrounding erythema.
- Rupture of bullae leaves a narrow rim of scale at the edge of shallow, moist, red erosions (scalded skin appearance; Figs. 3-8, 3-9 and 3-10)
- Intact or ruptured bullae are round or oval in shape.
- Nikolsky's sign absent (unlike staphylococcal scalded skin syndrome)
- More commonly distributed in covered areas (*unlike impetigo due to GABHS*)
- Common sites: trunk, perineum, buttocks, extremities
- Lesions occur on intact skin (*unlike impetigo due to GABHS*).
- No seasonal predilection; seen all year round (*unlike impetigo due to GABHS*)
- Associated lymphadenopathy and fever uncommon (*unlike impetigo due to GABHS*)
- Lesions heal without scarring.

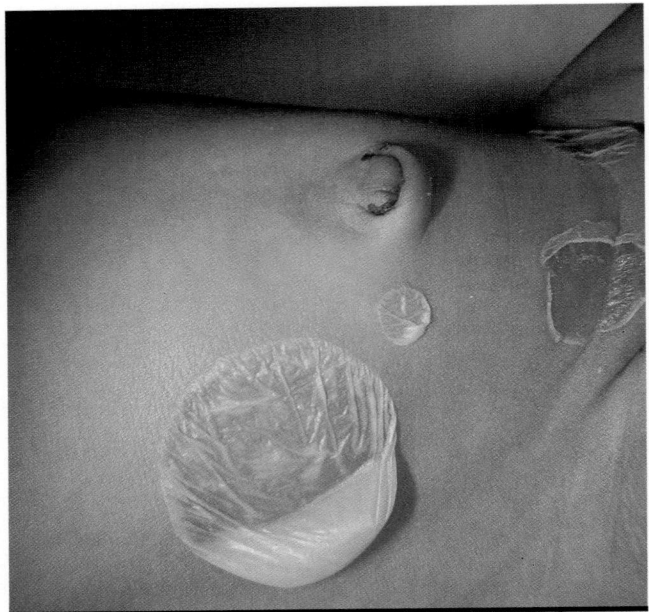

Figure 3-8. Bullous Impetigo

An intact bullous lesion filled with purulent material is seen in a 10-day-old neonate. He also had several round, ruptured erosions with a moist, red surface, that were surrounded by a narrow ring of scale.

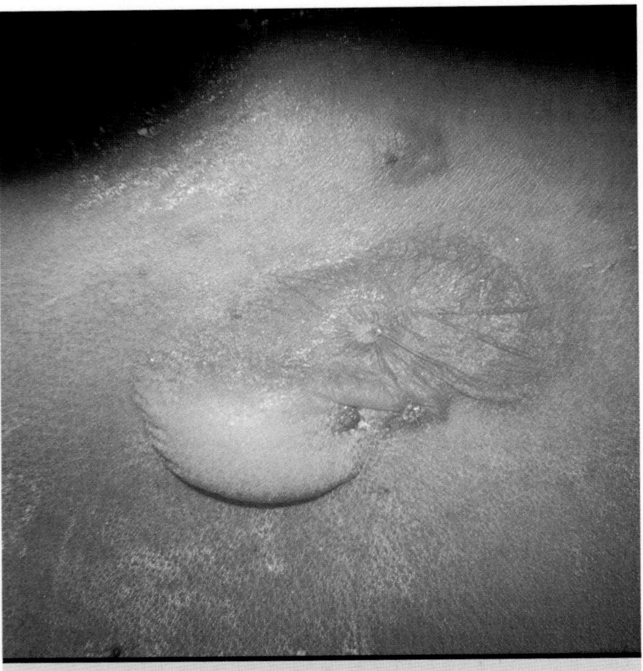

Figure 3-9. Bullous Impetigo

A child with chickenpox and a bullous lesion (secondary bacterial infection) filled with purulent material from which *S. aureus* was cultured.

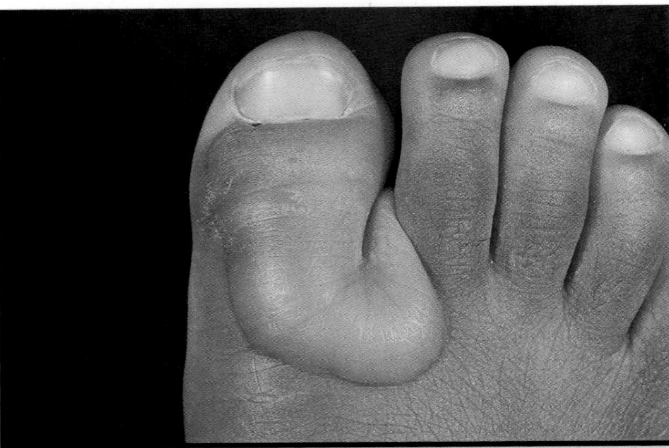

Figure 3-10. Bullous Impetigo

A 7-month-old infant was referred to ED with this lesion that was thought to be an inflicted burn injury (child abuse). Aspiration of the lesion showed gram-positive cocci in clusters on Gram's stain and culture was positive for *S. aureus*. Posttraumatic paronychia due to *S. aureus* should also be considered in the differential diagnosis.

BOX 3-10. DIFFERENTIAL DIAGNOSIS OF BULLOUS IMPETIGO

- Impetigo due to GABHS
- Bullous arthropod bites (Fig. 3-11)
- Poison ivy
- Child abuse (abusive burn injury)
- Autoimmune blistering disease (e.g., linear IgA dermatosis, pemphigus)
- Epidermolysis bullosa

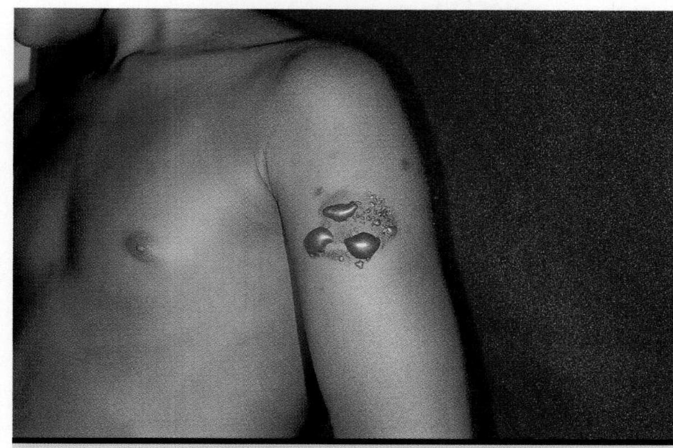

Figure 3-11. Bullous Arthropod Bites

Multiple lesions on upper extremity (exposed area) due to arthropod bites in a child. These lesions can be mistaken for either second-degree burns or bullous impetigo.

BOX 3-11. COMPLICATIONS OF BACTERIAL AND BULLOUS IMPETIGO

Complications	Associated Organism (Comment)
Sepsis	SA, GABHS
Osteomyelitis	SA, GABHS
Septic arthritis	SA, GABHS
Endocarditis	SA, GABHS
Pneumonia	SA, GABHS
Cellulitis	SA, GABHS (common with nonbullous impetigo)
Lymphangitis	GABHS
Lymphadenitis	SA, GABHS
Guttate psoriasis	GABHS
Staphylococcal scalded skin syndrome	SA (common during infancy)
Toxic shock syndrome	SA, GABHS
Acute poststreptococcal glomerulonephritis	GABHS

Abbreviations: GABHS, group A beta-hemolytic streptococci (*Streptococcus pyogenes*); SA, *Staphylococcus aureus*.
(Reproduced with permission from: Mancini AJ: Bacterial skin infections in children: The common and the not so common. *Pediatr Ann* 2000;29:28. SLACK Incorporated)

DIAGNOSIS

ECTHYMA

Definition and Etiology

1. Ecthyma is a skin infection caused by group A beta-hemolytic streptococci (*Streptococcus pyogenes*) and/or *Staphylococcus aureus.*
2. Unlike impetigo, which is the most superficial of the pyodermas, ecthyma involves deeper layers of the skin (the entire thickness of the epidermis to the upper reaches of the dermis).

Associated Clinical Features

1. Ecthyma is seen in children of all ages, and is seen more frequently during summer.
2. There is frequently a history of preceding minor skin trauma (e.g., abrasions, insect bites). Other predisposing factors include conditions associated with pruritus (e.g., scabies, pediculosis), poor hygiene, and malnutrition. Extensive involvement with complicating bacteremia has been reported in a patient with AIDS.
3. Ecthyma is diagnosed clinically and usually no laboratory tests are required. Culture of the exudate (beneath an unroofed crust) reveals GABHS and *S. aureus.*
4. Antistreptolysin O titer (ASLO) elevation after streptococcal impetigo and ecthyma is minimal or absent; however, titers of anti-DNAase B and antihyaluronidase increase significantly.
5. Ecthyma may progress to cellulitis or lymphangitis if left untreated. Poststreptococcal glomerulonephritis is also a rare complication.

Emergency Department Treatment and Disposition

1. General measures include washing the affected area with antibacterial soap (e.g., Betadine), and removal of the crust (facilitated by softening the crust by soaking with a wet cloth compress).
2. Topical mupirocin therapy is used until all lesions have cleared.
3. Patients with ecthyma should be treated with a 10-day course of an oral antibiotic that provides coverage for both *S. pyogenes* and *S. aureus* (e.g., dicloxacillin or cephalexin).
4. Even though rare cases of erythromycin-resistant *S. aureus* have been seen, for most patients erythromycin is still a cheaper alternative therapy (especially in patients with penicillin allergy). Azithromycin given over 5 days as a once-daily regimen is also an effective alternative therapy.

Clinical Pearls: Ecthyma

1. Lesions of ecthyma begin in a similar fashion as impetigo due to GABHS, but penetrate through the entire thickness of the epidermis to the upper reaches of dermis. Thick crusts and underlying ulcers differentiate ecthyma from the impetigo due to GABHS.
2. Ecthyma lesions are discrete, round, "punched-out" ulcers covered with dark greenish yellow crusts that extend deeply into the epidermis (Fig. 3-12).
3. Ecthyma can be mistakenly attributed to cigarette burns of child abuse (Fig. 3-13).

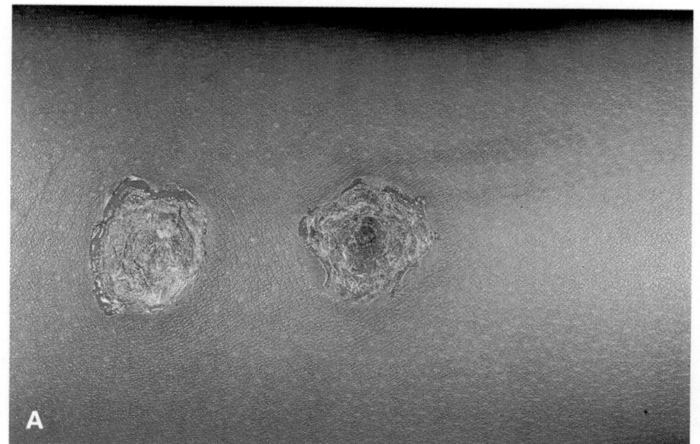

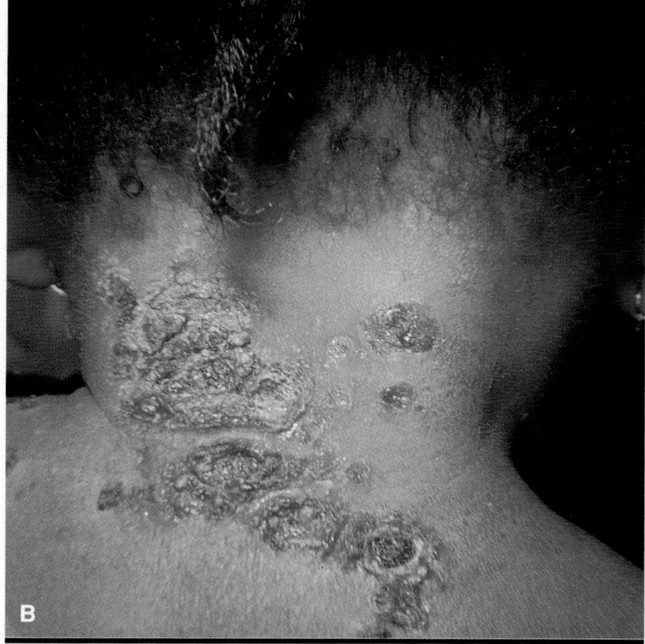

Figure 3-12. Ecthyma

A. Discrete, round lesions with a dark crust in the center surrounded by a rim of shallow ulceration are seen on the arm of an infant. *B*. Multiple ecthyma lesions on the neck.

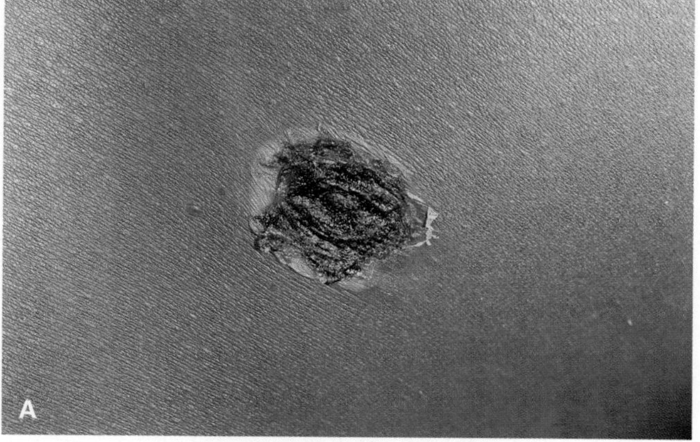

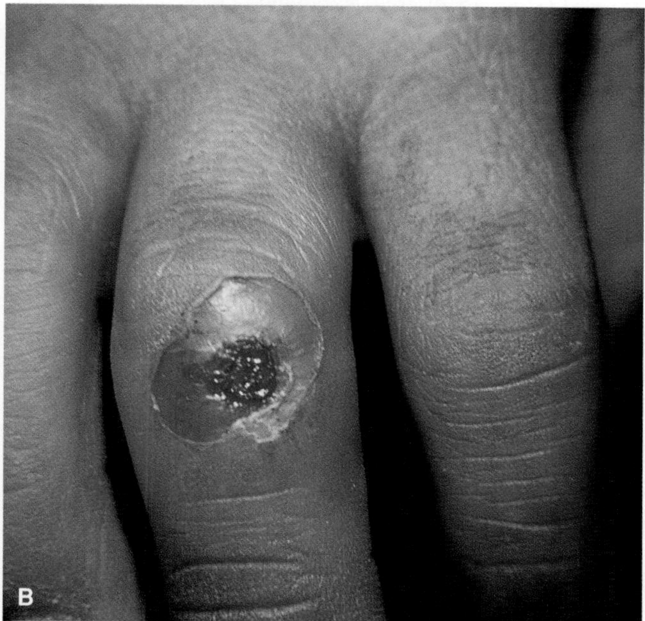

Figure 3-13. Ecthyma versus Cigarette Burn

Ecthyma (*A*) may be confused with cigarette burns (*B*). Ecthyma lesions are frequently of different sizes and are associated with crusting, while cigarette burns are uniform in size with an average diameter of about 8 to 10 mm. (Photo B reproduced with permission from: American Academy of Pediatrics: *The Visual Diagnosis of Child Physical Diagnosis*. The C. Henry Kempe National Center on Child Abuse and Neglect. EIK Grove Village, IL, American Academy of Pediatrics, 1994, p. 25.)

BOX 3-12. CLINICAL FEATURES OF ECTHYMA

- Lesions begin as vesicles or vesiculopustules with an erythematous base.
- Lesions rupture to form crusts and erode through the epidermis into the dermis, forming indolent "punched-out" ulcers with elevated margins.
- Ulcers become elevated and obscured by thick, dark greenish-yellow tightly adherent crusts that contribute to the persistence of the infection.
- Lesions are discrete and round.
- Most common site: lower legs
- Lesion may be spread by autoinoculation
- Lesion may heal with scarring (*unlike impetigo due to GABHS*)

BOX 3-13. DIFFERENTIAL DIAGNOSIS OF ECTHYMA

- Impetigo due to GABHS (early vesiculopustular phase of ecthyma)
- Cigarette burns (due to child abuse)
- Ecthyma gangrenosum (*Pseudomonas aeruginosa* infection)

DIAGNOSIS

ERYSIPELAS

SYNONYMS

St. Anthony's fire
Ignis sacer

Definition

Erysipelas is a distinct infection of the skin involving the uppermost layers of the subcutaneous tissue and cutaneous lymphatic vessels. In contrast to erysipelas, cellulitis extends more deeply into the subcutaneous tissues.

Etiology

Erysipelas is caused by group A beta-hemolytic streptococci (GABHS) in the great majority of the cases. Rarely it is caused by groups G, C, and B streptococci.

Associated Clinical Features

1. It is most frequently seen in infants, young children, older adults, and debilitated patients.
2. The organism gains access to the deeper layers of the skin through lesions such as abrasions, lacerations, wounds, chronic ulcers, or other breaks in the skin. Predisposing factors also include lymphedema, local lymphatic dysfunction, venous stasis, diabetes mellitus, malnutrition, and immunocompromised states. Erysipelas usually occurs proximal to the portal of entry into the skin.
3. The clinical presentation is so characteristic that erysipelas is usually diagnosed clinically and no laboratory tests are required.
4. Leukocytosis with a left shift may be present. Group A beta-hemolytic streptococci (GABHS) cannot be cultured from the surface of the skin lesion. It may rarely be cultured from blood (~5% of patients), or by aspiration from the advancing margin of the lesion. Antistreptolysin O (ASLO) titer or streptozyme may help to confirm the diagnosis, but these tests rarely help during acute management.
5. As erysipelas produces lymphatic obstruction, recurrences frequently occur at the same site. Impairment of lymphatic drainage occurs with each recurrence, leading to lymphedema, which predisposes to further infections and permanent swelling.
6. Complications are the same as with any GABHS infection (see Box 3-3).

Emergency Department Treatment and Disposition

1. The rapid spread of infection (especially on the face) coupled with the systemic signs usually requires hospitalization for intravenous antibiotics for at least 48 to 72 hours.
2. Penicillin G can be used as most cases are due to GABHS. Penicillinase-resistant penicillins (nafcillin or oxacillin)

are commonly used as an alternative to cover for *S. aureus* (with a possible differential diagnosis of cellulitis in mind).

3. Erythromycin or cephalexin clindamycin, is used if the patient is allergic to penicillin.
4. Patients with milder presentations may be treated as outpatients with oral therapy and close follow-up.
5. Rest, immobilization, elevation of the affected part, and cool, wet dressings are other forms of supportive therapy.
6. The prognosis is excellent with early institution of antibiotic therapy. Extension to deeper soft tissues is rare and surgical débridement is not necessary.

Clinical Pearls: Erysipelas

1. Erysipelas is a rapidly-spreading, fiery red infection of the skin with a sharp advancing border that is raised and well demarcated from the adjacent normal tissue.
2. The great majority of cases of erysipelas are caused by GABHS.

BOX 3-14. CLINICAL FEATURES OF ERYSIPELAS

- Usually abrupt onset with constitutional symptoms (fever, chills, malaise, headache)
- Common sites (may occur anywhere):
  - (1) Face (5 to 20% of cases; usually associated with pharyngitis)
  - (2) Extremities (70 to 80% of cases; usually associated with a wound)
- Initiating lesion frequently inconspicuous
- Spreads peripherally with a raised, advancing border
- Fiery red or salmon in color (Fig. 3-14)
- Lesion hot, tender, tense, indurated plaque, sometimes with peau d'orange appearance
- Lesion well circumscribed with a sharp demarcated border distinguishing it from the surrounding normal tissue
- Marked involvement of superficial lymphatics (reddish lymphatic streaks projecting out from margins of the lesion toward regional nodes)
- Intense edema may lead to formation of vesicles or tense bullae (bullous erysipelas) that later rupture and crust.
- May create a "butterfly" appearance on the face with involvement of both cheeks and the bridge of the nose (Fig. 3-15)
- Rash appears with or without local lymphadenopathy
- Desquamation of involved skin may occur 5 to 10 days into the illness.

Clinical pearl:

Erysipelas is commonly referred as St. Anthony's fire because it spreads rapidly like a fire, affecting a very large area of the skin within a short period of time.

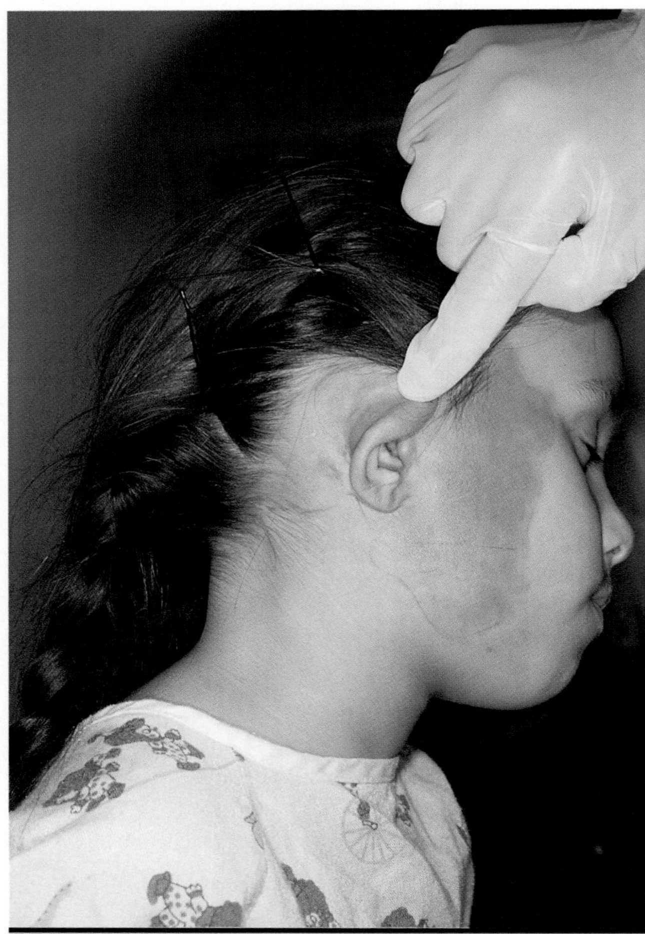

Figure 3-14. Erysipelas

A rapidly spreading, tender, salmon-colored rash accompanied by high fever was seen on the face of this 8-year-old girl. She had scratch marks on her cheek (portal of entry). The sharp demarcation between the salmon-red erythema and the normal surrounding skin is evident. Marking the margins of the erythema with ink helps in following the clinical course (progression or regression) of the infection. A marked improvement was seen after 2 days of IV antibiotic therapy. Mild desquamation of the involved skin was also apparent.

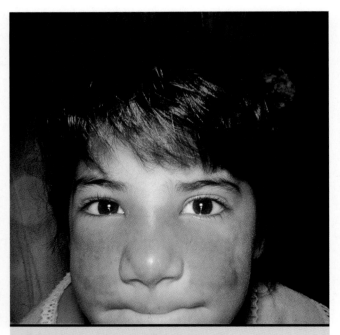

Figure 3-15. Butterfly Rash of Erysipelas

A rapidly spreading (<12-hour duration), tender, fiery red, indurated rash on the face was seen in this 7-year-old girl. She had temperature of 40°C with leukocytosis. The sharp demarcation between the salmon-red erythema and the normal surrounding skin is evident. Erysipelas may create a "butterfly" appearance (mimicking the rash of systemic lupus erythematosus) on the face with involvement of both cheeks and the bridge of the nose. She gave a history of falling off the monkey bar 2 days prior to this appearance of this rash. Within 6 months after this infection, she presented with another episode of erysipelas at the same site. (Reproduced with permission from: Shah BR, Santucci K, Tunnessen W: Erysipelas. *Arch Pediatr Adolesc Med* 1995;149:55.)

BOX 3-15. DIFFERENTIAL DIAGNOSIS OF ERYSIPELAS

- Cellulitis (Fig. 3-16)
- Erysipelas-like presentation due to other bacterial infection (e.g., other streptococci [groups G, B, and C], *Streptococcus pneumoniae, S. aureus, Yersinia enterocolitica*)
- Butterfly rash of systemic lupus erythematosus
- Necrotizing fasciitis
- Deep vein thrombosis or thrombophlebitis
- Contact dermatitis
- Giant urticaria
- Angioneurotic edema
- Erysipelas-like lesions of familial Mediterranean fever

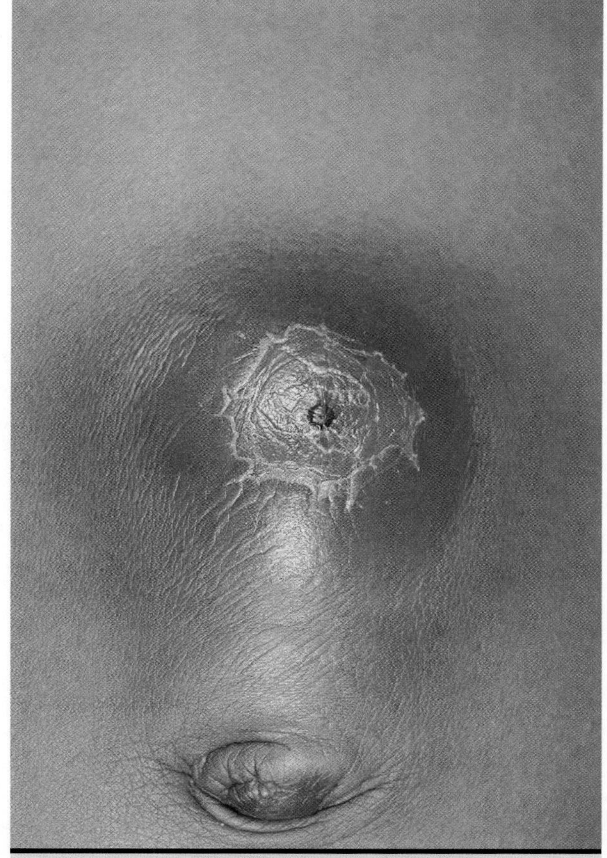

Figure 3-16. Cellulitis

Unlike erysipelas, the borders of cellulitis are ill-defined because of the deeper tissue involvement. Cellulitis also spreads more slowly. Common organisms causing cellulitis include GABHS, *Staphylococcus aureus*, *Streptococcus pneumoniae*, and *Haemophilus influenzae*.

BOX 3-16. BACTERIAL SKIN INFECTIONS

- Impetigo contagiosum
  (1) Vesiculopustular lesions
  (2) Honey-colored crust
- Bullous impetigo
  (1) Flaccid round or oval- shaped bullae filled with clear fluid or pus
  (2) Rupture of bullae leaves a narrow rim of scale at the edge of a shallow, moist, red erosion (scalded skin appearance)
- Ecthyma
  (1) Infection involves deeper layers of dermis
  (2) Discrete, round, elevated lesions covered by a dark crust and surrounded by a rim of shallow ulceration
- Erysipelas
  (1) Infection of superficial skin with marked involvement of superficial lymphatics
  (2) Fiery red, painful, rapidly enlarging well-circumscribed lesion with a sharp demarcated border separating it from the surrounding normal tissue
- Cellulitis
  (1) Deeper infection involving the dermis and subcutaneous tissues
  (2) Poorly demarcated borders
- Necrotizing fasciitis
  (1) Life-threatening infection of fascia and subcutaneous tissues
  (2) Begins as erythematous, indurated, tender, ill-defined plaque
  (3) Dusky purple or brown discoloration of affected area
  (4) Vesicles/bullae filled with or without maroon or violaceous fluid in the center of the affected area
- Follicular impetigo
  (1) Inflammation of hair follicles
  (2) Scattered small pustular or papular lesions
- *Furuncle:* tender deep-seated nodule (abscess) around a hair follicle with signs of "pointing"
- *Carbuncle*: several confluent furuncles with openings on the surface

DIAGNOSIS NECROTIZING FASCIITIS

SYNONYMS

Streptococcal gangrene
Flesh-eating bacteria or flesh-eating bacteria syndrome
Hospital gangrene
Necrotizing erysipelas or necrotizing cellulitis

Definition

Necrotizing fasciitis (NF) is a life-threatening bacterial infection of the fascia and subcutaneous tissues. When muscle is involved, the term bacterial myonecrosis is used.

Etiology

1. *Streptococcus pyogenes* or group A beta-hemolytic streptococci (rarely groups B, C, and G)
2. *Staphylococcus aureus*
3. *Pseudomonas aeruginosa*
4. Anaerobes (e.g., *Bacteroides*, *Peptostreptococcus*, *Clostridium* spp.)
5. Polymicrobial infection (gram-negative bacilli [*Escherichia coli*, *Proteus* spp.] and anaerobic bacteria)

Associated Clinical Features

1. About 80% of cases of NF occur as an extension from a localized nearby skin infection.
2. Infection expands along fascial planes leading to edema, vascular injury, and thrombosis resulting in widespread necrosis of the superficial fascia, adjoining tissues, and deeper layer of dermis (Fig. 3-17). Associated compression or destruction of nerves innervating skin results in anesthesia.
3. Laboratory tests are nonspecific and may show leukocytosis with immature forms, anemia, hyponatremia, hypocalcemia, hypoproteinemia, an abnormal coagulation profile, and elevated values of BUN, creatinine, and liver enzymes.
4. Fine-needle aspiration from the involved area may show the presence of pus and bacteria on Gram's stain. Aspirated material and blood culture should be sent for both aerobic and anaerobic pathogens.

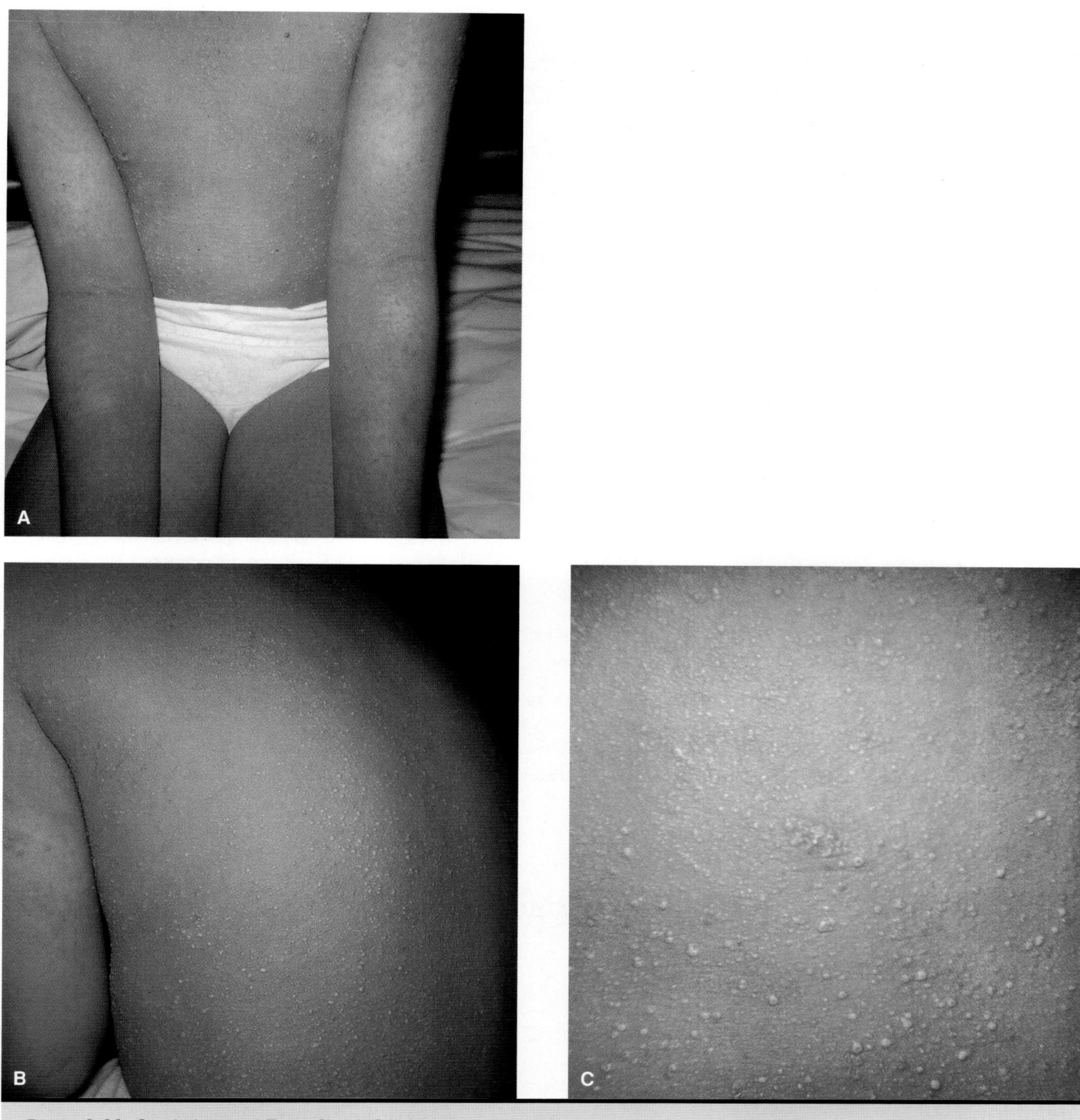

Figure 3-22. Staphylococcal Toxic Shock Syndrome

A., B. Generalized erythroderma and innumerable pustular lesions were seen on the skin of this child who presented with hypotension and multiorgan failure. Her blood culture was positive for *S. aureus* (blood culture is positive in $<5\%$ of patients with staphylococcal TSS). *C.* Close-up showing pustular lesions. Culture from these lesions was negative for *S. aureus*.

BOX 3-24. DIFFERENTIAL DIAGNOSIS: STAPHYLOCOCCAL TOXIC SHOCK SYNDROME VERSUS STREPTOCOCCAL TOXIC SHOCK SYNDROME

Characteristic	Staph-TSS	Strep-TSS
Age	15–35	20–50
Sex	More women	Either
Severe pain in skin	Common	Rare
Hypotension	100%	100%
Blood culture (+)	<5%	>50%
Clinical features		
Erythroderma	Very common	Less common
Profuse watery diarrhea, vomiting	Frequent	Less common
Conjunctival injection	Frequent	Less common
Severe myalgias	Frequent	Less common
Local soft tissue infection		
Cellulitis, abscess	Rare	Common
Necrotizing fasciitis, myositis	Rare	Common
Predisposing factors	Tampons, nasal packing	Skin trauma, varicella
Mortality	<30%	30–70%
Recurrence	Seen (menses associated)	Not seen

(Reproduced with permission from: Shah BR: Toxic shock syndrome. In: Perkin RM, Swift JD, Newton D (eds). *Pediatric Hospital Medicine*. Lippincott Williams & Wilkins, Philadelphia, 2003, page 525.)

DIAGNOSIS STAPHYLOCOCCAL SCALDED SKIN SYNDROME

SYNONYMS

Ritter's disease (SSSS of the newborn or pemphigus neonatorum)
Lyell's disease

Definition

1. Staphylococcal scalded skin syndrome (SSSS) is the most severe manifestation of infection caused by certain *Staphylococcus aureus* strains that produce an exfoliative toxin, and is characterized by widespread bullae and exfoliation.
2. When Lyell described toxic epidermal necrolysis (TEN) that mimicked SSSS in many ways, it led to some confusion in the terminology. This entity, referred as Lyell's disease, was subsequently differentiated into two subtypes: one that is seen most frequently in adults secondary to drug hypersensitivity (now referred as TEN), and the other occurring in infants secondary to staphylococcal infection (now referred as SSSS, which also represents what was formerly known as Ritter's disease).

Etiology

1. *S. aureus* strains belonging to phage 2 (types 71, 55, 3A, 3B, 3C) produce an epidermolytic toxin called *exfoliative toxin*. The toxin is antigenic and elicits an antibody response when elaborated. Two distinct *S. aureus* exfoliative toxins (ET A and ET B) have been identified.
2. These toxins are capable of causing clinical diseases that include bullous impetigo, generalized scarlatiniform eruption without exfoliation (staphylococcal scarlatina), and exfoliative disease (SSSS).
3. *S. aureus* colonizes mucous membranes of the nasopharynx, eyes, and other areas (e.g., umbilical stump, circumcision sites), producing a localized infection. Toxin produced in

these areas circulates and acts specifically at the zona granulosa of the epidermis, leading to characteristic exfoliation.

4. Besides SSSS, other toxin-mediated syndromes caused by *S. aureus* include toxic shock syndrome (see TSS, Figs. 3-21 and 3-22). and food poisoning.

Associated Clinical Features

1. Most commonly seen in infants and young children:
   a. 90% of those infected are <6 years of age, and 62% are <2 years of age.
   b. Lack of specific antibody to exfoliative toxin and renal immaturity that leads to poor clearance of the toxin are contributing factors in the younger age group.
   c. Epidermolytic toxin antibody is present in about 75% of normal people over the age of 10 years, a fact that explains the rare occurrence of SSSS in adults.
2. Infection in older children and adults is related to a decreased renal clearance of the toxin (e.g., patients with renal insufficiency, patients on hemodialysis) or in association with lymphoma or immunosuppression (e.g., HIV infection).
3. An associated staphylococcal infection such as impetigo or purulent conjunctivitis may be present.
4. Diagnosis of SSSS may not be suspected early in the course, as the eruption may resemble scarlet fever. Some cases of SSSS do not progress beyond the staphylococcal scarlatina stage (forme fruste of SSSS). These cases are referred as staphylococcal scarlet fever or staphylococcal scarlatina.
5. Culture from colonized sites like mucous membranes of nasopharynx, conjunctiva, or umbilical stump may be positive for *S. aureus*. Cultures of the skin are negative for staphylococci. Cultures of the intact bullae are also negative (*unlike those of bullous impetigo*). Blood culture is often negative in children and positive in adults.
6. A rapid, quantitative measure of exfoliative toxin directly from the serum (e.g. F [ab′] [2] fragment ELISA) may become commercially available in the future and will allow confirmation of the diagnosis with a blood test.
7. A skin biopsy specimen (or a frozen section of an induced peel for a more rapid diagnosis) will help to distinguish between SSSS and TEN.
   a. Splitting of the epidermis is in the stratum granulosum near the skin surface (partial split of upper epidermis) in SSSS.
   b. Bulla is subepidermal and associated with full-thickness necrosis of epidermis in TEN.
8. Complications include fluid and electrolyte losses leading to hypovolemia, faulty temperature regulation, cutaneous infection (cellulitis), pneumonia, and septicemia.
9. Long-term complications are rare because the skin lesions are superficial and heal rapidly without scarring. Overall mortality varies between 1 and 10%. Mortality in adults is about 60% despite aggressive treatment, usually because of serious underlying illness.

Consultation

Dermatology (if diagnosis unclear between SSSS and TEN)

Emergency Department Treatment and Disposition

1. All patients with SSSS with widespread erosions and denuded skin require hospitalization, including close monitoring for fluid and electrolyte deficits (caused by loss of the epidermal barrier).
2. Intravenous antibiotic therapy:
   a. Start penicillinase-resistant beta-lactam antibiotic (e.g., oxacillin or nafcillin) therapy.
   b. Patients allergic to penicillin can be treated with a cephalosporin such as cefuroxime (if patient not allergic to cephalosporin), or clindamycin or vancomycin.
   c. Usual duration of therapy is 5 to 7 days.
   d. Bacteremic or immunocompromised patients require a longer duration of therapy.
3. Skin care includes:
   a. Gently moistening and cleaning the skin with isotonic saline or Burow's solution
   b. Applying an emollient to provide lubrication and to reduce discomfort
   c. Avoid wet dressing, as it may cause further drying and cracking.
   d. Application of a topical antibiotic is not necessary.
4. Corticosteroids are contraindicated because they interfere with host defense mechanisms.
5. Patients with localized SSSS can be treated with oral antibiotic therapy (e.g., dicloxacillin or a first- or second-generation cephalosporin) with very close follow-up.

Clinical Pearls: Staphylococcal Scalded Skin Syndrome

1. Radial sunburst crusting and fissuring around the orifices (mouth, eyes, nose) are hallmarks of SSSS (Fig. 3-23).
2. Early distinction between SSSS and TEN is extremely important because therapy for SSSS includes antistaphylococcal antibiotics, whereas in TEN *discontinuation of treatment with the offending drug* and aggressive supportive therapy in a burn unit may be lifesaving.
3. Cultures from the affected skin/bulla are negative for *S. aureus* in SSSS, while cultures from the colonized sites such as mucous membranes of the nasopharynx, conjunctiva, or umbilical stump may be positive.
4. The hallmark of SSSS is the toxin-mediated cleavage of the stratum granulosum layer of the epidermis.
5. SSSS is a potentially serious but highly treatable infection.

BOX 3-25. CLINICAL FEATURES OF STAPHYLOCOCCAL SCALDED SKIN SYNDROME

- Incubation period: usually 1 to 10 days
- Sudden onset of fever, irritability
- Prominent crusting around the eyes and mouth occurs early.
- May have pharyngitis, conjunctivitis, or superficial erosions of lips
- Intraoral mucosal surfaces spared
- Rash
  (1) No prodromal period at the time of onset of rash
  (2) Exquisite tenderness of the skin (e.g., infant cries when held)
  (3) Begins as diffuse erythematous scarlatiniform eruption with sandpaperlike texture
  (4) Rash accentuated in the perioral and flexural areas.
  (5) Within 24 to 48 hours the skin wrinkles and flaccid bullae develop, followed by exfoliation in sheets revealing a moist, red, shiny scalded-looking surface.
  (6) Borders of exfoliating skin are rolled like wet tissue paper.
  (7) Nikolsky sign positive (slight rubbing of normal-looking adjacent skin results in blistering)
  (8) Exfoliation can spread to cover the entire body surface area in the most severe form.
  (9) Drying of exfoliated areas with flaky desquamation lasting 3 to 5 days
  (10) Hair and nails may also be shed.
  (11) Healing of rash occurs without scarring in 7 to 14 days. (see Figs. 3-23 to 3-27)

(Modified and reproduced with permission from: Shah BR: Staphylococcal scalded skin syndrome. In: Perkin RM, Swift JD, Newton DA (eds). *Pediatric Hospital Medicine. Textbook of Inpatient Management.* Lippincott Williams & Wilkins, Baltimore, 2003, p. 520.)

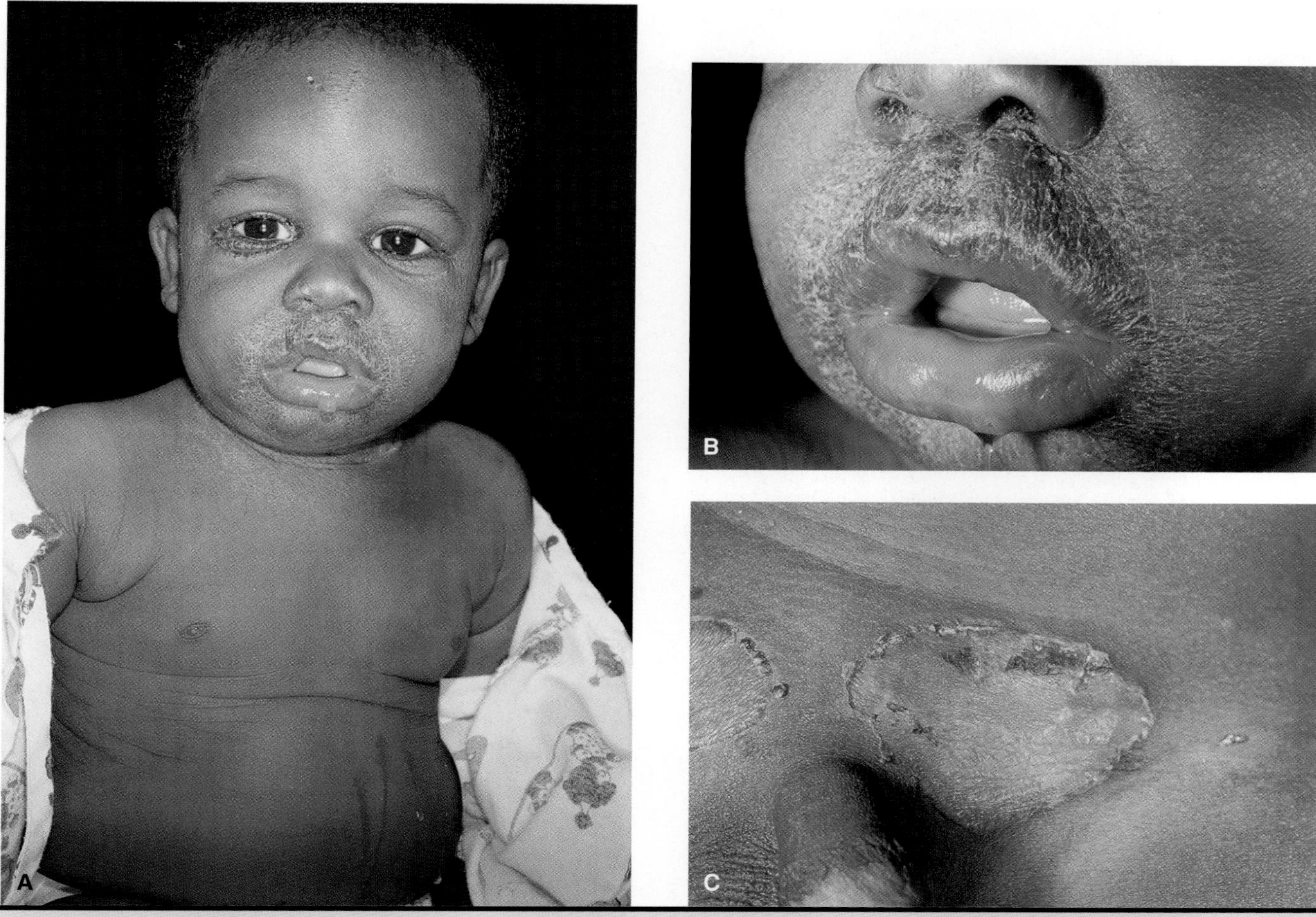

Figure 3-23. Staphylococcal Scalded Skin Syndrome.

A., B. Radial sunburst crusting and fissuring around the orifices (mouth, eyes, nose) are hallmarks of SSSS (first day of rash in this patient). Note the absence of any mucous membrane involvement of the mouth or eyes (unlike the prominent mucous membrane involvement seen in TEN or Stevens-Johnson syndrome). Within 24 hours after these photographs were taken, the skin over the trunk and perineum (*C*) started wrinkling and flaccid bullae developed, followed by exfoliation in sheets revealing a red scalded-looking surface. In SSSS, *S. aureus* is not cultured from the areas of desquamation.

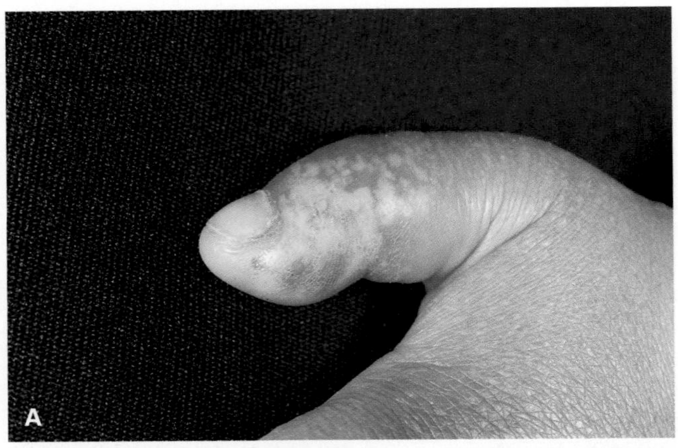

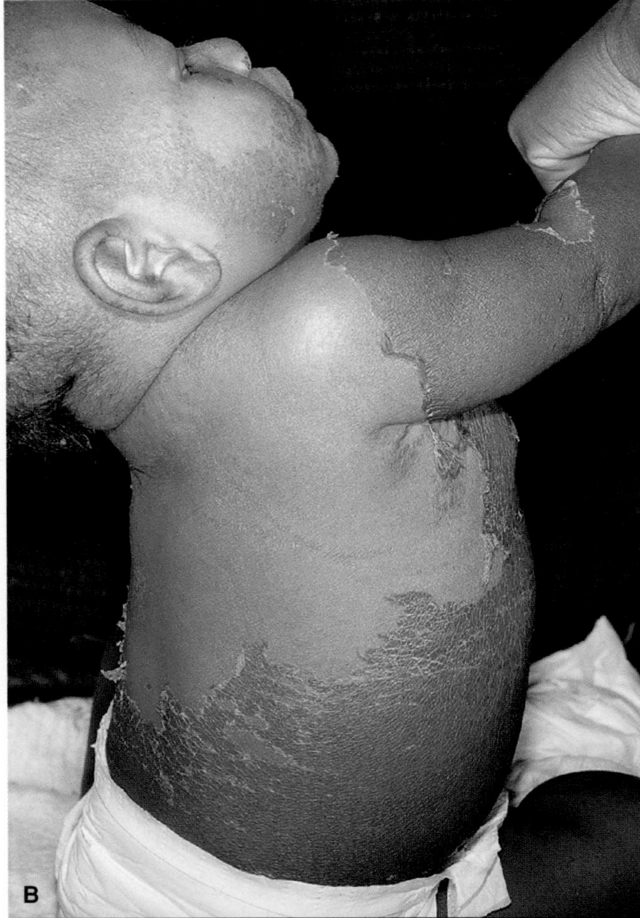

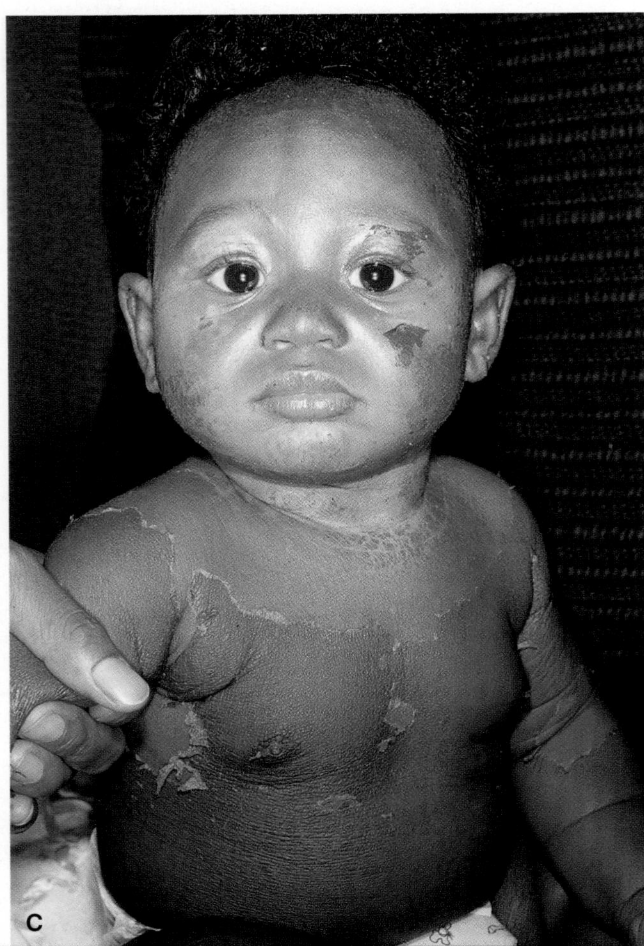

Figure 3-24. Staphylococcal Scalded Skin Syndrome

A. A 15-month-old infant presented with pustular lesions with cellulitis on the thumb. He also had fever and generalized scarlatiniform rash associated with skin tenderness. Subsequently he developed exfoliation in sheets, revealing a scalded-looking surface. Photographs taken on the third day after hospitalization (*B.*, *C*) show drying of exfoliated areas with flaky desquamation. Note the absence of any mucous membrane involvement.

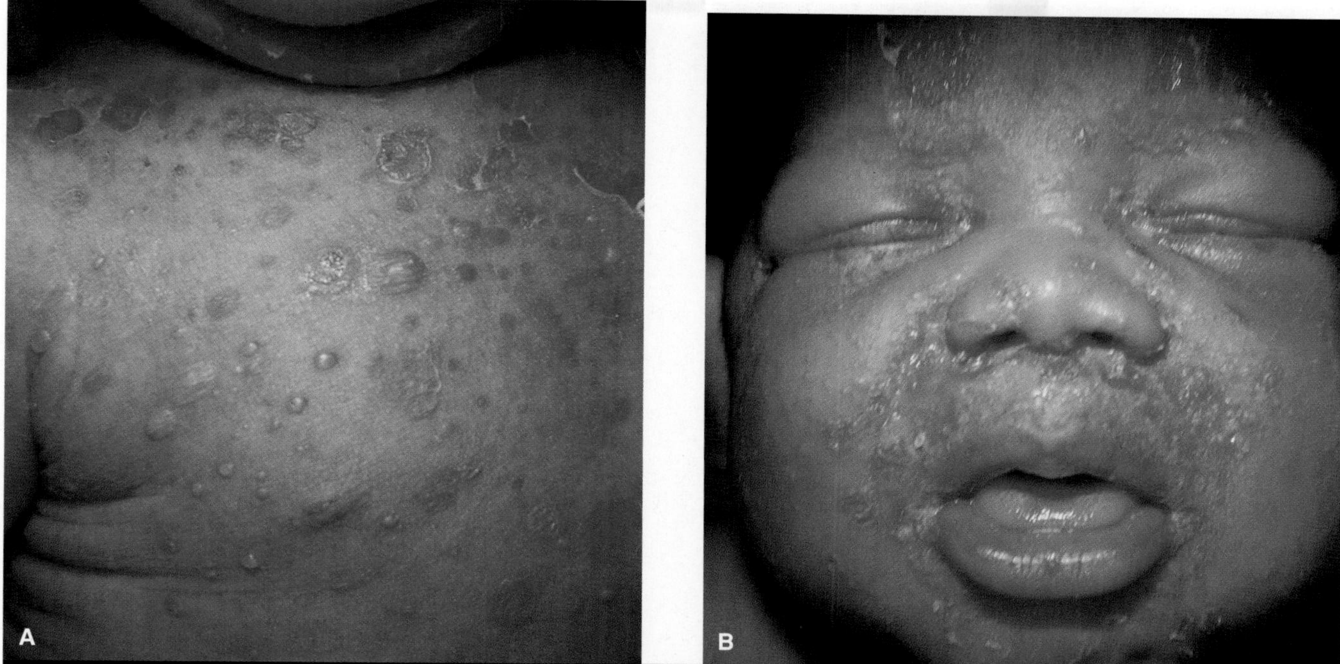

Figure 3-25. Staphylococcal Scalded Skin Syndrome in a Neonate (Ritter's Disease)

Following circumcision at birth, this 1-week-old neonate presented with extreme irritability, fever, and a combination of numerous pus-filled intact bullae on the trunk with some lesions exfoliating, and prominent involvement with some denuded areas around the eyes, nose, and mouth. Purulent conjunctivitis (pus seen here at the medial canthus) was also present. Within 48 hours after this photo was taken, there was generalized exfoliation over the entire body. Pus from the intact bullae was positive for *S. aureus*.

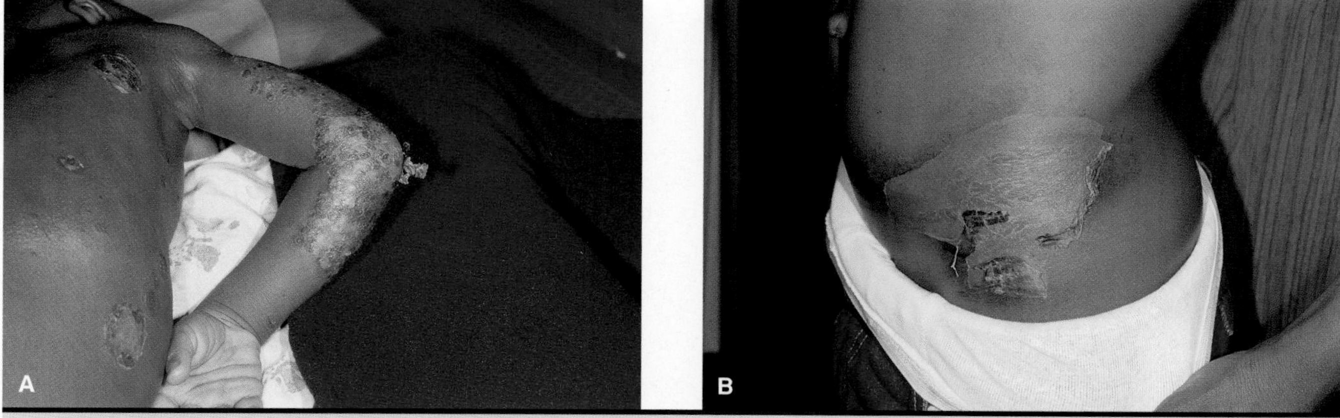

Figure 3-26. Staphylococcal Scalded Skin Syndrome

A. A combination of several well-circumscribed drying lesions with desquamation (these lesions were bullous impetigo filled with pus) are seen on the trunk, and a large denuded area with thick white and brown flaky desquamation is seen on the arm. *B*. One large flaccid bullous lesion followed by a denuded area with exfoliation was seen in this patient (localized SSSS). He was referred to the ED to rule out child abuse (inflicted burn injury).

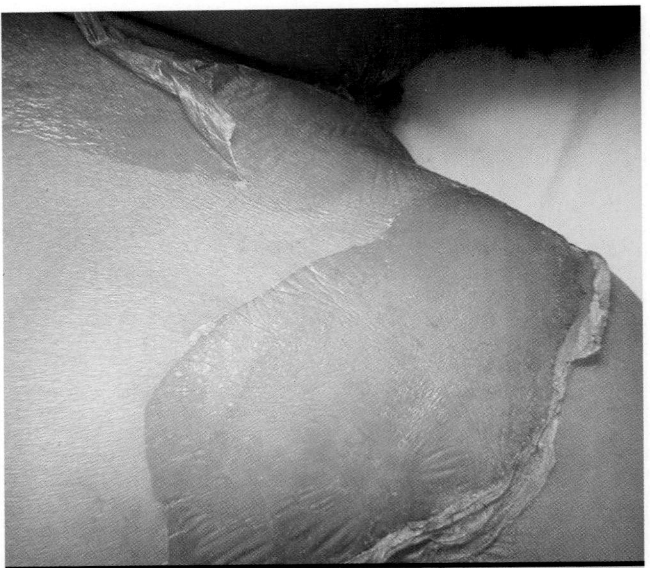

Figure 3-27. Staphylococcal Scalded Skin Syndrome

Large areas of exfoliation revealing a scalded-looking surface in a patient with SSSS. Note that the borders of the exfoliating skin roll up like wet tissue paper.

BOX 3-26. DIFFERENTIAL DIAGNOSIS OF STAPHYLOCOCCAL SCALDED SKIN SYNDROME

- Streptococcal scarlet fever
- Staphylococcal scarlet fever
  (1) Sandpaper rash with Pastia's sign present
  (2) Skin tenderness and a positive Nikolsky's sign
  (3) Absence of strawberry tongue
  (4) Absence of exudative tonsillopharyngitis and palatal petechiae
- Bullous impetigo
- Stevens-Johnson syndrome or toxic epidermal necrolysis
- Toxic shock syndrome
- Other drug eruptions
- Epidermolysis bullosa
- Pemphigus

Differential diagnosis of positive Nikolsky's sign:

- Staphylococcal scalded skin syndrome
- Toxic epidermal necrolysis
- Stevens-Johnson syndrome
- Pemphigus vulgaris

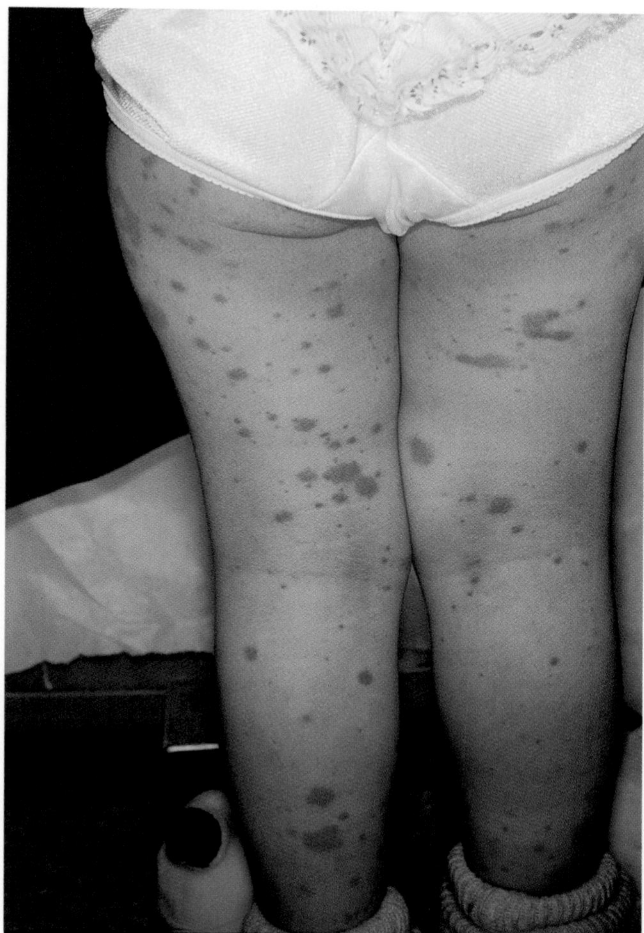

Figure 3-32. Henoch-Schönlein Purpura (Differential Diagnosis of Meningococcemia)

Symmetrically distributed palpable purpuric lesions on both lower extremities and buttocks (usually below the waist) are characteristic features of HSP. Other associated signs and symptoms (e.g., arthralgia/arthritis, abdominal pain, microscopic or gross hematuria) also help in differentiating HSP from meningococcemia. Patients with HSP are also usually afebrile and the platelet count is usually elevated or normal.

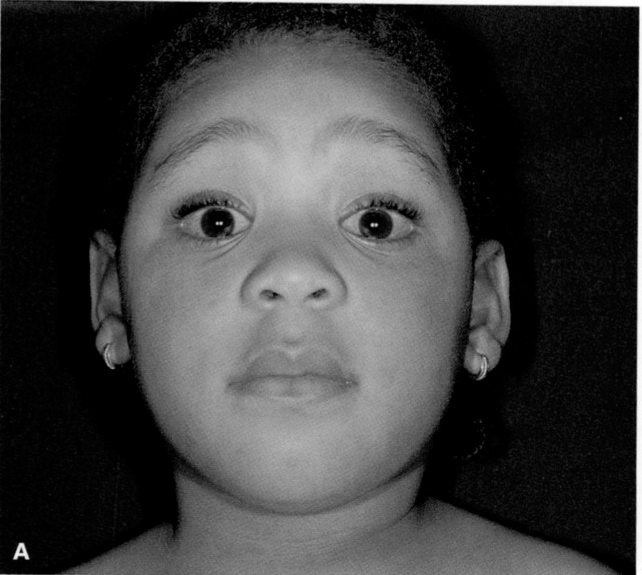

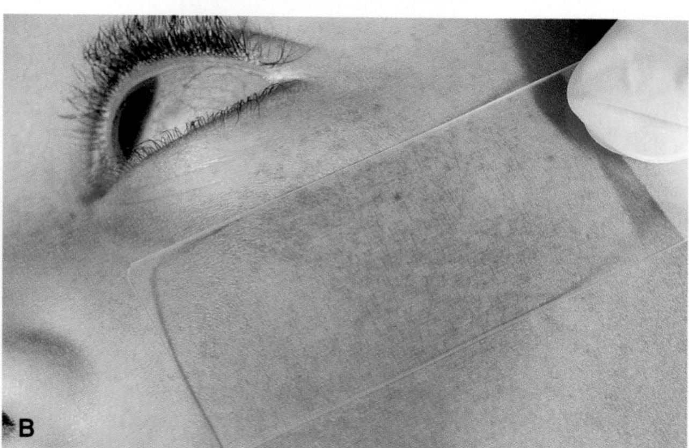

Figure 3-33. Petechiae from Other Etiology (Differential Diagnosis of Meningococcemia)

Petechiae on the face and upper thorax occur commonly in healthy children following intractable episodes of coughing, vomiting, or crying. Meningococcal infections would not cause petechiae only limited to the face. An absence of generalized distribution in an otherwise well-appearing child and significant contributory history (e.g., severe bouts of vomiting) help in differentiating meningococcemia from other etiologies of petechiae. Sudden eruption of a petechial rash on the face associated with subconjunctival hyperemia were the presenting complaints of this girl. This rash appeared following several violent episodes of vomiting due to food poisoning. Her rash was present only on the face, she was afebrile, and the remainder of her examination was normal.

BOX 3-30. COMPLICATIONS OF MENINGOCOCCEMIA

- Disseminated intravascular coagulation
- Purpura fulminans
  (1) Tissue necrosis
  (2) Gangrene and autoamputation of distal extremities
- Cardiac
  (1) Myocarditis
  (2) Pericarditis
  (3) Congestive heart failure
  (4) Conduction abnormalities
- Pulmonary
  (1) Pneumonia
  (2) Lung abscess
- Neurologic sequelae from meningitis
  (1) Sensorineural deafness
  (2) Subdural effusion or empyema
  (3) Brain abscess
  (4) Obstructive hydrocephalus
  (5) Seizures
  (6) Hemiparesis or quadriparesis
- Waterhouse-Friderichsen syndrome
  (1) Bleeding into adrenals
  (2) Shock, coma, and death
- Eye: endophthalmitis
- Immune-complex mediated late complications (seen 4 to 9 days after onset of illness)
  (1) Arthritis (usually monarticular)
  (2) Cutaneous vasculitis

(Modified and reproduced with permission from: Shah BR: Meningococcemia. In: Perkin RM, Swift JD, Newton DA (eds). *Pediatric Hospital Medicine. Textbook of Inpatient Management*. Baltimore, Lippincott Williams & Wilkins, 2003, p. 509.)

DIAGNOSIS ROCKY MOUNTAIN SPOTTED FEVER

Definition and Etiology

1. Rocky Mountain spotted fever (RMSF) is an acute febrile exanthematous illness caused by *Rickettsia rickettsii*.
2. *Rickettsia rickettsii* is transmitted by any of the following vectors:
   a. Dog tick: *Dermacentor variabilis* (Eastern United States)
   b. Wood tick: *Dermacentor andersoni* (western United States)
   c. Lone star tick: *Amblyomma americanum*
3. These ticks are systemically infected with the organism and transmit it to humans and other vertebrates while feeding. They inoculate rickettsiae into the dermis from which the organisms disseminate hematogenously. Rickettsiae multiply in the endothelial lining of small blood vessels, leading to widespread vasculitis.
4. Transmission from human to human via blood transfusion from a patient incubating the disease or through an accidental needlestick contaminated with infected blood has been reported rarely.

Associated Clinical Features

1. RMSF is the second most common (after Lyme disease) reported tick-borne infection in the United States.
2. RMSF is a misnomer; cases are reported from all parts of the United States. It is endemic in southeastern states, central states, and Rocky Mountain states. The top ten states reporting RMSF include North Carolina, Oklahoma, Wyoming, Arkansas, Mississippi, Tennessee, South Carolina, South Dakota, Georgia, and Maryland.
3. For all ages, risk factors for RMSF include exposure to dogs, residence in wooded areas, and male gender.
4. The tick bite is painless and often goes unrecognized. About 60% of cases are preceded by the removal of an attached and engorged tick.
5. Laboratory abnormalities include a normal or low WBC (first 4 to 5 days) with bandemia, thrombocytopenia, and anemia. Hyponatremia, hypoalbuminemia, elevated serum values of CPK and liver enzymes may be seen. CSF exam may be normal or show pleocytosis with an elevated protein and normal glucose values.
6. Culture of *R. rickettsii* is usually not attempted (due to danger of transmission to lab personnel).
7. Weil-Felix serologic test (*Proteus vulgaris* OX-19 and OX-2 agglutinins)
   a. The test becomes positive 10 to 14 days after onset of illness.
   b. Testing is *not* recommended, as it is nonspecific and insensitive.

   c. Many false positive results (e.g., *Proteus* infections, leptospirosis)

8. Polymerase chain reaction demonstrates presence of *R. rickettsii* DNA in blood and biopsy specimens early in the course of illness (unfortunately, this test is not widely available).

9. Specific serologic antibody titers showing a fourfold or greater rise in titer between the acute and convalescent phases are diagnostic.
   a. Examples of the most sensitive and specific tests include indirect immunofluorescent antibody, indirect hemagglutination, or enzyme immunoassay tests.
   b. Examples of highly specific but insensitive tests include complement fixation or microagglutination tests.

Consultation

Dermatology consultation may be obtained after initial stabilization. Diagnosis of RMSF can be confirmed rapidly (usually between 4 and 8 days) in patients with a rash. Immunofluorescent staining of skin biopsy samples demonstrate immunofluorescent rickettsiae.

Emergency Department Treatment and Disposition

1. RMSF is a curable but potentially fatal disease. An important factor in patient survival is early diagnosis and therapy.

2. Hospitalize critically ill patients after stabilization of vital signs including restoration of fluid and electrolyte abnormalities.

3. Empiric therapy for RMSF is *started based on clinical findings and therapy is not withheld while awaiting confirmation by the serology tests* (it takes 7 to 10 days into the course of illness to yield results). Patients should also receive an antibiotic (e.g., a third-generation cephalosporin) against *N. meningitidis* while awaiting culture results.

4. Doxycycline (*drug of choice*) given intravenously (critically ill patients) or orally:
   a. Dose: two loading doses of 2.2 mg/kg per dose given at 12-hour intervals on the first day followed by 2.2 mg/kg per day given in two doses; maximum 300 mg/dose
   b. Duration: usually for 7 to 10 days or until the patient is afebrile for at least 2 to 3 days
   c. May be used in all age groups
   d. Tetracycline staining of teeth is dose-related; doxycycline is less likely to cause dental staining than other tetracyclines

5. Other alternatives include tetracycline (for patients >8 years of age) or chloramphenicol (less effective than tetracycline).

6. *Do not use* sulfonamide antibiotics. Worsening of the disease and adverse outcome (including death) have been associated with its use in patients with RMSF.

Prevention

1. Avoid tick-infested areas.

2. Wear protective clothing that covers arms, legs, and other exposed areas.

3. Apply insect or tick repellents to clothes and exposed body parts.
   a. For clothes: permethrin spray to decrease tick attachment
   b. For skin: DEET (N,N-diethyl-meta-toluamide) application

4. Thoroughly inspect body, clothing, and pets for ticks after outdoor activity during tick season.

5. To remove a tick:
   a. Grasp the tick with fine tweezers close to the skin and pull gently straight out without twisting.
   b. If fingers are used, protect them with tissue and avoid squeezing the body of the tick; thoroughly wash hands after removal.

Clinical Pearls: Rocky Mountain Spotted Fever

1. RMSF rash usually appears first on the wrists and ankles, often spreading within hours proximally to the trunk (Fig. 3-34).

2. The classic triad of fever, rash, and history of tick bite is present in only 60 to 70% of patients. Neither absence of tick exposure nor absence of rash excludes the diagnosis.

3. The most significant risk factor for death from RMSF is a delay in initiation (beyond day 6 of illness) of appropriate antibiotic therapy.

4. It is difficult to distinguish RMSF from meningococcemia with clinical presentation alone.

5. The clinician must maintain a high index of suspicion for RMSF in endemic areas (especially during spring and summer), even in the absence of a history of tick attachment, absence or delayed appearance of rash, or absence of headache.

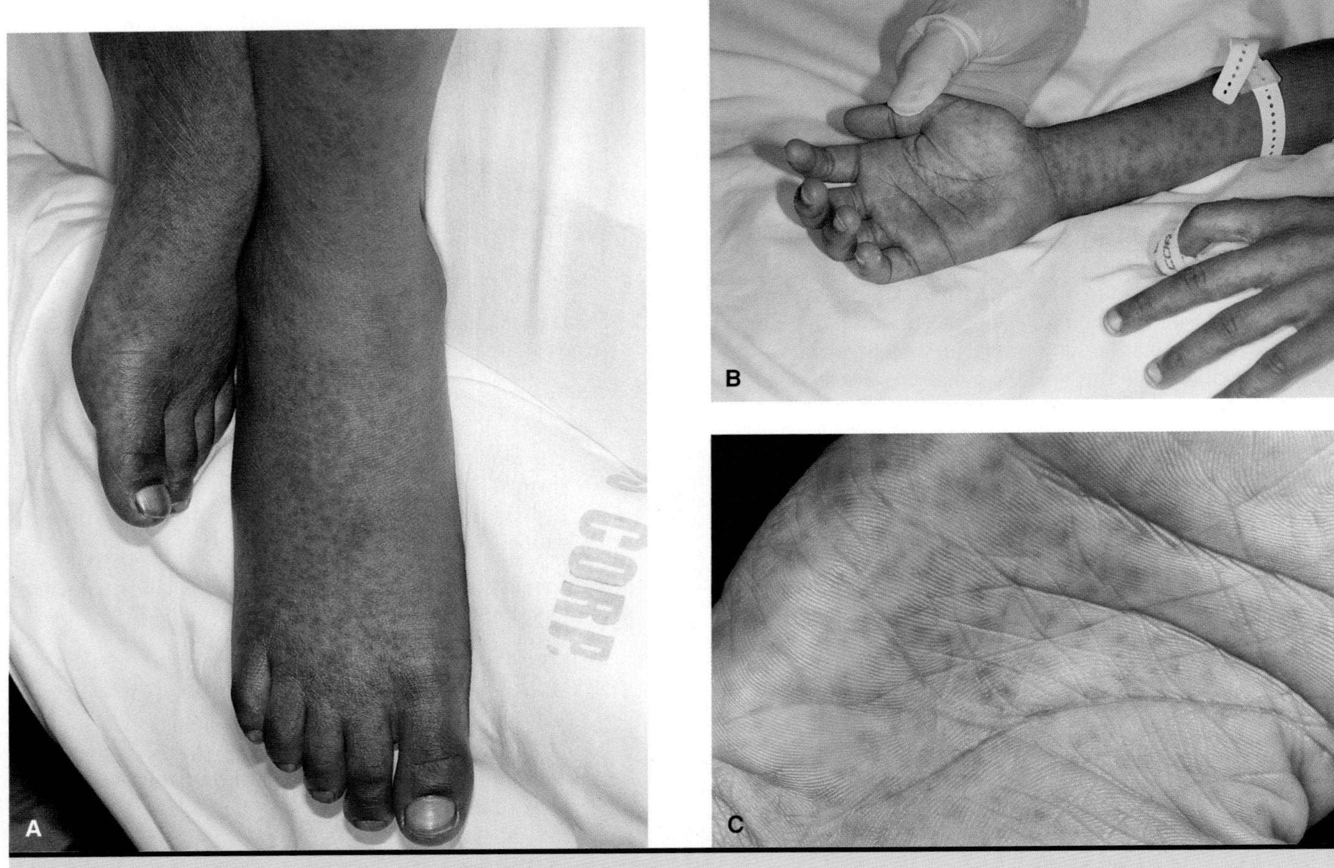

Figure 3-34. Rocky Mountain Spotted Fever

A., B., C. Erythematous maculopapular eruption that started on the distal extremity and subsequently become petechial was seen in this 12-year-old boy. He also had fever, severe headache, and myalgia. He gave a history of camping outdoors during his summer vacation in North Carolina 12 days prior to onset of this rash. These photographs were taken on the fifth day of the illness. As seen here the palms and soles are nearly always affected in RMSF. He also had edema of both hands and feet.

BOX 3-31. CLINICAL FEATURES OF ROCKY MOUNTAIN SPOTTED FEVER

- Highest incidence of RMSF: in children between 5 to 9 years of age
- Seasonal incidence with most cases seen during period of maximal exposure to ticks (April through October)
- Incubation period: 1 week (range 2 to 14 days)
- Prodromal period with nonspecific symptoms (*often mimics viral infection*)
  - (1) Severe headache (*thought to be classic*)
  - (2) Myalgias with bilateral calf pain (*thought to be classic*)
  - (3) Photophobia
  - (4) Abdominal pain, vomiting, diarrhea
  - (5) Abrupt onset of fever and chills
- Rash
  - (1) Seen 2 to 4 days after onset of illness
  - (2) Severity varies from mild evanescent to covering the entire body
  - (3) Starts from flexors of wrists and ankles
  - (4) Within hours spreads to involve arms, legs, and centrally towards trunk
  - (5) Starts as erythematous maculopapular eruption that blanches on pressure
  - (6) Within 1 to 3 days rash becomes petechial (~50% of cases)
  - (7) May become confluent with areas of necrosis at sites of maximal involvement
  - (8) Involvement of the scrotum and vulva is a diagnostic clue
  - (9) Palms and soles nearly always affected
  - (10) Centripetal spread is the hallmark
  - (11) Pigmentation during convalescence
  - (12) Desquamation seen over severely affected areas
- "Spotless RMSF"
  - (1) Rash absent in 5% of children
  - (2) Rash absent in 10% of adults
- Other findings (variable frequency)
  - (1) Conjunctivitis
  - (2) Lymphadenopathy
  - (3) Hepatosplenomegaly
  - (4) Jaundice
  - (5) Periorbital or peripheral edema

BOX 3-32. DIFFERENTIAL DIAGNOSIS OF ROCKY MOUNTAIN SPOTTED FEVER

(See also Box 3-29, Differential Diagnosis of Meningococcemia)

- Meningococcemia
- Bacterial sepsis from other pathogens (e.g., *S. pneumoniae, H. influenzae* type b)
- Henoch-Schönlein purpura
- Maculopapular rash from other viral exanthems (e.g., echovirus, Epstein-Barr virus, cytomegalovirus)
- Toxic shock syndrome
- Idiopathic thrombocytopenic purpura
- Measles or atypical measles
- Drugs (e.g., sulfonamides, penicillins)
- Secondary syphilis
- Kawasaki disease
- Lyme disease
- Ehrlichiosis
- Dengue fever
- Leptospirosis
- Hemolytic uremic syndrome

BOX 3-33. COMPLICATIONS OF ROCKY MOUNTAIN SPOTTED FEVER

- Hematologic: disseminated intravascular coagulation
- Gangrene: fingers, toes, nose, scrotum, vulva
- Multiorgan dysfunction
  (1) Acute respiratory distress syndrome
  (2) Renal failure
  (3) Myocarditis/heart failure
  (4) Hepatocellular dysfunction
- Neurologic manifestations/sequelae
  (1) Delirium, confusion, or stupor
  (2) Seizures
  (3) Meningismus
  (4) Blindness, deafness
  (5) Paralysis
  (6) Intellectual impairment
  (7) Peripheral neuropathy
  (8) Bladder/bowel incontinence

DIAGNOSIS CAT-SCRATCH DISEASE

Definition and Etiology

1. Cat-scratch disease (CSD) is a zoonotic bacterial infection caused by *Bartonella henselae* following a cat scratch (especially kittens or feral cats). *B. henselae* are fastidious, slow-growing, gram-negative bacilli.
2. Infection is transmitted by cutaneous inoculation. The precise mechanism of cat-to-human transmission remains unclear. Transmission between cats occurs by the cat flea (*Ctenocephalides felis*).

Associated Clinical Features

1. Domestic cats represent the single largest category of companion animals in the United States. CSD is very common with about 25,000 estimated cases per year in the United States.
2. CSD occurs in persons of all ages. The highest age-specific incidence is among children <10 years old.
3. CSD occurs predominantly in the fall and winter and usually occurs sporadically. Even though many siblings may play with the same kitten, only one family member is usually affected. Occasionally clusters of CSD may be seen in the same family within weeks of one another.
4. A definite history of a cat scratch or bite is present in >50% of cases.
5. CSD can be diagnosed by any of the following tests:
   a. Indirect fluorescent antibody (IFA) test for detection of serum antibody to antigens of *Bartonella* species (this test is available through the Centers for Disease Control and Prevention)
   b. Polymerase chain reaction assay (available in some commercial laboratories)
   c. Histopathology of nodes shows nonspecific inflammatory reactions including granulomata and stellate necrosis. Bacilli are best demonstrated by Warthin-Starry silver impregnation stain (test is not specific for *B. henselae*).
6. Ultrasonography is helpful in assessing lymph nodes' size and suppuration.
7. Hypercalcemia may be seen with CSD lymphadenopathy due to endogenous production of vitamin D associated with granuloma formation.
8. *B. henselae* also have been identified as the causative agent of bacillary angiomatosis and peliosis hepatitis (infections that have been reported primarily in patients infected with human immunodeficiency virus).

Emergency Department Treatment and Disposition

1. CSD is a self-limited infection and management is primarily symptomatic.
2. Lymphadenopathy may persist for 2 to 4 months. Rarely, it may last considerably longer but spontaneous resolution is the rule.
3. Direct needle aspiration of pus may be required to relieve discomfort with suppurative nodes. Surgical excision generally is unnecessary.
4. Antibiotic therapy
   a. May be considered for acutely or severely ill patients with systemic symptoms (e.g., patients with large painful adenopathy or hepatosplenomegaly or immunocompromised hosts)

b. No well-controlled randomized clinical trials have been performed that clearly demonstrate a clinically significant benefit of antimicrobial therapy for CSD.
c. Choices include several oral antibiotics (e.g., azithromycin, rifampin, trimethoprim-sulfamethoxazole, and ciprofloxacin) and parenteral antibiotics (e.g., gentamicin)

5. Educate families about the following information:
   a. Cats are usually healthy and require no treatment.
   b. The best way to prevent this infection is to avoid playing roughly with cats and kittens.
   c. It is not necessary to get rid of the cat because of the diagnosis.
   d. Declawing the cat helps lower the risk of getting infected through a cat scratch.
   e. Careful hand washing after handling the cat is another way to prevent infection.
   f. Rid the cat of fleas (infection rate is about 30 times higher in kittens with fleas than in kittens without fleas).
   g. Persons with immune deficiencies should avoid contact with cats that scratch or bite (especially cats <1 year of age). Immediately washing sites of cat scratches or bites and not allowing cats to lick open cuts or wounds are other preventive measures.

Clinical Pearls: Cat-Scratch Disease

1. CSD is a relatively common and occasionally serious zoonotic infection. A history of contact with a cat or scratch from a cat is an important clue.
2. Chronic regional lymphadenitis is the hallmark of CSD. *B. henselae* is one of the most common causes of chronic lymphadenopathy in children.
3. Consider the diagnosis of CSD in patients with adenopathy, fever, malaise, and history of feline contact.

BOX 3-34. CLINICAL FEATURES OF CAT-SCRATCH DISEASE

- Incubation period
  (1) From time of scratch to appearance of primary skin papule: 7 to 12 days
  (2) From skin lesion to appearance of regional lymphadenopathy: 5 to 50 days (usually 1 to 4 weeks)
- Site of bacterial inoculation: Scratch or bite or one or more small red papules or pustules (*often overlooked because of small size*)
- Typical CSD presentation (89% of cases)
  (1) Regional lymphadenopathy
  (2) Low-grade fever (~33 to 60% of cases)
  (3) Other signs and symptoms: malaise, anorexia, fatigue, and headache
- Atypical CSD (11% of cases)
  A. Parinaud oculoglandular syndrome
     (1) Involvement of conjunctiva with granuloma but without any discharge or pain
     (2) Involvement of ipsilateral preauricular lymph node
     (3) May involve ipsilateral submandibular or cervical lymphadenopathy
  B. Rare manifestations
     (1) Persistent fever
     (2) Skin rashes (erythema nodosum, maculopapular rashes, erythema multiforme)
     (3) Aseptic meningitis
     (4) Encephalitis
     (5) Status epilepticus
     (6) Hepatitis
     (7) Weight loss
     (8) Abdominal pain
     (9) Pneumonia
     (10) Microabscesses in liver and spleen
     (11) Osteolytic lesions
     (12) Thrombocytopenic purpura

BOX 3-35. LYMPHADENOPATHY IN CAT-SCRATCH DISEASE

- Most prominent and common manifestation (>90% of typical cases)
- Usually involves nodes that drain the site of inoculation
- Usually single lymph node involvement; may involve several nodes at same regional site
- Occasionally lymph nodes at multiple sites (other than regional site) may be involved
- Size: usually 1 to 5 cm in size (although they may become much larger)
- Sites: 80% upper extremities, neck, head (in following order)
  (1) Axilla (Fig. 3-35)
  (2) Cervical
  (3) Submandibular
  (4) Preauricular
  (5) Epitrochlear
  (6) Femoral
  (7) Inguinal nodes
- Signs of inflammation: tender, warm, erythematous, and indurated
- Spontaneous suppuration seen in about 10 to 40% of cases
- Duration of lymphadenopathy usually 1 to 2 months (rarely may persist up to 1 year)

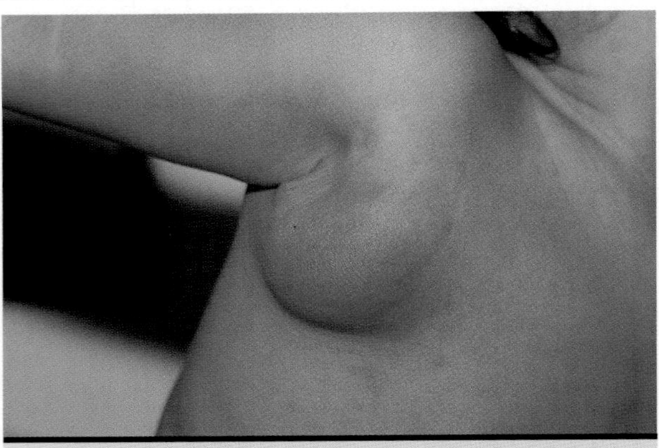

Figure 3-35. Cat-Scratch Disease

Axillary lymphadenitis of 3 weeks' duration in a 4-year-old child. He received a kitten as a Christmas gift 2 months prior to the onset of this swelling. He gave a history of playing roughly and receiving several scratches on his arm by the kitten. His lymphadenopathy was tender, erythematous, and warm and required needle aspiration to relieve the symptoms (usually needle aspiration of suppurative nodes is preferred over incision and drainage to avoid prolonged drainage and possible scarring).

BOX 3-36. DIFFERENTIAL DIAGNOSIS OF CAT-SCRATCH DISEASE

- Differential diagnosis of unilateral lymphadenopathy
  (1) Bacterial adenitis (Fig. 3-2)
  (2) Viral infections (e.g., infectious mononucleosis)
  (3) Malignancy (e.g., lymphoma)
  (4) Typical or atypical mycobacterial infection
  (5) Tularemia
  (6) Brucellosis
  (7) Histoplasmosis
  (8) Toxoplasmosis
  (9) Lymphogranuloma venereum

DIAGNOSIS

CHICKENPOX

SYNONYM

Varicella

Definition and Etiology

1. Chickenpox is a highly contagious acute exanthematous illness caused by varicella-zoster virus (VZV; a member of the human herpes virus group).
2. Humans are the only source of this infection. Humans get infected when VZV comes in contact with either mucosa of upper respiratory tract or conjunctiva.
3. Person-to-person transmission occurs primarily by direct contact with patients with chickenpox or herpes zoster. Chickenpox occasionally occurs by airborne spread from respiratory tract secretions.
4. During maternal varicella infection, transplacental passage of VZV can result in in utero infection.

Associated Clinical Features

1. Chickenpox is most commonly seen during late winter and early spring.
2. Diagnosis is usually made clinically and laboratory tests are rarely required. Tests that aid in making the diagnosis include:
   a. Tzanck smear (Fig. 3-49)
   b. Viral culture from the base of a new vesicle (first 3 to 4 days of eruption)
   c. Serologic testing for IgG antibody in acute and convalescent serum samples (e.g., fluorescent antibody to membrane assay [FAMA] is most sensitive and specific)
   d. Polymerase chain reaction in body fluid or tissue

Emergency Department Treatment and Disposition

1. Chickenpox is a benign, self-limiting disease with a low rate of complications in otherwise healthy children, and oral acyclovir is not recommended for routine use in such children.
2. Antiviral therapies that can be used to treat varicella include intravenous or oral acyclovir, valacyclovir, famciclovir, and foscarnet. The decision to use therapy, which route, and how long would be determined by the specific host factors and extent of the infection.
3. Acyclovir (given within 24 hours of onset of rash) can be considered in otherwise healthy children at increased risk for moderate to severe varicella, including:
   a. Patients >12 years of age
   b. Patients receiving long-term salicylate therapy
   c. Patients with chronic pulmonary disorders
   d. Patients with chronic skin disorders
   e. Patients receiving short, intermittent, or aerosolized courses of corticosteroids
   f. Acyclovir is given orally (dose: 80 mg/kg per day in four divided doses for 5 days [maximum dose 3200 mg/day])
4. Immunocompromised patients usually need hospitalization for IV antiviral therapy and very close monitoring. Oral acyclovir is not recommended to treat such children because of poor oral bioavailability.
5. Chickenpox is highly contagious. Patients are most contagious from 1 to 2 days before the onset of rash until all the lesions have turned into dried crusts.
6. Secondary cases occur in 98% of susceptible persons when exposed to an index case. Varicella-zoster immune globulin (passive immunoprophylaxis; given as soon as possible after exposure [within 96 hours]) is recommended for susceptible persons at risk of developing severe varicella. Refer to American Academy of Pediatrics 2003 *Red Book* for details. Candidates for prophylaxis include:
   a. Immunocompromised children
   b. Neonates whose mothers had onset of varicella within 5 days before delivery or within 48 hours after delivery
7. Children with varicella should not receive salicylates because of an association with Reye's syndrome.
8. For the pruritus and discomfort, a child may be prescribed colloidal oatmeal baths and antipruritic lotions like pramoxine. Be careful when prescribing antipruritic medications that cause drowsiness, as this side effect may mask lethargy and drowsiness related to complications of chickenpox (e.g., meningoencephalitis).

Clinical Pearls: Chickenpox

1. Varicella-zoster virus remains in a latent state in the dorsal root ganglion cells, and may get reactivated (as the immunity wanes) resulting in herpes zoster.
2. Chickenpox is one of the most important risk factors for invasive group A streptococcal diseases (e.g., streptococcal toxic shock syndrome, necrotizing fasciitis).
3. Chickenpox is more severe in adolescents, adults, and immunocompromised hosts.
4. A single dose of live attenuated varicella vaccine is now routinely given to all healthy children between 12 months and 13 years of age. In persons >13 years of age, two doses are given 4 to 8 weeks apart.

BOX 3-37. CLINICAL FEATURES OF CHICKENPOX

- Incubation period
  (1) Average 14 to 16 days (range 10 to 21 days)
  (2) Shortened in immunocompromised patients
  (3) Between 1 and 16 days of life in neonates born to mothers with active chickenpox around time of delivery
- Prodromal period usually absent in children
- Rash and constitutional symptoms (low grade fever, headache, malaise) occur simultaneously
- Skin eruption
  (1) Vesicular rash typically consisting of about 250 to 500 lesions (Figs. 3-36 and 3-37)
  (2) Centripetal distribution (more lesions on torso than face and extremities, unlike smallpox) (Figs. 3-39 and 3-40)
  (3) Lesions also seen on scalp and mucous membranes (e.g., conjunctiva, oropharynx, vagina)
  (4) Lesions go through stages: macule to papule to vesicle to pustule, followed by crusting
  (5) Classic lesion: a vesicle surrounded by erythema ("a dew drop on a rose petal"; Fig. 3-37)
  (6) Lesions either round or oval with central umbilication as healing occurs
  (7) Different stages of lesions seen together in the same anatomic area (unlike smallpox)
  (8) Rash may be more confluent wherever skin is abraded (e.g., diaper area)
  (9) With or without pruritus
  (10) Duration of eruption: 5 to 7 days
  (11) Healed lesions may leave residual hypopigmentation but scarring is uncommon
- Varicella in immunocompromised patients
  (1) Hemorrhagic varicella (more common than in immunocompetent hosts)
  (2) Progressive severe varicella with continuing eruption of lesions and high fever persisting into second week of illness
  (3) Complications such as pneumonia, encephalitis, and hepatitis
  (4) Chronic or recurrent varicella and disseminated herpes zoster with new lesions appearing for months (in children with HIV infection)
  (5) Severe (and fatal) varicella in otherwise healthy children receiving intermittent courses of corticosteroids (e.g., for asthma or other illness [especially when steroids are given during incubation period of chickenpox])

BOX 3-41. OTHER MANIFESTATIONS OF HERPES ZOSTER

- Ramsay Hunt syndrome
  (1) Herpes zoster affecting geniculate ganglion (facial or auditory nerves)
  (2) Vesicular eruption on pinna, auditory canal, tympanic membrane, anterior two-thirds of tongue
  (3) Ipsilateral Bell's palsy, tinnitus, deafness, vertigo, hearing loss, otalgia
  (4) Decreased taste on anterior two-thirds of tongue
- Herpes zoster ophthalmicus
  (1) Herpes zoster affecting the ophthalmic branch of the trigeminal nerve
  (2) Seen in ~10 to 15% of cases
  (3) Vesicular eruption on eyelids
  (4) Other findings may include conjunctivitis, keratitis, iridocyclitis, secondary glaucoma, ocular muscle palsies, ptosis, mydriasis, panophthalmitis
- Hutchinson's sign
  (1) Involvement of nasociliary division of the ophthalmic nerve
  (2) Vesicles on the side and the top of the nose
- Involvement of the maxillary branch of the trigeminal nerve

  Sites of eruption: palate, uvula, tonsillar fossa
- Involvement of the mandibular branch of the trigeminal nerve

  Sites of eruption: buccal mucosa, floor of the mouth, anterior part of the tongue
- Disseminated zoster
  (1) Seen in patients with persistent depression of cell-mediated immunity to VZV (e.g., following bone marrow transplantation)
  (2) Localized dermatomal rash, then viremia leading to generalized rash
  (3) Fever
  (4) Visceral dissemination (pneumonia, hepatitis, meningoencephalitis)
- Zoster sine herpete (zoster without rash)

  Dermatomal pain and serologic or virologic evidence of zoster in a patient who fails to develop zoster rash

BOX 3-42. DIFFERENTIAL DIAGNOSIS OF HERPES ZOSTER

- Dermatomal herpes simplex (HSV) infections (e.g., anogenital herpes; shingles that recurs in sacral area is almost always HSV type 2 infection)
- Contact dermatitis
- Grouped arthropod bites
- Localized bacterial (e.g., localized cellulitis) or viral skin infections
- Vaccinia autoinoculation
- Burns

DIAGNOSIS OROPHARYNGEAL HERPES SIMPLEX VIRUS INFECTION

SYNONYM

Fever sores or cold sores for herpes labialis

Definition and Etiology

1. Oropharyngeal herpes virus infections manifest as acute herpetic gingivostomatitis (Fig. 3-46), herpes labialis (Figs. 3-47 and 3-48), or pharyngitis (exudative or nonexudative). These infections are caused by herpes simplex virus (HSV).
2. Two known variants of HSV cause human infections:
   a. Herpes simplex virus type 1 (HSV-1; usually infections above the waist)
   b. Herpes simplex virus type 2 (HSV-2; usually infections below the waist)
   c. Either type of virus (HSV-1 or HSV-2) can be found in either site, depending on the source of infection.
3. Herpes virus is transmitted by skin-to-skin, mucosa-to-mucosa, or skin-to-mucosa contact.

Associated Clinical Features

1. Most primary HSV infections are asymptomatic.
2. After the primary infection, the virus persists for life in a latent form in a sensory ganglion (e.g., site of latency for oropharyngeal herpes is the trigeminal ganglia). Reactivation resulting in clinical disease may follow any of the triggering factors (e.g., febrile illnesses, sun exposure, emotional or physical stress, debilitating activities, or trauma).
3. Recurrent orofacial herpes affects 25 to 50% of the general population.
4. In college-aged adolescents, primary HSV manifests as pharyngitis (shallow tonsillar ulcers with or without gray exudates), and may be caused by either HSV-1 or HSV-2 (seen especially with oral-genital sexual practices).
5. The diagnosis is usually made clinically.
6. The diagnosis may be suggested by Tzanck smear (Fig. 3-49).
   a. Rapid test

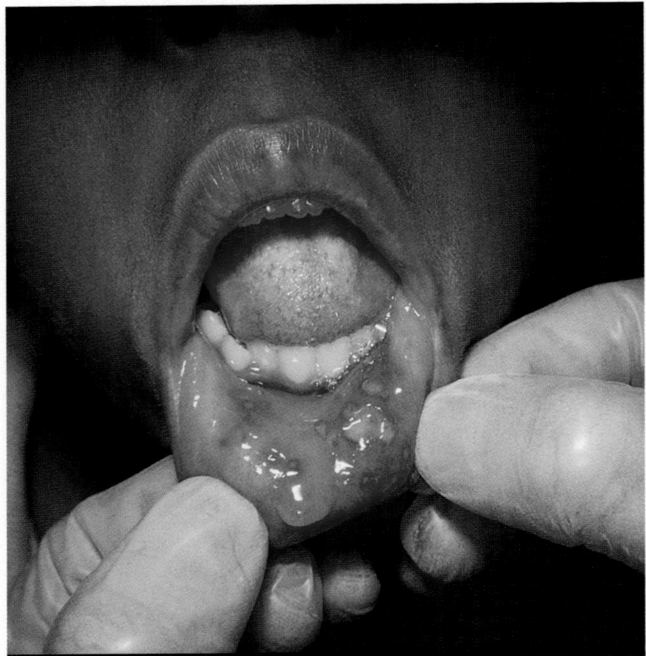

Figure 3-46. Herpetic Gingivostomatitis

A child presenting with high fever, refusal to eat, and sores in the mouth.

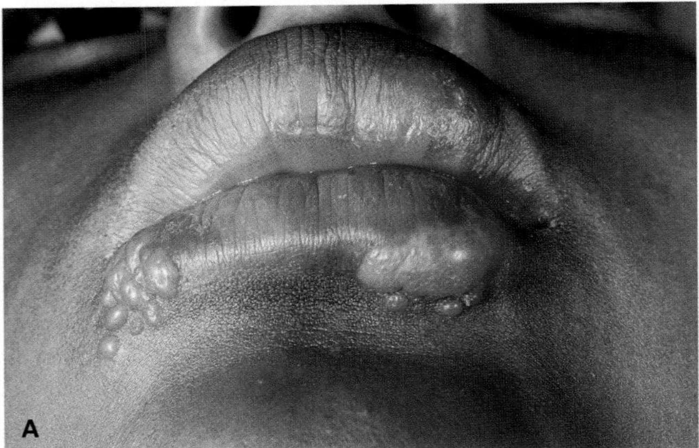

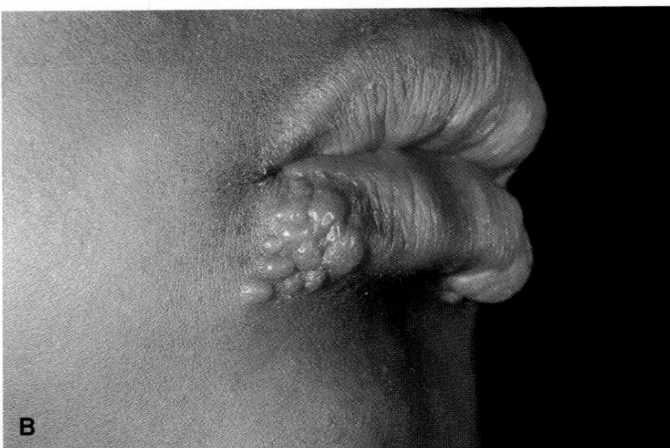

Figure 3-47. Herpes Labialis

A., *B.* Grouped vesicles on an erythematous base on the mucocutaneous junction of the lip. This patient had recurrent herpes labialis that was followed by erythema multiforme minor.

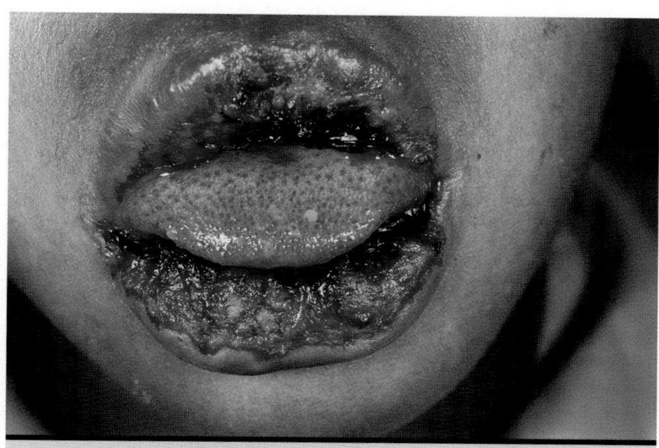

Figure 3-48. Herpes Labialis

Recurrent herpetic lesions that began with vesicles and healed with crusting were seen in this patient with HIV infection. This patient also had lesions on the tongue and buccal mucosa.

b. Scrape the base of a fresh vesicle, smear thinly on a slide, dry, and stain with either Wright's or Giemsa's stain (smears from crusted lesions are least helpful).
c. A positive test shows multinucleated giant keratinocytes.
d. Test positive in about 75 to 80% of HSV and varicella zoster virus (VZV) infections
e. A positive test cannot differentiate between HSV (HSV-1, HSV-2) and VZV infections.

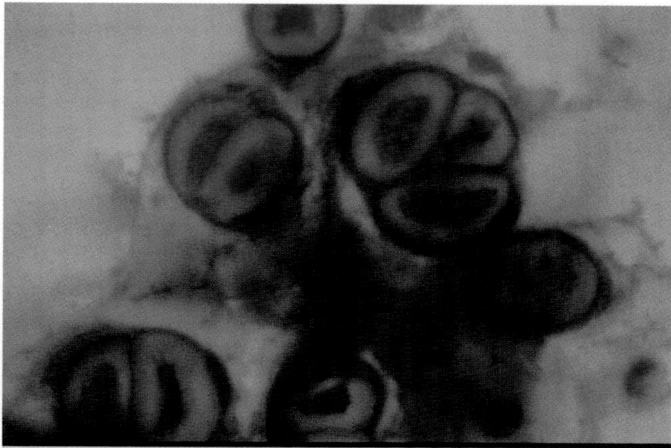

Figure 3-49. Tzanck Smear of Herpetic Infection

Giemsa stain of vesicle contents demonstrating multinucleated giant cells (fused virally-infected keratinocytes) are indicative of a herpetic infection. (Reproduced with permission from: Kane KS, Ryder JB, Johnson RA, Baden HP, Stratigos A: Herpes simplex virus. In: *Color Atlas & Synopsis of Pediatric Dermatology*. New York, McGraw-Hill, 2002, p. 544.)

7. The gold standard test for HSV is culture. HSV grows readily in cell culture in 24 hours to 7 days. The sample should be obtained either from vesicle fluid or by scraping the base of a fresh lesion (not from a crusted lesion).
8. Polymerase chain reaction (PCR) detection of viral DNA
   a. Rapid and extremely sensitive test
   b. Able to differentiate between HSV-1, HSV-2, and VZV infections

Emergency Department Treatment and Disposition

1. Immunocompromised patients
   a. Ill patients with oropharyngeal HSV infection will need hospitalization for intravenous acyclovir (or foscarnet in patients known to have acyclovir-resistant HSV isolates).
   b. Topical, oral, or IV acyclovir diminishes the duration of viral shedding, and improves time to cessation of pain and to total healing of HSV lesions.
   c. Prophylactic oral or IV acyclovir significantly reduces the incidence of symptomatic HSV infection.
2. Immunocompetent patients
   a. Limited data are available on the efficacy of acyclovir on the course of primary or recurrent oropharyngeal HSV infections (especially in children).
   b. Acyclovir is not recommended as a routine therapy.
3. Herpetic gingivostomatitis
   a. Patients may refuse to eat or drink because of pain. Supportive therapy should include antipyretics, hydration (either oral, or if indicated, intravenous) and dietary modifications (e.g., cool drinks, popsicles, soft diet, *avoid citrus juices*).
   b. Oral anesthetic agents (e.g., lidocaine viscous) *should not* be used because of risk of absorption from the oral mucosa and subsequent risk of lidocaine toxicity.
4. Herpes labialis
   a. Topical acyclovir is not efficacious in the treatment of herpes labialis.
   b. No data exist on the treatment of children or adolescents with herpes labialis.
   c. No data support the use of long-term suppressive treatment with acyclovir for the prevention of herpes labialis (in adults, acyclovir given orally for 5 days reduces the duration of pain and time to crusting by about one-third, if the treatment is started during the prodromal or erythematous stages of recurrent infection).

Clinical Pearls: Oropharyngeal HSV Infection

1. The mouth is the most common site of HSV-1 infections.
2. The hallmark of HSV skin infection is painful, grouped vesicles on an erythematous base.

3. The most common manifestation of recurrent HSV infection is herpes labialis.
4. HSV is the most common etiology of erythema multiforme (EM; about 60% cases). Recurrent HSV infections (e.g., herpes labialis) may be associated with recurrent episodes of EM.
5. Herpetic gingivostomatitis may be confused with herpangina. Vesicles are usually not seen on the buccal mucosa and anterior portion of the mouth in herpangina.

BOX 3-43. CLINICAL FEATURES OF ACUTE HERPETIC GINGIVOSTOMATITIS

- Most common clinical manifestation of first-episode HSV infection in children
- Usually caused by HSV-1
- Most common age: children 1 to 3 years of age
- High fever (often up to 40°C)
- Foul breath
- Inability to eat or drink, leading to dehydration
- Drooling
- Irritability
- Lesions
  (1) Begin as vesicles that rapidly rupture, then turn into shallow gray ulcers on an erythematous base
  (2) Ulcers 1 to 3 mm size, extremely painful, friable and bleed easily
  (3) Sites: anterior tongue, buccal mucosa, gums, hard and soft palate (any part of the oral lining may be involved)
  (4) Lesions may extend to the lips, chin, or neck (even in an immunocompetent child)
  (5) Lesions evolve for 4 to 5 days
- Gums swollen, ulcerated, erythematous, friable, and bleed easily (e.g., during examination)
- Gingivitis may precede appearance of mucosal vesicles
- Tender cervical and submandibular/submental lymphadenopathy
- Self-limited illness; usually resolves in additional 5 to 7 days

BOX 3-44. CLINICAL FEATURES OF HERPES LABIALIS ("FEVER BLISTERS" OR "COLD SORES")

- Usually caused by HSV-1
- Prodrome of pain, burning, tingling, or itching lasting a few hours
- Systemic symptoms unusual
- Eruption
  (1) Lesion begins within 24 to 48 hours after prodrome
  (2) Begins as papule, then becomes a vesicle, then an ulcer, which then crusts over
  (3) Painful (especially during vesicular stage)
  (4) Single or grouped vesicles
  (5) Typical site: vermilion border of lip, mucocutaneous junction of perioral region
  (6) Lesions usually localized in a nondermatomal distribution
  (7) Crusting of lesions within 3 to 4 days
  (8) Complete healing within 5 to 10 days
- Recurrences at the same location or closely adjacent areas tend to occurs.

BOX 3-45. DIFFERENTIAL DIAGNOSIS OF OROPHARYNGEAL HERPES SIMPLEX VIRUS INFECTION

- Acute herpetic gingivostomatitis and herpes labialis
  (1) Herpangina (Coxsackie virus, echovirus; vesicles/ulcers on anterior pillars, posterior palate, and pharynx)
  (2) Hand-foot-and-mouth disease (coxsackie virus)
  (3) Aphthous stomatitis (recurrent ulcers with rim of erythema and gray exudates)
  (4) Herpes zoster involving the face (zoster ophthalmicus)
- Herpes pharyngitis
  (1) Acute tonsillopharyngitis from other etiology (viral [e.g., adenovirus, influenza virus], bacterial [*Streptococcus pyogenes*])
  (2) Acute exudative tonsillopharyngitis from other etiology (e.g., *Streptococcus pyogenes*, adenovirus, Epstein-Barr virus)

DIAGNOSIS

HERPETIC WHITLOW

Definition and Etiology

Herpetic whitlow is a cutaneous infection of the terminal phalanx of the fingers or thumb caused by herpes simplex virus (usually HSV-1 or HSV-2) (Fig. 3-50).

Associated Clinical Features

1. Herpetic whitlow may occur in infants and young children, and the first episode may accompany herpetic gingivostomatitis.
2. Herpetic whitlow is an occupational hazard in the dental and medical professions. Physicians, dentists, dental hygienists, and nurses get inoculated inadvertently by HSV on their hands while examining the mouth or genital regions of patients.
3. After the primary infection, herpes virus remains dormant in the sensory ganglia (see Fig. 3-41), and can recur in the same location.
4. Diagnosis is usually made clinically. A needle aspiration of the lesion for HSV culture and Tzanck smear will confirm the diagnosis.

Emergency Department Treatment and Disposition

1. Herpetic whitlow usually resolves without any specific therapy.
2. *Do not* incise or drain herpetic whitlow; surgical débridement may exacerbate the condition.
3. Supportive therapy includes antipyretics and analgesics for pain as indicated.
4. Topical pencyclovir cream applied to affected areas every 2 hours may be used.
5. Acyclovir may be used for severe infections.
   a. Oral dose for immunocompetent children: 1200 mg/24 hours divided every 8 hours for 7 to 10 days
   b. Max dose of oral acyclovir in children: 80 mg/kg per 24 hours

Clinical Pearls: Herpetic Whitlow

1. Grouped umbilicated vesiculopustular lesions on an erythematous base on the distal fingertips or thumb.
2. Herpetic whitlow is commonly confused with a bacterial paronychia or felon (Fig. 3-51).

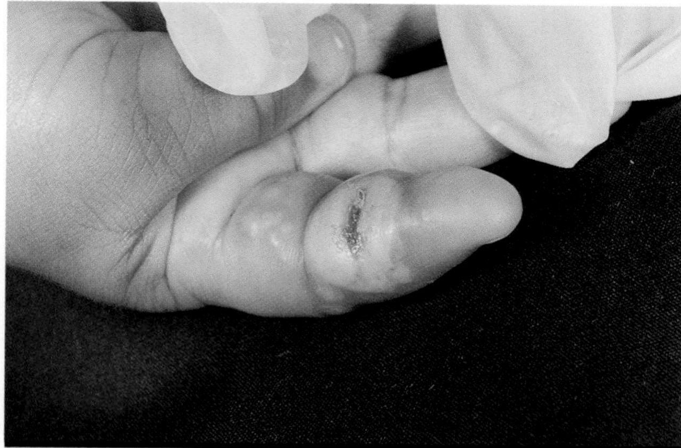

Figure 3-50. Herpetic Whitlow

A 4-month-old infant presenting with clusters of vesiculopustular lesions on an erythematous base on the finger. This infant's mother had "cold sores" 7 days prior to developing this rash. Culture of the lesion was positive for HSV-1.

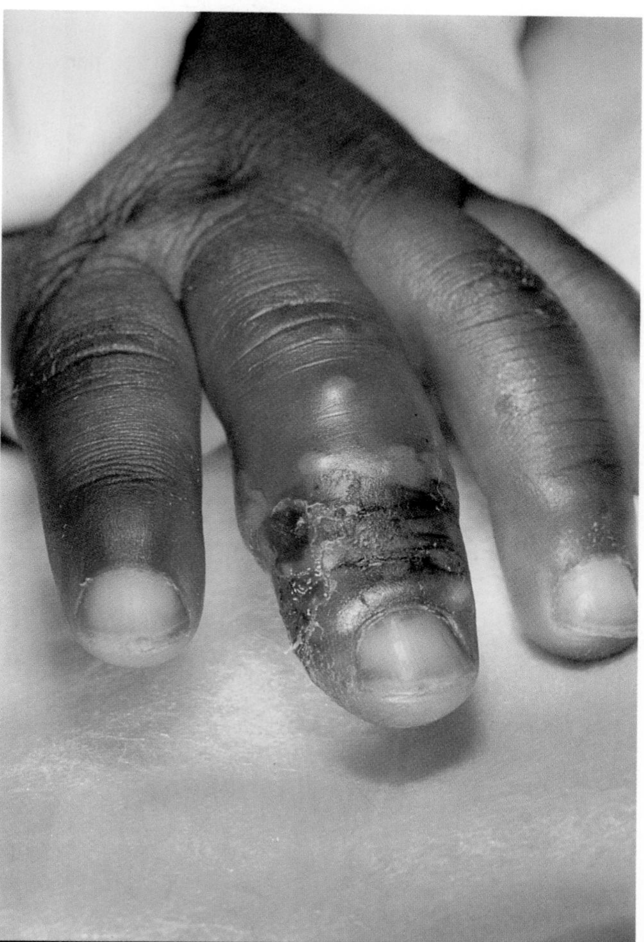

Figure 3-51. Herpetic Whitlow

Herpes simplex virus infection like this often gets mistaken for paronychia.

BOX 3-46. CLINICAL FEATURES OF HERPETIC WHITLOW

- Skin lesion
  - (1) Abrupt onset
  - (2) Pain or paresthesia at the site
  - (3) Initially begins as groped vesicles and/or pustules on an erythematous base
  - (4) Subsequently becomes a painful, erythematous, swollen lesion (thus may get mistaken for a bacterial infection)
  - (5) Sites
    Terminal phalanx of finger (69%)
    Thumb (21%)
    May involve one or more fingertips
  - (6) Lesions usually persist for 7 to 10 days (range, 1 to 3 weeks)
- Fever may accompany lesion
- Lymphangitis may accompany lesion
- Regional lymphadenopathy may accompany lesion
- Recurrences
  - (1) Seen in about 20% of cases
  - (2) Seen at same site

BOX 3-47. DIFFERENTIAL DIAGNOSIS OF HERPETIC WHITLOW

- Paronychia
- Felon
- Contact dermatitis
- Dyshidrotic eczema

DIAGNOSIS ROSEOLA INFANTUM

SYNONYMS

Exanthem subitum
Sixth disease
Roseola

Definition and Etiology

1. Roseola infantum is an acute exanthematous illness caused by human herpesvirus-6 (HHV-6) or HHV-7 and is characterized by a rash that appears after 3 to 4 days of high fever.
2. The most common etiologic agents are HHV-6 (~66% of cases) and HHV-7 (~23% of cases). Other viruses (e.g., echovirus) account for the remainder of cases.

Associated Clinical Features

1. Humans are the only known natural hosts for HHV-6 and HHV-7. Most cases of roseola infantum occur without a known exposure. Secondary cases occur with an incubation period of about 10 days.
2. Infants can experience HHV-6–associated roseola followed by HHV-7–associated roseola.
3. There is no seasonal predilection in roseola and cases occur throughout the year, unlike some viral exanthems (e.g., enteroviruses during the summer months and adenoviruses during the winter months).
4. The diagnosis of roseola is made clinically based on the age, classic history, and clinical findings displayed over a short period of time. Classic roseola is rarely confused with other viral exanthems.
5. Cerebrospinal fluid (CSF) examination in infants with HHV-6-associated febrile seizures is usually normal.
6. Polymerase chain reaction amplification tests in serum or CSF for HHV-6 and HHV-7 confirm the diagnosis. Serologic tests for HHV-6 are also available. Seroconversion or fourfold increases of HHV-6 IgG antibodies in serum

during the acute and convalescent phases establish primary HHV-6 infection. A single positive HHV-6 IgG test is of no diagnostic value (due to a high seroprevalence of HHV-6 in the general population).

7. Central nervous system complications include febrile seizures during the febrile prodromal stage (most frequent complication, seen in 8 to 13%), meningoencephalitis or encephalitis, and hemiplegia.

Emergency Department Treatment and Disposition

1. Many infants undergo sepsis work-up, receive antibiotic therapy while awaiting culture results, and hospitalization (especially infants presenting with a bulging anterior fontanelle) during the pre-eruptive, highly febrile stage of roseola. A diagnosis of roseola is often established in these infants retrospectively when they develop the rash (Fig. 3-52). No therapy is required during this stage except reassuring the family about the benign natural course and excellent prognosis of roseola.
2. A majority of infants appear quite comfortable during the pre-eruptive febrile stage of roseola and require only supportive care (e.g., management of fever, adequate hydration).

Clinical Pearls: Roseola Infantum

1. Roseola infantum is the most common exanthem of infants <2 years of age.

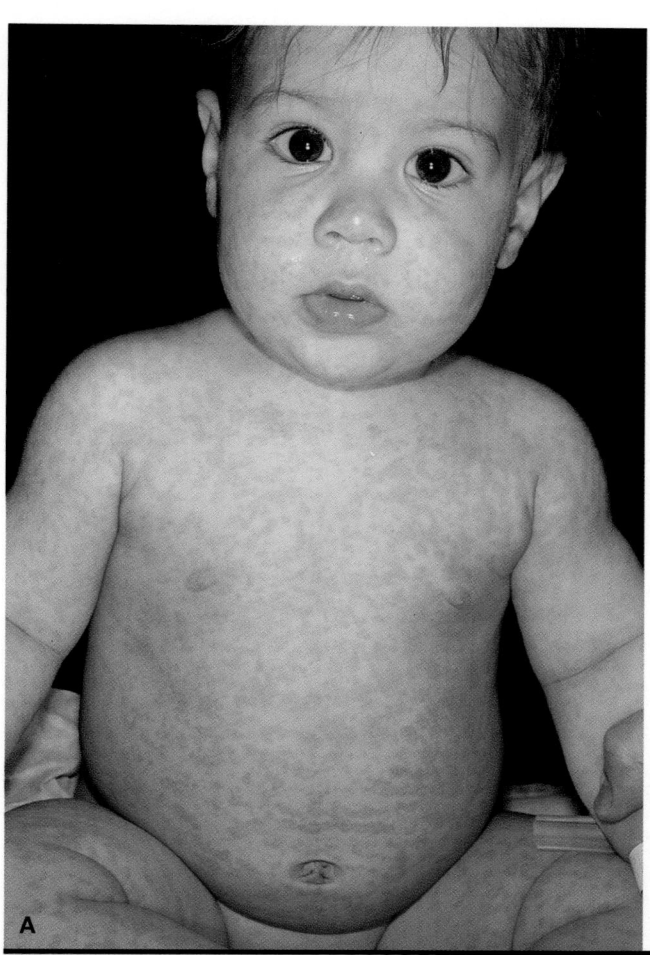

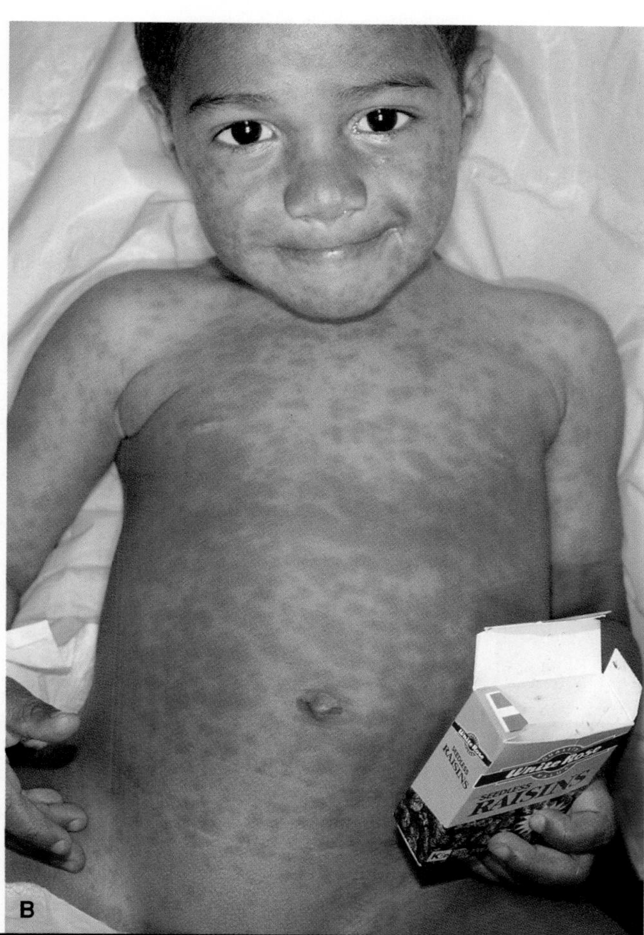

Figure 3-52. Roseola Infantum

A. Diffuse erythematous maculopapular eruptions that developed after 3 days of intermittently high fever (spiking up to 40°C) in this well-appearing 8-month-old infant. He was hospitalized with a clinical impression of sepsis because he presented with a bulging fontanelle associated with fever. All the cultures were negative including CSF examination. Subsequently he developed this rash and a diagnosis of roseola infantum was made. Note the absence of conjunctival injection and red lips (characteristic features that are often seen in a highly febrile infant with Kawasaki disease). *B*. Diffuse erythematous maculopapular eruption that developed after 4 days of high fever (spiking up to 40°C) in this very happy looking 18-month-old toddler. He was treated for occult bacteremia as an outpatient. He continued to spike fever in spite of antibiotic therapy and all his cultures (blood and urine) were negative. He was rushed to the ED when this rash appeared on the fifth day (he was afebrile). A diagnosis of roseola infantum was made (*Important: A toddler should not be allowed to eat raisins due to the risk of choking and foreign body aspiration*).

2. The *sine qua non* of roseola is the appearance of rash at defervescence; thus roseola often gets diagnosed retrospectively once the typical febrile course has been observed and the rash has appeared at defervescence.
3. Roseola rash is frequently misdiagnosed as drug hypersensitivity rash, as these infants are frequently receiving antibiotics prescribed during the febrile pre-eruptive phase of roseola. A detailed history of the appearance of rash in relation to the fever will establish the diagnosis of roseola.

BOX 3-48. CLINICAL FEATURES OF ROSEOLA INFANTUM

- About 95% of cases are seen in infants between 6 and 36 months of age.
- Most cases occur in infants <2 years old (peak between 6 and 15 months)
- Incubation period: 7 to 15 days (average: 10 days)
- Prodromal period: usually asymptomatic or mild rhinorrhea, pharyngeal and conjunctival injection
- Clinical illness: fever followed by rash

A. Fever

(1) Abrupt onset rising rapidly up to 39° to 41°C
(2) Fever may be present consistently or intermittently for 3 to 6 days
(3) *Most infants look well* during the febrile period (mild irritability in some).
(4) Fever drops precipitously to normal after 3 to 6 days in the majority of cases.
(5) Other features during febrile period:
Bulging anterior fontanelle (26%)
Lymphadenopathy (cervical, occipital)

B. Rash

(1) *Rash appears with defervescence within 12 to 24 hours* (a hallmark of the disease; rarely the rash appears before the fever has subsided completely or not until after 1 afebrile day)
(2) Pink to rose-colored macules or maculopapules that blanch on pressure
(3) *Nonpruritic* (unlike drug hypersensitivity)
(4) First seen on the trunk, then spreads to the face, neck, and proximal extremities
(5) *Does not* become vesicular, pustular, or petechial
(6) Remains discrete in a majority (rarely confluent)
(7) Evanescent rash lasting from a few hours to 1 to 3 days
(8) Clears completely *without* pigmentation or desquamation

BOX 3-49. DIFFERENTIAL DIAGNOSIS OF ROSEOLA INFANTUM: CONDITIONS ASSOCIATED WITH MACULOPAPULAR ERUPTIONS

- Viral infections
  (1) Enteroviral infections (e.g., coxsackie, echovirus)
  (2) Infectious mononucleosis
  (3) Cytomegalovirus infection
  (4) Rubella
  (5) Erythema infectiosum
  (6) Toxoplasmosis
  (7) Measles
  (8) Atypical measles
  (9) Hepatitis B virus
- Bacterial infections
  (1) Scarlet fever
  (2) Meningococcemia
  (3) Staphylococcal scalded skin syndrome
- Drugs
- Stevens-Johnson syndrome/toxic epidermal necrolysis
- Other
  (1) Kawasaki disease
  (2) Tick fever

DIAGNOSIS

MEASLES

Synonyms

Rubeola
First disease

Definition and Etiology

Measles is a highly contagious exanthematous illness caused by a paramyxovirus (an RNA virus).

Associated Clinical Features

1. Other signs and symptoms of measles include vomiting, diarrhea, abdominal pain, anorexia, malaise, splenomegaly, and lymphadenopathy (cervical, postauricular, occipital).
2. Findings of modified measles
   a. Illness similar but milder than typical measles (e.g., afebrile course, rash may only last 1 to 2 days and does not become confluent)
   b. Seen in infants <9 months of age because of the presence of a transplacental antibody or as a result of administration of immunoglobulin to an exposed individual
3. Findings of atypical measles
   a. Seen in patients who received killed vaccine between 1963 and 1967 and subsequently got exposed to wild measles virus (hypersensitivity reaction)
   b. Seen in young adults (second and third decades of life)
   c. Rash begins on distal extremities, may be pronounced on wrists and ankles, and progresses in a cephalad direction
   d. Rash may be erythematous, maculopapular, vesicular, petechial, or purpuric
   e. Pulmonary involvement (e.g., nodular pneumonia, hilar adenopathy, pleural effusion)
4. Diagnosis of measles is usually made from a typical clinical presentation. The following tests may help in arriving at the diagnosis:
   a. Leukopenia with a relative lymphocytosis (uncomplicated measles)
   b. CSF examination in suspected encephalitis shows mild pleocytosis with predominance of lymphocytes with increased protein and normal glucose values.
   c. Isolation of virus from urine, blood, or nasopharyngeal aspirate (through public health laboratory or CDC)
   d. Measles IgM antibody in the serum during the acute phase (4 days after the appearance of the rash) confirms the diagnosis.
   e. A significant rise in measles IgG antibody (e.g., enzyme immunoassay [EIA]) titers drawn during acute (within 4 days after rash) and convalescent stage (2 to 4 weeks later)
5. Complications of measles include
   a. Otitis media
   b. Pneumonia (interstitial pneumonitis from measles virus or bronchopneumonia from secondary bacterial infection)
   c. Cervical adenitis
   d. Encephalomyelitis (incidence: 1/1000 cases of measles)
   e. Laryngotracheobronchitis
   f. Myocarditis, pericarditis
   g. Exacerbation of tuberculosis
   h. Transient loss of hypersensitivity to tuberculin skin test
   i. Black measles (hemorrhagic measles, purpura fulminans with disseminated intravascular coagulation)
   j. Corneal ulceration, blindness
   k. Subacute sclerosing panencephalitis

Emergency Department Treatment and Disposition

1. Measles is a self-limiting disease in normal children and treatment is purely supportive.
2. Patients are contagious from 3 to 5 days before the rash to 4 days after the appearance of the rash. Immunocompromised patients are contagious for the duration of the illness (prolonged excretion of the virus in respiratory tract secretions). Measures should be undertaken to prevent their exposure to susceptible persons.
3. Hospitalize infants, malnourished children, or patients with complications (e.g., pneumonia, croup, encephalitis).
4. Vitamin A therapy in children with measles has been associated with a reduction in morbidity and mortality. Current recommendations include:
   a. Children living in developing countries
   b. Consider for children in the United Sates with any of the following:
      1) Children between 6 and 24 months of age hospitalized with measles-related complications
      2) Children with immunodeficiency, ophthalmologic evidence of vitamin A deficiency, impaired intestinal absorption, moderate to severe malnutrition, or recent immigration from areas with a high mortality rates for measles
   c. Dose of vitamin A:
      1) A single dose given orally
      2) 200,000 IU for infants 1 year of age and older
      3) 100,000 IU for infants between 6 and 12 months of age
      4) A repeat dose is given the next day followed by another dose at 4 weeks with any ophthalmologic evidence of vitamin A deficiency.
5. Immune globulin (IG) to prevent or modify measles in a susceptible person (given within 6 days of exposure); examples include:

a. Susceptible household contacts of a patient with measles
b. Immunocompromised persons
c. Infants 6 months to 1 year of age
d. Infants <5 months of age who are not protected by passive immunity (e.g., either born to mothers who develop measles or mothers without measles immunity)
e. Pregnant women

Clinical Pearls: Measles

1. Measles is characterized by a prominent prodrome of cough, coryza, and conjunctivitis (*the 3 C's*) followed by confluent erythematous maculopapular (morbilliform) rash.
2. Measles vaccine is given (usually as measles, mumps, rubella [MMR]) routinely to healthy infants between 12 and 15 months of age, followed by a second dose at school entry between 4 and 6 years of age. Children not reimmunized at school entry should receive the second dose by 11 to 12 years of age.
3. Mortality from measles is increased in children <5 years of age and in immunocompromised children (especially children with leukemia, HIV infection, and malnutrition). Characteristic measles rash may also not develop in immunocompromised patients.

BOX 3-50. CLINICAL FEATURES OF MEASLES

- Incubation period: 10 to 12 days
- Prominent prodrome
  (1) Fever
  (2) The 3 C's: *c*ough, *c*oryza, *c*onjunctivitis (exudative conjunctivitis) (Fig. 3-53)
  (3) Significant photophobia
- Enanthem (Koplik's spots; see below) (Fig. 3-54)
- Rash (exanthem)
  (1) Erythematous maculopapular lesions
  (2) Starts along the hairline, then proceed downwards (cephalocaudally) until it reaches the feet
  (3) Starts on the third day of illness
  (4) Peaks at height of fever/constitutional symptoms (between fourth and sixth day of illness)
  (5) Confluent in upper part of the body
  (6) Erythematous rash that blanches on pressure in the beginning
  (7) Involves the palms and soles
  (8) Rash undergoes brown staining that does not blanch after 3 to 4 days (represents capillary hemorrhage)
  (9) Rash starts resolving in order of appearance between the seventh and ninth day of illness
- Desquamation (follows disappearance of the rash)
  (1) Fine branny desquamation seen over sites of most extensive involvement
  (2) No desquamation seen over hands or feet (*unlike scarlet fever*)
- Koplik's spots
  (1) Pathognomonic enanthem of measles
  (2) Seen 2 days before and 2 days after rash
  (3) Transient nature; its absence does not exclude diagnosis
  (4) Common site of appearance: opposite lower molars
  (5) May spread to involve the entire buccal and labial mucosa
  (6) Seen as white papular dots on an erythematous buccal mucosa
  (7) Described as "salt grains sprinkled on a red background"

BOX 3-55. DIFFERENTIAL DIAGNOSIS OF MUMPS

Differential diagnosis of mumps parotitis

- Parotitis from other etiology
  - A. Viral parotitis
    - (1) HIV
    - (2) Influenza virus types 1 and 3
    - (3) Parainfluenza virus
    - (4) Enteroviruses (e.g., coxsackie virus)
    - (5) Cytomegalovirus
    - (6) Lymphocytic choriomeningitis virus
  - B. Suppurative (bacterial) parotitis
    - (1) *Staphylococcus aureus*
    - (2) *Streptococcus pyogenes*
    - (3) Gram-negative bacilli
    - (4) Anaerobes
    - (5) Nontuberculous mycobacteria
- Anterior cervical adenitis
- Preauricular adenitis
- Other causes of parotid swelling
  - (1) Sarcoidosis
  - (2) Sjögren's syndrome
  - (3) Parotid duct stone
  - (4) Chronic wind instrument use
  - (5) Pneumoparotitis (e.g., playing wind instrument, glass blowing, scuba diving)
  - (6) Tumor of the parotid gland
  - (7) Diabetes mellitus
  - (8) Cirrhosis
  - (9) Malnutrition
  - (10) Drug reactions (e.g., phenylbutazone, thiouracil, iodides)
  - (11) Starch ingestion

Differential diagnosis of mumps orchitis

- Epididymo-orchitis from other etiology (e.g., STDs)
- Testicular torsion (especially when orchitis precedes parotitis or occurs in the absence of parotitis)

Differential diagnosis of mumps meningoencephalitis

- Meningoencephalitis from other viruses (e.g., enterovirus)

DIAGNOSIS INFECTIOUS MONONUCLEOSIS

SYNONYM

Glandular fever

Definition

Infectious mononucleosis (IM) is a usually benign, self-limited disease of children and young adults caused, in the vast majority, by Epstein-Barr virus (EBV). It derives its name from the mononuclear lymphocytosis with atypical lymphocytes that accompanies the illness.

Etiology

1. Epstein-Barr virus, a DNA virus, belonging to the herpes group of viruses, and causes >90% of IM cases.
2. About 5 to 10% of IM-like illnesses are caused by primary infection with cytomegalovirus, *Toxoplasma gondii*, adenovirus, viral hepatitis, and HIV.

Associated Clinical Features

1. IM occurs in all age groups, but the clinical expression depends on the age of the patient. In young children, primary EBV infection is often clinically asymptomatic or indistinguishable from other childhood infections. IM presents in a more classic way in adolescents and young adults.
2. IM is transmitted in oral secretions by close contact such as kissing (hence the name "kissing disease") or exchange of saliva from child to child (e.g., child care centers). The period of communicability is indeterminate.
3. The diagnosis of IM is usually made by the presence of typical clinical findings with atypical lymphocytosis in the peripheral blood, and confirmed by serologic testing.
4. Laboratory tests that suggest the diagnosis include:
   a. CBC usually shows leukocytosis with predominant lymphocytosis; atypical lymphocytes usually account for 20 to 40% of the total number (in other viral infec-

tions [e.g., rubella, hepatitis] the percentage is usually <10%). Mild thrombocytopenia (50,000 to 200,000 cells/mm^3) may also be seen (>50% of patients).

b. Monospot test (heterophile) is usually negative in young children <4 years of age; by 4 years of age, 80% of children undergoing primary EBV infection are heterophile antibody-positive.

c. EBV serology (Box 3-57)

5. Complications of IM include:
   a. Upper airway obstruction
   b. Splenic rupture (a rare but serious complication leading to hemorrhage, shock, and death; incidence highest in second or third week of illness; may be first sign of IM)
   c. Hematologic (thrombocytopenia, agranulocytosis, hemolytic anemia, aplastic anemia)
   d. Myocarditis, pericarditis
   e. Orchitis
   f. Disseminated lymphoproliferative disease
   g. Chronic fatigue syndrome

Consultations

Hematology (indicated for patients with extremely high or low white blood cell counts, moderate thrombocytopenia, and anemia; a bone marrow examination is warranted in such patients to exclude the possibility of leukemia, especially *before* giving corticosteroid therapy)

Emergency Department Treatment and Disposition

1. IM is a self-limited illness in the vast majority of patients and greater than 95% of cases recover spontaneously without any specific therapy.
2. Indications for hospitalization include IM associated with complications (e.g., patients presenting with upper airway obstruction requiring a nasopharyngeal airway).
3. Corticosteroid therapy
   a. *Not routinely* recommended
   b. Short course may be considered in the following situations (no controlled data to show efficacy in any of these conditions)
      1) Upper airway obstruction
      2) Hematologic (severe thrombocytopenia or hemolytic anemia)
      3) CNS (advocated by some in meningitis, seizures)
      4) Cardiac (myocarditis or pericarditis)
      5) Massive splenomegaly
   c. Dose: prednisone 1 mg/kg per 24 hours (maximum 20 mg/24 hours if >10 kg) given orally for 7 days with subsequent tapering
4. Family and patient education
   a. Avoid contact sports or heavy lifting, especially during the first 2 to 3 weeks of illness, particularly if splenomegaly is present or until spleen size returns to normal.
   b. Seek immediate medical attention if any of the following occurs:
      1) Sudden onset of abdominal pain (especially left-sided)
      2) Vomiting and abdominal pain (signs of peritoneal irritation)
      3) Pallor, lethargy, and fatigue (signs of hemorrhage)

Clinical Pearls: Infectious Mononucleosis

1. Classic IM is an acute illness characterized by a triad of fever, exudative pharyngitis, and cervical adenopathy (Figs. 3-58, 3-59, and 3-60).
2. The spectrum of IM varies widely, ranging from asymptomatic infection to fatal infection. Most patients with IM recover uneventfully over a 2- to 3-week period.
3. The most frequent causes of death from IM in otherwise apparently healthy persons include neurologic complications, splenic rupture, or upper airway obstruction.
4. Streptococcal pharyngitis clinically mimics IM; tender tonsillar and cervical adenopathy and absence of hepatosplenomegaly are some features that help in differentiating the two. Failure of a patient with streptococcal pharyngitis to improve within 48 to 72 hours after antibiotic therapy should raise a suspicion of IM.
5. Ampicillin or Amoxicillin given to patients with IM, causes nonallergic morbilliform rashes in a significant proportion of patients with IM (Fig. 3-61). This rash often is mistaken for as penicillin allergy.

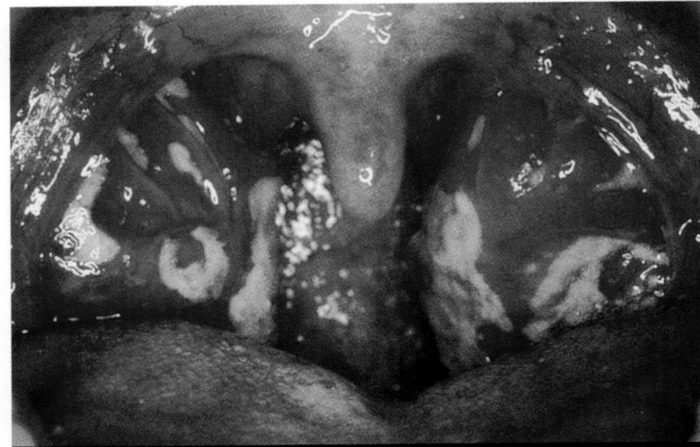

Figure 3-58. Exudative Tonsillopharyngitis of Infectious Mononucleosis

Marked white exudates on the tonsils of a child with infectious mononucleosis. (Reproduced with permission from: Mei Kane KS, Ryder JB, Jonson RA et al: Epstein-Barr virus. *Color Atlas & Synopsis of Pediatric Dermatology*. New York, McGraw-Hill, 2002, p. 576.)

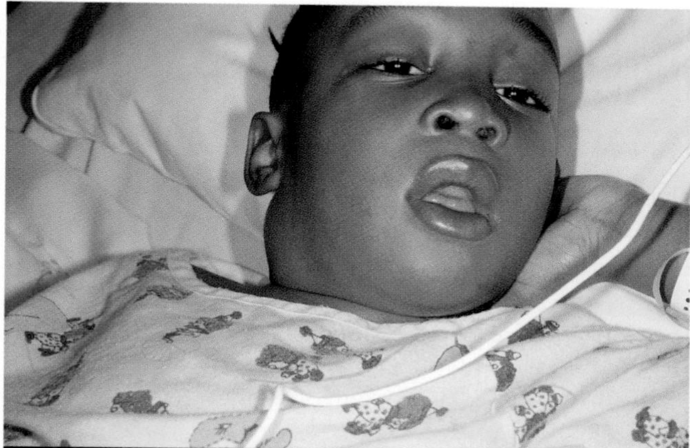

Figure 3-59. Infectious Mononucleosis

Cervical lymphadenopathy, difficulty breathing, fever, and sore throat were the presenting complaints in this 8-year-old child. He had 25% atypical lymphocytes on peripheral blood, and his monospot was also positive.

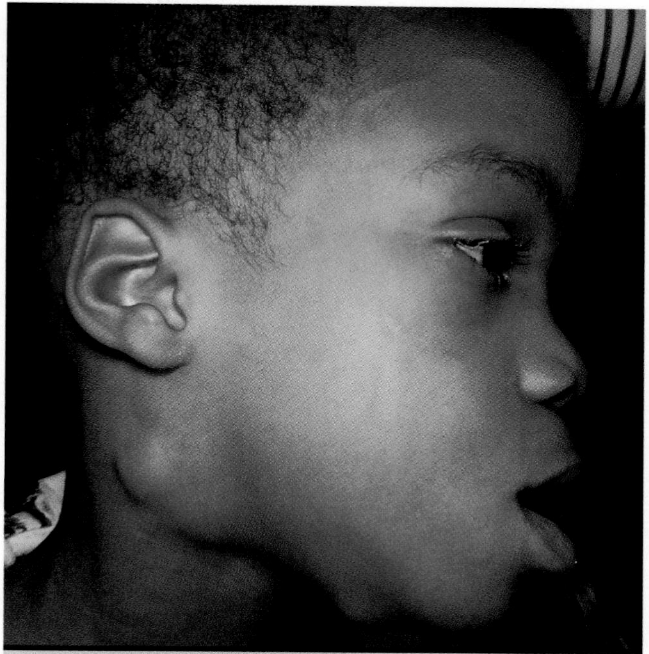

Figure 3-60. Infectious Mononucleosis

Cervical lymphadenopathy, "worsening of his snoring and mouth breathing," sore throat, and low-grade fever were the presenting complaints in this 9-year-old child. He had 30% atypical lymphocytes on peripheral blood, and his monospot was also positive. (For upper airway obstruction due to IM in a patient demonstrating mouth breathing, subcostal and intercostal retractions, stridor, and a significant drop in oxygen saturation during sleep, see Fig. 6-22).

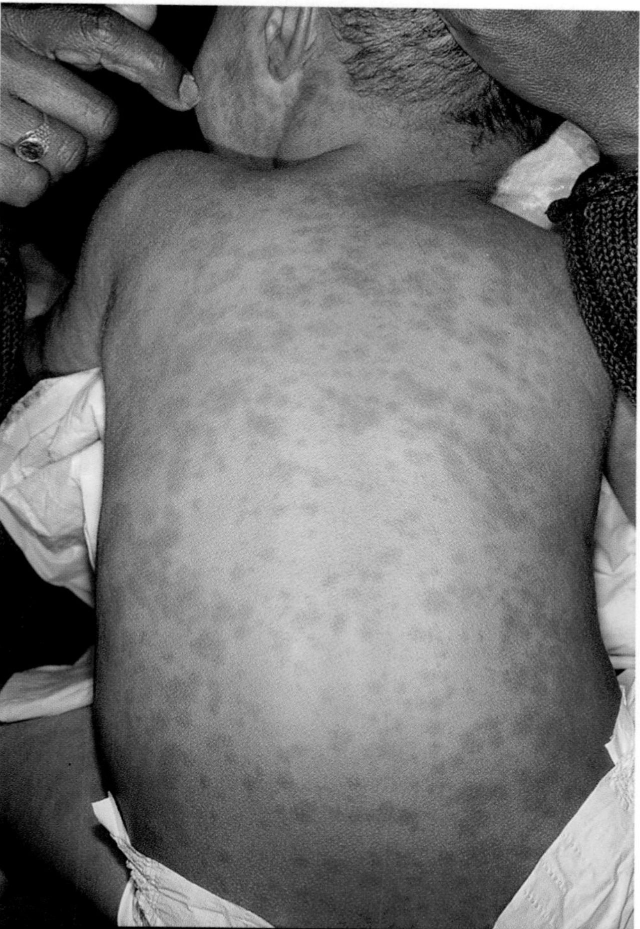

Figure 3-61. Infectious Mononucleosis

This generalized erythematous papular rash was precipitated by amoxicillin, which was given to this patient 3 days earlier for exudative tonsillopharyngitis presumed to be "strep throat." He continued to have fever and sore throat while receiving amoxicillin. He had splenomegaly, atypical lymphocytosis on peripheral smear, negative monospot, and positive EBV antibody titers. This rash is not an allergic reaction to penicillin (true penicillin allergic skin manifestations include urticaria, erythema multiforme minor and Stevens-Johnson syndrome/toxic epidermal necrolysis; see Figs. 7-5 to 7-9).

BOX 3-56. CLINICAL FEATURES OF INFECTIOUS MONONUCLEOSIS

- Incubation period: 30 to 50 days
- Fever >90% of cases (associated with myalgias, headache, anorexia, chills)
- Sore throat
- Moderate to severe pharyngitis with marked tonsillar enlargement
- Exudative pharyngitis (>50% of cases)
- Associated group A beta-hemolytic streptococcal pharyngitis (about 5 to 25% of cases)
- Lymphadenopathy
  - (1) Usually bilateral anterior and posterior cervical adenopathy (80 to 90% of patients)
  - (2) Mildly tender to palpation (*unlike acute cervical adenitis*)
  - (3) Other sites: submandibular, axillary, inguinal, epitrochlear
- Hepatic
  - (1) Transient elevations of hepatocellular enzyme (~80 to 90% of cases)
  - (2) Hepatomegaly (~10 to 15% of cases)
  - (3) Icteric hepatitis (~5% of cases)
- Splenomegaly (moderate enlargement in ~50% of cases)
- Skin rash
  - (1) Seen in 5 to 15% of cases
  - (2) Either morbilliform, scarlatiniform, macular, petechial, urticarial, or erythema multiforme–like
- Ampicillin (or other penicillin)–related rash in IM
  - (1) Administration of penicillin produces rash in 40% and ampicillin in 90 to 100% of patients with IM
  - (2) Rash may be pruritic
  - (3) Erythematous or copper-colored maculopapular rash
  - (4) Begins 5 to 10 days after the drug is begun
  - (5) Lasts up to 1 week
  - (6) Involvement extensive on trunk and involves palms and soles
  - (7) Rash is not a hypersensitivity reaction to antibiotic
- Periorbital eyelid edema
- Palatal petechiae (at the junction of hard and soft palates)
- Hematologic
  - (1) Greater than 50% mononuclear cells
  - (2) Greater than 10% atypical lymphocytes
  - (3) Mild thrombocytopenia
- Central nervous system manifestations
  - (1) Encephalitis or aseptic meningitis
  - (2) Bell's palsy
  - (3) Guillain-Barré syndrome
  - (4) Acute cerebellar ataxia
  - (5) Optic neuritis
  - (6) "Alice in Wonderland" syndrome
  - (7) Acute hemiplegia
  - (8) Cranial nerve palsies
- Serology
  - (1) Transient appearance of heterophile antibodies
  - (2) Permanent emergence of antibodies to EBV

BOX 3-57. SERUM EPSTEIN-BARR VIRUS ANTIBODIES IN INFECTIOUS MONONUCLEOSIS

Infection	*VCA-IgG*	*VCA-IgM*	*EA (D)*	*EBNA*
No previous infection	−	−	−	−
Acute infection	+	+	+/−	−
Recent infection	+	+/−	+/−	+/−
Past infection	+	−	−	+

VCA-IgG indicates IgG class antibody to viral capsid antigen.
VCA-IgM indicates IgM class antibody to VCA.
EA (D), early antigen diffuse staining; EBNA, EBV nuclear antigen
(Reproduced with permission from: American Academy of Pediatrics. Epstein-Barr virus infections. In: Pickering LK, (ed). *2003 Red Book: Report of the Committee on Infectious Diseases,* 26th ed. Elk Grove Village, IL, American Academy of Pediatrics, 2003, p. 273.)

BOX 3-58. DIFFERENTIAL DIAGNOSIS OF INFECTIOUS MONONUCLEOSIS

- Streptococcal pharyngitis
- Infectious mononucleosis-like illness caused by cytomegalovirus
- Leukemia
- Other viral exanthems (e.g., rubella)
- Viral hepatitis
- Acquired toxoplasmosis
- HIV infection
- Kawasaki disease
- Diphtheria

DIAGNOSIS ERYTHEMA INFECTIOSUM

SYNONYM

Fifth Disease

Definition and Etiology

Erythema infectiosum (EI) is a childhood exanthematous illness caused by human parvovirus B19.

Associated Clinical Features

1. Sporadic cases of EI are seen throughout the year, while seasonal peaks occur in late winter and spring.
2. EI is usually diagnosed clinically based on the typical exanthem.
3. Serologic tests that help in confirming the diagnosis in immunocompetent patients include:
   a. The presence of anti-B19 IgM antibody on a single serum specimen confirms acute or recent infection. Patients with EI are almost always IgM-antibody positive; IgM antibodies are detected shortly after acute infection and persist for 6 to 8 weeks.
   b. IgG antibodies are detected a few days after IgM antibodies and persist for years (a lifetime in some). Seroconversion from IgG-negative to IgG-positive on paired sera confirms a recent infection.
4. Complications of parvovirus B19 infection include:
   a. Aplastic crisis seen in patients with sickle cell disease and other forms of congenital hemolytic anemia
   b. Arthropathy
      1) Commonly seen in adolescents and adults (60 to 80% of cases); rare in children <9 years old (10% of cases)
      2) More common in females than in males
      3) Symmetrical peripheral polyarthropathy
      4) Usual joints: hands, wrists, knees, and ankles
      5) Presentation includes arthralgias with morning stiffness to arthritis
      6) Symptoms resolve in a majority of patients within 2 to 4 weeks
   c. Neurological complications include meningitis, encephalitis, and peripheral neuropathy
   d. Thrombocytopenic purpura
   e. Infection during pregnancy leading to intrauterine infection of the fetus may result in fetal wastage and hydrops fetalis.
   f. Chronic parvovirus B19 infection may cause severe anemia in patients infected with HIV.

Emergency Department Treatment and Disposition

1. EI is a self-limited illness and only supportive therapy is required for immunocompetent patients.
2. Children with EI *do not* need isolation and exclusion from school or day care. Rash represents an immune-mediated postinfectious phenomenon and children are no longer contagious by the time rash is noted.
3. Educate the family about the usual benign course of EI and possible recurrence of the rash.
4. No specific therapy is necessary for arthritis except therapy directed at the relief of pain.
5. Patients with hemolytic anemias (e.g., sickle cell disease) who present with B19-induced red cell aplasia require close monitoring and possible transfusion (see Fig. 11-1).
6. Inform pregnant health care professionals about the potential risks to the fetus from parvovirus B19 infections and about preventive measures that may decrease these risks (e.g., strict infection control procedures or not caring for immunocompromised patients with chronic parvovirus infection).

Clinical Pearls: Erythema Infectiosum

1. Slapped-cheek appearance in an otherwise well-appearing child is pathognomonic of EI (Fig. 3-62).
2. Slapped-cheek appearance followed by a lacy exanthem on the torso and extremities are classic features of EI (Figs. 3-63 and 3-64).
3. The rash of EI can fluctuate in intensity and recur for weeks to months with environmental changes (e.g., temperature fluctuations or exposure to sunlight).

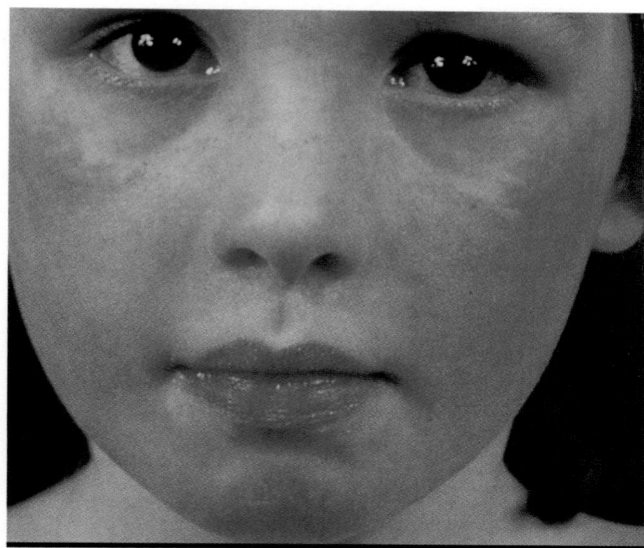

Figure 3-62. Slapped-Cheek Appearance of Erythema Infectiosum

Slapped-cheek appearance in a child with parvovirus B19 infection. (Reproduced with permission from: Mei Kane KS, Ryder JB, Jonson RA et al: Human parvovirus B19. *Color Atlas & Synopsis of Pediatric Dermatology*. New York, McGraw-Hill, 2002, p. 579).

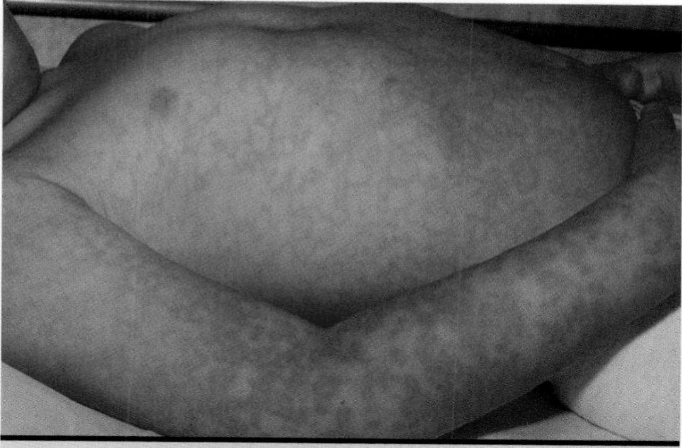

Figure 3-63. Erythema Infectiosum

Lacy, reticulated rash on the body of a child with EI. (Reproduced with permission from: Shah BR, Laude TL: Erythema infectiosum. In: *Atlas of Pediatric Clinical Diagnosis*. Philadelphia, WB Saunders, 2000, p. 70).

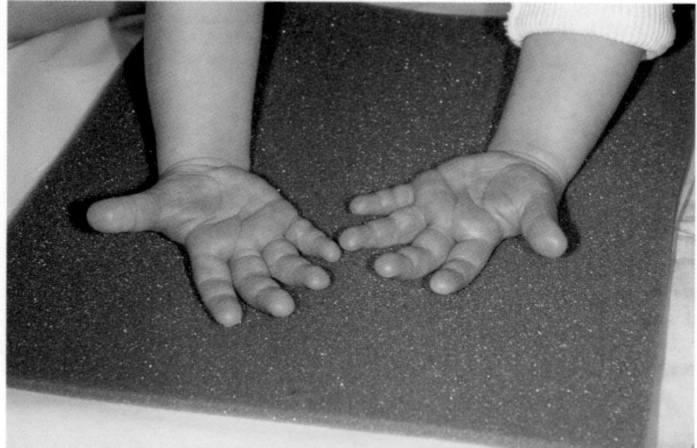

Figure 3-64. Papular Purpuric "Gloves and Socks" Syndrome in Parvovirus B19 Infection

This papular purpuric "gloves and socks" syndrome is characterized by petechiae on the hands and feet that appear in a distinct glove-and-socks distribution. It is usually seen in older children and adolescents.

BOX 3-59. CLINICAL FEATURES OF ERYTHEMA INFECTIOSUM

- Most commonly seen in school-aged children
- About 70% of cases occur between 5 and 15 years of age
- Incubation period: 4 to 28 days (average 16 days; rash and joint symptoms occur 2 to 3 weeks after infection)
- Usually prodromal period absent or very mild (myalgia, headache, malaise)
- Usually patient *afebrile* (or very low-grade fever)
- *No* enanthem
- First sign of illness is rash

Three stages of rash in the following sequence:

Stage 1: Red flushed cheeks (sunburn-like malar flush) with circumoral pallor (slapped-cheek appearance) lasting 1 to 4 days

Stage 2:

(1) Symmetric, erythematous maculopapular rash

(2) Starts on the trunk, moving peripherally to involve the arms, buttocks, and thighs

(3) Palms and soles usually spared

(4) Rash more prominent on extensor surfaces

(5) Central clearing of macular rash leading to lace-like or reticulated pattern as it fades

(6) Rash often pruritic

(7) Arthralgias/arthritis may be present in adolescents and adults

(8) Spontaneous resolution of rash without desquamation (within ~3 weeks)

Stage 3: Recurrent waxing and waning of rash for weeks or sometimes months precipitated by a variety of stimuli (e.g., sunlight, vigorous exercise, hot shower, stress)

BOX 3-60. DIFFERENTIAL DIAGNOSIS OF ERYTHEMA INFECTIOSUM

Differential diagnosis of EI rash

- Rubella
- Enteroviral infections
- Drug eruptions
- Scarlet fever
- Measles
- Roseola infantum

Differential diagnosis of arthralgia/arthritis of EI:

- Collagen vascular diseases (e.g., juvenile rheumatoid arthritis, systemic lupus erythematosus)

BOX 3-61. HISTORICAL CLASSIFICATION OF CHILDHOOD EXANTHEMS

- First disease = Measles
- Second disease = Scarlet fever
- Third disease = German measles
- Fourth disease = Filatov-Dukes disease (a variant of scarlet fever [not recognized at the present time])
- Fifth disease = Erythema infectiosum
- Sixth disease = Roseola infantum

DIAGNOSIS HAND-FOOT-AND-MOUTH DISEASE

Definition and Etiology

1. Hand-foot-and-mouth disease (HFMD) is a clearly recognizable viral infection caused by coxsackie virus (nonpolio enteroviruses).
2. Coxsackie A16 and A5 are the most common serotypes, while A9, A6, and A10 are occasional serotypes causing HFMD. The same clinical picture also has been reported with coxsackie virus B1, B3, and enterovirus 71.

Associated Clinical Features

1. HFMD is more common in children than adults.
2. It tends to be more severe in children <5 years of age.
3. It is commonly seen during late summer and early fall in temperate climates (the seasonal pattern is less evident in the tropics), and often occurs in epidemics.
4. It is a highly contagious illness; modes of transmission include oral-oral, fecal-oral, respiratory routes, and from fomites.
5. The diagnosis is made clinically, especially with a typical distribution of the skin lesions, and no laboratory tests are usually performed.
6. Virus can be isolated from the vesicle, oropharyngeal and rectal swabs, and stool (*viral shedding may continue for 6 to 12 weeks following an asymptomatic infection, making enterovirus isolation from stool as a cause of illness less specific*). A rise in virus-specific neutralizing antibody titers demonstrated between acute and convalescent titers also helps in confirming the diagnosis.
7. Rare complications reported with coxsackie A virus include myocarditis, meningoencephalitis, aseptic meningitis, and paralytic disease.

Emergency Department Treatment and Disposition

1. HFMD is a self-limited disease in the majority, and treatment is supportive with antipyretics/analgesics (as indicated) with attention to adequate hydration. Young infants with extensive involvement around the mouth may become dehydrated because of poor oral intake. Soft diet and cool, noncitrus liquids are often well tolerated in the presence of oral ulcerations.
2. *Do not* use lidocaine viscous topically for the relief of pain associated with mouth lesions. Systemic toxicity can occur due to absorption of the lidocaine from the buccal mucosa.
3. Special attention to personal hygiene including hand washing is important to prevent spread of the enteroviruses.
4. Prognosis is excellent, with resolution of skin lesions *without* scarring.

Clinical Pearls: Hand-Foot-and-Mouth Disease

1. The characteristic features of HFMD are vesicular lesions in the mouth and distal extremities (as the name implies) (Fig. 3-65).
2. Skin lesions of HFMD are seen in almost 100% of affected preschool-aged children, 38% of infected school-aged children, and only in 11% of infected adults.
3. Although commonly distributed over the hands, feet, and mouth, lesions may also be seen outside of those areas, especially in young infants (Fig. 3-66).

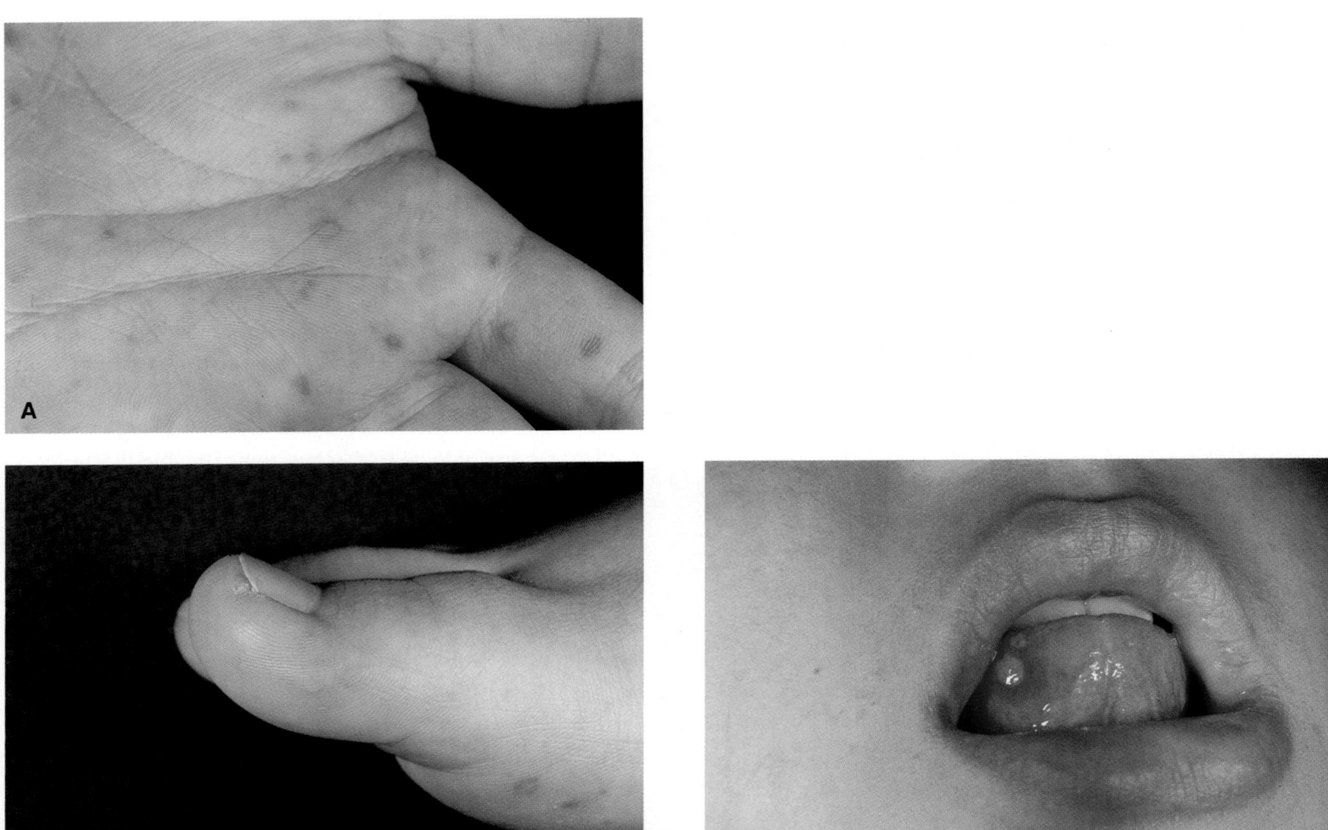

Figure 3-65. Hand-Foot-and-Mouth Disease

Typical elliptical or oval-shaped papulovesicular lesions with erythematous rims are seen on the hand and foot (*A*, *B*), and ulcers surrounded by a rim of erythema are seen in the mouth (*C*).

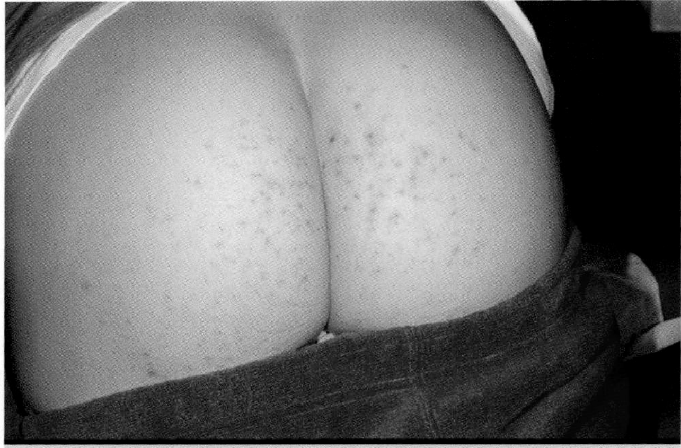

Figure 3-66. Hand-Foot-and-Mouth Disease

A nonvesicular maculopapular rash is seen on the buttocks in the same child seen in Fig. 3-65. The buttocks are the most common sites and the rash may be petechial. Similar lesions may also be seen on the upper thighs and knees (the arms, legs, and face are less commonly involved).

BOX 3-70. CLINICAL FEATURES OF ASCARIASIS

- Asymptomatic (vast majority of patients)
- Pulmonary signs and symptoms (*during larval migration stage through the lungs*)
  - (1) Fever
  - (2) Shortness of breath/dyspnea
  - (3) Substernal pain
  - (4) Wheezing/asthma
  - (5) Hemoptysis
  - (6) Rales
  - (7) Eosinophilia (peripheral blood)
  - (8) Löffler's pneumonia or Löeffler's syndrome (transient pulmonary infiltrates)
- Gastrointestinal signs and symptoms (*due to adult worms inhabiting lumen of small intestine*)
  - (1) Abdominal pain (persistent or recurrent)
  - (2) Abdominal distension
  - (3) Vomiting (with or without bile)
  - (4) Diarrhea
  - (5) Passing worms in vomitus or in stools during an attack
  - (6) Malabsorption (e.g., steatorrhea, diminished vitamin A absorption)
  - (7) Pancreatic-biliary ascariasis
  - (8) Abdominal or right upper quadrant pain
  - (9) Ascending cholangitis (migration to the common bile duct)
  - (10) Acute pancreatitis (migration to the pancreatic duct)
  - (11) Gallstones (dead worms are nidi for stone)
  - (12) Obstructive jaundice (rare)
  - (13) Acute intestinal obstruction (seen in children with heavy infection)
  - (14) Acute appendicitis (migration to appendix)
  - (15) Perforation, peritonitis
  - (16) Diverticulitis (migration to the diverticula)
  - (17) Volvulus
  - (18) Intussusception
- Allergic reactions (*due to absorption of toxins from products of living or dead worms*)
  - (1) Asthma
  - (2) Hay fever
  - (3) Urticaria
  - (4) Conjunctivitis

BOX 3-71. DIFFERENTIAL DIAGNOSIS OF ASCARIASIS

- Pulmonary ascariasis with eosinophilia
  - (1) Asthma
  - (2) Löffler's syndrome from other parasites (e.g., toxocariasis, strongyloidiasis, hookworm, paragonimiasis)
  - (4) Eosinophilic pneumonia
- Ascariasis-induced GI diseases
  - (1) Pancreatitis (from other etiology)
  - (2) Appendicitis (from other etiology)
  - (3) Cholecystitis (from other etiology)
  - (4) Diverticulitis
  - (5) Duodenitis
  - (6) Esophagitis

ACUTE EXANTHEMS: SCHEMATIC DIAGRAMS AND DRAWINGS

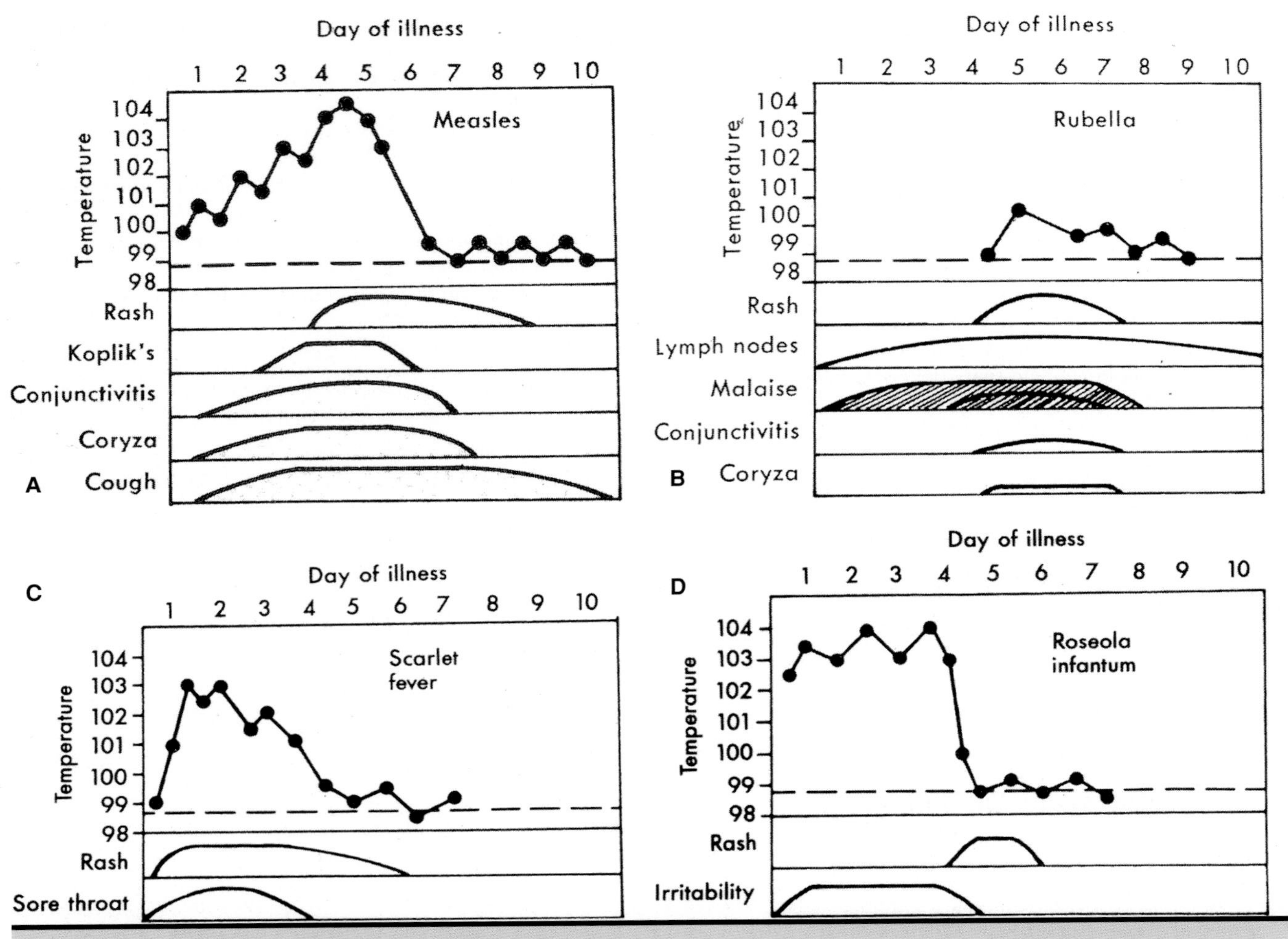

Figure 3-73. Schematic Diagrams Illustrating Differences Between Four Acute Exanthems Characterized by Maculopapular Eruptions

A. Measles. Clinical course of a typical case of measles. The rash appears 3 to 4 days after onset of fever, conjunctivitis, coryza, and cough. Koplik's spots develop 2 days before the rash. *B*. Rubella. Clinical course of a typical case of rubella in children and adults. Lymph nodes begin to enlarge 3 to 4 days before the rash. Prodromal symptoms (malaise) are minimal in children. In adults there may be a 3- to 4-day prodrome. Conjunctivitis and coryza, if present, are usually minimal and accompany the rash. *C*. Scarlet fever. Clinical course of a typical case of untreated uncomplicated scarlet fever. The rash usually appears within 24 hours of onset of fever and sore throat. *D*. Exanthem subitum (roseola infantum). Clinical course of a typical case of roseola infantum. A 3- to 4-day prodrome of an abrupt onset of high fever and irritability precedes the rash of roseola infantum, which appears as the temperature falls to normal by crisis. (Modified and reproduced with permission from: Katz SL et al (eds.): *Krugman's Infectious Diseases of Children*, 10th ed. St. Louis, Mosby-Year Book, 1998, p. 708).

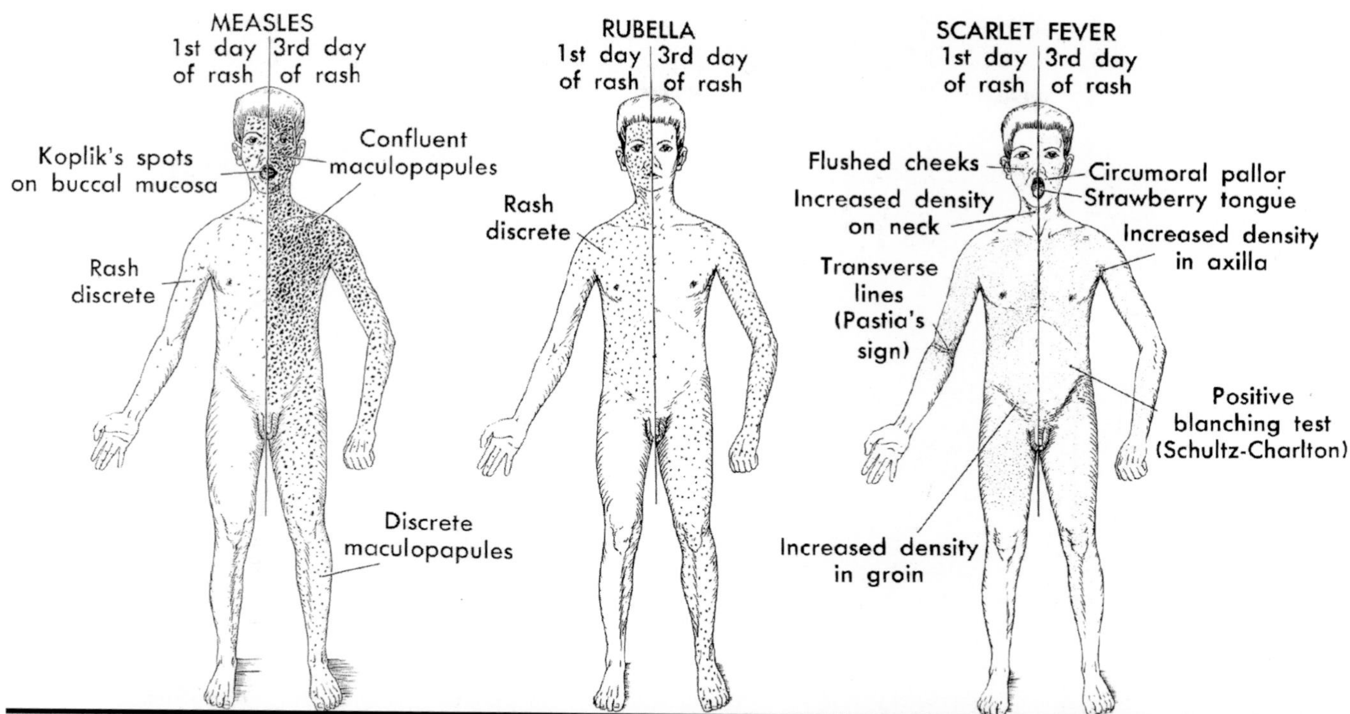

Figure 3-74. Schematic Drawings Illustrating Differences in Appearance, Distribution, and Progression of Measles, Rubella, and Scarlet Fever.

(Reproduced with permission from: Katz SL et al (eds.): *Krugman's Infectious Disease of Children*, 10th ed. St. Louis, Mosby-Year Book, 1998, p. 710).

Suggested Readings

American Academy of Family Physicians: Cat scratch disease. Patient handout. 2002.

American Academy of Pediatrics: Varicella-zoster infections. In: Pickering LK (ed). *2000 Red Book: Report of the Committee on Infectious Disease*, 25th ed. Elk Grove Village, IL, American Academy of Pediatrics.

Gershon AA, LaRussa P: Varicella-zoster virus infections. In: Katz SL et al (eds). *Krugman's Infectious Diseases of Children*, 10th ed. St. Louis, Mosby-Year Book, 1998, p. 620.

Habif TP. Bacterial infections. In: *Clinical Dermatology*, 3rd ed. St. Louis, Mosby-Year Book, 1996, p. 264.

Jain A, Daum RS: Staphylococcal infections in children: Part 3. *Pediatr Rev* 1999;20:261.

Katz SL et al (eds): Rubella (German measles). In: *Krugman's Infectious Diseases of Children*, 10th ed. St. Louis, Mosby-Year Book, 1998, p. 710.

Koch WC, Adler SP: Parvovirus infections. In: Katz SL et al (eds). *Krugman's Infectious Diseases of Children*, 10th ed. St. Louis, Mosby-Year Book, 1998, p. 326.

Kohl S: Postnatal herpes simplex virus. In: Oski FA. DeAngelis ??, Feigin ??, McMillan ??, Warshaw ??. *Principles and Practice of Pediatrics*, 2nd ed. CITY?, Lippincott, 1994, p. ???.

Ladhni S: Clinical, microbial, and biochemical aspects of the exfoliative toxins causing staphylococcal scalded syndrome. *Clin Microbiol Rev* 1999;12:224.

Ladhani S: Development and evaluation of detection systems for staphylococcal exfoliative toxin A responsible for scalded-skin syndrome. *J Clin Microbiol* 2001;39:2050.

Leach CT: Roseola (human herpesvirus types 6 and 7). In: Behrman RE, Kliegman RM, Jenson HB (eds). *Infectious Diseases. Nelson Textbook of Pediatrics*, 16th ed. Philadelphia, WB Saunders, 2000, p. 984.

Manders SM: Toxin-mediated streptococcal and staphylococcal disease. *J Am Acad Dermatol* 1998;39:383.

Nielsen HE, Andersen J, Bottiger B et al: Diagnostic assessment of haemorrhagic rash and fever. *Arch Dis Child* YEAR?;85:160.

Slavin KA, Frieden IJ: Picture of the month. Hand-foot-mouth disease. *Arch Pediatr Adolesc Med* 1998;152:505.

Stewart C: Skin and soft tissue infection update: Presentation, diagnosis, and syndrome–specific antibiotic management, in emergency medicine reports. *Am Health Consultant* 2000;VOL:21 NOS.2000.

Swartz MN: Cellulitis and subcutaneous tissue infections. In: Mandell GL (ed). *Principles and Practice of Infectious Diseases*, 5th ed. Philadelphia, Churchill Livingstone, 2000, p. 1037.

Weber DJ, Cohen MS, Fine JD: The acutely ill patient with fever and rash. In: Mandell GL, Bennett JE and Dolin R (eds). *Principles and Practice of Infectious Diseases*, 5th ed. Philadelphia, Churchill Livingstone, 2000, p. 639.

Wells LC, Smith JC, Weston VC, Collier J, Rutter N: The child with a non-blanching rash: how likely is meningococcal disease? *Arch Dis Child* 2001;85:218.

Wong VK, Hitchcock W, Mason WH: Meningococcal infection in children: a review of 100 cases. *Pediatr Infect Dis* 1989;8:224.

CHAPTER 4

SEXUAL ABUSE, GYNECOLOGY, AND SEXUALLY TRANSMITTED DISEASES

Binita R. Shah / Sarah Rawstron / Amy Suss
Edited by Binita R. Shah

DIAGNOSIS — SEXUAL ABUSE AND SEXUALLY TRANSMITTED DISEASES

Definition

1. Sexual abuse is engaging a child in sexual activities with any of the following:
   a. Sexual activities the child cannot comprehend
   b. Sexual activities for which the child is not developmentally prepared, and cannot give consent
   c. Sexual activities that violate the law or taboos of society
2. Sexual abuse includes a wide range of activities, from nontouching abuses (e.g., exhibitionism, voyeurism) to activities with direct genital, anal, or oral-genital contact, and using a child in fabricating pornographic materials that portray rape or seduction.

Associated Clinical Findings

1. About 1% of children experience some form of sexual abuse each year, resulting in the sexual victimization of 12 to 25% of girls and 8 to 10% of boys by 18 years of age.
2. About 80 to 90% of abused children are female, with a mean ages of 7 to 8 years.
3. Perpetrators are male in 75 to 90% of cases and usually involve adults or minors known to the child (either a family member or nonfamily member).
4. Abuse by family members or known acquaintances usually involves multiple episodes over periods of time ranging from weeks to years (as opposed to abuse by strangers or unknown assailants that usually involve only a single episode).
5. While conducting the interview:
   a. Interview the child alone if possible (usually children <3 years of age are not interviewed).
   b. Use nonleading questions (e.g., "Tell me more" and ". . . and then what happened . . .").
   c. Do not show emotions such as disbelief or shock while listening to the child's account.
6. Physical examination:
   a. The patient needs immediate examination if:
      1) Presenting within 72 hours of the alleged sexual abuse
      2) Presenting with acute injury or bleeding
      3) Presenting with vaginal discharge and the possible presence of sexually transmitted diseases (STDs)
      4) There is a possibility of pregnancy with a history of penile vaginal penetration in an adolescent who has reached menarche.
   b. Emergency examination is usually not necessary in the absence of the aforementioned findings, and the exam can be scheduled at the earliest time that is convenient for the child, the investigative team, and the physician.
   c. Perform a thorough physical examination from head to toe (the child may also be a victim of physical abuse or neglect), including the child's developmental, emotional, and behavioral status.
   d. Give special attention to areas that are involved in sexual activity (mouth, breasts, genitals [labia majora and minora, clitoris, urethra and periurethral tissue, hymen, hymenal opening, fossa navicularis, posterior fourchette, penis, scrotum], perineum, medial aspects of the thighs, buttocks, anus.
   e. Do not use perform speculum or digital examinations in a prepubertal child. Digital rectal examination is also usually not necessary.
   f. *Do not use terminology such as "The hymen is intact" to describe the findings.*
   g. *Do not use diagnostic terms such as "There is no evidence of sexual abuse" or "Sexual abuse can be ruled out."*

   h. Use drawings and photographs to supplement written documentation and secure all the records for possible use in civil or criminal court proceedings. Use dolls or line drawings for illustration when interviewing 3- to 6-year-old children.

7. The American Academy of Pediatrics Committee on Child Abuse and Neglect Recommendations (1999):
   a. Routine cultures and screening of all sexually abused children for gonorrhea, syphilis, HIV, or other STDs are not recommended.
   b. The yield of positive cultures is very low in asymptomatic prepubertal children, especially those with a history of fondling only.
   c. Appropriate cultures and serologic tests are recommended "when epidemiologically indicated or when history and/or physical findings suggest the possibility of oral, genital, or rectal contact" (Fig. 4-5).
8. Order cultures for *Neisseria gonorrhoeae* on special culture media.
   a. Girls: specimens should be collected from the vagina, rectum, and pharynx; a cervical specimen is not recommended for prepubertal girls.
   b. Boys: take a urethral swab culture if
      1) Urethral discharge
      2) Dysuria
      3) Positive urine leukocyte esterase
      4) Presence of erythema
9. Order cultures for *Chlamydia trachomatis*
   a. Girls: specimens collected from vagina and anus
   b. Boys: specimens collected from anus and urethra (if urethral discharge is present)
   c. Cultures for *C. trachomatis* are not recommended from the following sites:
      1) Intraurethral specimen in the absence of urethral discharge in prepubertal boys (low yield, traumatic experience for patient)
      2) Pharyngeal specimen for either sex (low yield, persistence of perinatally acquired infection beyond infancy)
10. Rape kit protocol modified for child sexual abuse:
    a. When the alleged sexual abuse has occurred within 72 hours, and
    b. The child provides a history of sexual abuse including ejaculation
11. Serologic test for syphilis (VDRL)
12. Serologic test for hepatitis B (hepatitis B surface antigen and antibody)
13. HIV serology (as indicated)

Emergency Department Treatment and Disposition

(see also page child abuse section for legal reporting issues)

1. Attention to all acute injuries that may require immediate intervention
2. Use a multidisciplinary approach involving local or regional child abuse consultants and a social worker.
3. Once sexual abuse is identified, all siblings of the sexual abuse victim should be examined.
4. Treatment for STDs and reporting requirements (see Box 4-4)
   a. Presumptive treatment for children who have been sexually abused is usually not done.
      1) Lower risk for ascending infection in girls than in adolescents
      2) Close follow-up can be arranged.
   b. Treatment is given once the specific diagnosis is confirmed.
5. Schedule a follow-up visit in about 2 weeks (after the most recent sexual exposure):
   a. For collection of additional specimens (infecting pathogens may not be present in sufficient quantities, initially resulting in negative cultures following a very recent exposure)
   b. For a repeat physical examination
6. To allow sufficient time for antibody production, schedule a follow-up visit in about 12 weeks (after the most recent sexual exposure) to collect sera for antibody titers.
7. Recommendations for mental health assessment and treatment should be considered as indicated.

Clinical Pearls: Sexual Abuse and Sexually Transmitted Diseases

1. A normal physical examination does not exclude child sexual abuse; diagnostic findings of sexual abuse are seen in only 3 to 16% of victims.
2. Physical examination of sexually abused children should not result in subjecting them to additional emotional trauma.
3. The diagnosis of child sexual abuse is often made on the basis of a child's history; a child's statement that he or she was sexually abused is often the most important evidence of molestation.
4. Presume sexual abuse until proven otherwise in a child presenting with an STD.

BOX 4-1. SIGNS AND SYMPTOMS SUGGESTIVE OF CHILD SEXUAL ABUSE

- Behavioral changes:
  (1) Appetite disturbances
  (2) Abdominal pain
  (3) Suicidal attempts or ideation
  (4) Withdrawal or depression
  (5) Poor school performance
  (6) Precocious sexual behavior
  (7) Sleep disturbances and nightmares
  (8) Enuresis
  (9) Encopresis
  (10) Phobias
- Genitourinary- and anogenital-related signs and symptoms:
  (1) Anal or genital pain
  (2) Vaginal discharge
  (3) Urethral discharge
  (4) Genital or anal bleeding
  (5) Painful urination
  (6) Painful defecation
  (7) Infections
  Recurrent urinary tract infections
  Recurrent vulvovaginitis
  Sexually transmitted diseases

BOX 4-2. CLINICAL FINDINGS SUGGESTIVE OF SEXUAL ABUSE

- Hymenal findings

A. Hymenal injuries
  (1) Most common sites of injures: between the 3 o'clock and 9 o'clock positions
  (2) Types of injuries: laceration, transection, disruption (strongly suggest abuse)
  (3) Notches or midline scarring in the lower portion of the hymen
  (4) Posterior or lateral concavities (indentations in hymenal tissues)

B. Hymenal diameter more than two standard deviations above normal for age in the presence of other findings

- Anal injuries
  (1) Fresh anal injuries (e.g., laceration) without adequate accidental history
  (2) Anal dilation >15 mm transverse with gentle buttock traction (in absence of stool in rectal vault this finding strongly suggests abuse)
- Injuries in posterior fourchette (*strongly suggest abuse*; Fig. 4-4)
- Bruising of inner thighs or genitalia or bite marks
- Oral cavity (frequent site of sexual abuse in children)
  (1) Unexplained erythema or petechiae of the palate (especially at the junction of the hard and soft palates)
  (2) Oral or perioral condylomata acuminata

Clinical pearls:

- All girls are born with hymens (in the absence of congenital anomalies) and normal hymens have different configurations (e.g., fimbriated, crescentic, annular).
- Acquired imperforate hymen or labial agglutination may result from sexual abuse (see Box 2-26).
- Hymenal diameter increases with age and it is also dependent on position, degree of traction, and degree of the child's relaxation during the examination.
- The hymenal orifice diameter alone should not be used as a screening test for the presence of sexual abuse.
- Hymenal notches between the 9 o'clock and 3 o'clock positions, bumps, tags, and vestibular bands are normal findings.
- Masturbation, tampons, or accidents (e.g., straddle injury) are *not* likely to cause injury to the hymen or internal genital structures.

BOX 4-3. SEXUAL ABUSE AND SEXUALLY TRANSMITTED DISEASES

- Modes of transmission of STDs (any of the following):
  (1) Transplacental
  (2) Perinatal
  (3) Sexual abuse
  (4) Consensual sexual intercourse
  (5) Accidental
- STDs may be transmitted during sexual assault and evidence of an STD may be the first indication that child sexual abuse has occurred.
- STDs in sexually abused children (Figs. 4-1, 4-2, 4-3 and 4-5):
  (1) Prevalence ranges from 2 to 7% in girls and 0 to 5% in boys.
  (2) Most common STDs: gonorrhea, chlamydia, human papillomavirus (condylomata acuminata)
  (3) Infrequent STDs: syphilis, infections caused by HIV, herpes simplex virus, trichomoniasis, *Ureaplasma urealyticum,* vaginosis

Clinical findings specific for sexual abuse:

- Presence of sperm or semen in the mouth, vagina, or anus
- Presence of acid phosphatase in sperm sample (acid phosphatose is normally secreted by prostate gland and normally is not found in the vagina)
- Pregnancy in a preadolescent or young adolescent
- Evidence of the following STDs (in the absence of perinatally-acquired infection or transfusion; sexually acquired HIV infection or HIV infection acquired through needle sharing):
  (1) Positive culture for gonorrhea
  (2) Positive test for syphilis
  (3) Positive test for HIV infection

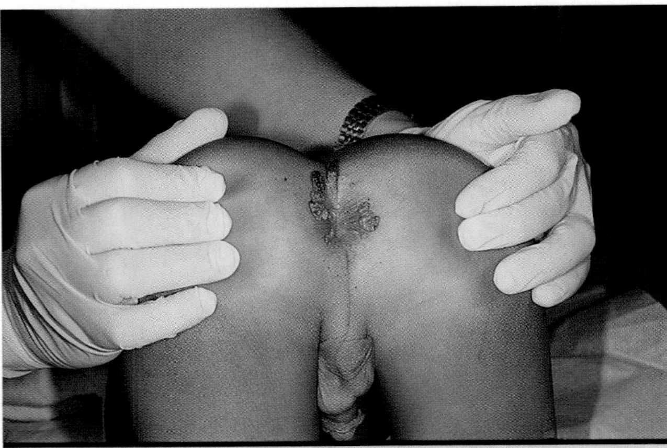

Figure 4-1. Condylomata Acuminata (Genital Warts due to Sexual Abuse)

Lesions are seen in the perianal area of this 3-year-old male child who was abused by his maternal uncle. Genital warts are soft, flesh-colored, elongated lesions that develop around mucocutaneous junctions and intertriginous areas (e.g., perianally, the mucosae of female genitalia). Condylomata acuminata must be differentiated from condylomata lata (see Fig. 4-3), as both occur in the same areas.

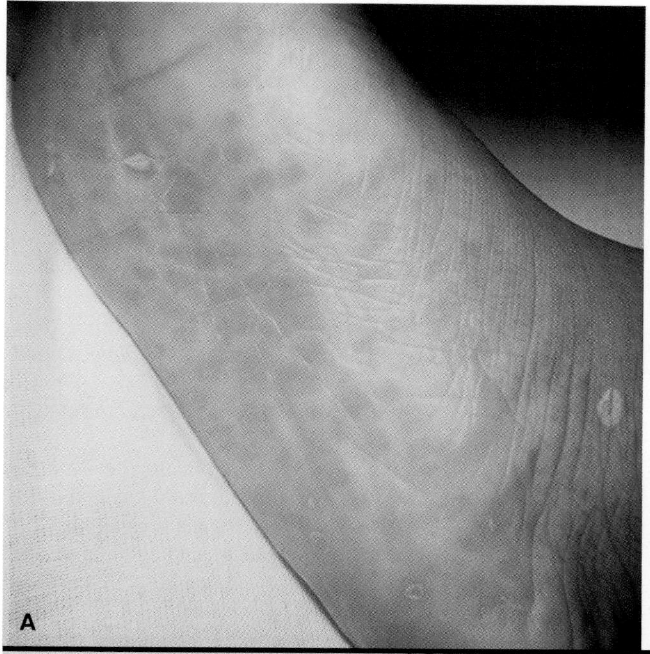

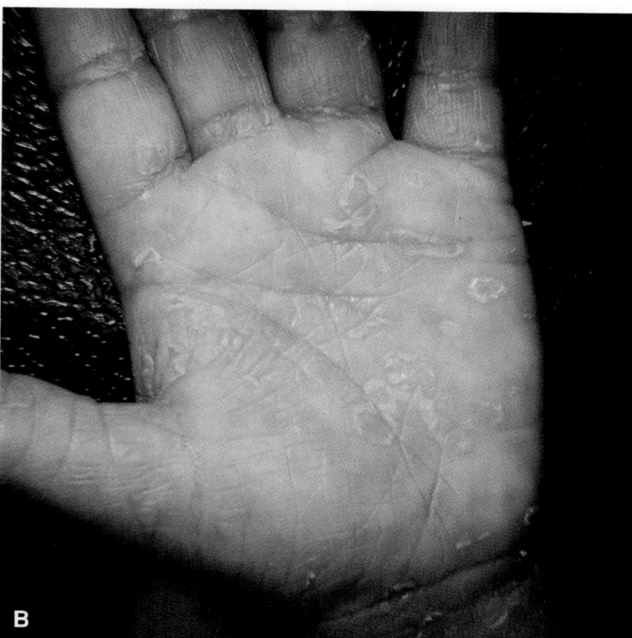

Figure 4-14. Secondary Syphilis

Copper-colored lesions on the palms and soles are characteristic findings of secondary syphilis. These erythematous papulosquamous nonpruritic lesions were present on the palms and feet in a 6-year-old girl who was placed in different foster homes since birth and was sexually abused on numerous occasions. Both her VDRL and FTA-ABS tests were positive.

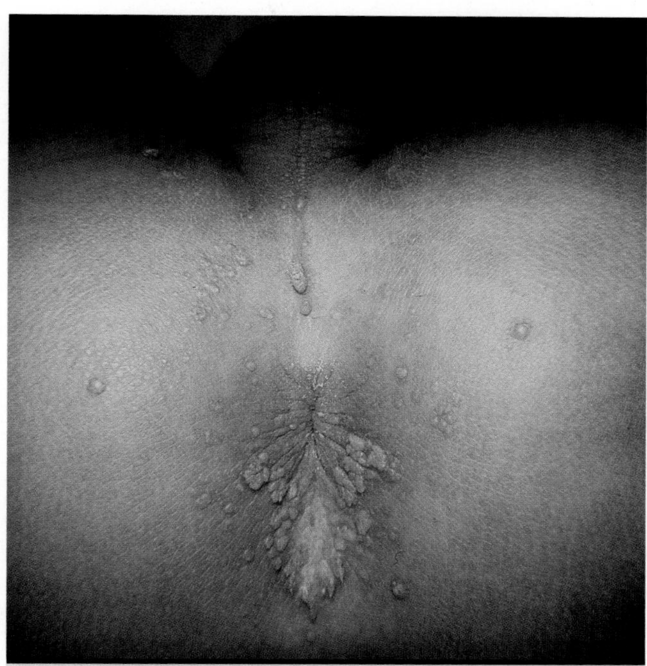

Figure 4-15. Condyloma Lata

Flat-topped round to oval plaques (formed by papules that coalesce) with a wide base are seen around the anogenital area (see also Fig. 4-3). Unlike condylomata acuminata, these lesions are flat and not covered by digitate vegetations. These lesions were seen in a 5-year-boy who was repeatedly sexually abused by his stepfather.

BOX 4-11. DIFFERENTIAL DIAGNOSIS OF PRIMARY AND SECONDARY SYPHILIS

- *Primary syphilis:*
  - (1) Chancroid (chancre of chancroid is soft and painful)
  - (2) Lymphogranuloma venereum
  - (3) Trauma
  - (4) Fixed drug eruption
  - (5) Secondary bacterial infection of herpetic lesions
  - (6) Reiter's syndrome
- *Secondary syphilis:*
  - (1) Pityriasis rosea
  - (2) Tinea versicolor
  - (3) Guttate psoriasis
  - (4) Erythema multiforme
  - (5) Drug eruptions
  - (6) Lichen planus
  - (7) Viral eruptions
  - (8) Id reaction

DIAGNOSIS GONORRHEA

SYNONYM

Clap

Definition and Etiology

Gonorrhea is one of the most common reportable sexually transmitted diseases (STDs) in the United States with an estimated 600,000 new cases every year. *Neisseria gonorrhoeae* is a fastidious gram-negative organism that occurs in pairs that are usually located within or associated with polymorphonuclear (PMN) leukocytes. There are >70 different strains of *N. gonorrhoeae*.

Associated Clinical Features

1. About 75 to 90% of all gonococcal infections in women and 10 to 40% of infections in men are asymptomatic.
2. About 60% of all cases of gonorrhea in men and women occur between the ages of 15 and 24 years with twice as many cases occurring in those aged 15 to 19. The reasons for the high incidence in this age group include biological and psychosocial factors such as increased rates of sexual activity, lack of condom use, a high incidence of asymptomatic carriers, and lack of compliance with therapy.
3. Clinical manifestations are similar to those of *Chlamydia trachomatis,* and both frequently occur in the same individual. Susceptible sites are usually mucosal columnar epithelial areas (e.g., the cervical transition zone in adolescent girls).
4. Extragenital sites of gonococcal infection include the pharynx, rectum, and conjunctiva.
5. Newborns of mothers with gonococcal infection are at risk for ophthalmia neonatorum, scalp abscesses at the sites of fetal monitors, rhinitis, pneumonia, or anorectal infections.
6. Disseminated gonococcal infection (DGI)
   a. Certain strains of *N. gonorrhoeae* are more likely to disseminate.
   b. About 0.5 to 3% of individuals with gonorrhea develop DGI.
   c. Most commonly characterized by arthritis/arthralgia, tenosynovitis, and dermatitis
   d. DGI is more prevalent in females (ratio 4:1), in particular pregnant females and those who had menses within the previous 7 days (probably due to hormonal influences or alterations in the pH of vaginal secretions).
   e. Other risk factors for DGI include pharyngeal gonorrhea, complement deficiency, and other immune system diseases such as systemic lupus erythematosus.
   f. Blood cultures should be done in the first few days of illness despite the fact that only 20 to 30% will be positive. Blood cultures are rarely positive by the time the infection has invaded a joint.
   g. Gonococcal infections have been found on mucosal surfaces 80% of the time despite negative blood, skin, and joint cultures.
   h. Other DGI complications include meningitis, endocarditis, osteomyelitis, pneumonia, and hepatitis.
7. Diagnosis of gonorrhea
   a. Gram's stain (gram-negative intracellular diplococci) and culture (e.g., Thayer-Martin culture plate, chocolate agar)
   b. Nucleic acid amplification techniques (NAATs) with sensitivities and specificities >95%
   c. Specimen swabs can be taken from nonsterile areas such the urethra, vagina, cervix, rectum, and pharynx. Specimens obtained from sterile areas such as blood or spinal or synovial fluid should be plated onto nonselective chocolate agar, as the role of NAATs for these sites has not been adequately studied.
   d. NAAT testing can also be done on urine samples. As opposed to urethral swabs, this noninvasive urine sampling is preferred by asymptomatic sexually-active males.
8. Long-term sequelae of gonorrhea in females includes tubal scarring, infertility, and ectopic pregnancy.

Consultation

Social services if sexual abuse is suspected

Emergency Department Treatment and Disposition

1. Patients infected with *N. gonorrhoeae* often are coinfected with *C. trachomatis*. Thus, patients treated for gonococcal infection also need to be treated for uncomplicated chlamydia infection. Either azithromycin 1 gram orally in a single dose or doxycycline 100 mg orally twice a day for 7 days should be given in patients in whom chlamydial infection is not ruled out.
2. Recommendations for the treatment of uncomplicated gonococcal infections from the Centers for Disease Control (CDC) 2002 STD Guidelines include:
   a. Cephalosporins: cefixime 400 mg orally in a single dose or ceftriaxone 125 mg IM in a single dose *or*
   b. Quinolones:
      1) Fluoroquinolones are not recommended for persons aged <18 years because studies have indicated that they can damage articular cartilage in some young animals. However, no joint damage attributable to quinolone therapy has been observed in children treated with prolonged ciprofloxacin regimens. Thus, children who weigh >45 kg can be treated with any regimen recommended for adults.

2) Due to quinolone-resistant *N. gonorrhoeae* (QRNG), quinolones should *not* be used for treating infections acquired in Asian or Pacific regions and should be avoided for treating infections acquired in California and other areas with increased prevalence of QRNG.
3) Dosage: ciprofloxacin 500 mg orally in a single dose *or* ofloxacin 400 mg orally in a single dose *or* levofloxacin 250 mg orally in a single dose

3. Hospitalization is recommended for all patients with DGI for IV therapy.
4. Refer to STD guidelines published by the CDC for the current treatment of complicated gonococcal infections, including extragenital sites, DGI, and infections acquired during pregnancy.
5. Patients should be instructed to refer their sex partners for evaluation and treatment. Follow-up referrals for counseling and patient education should be provided. *Treatment failures most often represent reinfection.*

Clinical Pearls: Gonorrhea

1. Many infections are asymptomatic (thus screening is important).
2. Symptomatic males present with genitourinary infection with complains of dysuria, urinary frequency, and purulent urethral discharge.
3. Symptomatic women complain of abnormal vaginal discharge (Fig. 4-16), intermenstrual bleeding, menorrhagia, or dysuria. Symptoms are related to those found with cervicitis, urethritis, bartholinitis/Bartholin gland abscess (Fig. 4-17), pelvic inflammatory disease (PID), perihepatitis, and tubo-ovarian abscess (TOA).
4. DGI is characterized by symptoms of arthritis/arthralgia, tenosynovitis, and dermatitis (arthritis-dermatitis syndrome).

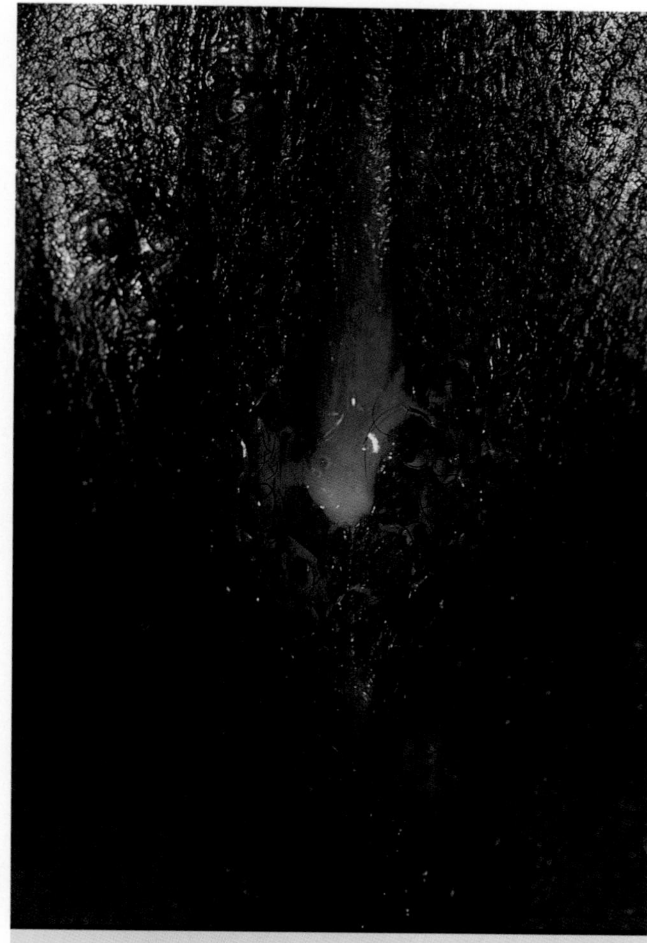

Figure 4-16. Gonorrhea

Dysuria and vaginal discharge were the presenting complaints of this sexually-active adolescent female. Culture was positive for *N. gonorrhoeae*.

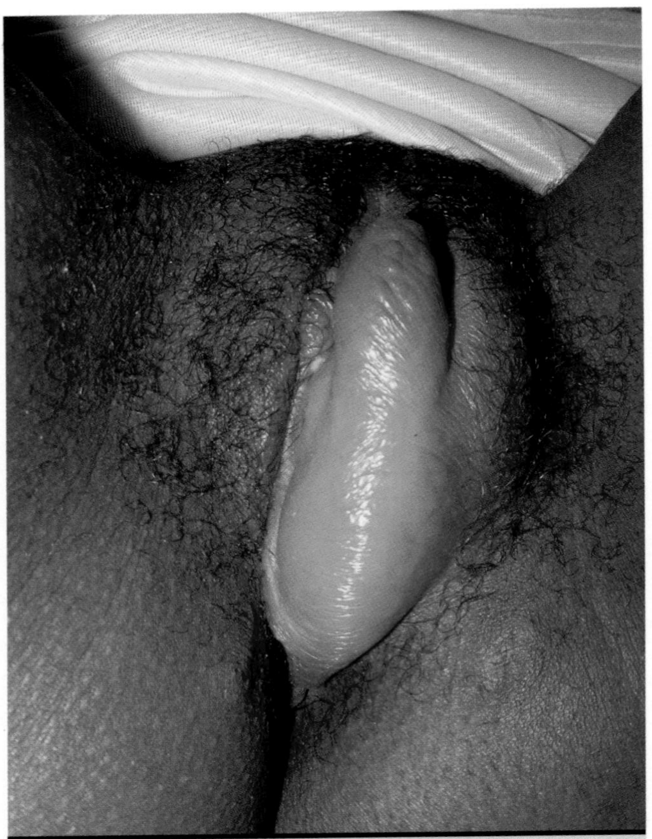

Figure 4-17. Bartholin Gland Abscess: Gonococcal Infection

Bartholin's glands are located bilaterally at the posterior introitus and drain through ducts that empty into the vestibule at approximately the 4 o'clock and 8 o'clock positions. These glands are normally pea-sized and are neither palpable nor visible unless infected or inflamed. A Bartholin gland abscess is a Bartholin glandular or ductal cyst infection usually caused by polymicrobial agents including *Neisseria gonorrhoeae, Chlamydia trachomatis, Escherichia coli, Proteus mirabilis,* and anaerobes including *Bacteroides fragilis* and *Peptostreptococcus* spp. Patients with a Bartholin gland abscess usually present with unilateral swelling and pain at the lower lateral vaginal opening, and its occurrence is associated with difficulty in sitting and walking. An extremely tender, fluctuant, ovoid to spherical mass with surrounding edema and erythema of the labia majora is seen on physical examination. There are usually no systemic symptoms. Bartholin gland abscess requires incision and drainage. The culture of this abscess grew *N. gonorrhoeae* (about 10 to 15% of the time *N. gonorrhoeae* is the causative agent in Bartholin gland abscess).

BOX 4-12. CLINICAL FEATURES OF GONORRHEA IN MALES

Genitourinary infection (most common clinical manifestations):

- Urethritis
  - (1) Incubation period: 2 to 5 days
  - (2) Dysuria, urethral discharge
  - (3) Spread of infection, (prostatitis or epididymitis)
- Prostatitis
  - (1) May be asymptomatic
  - (2) Symptoms: chills, fever, malaise, myalgia, rectal pain and discomfort, lower back pain, lower abdominal pain, suprapubic discomfort
- Epididymitis
  - (1) Seen in 10 to 30% of untreated males
  - (2) Urethral discharge, dysuria
  - (3) Scrotal pain and tenderness
  - (4) Scrotal swelling and erythema
  - (5) Inguinal pain, flank pain (severe cases)
  - (6) Swelling and pain of spermatic cord

BOX 4-13. CLINICAL FEATURES OF GONORRHEA IN FEMALES

- Incubation period: symptoms usually develop within 10 days of exposure.
- Cervicitis
  - (1) Increased vaginal discharge
  - (2) Dyspareunia
  - (3) Friability of cervix
- Urethritis
  - (1) Dysuria, urinary frequency
  - (2) Exudate from urethra
  - (3) Suprapubic pain
- Bartholinitis/Bartholin gland abscess
  - (1) Purulent exudate from gland
  - (2) Labial swelling/pain
- Pelvic inflammatory disease (endometritis, salpingitis)
  - (1) Lower abdominal pain
  - (2) Intermenstrual bleeding or menorrhagia
  - (3) Dyspareunia
  - (4) Cervical motion tenderness or adnexal mass/tenderness
  - (5) Perihepatitis (complication of PID)
  - (6) Tubo-ovarian abscess (complication of PID)

BOX 4-14. CLINICAL FEATURES OF DISSEMINATED GONOCOCCAL INFECTION (DGI)

Arthritis-dermatitis syndrome:

- Arthritis
  (1) Most common systemic complication of gonorrhea
  (2) Usually occurs within 1 month of exposure
  (3) About 25% complain of pain in a single joint
  (4) Up to 75% will have migratory polyarthralgia or tenosynovitis (e.g., extensor and flexor tendons of the hands and feet).
  (5) Most common site of purulent gonococcal arthritis: knee
  (6) All joints including wrist, ankle, metacarpophalangeal joint, hip, and shoulder can be affected.
  (7) About 60% of patients present without a detectable synovial effusion.
  (8) Synovial fluid cultures positive in about 25% of patients.
- Skin lesions
  (1) Second most common systemic complication of gonorrhea
  (2) Rash seen in 50 to 75% of cases with variable clinical presentations.
  (3) Most common: tender erythematous macules, papules, pustules, or vesicles
  (4) Lesions may become hemorrhagic.
  (5) Location: distal portions of the extremities including palms, fingers, and soles
  (6) Gram's stain and cultures usually negative
  (7) Lesions represent septic emboli.
- Other signs and symptoms:
  (1) Fever, chills, and leukocytosis
  (2) Up to 40% or patients are afebrile

BOX 4-15. DIFFERENTIAL DIAGNOSIS OF GONORRHEA

Differential diagnosis of gonococcal arthritis

- Meningococcemia
- Endocarditis
- Infectious arthritis
- Reiter's syndrome
- Ankylosing spondylitis
- Systemic lupus erythematosus
- Drug allergy

Differential diagnosis of gonococcal meningitis

- Meningococcal infection (*gonococcal meningitis may be indistinguishable from meningococcal infection*)

DIAGNOSIS GENITAL HERPES

SYNONYM

Herpes genitalis

Definition and Etiology

1. Genital herpes is caused by a large DNA virus, the herpes simplex virus (HSV), with two serotypes, herpes simplex virus type 1 (HSV-1) and herpes simplex virus type 2 (HSV-2).
2. Approximately 70 to 95% of genital infections are caused by HSV-2.
3. The virus gains entry to the body via mucosal surfaces or abraded skin and replicates in the epidermal and dermal cells of a susceptible host. After replication, the virus spreads via contiguous cells to mucocutaneous projections of sensory nerves.
4. Transmission is through sexual contact, either genital-genital or oral-genital, and by mucosal contact with infected secretions. Viral shedding is highest while genital lesions are present.

Associated Clinical Features

1. Incidence of HSV infection increases rapidly after puberty, reaching a peak in the third decade of life.
2. Asymptomatic viral shedding occurs after resolution of symptoms. Court cases have established that physicians have an obligation to inform their patients about the risk of transmitting HSV during asymptomatic periods.
3. Recurrences are less symptomatic than primary infections and are more likely to cause anxiety and sexual dysfunction. Recurrent herpes, like primary herpes, tends to be more severe in women.
4. Clinical history and examination for typical lesions is important for diagnosis (Fig. 4-18). A history of prior episodes or recent contact with an infected partner is helpful but not necessary to establish a diagnosis.
5. Laboratory diagnosis includes:
   a. Tzanck smear showing multinucleated giant cells (see Fig. 3-49). This test is rapid and inexpensive but its sensitivity ranges from 30 to 80%.
   b. Viral culture is the gold standard and it differentiates between HSV-1 and HSV-2. The sensitivities in various stages are vesicle, 94%; pustule, 87%; ulcer, 70%; crusting, 27%.
   c. An enzyme-linked immunosorbent assay (ELISA) is available, with a sensitivity of 70 to 90%, but it does not differentiate between virus types.
   d. DNA probes and nucleic acid amplification techniques are highly sensitive and specific but not widely available.
   e. Both type-specific and nonspecific antibodies to HSV develop during the first few weeks following infection and persist indefinitely. The sensitivities of these tests for detection of HSV-2 vary from 80 to 90%, and false-negative results may occur, especially at early stages of infection. Because false-negative HSV cultures can occur, especially in patients with recurrent infection or with healing lesions, type-specific serologic tests are useful in confirming a clinical diagnosis of herpes.

Consultation

Social services if sexual abuse is suspected

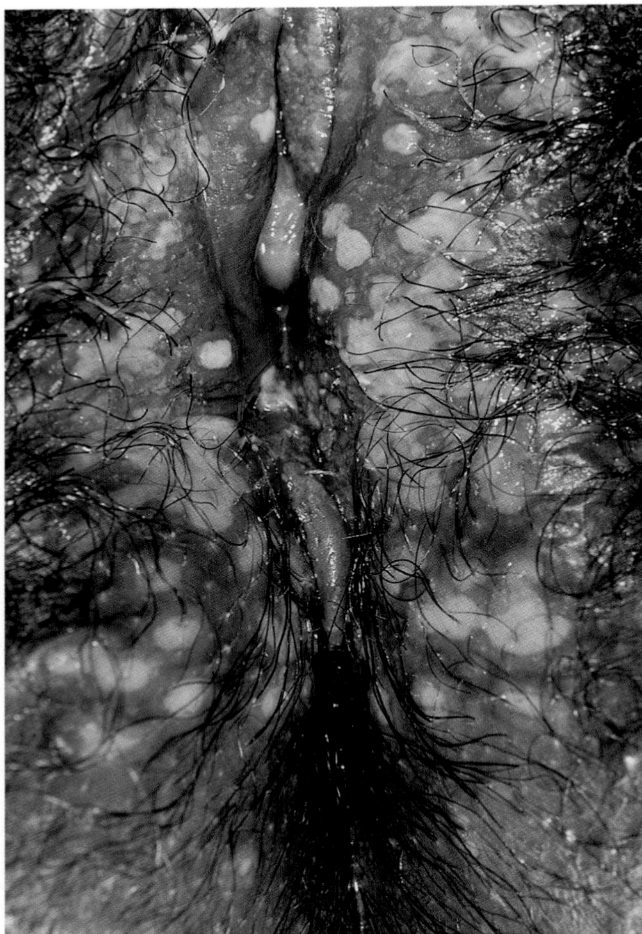

Figure 4-18. Herpetic Vulvovaginitis

A sexually-active adolescent female patient presented with dysuria, urinary retention, and these ulcerated lesions that were surrounded by erythema and edema. Note some of the lesions have coalesced, producing large ulcerated areas and bleeding. This was her first episode of HSV infection.

DIAGNOSIS

ECTOPIC PREGNANCY

SYNONYM

Tubal pregnancy

Definition and Etiology

1. Ectopic pregnancy is the implantation of a fertilized egg in the fallopian tube instead of the endometrium (uterus).
2. The precise cause of ectopic pregnancy is unclear, but several theories such as slowed tubal motility, abnormal or damaged fallopian tubes, defects in the ovum, and endometrial abnormalities have been suggested.

Associated Clinical Features

1. Most common risk factors for tubal abnormalities
   a. Previous tubal infections (e.g., pelvic inflammatory disease)
   b. Previous ectopic pregnancy
   c. Prior tubal surgery
   d. Tubal adhesions from previous appendicitis or abdominopelvic surgery
2. Other risk factors include vaginal douching and smoking (which more than doubles the risk for ectopic pregnancy).
3. Diagnosis of ectopic pregnancy can be evaluated using serial measurement of serum β-human chorionic gonadotropin (β-hCG).
   a. Serum levels of β-hCG should increase by at least 66% every 48 hours in a normal pregnancy within the first 30 days after implantation.
   b. If β-hCG levels are unchanged or increasing more slowly than normal, the pregnancy is abnormal (it may be an abnormal intrauterine pregnancy or it may be an ectopic pregnancy).
   c. Pregnancies that have lower than normal β-hCG levels are more likely to be ectopic.
4. Ectopic pregnancies are diagnosed by transvaginal ultrasound if:
   a. Absence of intrauterine pregnancy and
   b. β-hCG levels are in the so-called discriminatory zone (the accepted β-hCG levels in which an intrauterine pregnancy is first visible on ultrasound).

Consultation

Surgery or obstetrics/gynecology

Emergency Department Treatment and Disposition

1. Ectopic pregnancy is a surgical emergency.
2. Stabilization of vital signs is needed in a patient presenting with circulatory impairment. The patient will require large-bore IV lines and fluid resuscitation.
3. Transfusion may be started if clinically indicated, but surgery should not be delayed by the need to give the patient a transfusion. Often the patient is losing blood internally at a faster rate than it is possible to replace it by transfusion.
4. Emergency surgery is necessary to stop the bleeding and try to preserve at least a portion of the affected fallopian tube, if it is not completely ruptured. An oophorectomy is not indicated unless the ovary is bleeding uncontrollably or has other pathology.
5. In those cases in which an ectopic pregnancy is probable or possible, the work-up and management depends on the woman's risk factors, her serial measurements of serum β-hCG levels, and results of transvaginal ultrasonography over a period of days.
6. A patient with suspected ectopic pregnancy should be followed in consultation with an obstetrician as an outpatient if she is stable (e.g. patient asymptomatic with normal vital signs and normal hematocrit values), and is reliable for outpatient follow-up and monitoring.

Clinical Pearls: Ectopic Pregnancy

1. Ectopic pregnancies must be considered in the differential diagnosis of the pregnant adolescent with pelvic pain, particularly early in gestation if such pain is associated with abnormal uterine spotting or bleeding.
2. Patients with an acutely ruptured ectopic pregnancy present with sudden onset of extreme sharp or stabbing unilateral pain as well as shoulder pain. Other acute symptoms include dizziness or loss of consciousness from acute intraperitoneal hemorrhage.
3. Diagnosis of ectopic pregnancy can be evaluated using serial measurement of serum β-hCG.
4. Ectopic pregnancies are diagnosed by transvaginal ultrasound if there is no intrauterine pregnancy (Fig. 4-23).

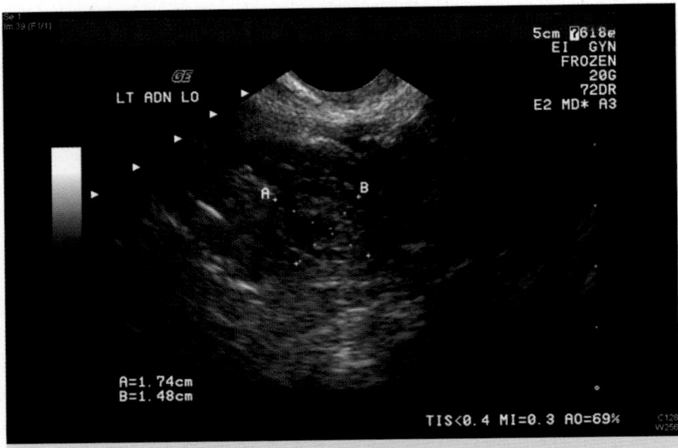

Figure 4-23. Ectopic (Tubal) Pregnancy

A complex heterogenous mass is seen in the left adenexa. With a positive pregnancy test, this is highly suggestive of an ectopic pregnancy.

BOX 4-25. CLINICAL FEATURES OF ECTOPIC PREGNANCY

- Signs and symptoms of acutely ruptured ectopic pregnancy:
  (1) Sudden onset of extreme sharp or stabbing unilateral pain
  (2) Sudden onset of shoulder pain (referred from subdiaphragmatic irritation)
  (3) Other acute signs and symptoms: dizziness or loss of consciousness (due to acute intraperitoneal hemorrhage)
- Abnormal menses (patient may have missed a period and/or experienced abnormal vaginal bleeding or spotting)
- Vague pelvic pain before the onset of acute symptoms
- Pregnancy symptoms (e.g., nausea, vomiting, or other symptoms of early pregnancy)
- Subacute presentations of a probable or possible ectopic pregnancy
  (1) Any pregnant patient with cramping
  (2) Abnormal vaginal spotting or bleeding
  (3) Lower abdominal/adnexal pain or mass

BOX 4-26. DIFFERENTIAL DIAGNOSIS OF ECTOPIC PREGNANCY

- Pelvic inflammatory disease
- Normal intrauterine pregnancy
- Threatened or spontaneous pregnancy
- Appendicitis
- Hemorrhagic corpus luteum cyst
- Torsion of the adnexa (fallopian tube and/or ovary)
- Ruptured ovarian cyst
- Acute gastroenteritis
- Endometriosis
- Diverticulitis

Suggested Readings

American Academy of Pediatrics: Syphilis. In: Pickering LK (ed). *Red Book: 2003 Report of the Committee on Infectious Diseases*, 26th ed. American Academy of Pediatrics, Elk Grove Village, IL, 2003, p. 595.

Centers for Disease Control and Prevention: Sexually transmitted diseases treatment guidelines 2002. *Morb Mortal Wkly Rep* 2002;51:RR-6.

Emans SJ, Laufer MR, Goldstein D (eds). *Pediatric and Adolescent Gynecology*, 4th ed. Lippincott-Raven, Philadelphia, 1998.

Neinstein LS (ed): *Adolescent Health Care: A Practical Guide*, 4th ed. Lippincott Williams & Wilkins, Baltimore, 2002.

CHAPTER 5

CARDIOLOGY

Binita R. Shah
Edited by Sudha M. Rao

DIAGNOSIS ASYSTOLE

Definition

1. Asystole is a *pulseless arrest* associated with absent cardiac electrical activity.
2. Asystole is one of the examples of collapse rhythms (the others being ventricular fibrillation [VF], pulseless ventricular tachycardia [VT], and pulseless electrical activity [PEA]).

Associated Clinical Features

1. All collapse rhythms including asystole are characterized by an absence of signs of circulation.
   a. Absence of *adequate* breathing (there may be agonal breathing)
   b. Absence of central pulses and unobtainable blood pressure
   c. Lack of response to any stimulation
2. Asystole must be confirmed in more than one electrocardiogram (ECG) lead, as artifacts or very subtle VF can be mistaken for asystole.
   a. Suspect asystole with risk factors for hypoxemia/ischemia (e.g., apnea, drowning, trauma).
   b. Suspect VF with prior known risk factors for cardiac disease.
3. ECG findings: absent cardiac electrical activity seen as a flat (straight) line (Fig. 5-1).

Emergency Department Treatment and Disposition

1. Assess, confirm asystole, and begin cardiopulmonary resuscitation (CPR).
2. Support ABCs (airway, breathing, and circulation) including tracheal intubation with 100% O_2 therapy, vascular access, and continuous cardiac and pulse oximetry monitoring.
3. Identify and treat the reversible causes of pulseless arrest.
4. Epinephrine is the drug of choice for asystole.
5. Defibrillation and transthoracic pacing are *not* effective for asystole.
6. With successful resuscitation and postresuscitation stabilization, the patient is transferred to the pediatric intensive care unit (PICU) for subsequent management.
7. With unsuccessful resuscitative outcome:
   a. Family members need to be informed as soon as possible by the heath care provider (usually the most senior physician involved in the resuscitation) with a very caring and concerned attitude. This communication should preferably take place in a private setting and all the questions raised by the family members should be answered honestly and in a language that they can understand (not with complex medical terminology).
   b. If indicated, report the case to the medical examiner for autopsy (e.g., for suspicious deaths or infants/children

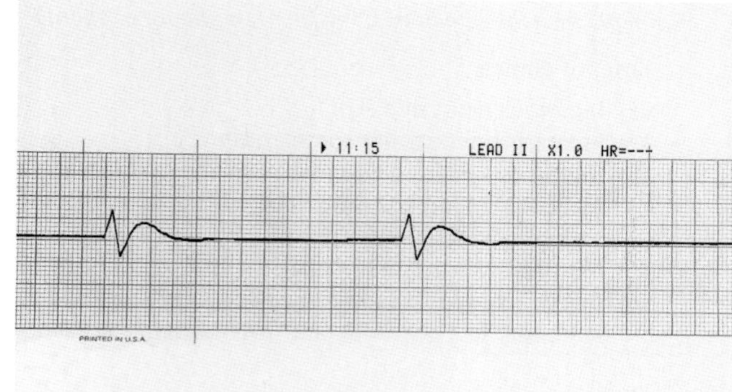

Figure 5-1. Asystole

Terminal agonal rhythm with QRS complex (terminal ventricular activity) followed by asystole (absence of any organized electrical activity [flat line]) is seen on the ECG tracing of a 3-month-old infant who was found unresponsive in the crib. He had absent pulses and no signs of circulation.

presenting with cardiopulmonary arrest without any underlying chronic preexisting conditions [e.g., AIDS or malignancy]).

Clinical Pearls: Asystole

1. Asystole is the most common rhythm seen in infants/children presenting with out-of-hospital arrest.
2. A flat line on ECG can also be caused by a loose ECG lead; *absence of signs of circulation (absent pulse and respiration and lack of response to stimulation) must be confirmed clinically*.
3. Confirm asystole in more than one ECG lead to identify any artifact or subtle VF that can be mistaken for asystole.

BOX 5-1. POTENTIALLY TREATABLE AND REVERSIBLE CAUSES OF PULSELESS ARREST OR COLLAPSE RHYTHMS: ASYSTOLE, PULSELESS ELECTRICAL ACTIVITY, VENTRICULAR FIBRILLATION, AND PULSELESS VENTRICULAR TACHYCARDIA

"H"s and "T"s of CPR

- 8 "H"s
  - (1) Hypoxemia (severe)
  - (2) Hypovolemia (severe)
  - (3) Hypothermia (profound)
  - (4) Hyperkalemia or hypokalemia
  - (5) Hydrogen ion disturbance (severe acidosis)
  - (6) Hypoglycemia
  - (7) Hypocalcemia
  - (8) Hypomagnesemia
- 4 "T"s
  - (1) Tamponade (cardiac)
  - (2) Tension pneumothorax
  - (3) Toxins/poisons/drug overdose:
    - Tricyclic antidepressants
    - Beta-blockers
    - Calcium channel blockers
  - (4) Thromboembolism

(Modified and Reproduced with permission from Hazinski MF et al (eds): PALS Provider Manual. American Heart Association, Dallas, Texas, 2002, p. 189.)

BOX 5-2. DRUG THERAPY OF ASYSTOLE AND PULSELESS ELECTRICAL ACTIVITY

Epinephrine (the queen of CPR [the king being oxygen])

- Drug of choice
  - (1) Increases heart rate (HR)
  - (2) Increases myocardial contractility
  - (3) Increases systemic vascular resistance (SVR)
  - (4) Increases blood pressure (due to increase in SVR and myocardial contractility)
  - (5) Increases cardiac automaticity
  - (6) Increases myocardial oxygen consumption (due to increases in HR, SVR, and myocardial contractility)
  - (7) Increases coronary perfusion pressure
- For intravenous or intraosseous route
  - (1) *Initial* dose: 0.01 mg/kg (0.1 mL/kg) of *1:10,000* dilution
  - (2) *Subsequent* doses: Consider higher doses of 0.1 mg/kg (0.1 mL/kg) of *1:1000* dilution
  - (3) Subsequent doses repeated every 3 to 5 minutes
- For endotracheal route
  - (1) All doses diluted to a minimum volume of 3 to 5 mL for instillation
  - (2) *Initial* dose: 0.1 mg/kg (0.1 mL/kg) of *1:1000* dilution
  - (3) *Subsequent* doses 0.1 mg/kg (0.1 mL/kg) of *1:1000* dilution
  - (4) Subsequent doses repeated every 3 to 5 minutes
- High-dose epinephrine
  - (1) *Not used routinely* (does not improve the outcome)
  - (2) May be considered for special situations that suggest catecholamine-resistant states (e.g., anaphylaxis, drug overdose [alpha- or beta-blockers], patients already receiving high-dose pressors)
  - (3) Dose: 0.1 to 0.2 mg/kg (0.1 to 0.2 mL/kg) of *1:1000* dilution
  - (4) Adverse effects of high-dose epinephrine: increased myocardial oxygen consumption during CPR, post-arrest hyperadrenergic state with post-arrest myocardial dysfunction

BOX 5-3. DIFFERENTIAL DIAGNOSIS OF ASYSTOLE

- Loose ECG lead leading to artifact (flat line)
- Very subtle VF

DIAGNOSIS PULSELESS ELECTRICAL ACTIVITY

SYNONYM

Electromechanical dissociation

Definition

1. Pulseless electrical activity (PEA) is a rhythmic display of electrical activity (other than ventricular fibrillation [VF] or pulseless ventricular tachycardia [VT]) *without* a palpable arterial pulse.
2. PEA is an example of a collapse rhythm (the others being asystole, VF, and pulseless VT).

Associated Clinical Features

1. All collapse rhythms including PEA are characterized by an absence of signs of circulation.
   a. Absence of *adequate* breathing (there may be agonal breathing)
   b. Absence of central pulses and unobtainable blood pressure
   c. Lack of response to stimulation
2. It is important to identify treatable (and thus reversible) causes of PEA. Such etiologies (see Box 5-1) should be suspected based on the preceding events that led to cardiopulmonary failure/arrest. Examples include:
   a. Severe hypovolemia
      1) Suspect in patients with a history of volume loss (e.g., diarrhea, vomiting, or blood loss)
      2) Suspect in patients who presented with signs of moderate to severe dehydration
   b. Tension pneumothorax (the diagnosis must be established by physical examination [*without a preliminary chest radiograph*] prompted by a high index of suspicion).
      1) Suspect in ventilated patients receiving high inspiratory volumes under positive pressure to potentially injured lung parenchyma
      2) Suspect with asymmetrical chest wall movement (affected side versus normal side)
      3) Suspect with absent breath sounds (affected side)
      4) Suspect with tracheal deviation (opposite side)
      5) Suspect with distended neck veins
      6) Suspect with hyperresonance (affected side)
   c. Cardiac tamponade
      1) Suspect with penetrating or crush injuries, placement of a central venous catheter, and after cardiac catheterization or open heart surgery
      2) Suspect with the diagnostic triad of shock, distended neck veins (with massive hepatomegaly), and muffled heart sounds

Emergency Department Treatment and Disposition

1. Begin cardiopulmonary resuscitation as for asystole (see Box 5.2).
2. Identify and correct reversible causes of PEA. (*Important:* Many cases of PEA involve obstruction of venous return to the heart [obstructive shock] or hypovolemia.)
   a. Hypovolemia: volume expansion (20 mL/kg of crystalloid infusion and repeat as indicated)
   b. Tension pneumothorax: needle decompression followed by tube thoracostomy (Fig. 5-2)
   c. Cardiac tamponade: large fluid bolus *and* pericardiocentesis
   d. Specific antidote for ingestions leading to PEA
3. Use of drug therapy (epinephrine) is the same as for asystole (see Box 5-2).

Clinical Pearls: Pulseless Electrical Activity

1. PEA is reversible if the underlying cause is identified early and treated appropriately (see Box 5-1).
2. PEA quickly degenerates into asystole or an agonal ventricular rhythm if not treated emergently.

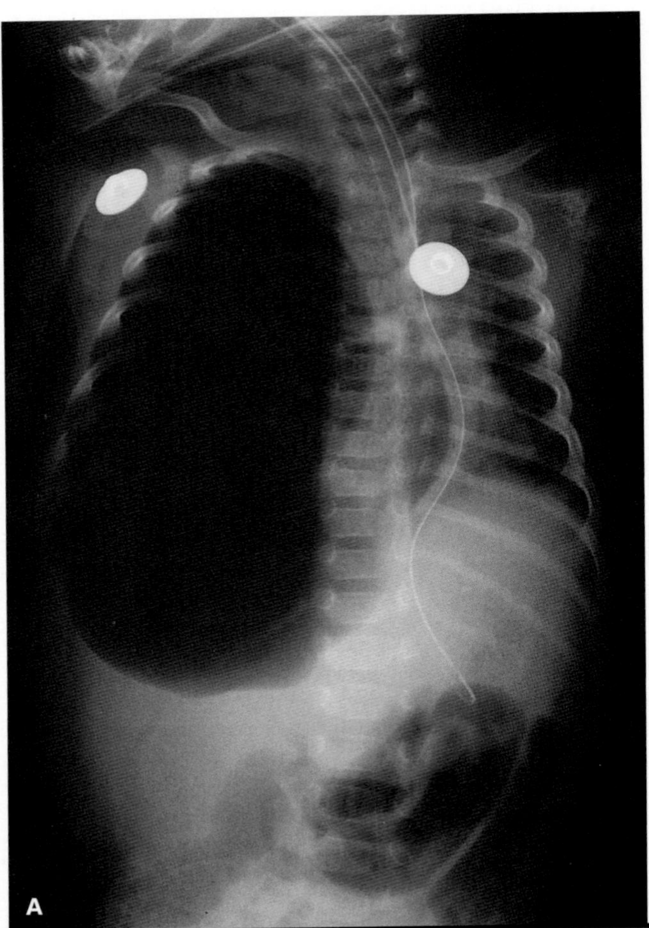

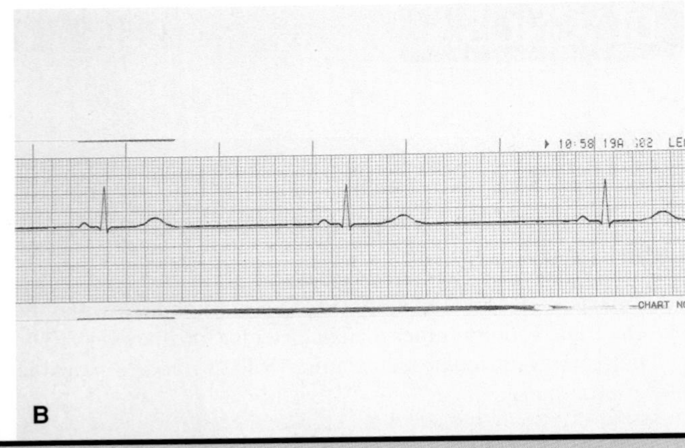

Figure 5-2. Tension Pneumothorax: A Treatable Cause of Pulseless Electrical Activity

A. A 4-month-old infant was brought to the ED in cardiopulmonary arrest (the patient was being bagged with 100% oxygen and receiving chest compressions upon admission). He had diminished breath sounds on the right side. Electrical activity was seen on the monitor but there were no palpable pulses (PEA). CPR was continued (including intubation), and several rounds of epinephrine were given with no response. Tension pneumothorax was not recognized prior to his death, and was recognized only on the postmortem radiograph. The only physical findings were a bruise on the lower eyelid and bilateral retinal hemorrhages. At autopsy he was found to have bilateral subdural hematomas. Subsequently the mother confessed to shaking him violently because he would not stop crying. *B.* Rhythmic display of organized electrical activity was seen on the monitor, but the patient had absent palpable arterial pulses and signs of perfusion. (*Important: Always consider treatable or reversible causes of PEA.*)

DIAGNOSIS BRADYCARDIA

Definition

1. Bradycardia is defined as a heart rate below the normal range for age (see Box 5-4).
2. Clinically significant bradycardia is defined as a heart rate <60 beats per minute (bpm) associated with poor systemic perfusion (Fig. 5-3).

Associated Clinical Features

1. Signs of circulatory impairment (poor end-organ perfusion) include:
   a. Skin perfusion: color pale, cyanotic, or mottled, cool extremities, prolonged capillary refill
   b. Peripheral pulses: thready, weak, or absent
   c. Discrepancy in volume between peripheral and central pulses
   d. CNS: irritable, lethargic, confused, or decreased level of consciousness
   e. Diminished response to pain
   f. Respiratory difficulty
   g. Decreased pulse pressure of >20 mmHg
   h. Hypotension (decompensated shock)
   i. Decreased or no urine output

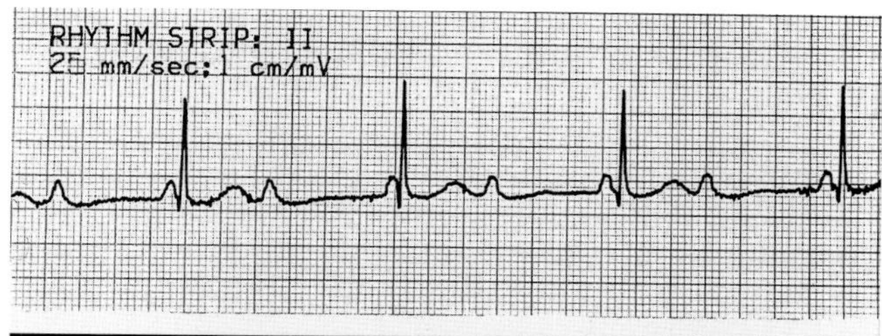

Figure 5-6. Third-Degree (Complete) Heart Block

CHB seen in a 5-month-old infant born to a mother with SLE. The mother was asymptomatic at the time of birth of this infant, and her diagnosis was entertained only after the diagnosis of CHB in the infant.

BOX 5-13. THIRD-DEGREE ATRIOVENTRICULAR HEART BLOCK

Characteristic features:

- Failure of conduction of atrial impulses to the ventricles
- AV dissociation (the atria and ventricles beat *completely independently* and P waves and QRS complexes have *no* constant relationship)
- The ventricles are paced by an escape pacemaker at a rate slower than the atrial rate.
- The QRS duration may be prolonged or may be normal if the heartbeat is initiated high in the bundle of His (generally, the lower the location of the pacemaker within the ventricular conduction system, the slower the heart rate and the wider the QRS complexes).

BOX 5-14. ETIOLOGY OF THIRD-DEGREE ATRIOVENTRICULAR BLOCK

Some examples of congenital or acquired diseases leading to complete heart block include:

- Infants born to mothers with systemic lupus erythematosus (SLE), rheumatoid arthritis, dermatomyositis, or Sjögren's syndrome (autoimmune destruction of AV tracts by maternally-derived IgG antibodies)
- Complex congenital heart anomaly (e.g., common AV canal)
- Abnormal embryonic development of the conduction system
- Postsurgical repair of congenital heart disease involving the ventricular septum
- Myocarditis
- Long QT syndrome
- Lyme disease (87% incidence of AV block in patients with carditis with Lyme disease)
- Digoxin toxicity
- Myocardial tumors
- Myocardial abscess due to endocarditis

DIAGNOSIS LONG QT SYNDROME

SYNONYM

Prolonged QT syndrome

Definition

1. Long QT syndrome (LQTS) is characterized by a pathologically prolonged corrected QT interval.
2. The corrected QT interval (QTc) is calculated using the formula shown in Box 5-15.

Associated Clinical Features

1. The condition may be acquired, but more often is congenital and inherited (Box 5-16; Fig. 5-7). Several genes have been identified and the genotype influences the clinical course (e.g., the risk of arrhythmia is significantly higher among those who have mutations at the LQT1 or LQT2 locus, and the percentage of lethal cardiac events is significantly higher with mutations at the LQT3 locus).

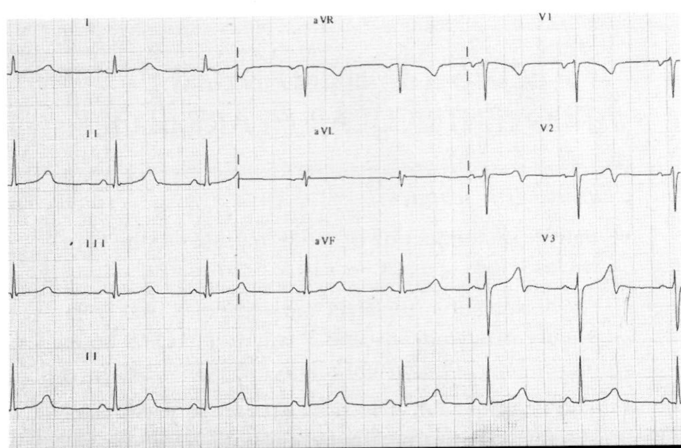

Figure 5-7. Long QT Syndrome

A QT interval of 0.48 seconds is seen in a 10-year-old patient presenting with syncope following exercise. This patient had two prior episodes of syncope, but never had an ECG performed for evaluation of his syncope. His family history was positive for heart disease (his father died an unexplained death at 35 years of age); his family history was negative for deafness. (*Important: ECG and a thorough family history are important elements of evaluation of syncope in the ED.*)

2. Prolongation of the QTc interval results from a prolongation of the refractory period of the myocardium (during which the atrium is still firing at its regular pace), leading to torsades de pointes ("R-on-T phenomenon"; a malignant form of ventricular tachycardia [VT]).
3. Common presenting signs and symptoms of LQTS include:
   a. Syncope or presyncope (about 26% of cases)
      1) May have recurrent episodes
      2) Often precipitated by exercise, fright, or being startled
   b. Seizures (about 10% of cases)
   c. Palpitations
   d. Episodes of paroxysmal VT
      1) VT often has torsades de pointes morphology
      2) VT can progress to ventricular fibrillation and sudden death
      3) Precipitating factors: stress, emotional lability
   e. Cardiac arrest (about 10% of cases)
   f. Incidental ECG finding
4. Family history may be positive for:
   a. Occurrence of sudden death in young relatives
   b. Syncope with exercise or emotional stress
   c. Seizures
   d. Arrhythmias
   e. Hearing impairment
5. *Patients with LQTS may have a normal ECG in the ED.* Other ECG features include low heart rate for age, notched T waves and T-wave alternans. Presence of other family members with LQTS, stress testing (exertional LQTS), or 24-hour Holter monitoring (intermittent LQTS) may help in arriving at the final diagnosis.
6. LQTS in association with hypertrophic cardiomyopathy accounts for up to half of the cases of sudden cardiac death.

Consultation

Cardiology

Emergency Department Treatment and Disposition

1. Treatment of VT associated with LQTS:
   a. Support airway, breathing, and circulation (ABCs) and provide oxygen and ventilation as needed.
   b. Lidocaine: 1 mg/kg per dose via intravenous bolus (IV) *or*
   c. Amiodarone: 5 mg/kg per dose IV over 20 to 60 minutes *or*
   d. Procainamide: 15 mg/kg per dose IV over 30 to 60 minutes
   e. If the above medical therapy fails:
      1) Synchronized cardioversion for stable patients with VT with palpable pulses (for details, see page 220)
      2) Defibrillation for patients with pulseless VT (for details, see Box 5-29)
2. Long-term goals of therapy of LQTS:
   a. Beta-blockade (propranolol is drug of choice)
      1) To prevent VT from progressing to ventricular fibrillation and sudden death
      2) Blunt heart rate response to exercise
      3) Therapy continued for life
   b. A pacemaker may be required in some patients to overcome profound bradycardia (a common association).
   c. Exercise restriction
   d. Avoid drugs that are known to cause prolongation of the QT interval (see Box 5-16).
   e. Teach parents cardiopulmonary resuscitation (as exercise restriction and drug therapy may be ineffective for some children).
   f. An implantable cardioverter-defibrillator may be considered in patients with continued episodes of syncope in spite of therapy, and in those with a prior history of cardiac arrest.

Clinical Pearls: Long QT Syndrome

1. *Patients with LQTS may have a normal ECG in the ED.*
2. Congenital long QT syndrome results in a mortality rate in excess of 90% if not diagnosed and properly treated.
3. Children with LQTS are predisposed to episodic ventricular arrhythmias, torsades de pointes, syncope, and generalized seizures.
4. Patients with LQTS may develop fatal ventricular arrhythmias, especially if exposed to some medications such as antihistamines, macrolide antibiotics, phenothiazines, or cisapride (see Box 5-16).

5. All family members of a patient with LQTS should undergo a 12-lead ECG (and cardiac evaluation as indicated).
6. Any patient presenting with VT (especially torsades de pointes or a polymorphic type) should have a corrected QT interval determined while in sinus rhythm.

BOX 5-15. THE QTc INTERVAL

- Formula (Bazett's equation) for calculating the corrected QT interval:

$$QTc = \frac{QTm}{\sqrt{R\text{-}R}}$$

  where QTc = corrected QT interval in seconds; QTm = measured QT interval in seconds; and R-R = interval between previous two consecutive R waves on the ECG in seconds
- Normally the QT interval is heart-rate dependent
- The above formula corrects the measured QT interval to a heart rate of 60 bpm, at which the normal R-R interval is 1 second. Since the square root of 1 = 1, the QTc equals the QTm at a heart rate of 60 bpm, with a normal QT interval range of 0.35 to 0.44 second.
- Pronged QT interval: any QTc >0.44 seconds
- Longer QTc is associated with a higher risk of symptoms (most patients with LQTS have a QTc >0.5 second)
- The QT interval normally shortens with exercise.
- In patients with LQTS, the QT interval does not shorten appropriately with exercise.

BOX 5-16. ETIOLOGY OF PROLONGED QT INTERVAL

Congenital (about 50% of cases):

- Two clinical syndromes with LQTS (in the absence of structural heart disease):
  (1) Romano-Ward syndrome: autosomal dominant inheritance *without* deafness
  (2) Jervell and Lange-Nielsen syndrome: autosomal recessive inheritance *with* sensorineural deafness

Acquired:

- Heart disease
  (1) Myocarditis
  (2) Mitral valve prolapse
- Electrolyte abnormalities
  (1) Hypokalemia
  (2) Hypocalcemia
  (3) Hypomagnesemia
- Medications
  (1) Tricyclic antidepressants (e.g., imipramine, amitriptyline, desipramine, nortriptyline)
  (2) Phenothiazines (e.g., thioridazine, pimozide)
  (3) Other psychotropic drugs (e.g., haloperidol, risperidone, lithium carbonate)
  (4) Gastrointestinal prokinetics (e.g., cisapride)
  (5) Antihistamines (e.g., diphenhydramine, terfenadine, astemizole)
  (6) Antiarrhythmics (e.g., quinidine, procainamide, amiodarone)
  (7) Antibiotics (e.g., trimethoprim, erythromycin, clarithromycin, azithromycin, sulfamethoxazole)
  (8) Antifungals (e.g., fluconazole, ketoconazole)
  (9) Epinephrine
- Other
  (1) CNS pathology
  (2) Ischemia
  (3) Anorexia/bulimia

DIAGNOSIS SYNCOPE

Synonym

Fainting spell

Definition

Syncope is a sudden and brief loss of consciousness accompanied by a loss of postural tone, from which recovery is spontaneous. All forms of syncope result from a sudden decrease or brief cessation of cerebral blood flow.

Associated Clinical Features

1. Vasovagal syncope (synonyms: neurocardiogenic syncope, neurally-mediated syncope, vasodepressor syncope, fainting spell)
    a. Largest group of disorders causing syncope
    b. Examples: emotional fainting, situational syncope (e.g., in response to cough [cough syncope], micturition, or defecation), syncope with panic, syncope associated with exercise in athletes *without heart disease*
    c. Usually seen in adolescents
    d. Most episodes occur after prolonged standing (e.g., crowded, warm environment), or with noxious stimuli, strong emotions, or fatigue.
2. Orthostatic syncope
    a. Most episodes occur while the patient is standing or during a rapid change from a supine or sitting position to standing.
    b. Orthostatic blood pressure (BP) should be measured 3 minutes after the patient stands up following a supine period of 5 minutes (orthostatic changes present if BP changes >15 mmHg and HR changes >10 bpm).
    c. Predisposing events: dehydration, acute blood loss, vasodilator drugs
3. Cardiac syncope (Box 5-18)
    a. Results from hypoxemia due to cyanotic heart disease or decreased cardiac output secondary to arrhythmia, obstructive lesion, or myocardial dysfunction
    b. Syncope occurs during physical exertion (e.g., long QT syndrome; see Fig. 5.7).
    c. Syncope occurs suddenly without warning.
4. Breath-holding spell
    a. Most commonly seen between 1 and 5 years of age (peaks around 2 years of age)
    b. Resolves spontaneously by school age
    c. Types: cyanotic type (about 80%) and pallid type (about 20%)
    d. Provoking events: pain, anger, frustration
    e. Vigorous crying followed by forced expiration, apnea (breath-holding spell), and unconsciousness
    f. Occurs due to decreased cardiac output
    g. Generalized clonic jerks, opisthotonus, and bradycardia may occur; incontinence absent
    h. Normal physical examination (including cardiac and neurological)
5. Routine basic laboratory tests (e.g., CBC, electrolytes, glucose) are rarely helpful. Additional tests are guided by the history and examination (e.g., toxicology screen, carboxyhemoglobin, tilt table testing for patients with orthostatic syncope). Pregnancy should be excluded in adolescent girls.
6. A 12-lead ECG (with rhythm strip) is recommended in all patients (in spite of its low yield) because findings can lead to specific therapy (e.g., pacemaker for complete heart block [see Fig. 5-6], beta-blocker for long QT syndrome [see Fig. 5-7]).
7. Arrhythmias that lead to syncope may not be present during ED evaluation. The patient may need 24-hour Holter monitoring if indicated based on the history or examination.

Consultations

1. Cardiology (if cardiac syncope is likely based on history, examination, or abnormal ECG findings, or syncope is associated with chest pain, arrhythmias, or palpitations, or if there is a family history of sudden death)
2. Neurology (if seizures cannot be excluded based on the history and examination, or if there is a neurological abnormality found on focal neurological examination)

Emergency Department Treatment and Disposition

1. Determine the degree of hemodynamic stability including orthostatic BP and HR measurements.
2. Specific treatment of syncope depends on the underlying etiology (e.g., structural cardiac disease, long QT syndrome).
3. Vasovagal syncope
    a. Reassurance and education about the benign nature of syncope
    b. Identify and avoid precipitating factors (e.g., dehydration, ensure intake of salty foods during intense physical activity).
    c. Learn to recognize prodromal symptoms and assume a sitting or supine position with elevation of the feet.
    d. Rare patients with severe vasovagal episodes that fail to respond to simple measures may need beta-blocker therapy (e.g., propranolol; reduces stimulation of cardiac mechanoreceptors) or transdermal scopolamine (reduces vagal tone).
4. Orthostatic syncope
    a. Appropriate fluid therapy in patients with volume depletion

   b. Encourage patients to get up slowly after lying or sitting.
   c. Discontinue or reduce the dose of any medication that may be responsible for orthostasis.

5. Indications for admission of patients presenting with syncope:
   a. Recurrent syncope (undetermined etiology)
   b. Cardiac syncope (e.g., prolonged QT interval, tachyarrhythmia, or symptoms suggestive of arrhythmias [e.g., syncope associated with palpitations, exertional syncope], atrioventricular block, valvular or congenital heart disease (Fig. 5-8), pacemaker malfunction, congestive heart failure, cyanotic spells)

Clinical Pearls: Syncope

1. Syncope is a symptom, not a disease.
2. A thorough history and physical examination are essential for the evaluation of syncope and may lead to or suggest a diagnosis that can be evaluated with directed testing.
3. Vasovagal syncope is the most common cause of fainting in children and adolescents, and accounts for greater than 50% of cases of childhood syncope.
4. Distinguishing syncope from seizure can be difficult (Box 5-17).
5. Dizziness, vertigo, and presyncope do not result in loss of consciousness or postural tone.

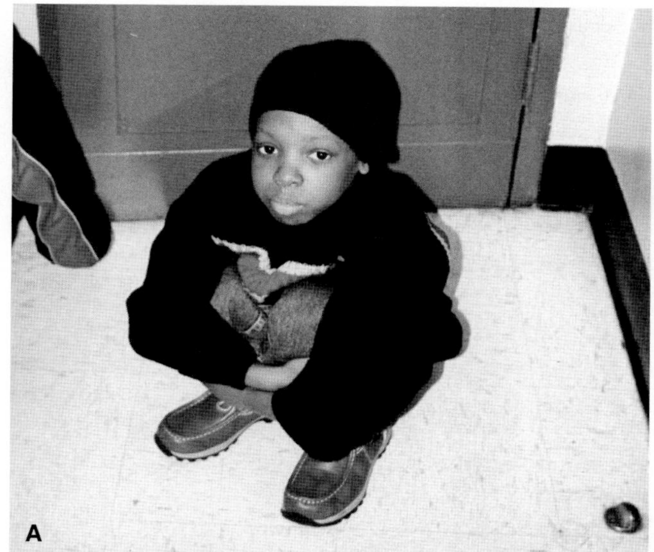

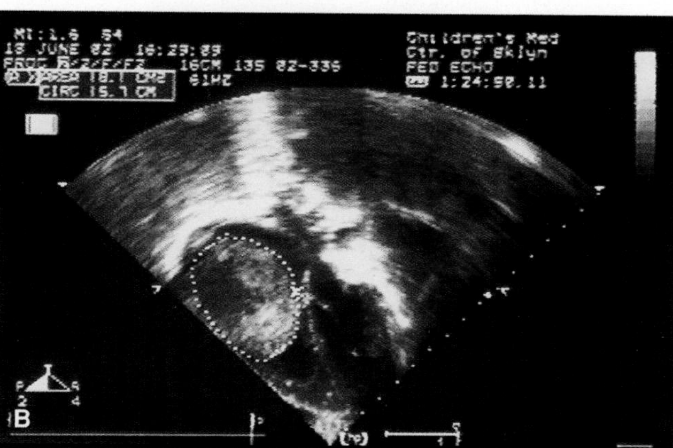

Figure 5-8. Right Atrial Mass Obstructing Right Ventricular Inflow Tract

A. Squatting position assumed by the patient in the ED while "feeling tired" after coming back from the radiology department. This 10-year-old previously healthy boy presented with syncope and weakness, increasing tiredness, and shortness of breath of 2 weeks' duration. His vital signs showed hypotension with blood pressure of 87/63 mmHg (*Remember:* the median [50th percentile] systolic BP for children older than 1 year is 90 + [2 × age in years], and the lower limit [5th percentile] is 70 + [2 × age in years]). His heart rate was 90 bpm and cardiac examination was normal, except for hepatomegaly and prominent hepatojugular reflux. His ECG showed right atrial enlargement and his chest radiograph showed mild cardiomegaly. *B*. Right atrial mass obstructing right ventricular inflow tract is seen on echocardiography. This mass, measuring 6.5 × 5.5 × 4 cm, was resected and was found to be precursor B lymphoblastic lymphoma/leukemia (localized intracardiac lymphoblastic lymphoma; he is currently being treated with chemotherapy).

BOX 5-17. DIFFERENTIAL DIAGNOSIS: SYNCOPE VERSUS SEIZURES

	Syncope	*Seizures*
Precipitants of episodes: Pain, exercise, stressful event, micturition, defecation	Usually present	Absent
Symptoms before or during episode	Sweating, nausea, feeling of "passing out"	Aura may be present
Disorientation after event	Absent	Present
Slowness in regaining consciousness	Absent	Present
Confusion on awakening	Absent or mild	Marked
Period of unconsciousness	Usually seconds	Minutes or longer
Unconsciousness >5 minutes	Absent	May be present
Rhythmic movements: Tonic-clonic movements, myoclonic jerks	Occasionally seen	Commonly seen
Incontinence during episode	Absent	May be present
Electroencephalogram	Normal	May be abnormal

BOX 5-18. ETIOLOGY OF SYNCOPE

Cardiac syncope (cardiac lesions producing syncope):

- Tetralogy of Fallot
- Long QT syndrome
- Hypertrophic cardiomyopathy
- Valvular heart disease
  (1) Critical aortic stenosis
  (2) Tricuspid stenosis
  (3) Mitral stenosis
- Bradydysrhythmia
  (1) Sick sinus syndrome
  (2) Heart block (second- and third-degree)
  (3) Pacemaker malfunction
- Tachydysrhythmia
  (1) Ventricular tachycardia
  (2) Supraventricular tachycardia
  (3) Torsades de pointes
- Pericardial disease
- Myocardial ischemia/infarction
- Myxoma
- Aortic dissection
- Pulmonary embolism
- Pulmonary hypertension

Noncardiac syncope:

- Autonomic dysfunction
  (1) Vasovagal
  (2) Orthostatic
  (3) Breath-holding spell
  (4) Situational (cough, micturition)
- Metabolic (e.g., hypoglycemia)
- Hypoxia
- Carbon monoxide poisoning
- Neuropsychiatric syncope
  (1) Hyperventilation syndrome
  (2) Atonic seizures (drop attacks)
  (3) Hysterical syncope

DIAGNOSIS SINUS TACHYCARDIA

Definition

1. Sinus tachycardia (ST) is defined as a rate of sinus node discharge that is higher than normal for the patient's age (see Box 5-4).
2. The usual upper limit of ST in infants and young children (up to 5 years old) is a heart rate up to 200 bpm. The upper limit of ST in older children is a heart rate up to 180 bpm.

Associated Clinical Features

1. Tachycardia is a physiological response to the body's need for increased cardiac output (CO) or oxygen delivery (tachycardia is the first sign of hypovolemia: CO = SV × HR; thus to maintain cardiac output, a compensatory increase in HR occurs, as the child's ability to increase stroke volume [SV] is limited).
2. ST is a nonspecific sign of an underlying condition rather than a true arrhythmia.
3. Electrocardiogram
   a. All P waves are normal in configuration (upright in lead II).
   b. All QRS complexes are preceded by a P wave.
   c. P-, QRS-, and T-wave morphology are normal.

Emergency Department Treatment and Disposition

1. Continuous cardiac and pulse oximetry monitoring helps when monitoring patients presenting with ST that is near the range of supraventricular tachycardia (SVT) (e.g., HR approaching 200 bpm; Fig. 5-9).
2. Treatment of ST involves treatment of the underlying cause:
   a. Antipyretics for fever
   b. Oxygen therapy for hypoxia
   c. Fluid therapy for hypovolemia
   d. Pain management
3. Do not attempt to decrease the heart rate by pharmacologic or electrical intervention. ST usually resolves once the stressor ceases. The heart rate will return to normal levels with appropriate treatment of the underlying cause.

Clinical Pearls: Sinus Tachycardia

1. ST is the most common rhythm disturbance in children.
2. Treatment of ST involves treatment of the underlying cause.
3. Persistent ST without an apparent inciting cause may be indicative of occult cardiac disease (e.g., myocarditis) or an unrecognized noncardiac condition (e.g., hypovolemia).

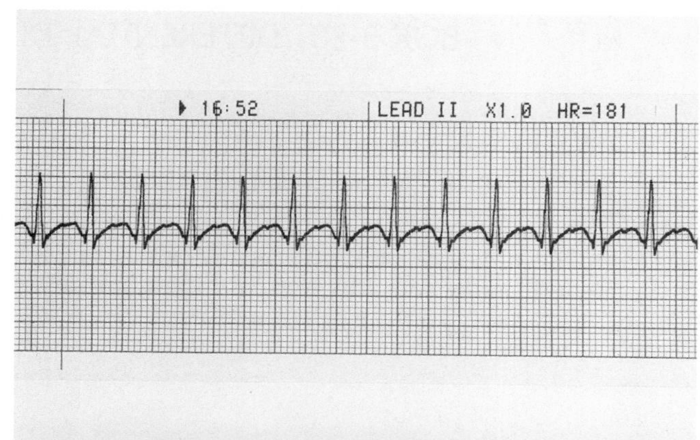

Figure 5-9. Sinus Tachycardia

A heart rate of 187 bpm was seen in an 8-month-old infant with fever and several episodes of vomiting and diarrhea. In ST, even though there may be some variation in the R-R interval, there is a constant PR interval with a normal P-QRS-T–wave sequence. The P-wave axis is normal (i.e., the P waves are normal in configuration) and the QRS duration is normal (<0.08 second). This patient's heart rate decreased to 120 bpm after reduction of fever and rehydration.

BOX 5-19. ETIOLOGY OF SINUS TACHYCARDIA

- *Common causes of ST:*
  (1) Fever
  (2) Crying
  (3) Anxiety
  (4) Exercise
  (5) Pain
- *Serious causes of ST:*
  (1) Hypovolemia
  (2) Hypoxia
  (3) Sepsis
  (4) Anemia
  (5) Toxins and drugs (e.g., amphetamines, antihistamines, atropine/anticholinergics, cocaine, phencyclidine, tricyclic antidepressants, ephedrine/pseudoephedrine, theophylline, iron, organophosphates, thyroxine, carbon monoxide and cyanide poisoning)
  (6) Myocarditis
  (7) Hyperthyroidism/thyroid storm
  (8) Pericardial tamponade
  (9) Tension pneumothorax

BOX 5-20. DIFFERENTIAL DIAGNOSIS: SINUS TACHYCARDIA

Sinus tachycardia (ST) versus supraventricular tachycardia (SVT; see Box 5-21)

- Sometimes it is difficult to differentiate between the two.
- Beat-to-beat variation is seen in ST, but not in SVT (e.g., HR varies with activity in ST, but not in SVT).
- Infants
  (1) HR >220 bpm = probable SVT
  (2) HR <200 bpm = ST
- Children
  (1) HR >180 bpm = probable SVT
  (2) HR <180 bpm = ST

DIAGNOSIS SUPRAVENTRICULAR TACHYCARDIA

SYNONYM

Paroxysmal atrial tachycardia

Definition

1. Supraventricular tachycardia (SVT) is defined as:
   a. Heart rate in infants and young children >220 bpm (range: 220 to 320 bpm; Fig. 5-10)
   b. Heart rate in older children >180 bpm (range: 180 to 250 bpm)
2. SVT is the most common dysrhythmia seen in the pediatric age group.

Etiology

1. SVT is most commonly caused by a reentry mechanism involving atrioventricular [AV] nodal reentry, accessory pathways, or increased automaticity.
2. SVT due to accessory pathway conduction (e.g., Wolff-Parkinson-White syndrome [WPW syndrome]) is the predominant mechanism in the fetus and young infant. AV nodal reentry typically appears in 5- to 10-year-old children, and is the predominant mechanism in adults.
3. Primary atrial tachycardia (e.g., atrial flutter or fibrillation) accounts for 10 to 15% of SVT at all ages.
4. Associated structural heart disease (e.g., Ebstein's anomaly, corrected transposition of the aorta) is present in about 20% of cases.
5. Other etiologies include drugs (e.g., cold medications containing sympathomimetics), hyperthyroidism, myocarditis, cardiomyopathy, or infections.

Associated Clinical Features

1. Usual presentation:
   a. Infants usually present with nonspecific symptoms of poor feeding, irritability, or restlessness.

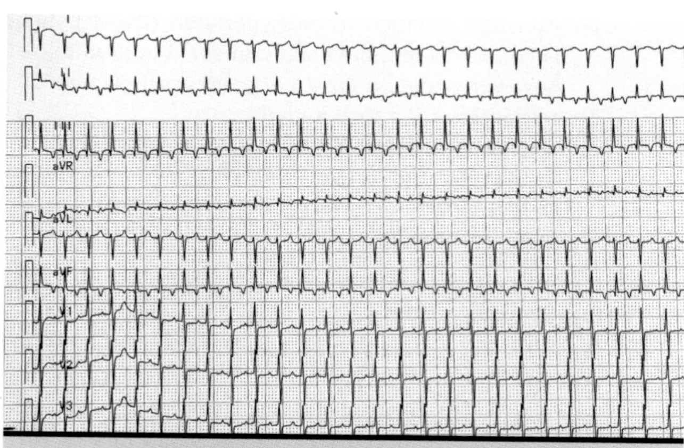

Figure 5-10. Supraventricular Tachycardia

A ventricular rate of 250 bpm with a narrow QRS complex in a 12-day-old neonate who presented with poor feeding and irritability of several hours' duration. The patient had good capillary refill and peripheral perfusion with a BP of 104/73. The patient received one dose of IV adenosine followed by conversion to regular sinus rhythm.

b. If SVT persists for many hours at rapid rates, signs of congestive heart failure (e.g., tachypnea, tachycardia, hepatomegaly) or cardiogenic shock/cardiovascular collapse (e.g., an acutely ill infant with prolonged capillary refill, thready pulses, poor tissue perfusion, ashen color, and metabolic acidosis) develop.
c. About 20% of infants may be completely asymptomatic and SVT may be detected during a routine examination.
d. Older children may present with pounding or racing heartbeat, dizziness, diaphoresis, or tiredness.
e. Episodes of SVT are often paroxysmal; older children may give a history of episodes of a racing heartbeat that starts and stops suddenly.
f. Chest pain is not a usual presenting symptom of SVT.

2. Clinically the heart rate may be too rapid to count.
3. Most common age at presentation:
   a. Most first episodes of childhood SVT occur in the first 2 months of life.
   b. About 60% of cases: infants <4 months of age
   c. About 80% of cases: infants <12 months of age
4. Electrocardiography is required to confirm the diagnosis:
   a. P waves may not be visible (obscured by the ST segment).
   b. QRS complex
      1) Narrow QRS complex in 90% of cases
      2) Wide QRS complex in 10% of cases (aberrant SVT)
   c. With persistent tachycardia, ST- and T-wave changes consistent with myocardial ischemia may be seen.
   d. Features of WPW syndrome may be seen once the episode of SVT terminates, and may include a short PR interval, a delta wave (slow upstroke of QRS complex), and a wide QRS complex.
5. A chest radiograph may show the presence of cardiomegaly, suggesting CHF or underlying structural heart disease.

Consultation

Cardiology consultation (*once the patient is stabilized*) for:

1. Echocardiography in patents with a first episode of SVT (to rule out associated structural heart disease)
2. Beginning chronic maintenance therapy (e.g., digoxin, propranolol, procainamide, or amiodarone) as indicated in patients with either a first episode or recurrent episodes of SVT
3. Possible electrophysiology testing and radiofrequency catheter ablation for patients with refractory SVT, those requiring multiple medications, or those with undesirable side effects from medications

Emergency Department Treatment and Disposition

1. Evaluation of the hemodynamic status and stabilization as indicated; high-flow oxygen, continuous cardiac, blood pressure, and pulse oximetry monitoring
2. SVT without circulatory compromise (stable patient):
   a. Vagal maneuvers that heighten the vagal tone to the AV node
      1) Diving reflex: application of an ice bag to the face in infants or submersion of the face in ice cold water in older children (*Caution: Application of ice to infants should be brief [10 to 20 seconds max], and a cloth or plastic barrier should be used to avoid the occurrence of fat necrosis. Avoid repeated applications of ice to the same location.*)
      2) Valsalva maneuver: Ask the patient to strain as if attempting straining at stool.
      3) Unilateral carotid massage: Massage at the junction of the carotid artery and the mandible.
      4) Ocular pressure should not be used (due to the risk of retinal detachment).
   b. Adenosine (Box 5-22; Figs. 5-11 and 5-12)
   c. Verapamil
      1) Do not use in infants <1 year of age (life-threatening side effects include profound bradycardia, hypotension, and cardiac arrest).

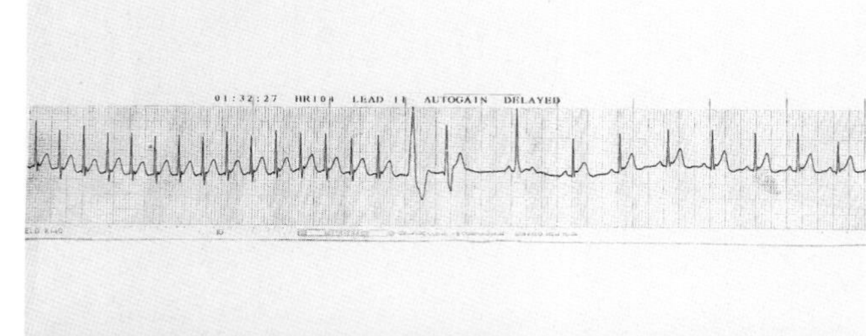

Figure 5-11. Supraventricular Tachycardia

Following one dose of IV adenosine, an abrupt change from SVT to one premature ventricular contraction followed by sinus rhythm is seen.

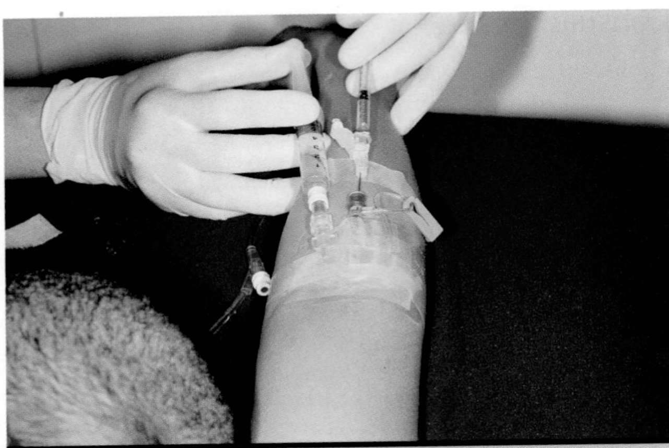

Figure 5-12. Two-Hand/Two-Syringe Technique for Administration of Adenosine

Because of its extremely short half-life, adenosine must be given as a *rapid* IV bolus (inject in 1 to 3 seconds to maximize the concentration that reaches the heart). While maintaining pressure on the plunger of the syringe containing the adenosine, *simultaneously* inject a rapid bolus of 3 to 5 mL of normal saline to accelerate delivery to the heart. Injection should be made close to the hub of the catheter, so that it is done closest to the patient. Intravenous tubing above the injection port should be clamped before the adenosine/normal saline push, and it should be unclamped after the injection.

2) Do not use in children with CHF, myocardial depression, or those receiving beta-blockers.

3. SVT with circulatory compromise or severe CHF (unstable patient with shock, acidosis):
   a. Adenosine (Box 5-22) if immediate vascular access is available
   b. Synchronized cardioversion (synchronization of the delivered energy with the ECG reduces the possibility of inducing VF, which can occur if the energy is delivered during the relative refractory period of the ventricle)
      1) Consider sedation in older children (if the patient is conscious and time and clinical condition allow; however, sedation *must not* delay cardioversion).
      2) Initial dose: 0.5 to 1 joule/kg
      3) Double the dose if SVT persists.
      4) *Reconsider the diagnosis of SVT if conversion to sinus rhythm does not occur; patient may actually have sinus tachycardia.*
4. Admit to the ICU to monitor for recurrences of SVT and for further management.
   a. Any patient presenting with hemodynamic instability
   b. Any patient with a first episode of SVT (e.g., for parental and patient education, and to begin maintenance therapy, especially in neonates and infants with possible recurrences of SVT)
5. Patients known to have SVT can be discharged home once converted to sinus rhythm; make a follow-up appointment with the cardiologist or primary care physician.

Clinical Pearls: Supraventricular Tachycardia

1. SVT is the most common dysrhythmia seen in the pediatric age group.
2. Aberrant SVT presents with a wide QRS complex and may resemble VT. If uncertain, all wide-complex tachycardias are assumed to be VT.
3. A diagnosis of sepsis may be mistakenly made in an infant with SVT presenting with poor feeding, irritability, rapid breathing, or shock.
4. Heart rates >220 bpm are highly unusual for ST and probably suggest SVT.
5. Do not delay cardioversion in severely compromised patients while trying to establish vascular access.
6. Do not prescribe sympathomimetics (common in over-the-counter decongestants) for the treatment of upper respiratory infections in children with SVT, and advise patients also to avoid caffeine.

BOX 5-21. DIFFERENTIAL DIAGNOSIS: SINUS TACHYCARDIA VERSUS SUPRAVENTRICULAR TACHYCARDIA

Sinus Tachycardia	*Supraventricular Tachycardia*
History of volume loss (vomiting, diarrhea, blood loss), fever, hypoxia	History nonspecific (e.g., irritability, poor feeding, excessive crying)
Signs of dehydration or hypovolemic shock or sepsis (depending on underlying etiology)	Signs of cardiogenic shock (tachypnea, sweating, pallor, or hypothermia)
Rate greater than normal for age (usually <220 bpm)	Rate >220 bpm in infants; rate >180 bpm in older children
Regular rhythm	Usually regular rhythm (associated AV block extremely rare)
Beat-to-beat variation (e.g., HR decreases with sleep or when quiet)	*No* beat-to-beat variation; monotonous/fixed rate
Normal P-wave axis	P-wave axis usually abnormal
P wave may not be identifiable (with very high ventricular rate)	P wave may not be identifiable (with very high ventricular rate)
Some variation in RR interval may be present	Monotonous/fixed RR interval
Normal QRS duration	Normal QRS duration in >90% of cases
Heart rate slows gradually with treatment (e.g., O_2 therapy for hypoxia or fluids for dehydration)	Abrupt termination to sinus rhythm (either spontaneously or with treatment)
Normal P-QRS-T–wave sequence	

BOX 5-22. ADENOSINE AND SUPRAVENTRICULAR TACHYCARDIA

- Drug of choice in stable patients or acutely ill patients *with readily available* vascular access
- Relatively safe drug that can be *given to infants and children of all ages,* including full-term and preterm newborn infants
- May also be used in children with WPW syndrome or other AV bypass tracts
- After its administration:
  (1) It transiently depresses sinus and AV nodes, leading to slowed conduction and interruption of the reentry pathway
  (2) *Be prepared to expect brief periods of sinus arrest (asystole).*
  (3) Also be prepared to treat other hemodynamically compromising cardiac effects such as bradycardia, AV block, atrial fibrillation, atrial flutter, ventricular tachycardia, or ventricular fibrillation.
- Untoward effects are brief (ultra-short half-life [< 10 seconds]):
  (1) Dyspnea, flushing, chest pain/discomfort, headache, episodes of apnea
  (2) Bronchospasm (asthma is not a contraindication to adenosine use; however, be prepared to treat immediate or delayed bronchospasm)
- Dose and route of administration:
  (1) Initial dose 0.1 to 0.3 mg/kg (*maximum first dose: 6 mg*)
  (2) If initial dose is unsuccessful, may double and repeat dose once (*maximum second dose: 12 mg*)
  (3) Maximum single dose: 12 mg
  (4) Use rapid IV bolus followed by normal saline flush (see two-hand technique, Fig. 5-12).
  (5) May be given intraosseously
  (6) Adolescents ≥50 kg: 6 mg rapid IV push; if no response after 1–2 min, give 12 mg rapid IV push. May repeat a second 12 mg dose after 1–2 min, if required.

DIAGNOSIS PREMATURE VENTRICULAR CONTRACTIONS

SYNONYMS

Ventricular premature contraction (VPC)
Ventricular extrasystoles
Premature ventricular beats

Definition

Premature ventricular contractions (PVCs) are premature, wide, and bizarre-shaped QRS complexes originating from ventricular tissue.

Associated Clinical Features

1. PVCs are commonly seen in asymptomatic healthy adolescents (without structural heart disease). They can be seen in any age group including newborns.
2. Presenting signs and symptoms include:
   a. Palpitations or "skipped beats"
   b. Chest discomfort, chest pain, and difficulty breathing
   c. Irregular heartbeat detected during routine examination
   d. Incidental detection during ECG recording
   e. Syncope or dizziness
   f. Frequent PVCs in the presence of compromised cardiac function may produce signs of CHF.
3. ECG findings include:
   a. Widened, bizarre QRS complexes that are *not* preceded by P waves
   b. P wave may show AV dissociation or retrograde conduction or may be absent
   c. T-wave polarity usually opposite to the major QRS deflection
   d. A compensatory pause often follows a PVC.
   e. A rhythmic pattern of PVC with a fixed ratio with normal beats is referred to as bigeminy (1:1), trigeminy (2:1), or quadrigeminy (3:1).
   f. Presence of unifocal PVCs or multifocal PVCs (Box 5-24)
   g. Nonsustained ventricular tachycardia (VT) consists of three or more PVCs that last for 10 seconds or less.
4. PVCs do not lead to any radiographic findings; underlying heart disease may have abnormal radiographic findings (e.g., cardiomegaly in cardiomyopathy).
5. A 24-hour Holter monitor, exercise stress testing, and echocardiography may be considered per consultation with the cardiologist.

Consultation

Cardiology consultation for "serious" PVCs (Box 5-24)

Emergency Department Treatment and Disposition

1 Patients with "benign" PVCs do not require any treatment. Reassurance about their benign nature and education about avoiding stimulants (e.g., excess caffeine intake, sympathomimetic agents) is discussed with the patient and family.
2. Cardiology consultation and hospitalization for monitoring and management for:
   a. Patients with "serious" PVCs
   b. Patients presenting with cardiac symptoms (e.g., syncope, chest pain) with PVCs
   c. Patients with new onset of PVCs with underlying heart disease
   d. Treatment may include lidocaine, procainamide, propranolol, or amiodarone.

Clinical Pearls: Premature Ventricular Contraction

1. "Benign" PVCs are commonly seen in healthy adolescents and children.
2. If a PVC falls on the T wave of the preceding normal complex (R-on-T phenomenon), it may initiate ventricular tachycardia.

BOX 5-23. ETIOLOGIES AND DIFFERENTIAL DIAGNOSIS OF PREMATURE VENTRICULAR CONTRACTIONS

- Benign PVCs (see Box 5-24)
- *Drugs/ingestions:*
  (1) Sympathomimetic agents
  (2) Tricyclic antidepressants
  (3) Digoxin
  (4) Caffeine
  (5) Tobacco
- *Electrolyte imbalance:*
  (1) Hypokalemia
  (2) Hypocalcaemia
- *Underlying heart disease:*
  (1) Mitral valve prolapse
  (2) Myocarditis (e.g., viral)
  (3) Lyme myocarditis
  (4) Cardiomyopathy
  (5) Coronary artery disease
  (6) Cardiac tumors
  (7) Hemochromatosis

BOX 5-24. BENIGN VERSUS SERIOUS PREMATURE VENTRICULAR CONTRACTIONS

Benign PVCs:

- Healthy adolescents and children
- Usually asymptomatic
- *Without* underlying heart disease
- Unifocal (uniform [of the same morphology]; Fig. 5-13)
- Consistent interval from the preceding QRS
- Infrequent
- Usually single
- Corrected QT interval normal
- *Not* associated with R-on-T phenomenon
- PVCs suppressed by exercise

Serious PVCs:

- Symptomatic
- Associated with underlying heart disease
- Multifocal (multiform [of more than one morphology]; Fig. 5-14)
- Varying intervals from the preceding QRS
- Associated with prolonged QTc interval
- Associated with R-on-T phenomenon
- Pairs of PVCs or runs of PVCs (three or more PVCs [ventricular tachycardia])
- Exercise either has no effect or increases frequency of PVCs

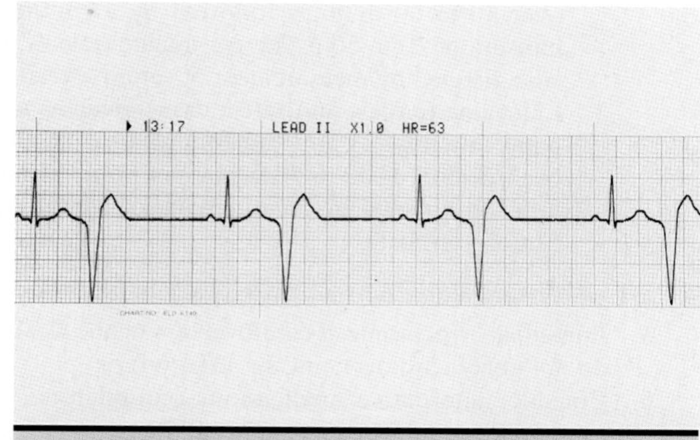

Figure 5-13. Unifocal Premature Ventricular Contraction

Note the uniform morphology of PVCs seen in a healthy 16-year-old adolescent on a routine examination.

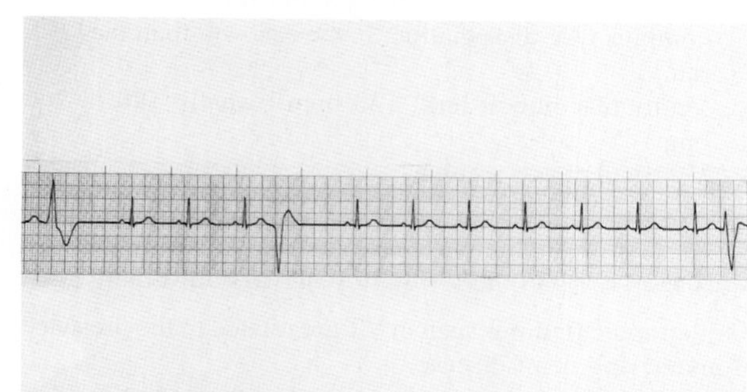

Figure 5-14. Multifocal Premature Ventricular Contraction

Note the multiform morphology of PVCs seen in a child with cardiomyopathy.

DIAGNOSIS VENTRICULAR TACHYCARDIA

Definition

Ventricular tachycardia (VT) is defined as three or more consecutive premature ventricular contractions (PVCs).

Associated Clinical Features

1. Ventricular tachycardia is uncommon in the pediatric age group.
2. Heart rate in VT varies from near normal to more than 200 bpm.
3. Stroke volume and cardiac output may become compromised with rapid ventricular rates, and VT may deteriorate into pulseless VT or VF.
4. Presenting signs and symptoms of VT include:
    a. Sudden onset of rapid heartbeat and palpitations
    b. Chest pain

   c. With slower tachycardia: fatigue, lethargy, or symptoms of CHF
   d. Syncope
   e. Occasionally asymptomatic
   f. Cardiac arrest
   g. Signs of circulatory impairment (poor end-organ perfusion)
      1) Skin perfusion: color pale, cyanotic, or mottled, cool extremities, prolonged capillary refill
      2) Peripheral pulses: rapid, thready, weak, or absent
      3) Discrepancy in volume between peripheral and central pulses
      4) CNS: irritable, lethargic, confused, or decrease in level of consciousness
      5) Diminished response to pain
      6) Respiratory difficulty
      7) Pulse pressure decrease of >20 mmHg
      8) Hypotension (decompensated shock)
      9) Decreased or no urine output

5. Electrocardiographic findings of VT include:
   a. P waves usually not identifiable
   b. If P waves are present, they are not related to the QRS complex (AV dissociation; P wave slower than the QRS rate)
   c. Ventricular rate at least 120 bpm (usually 120 to 200 bpm)
   d. Ventricular rate regular
   e. Wide QRS complex (>0.08 second [*QRS width is age dependent in children*]; Fig. 5-15)
   f. T waves usually opposite in polarity to QRS complex

6. Radiographic findings seen in VT are related to the presence of underlying heart disease.

Consultation

Cardiology (usually after initial stabilization)

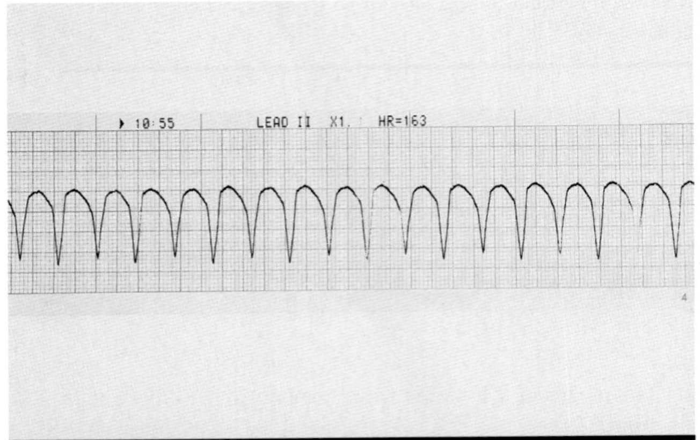

Figure 5-15. Ventricular Tachycardia

Ventricular rhythm is rapid and regular. Note QRS widening of >0.08 second and absence of atrial depolarization.

Emergency Department Treatment and Disposition

1. Assess and support ABCs as needed (provide 100% oxygen, ventilation as needed, continuous cardiac and pulse oximetry monitoring)

2. During evaluation identify and treat possible contributory causes (see Box 5-1 for "H"s and "T"s of CPR).

3. VT *with palpable pulses and adequate perfusion:*
   a. Consult a pediatric cardiologist.
   b. Synchronized cardioversion: 0.5 to 1 joule/kg (consider sedation; may double dose if initial dose ineffective) *or*
   c. Consider alternative medications (any of the following; *do not* give amiodarone and procainamide together):
      1) Amiodarone given intravenously at a loading dose of 5 mg/kg over 20 to 60 minutes followed by a continuous infusion at rates of 5 to 10 μg/kg per minute (5 to 10 mg/kg per day) *or*
      2) Procainamide given IV at a loading dose of 15 mg/kg over 30 to 60 minutes followed by a continuous infusion of 30 to 50 μg/kg per minute (rate of infusion directed by measurement of serum levels) *or*
      3) Lidocaine (easiest and safest drug) given as an IV bolus at a dose of 1 mg/kg followed by a continuous infusion of 30 to 50 μg/kg per minute (rate of infusion directed by measurement of serum levels [2 to 5 μg/mL])

4. VT *with palpable pulses and poor systemic perfusion:*
   a. Immediate synchronized cardioversion (same as above; do not delay cardioversion for sedation) *or*
   b. Consider alternative medications (amiodarone, procainamide, or lidocaine; same as above)

5. VT *without palpable pulses and poor systemic perfusion (pulseless VT):*
   a. Begin CPR and attempt defibrillation.
   b. Treatment same as for ventricular fibrillation/pulseless arrest (see Box 5-29)

6. Following stabilization, all patients require hospitalization in the PICU for continuous monitoring and subsequent management.

Clinical Pearls: Ventricular Tachycardia

1. Ventricular tachycardia may degenerate into ventricular fibrillation.

2. Aberrant SVT presents with a wide QRS complex and may resemble VT. *If uncertain, all wide-complex tachycardias are assumed to be VT unless proved otherwise.*

3. Both amiodarone and procainamide prolong the QT interval, and when given rapidly together can cause vasodilatation, hypotension, and increase the risk of heart block and polymorphic VT.

BOX 5-25. ETIOLOGY OF VENTRICULAR TACHYCARDIA

- Structural congenital heart disease or post–cardiac surgery (most common etiologies)
  (1) Tetralogy of Fallot
  (2) Eisenmenger's syndrome
  (3) Aortic stenosis
  (4) Transposition of the great arteries
  (5) Anomalies of coronary arteries
- Cardiac catheterization (mechanical irritation)
- Prolonged QT syndrome (see Fig. 5-7)
- Myocarditis (e.g., viral)
- Cardiomyopathy (e.g., dilated, hypertrophic)
- Pulmonary hypertension
- Arrhythmogenic RV dysplasia
- Cardiac tumors
- Drugs or poisons (see Box 5-26)
- Possible contributory causes: "H"s and "T"s of CPR (see Box 5-1)

BOX 5-26. DRUGS THAT CAUSE VENTRICULAR TACHYCARDIA AND SUPRAVENTRICULAR TACHYCARDIA

(1) Anticholinergics
(2) Antihistamines
(3) Catecholamine infusion
(4) Digitalis toxicity
(5) Tricyclic antidepressants
(6) Phenothiazines
(7) Sympathomimetics (e.g., beta-agonists, alpha-agonists, cocaine, amphetamines, phencyclidine)
(8) Sedative hypnotics (e.g., chloral hydrate, ethanol)
(9) Antidysrhythmics (classes I through IV)
(10) Thyroid hormone
(11) Carbamazepine

BOX 5-27. DIFFERENTIAL DIAGNOSIS OF VENTRICULAR TACHYCARDIA

- Supraventricular tachycardia (SVT) with aberrant conduction (due to bundle-branch block or WPW syndrome)
  (1) Seen in 10% of children with SVT
  (2) Presents with wide QRS complex and *may resemble VT*
  (3) The ability to terminate tachycardia with vagal maneuvers *does not* distinguish SVT from VT.
  (4) Hemodynamic stability also *does not* predict SVT versus VT (e.g., a patient without signs of circulatory impairment with a wide-complex tachycardia is more likely to have VT, and should not be assumed to have SVT).
  (5) *Erroneously treating VT as SVT can be devastating (VT deteriorates into pulseless VT/VF).*

DIAGNOSIS VENTRICULAR FIBRILLATION

Definition

Ventricular fibrillation (VF) is disorganized, chaotic ventricular electrical activity resulting in quivering myocardium that is incapable of producing adequate stroke volume (Fig. 5-16).

Associated Clinical Features

1. VF is an uncommon terminal rhythm in the pediatric age group. It is a more common arrest rhythm in adolescents than in infants. It is reported in about 3 to 20% of out-of-hospital pediatric and adolescent cardiac arrest victims.
2. VF leads to pulseless arrest (or collapsed rhythm). Other causes of pulseless arrest include pulseless VT, asystole, and pulseless electrical activity.
3. Patients with VF are pulseless, unresponsive, and have no signs of perfusion.

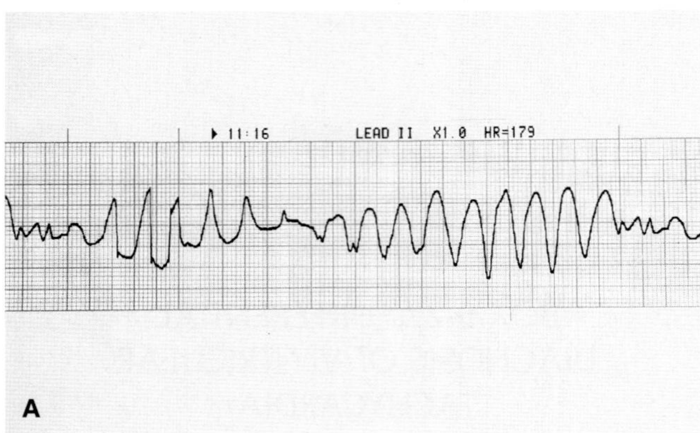

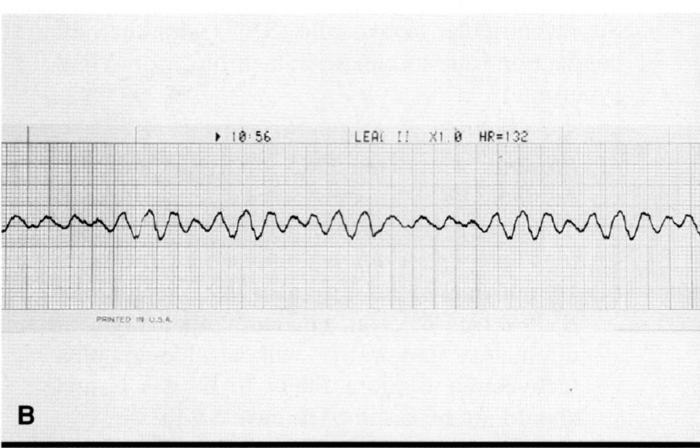

Figure 5-16. Ventricular Fibrillation

A. Coarse ventricular fibrillation: Chaotic, disorganized ventricular electrical activity without identifiable QRS or T waves. *B.* Fine ventricular fibrillation: Fine VF can be mistaken for asystole.

4. Ventricular tachycardia (VT) can degenerate into VF, either as a terminal event or with R-on-T phenomenon.
5. Electrocardiographic findings of VF include:
   a. VF can be either coarse with high amplitude or fine in appearance.
   b. Waveforms vary in size, shape, and rhythm.
   c. No identifiable QRS or T waves are present.
6. The survival rate for VF or pulseless VT is higher than the survival rate for asystole.

Consultation

Cardiology (usually after initial stabilization)

Emergency Department Treatment and Disposition

1. During evaluation of pulseless arrest, identify and treat possible contributory causes (see Box 5-1).
2. Even though lidocaine was used in the past for treatment of ventricular arrhythmias in children, data suggest that it is not very effective unless the arrhythmia is associated with focal myocardial ischemia.
3. Administration of amiodarone in children with VF and pulseless VT carries a Class Indeterminate recommendation (meaning there is not enough evidence to recommend or discourage its use in children).
4. Any patient who survives following stabilization requires hospitalization in a PICU for continuous monitoring and subsequent management.

Clinical Pearls: Ventricular Fibrillation

1. Ventricular fibrillation and pulseless VT are examples of pulseless arrest and are treated in the same manner.
2. Prompt defibrillation is the *definitive treatment* for both VF and pulseless VT.
3. The paddles selected for defibrillation (and cardioversion) should be the largest size that allows good chest contact over the entire paddle surface area and good separation between the two paddles. Infant paddles are used for infants <1 year or <10 kg, and adult paddles are used for patients older than 1 year or those weighing >10 kg.
4. Epinephrine increases the vigor and intensity of VF, improving the chance for successful defibrillation.
5 Epinephrine should be given for VF that is unresponsive to defibrillation attempts or CPR until a defibrillator is available.

BOX 5-28. PULSELESS ARREST OR COLLAPSE RHYTHMS

(1) Asystole

(2) Pulseless electrical activity

(3) Pulseless ventricular tachycardia

(4) Ventricular fibrillation

- Patients with known risk factors for cardiac disease preceding the arrest are more likely to have pulseless VT or VF as a cause of their collapse rhythm.
- Patients with risk factors for hypoxia preceding arrest (e.g., patients with apnea, asphyxia, trauma, or drowning) are more likely to have asystole as a cause of their collapse rhythm.
- For reversible and treatable causes of pulseless arrest ("H"s and "T"s of CPR) see Box 5-1.

BOX 5-29. MANAGEMENT OF PULSELESS VENTRICULAR TACHYCARDIA OR VENTRICULAR FIBRILLATION

Defibrillation Sequence:

- Ventilate with 100% oxygen, attach monitors and defibrillator, and create vascular access, *but these steps should not delay rapid defibrillation.*
- Assess and confirm that rhythm is VF/VT.
- Perform defibrillation up to three times if required:
  (1) First shock: 2 joules/kg
  (2) Second shock (if no response): 4 J/kg
  (3) Third shock (if no response): 4 J/kg
- Give epinephrine, if no response after 3 attempts at defibrillation
  (1) *Initial* IV/IO dose: 0.01 mg/kg (0.1 mL/kg) of *1:10,000 dilution*
  (2) Initial ET route dose: 0.1 mg/kg (0.1 mL/kg) of *1:1000 dilution* (all doses diluted to a minimum volume of 3 to 5 mL for instillation)
  (3) Subsequent doses: 0.1 mg/kg (0.1 mL/kg) of *1:1000 dilution*
  (4) Subsequent doses repeated every 3 to 5 minutes
  (5) Perform defibrillation within 30 to 60 seconds after each dose.
- Consider antiarrhythmic medications as indicated:
  (1) Amiodarone (dose: 5 mg/kg bolus given IV/IO) *or*
  (2) Lidocaine (dose: 1 mg/kg bolus IV/IO/ET) *or*
  (3) Magnesium (dose: 25 to 50 mg/kg IV/IO for torsades de pointes)
  (4) Perform defibrillation within 30 to 60 seconds after each dose.
- Identify and treat possible reversible causes ("H"s and "T"s of CPR; see Box 5-1)

DIAGNOSIS HYPERCYANOTIC SPELL OF TETRALOGY OF FALLOT

SYNONYMS

Tetralogy spells
"Tet spells"
Hypoxemic spell or paroxysmal hypoxemia

Associated Clinical Features

1. Tetralogy of Fallot (TOF) consists of a spectrum of anatomic abnormalities ("tetrad") that includes:
   a. A large unrestrictive malaligned ventricular septal defect (VSD)
   b. Right ventricular (RV) outflow tract obstruction (infundibular pulmonary stenosis); the severity of pulmonic stenosis ranges from mild to severe pulmonary stenosis or to pulmonary atresia
   c. RV hypertrophy
   d. Dextroposition (overriding) of the aorta
2. Clinical presentation of TOF (depends on the nature and degree of infundibular pulmonary stenosis):
   a. An ejection systolic murmur is normally heard at the mid-upper left sternal border (murmur of pulmonary stenosis) and may radiate toward the back.
   b. The loudness of the murmur depends on the volume of blood flowing across the outflow tract.
   c. Varying degrees of cyanosis due to right-to-left shunt resulting in an oxygen saturation of 75 to 85%
   d. *Cyanosis shows minimal improvement with O_2 supplementation.*
   e. Increased RV impulse at the lower left sternal border (due to RV hypertrophy)
   f. Loud single heart sound (pulmonary closure sound very soft)
   g. Digital clubbing (Fig. 5-17)
   h. Hypercyanotic spell of TOF (see Box 5-30)
      1) Cyanotic spells in infants and children with TOF are referred as *hypercyanotic spells.*
      2) Increased RV outflow tract obstruction exaggerates a right-to-left shunt, resulting in a decrease in pulmonary blood flow and a hypercyanotic spell (nearly all of the blood in the RV crosses through the VSD and enters the aorta).
3. Complete blood count shows polycythemia (compensatory due to chronic hypoxemia).
4. The ECG shows RV hypertrophy with right axis deviation.
5. Radiography:
   a. Infants: normal chest radiograph or may show only decreased pulmonary vascular markings
   b. Older children: "Boot-shaped heart" (Fig. 5-18)
   c. About 25% of patients with TOF have a right-sided aortic arch.

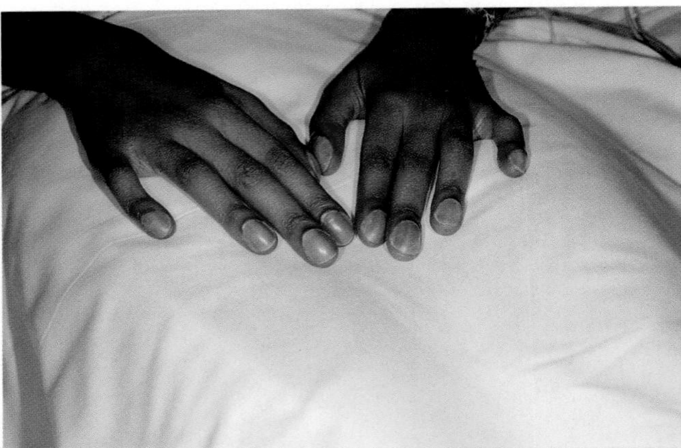

Figure 5-17. Clubbing and Cyanotic Nail Beds

This 12-year-old patient with TOF had a hemoglobin value of 22.5 g/dL, a hematocrit of 69.2%, an O_2 saturation of 75%, and a Po_2 of 45 mmHg on room air.

Consultation

Cardiology (usually after stabilization and management of the hypercyanotic spell)

Emergency Department Treatment and Disposition

1. Hospitalize:
   a. Any patient with a hypercyanotic spell requiring more than O_2 therapy and positional interventions to abate the spell

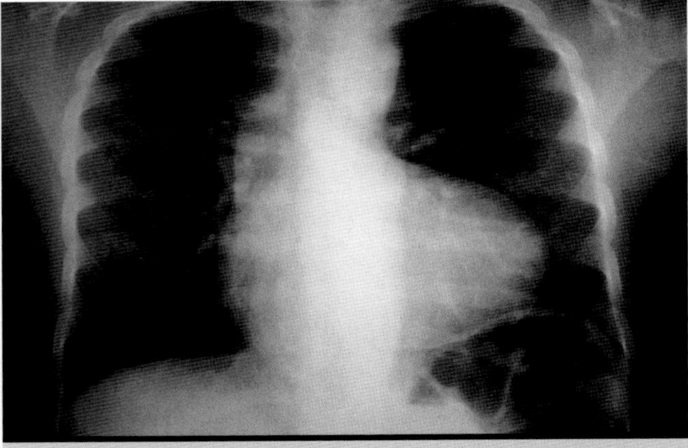

Figure 5-18. "Boot-Shaped Heart" in Tetralogy of Fallot

Frontal radiograph of the chest of the same patient shown in Fig. 5-17 at the age of 6 years, showing a typical boot-shaped heart (uplifted apex due to the RV enlargement associated with concavity of the upper left heart border due to a small or absent main pulmonary artery segment). There are also decreased pulmonary vascular markings.

BOX 5-30. HYPERCYANOTIC SPELL OF TETRALOGY OF FALLOT

Characteristic presenting features:

- Spells usually occur in the morning shortly after awakening (but may occur anytime).
- Spells are self-limited and usually last <15 to 30 minutes.
- Spells may occur spontaneously.
- Spells precipitated by stress, dehydration, injury, sudden fright, or anything that makes the infant cry
- Profound cyanosis (or history of increasing cyanosis) in a child with prior history of heart disease
- Prior history of squatting or knee-chest position with exertion

During the spell the infant or child may present with any of the following:

(1) Irritability/crying/agitation (signs of hypoxemia)
(2) Lethargy
(3) Profound cyanosis (Fig. 5-19)
(4) Unconsciousness
(5) Syncope (recurrent or prolonged [see Box 5-18; cardiac lesions producing syncope])
(6) Seizures
(7) Cerebrovascular accidents (associated with polycythemia)
(8) *Notable absence or decrease in intensity of a previously heard heart murmur* (due to decreased antegrade flow into the pulmonary arteries)
(9) Increased rate and depth of respiration (*hyperpnea, an important feature*)
(10) Increased right-to-left shunting during the spell, leading to hypoxemia, hypercapnia, and acidosis, leading to a decrease in systemic vascular resistance (SVR), which may further exaggerate the right-to-left shunt; hypoxia and acidosis stimulate the respiratory center to maintain and deepen the hyperpnea.

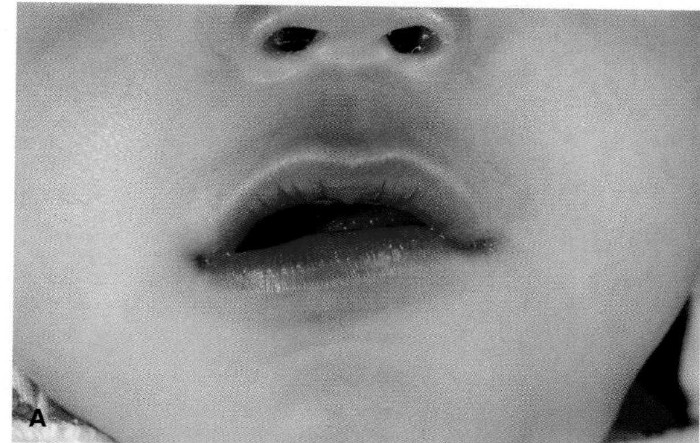

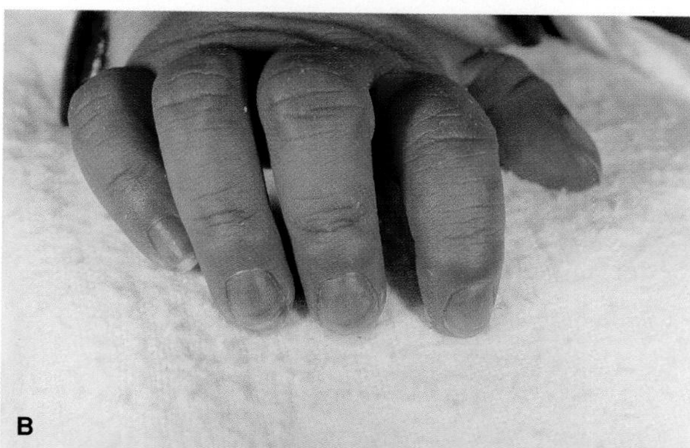

Figure 5-19. Cyanotic Congenital Heart Disease

A. Cyanosis of the lips. *B*. Cyanosis of the nail beds. A 4-month-old infant with a known case of TOF presented with a hypercyanotic spell (lethargy and extreme cyanosis with *hyperpnea and notable absence of a heart murmur*). These photographs were taken after stabilization.

b. Any patient who presents with complications related to prolonged hypoxemia (e.g., seizures)

2. Maintenance medical therapy may be required to control the recurrent hypercyanotic spells (e.g., propranolol therapy while awaiting surgical intervention).
3. Surgical interventions include a palliative shunt (systemic-to-pulmonary artery to provide sufficient pulmonary blood flow) or definitive repair (closure of VSD and relief of RV outflow tract obstruction).

Clinical Pearls: Hypercyanotic Spell of Tetralogy of Fallot

1. Two hallmarks of TOF are a pulmonary stenosis murmur and cyanosis.
2. Hypercyanotic spells of TOF are very dramatic in their presentation. Failure to recognize the spell and to intervene immediately may result in hypoxic seizures, profound metabolic acidosis, cerebrovascular accident (due

BOX 5-31. MANAGEMENT OF HYPERCYANOTIC SPELL OF TETRALOGY OF FALLOT

Interventions should be done in the following order, as indicated.

Standard initial therapeutic interventions that result in prompt abatement of the spell:

- Give 100% O_2 via a nonrebreathing facemask.
- Try to calm the child.
- Have the child assume the knee-chest position (knees flexed and drawn-up close to the child's chest and pressing on the abdomen); this increases SVR in the lower extremities, promoting increased venous return to the heart and increased pulmonary blood flow.
- Morphine sulfate: 0.1 to 0.2 mg/kg per dose given IM, SC, or IV
- Maintenance rate of IV fluids or correct hypovolemia if present (to maintain RV output and pulmonary blood flow)
- Correct hypoglycemia if present (hypoglycemia may contribute to a spell).

Additional interventions if above measures fail:

- Sodium bicarbonate
  (1) To correct metabolic acidosis that occurs after prolonged hypoxemia
  (2) Sodium bicarbonate can be given empirically without documented metabolic acidosis.
  (3) Dose: 2 to 3 mEq/kg IV (adequate ventilation must be ensured)
- Propranolol (beta-blocker)
  (1) To decrease the dynamic contraction of the infundibulum
  (2) Dose: 0.2 mg/kg per dose given IV over 5 minutes
- Phenylephrine (alpha-agonist)
  (1) To increase SVR
  (2) Dose: given IV at rate of 2 to 10 μg/kg per minute
- Alternative beta-blocker: esmolol (ultrashort-acting agent)
- Additional vasopressors: methoxamine or metaraminol
- Endotracheal intubation, mechanical ventilation, neuromuscular blockade to reduce O_2 consumption due to increased work of breathing
- *Important: Do not use epinephrine or norepinephrine to abate the spell.*

to polycythemia/hyperviscosity), deterioration in cardiac rhythm, and death.

3. Increasing cyanosis in a child with a prior history of heart disease or prior history of squatting with exertion is an important clue indicating a potential hypercyanotic spell.
4. A notable absence or lessening of a previously heard heart murmur in a cyanotic child is the most important clue suggesting a hypercyanotic spell.

BOX 5-32. CYANOTIC CONGENITAL HEART DISEASE

5 "T"s:

- *T*etralogy of Fallot
- *T*runcus arteriosus
- *T*ransposition of the great arteries
- *T*ricuspid atresia
- *T*otal anomalous pulmonary venous connection

Important: Tetralogy of Fallot is the most common cause of congenital cyanotic heart disease in children.

DIAGNOSIS

DUCTAL-DEPENDENT CARDIAC LESIONS/ HYPOPLASTIC LEFT HEART SYNDROME

Definition

1. Hypoplastic left heart syndrome (HLHS) refers to a spectrum of congenital heart defects that have in common a very small LV and other associated anatomic abnormalities (Box 5-34).
2. There is inadequate antegrade flow to support the systemic circulation because of the hypoplasia of the left heart. Since systemic circulation is supported by the right side of the heart through the ductus arteriosus, these lesions are referred to as ductal-dependent lesions.
3. Right-sided ductal-dependent congenital heart defects also occur in which the pulmonary circulation is dependent on patency of the ductus arteriosus.

Associated Clinical Features

1. HLHS is discussed here as a representative of ductal-dependent congenital heart defects, as it is one of the most serious cardiac anomalies presenting in infancy, and accounts for 25% of cardiac deaths in the first week of life.
2. A neonate born with HLHS appears normal at birth (with normal Apgar scores) because systemic perfusion and oxygenation are normal in utero. Typically on day 2 or 3 of life, the patient develops signs of poor systemic perfusion as the ductus arteriosus closes (Fig. 5-20).
3. All patients with HLHS have a single, loud second heart sound and variable heart murmurs that are usually not diagnostic.
4. The ECG may show right atrial enlargement (~30 to 40%), right ventricular hypertrophy (~80 to 90%) and diminished left ventricular forces (~30 to 40%).
5. Radiograph typically shows marked cardiomegaly with normal to increased pulmonary markings.

Consultation

Cardiology consultation (after initial stabilization) to confirm the diagnosis by two-dimensional echocardiography and subsequent referral for surgical management

Emergency Department Treatment and Disposition

1. All ductal-dependent cardiac lesions present in a similar fashion (like HLHS) and the initial medical management is *identical* in all.

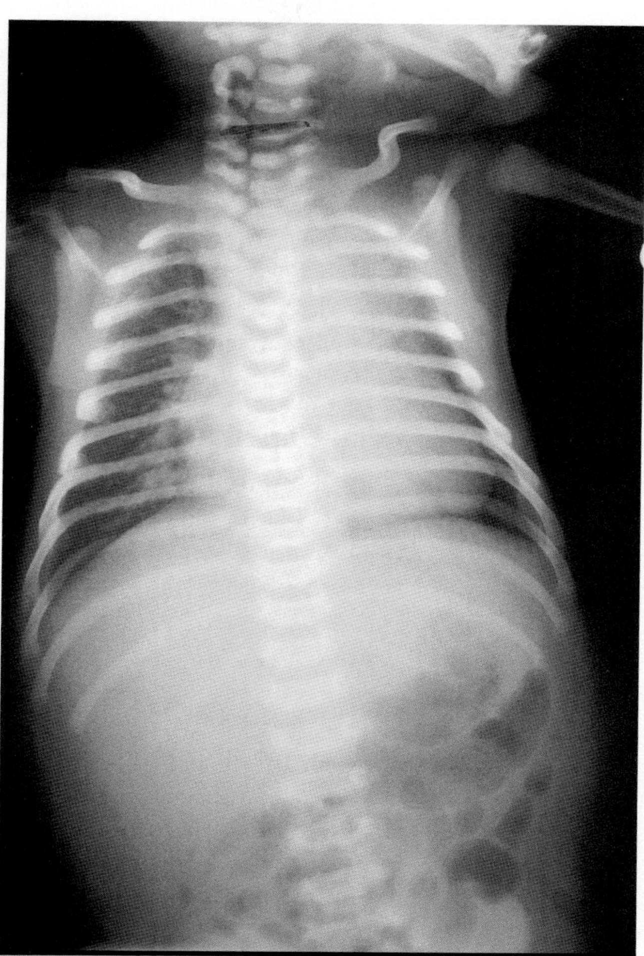

Figure 5-20. Cardiomegaly: Critical Coarctation of the Aorta (Ductal-Dependent Cardiac Lesion)

A 21-day-old neonate presented with extreme cyanosis, severe respiratory distress, tachycardia, wheezing, and shock with poor systemic perfusion and hepatomegaly. He had marked acidosis (arterial pH 6.86, Pco_2 47 mmHg, Po_2 35.7 mmHg, base deficit of −22.4, and total bicarbonate of 6.7). His wheezing and respiratory distress were thought to be due to bronchiolitis. With the cardiomegaly seen on the chest radiograph, the possibility of a ductal-dependent cardiac lesion with cardiogenic shock was entertained. The patient was started on PGE_1 infusion and a diagnosis of critical coarctation of the aorta was confirmed by 2-D echocardiography. *A ductal-dependent cardiac lesion must be considered in any neonate up to 28 days of age with sudden onset of shock, severe hypoxemia, acidosis, cyanosis, and CHF.*

2. Support the ABCs and provide continuous cardiac and pulse oximetry.
3. Maintain ductal patency with an infusion of prostaglandin E_1 (PGE_1) (Box 5-35; Fig. 5-21).
4. Treat metabolic acidosis by fluid therapy and sodium bicarbonate (acidosis leads to increased systemic vascular resistance, and in turn increases pulmonary blood flow).
5. Avoid any maneuvers that decrease pulmonary vascular resistance and pulmonary pressure as these will steal blood flow from the systemic circulation (e.g., supplemental O_2 therapy [O_2 acts as pulmonary vasodilator] and hyperventilation [low P_{CO_2} acts as pulmonary vasodilator]). Aim at the "ideal arterial blood gas with 7.4/40/40" (pH 7.4, P_{O_2} 40 mmHg, P_{CO_2} 40 mmHg). This is usually achieved with low (or no) mechanical ventilatory support on room air.
6. After initial stabilization all patients require admission to the PICU for subsequent management.

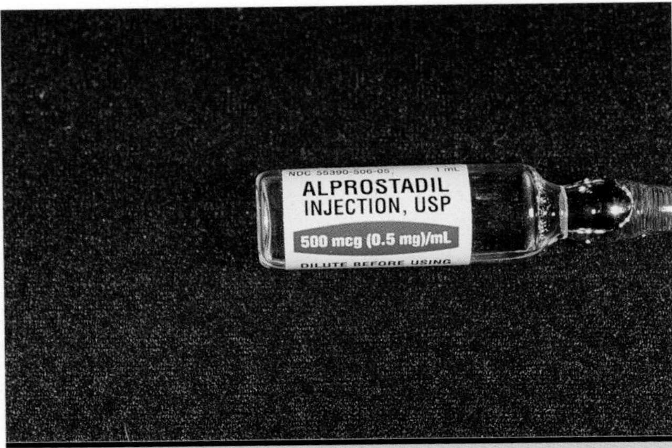

Figure 5-21. Prostaglandin E_1 for Intravenous Infusion

Neonates presenting with shock should be treated as having ductal-dependent lesions until proved otherwise; PGE_1 infusion, by maintaining patency of the ductus arteriosus, is *life-saving* in such infants.

Clinical Pearls: Ductal-Dependent Cardiac Lesions/Hypoplastic Left Heart Syndrome

1. A ductal-dependent cardiac lesion must be considered in any neonate (*up to 28 days old*) with sudden onset of shock, severe hypoxemia, acidosis, or intense cyanosis (systemic circulatory collapse).
2. Neonates presenting with shock should be treated as having ductal-dependent lesions until proved otherwise; PGE_1 infusion, by maintaining patency of the ductus arteriosus, is *life-saving* in such infants.

BOX 5-33. CLINICAL FEATURES OF DUCTAL-DEPENDENT CARDIAC LESIONS/HYPOPLASTIC LEFT HEART SYNDROME

Typical age at presentation:

- Neonates usually present within the first few days of life (when the ductus closes).
- Neonates may present as late as 1 or 2 weeks of life, and sometimes even older.

Typical presentation in the first 7 to 10 days of life:

- Signs of shock
  (1) Skin perfusion: cyanotic or mottled, cool extremities, prolonged capillary refill
  (2) Peripheral pulses: rapid, thready, weak, or absent
  (3) Discrepancy in volume between peripheral and central pulses
  (4) CNS: irritable, lethargic, poor feeding, or unresponsiveness
  (5) Diminished response to pain
  (6) Respiratory distress (compensation for severe metabolic acidosis and increased pulmonary blood flow)
  (7) Hypotension (decompensated shock)
  (8) Metabolic acidosis due to poor tissue perfusion
  (9) Decreased or no urine output
- Multisystem organ failure (e.g., acute renal failure/acute tubular necrosis, seizures)

Typical presentation between 2 and 6 weeks (ductus remains patent naturally in some patients):

- Signs of congestive heart failure (as pulmonary vascular resistance falls)
  (1) Feeding difficulty and poor weight gain
  (2) Tachypnea, rales, or wheezing
  (3) Tachycardia, gallop rhythm
  (4) Hepatomegaly
  (5) Pulses mildly to moderately decreased or increased

BOX 5-34. DIFFERENTIAL DIAGNOSIS OF DUCTAL-DEPENDENT CARDIAC LESIONS

- Sepsis/septic shock
- Ductal-dependent systemic blood flow
  (1) Hypoplastic left heart syndrome (very small LV with other associated anatomical defects)
  Mitral atresia and aortic atresia with extreme hypoplasia or absence of identifiable LV
  Severe aortic stenosis or atresia with patent mitral valve
  Mitral valve stenosis or hypoplasia with aortic valve hypoplasia
  Common atrioventricular canal with hypoplasia of LV
  (2) Critical coarctation of the aorta
  (3) Aortic arch interruption
- Ductal-dependent pulmonary blood flow
  (1) Pulmonary atresia with intact ventricular septum
  (2) Tricuspid atresia
  (3) Critical pulmonary stenosis

BOX 5-35. DUCTAL-DEPENDENT CARDIAC LESIONS AND PROSTAGLANDIN E_1 (PGE_1)

PGE_1 infusion:

- Mechanism of action: vasodilator (especially of ductal tissue)
- Indications: to maintain or reopen the ductus arteriosus in neonates with CHD when adequate systemic or pulmonary blood flow depends on ductal patency
- Contraindications: *almost none* except total anomalous pulmonary venous connection
- Given as a continuous infusion
- Very short half-life (about 90% is metabolized in one pass through a normal lung)
- Initial dose
  (1) 0.05 to 0.10 μg/kg per minute after an initial bolus of 0.10 μg/kg
  (2) Titrate maintenance dose to clinical effect
- Side effects
  (1) Vasodilator effects include hypotension, flushing, and peripheral edema.
  (2) Apnea
  (3) Hyperpyrexia
  (4) Jitteriness or convulsions
  (5) Rhythm disturbances (e.g., bradycardia)
  (6) Metabolic (hypoglycemia, hypocalcemia)
  (7) Renal failure
  (8) Coagulopathies
  (9) Diarrhea
  (10) Rash

Clinical pearl

- *Be prepared to support life-threatening side effects (e.g., apnea, bradycardia, and hypotension) while initiating PGE_1* therapy.

DIAGNOSIS INFECTIVE ENDOCARDITIS

Definition

1. Infective endocarditis (IE) is a microbial infection of the endocardial/endothelial surface.
2. Endocarditis may be classified as acute or subacute or as native valve endocarditis, prosthetic valve endocarditis, or endocarditis in intravenous drug abusers.

Etiology

1. Gram-positive cocci account for 90% of culture-positive endocarditis.
2. About 5 to 7% of cases of endocarditis are culture-negative.
3. Etiological agents include:
   a. *Streptococcus viridans* (the most common etiology of endocarditis; between 32 and 43%) in all age groups
   b. *Staphylococcus aureus* (second most common etiology; between 27 and 33%)
   c. Coagulase-negative *S. epidermidis* (2 to 12%)
   d. *Enterococcus* species (4 to 7%)
   e. *Streptococcus pneumoniae* (3 to 7%)
   f. HACEK group (*Haemophilus* species, *Actinobacillus actinomycetemcomitans*, *Cardiobacterium hominis*, *Eikenella corrodens*, and *Kingella kingae*; 4 to 5%)
   g. Fungi (*Candida* species, *Aspergillus* species)

Associated Clinical Features

1. Endocarditis in childhood is seen in patients with preexisting congenital heart disease (CHD). High-risk group includes patients with complex cyanotic congenital heart disease (e.g., single ventricle, transposition of the great arteries, tetralogy of Fallot), and post–cardiac surgery (e.g., palliative shunt procedures, prosthetic valves). Moderate-risk group includes patients with an uncorrected ventricular septal defect, patent ductus arteriosus, atrial septal defect, bicuspid aortic valve, and rheumatic valvular disease.
2. Endocarditis can also occur without underlying CHD. Predisposing factors in such cases include infected indwelling central venous catheters. Unlike in adults, intravenous drug abuse is not a common predisposing factor in younger children.
3. Bacteremia may occur during severe burns, any bacterial infection (e.g., cellulitis, pneumonia, urinary tract infection), or following any dental or surgical procedures, any instrumentation of mucosal surfaces, or spontaneously following activities such as brushing teeth.
4. Blood cultures are positive in >95% of cases of IE, and remain the gold standard for making the diagnosis. Ideally, at least three sets of blood cultures (from separate venipuncture sites and with as large a quantity of blood as possible) should be obtained.
5. Additional laboratory abnormalities seen in IE include normocytic normochromic anemia, leukocytosis, elevated ESR, microscopic hematuria, proteinuria, and decreased complement value.
6. The Duke criteria are a combination of major and minor criteria that help in arriving at the diagnosis of IE. Definitive clinical diagnosis of IE can be made when two major or one major and three minor criteria or five minor criteria are present.
   a. Major criteria:
      1. Positive blood culture (two separate blood cultures positive): *Streptococcus viridans*, *Streptococcus bovis*, HACEK group, *S. aureus*, or enterococci
      2. Microorganism consistent with IE from persistently positive blood culture (two or more positive blood cultures drawn at least 12 hours apart, or all of three or a majority of four or more separate cultures of blood [first and last samples drawn at least 1 hour apart])
      3. Evidence of endocardial involvement (positive echocardiography):
         i. Oscillating intracardiac vegetations on valve or supporting structures, in the path of regurgitant jets, or on implanted material, or abscess or new partial dehiscence of prosthetic valve (Fig. 5-22)
         ii. New valvular regurgitation
   b. Minor criteria:
      1. Predisposing structural cardiovascular lesion or intravenous drug abuse

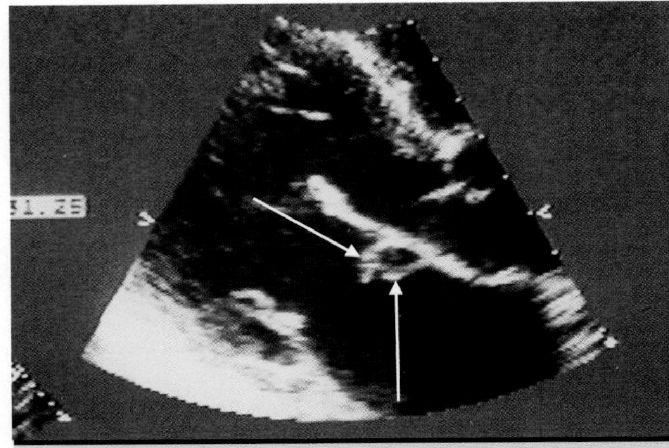

Figure 5-22. Vegetations on the Mitral Valve

Transthoracic echocardiogram parasternal long axis view showing echogenic shadow on the anterior mitral valve leaflet suggestive of a vegetation.

   2. Fever >38°C (100.4°F)
   3. Vascular phenomena (major arterial emboli, septic pulmonary emboli, mycotic aneurysm, intracranial hemorrhage, conjunctival hemorrhages, Janeway lesions)
   4. Immunologic phenomena (glomerulonephritis, Osler's nodes (Fig. 5-23), Roth's spots, positive rheumatoid factor)
   5. Microbiological evidence (positive blood culture that does not meet a major criterion as noted above)
   6. Echocardiographic findings (consistent with IE but do not meet a major criterion as noted above)

7. Two-dimensional transthoracic echocardiography (TTE) is used for detecting the presence of vegetations. The sensitivity of TTE in children is about 80%; thus, a negative TTE does not exclude endocarditis. Transesophageal echocardiography may be used if TTE is negative.

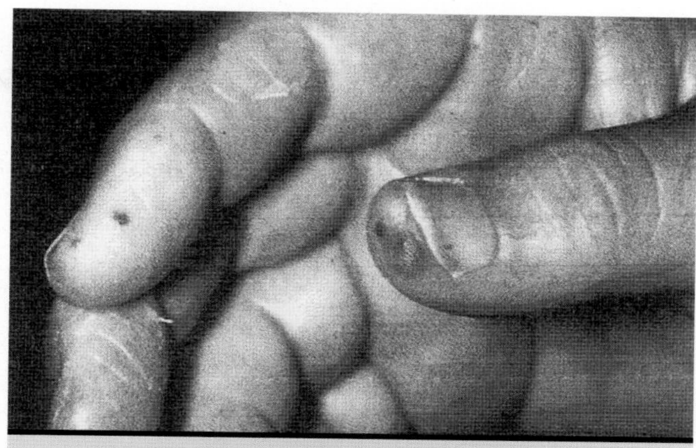

Figure 5-23. Osler's Nodes

Subcutaneous, purplish, tender nodules in the pulp of fingers. (Courtesy of the Armed Forces Institute of Pathology, Bethesda, Maryland.)

Consultations

Cardiology and infectious disease specialist

BOX 5-36. CLINICAL FEATURES OF INFECTIVE ENDOCARDITIS IN CHILDREN

- Fever (most common symptom), prolonged low-grade fever, rigors, diaphoresis
- Fatigue, nausea, vomiting, abdominal pain, anorexia, weight loss, malaise
- Splenomegaly (less common than in adults)
- Arthralgias or arthritis
- Chest pain
- Congestive heart failure (valve destruction, regurgitation)
- Valvulitis (new or changing murmurs)
- Cardiac arrhythmias
- Roth's spots (less common than in adults)
  (1) Small, pale, retinal lesions with areas of hemorrhage
  (2) Usually located near the optic disc
- Subungual splinter hemorrhages (less common than in adults; Fig. 5-24)
- Embolic events (CNS, kidneys, spleen, skin, lungs)
- CNS signs and symptoms of cerebral infarction
  (1) Seizures
  (2) Changing mental status
  (3) Ataxia
  (4) Aphasia
  (5) Acute hemiplegia
  (6) Focal neurological deficits
  (7) Sensory loss

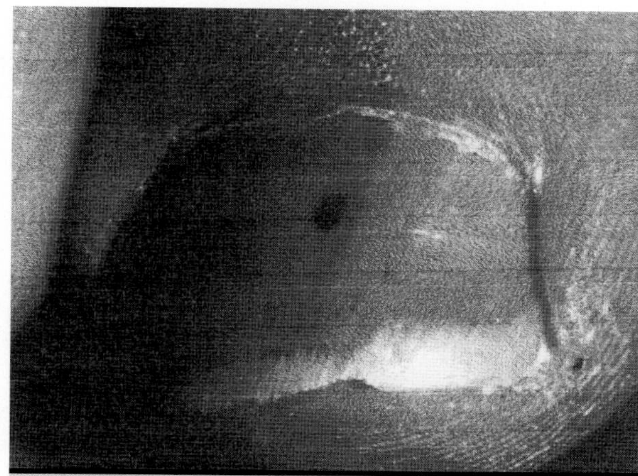

Figure 5-24. Splinter Hemorrhages

Note splinter hemorrhages along the distal aspect of the nail plate due to emboli from subacute bacterial endocarditis. (Courtesy of the Armed Forces Institute of Pathology, Bethesda, Maryland.)

Emergency Department Treatment and Disposition

1. All suspected cases of IE require hospitalization (intensive care setting, if indicated, in acutely ill patients) for confirmation of the diagnosis, IV antibiotic therapy, and continuous cardiac monitoring.
2. Antibiotic therapy is guided by the identification of the pathogen and sensitivity. It is best not to administer the antibiotics in the ED while awaiting collection of more blood culture samples and culture results. Duration of therapy varies from 2 to 6 weeks.

Clinical Pearls: Infective Endocarditis

1. Suspect endocarditis in any patient with a heart murmur and persistent unexplained high fever, especially if there is a cardiovascular lesion or condition that increases the risk of bacteremia, or in any febrile intravenous drug abuser (even in the absence of a heart murmur).
2. Prophylactic antibiotics can prevent endocarditis during procedures. Follow the recommendations for prophylaxis published by the American Heart Association (see Dajani et al, 1997 reference).
3. Patients with CHD presenting to the ED with evidence of soft tissue infections (e.g., abscess) must receive appropriate antibiotic coverage prior to débridement or incision and drainage.
4. The Duke criteria help in establishing the diagnosis of this life-threatening infection.

BOX 5-37. DIFFERENTIAL DIAGNOSIS OF INFECTIVE ENDOCARDITIS

- Malignancy
- Collagen vascular diseases
- Other infections affecting the heart (e.g., acute rheumatic fever)

BOX 5-38. DERMATOLOGICAL MANIFESTATIONS OF INFECTIVE ENDOCARDITIS

- Skin lesions are reported to occur in 15 to 50% of cases of IE.
- Types of skin lesions include petechiae, Osler's nodes, and Janeway's lesions.

A. Petechiae (less common in children than in adults; Fig. 5-25)
   (1) Most common skin manifestation
   (2) Seen in about 30 to 50% of patients
   (3) Occur in small crops
   (4) Pinpoint, reddish-brown macular lesions that do not blanch on pressure
   (5) Usually transient
   (6) Common sites: mucous membranes of the mouth, conjunctiva, upper part of the chest, extremities

B. Osler's nodes (less common in children than in adults)
   (1) Erythematous indurated nodules with pale centers
   (2) Tender (pain may be elicited by palpating the tips of the digits)
   (3) Pea-sized slits
   (4) Few in number
   (5) Transient in nature (clears after 1 to 2 days of antibiotic therapy)
   (6) Resolves without necrosis or suppuration
   (7) Sites: pads of fingers and toes (most common site), thenar and hypothenar eminences, sides of the fingers, arms

C. Janeway's lesions (peripheral embolization; less common in children than in adults)
   (1) Painless
   (2) Small erythematous macules or small nodular hemorrhages
   (3) Site: palms or soles

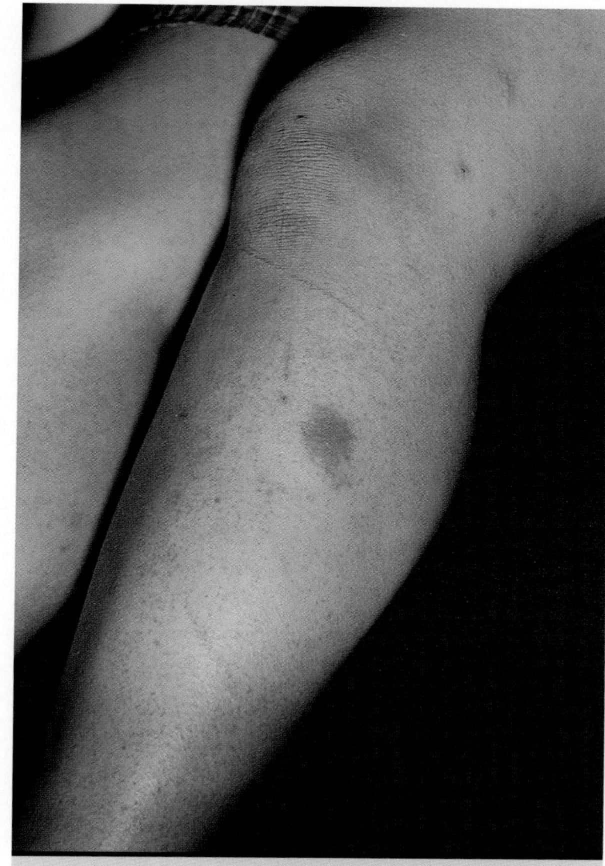

Figure 5-25. Petechiae

Infective endocarditis presenting as persistent fever and petechiae on the lower extremities in a patient with VSD. Blood culture was positive for *S. pneumoniae*. Occasionally a patient with IE presents with numerous petechiae on the lower extremities (as shown here), and may mimic a primary vasculitis.

Suggested Readings

Bernstein D: Bradyarrhythmias. In: Behrman RE, Kliegman RM, Jenson HB (eds). *The Cardiovascular System. Nelson Textbook of Pediatrics,* 16th ed. WB Saunders, Philadelphia, 2000, p. 1422.

Bolton E: Disturbances of cardiac rhythm and conduction. In: Tintinalli JE, Kelen GD, Stapcznski JS (eds). *Emergency Medicine. A Comprehensive Study Guide,* 5th ed. McGraw-Hill, New York, 2000, p. 182.

Dajani AS, Taubert KA, Wilson W, et al: Prevention of bacterial endocarditis: Recommendations by the American Heart Association. *JAMA* 1997;277:1794.

Delgado CA: Syncope. In: Fleisher GR, Ludwig S (eds). *Textbook of Emergency Medicine,* 4th ed. Lippincott Williams & Wilkins, Baltimore, 2000, p. 593.

Ferrieri P, Gewitz MH, Gerber MA et al: Unique features of infective endocarditis in childhood. *Pediatrics* 2002;109:931.

Gewitz MH, Vetter VL: Cardiac emergencies. In: Fleisher GR, Ludwig S (eds). *Textbook of Pediatric Emergency Medicine,* 4th ed. Lippincott Williams & Wilkins, Baltimore, 2000, p. 684.

Gewitz MH, Vetter VL: Hypoxemic attacks. In: Fleisher GR, Ludwig S (eds). *Cardiac Emergencies. Textbook of Pediatric Emergency Medicine,* 4th ed. Lippincott Williams & Wilkins, Baltimore, 2000, p. 694.

Gewitz MH, Woolf PK: Ventricular premature contractions. In: Crain E, Gershel J (eds). *Cardiac Emergencies. Clinical Manual of Emergency Pediatrics.* McGraw-Hill, New York, 1997, p. 32.

Kapoor WN: Syncope. *N Engl J Med* 2000;343:1856.

Hazinski MF, Cummins R, Field JM (eds). American Heart Association. *2000 Handbook of Emergency Cardiovascular Care for Health Care Providers.* Dallas, Texas, 2000.

Law IH, Atkins DL: Tachyarrhythmias. In: Finberg L, Kleinman RE (eds) *Saunders Manual of Pediatric Practice*, 2nd ed. WB Saunders, Philadelphia, 2002, p. 652.

Losek JD, Endom E, Dietrich A et al: Adenosine and pediatric supraventricular tachycardia in the emergency department: multicenter study and review. *Ann Emerg Med* 1999;33:185.

Narchi H: The child who passes out. *Pediatr Rev* 2000;21:384.

Rhythm disturbances: In: *PALS Provider Manual.* American Heart Association, American Academy of Pediatrics, Dallas, Texas, p. 185.

Weinberg PM, Cohen MS: Hypoplastic left heart syndrome. Cardiology. In: Finberg L, Kleinman RE (eds). *Saunders Manual of Pediatric Practice,* 2nd ed. WB Saunders, Philadelphia, 2002, p. 617.

CHAPTER 6

RESPIRATORY DISORDERS

Binita R. Shah

DIAGNOSIS FOREIGN BODY ASPIRATION

Definition

Foreign body aspiration (FBA) is accidental inhalation of foreign material into the airways which may result in asphyxiation or severe lung damage.

Associated Clinical Features

1. Most common ages:
   a. Toddler through preschool ages: about 85% of FBA
   b. Children >5 years: <15% of FBA
2. Foreign bodies (FBs) entering the tracheobronchial tree must run through protective anatomical barriers consisting of the epiglottis, upper laryngeal inlet, false cords, true vocal cords, and cough reflex.
3. Most common location of foreign body:
   a. Right and left main stem bronchial FBAs occur with roughly equal frequency in children (unlike FBAs in adults).
   b. Children have symmetrical angles of both the right and left main stem bronchi at the carina until about 15 years of age; the fully developed aortic knob then displaces the left main stem bronchus, creating a more obtuse angle at the carina, predisposing adolescents and adults to higher incidence of FBA in the right main bronchus, bronchus intermedius, or right lower lobe bronchus.
4. Radiographic studies that may help (should *only* be done with very close monitoring of the patient and if the patient is not in extreme respiratory distress):
   a. AP and lateral chest and neck radiographs (routinely performed first)
   b. Inspiratory and expiratory AP chest x-ray (air trapping, obstructive emphysema, mediastinal shift may be seen during expiration)
   c. Right and left decubitus films
   d. Fluoroscopy during inspiration and expiration
      1) Helps to localize the FB (the obstructed lung remains expanded during expiration, but the heart and mediastinum shift to the opposite side as the unobstructed lung empties; the diaphragm also remains low and flat on the obstructed side, while its excursion is free and exaggerated on unobstructed side)
      2) Detects complete obstruction of bronchus producing atelectasis (the heart and mediastinum are drawn toward the obstructed side and remain there during both phases of respiration; the diaphragm on the obstructed side remains high, but the diaphragm on the unobstructed side moves normally)
4. Complications of FBA (related to delay in diagnosis and treatment):
   a. Pneumonia, lung abscess (obstruction leading to retained secretions that promote bacterial superinfection), atelectasis, pneumothorax, bronchiectasis, and perforation of the tracheobronchial tree
   b. Arachidic bronchitis (produced by organic foreign bodies such as peanuts and characterized by cough, septic fever, dyspnea, and a spidery pattern on x-ray)
   c. Nonobstructing metallic objects may remain within the tracheobronchial tree for extended periods of time with little tissue damage.

Consultations

Radiology, surgery, anesthesiology and pulmonary (as indicated)

Emergency Department Treatment and Disposition

1. Assess the patency of airway and breathing. Recommendations for a choking infant or child include:
   a. Infants <1 year: repetitive use of four back blows (with the heel of the hand between the scapulas) and four chest thrusts (technique and hand positioning same as for closed cardiac compression) with infant in a head-down position (head lower than trunk)
   b. Child >1 year: 6 to 10 abdominal thrusts (Heimlich maneuver) using the heel of one hand and pushing

upward and inward from midabdomen, performed with a patient in a supine position

c. Do not perform blind oropharyngeal finger sweeping; grasp and remove the visualized foreign body.

2. No emergency measures need to be taken if the child is able to speak, cough, or cry (all these findings suggest absence of complete obstruction requiring emergent intervention). Provide supplemental O_2 therapy while continuously monitoring the patient on cardiac and pulse oximetry and placing the child in the sniffing position (allows maximal airway patency).

3. If the diagnosis is suspected by history, examination, and radiographic findings, prepare the patient for the operating room for extraction of the foreign body via rigid bronchoscopy under general anesthesia (allows ventilation throughout the procedure and provides a larger working area for extraction of the FB through the instrument [e.g., high-resolution optical telescope]). Flexible fiberoptic bronchoscopy may be employed if history and physical examination are equivocal.

4. Following the procedure, the patient is usually admitted to the ICU for close observation. Pulmonary toilet, bronchodilator therapy, and antibiotic therapy are given as indicated.

5. Rarely, the patient may need open thoracotomy for the removal of a FB that cannot be removed by bronchoscopy.

6. All patients with a strong suspicion of FBA (history and examination but negative initial radiographs) should be hospitalized.

7. Hospitalize for continuous monitoring all patients who present with respiratory symptoms after expulsion of a FB from the airway.

Clinical Pearls: Foreign Body Aspiration

1. The most common objects aspirated by children are food products (Figs. 6-1, 6-2, and 6-3).

2. Beans and seeds absorb water over time, and with subsequent swelling may rapidly change from a partial to a complete bronchial obstruction.

3. Up to 50% of patients with FBA may not have a contributory history. With a history of a choking episode, a diagnosis of FBA must not be excluded, even in the absence of clinical or radiologic findings.

4. Consider FBA in a patient with any unexplained new onset of pulmonary symptoms (e.g., wheezing, stridor) or unexplained persistent or recurrent pulmonary findings (e.g., pneumonia, lung abscess) regardless of the history of an aspiration event.

5. Rigid bronchoscopy under general anesthesia is the therapeutic intervention of choice for the extraction of airway FBs.

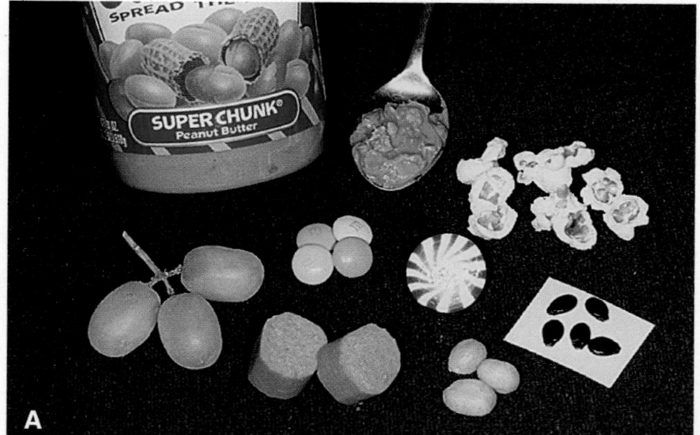

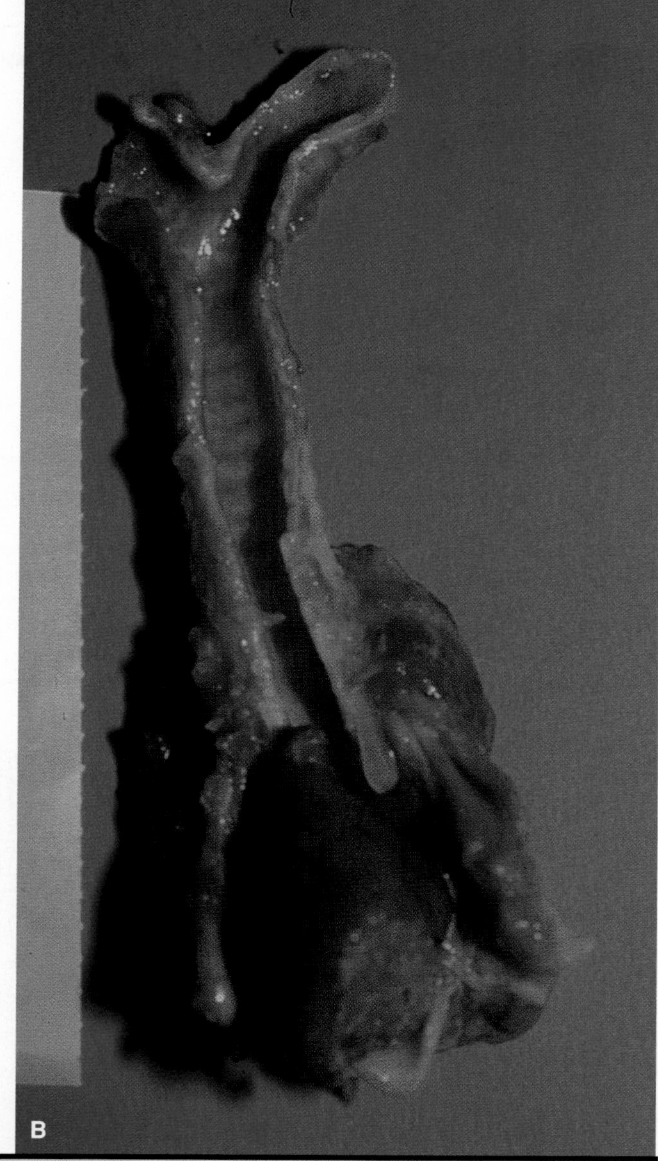

Figure 6-1. Foreign Body Aspiration

A. The most commonly aspirated food products by infants and children include peanuts, chunky peanut butter, hot dogs, popcorn, seeds, grapes, raisins, carrots, meat, and hard candies. Children too young to chew and swallow carefully (usually <5 years of age) should not be given these foods. Similarly, toys containing small or loosely attached parts should not be given to children who are still putting such objects into their mouths. *B*. A piece of hot dog is seen lodged in the trachea of a 2.5-year-old child presenting in cardiopulmonary arrest. Children <5 years old should not be given foods such as hot dogs. For young children, hot dogs should be cut longitudinally and not into round pieces.

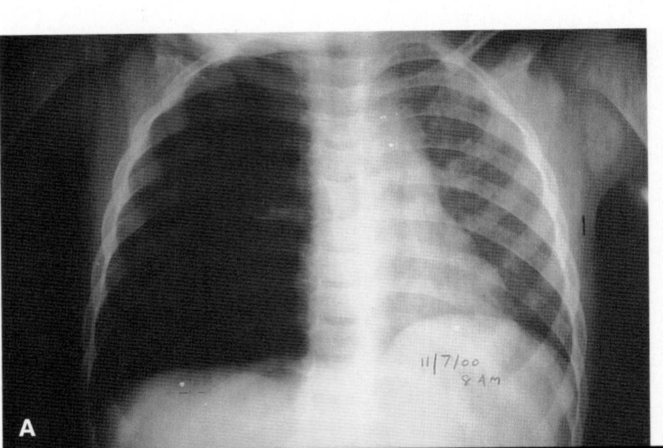

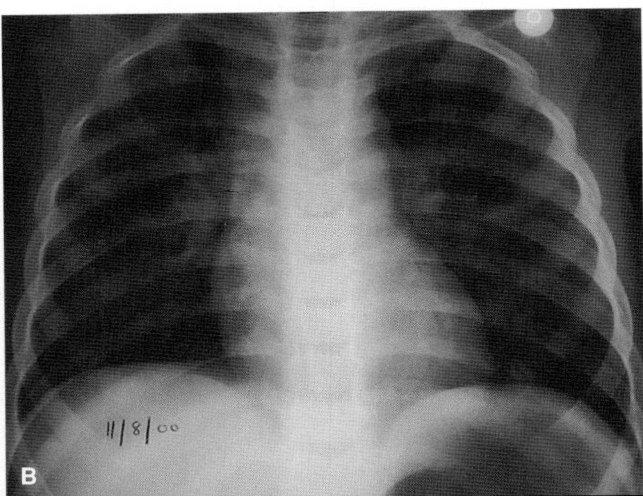

Figure 6-2. Radiolucent Foreign Body Aspiration

A. Frontal chest radiograph showing unilateral hyperinflation of the right lung with a slight mediastinal shift to the left. Flattening of the right hemidiaphragm is also seen. This 2.5-year-old child presented with a history of coughing and a first episode of wheezing 20 hours following a history of choking while eating peanuts. He had tachypnea (RR 40/min) with mild retractions, wheezing, and diminished breath sounds on the right side. *B*. Normal expansion of both lung fields. Unilateral hyperinflation seen in radiograph *A* is no longer appreciated after extraction of the peanut fragment from the right lower lobe bronchus by rigid bronchoscopy.

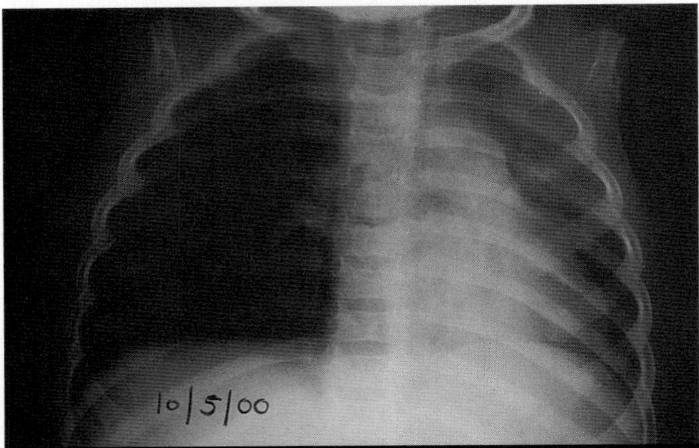

Figure 6-3. Radiolucent Foreign Body Aspiration

Frontal chest radiograph shows hyperinflation and hyperlucency of the right lung with a mediastinal shift to the left. This 13-month-old infant presented with a new onset of wheezing and coughing after choking while eating a chunky peanut butter sandwich.

BOX 6-1. CLINICAL FEATURES OF FOREIGN BODY ASPIRATION

Symptoms and signs of FBA:

- Sudden episode of choking or gagging while eating or playing, followed by:
  - (1) Wheezing (e.g., bypass valve with passage of air in both directions with slight obstruction)
  - (2) Coughing (may be paroxysmal or violent during aspiration event)
  - (3) Stridor
  - (4) Cyanosis
  - (5) Hoarseness
  - (6) Aphonia or dysphonia
  - (7) Tachypnea/respiratory distress
  - (8) Diminished breath sounds (distal to obstruction) on affected side
  - (9) Hyperresonance (hyperinflation) or dull percussion (atelectasis) of the lung on the affected side
  - (10) Blood-streaked sputum (older children)
- Asymptomatic period (after initial symptoms that may be forgotten, the symptom-free interval may last from hours to weeks [e.g., with nonobstructing nonirritating FB])
- Fever (FB contaminated, causing chemical irritation, or present for a long period may lead to complications; e.g., pneumonia)
- Refractory asthma (that does not respond to conventional therapy)
- Recurrent or persistent pneumonia

Commonly aspirated FBs:

- Foods: peanuts/nuts (*account for more than half of FBAs*), popcorn, raisins, sunflower seeds, hot dogs, beans, bones [fish, chicken])
- Nonfood items: crayons, toy parts, tacks, pins, pen tops, nails/screws, bullets, teeth, staples, rocks/ stones, coins, springs, earrings, styrofoam cup fragments, pencil lead

BOX 6-2. RADIOGRAPHIC FINDINGS OF FOREIGN BODY ASPIRATION

- Normal findings (usually seen when x-rays are obtained within 24 hours of FBA)
- Radiopaque foreign body (only a small number of foreign bodies are radiopaque; Fig. 6-4)
- Localized hyperinflation (e.g., check valve or ball valve obstruction that allows air entry during inspiration but not air exit during expiration)
- Atelectasis (e.g., stop valve obstruction [complete obstruction] without any air entry or exit; lung collapse develops as air distal to the obstruction gets absorbed)
- Mediastinal shift
- Pneumonia
- Findings of retained FB (prolonged period)
  - (1) Obstructive emphysema
  - (2) Pneumonia (recurrent or persistent)
  - (3) Lung abscess
  - (4) Bronchiectasis

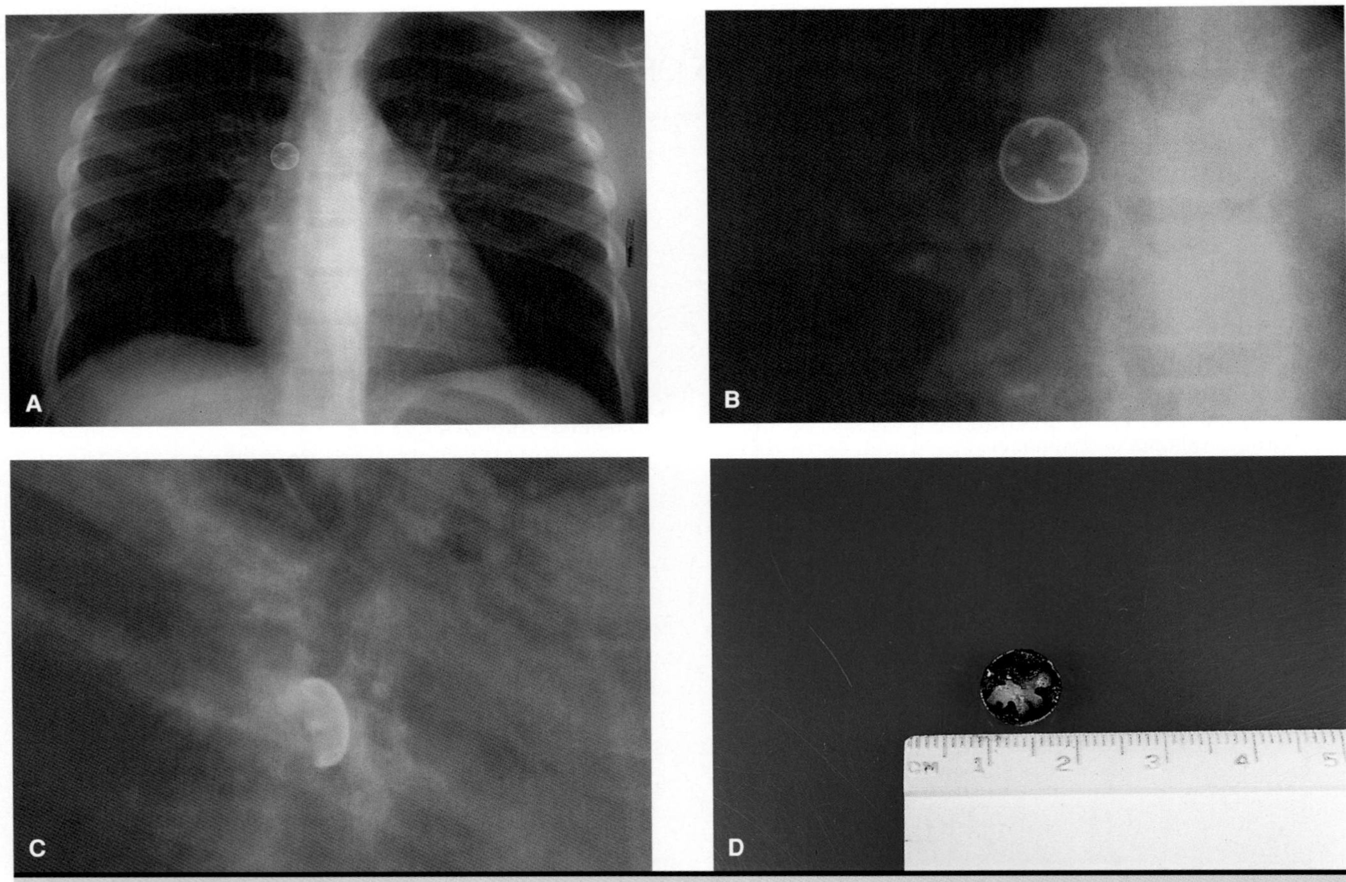

Figure 6-4. Radiopaque Foreign Body Aspiration

A. A round radiopaque density is seen in the area of right main stem bronchus. There is no mediastinal shift, air trapping, pneumothorax, or distal atelectasis. This 4-year-old patient presented with a history of worsening cough of 6 days' duration and first episode of wheezing. Three days prior to this visit to ED, she was seen by her primary care physician, who prescribed cough medicine. *B., C*. Close-ups of the FB in AP and lateral projections. *D*. Close-up of the brown metal button measuring 1 × 1 × 0.5 cm that was removed from the right bronchus by direct bronchoscopy.

BOX 6-3. DIFFERENTIAL DIAGNOSIS OF FOREIGN BODY ASPIRATION

- Wheezing from other etiology (e.g., asthma, bronchiolitis)
- Acute pneumonia from other etiology (e.g., bacterial or viral)
- Stridor from other etiology (e.g., croup, retropharyngeal abscess)
- Recurrent or persistent pneumonia from other etiology (e.g., cystic fibrosis)
- Unilateral inflammation from other etiology (e.g., congenital lobar emphysema)

DIAGNOSIS CROUP

SYNONYMS

Laryngotracheobronchitis
Viral croup

Definition

Croup is an acute viral inflammation of the larynx, trachea, and bronchi (laryngotracheobronchitis, as the name implies) resulting in varying degrees of upper airway obstruction.

Etiology

1. Parainfluenza virus types 1 and 3 are the most common etiology (about 75% of cases).
2. Other viruses include influenza viruses A and B, respiratory syncytial virus, adenovirus, enteroviruses, rhinovirus, herpes simplex virus, and measles.

Associated Clinical Features

1. Seen almost exclusively in children <5 years of age (most common ages: 6 months to 2 years)
2. Most commonly seen between late fall and early winter months (in association with community outbreaks of parainfluenza or influenza viruses)
3. Croup is diagnosed clinically by history and physical examination and usually no specific laboratory tests are required.
4. Arterial blood gas analysis will confirm the impending or frank respiratory failure, but clinical evaluation is sufficient to identify patients who will need intubation and assisted ventilation.
5. Radiographs
   a. *Not* routinely indicated for the diagnosis of croup
   b. When the diagnosis is unclear, neck and chest radiographs may be helpful to exclude other conditions (e.g., a lateral neck radiograph may help to exclude retropharyngeal abscess or the presence of a foreign body).
   c. Narrowing of the upper airway is seen as a "steeple" sign on a anteroposterior view of the neck in croup (Fig. 6-5).

Emergency Department Treatment and Disposition

1. Principles of therapy in croup include supportive therapy (assuring adequate hydration and control of fever) and reducing airway obstruction.
2. Mild cases of croup, with a reliable caretaker (capable of determining the signs of worsening respiratory distress), can be managed as outpatients with a close follow-up. Cool or warm mist delivered by a humidifier is recommended. Warm steam created in the bathroom with a hot shower running is also very helpful in relieving the obstruction (soothing inflamed mucosa and thinning secretions).
3. Patients presenting with moderate to severe respiratory distress (if possible, allow a parent to hold the infant in her lap while offering therapy in order to reduce the child's agitation, which may worsen the obstruction]):
   a. Humidified oxygen as indicated by pulse oximetry
   b. Corticosteroids (reduces subglottic edema) given as
      1) Dexamethasone (0.6 mg/kg orally or intramuscularly as a single dose) *or*
      2) Aerosolized budesonide (dose: 2 to 4 mg)
   c. Nebulized racemic epinephrine 2.25% solution (mucosal vasoconstriction will help reduce edema)
      1) Dose: 0.25 mL for <10 kg, 0.5 mL for 10 to 20 kg, and 0.75 mL for >20 kg, mixed with 3.5 mL of normal saline and given over 10 minutes
      2) Observe patient for at least 2 hours (rebound after nebulized epinephrine therapy is a myth; patients

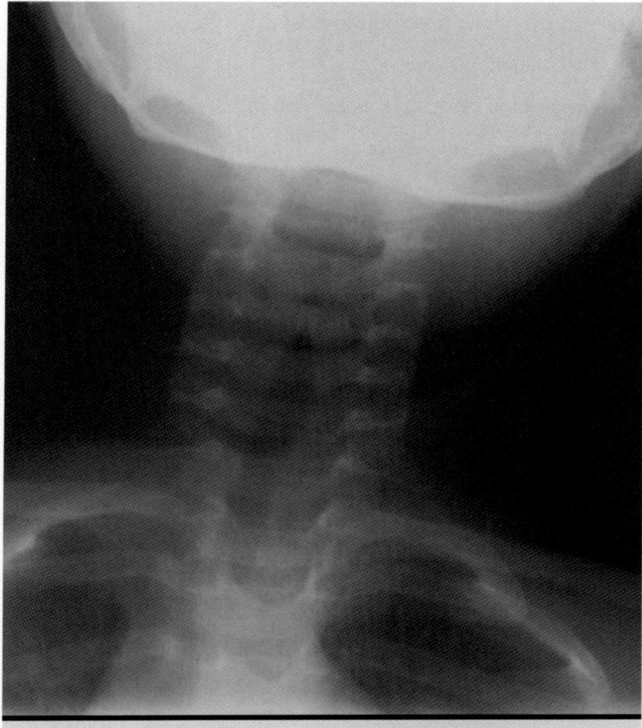

Figure 6-5. Laryngotracheobronchitis (Croup)

Anteroposterior radiograph of the neck showing typical steeple sign (subglottic narrowing) in a patient with croup.

do not get worse but may return to their baseline after receiving therapy [possible need for additional therapy]).

d. Nebulized L-epinephrine 1:1000 (if racemic epinephrine not available)
   1) 2.5 mL for child <10 kg, 5 mL for child >10 kg

4. Indications for hospitalization include:
   a. Persistent or worsening signs of respiratory distress despite therapy
   b. Signs of impending or frank respiratory failure or compensated respiratory failure
   c. Stridor at rest
   d. Unreliable caretaker
   e. Poor oral fluid intake

5. Indications for intubation (and ICU admission) include patients who fail to respond to racemic epinephrine and dexamethasone, and in whom progressive hypoxia, cyanosis, hypercarbia, and increasing respiratory distress and tachycardia develop (signs of respiratory failure).

6. Duration of illness usually ranges from a few to several days. Rarely, it may persist for several weeks. Recurrences may be seen from 3 to 6 years of age and decrease with growth of the airway.

Clinical Pearls: Croup

1. Croup is the most common form of acute upper airway obstruction in infants and children.
2. Inspiratory stridor, hoarseness, and barking cough are characteristic features of croup.
3. Drooling, dysphagia, high fever, and toxic appearance are notably absent in viral croup and suggest another diagnosis (e.g., epiglottitis).
4. Croup is a clinical diagnosis made by history and physical examination. Attempts to perform laboratory tests often lead to more agitation and worsening of the airway obstruction and respiratory distress.

BOX 6-4. CLINICAL FEATURES OF CROUP

- Low-grade fever, rhinorrhea
- Hoarseness
- Barking cough (seal-like cough)
- *Not* toxic appearing
- *Absence of* drooling
- Varying degrees of upper airway obstruction, and these signs and symptoms:
  (1) Tachypnea
  (2) Tachycardia (hypoxia, fever)
  (3) Inspiratory stridor with or without expiratory stridor (present with increasing obstruction)
  (4) Stridor at rest
  (5) Use of accessory muscles (flaring of nares, intercostal, subcostal, suprasternal and/or supraclavicular retractions)
  (6) Decreased air entry
  (7) Wheezing may be present
  (8) Restlessness, agitation, or cyanosis (signs of hypoxia; impending/frank respiratory failure)
  (9) Hypotonia (sign of CO_2 retention; impending/frank respiratory failure)
  (10) Difficult to arouse or lethargic (sign of CO_2 retention; impending/frank respiratory failure)
- Signs and symptoms greatly aggravated by crying or handling the patient

BOX 6-5. DIFFERENTIAL DIAGNOSIS OF CROUP

- Epiglottitis (see Fig. 6-6)
- Spasmodic croup
  (1) Sudden onset of stridor and croupy cough
  (2) Usually occurs in the middle of the night
  (3) Notable absence of fever, drooling, dysphagia, toxicity
  (4) History of recurrence
  (5) Warm steam, vomiting, or changing the environment usually aborts symptoms.
- Bacterial tracheitis
- Retropharyngeal abscess (see Fig. 9-4)
- Foreign body ingestion/aspiration (see Figs. 15-1 to 15-5)
- Acute allergic reactions
- Laryngomalacia
- Subglottic stenosis (congenital or acquired)
- Diphtheria

BOX 6-6. DIFFERENTIAL DIAGNOSIS OF STRIDOR

Inflammatory causes:

- Laryngotracheobronchitis
- Epiglottitis
- Retropharyngeal abscess
- Bacterial tracheitis
- Diphtheria
- Papillomatosis
- Inhalation injury
- Peritonsillar abscess

Congenital causes:

- Laryngomalacia
- Tracheomalacia
- Tracheal stenosis
- Vocal cord paralysis
- Vascular ring
- Laryngeal or tracheal webs
- Laryngeal papilloma
- Tracheoesophageal fistula
- Cystic hygroma
- CNS malformation

Noninflammatory causes:

- Foreign body (airway, esophageal)
- Postintubation (edema, stenosis, granuloma)
- Ingestion (e.g., caustic)
- Gastroesophageal reflux
- Hypocalcemic tetany
- Facial trauma
- Retropharyngeal hematoma
- Laryngeal/tracheal fracture or swelling
- Anaphylaxis (angioedma, laryngospasm)
- Hereditary angioneurotic edema
- Tumors (e.g., rhabdomyosarcoma, lymphoma, lymphangioma)
- Kartagener's syndrome
- Hysterical stridor

DIAGNOSIS EPIGLOTTITIS

SYNONYMS

Supraglottitis
Bacterial croup

Definition

Epiglottitis is an acute life-threatening inflammation of supraglottic structures with involvement of the epiglottis, aryepiglottic folds (false vocal cords), arytenoids, and vallecula.

Etiology

1. Bacterial
   a. *Haemophilus influenzae* type b (HIB; most common pathogen until the advent of HIB vaccine)
   b. *Streptococcus pneumoniae*
   c. *Staphylococcus aureus*
   d. *Streptococcus pyogenes* (group A beta-hemolytic streptococci)
   e) Group B and C streptococci
   f) *Haemophilus parainfluenzae*
   g. *Neisseria meningitidis*
   h. *Neisseria gonorrhoeae* (sexually active adolescents and adults)
2. Noninfections etiology
   a. Direct trauma
   b. Thermal injury (e.g., scalding burns of face, drinking hot liquids)

Associated Clinical Features

1. Age at presentation
   a. Usually seen in children 2 to 7 years of age (peak incidence: 3.5 years)

b. Typically patients with epiglottitis are older than patients with croup.
c. Any age can be affected including adults (infrequently).

2. Laboratory studies such as CBC (usually leukocytosis with a left shift), blood culture (positive in ~90% of cases), and culture of epiglottis (positive in ~70% of cases) are done only after securing the airway.
3. Diagnosis is confirmed by direct visualization of supraglottic structures by laryngoscopy. Edema with intense erythema of epiglottis (often described as cherry-red appearance) and surrounding structures including arytenoids and aryepiglottic folds and vocal cords are seen.
4. Lateral neck radiograph
   a. Usually not done routinely to confirm the diagnosis and should not delay definitive treatment
   b. Usually obtained only when the diagnosis of epiglottitis is uncertain
   c. Usually obtained to exclude other conditions (e.g., retropharyngeal abscess or presence of foreign body) once epiglottitis has been excluded by direct visualization
   d. An enlarged epiglottis is seen as a "thumbprint" sign with thickened aryepiglottic folds, hypopharyngeal distension, and a normal subglottis (Fig. 6-6).
5. A chest radiograph is performed after intubation to confirm appropriate placement of the endotracheal tube and to exclude pneumonia (most commonly associated illness).

Consultations

Follow the institution's emergency protocol for handling patients with suspected epiglottitis. Usually pediatric surgery or otolaryngology (stand by in operating room if emergency tracheostomy is required), anesthesiology, and pediatric intensivist are part of the team.

Emergency Department Treatment and Disposition

1. Make emergent arrangements to bring the patient to the OR to confirm the diagnosis and control the airway, followed by admission to the ICU for continuous monitoring.
2. Establishment of an airway by endotracheal intubation (or tracheostomy if attempts at intubation fail) is indicated in patients with epiglottitis once the diagnosis is confirmed by direct visualization, regardless of the degree of apparent respiratory distress. Average length of intubation is about 24 to 48 hours.
3. Empiric IV antibiotic therapy while awaiting culture/sensitivity results:
   a. Ceftriaxone (dose: 75 to 100 mg/kg per day divided every 12 to 24 hours) *or*
   b. Cefuroxime (dose: 100 to 150 mg/kg per day divided every 8 hours)
   c. Usual duration is between 7 and 10 days

Clinical Pearls: Epiglottitis

1. Epiglottitis is a life-threatening upper airway emergency requiring prompt intervention; *observation alone of a child with epiglottitis is inadvisable.*
2. Patients with epiglottitis usually prefer a tripod position. Because of an increased risk of airway obstruction, *do not* force the patient to lie in a supine position (a gravity-induced change in the position of the epiglottis in a supine posture may lead to total obstruction).
3. Examination of the pharynx with a tongue blade may induce reflex laryngospasm, leading to a complete airway obstruction; this exam *should not* be undertaken in a child with suspected epiglottitis without complete preparation for immediate endotracheal intubation under controlled conditions.
4. A diagnosis of epiglottitis is confirmed by direct visualization and *not* by a neck x-ray (performing an x-ray is dangerous, as the patient may develop laryngospasm leading to a complete airway obstruction during an attempt to forcefully hyperextend the neck for the radiograph).

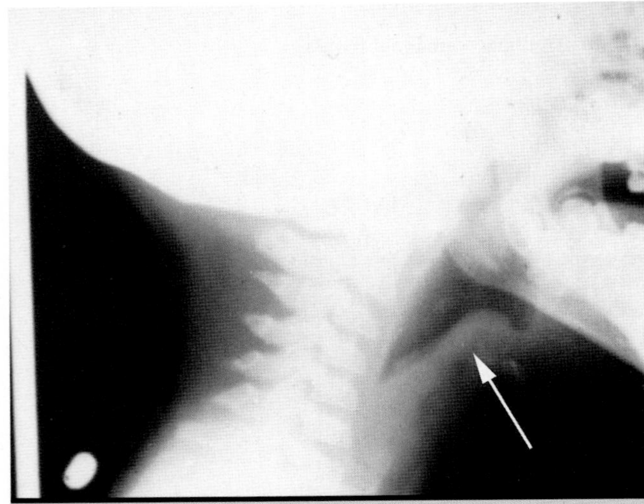

Figure 6-6. Epiglottitis

A lateral neck x-ray is usually obtained when the diagnosis of epiglottitis is unlikely and to exclude other causes of acute airway obstruction, such as retropharyngeal abscess or a foreign body in the aerodigestive tract. The patient must be accompanied to the x-ray department by a physician capable of intubating the airway, if required. Lateral x-ray shows the "thumbprint sign" (marked enlargement of the epiglottis with thickening and bulging of the aryepiglottic folds) in patients with epiglottitis. (Reproduced with permission from: Cordle R, Relich NC: Upper respiratory emergencies. In: Tintinalli JE, Kelen GD, Stapczynski JS (eds). *Emergency Medicine. A Comprehensive Study Guide,* 5th ed. McGraw-Hill, New York, 2000, p. 879.)

BOX 6-7. CLINICAL FEATURES OF EPIGLOTTITIS

- Absence of prodromal upper respiratory infection
- Sudden onset of high fever
- Aphonia or muffled voice/cry
- Drooling
- Dysphagia
- Sore throat (older child)
- Inspiratory stridor
- Varying degrees of moderate to severe respiratory distress (retractions [subcostal, intercostal, suprasternal, supraclavicular], nasal flaring)
- Varying degree of hypoxia (restlessness or agitation) or cyanosis
- Typical posture: "tripod position" (this position maximizes the size of the supraglottic airway)
  (1) Seen in an older child
  (2) Sitting position with arms providing support
  (3) Neck extended in sniffing position
  (4) Leaning forward with open mouth and a protruding tongue
- Fulminant course (rapid progression to shock-like state with pallor, cyanosis, unconsciousness)

BOX 6-8. DIFFERENTIAL DIAGNOSIS OF EPIGLOTTITIS

- Croup (laryngotracheobronchitis; see Fig. 6-5)
- Spasmodic croup
- Bacterial tracheitis (pseudomembranous tracheitis)
- Retropharyngeal abscess (see Fig. 9-4)
- Foreign body ingestion/aspiration (see Figs. 15-1 to 15-5)
- Acute allergic reactions (angioneurotic edema/anaphylaxis)
- Caustic ingestion
- Diphtheria (unimmunized child)

BOX 6-9. DIFFERENTIAL DIAGNOSIS OF INFECTIOUS CAUSES OF UPPER AIRWAY OBSTRUCTION

Clinically	***Epiglottitis***	***Croup***	***Spasmodic croup***	***Bacterial tracheitis***
Etiology	Bacterial	Viral	Viral or allergic	Bacterial
Age	2–7 years	1–3 years	1–3 years	5
Onset	Sudden	Gradual	Sudden at night	Gradual
Viral prodrome	Absent	Present	Usually absent	Present
Involvement	Supraglottic	Subglottic	Subglottic	Subglottic
Fever	High	Low-grade	Absent	High
Toxicity	Present	Absent	Absent	Present
Barking/brassy cough	Usually absent	Present	Present	Absent
Dysphagia	Present	Absent	Absent	Present
Drooling	Present	Absent	Absent	Present
Voice	Muffled	Hoarse	Hoarse	
Inspiratory/expiratory stridor	Present	Present	Present	Present
Stridor intensity	Moderate–severe	Mild–severe	Moderate–severe	Moderate–severe
Posture preference	Present (“tripod posture”)	Absent	Absent	Absent
Radiology	Enlarged epiglottis; thick aryepiglottic folds	Subglottic narrowing	Subglottic narrowing	Subglottic narrowing; irregular tracheal border
Endoscopy	Cherry-red epiglottis; aryepiglottic swelling	Deep red mucosa; subglottic narrowing	Pale mucosa; subglottic narrowing	Deep red mucosa; copious tracheal secretions

BOX 6-10. MANAGEMENT OF EPIGLOTTITIS

Do's and don'ts in the ED:

- *Do not* agitate the patient (e.g., avoid taking blood samples, including for blood gases, prior to establishing an airway).
- *Do not* force the patient to lie down (allow the patient to assume a position of comfort).
- *Do not* try to confirm the diagnosis by throat exam with a tongue blade (a tongue blade may induce reflex laryngospasm, causing complete airway obstruction and potentially respiratory arrest or even death).
- *Do not* send the patient for a lateral neck x-ray to confirm the diagnosis (hyperextension of the neck for the procedure may cause reflex laryngospasm, leading to complete airway obstruction and respiratory arrest or even death).
- *Do not* use a racemic epinephrine trial (delays definitive care and causes agitation).
- Administer oxygen in a nonthreatening manner (if possible, do not separate the child from the caregiver, and use their help).
- *Never* leave the child unaccompanied; be prepared to emergently intubate and ventilate the patient at all times while arranging for transfer to the operating room.
- Confirm the diagnosis by direct visualization of the epiglottis followed by endotracheal intubation (or tracheostomy if attempts to intubate fail) in the operating room.

DIAGNOSIS

BRONCHIOLITIS

Definition

Bronchiolitis is a lower respiratory tract disease of infants resulting from inflammatory obstruction of the small airways and predominantly caused by viruses.

Etiology

1. Respiratory syncytial virus (RSV)
   a. Most common etiology (up to 75% of cases)
   b. Yearly epidemics (winter to spring)
2. Parainfluenza viruses (types 3, 2, 1; second most common etiology)
3. Rhinoviruses
4. Adenoviruses
5. Influenza viruses
6. *Mycoplasma pneumoniae*
7. Enteroviruses

Associated Clinical Features

1. Age at presentation
   a. First 2 years of life
   b. Peak incidence: around 6 months (range 2 to 10 months)
2. The diagnosis of bronchiolitis is made clinically (e.g., clinical presentation, community outbreaks), and usually no laboratory tests are required. Nasopharyngeal secretions may be tested for the virus by antigen detection tests (e.g., immunofluorescence or enzyme immunoassay), PCR, or culture.
3. A chest radiograph is not routinely indicated either for diagnosis or management. Abnormalities observed on x-ray often do not correlate with the degree of clinical illness, and the infant may be severely ill despite minimal findings on the chest x-ray. Radiographs are obtained if complications are suspected or other diagnoses cannot be excluded (e.g., foreign body aspiration).
4. Infants who develop RSV or other respiratory viral infections with wheezing or bronchiolitis as their initial infection are more likely to have some form of recurrent lower respiratory tract disease. Adenovirus-induced bronchiolitis may also be associated with long-term complications including bronchiolitis obliterans and hyperlucent lung syndrome.

Emergency Department Treatment and Disposition

1. The mainstay of therapy of bronchiolitis is supportive and includes providing O_2 therapy to maintain the oxygen saturation level >95% and maintaining adequate hydration.

2. Hospitalize all infants with any of the following:
   a. RR >70/min (after maximal ED therapy has been given)
   b. SaO_2 <95%
   c. Prematurity with gestational age <34 weeks
   d. Underlying cardiopulmonary disease (e.g., bronchopulmonary disease)
   e. Atelectasis/pneumonia on chest x-ray
   f. Age <3 months
   g. When parents are uncomfortable dealing with the severity of illness, or if they are unreliable or have only limited resources at home (especially young infants <3 months with bronchiolitis)

3. Patients with respiratory distress with impending or frank respiratory failure are best cared for in an ICU setting with continuous cardiac and pulse oximetry monitoring. Mechanical ventilation may be necessary in some infants. High tidal volumes, high peak inspiratory pressures, and low respiratory rates are used to achieve effective minute ventilation.

4. Bronchodilator therapy (use remains controversial)
   a. Nebulized albuterol (0.5% solution; 0.25 mL in 3 mL NS over 10 to 15 minutes is a commonly used therapy that may offer some benefit)
   b. Nebulized racemic epinephrine therapy is shown to be more effective than albuterol therapy.

3. Other therapies that are commonly used despite a lack of evidence supporting their beneficial effects
   a. Mist therapy
   b. Corticosteroid therapy (*not* effective and *not* indicated in a previously healthy infant with RSV bronchiolitis)

4. Antibiotic therapy is not routinely indicated unless the patient has evidence of a bacterial superinfection.

5. Ribavirin (antiviral agent) may be considered on an individual basis in hospitalized patients with specific clinical conditions with RSV bronchiolitis.
   a. Administered as a small-particle aerosol for 8 to 12 hours each day
   b. Usual duration: 2 to 5 days
   c. Special clinical conditions include infants at high risk for developing severe RSV infection (e.g., underlying complicated congenital heart disease, bronchopulmonary disease, cystic fibrosis, immunodeficiency, or immunosuppressive therapy).

6. RSV intravenous immune globulin (RSV-IVIG) or monoclonal antibody to RSV (palivizumab) given intramuscularly just prior to and during RSV season is effective in preventing severe RSV disease in infants at high risk (infants <2 years old with bronchopulmonary disease, premature birth <35 weeks' gestation).

Clinical Pearls: Bronchiolitis

1. Bronchiolitis is the most common wheezing-associated respiratory illness in infants under 2 years of age (Fig. 6-7).

2. Neonates and infants <3 months of age may present with apnea or a sepsis-like picture.

3. In infants presenting with a first episode of wheezing, it is impossible to clinically differentiate bronchiolitis from asthma. Reversible bronchospasm, a prior history of wheezing episodes, eosinophilia, a history of eczema, and a strong family history of asthma or atopy (in immediate family members) suggest a diagnosis of asthma.

4. Signs and symptoms of congestive heart failure (e.g., tachypnea, tachycardia, wheezing, rales, respiratory distress, hepatomegaly) can be easily mistaken for bronchiolitis, and giving repeated doses of β-agonist therapy to such infants can have serious consequences.

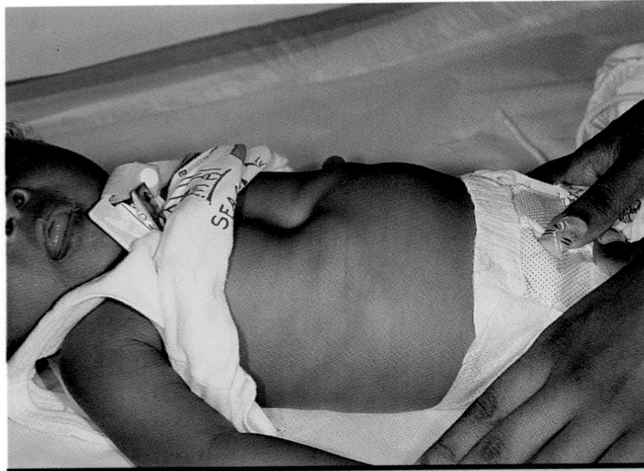

Figure 6-7. Bronchiolitis Presenting with Respiratory Distress

A 4-month-old infant presenting with new onset of wheezing associated with subcostal and intercostal retractions and pulling inward of the sternum with exacerbation of the pectus excavatum deformity is shown. Her chest radiograph showed hyperinflation, a hallmark finding of bronchiolitis.

BOX 6-11. CLINICAL FEATURES OF BRONCHIOLITIS

- Prodromal period (1 to 7 days)
- Signs and symptoms of upper respiratory infection (URI): low-grade fever, cough, serous rhinorrhea, sneezing, mild conjunctivitis
- Lower respiratory tract involvement: 2 to 3 days from onset of signs and symptoms of URI
- Tachypnea (RR ranges from 60 to 80 bpm or higher; shallow breathing)
- Tachycardia
- Signs of impending or frank respiratory failure
  (1) Varying degrees of respiratory distress (retractions [subcostal, intercostal, supraclavicular, suprasternal], flaring of nares)
  (2) Grunting (seen during expiratory phase and indicates small airway and/or alveolar collapse)
  (3) Signs of hypoxemia (cyanosis, air hunger, irritability or agitation)
  (4) Apneic spells (and respiratory arrest) in very young patients
  (5) Signs of CO_2 retention (e.g., poor muscle tone, lethargic or unresponsive)
  (6) Decreased or absent breath sounds
- Cough (may be paroxysmal mimicking pertussis)
- Wheezing (usually paroxysmal/intermittent) or prolonged expiration
- Rales may be present.
- Feeding difficulty (due to very rapid breathing)
- Dehydration (very rapid breathing [increased insensible water loss], poor oral intake)
- Otitis media (up to 30% of cases)
- Hepatosplenomegaly (due to hyperinflation)
- Radiographic findings
  (1) Hyperinflation (depressed diaphragms, hyperlucency of lungs, decreased costophrenic angle, increased AP diameter on lateral view)
  (2) Prominent bronchovascular markings/linear densities radiating out from the hila
  (3) Atelectasis of variable degree with or without infiltrates
  (4) Normal (about 10% of cases)
- Natural course
  (1) Typical course: 3 to 7 days
  (2) Most infants maximally ill 48 to 72 hours after onset of cough and tachypnea
  (3) Usual recovery period: 1 to 2 weeks

BOX 6-12. DIFFERENTIAL DIAGNOSIS OF BRONCHIOLITIS

- Asthma (indistinguishable, especially with first episode of wheezing)
- Foreign body aspiration (tracheobronchial)
- Esophageal foreign body (impingement on trachea)
- Congestive heart failure
- Myocarditis
- Pneumonia (e.g., bacterial, viral, chlamydial, mycoplasmal)
- Pertussis
- Cystic fibrosis
- Congenital malformations (e.g., congenital lobar emphysema, intrapulmonary cysts, vascular ring, tracheomalacia)
- Organophosphate poisoning

DIAGNOSIS BACTERIAL PNEUMONIA

Definition

Pneumonia is an inflammation of the lung (alveoli and terminal airspaces), caused most commonly by an infection.

Associated Clinical Features

1. Incidence of pneumonia varies inversely with age.
2. About 60 to 90% of cases of pneumonia are nonbacterial in origin.
3. Unlike viral pneumonia, there is no seasonal variation in bacterial pneumonia and it occurs throughout the year.
4. Bacterial pneumonia is often preceded by a viral respiratory infection. Other predisposing factors include skin infection (e.g., furunculosis or impetigo due to *S. aureus*) or underlying chronic illness for recurrent pneumonias, including cystic fibrosis or an immunologic deficiency.
5. *S. pneumoniae* is still the most common cause of bacterial pneumonia.
6. Pneumonia caused by *S. aureus* is a serious and rapidly progressive infection. Fortunately, it occurs less frequently than viral or pneumococcal pneumonia.
7. *H. influenzae* type b is an important cause of serious bacterial infection in infants and children who have not received *H. influenzae* type b vaccine. Pneumonia is second in frequency to meningitis in children with invasive *H. influenzae* disease.
8. Pneumonia due to *Streptococcus pyogenes* (group A beta-hemolytic streptococci [GABHS]) is uncommon, but certain viral infections, particularly those causing exanthems and epidemic influenza, predispose to these diseases, which are encountered most frequently in children 3 to 5 years of age.
9. Mycoplasma infection is usually characterized by gradual onset of headache, malaise, low-grade fever, hoarseness, cough with or without scant white, frothy sputum (usually a staccato cough), and typically absence of rhinorrhea. Other signs and symptoms may include rash (e.g., urticaria, erythema multiforme) and arthritis. Elevated cold agglutinins suggest *Mycoplasma* infection.
10. Diagnosis of pneumonia is suspected clinically and confirmed by chest radiograph. Lateral decubitus films may be requested if there is evidence of effusion on the AP and lateral views.
11. Complete blood cell count may show leukocytosis with a left shift. Eosinophilia is seen with *Chlamydia pneumoniae*. Significant leukocytosis with lymphocytosis is seen with *Bordetella pertussis* infection. Other laboratory tests include blood culture and arterial blood gas if indicated (may show hypoxemia with or without hypercapnia).
12. Tuberculin skin testing should be performed, especially in areas with a high incidence of tuberculosis.
13. In patients with empyema, pleural fluid typically reveals an exudate with polymorphonuclear cells, elevated protein, and a low glucose concentration; Gram's stain and cultures will identify the pathogen.
14. Complications of pneumonia include bacteremia, empyema, meningitis, pericarditis, cellulitis and suppurative arthritis, osteomyelitis, and metastatic infections.
15. Radiographic resolution of the infiltrate may not be complete for several weeks (3 to 4 weeks). There is no need to repeat the radiographs during the early course unless there is clinical deterioration.

Emergency Department Treatment and Disposition

1. Hospitalize a patient with any of the following:
   a. Presence of respiratory distress with or without hypoxia
   b. Toxic appearance (possible bacteremia that can lead to septicemia)
   c. Age <3 months (the course of illness in young infants is more variable and complications are more common)
   d. Immunocompromised child (e.g., sickle cell disease, HIV)
   e. Inability to maintain adequate hydration (failed oral therapy in the ED or protracted vomiting)
   f. Pneumonia with pleural effusion/empyema (may require diagnostic and therapeutic interventions)
   g. Unreliable caretaker
   h. Failed outpatient therapy
2. Intravenous antibiotics should be given to patients requiring hospitalization while awaiting culture results and sensitivity.
   a. Neonates (up to 2 months): broad-spectrum antibiotic (e.g., ampicillin and cefotaxime)
   b. Infants (preschool age): cefuroxime or ceftriaxone or ampicillin/sulbactam
   c. For suspected *S. aureus* pneumonia: semisynthetic penicillinase-resistant penicillin (e.g., nafcillin)
3. The majority of preschool-aged children (without the aforementioned indications for hospitalization) can be treated as outpatients with oral antibiotics (e.g., amoxicillin/clavulanic acid) with very close follow-up arranged with the PCP (e.g., daily follow-up until the fever resolves with clinical signs of improvement). The first dose of antibiotic may be given parenterally to such children.
4. Macrolide antibiotics (e.g., azithromycin or clarithromycin) are used in older children for clinically suspected *Mycoplasma pneumoniae* infection.
5. Thoracentesis is usually not necessary in patients with small pleural effusions (e.g., effusions seen on a lateral view of

the chest as blunting of the costophrenic angle). However, symptomatic patients with large effusions will require needle thoracentesis for both diagnostic as well as therapeutic reasons. A chest tube drain is usually required if pleural fluid has exudates (empyema).

6. If the initial response to antibiotics is good, oral treatment can be instituted to complete a 10- to 14-day course.

Clinical Pearls: Bacterial Pneumonia

1. The sine qua non of infectious pneumonia is tachypnea; however, tachypnea is a nonspecific sign and may be seen in a variety of other pathological processes (e.g., compensation for metabolic acidosis, sepsis, congestive heart failure).
2. *S. pneumoniae* is still the most common cause of bacterial pneumonia.
3. *M. pneumoniae* is the most common cause of bacterial pneumonia in school-aged children.
4. An abrupt onset and rapid progression of symptoms of pneumonia in very young infants should be considered to be due to staphylococci until proved otherwise.
5. Lower lobe pneumonia can present with signs of paralytic ileus and/or referred pain to the right lower quadrant (with right lower lobe pneumonia), mimicking acute abdomen.

BOX 6-13. VARIOUS ETIOLOGIES OF BACTERIAL PNEUMONIAS

Age	*Bacterial pathogens*
Neonates	Group B streptococci
	Escherichia coli
	Listeria monocytogenes
	Klebsiella pneumoniae
3 to 12 weeks	*Chlamydia trachomatis*
Infants through preschool	*Streptococcus pneumoniae*
	Haemophilus influenzae
	Staphylococcus aureus (30% of patients <3 months and 70% <1 year)
	Streptococcus pyogenes
	Moraxella catarrhalis
	Neisseria meningitidis
School age through adolescence	*Mycoplasma pneumoniae*
	S. pneumoniae
	Chlamydia pneumoniae
Any age aspiration pneumonia (e.g., neurologically impaired, during seizures)	Anaerobes

BOX 6-14. CLINICAL FINDINGS OF BACTERIAL PNEUMONIA

- Signs and symptoms in infants (*any of the following*)
  (1) Abrupt onset of fever
  (2) Restlessness, agitation (signs of hypoxia)
  (3) Signs of respiratory distress (tachypnea, tachycardia, grunting, air hunger, cyanosis, nasal flaring, retractions [supraclavicular, suprasternal, intercostal, subcostal])
  (4) Coughing without sputum production
  (5) Rales
  (6) Evidence of consolidation (may be difficult to demonstrate or absent)
  (7) Shock-like state
- Signs and symptoms in older children and adolescents (*any of the following*)
  (1) Abrupt onset of chills with fever
  (2) Pleuritic chest pain
  (3) Chest pain
  (4) Tachypnea and/or dyspnea
  (5) Splinting on the affected side (to minimize pleuritic pain)
  (6) Coughing with or without sputum (may be blood-tinged mucus)
  (7) Rales
  (8) Evidence of consolidation (dullness to percussion, diminished tactile and vocal fremitus, bronchial breathing, rales)
  (9) Evidence of effusion (dullness to percussion, diminished fremitus and breath sounds)
- Extrapulmonary findings
  (1) Nuchal rigidity or meningismus (right upper lobe pneumonia)
  (2) Abdominal distention (gastric dilation from swallowed air or ileus)
  (3) Right lower quadrant pain (diaphragmatic irritation with pain referred to abdomen [right lower lobe pneumonia]; mimics acute abdomen)
  (4) Paralytic ileus (absent bowel sounds, abdominal distension [lower lobe pneumonia]; mimics acute abdomen)
- Radiographic findings (infants/children/adolescents; Figs. 6-8 through 6-14)
  (1) Lobar or segmental consolidation (more common in older children)
  (2) "Round" pneumonia (circular-appearing pneumonia)
  (3) Interstitial pneumonitis (e.g., *Streptococcus pyogenes*)
  (4) Bilateral involvement (e.g., *S. aureus* pneumonia)
  (5) Effusion (pleural effusion or empyema [e.g., *S. aureus* pneumonia, *S. pneumoniae*)
  (6) Pneumatocele (e.g., *S. aureus* pneumonia)
  (7) Pyopneumothorax (e.g., *S. aureus* pneumonia)

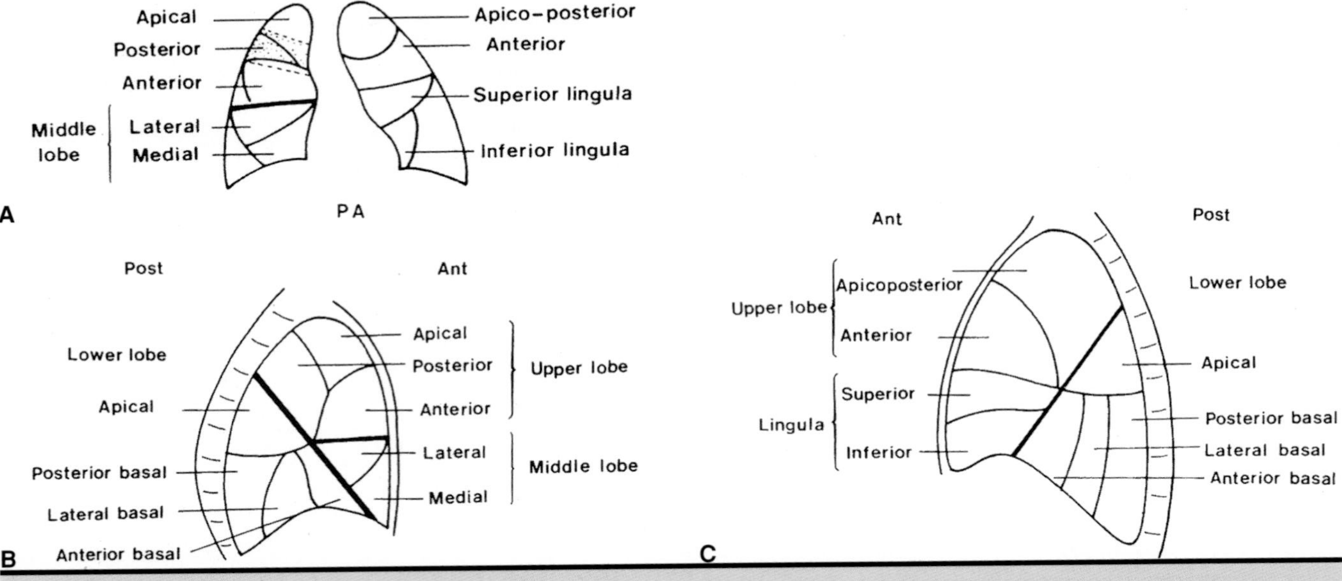

Figure 6-8. Schematic Lung Diagrams

Diagrams illustrating the approximate positions of the pulmonary segments as seen on the PA (*A*) and lateral radiographs (*B*, right lateral lung and *C*, left lateral lung). (Reproduced with permission from: Murfitt J: The normal chest: Methods of investigation and differential diagnosis. In: Sutton D (ed). *Textbook of Radiology and Medical Imaging,* 5th ed., International Student Edition. Churchill Livingstone, London, UK, 1992, p. 298.)

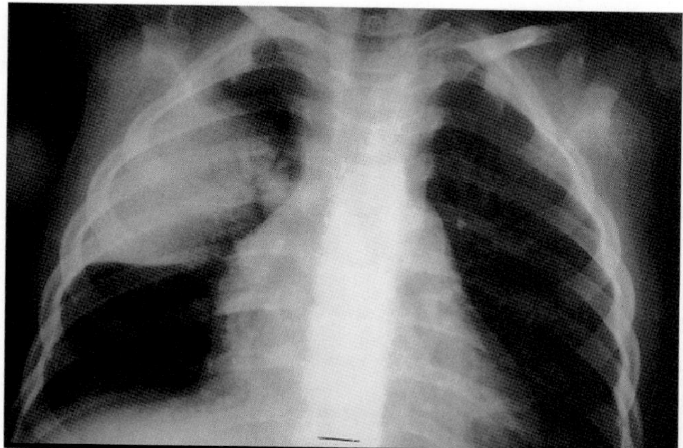

Figure 6-9. Lobar Consolidation in Pneumococcal Pneumonia

A frontal view of the chest showing right upper lobe pneumonia. There is anterior segment involvement. Note air bronchograms and the slight bulge in the minor fissure. This 7-year-old patient presented with fever, tachypnea, and leukocytosis (WBC 35,000/mm^3 with a left shift). Her blood culture was positive for *S. pneumoniae*. Bacteremia is present in 10 to 30% of patients with pneumococcal pneumonia.

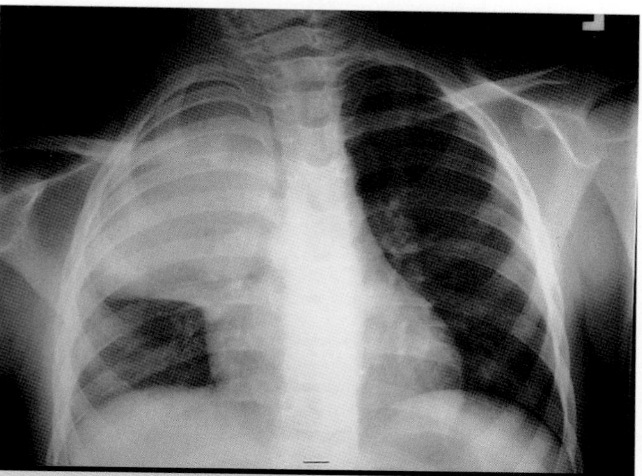

Figure 6-10. Lobar Consolidation in Pneumococcal Pneumonia

In this patient, apical, anterior, and posterior segments of the right upper lobe are involved.

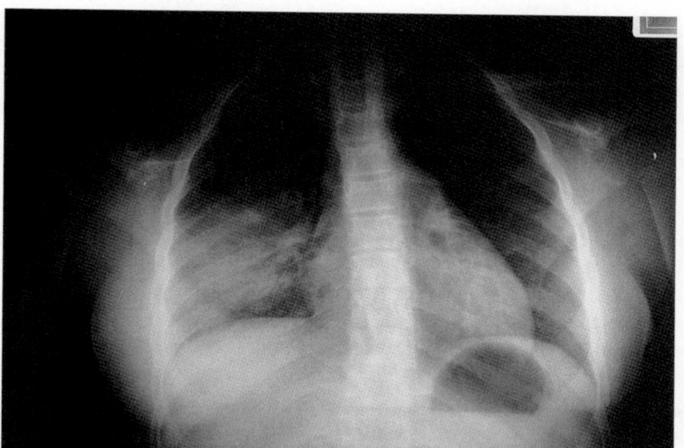

Figure 6-11. Lobar Consolidation in Pneumococcal Pneumonia

A frontal chest radiograph showing consolidation in the superior segment of the right lower lobe. There was a small area of consolidation in the right middle lobe that was better seen on the lateral projection.

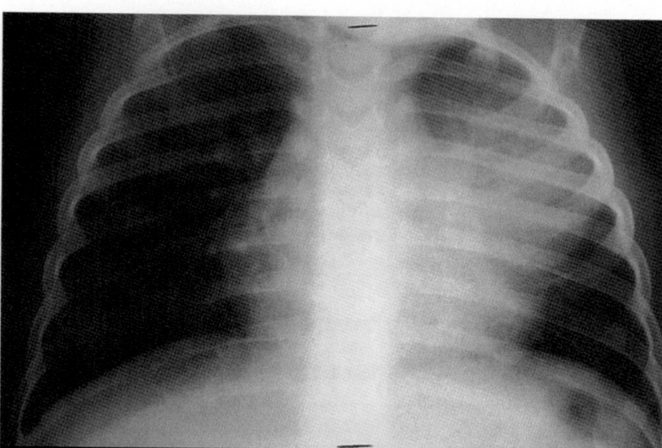

Figure 6-12. Left Upper Lobe Consolidation

A frontal chest radiograph showing left upper lobe consolidation involving the anterior and lingular segments. Obliteration of the left cardiac margin that occurs with lingular involvement is seen (likewise on the right, the right cardiac margin will be obliterated with right middle lobe consolidation).

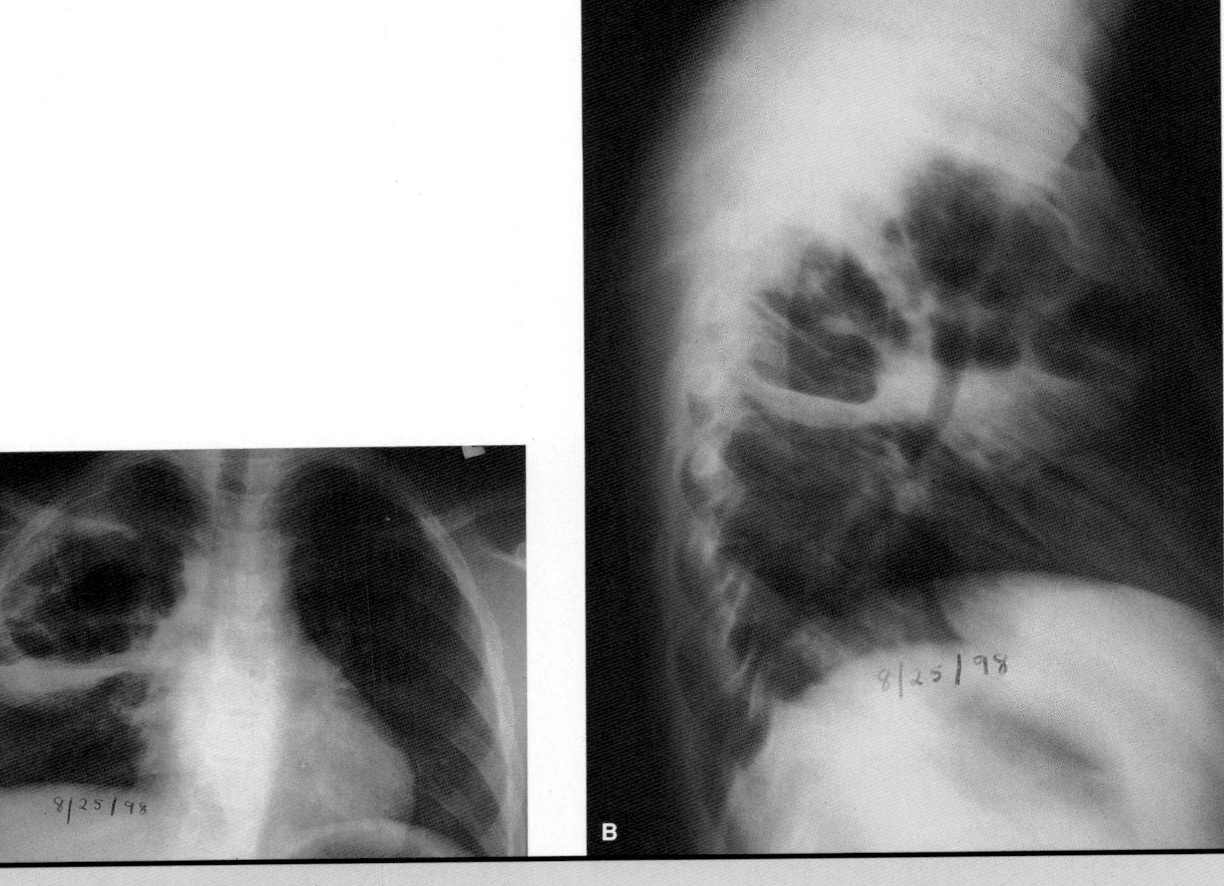

Figure 6-13. Staphylococcal Pneumonia

A., B. Frontal and lateral chest radiographs showing involvement of entire right upper lobe with multiple pneumatoceles, some of which have air-fluid levels. The minor fissure is displaced inferiorly ("bulging fissure"). This patient was diagnosed with cystic fibrosis after presenting with pneumonia. His blood culture was positive for *S. aureus*. A rapid progression of symptoms and a rapid progression from bronchopneumonia to effusion or pyopneumothorax with or without pneumatoceles are highly suggestive of staphylococcal pneumonia. Empyema, pyopneumothorax, and pneumatoceles are so common with staphylococcal pneumonia that they are considered part of the natural course of the illness and not complications. Other bacterial pneumonias that cause empyema or pneumatoceles include *S. pneumoniae,* group A streptococci, *Klebsiella, H. influenzae* (both type b and nontypable), and primary tuberculous pneumonia with cavitation. Aspiration of a radiolucent foreign body followed by pulmonary abscesses may occasionally lead to a similar clinical and radiologic picture.

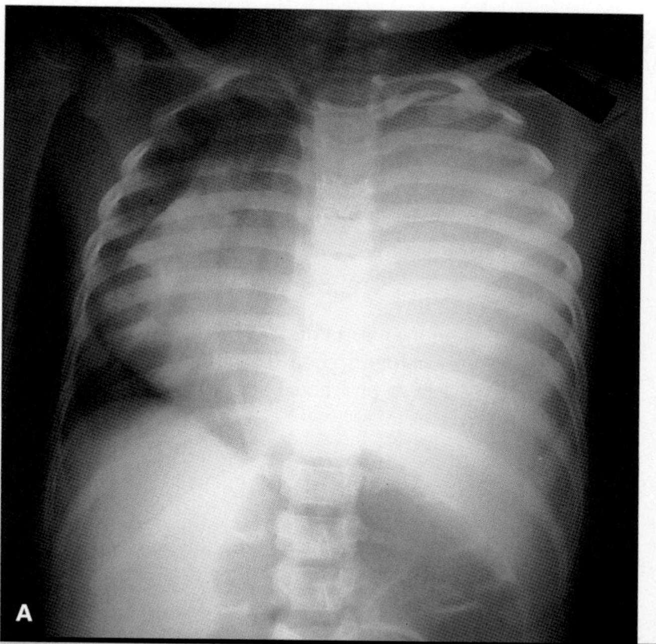

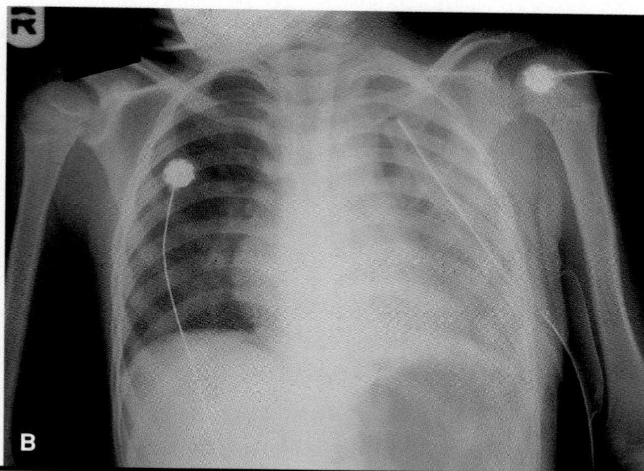

Figure 6-14. Empyema

A. Frontal view of the chest showing complete opacification of the left lung field and a mediastinal shift to the right in a 6-year-old boy who presented with high fever, respiratory distress, and hypoxia. He had an infected varicella lesion on his ear which was the portal of entry for invasive GABHS infection. About 700 mL of pus, which later grew GABHS, was drained from the pleural cavity. *B*. Frontal view of the chest in the same patient after chest tube insertion showing partial resolution of the previously noted empyema with re-expansion of the left lung. The mediastinal shift to the right had also resolved. (Photo A reproduced with permission from: Shah BR, Laude TA: Streptococcal toxic shock syndrome. *Atlas of Pediatric Clinical Diagnosis*. WB Saunders, Philadelphia, 2000, p. 90.)

BOX 6-15. DIFFERENTIAL DIAGNOSIS OF PNEUMONIA

- Pneumonias of varied etiology (bacterial, viral, noninfectious causes [e.g., chemical, aspiration, drug- or radiation-induced, hypersensitivity reactions])
- Bronchiolitis
- Atelectasis
- Foreign body aspiration
- Allergic bronchitis
- Congestive heart failure
- Pulmonary sequestration
- Lung abscess
- Acute appendicitis

DIAGNOSIS VIRAL PNEUMONIA

Definition and Etiology

1. Pneumonia is an inflammation of the parenchyma of the lung (alveoli and interstitial airspaces) most commonly caused by an infection.
2. The most common etiology of pneumonia in normal children includes respiratory viruses (see Box 6-16), *Mycoplasma pneumoniae,* and certain bacteria (see Box 6-13).
3. Less common infectious causes of pneumonia include nonrespiratory viruses (e.g., varicella-zoster virus), enteric gram-negative bacteria, mycobacteria, *Chlamydia, Rickettsia, Pneumocystis carinii,* and fungi.

Associated Clinical Features

1. There is a seasonal variation with viral pneumonias. Respiratory syncytial virus (RSV) infections are commonly seen during winter and early spring, parainfluenza infections are seen during fall, and influenza infections are seen during winter.
2. The peak incidence for viral pneumonia is between 2 and 3 years of age and decreases slowly thereafter.
3. The white blood cell count is either normal or slightly elevated with a predominance of lymphocytes in uncomplicated viral pneumonia.
4. Definitive diagnosis requires isolation of a virus from a specimen obtained from the respiratory tract. Rapid direct fluorescent antibody tests for RSV and adenovirus can be helpful.
5. Viral pneumonia cannot be definitely differentiated from mycoplasmal disease on clinical grounds, and may on occasion be difficult to distinguish from bacterial pneumonia. For other differential diagnoses see Box 6-15.
6. Most patients with viral pneumonia recover uneventfully without any sequelae. Secondary bacterial infections may complicate viral pneumonia (see Fig. 6-14). Rare complications include chronic lung disease leading to bronchiolitis obliterans (e.g., adenoviral infection).

Emergency Department Treatment and Disposition

1. A majority of patients with viral pneumonia can be managed as outpatients.
2. Treatment of viral pneumonia is mainly supportive, and includes:
   a. Monitoring for cardiac and oxygen status
   b. Providing humidified O_2 if indicated
   c. Maintaining good hydration
   d. Bronchodilator therapy, if indicated
   e. Chest physiotherapy
3. Hospitalize patients with any of the following:
   a. Presence of respiratory distress with or without hypoxia
   b. Impending or frank respiratory failure
   c. Age <3 months
   d. Immunocompromised child
   e. Inability to maintain good hydration (failed oral therapy in the ED or protracted vomiting)
   f. Unreliable caretaker

Clinical Pearls: Viral Pneumonia

1. Respiratory viruses are the most common etiology of pneumonia in the first few years of life.
2. RSV is the most common cause among viral pneumonias during infancy.

BOX 6-16. VIRAL ETIOLOGY OF PNEUMONIA

Age	*Etiologic agent*
Neonates	Cytomegalovirus
	Herpes simplex virus
	Rubella
Infants and preschoolers	Respiratory syncytial virus
	Adenovirus
	Influenza A and B
	Parainfluenza
	Rhinovirus
	Epstein-Barr virus
	Measles (unimmunized)
	Varicella (unimmunized)
	Rubella (unimmunized)
School-age and adolescents	Influenza
	Adenovirus
	Parainfluenza

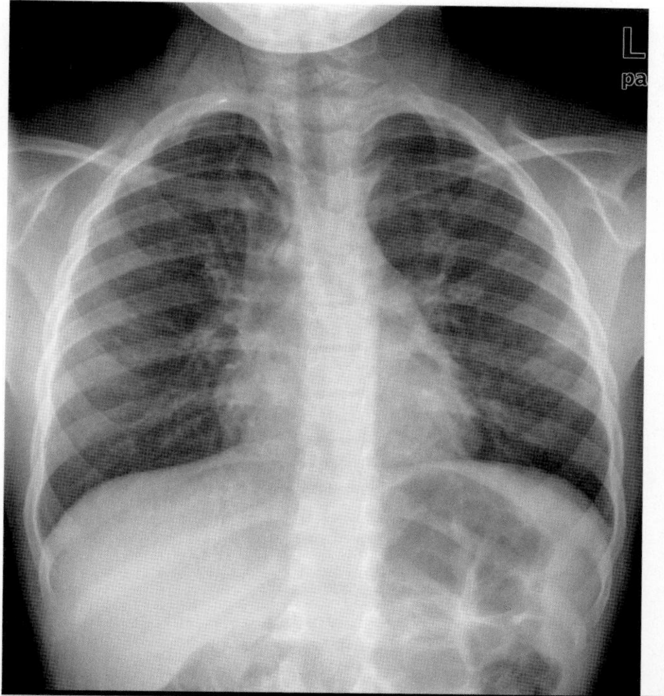

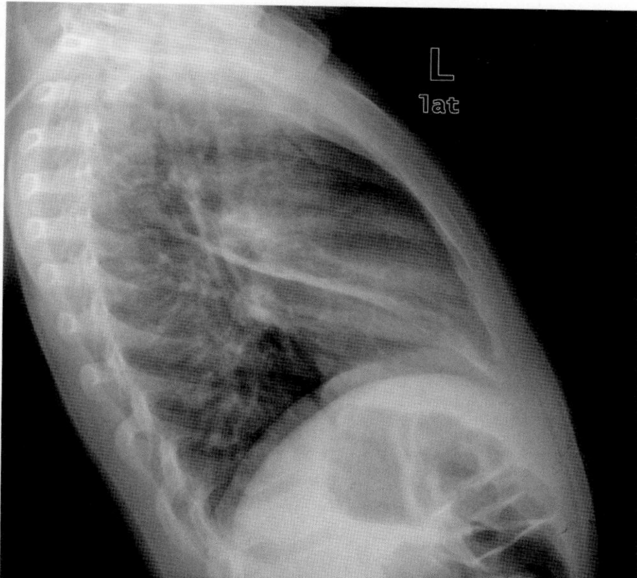

Figure 6-15. Viral Pneumonia

Frontal and lateral views of the chest show bilateral patchy infiltrates in an asthamatic child who presented with low-grade fever, tachypnea, coughing and wheezing. Nasopharyngeal aspirate was positive for adenovirus.

BOX 6-17. FINDINGS OF VIRAL PNEUMONIA

Clinical findings (any of the following):

- Preceding upper respiratory tract signs and symptoms (rhinitis, cough, low-grade fever)
- History of similar illness in other family members
- Tachypnea
- Tachycardia
- Signs of impending or frank respiratory failure
  (1) Varying degrees of respiratory distress (retractions [subcostal, intercostal, supraclavicular, suprasternal], flaring of nares, head bobbing, abdominal breathing)
  (2) Signs of hypoxemia (cyanosis, air hunger, irritability or agitation)
  (3) Signs of CO_2 retention (e.g., poor muscle tone, lethargic or unresponsive)
  (4) Decreased or absent breath sounds
- Grunting (seen during expiratory phase and indicates small airway and/or alveolar collapse)
- Rales
- Wheezing (often present)
- Poor oral intake/dehydration

Radiographic abnormalities:

- Perihilar infiltrate or bilateral diffuse interstitial infiltrates (Fig. 6-15)
- Hyperinflation may be present.
- Small effusion may occasionally be seen
- Lobar or segmental consolidation, large pleural effusion, and pneumatoceles (typical findings of bacterial pneumonias; see Figs. 6-9 through 6-14) are *not* seen

DIAGNOSIS

PERTUSSIS

SYNONYM

Whooping cough

Definition and Etiology

1. Pertussis is a respiratory tract infection produced by *Bordetella pertussis,* a gram-negative pleomorphic bacillus.
2. Pertussis is also called whooping cough because of the progressive, repetitive, and severe episodes of coughing that are followed by a forceful inspiration, which create the characteristic whooping sound.

Associated Clinical Features

1. Infants and young children are frequently infected by respiratory droplets from older siblings and adults who have mild or atypical pertussis (such as a URI or chronic cough without whoop).
2. Symptoms of pertussis may be also atypical in infants and partially immunized children.
3. Leukocytosis with absolute lymphocytosis (total count >50,000 cells/mm^3) may be seen at the beginning of the paroxysmal stage and may persist for 3 to 4 weeks (leukocytosis is usually not seen in young infants).
4. The chest radiograph may be normal or may show shaggy perihilar, patchy, or diffuse infiltrates.
5. Diagnosis is confirmed by culturing a nasopharyngeal sample on special media (e.g., Bordet-Gengou blood agar).
   a. Best samples are obtained during the catarrhal stage or early paroxysmal stage.
   b. May be recovered up to the second to third week of the paroxysmal stage (rarely positive after the fourth week)
   c. Negative cultures are seen in patients receiving antibiotics, those who were previously immunized, or during the late course of the illness.
4. Direct immunofluorescence assay (DFA) of nasopharyngeal secretions can also help in making the diagnosis (low specificity, variable sensitivity).
5. Complications of pertussis include (any of the following):
   a. Respiratory
      1) Otitis media
      2) Bronchopneumonia (aspiration of gastric contents and respiratory secretions during paroxysms of coughing, whooping, and vomiting; bacterial pathogens causing pneumonia include *Streptococcus pneumoniae*, *S. pyogenes*, *Haemophilus influenzae*, and *Staphylococcus aureus*)
      3) Atelectasis
      4) Subcutaneous emphysema, pneumothorax, and pneumomediastinum
   b. Hemorrhagic (subconjunctival bleeding, petechiae, epistaxis, hemoptysis; Fig. 6-16)
   c. Central nervous system (seizures, encephalopathy, anoxia, cerebral hemorrhages)
   d. Diaphragmatic rupture
   e. Umbilical and inguinal hernias
   f. Rectal prolapse

Emergency Department Treatment and Disposition

1. Hospitalize infants <1 year of age and patients with complications (e.g., apnea or cyanosis during episodes, pneumonia, respiratory distress) for continuous cardiac and pulse oximetry monitoring and supportive care. An intensive care setting is recommended for patients with severe disease.
2. Older patients without complications and milder disease can be followed closely as outpatients.

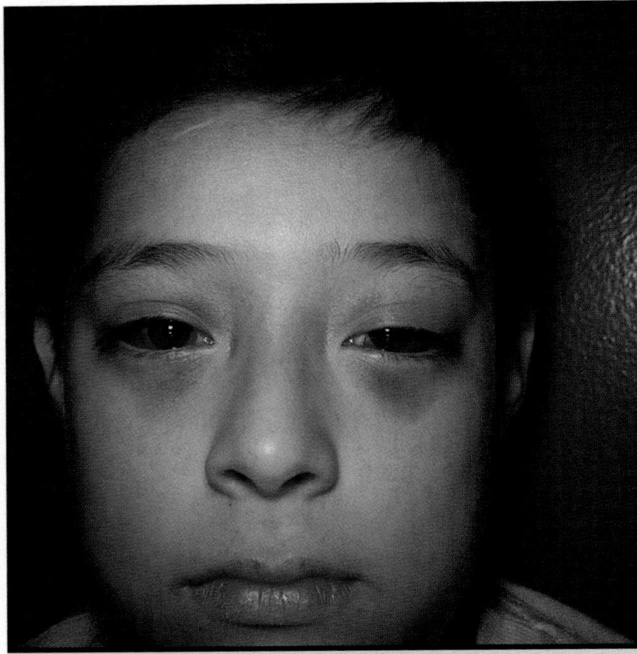

Figure 6-16. Bilateral Subconjunctival Hemorrhages and Ecchymoses; Pertussis

Violent episodes of coughing leading to hemorrhages (subconjunctival and periorbital) were the presenting complaints of pertussis in this 12-year-old unimmunized adolescent boy from El Salvador. Diagnosis of pertussis was confirmed by nasopharyngeal aspirate that was positive for *B. pertussis.* (*Important: These findings of subconjunctival hemorrhages and ecchymoses can be mistaken for inflicted injuries from child abuse.*)

3. In addition to standard precautions, respiratory droplet precautions are recommended for 5 days after initiation of antibiotic therapy or until 3 weeks after the onset of paroxysms without antibiotic therapy.
4. Supportive therapies include suctioning of secretions, humidified oxygen for hypoxia, and maintenance of adequate hydration and nutrition.
5. Erythromycin (drug of choice)
   a. Dose: 40 to 50 mg/kg per day divided qid and given orally for 14 days
   b. May abort or modify the course if started early during the catarrhal stage
   c. Eradicates *B. pertussis* from the upper respiratory tract
   d. Does not have any effect on the clinical course of a fully established disease (however, it is still given to prevent the spread of the disease)
6. Erythromycin given as soon as possible to an exposed person (preferably during the incubation period) will prevent or modify the course of the disease. Pertussis vaccine (follow standard immunization schedule) should also be given to unimmunized or incompletely immunized exposed children who are under 7 years of age.

Clinical Pearls: Pertussis

1. Pertussis means "violent cough," which is the hallmark of the disease. Prolonged paroxysmal coughing, inspiratory whoop, post-tussive vomiting, absolute lymphocytosis, or chronic cough are other characteristic features.
2. *Do not* use cough suppressants.
3. Pertussis is a life-threatening infection; pneumonia complicating pertussis is a leading cause of death, especially in infants and young children.
4. Pertussis is a highly contagious disease. About 90% of nonimmune household contacts acquire the disease. Erythromycin therapy decreases infectivity, limits the spread, and should be given to all household contacts and other close contacts (e.g., child care personnel) *regardless of age and immunization status (pertussis immunity is not absolute and may not prevent infection).*
5. Pertussis is a disease that is preventable by universal immunization with pertussis vaccine; a total of five doses is given starting at 2, 4, 6, and 15 to 18 months of age, followed by a booster dose at 4 to 6 years of age.

BOX 6-18. CLINICAL FEATURES OF PERTUSSIS

- Incubation period: 7 to 13 days
- Three stages (each lasting about 2 weeks; total duration may range from 6 to 10 weeks)
  (1) Catarrhal (1 to 3 weeks)
  (2) Paroxysmal (2 to 4 weeks)
  (3) Convalescent (1 to 2 weeks)

Catarrhal stage

(1) Low-grade fever, rhinorrhea, cough, mild conjunctival injection

(2) Indistinguishable from signs and symptoms of URI

Paroxysmal stage (characterized by paroxysms of coughing)

(1) Coughing is series of short expiratory bursts (little or no inspiration between cough) followed by a prolonged inspiratory gasp, which results in the typical whoop (inspiration through a partially closed glottis)
(2) Whoop may be absent in young infants, older children, and adults.
(3) Paroxysms are more frequent at night.
(4) Paroxysms occur spontaneously or are precipitated by external stimuli (e.g., noises or cold air).
(5) Paroxysms cause cyanosis and apnea (in infants <6 months of age), and facial flushing or frothing of mucus from mouth and nose.
(6) Paroxysm classically ends with an episode of vomiting.
(7) Patient appears exhausted after paroxysm
(8) Petechiae, subconjunctival hemorrhage (during paroxysms of cough)
(9) *Patient appears relatively well in between paroxysms.*

Convalescent stage: Waning of symptoms

BOX 6-19. DIFFERENTIAL DIAGNOSIS OF PERTUSSIS

- Pertussis-like syndrome (whooping cough syndrome) may be caused by:
  (1) Adenoviruses
  (2) *Bordetella parapertussis* (may cause pertussis as single agent or as a coinfection with *B. pertussis*)
  (3) *Bordetella bronchiseptica*
  (4) *Chlamydia trachomatis*
  (5) *Chlamydia pneumoniae*
  (6) *Mycoplasma pneumoniae*

DIAGNOSIS PULMONARY TUBERCULOSIS

Definitions and Etiology

1. Tuberculosis is an infection caused by *Mycobacterium tuberculosis,* which is an acid-fast bacillus (AFB).
2. Latent tuberculosis infection (LTBI) is defined as:
   a. A positive tuberculin skin test (TST)
   b. No physical findings of disease
   c. Chest radiograph either normal or showing granulomas or calcification in the lungs, regional lymph nodes, or both
3. Tuberculosis disease is defined as:
   a. Presence of signs and symptoms or radiographic manifestations caused by *M. tuberculosis* are apparent
   b. Disease may be pulmonary or extrapulmonary or both.

Associated Clinical Features

1. Incubation period from initial infection to positive TST is 2 to 12 weeks.
2. Risk of progression from LTBI to tuberculosis disease:
   a. Highest in infants and postpubertal adolescents
   b. Highest during the 6 months after infection and remains high for 2 years
   c. Other predisposing factors include human immunodeficiency virus (HIV) infection and other immunodeficiency states (e.g., immunosuppressive drugs, chronic steroids), malnutrition, malignancy (e.g., lymphoma), chronic diseases (e.g., diabetes), and IV drug use.
3. Reactivation or adult-type pulmonary TB is rare in children but can occur in adolescents.
4. Extrapulmonary manifestations of TB include diseases of meninges, bones, joints, middle ear, mastoid, and skin.
5. For additional details about TST guidelines, refer to the *Red Book,* 2003.
   a. Tuberculin reactivity appears 2 to 12 weeks after the initial infection (median interval 3 to 4 weeks).
   b. Usually a Mantoux test containing 5 tuberculin units (TU) of purified protein derivative (5 TU PPD) is used (Fig. 6-17).

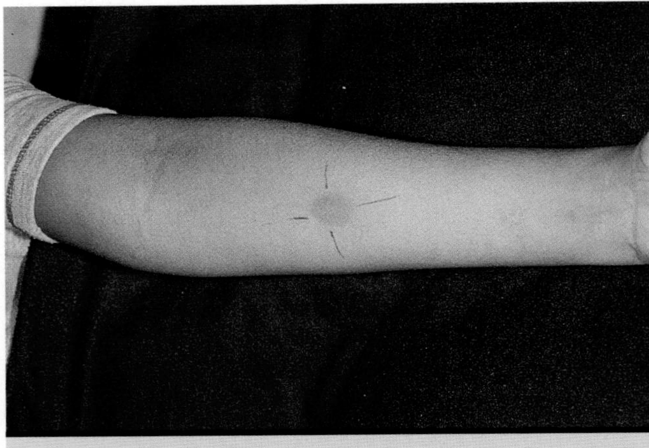

Figure 6-17. Positive Tuberculin Skin Test

A 5 TU PPD skin test result is assessed at 48 to 72 hours after administration. The diameter of induration (*and not erythema*) is measured perpendicularly to the long axis of the forearm (see text for criteria for a positive test).

c. For children at high risk, a reaction >5 mm is considered positive; examples include:
   1) Children with HIV infection or other immunosuppressed state
   2) Recent contact with an infectious person
   3) Clinical illnesses consistent with TB
d. For other high-risk groups, a reaction >10 mm is considered positive; examples include:
   1) Child <4 years of age
   2) Underlying medical conditions (e.g., lymphoma, diabetes mellitus, chronic renal failure)
   3) Children with increased exposure to TB disease (e.g., those born or whose parents were born in high-prevalence regions or those frequently exposed to adults who are HIV-infected, homeless, or users of illicit drugs)
e. For low-risk groups, a reaction >15 mm is considered positive; examples include:
   1) Children 4 years of age or older without any risk factors
   2) Children residing in communities where the prevalence of TB is low
f. In general, a TST reaction >10 mm in a bacille Calmette-Guérin (BCG)-vaccinated child or adult indicates infection with *M. tuberculosis* and necessitates further diagnostic evaluation and treatment.

6. Radiographic evaluation
   a. Chest radiograph recommended in all children with a positive TST reaction (regardless of child's BCG immunization status)
   b. Radiographic findings (any of the following; see Figs. 6-18 through 6-23)
      1) Lymphadenopathy (hilar, mediastinal)
      2) Infiltrate or atelectasis of a segment of the lobe or entire lobe
      3) Pleural effusion
      4) Cavitary lesion
      5) Miliary disease
      6) Residual calcification of primary focus or regional lymph nodes (appearance of calcification implies that the lesion has been present for at least 6 to 12 months)
7. Diagnosis of pulmonary TB is made by:
   a. Isolation of *M. tuberculosis* by culture from gastric aspirate, sputum, pleural fluid, cerebrospinal fluid, urine, other body fluids, or a biopsy specimen establishes the diagnosis.
   b. Early morning gastric aspirate obtained via nasogastric tube upon awakening and sent for smear for AFB and culture is the best method in a young child, older child, or adolescent who is coughing but is without sputum production.

Consultation

Pediatric pulmonologist

Emergency Department Treatment and Disposition

1. All patients with TB disease require hospitalization. Principles of management include:
   a. Use several drugs to achieve a relatively rapid cure.
   b. Prevent emergence of secondary drug resistance during therapy.
   c. Current recommendations of the American Academy of Pediatrics and Centers for Disease Control for treating intrathoracic tuberculosis in children is a regimen of isoniazid (INH) and rifampin (RIF) given for 6 months supplemented by pyrazinamide (PZA) during the first 2 months of therapy.
2. Patients with LTBI (asymptomatic with reactive TST, normal chest radiograph and physical examination) do not need hospitalization.
   a. Begin INH therapy and refer patient to PCP for ongoing follow-up.
   b. Current recommended regimen is daily INH therapy for 9 months.

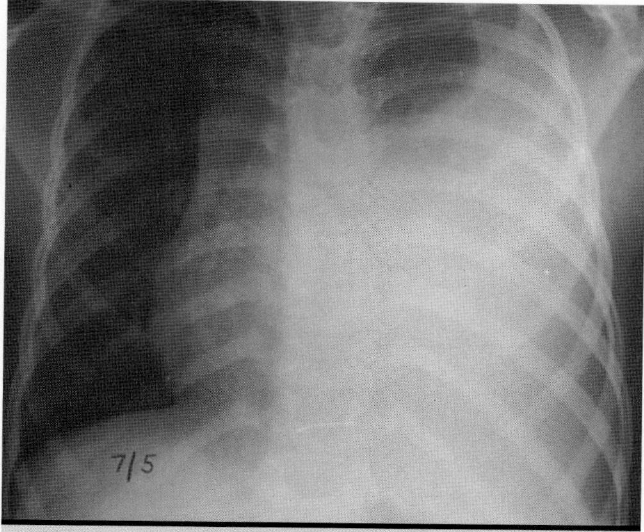

Figure 6-18. Pulmonary Tuberculosis with Pleural Effusion

Frontal chest radiograph showing opacification of the left middle and lower zones with obliteration of the left cardiac margin, left hemidiaphragm, and costophrenic angle (a hallmark for the presence of fluid [transudate or exudates]). There is a mediastinal shift to the right. This patient had a positive PPD test. The pleural fluid was straw colored and had a protein level of 2 g/dL, glucose of 40 mg/dL, and 5000 WBCs/mm^3 with predominant lymphocytes. Acid-fast smear of the fluid was negative, while the culture was positive for *M. tuberculosis*. The radiographic abnormality in TB effusion is often more impressive than would be suggested by either clinical findings or symptoms.

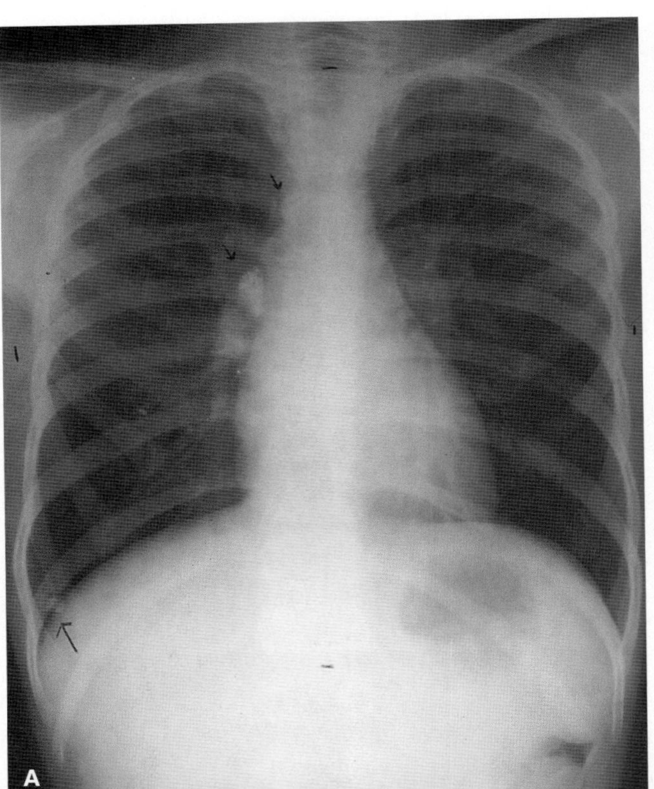

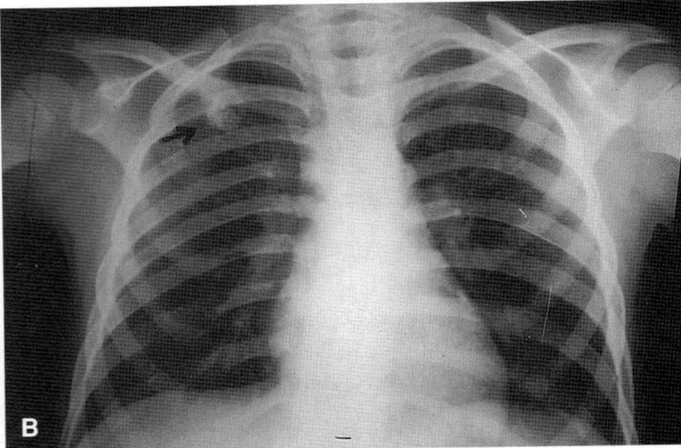

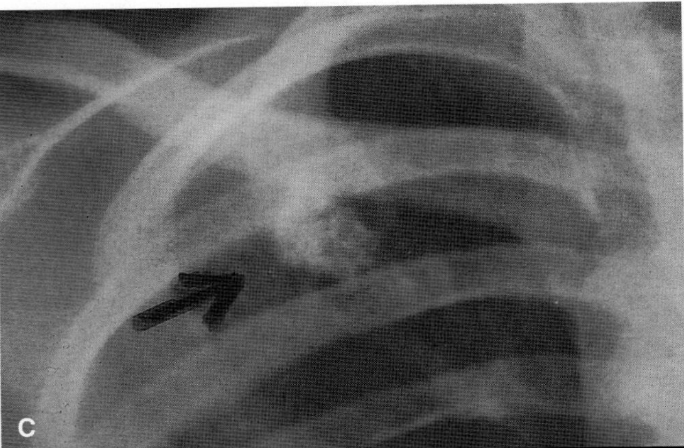

Figure 6-19. Childhood Pulmonary Tuberculosis with Lymph Node Calcifications (Ghon's Primary Complex)

A, *B* and *C*. The hallmark of childhood pulmonary TB is Ghon's complex (hilar lymphadenitis and parenchymal focus with or without lymph node calcification). A left-sided parenchymal focus often leads to bilateral hilar lymphadenopathy, whereas a right-sided focus is associated only with right-sided adenitis (because of the pattern of lymphatic circulation in the chest). Hilar adenopathy is inevitably present with childhood TB. However, it may not be detected on a plain x-ray in the absence of calcification. A CT scan detects both calcified and noncalcified lymph nodes.

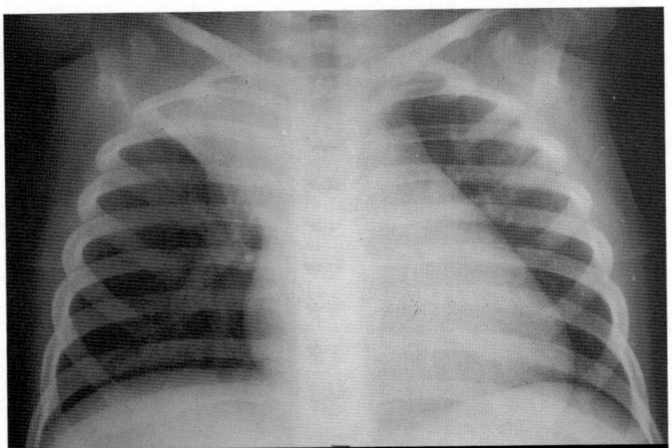

Figure 6-20. Endobronchial Tuberculosis

Frontal radiograph of the chest showing right upper lobe opacity with an elevation of the right fissure suggesting right upper lobe collapse. This infant presented with unilateral wheezing and coughing. His was cared by a babysitter who had cavitary pulmonary disease.

Clinical Pearls: Pulmonary Tuberculosis

1. A diagnosis of LTBI or TB disease in a child indicates recent transmission of *M. tuberculosis* in the community and mandates a thorough investigation to find the source.
2. Children younger than 12 years of age with primary pulmonary TB are not contagious (noncavitary pulmonary lesions, absent or minimal cough with sputum production, and little or no expectoration of bacilli).
3. Collapse/consolidation findings seen on radiograph in endobronchial TB are similar to those seen in foreign body aspiration.

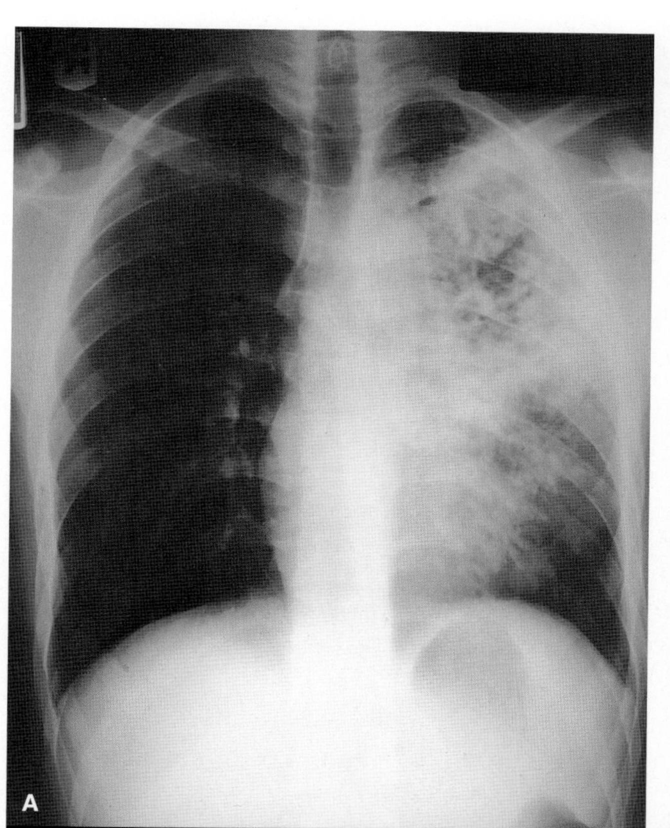

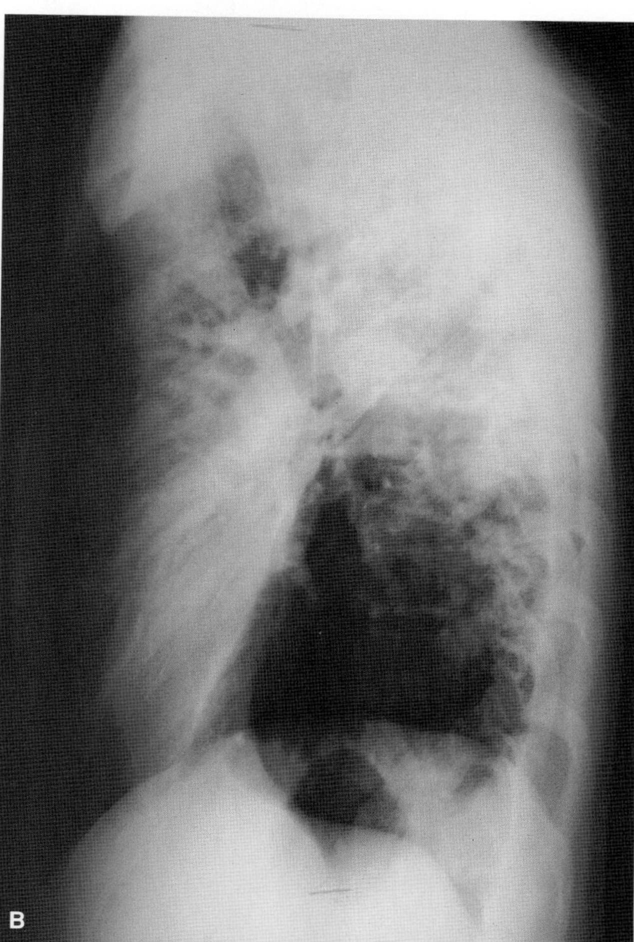

Figure 6-21. Reactivation Pulmonary Tuberculosis

A and *B*. Frontal and lateral chest radiographs showing extensive consolidation with air bronchograms in the left upper and lingular lobe in a 19-year-old boy. There is compensatory hyperinflation in the right lung with a shift of the mediastinum to the left. His sputum was positive for numerous AFB and subsequently culture was positive for *M. tuberculosis*. A CT scan showed consolidation of the entire left upper lobe with multiple areas of cystic bronchiectasis and confluent parenchymal destruction.

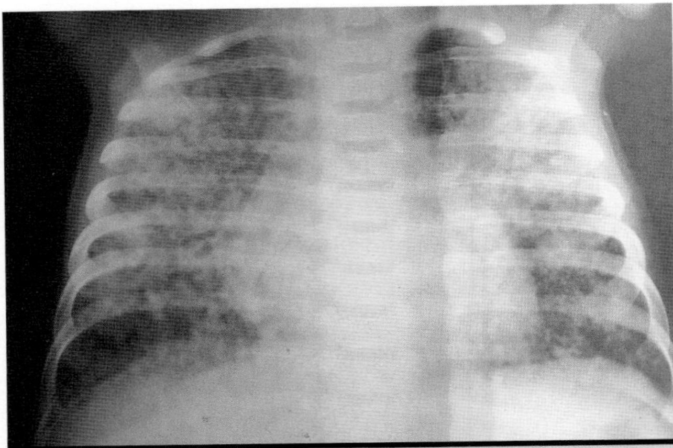

Figure 6-22. Miliary Tuberculosis

Frontal chest radiograph showing innumerable bilateral lung parenchymal opacities in an infant who presented with fever, hepatosplenomegaly, and failure to thrive.

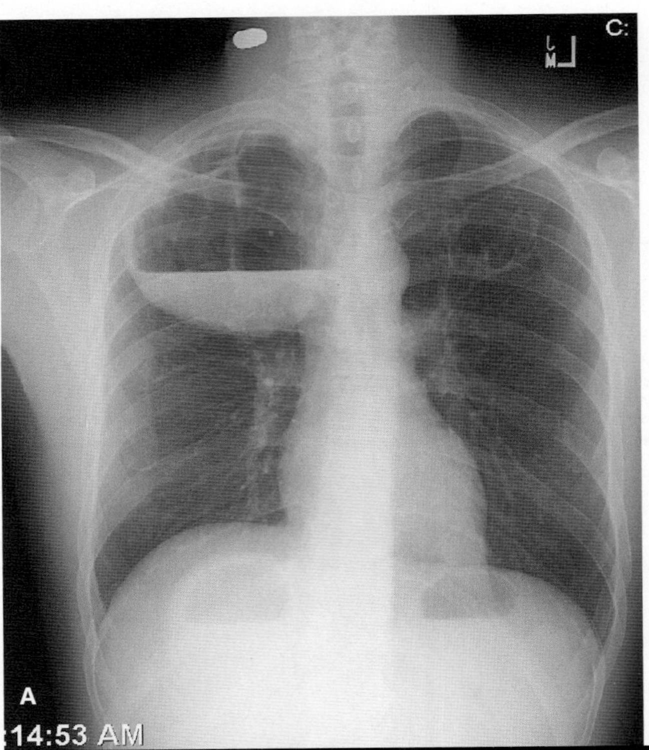

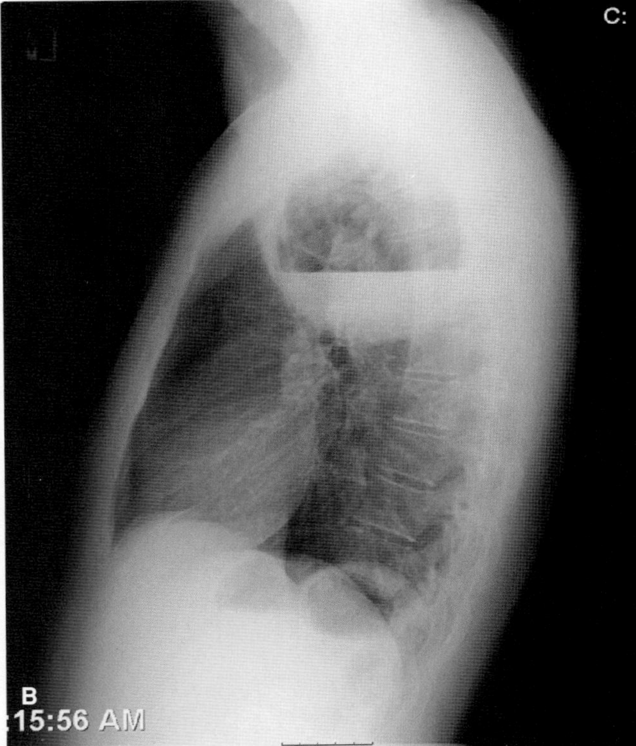

Figure 6-23. Reactivation Pulmonary Tuberculosis

A and *B*. Frontal and lateral chest radiographs showing a large cavitary lesion with an air-fluid level in the right upper lobe and a smaller cavitary focus (multiloculated) in the left upper lobe apical segment in an immunocompromised patient. The air-fluid level on the right represents a secondary infectious process leading to development of lung abscess. The most common form of reactivation TB is an infiltrate or cavity in the apex of the upper lobes. This patient had sputum smears positive for numerous AFB, and culture was positive for *M. tuberculosis*. Transmission of *M. tuberculosis* is usually by airborne mucus droplet nuclei from person to person. The risk of transmission increases when the patient has a sputum smear that is positive for AFB, an extensive upper lobe infiltrate or cavity (as seen here), and is having severe and forceful cough with copious production of thin sputum.

BOX 6-20. CLINICAL FINDINGS OF PULMONARY TUBERCULOSIS

- *Primary pulmonary complex*
  - (1) Involvement of parenchyma and regional lymph nodes (Ghon's complex [hilar lymphadenitis and parenchymal focus with or without lymph node calcification)
  - (2) Regional lymphadenitis much larger compared to relatively small lung focus
  - (3) Mild symptoms (low-grade fever, mild or absent cough)
  - (4) Lung exam normal
  - (5) Adenopathy (e.g., hilar, mediastinal) with normal lungs on chest x-ray
  - (6) Asymptomatic local pleural effusion (very common; consider as a component of primary complex)
- *Endobronchial TB*
  - (1) Seen commonly in infants
  - (2) Prominent cough
  - (3) Unilateral wheezing, rales, decreased breath sounds (depends on degree of obstruction)
  - (4) Lymphadenopathy with collapse/consolidation on chest x-ray
- *Progressive primary TB*
  - (1) Rare in children
  - (2) Enlargement, caseation, and liquefaction of primary focus, leading to cavity formation
  - (3) Fever with chills, weight loss, night sweats
  - (4) Productive cough, hemoptysis
  - (5) Chest pain
  - (6) Consolidation and cavitation at primary site on x-ray
  - (7) Dissemination (infiltrates at other sites on x-ray)
- *Miliary TB*
  - (1) Seen more commonly in infants
  - (2) Fever, weight loss
  - (3) Multiple small lesions seen in all lung fields
  - (4) Dissemination to other sites (e.g., liver, spleen, eyes)
- *Pleural effusion*
  - (1) Larger and clinically symptomatic effusions seen months to years after primary infection
  - (2) Uncommon in younger children
  - (3) Usually unilateral (rarely bilateral)
  - (4) Signs and symptoms include fever, shortness of breath, chest pain, dullness on percussion, and diminished breath sounds
  - (5) PPD positive in 70 to 80% of cases
- *Reactivation TB*
  - (1) Rare in children but can occur in adolescents
  - (2) Endogenous reactivation of the previous TB infection site
  - (3) This form remains localized to the lungs
  - (4) Extensive infiltrates or thick-walled cavities in upper lobes (high oxygen tension and blood flow)
  - (5) Highly contagious (sputum production and cough)

BOX 6-21. DIFFERENTIAL DIAGNOSIS OF PULMONARY TUBERCULOSIS

- Pneumonia of varied etiologies
- Bronchial asthma
- Foreign body aspiration
- Hilar and mediastinal adenopathy from another etiology (e.g., lymphoma)
- Pleural effusion/empyema from another etiology (e.g., staphylococcal pneumonia)
- Sarcoidosis

DIAGNOSIS OBSTRUCTIVE SLEEP APNEA SYNDROME

Definitions

1. Apnea is cessation of airflow at the level of the nostrils and mouth lasting for at least 10 seconds (20 seconds in premature infants). Hypopnea is a reduction but not a complete cessation of airflow.

2. Obstructive sleep apnea syndrome (OSAS) is a disorder of breathing during sleep characterized by prolonged partial airway obstruction and/or intermittent compiete obstruction that disrupts normal ventilation during sleep and normal sleep patterns (Fig. 6-24).

3. In OSAS, there is cessation of airflow at the nose and mouth despite apparent, often vigorous, inspiratory efforts. Central apnea (seen most commonly in the neonatal period) is cessation of airflow with *no* apparent respiratory effort.

Associated Clinical Features

1. Predisposing conditions for OSAS include:
   a. Adenotonsillar hyperplasia (most common cause)
   b. Nasal polyps (respiratory allergies, cystic fibrosis), nasal septal deviation, choanal stenosis, chronic rhinitis
   c. Obesity (e.g., Pickwickian syndrome)
   d. Mandibular hypoplasia (e.g., Pierre Robin anomaly)
   e. Down syndrome (hypotonia with collapse of pharyngeal tissues to hypopharynx during sleep)

3. If a history of nightly snoring or worsening snoring during upper respiratory tract infection is elicited in the ED, a more detailed history (e.g., labored breathing during sleep, observed apnea, restless sleep) needs to be obtained.

4. OSAS needs to be differentiated from habitual snoring. OSAS is very unlikely in the absence of habitual snoring.

5. Physical examination during wakefulness is often normal in children with OSAS and the patient needs to be observed during sleep.

6. Laboratory and radiology tests that help in making the diagnosis of OSAS include:
   a. Hemoglobin/hematocrit (Hgb/Hct; polycythemia due to chronic hypoxia)
   b. Serum electrolytes (compensatory metabolic alkalosis for hypoventilation)
   c. Lateral radiograph of the neck (for obstruction)
   d. Chest radiograph (evaluation for pneumonia and/or atelectasis related to aspiration and for cor pulmonale)
   e. Electrocardiogram and echocardiogram (evidence of cardiomegaly and cor pulmonale)

7. Diagnostic methods that have been used to make a diagnosis of OSAS include audiotaping or videotaping, pulse oximetry, abbreviated polysomnography, and full polysomnography. Nocturnal polysomnography is the only diagnostic technique shown to quantitate the ventilatory and sleep abnormalities associated with sleep-disordered breathing and is currently the gold standard.

8. Complications related to OSA include:
   a. Neurocognitive deficits (behavioral disturbances, poor school performance, attention deficit/hyperactivity disorder)
   b. Hypersomnolence
   c. Pulmonary hypertension and cor pulmonale (constriction of pulmonary arterioles due to repeated episodes of hypoxia or hypercarbia with respiratory acidosis)
   d. Systemic hypertension
   e. Pectus deformity
   f. Respiratory failure

Consultations

Pediatric pulmonologist, otolaryngologist, and cardiologist

Emergency Department Treatment and Disposition

1. Hospitalize in the ICU any patient presenting with:
   a. Cardiorespiratory failure
   b. Worsening of airway obstruction (e.g., during URI) for continuous cardiac and pulse oximetry monitoring, and to institute a temporary therapeutic intervention (while awaiting a more thorough evaluation by specialists) such as a nasopharyngeal airway to bypass the obstruction, or continuous positive airway pressure (CPAP) therapy.
   c. A short course of oral steroids should be given (e.g., prednisone 2 mg/kg per day for 5 days) to reduce pharyngeal lymphoid tissue that may worsen OSAS (e.g., in patients with infectious mononucleosis).

2. Patients not requiring hospitalization can be referred to their PCP.
   a. To arrange for polysomnography (the gold standard test) that will help in differentiating between primary snoring and OSAS
   b. To arrange for adenotonsillectomy if indicated (the first line of treatment for most children with OSAS)
   c. To arrange for CPAP (e.g., for patients with persistent OSAS after adenotonsillectomy)
   d. For follow-up for weight reduction for obese patients

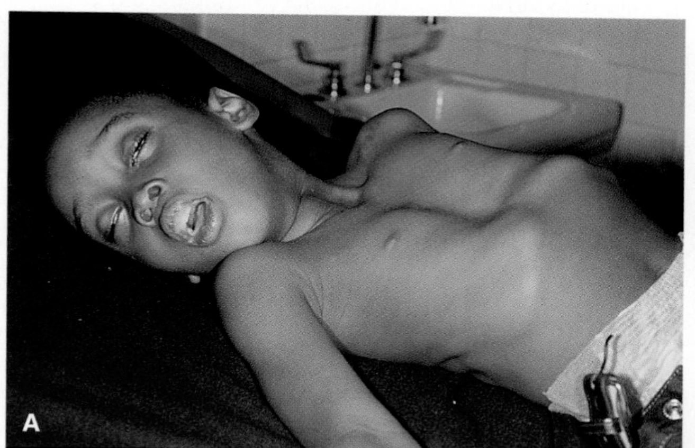

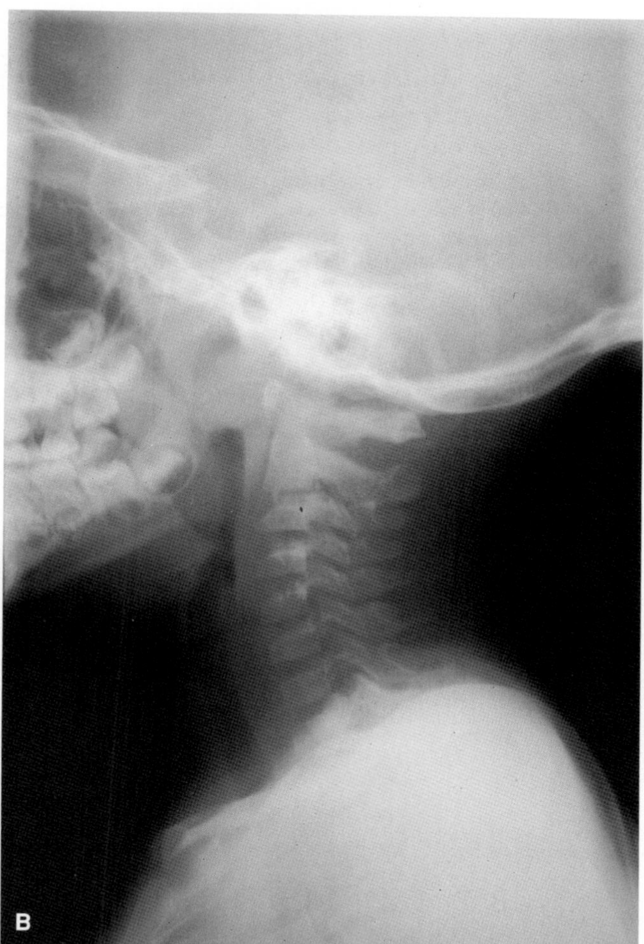

Figure 6-24. Obstructive Sleep Apnea Syndrome

A. A 4-year-old child presented with worsening of his long-standing history of breathing difficulty during sleep. His worsening of symptoms occurred during acute Epstein-Barr viral infection (infectious mononucleosis). He had numerous episodes of obstructive apnea during his sleep in the ED, resulting in a significant drop in oxygen saturation (pulse oximetry 96% while awake and 85% during sleep). This patient had supraclavicular, suprasternal, subcostal, and intercostal retractions. He had also developed pectus excavatum deformity. His Hgb/Hct values were 14.0/42.8, and his serum CO_2 value was 32. He was hospitalized and a nasopharyngeal airway was required to relieve his obstruction. *B*. Narrowing of the nasopharynx and hypopharynx. This lateral view of the airway shows hypertrophied adenoids and tonsils causing significant narrowing of the airway.

Clinical Pearls: Obstructive Sleep Apnea Syndrome

1. OSAS is a common condition in childhood and can result in severe complications including death if left untreated.
2. The two most common presenting symptoms of OSAS are snoring and sleep disturbances.
3. *Physical signs of obstruction are often not present when the child is awake; a child with suspected OSAS must be examined during sleep. Observation of pulse oximetry readings during sleep is helpful in the ED.*
4. In OSAS, there is a cessation of airflow at the nose and mouth (appreciated by using a stethoscope to listen for airflow at the nose and mouth) despite apparent, often vigorous, inspiratory efforts; however, these efforts are ineffective due to a lack of airway patency. Usually a condition of partial obstruction with some degree of airflow is maintained (by increased efforts) between periods of complete obstruction in OSAS.

BOX 6-22. CLINICAL FEATURES OF OBSTRUCTIVE SLEEP APNEA

- Common age at presentation
  (1) Peak incidence: preschool-aged children between 2 and 6 years old (tonsils and adenoids are largest in relation to airway size at these ages)
  (2) Seen in children of all ages (neonates to adolescents)
- Night symptoms
  (1) Breathing difficulty or apnea during sleep
  (2) Snoring
  (3) Restlessness
  (4) Enuresis
- Daytime symptoms
  (1) Excessive daytime somnolence
  (2) Morning headaches
  (3) Behavioral problems (e.g., attention-deficit disorder, excessive crankiness)
  (4) Feeling of being tired throughout the day
  (5) Learning problems, poor school performance
- Aspiration of pharyngeal secretions during obstructive episodes
  (1) Recurrent pneumonias
  (2) Chronic nocturnal cough
- Findings related to adenotonsillar hypertrophy
  (1) Mouth breathing
  (2) Adenoidal facies and orthodontic malformations
  (3) Nasal obstruction during wakefulness
  (4) Hyponasal speech
  (5) Difficulty swallowing
  (6) Frequent upper respiratory tract and/or middle ear infections
- Failure to thrive (poor caloric intake during the day and hypermetabolic state at night)
- Obesity (Pickwickian syndrome; adolescents/adults)

BOX 6-23. DIFFERENTIAL DIAGNOSIS OF OBSTRUCTIVE SLEEP APNEA

- Primary snoring
  (1) A clinically benign (*essentially asymptomatic*) condition
  (2) Snoring *without* obstructive apnea
  (3) Snoring *without* frequent arousals from sleep
  (4) Snoring *without* gas exchange abnormalities (normal alveolar ventilation and oxygenation)
  (5) Seen in 3 to 12% of preschool-aged children (as opposed to OSAS, which is seen in 2%)
  (6) Overall seen in 7 to 10% of children on a chronic basis
  (7) Overall seen in up to 20% of children on an intermittent basis
  (8) Snoring usually exacerbated by URI (*but no obstructive apnea*)

Suggested Readings

Abrunzo TJ, Santamaria JP: Emergencies of the oral cavity and neck. In: Strange GR et al (eds). *Pediatric Emergency Medicine. A Comprehensive Study Guide,* 2nd ed. McGraw-Hill, New York, 2002, p. 474.

Berger TJ, Shahidi H: Retropharyngeal abscess. eMedicine, DATE?, http://www.emedicine.com/ped/topic2682.htm

Conners GP: Pediatrics, foreign body ingestion. eMedicine, 2002, http://www.emedicine.com/EMERG/topic379.htm.

Friedman EM: Tracheobronchial foreign bodies. *Otolaryngol Clin North Am* 2000;33:179.

Lee SS, Schwartz RH, Bahadori RS: Retropharyngeal abscess: Epiglottitis of the new millennium. *J Pediatr* 2001;138:435.

Marcus CL, Chapman D, Ward SD, McColley SA: American Academy of Pediatrics. Clinical practice guideline: Diagnosis and management of childhood obstructive sleep apnea syndrome. *Pediatrics* 2002;109:704.

Munter DW: Foreign bodies, trachea. eMedicine, 2001, http://www.emedicine.com/EMERG/topic751.htm.

Orenstein DM: Foreign bodies in the larynx, trachea and bronchi. In: Behrman RE, Kliegman RM, Jenson HB (eds). *Nelson Textbook of Pediatrics*, 16th ed. WB Saunders, Philadelphia, 2002, p. 1279.

Rovin JD, Rodgers BM: Pediatric foreign body aspiration. *Pediatr Rev* 2000;21:86.

Santamaria JP, Schafermeyer R: Stridor: A review. *Pediatr Emerg Care* 1992;8:229.

BOX 7-3. DIFFERENTIAL DIAGNOSIS OF URTICARIA AND ANGIOEDEMA

- Erythema multiforme (see Fig. 7-5)
- Urticarial vasculitis
- Urticaria pigmentosa (mastocytosis; see Fig. 7-59)
- Hereditary angioedema

DIAGNOSIS SERUM SICKNESS

SYNONYMS

Inoculation reaction
Protein sickness

Definition and Pathogenesis

1. Serum sickness is a type III (immune complex) hypersensitivity reaction produced by exposure to a variety of agents and is characterized by fever, joint involvement, skin rash, and lymphadenopathy.
2. Exposure to antigens is followed by antibody response by the host. Circulating antibodies react to a newly introduced antigen to form antigen-antibody complexes that deposit in the vessel walls of various organs. This is followed by activation of the complement system and release of inflammatory complement cleavage products (e.g., C3a, C5a). C3a, a potent anaphylotoxin, induces mast cell degranulation to produce hives.

Etiology

1. Medications
   a. Antibiotics: penicillin, cephalosporins (e.g., cefaclor), streptomycin, sulfa drugs
   b. Other medications: hydantoins, thiouracil, cholecystographic dyes, aminosalicylic acid
2. Blood products (e.g., human gamma globulin)
3. Animal-derived serum (e.g., antitoxins for treatment of spider and snake envenomations [e.g., Crotalidae antivenin], antitoxins for clostridial intoxication [e.g., botulism, gas gangrene], anti-rabies serum)
4. *Hymenoptera* stings

Associated Clinical Features

1. Diagnosis of serum sickness is suspected based on history of an exposure to a foreign antigen.
2. CBC shows a variable degree of leukocytosis, elevated eosinophil counts and thrombocytopenia. The erythrocyte sedimentation rate (ESR) is also elevated.
3. Serum complement values (C3 and C4) are decreased and reach a nadir around the tenth day; C3a is usually increased. Circulating immune complexes are usually detectable, with peak levels around the tenth to twelfth day.
4. Proteinuria, microscopic hematuria, and hemoglobinuria may be present.
5. Skin biopsy is not necessary to make the diagnosis. Direct immunofluorescence studies of skin lesions reveal immune deposits of IgM, IgA, IgE, or C3 in the superficial small blood vessels.
6. Rare complications of serum sickness include anaphylaxis, carditis, glomerulonephritis, Guillain-Barré syndrome, and peripheral neuritis.

Emergency Department Treatment and Disposition

1. Discontinue the offending antigen if the patient is still receiving it.
2. Hospitalize patients with severe arthritis or serum sickness associated with complications.
3. The majority of patients can be treated as outpatients with antihistamines and nonsteroidal anti-inflammatory drugs (NSAIDs) as indicated.
4. Systemic corticosteroids may be used in severe cases (e.g., serum sickness associated with glomerulonephritis or peripheral neuropathy) and are very effective. Prednisone (dose: 1 to 2 mg/kg per day) is given for about 1 to 2 weeks (or until signs and symptoms remit).
5. Plasmapheresis (extracorporeal removal of circulating immune complexes) can be considered for severe serum sickness not responsive to the standard therapy.

Clinical Pearls: Serum Sickness

1. Serum sickness is a systemic, immune complex–mediated hypersensitivity vasculitis that occurs after exposure to a variety of agents. It is a classic example of a type III hypersensitivity reaction caused by antigen-antibody complexes.
2. Drugs are the most common cause of serum sickness.
3. Serum sickness is characterized by fever, rash, arthralgias, and lymphadenopathy.
4. Typical cutaneous reactions seen in serum sickness include urticaria or morbilliform eruptions (Fig. 7-4).
5. Serum sickness is self-limiting and resolves in 7 to 10 days without sequelae in most cases.

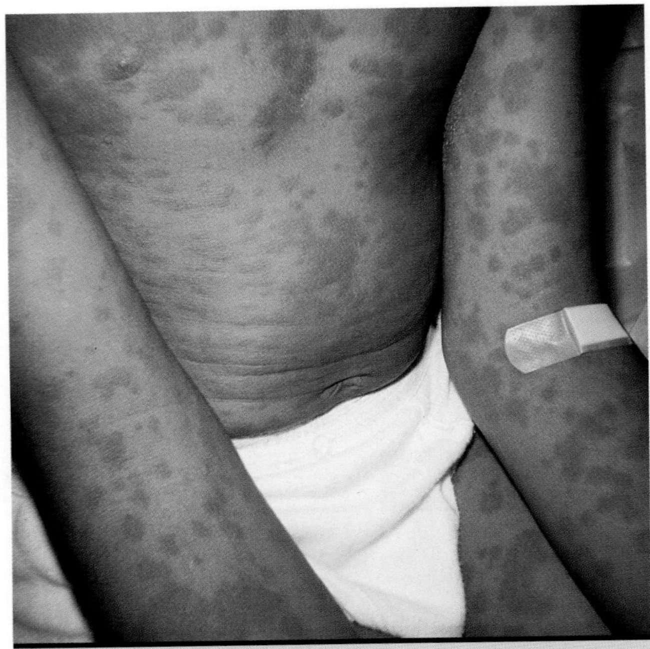

Figure 7-4. Serum Sickness

Generalized erythematous morbilliform eruption and swollen, tender knees were the presenting complaints in this adolescent patient who was receiving cefaclor for the past 8 days for a sinus infection. He also had myalgias, nausea, and mild diarrhea. Abnormal laboratory tests included an elevated ESR, thrombocytopenia, and 2 + proteinuria. Urticarial wheals are the most common type of rash (about 90%) seen with serum sickness. Other rashes that are seen include erythema multiforme-like lesions and scarlatiniform rash.

BOX 7-4. CLINICAL FEATURES OF SERUM SICKNESS

- Onset of symptoms
  (1) Typically within 7 to 14 days after exposure to the antigen (range, 7 to 21 days)
  (2) May present within 1 to 3 days *in an accelerated fashion* if there was a previous exposure to the foreign protein or a previous allergic reaction to the same foreign protein
- The site of injection of foreign material is red and swollen, usually 1 to 3 days before systemic symptoms set in.
- Skin lesions
  (1) Urticaria or morbilliform drug eruptions are usually limited to the trunk or may become generalized.
  (2) Faint erythema with a serpiginous border at the margins of palmar or plantar skin of the hands, feet, and toes
  (3) Intense pruritus
  (4) Lesion may become purpuric.
- Angioedema (e.g., face, neck)
- Facial flushing
- Diffuse lymphadenopathy (10 to 20%)
- Joint involvement
  (1) Arthralgia and/or arthritis (10 to 50% of cases)
  (2) Multiple joints (e.g., knees, wrists, ankles, fingers, toes)
- Other symptoms
  (1) Fever, malaise, myalgia
  (2) GI (diarrhea, nausea, abdominal cramps, occult blood in stool)
  (3) Proteinuria

BOX 7-5. DIFFERENTIAL DIAGNOSIS OF SERUM SICKNESS

- Drug-induced hypersensitivity reactions
- Anaphylaxis
- IgE-mediated urticarial reactions
- Acute rheumatic fever
- Systemic lupus erythematosus
- Viral infections (e.g., infectious mononucleosis)

DIAGNOSIS ERYTHEMA MULTIFORME MINOR

SYNONYM

von Hebra

Definition

1. Erythema multiforme (EM) minor is a distinctive acute hypersensitivity reaction following exposure to a sensitizing antigen, and is characterized by skin and mucous membrane lesions.
2. EM is subclassified (based on severity):
   a. EM minor: skin involvement alone or mucosal involvement limited to *one surface* and minimal systemic symptoms
   b. EM major: extensive skin and mucosal involvement [*two or more surfaces*] and significant systemic symptoms; entities under EM major include:
      1) Stevens-Johnson syndrome (see Box 7-10)
      2) Toxic epidermal necrolysis (see Box 7-12)

Associated Clinical Features

1. EM is most commonly seen between the ages of 10 and 30 years.
2. EM minor is a self-limiting, benign condition in the majority of patients. *There is usually no progression from EM minor to EM major.*
3. No permanent sequelae such as scarring or color changes follow EM minor.
4. The diagnosis of EM minor is usually made clinically.
5. Skin biopsy is not routinely performed to confirm the clinical diagnosis. Skin biopsy reveals dermal edema with a perivascular lymphocytic infiltrate, leukocytoclasis, and extravasated red blood cells. Necrotic keratinocytes lead to formation of subepidermal bullae.

Consultation

Dermatology (if the clinical diagnosis doubtful)

Emergency Department Treatment and Disposition

1. No specific therapy is required for EM minor. Acyclovir may be given if herpes simplex lesions are present.
2. Typical patients with EM minor are usually not severely ill and can be managed as outpatients with follow-up with a primary care provider.
3. Symptomatic relief (if indicated) may be offered by:
   a. Baths with colloidal oatmeal (e.g., Aveeno)
   b. Topical emollients (e.g., hydrated petrolatum, petroleum jelly, mineral oil, Aquaphor)
   c. Topical steroids (to be used *no more than* bid for 2 weeks)
      1) Low-potency steroids (e.g., 1 or 2.5% hydrocortisone) for face or groin
      2) Medium-potency steroids (e.g., mometasone furoate cream) on body or extremities
      3) Strong steroids (e.g., halobetasol propionate cream) may be used for older children and adolescents with severely affected areas.
   d. Systemic antihistamines may be used to control itching (e.g., hydroxyzine [dose: 2 to 4 mg/kg per day divided tid or qid] or diphenhydramine [dose: 5 mg/kg per day divided tid or qid])
   e. Systemic steroids may be considered for severe cases (e.g., prednisone 1 to 2 mg/kg per day divided once or twice daily for 5 to 14 days)

4. Identify and treat and/or eliminate the cause.
   a. Discontinue the drug, if suspected as the cause.
   b. Prophylactic oral acyclovir can be used for recurrent HSV-induced EM. Prompt treatment of HSV infections in such patients will prevent EM.

Clinical Pearls: Erythema Multiforme Minor

1. This disorder is referred as *multiforme* because the morphology of its lesions is so variable.
2. EM lesions are *fixed* (*unlike the evanescent nature of urticaria*); EM lesions may expand, but they remain on same body part for 4 to 7 days.
3. Target lesions are pathognomonic of EM; however, *not all* patients with EM minor have target lesions (Fig. 7-5).
4. Patients with HSV-associated EM may develop target lesions on the lips associated with lip necrosis that can mimic Stevens-Johnson syndrome.

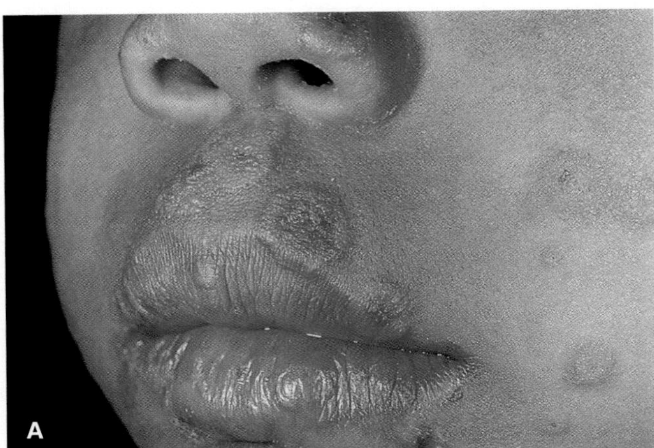

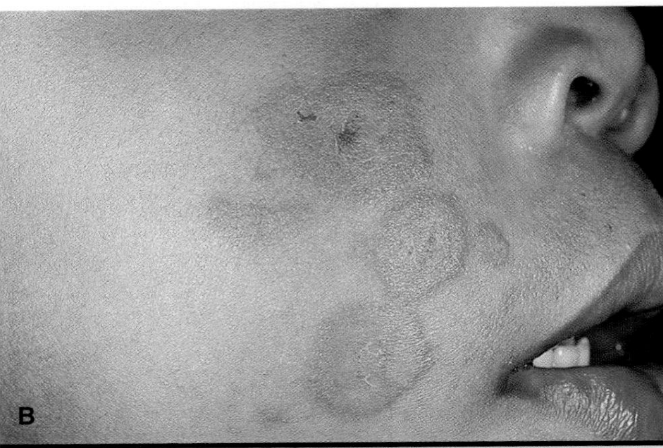

Figure 7-5. Erythema Multiforme Minor

A. Typical target lesions: annular/doughnut-shaped erythematous lesions with concentric rings of different appearance [outer erythematous and inner pale rings] are seen. *B*. A lesion with duskiness in the center is seen on the cheek. This 3-year-old child had herpes simplex labialis 5 days prior to the onset of EM.

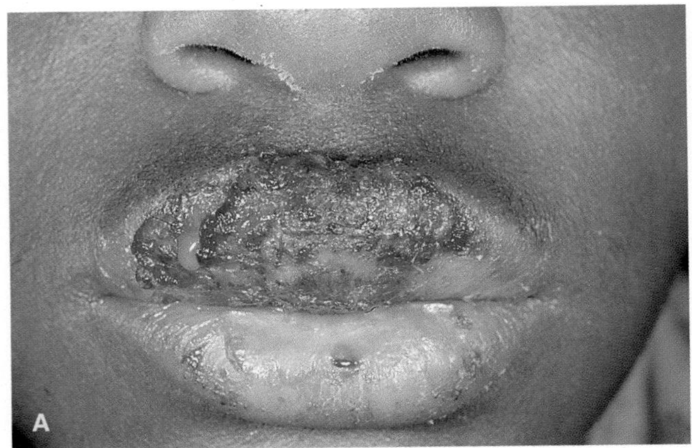

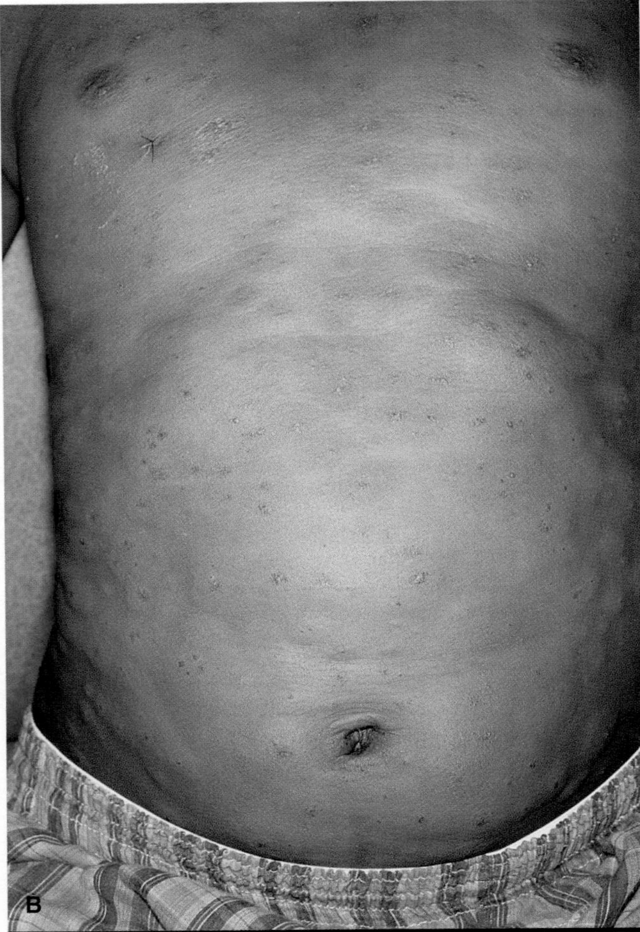

Figure 7-6. Herpes Simplex Labialis and Erythema Multiforme Minor

A. HSV is the most common etiology of EM minor, and recurrences of EM are common with recurrences of HSV infections. *B*. Numerous annular lesions with duskiness in the center are seen in this 11-year-old patient who developed this rash 3 days after developing cold sores.

BOX 7-6. ETIOLOGY OF ERYTHEMA MULTIFORME MINOR

- Infections
  (1) Viral (e.g., herpes simplex, EBV)
  (2) Bacterial (e.g., Group A streptococci)
  (3) *Mycoplasma pneumoniae*
  (4) Fungal (e.g., *Histoplasma*)
- Drugs
  (1) Sulfonamides
  (2) Penicillin
  (3) Cephalosporins
  (4) Quinolones
- EM and herpes simplex virus (HSV)
  (1) Most common etiology (about 60% of cases)
  (2) Preceded by either HSV labialis or HSV genitalis (less common)
  (3) Cold sores precede EM by 3 to 14 days.
  (4) Recurrences of EM common with recurrences of HSV.

BOX 7-7. CHARACTERISTICS OF ERYTHEMA MULTIFORME MINOR

- *Primary lesions:*
  (1) Dull red to dusky macules, papules, vesicles, bullae, or urticarial plaques
  (2) *Variable multiforme appearance;* however, in most patients a single type of lesion predominates
- *Pathognomonic target (or iris or bull's-eye) lesions:*
  (1) Annular or doughnut-shaped (plaques of variable size and shape)
  (2) Papules with erythematous outer border and inner pale ring with a blister or a dusky/necrotic central area (represents necrosis of keratinocytes in areas of active involvement)
  (3) Target lesions may coalesce and develop annular or serpiginous borders.
- *Sites of skin lesions:*
  (1) *Symmetrical eruption*
  (2) Extensor surfaces of arms, legs and back of hands
  (3) *Predilection for palms, soles*
  (4) Predominantly acral distribution
  (5) Trunk, face, neck
- *Mucous membrane involvement:*
  (1) Either absent or limited to only one mucosal surface (the mouth is involved in 50% of cases)
  (2) About 25% of cases of EM are confined to the oral mucosa (involving the vermilion border of the lips and buccal mucosa and tongue; *the gingivae are spared*)
- *Natural course:*
  (1) Individual lesions last about 1 week.
  (2) The eruption may continue to appear in crops for 2 to 3 weeks.
  (3) Duration from onset to healing: 1 to 4 weeks
  (4) Lesions heal without scarring.

BOX 7-8. DIFFERENTIAL DIAGNOSIS OF ERYTHEMA MULTIFORME MINOR

- *EM minor associated with vesiculobullous plaques*
  (1) Herpetic gingivostomatitis
  (2) Bullous pemphigoid
  (3) Pemphigus vulgaris
  (4) Viral exanthema (e.g., hand-foot-and-mouth disease, chickenpox)
  (5) Linear IgA dermatosis
- *EM minor with maculopapular or urticarial presentation*
  (1) Urticaria from other etiology
  (2) Contact dermatitis
  (3) Viral exanthems
  (4) Secondary syphilis
  (5) Pityriasis rosea
- *EM with target lesions*
  (1) Erythema annulare centrifugum
  (2) Other annular rashes (e.g., erythema chronicum migrans, dermatophyte infections)

DIAGNOSIS STEVENS-JOHNSON SYNDROME

SYNONYM

Erythema multiforme major

Definitions

1. Stevens-Johnson syndrome (SJS) is a severe life-threatening form of an adverse drug reaction (most commonly; rarely other etiologies) involving the skin and least two mucous membranes.
2. It is now believed that toxic epidermal necrolysis (TEN; see Figs. 7-8 and 7-9) is a disease spectrum beginning with SJS (SJS is a minimal form of the TEN spectrum), and both diseases could be induced by the same drugs.
3. SJS and TEN represent the same drug-induced acute inflammatory process that varies in severity. A three-grade classification that has been proposed as follows:
   a. *SJS:* mucosal erosions with widespread purpuric macules and epidermal detachment <10% body surface area (BSA)
   b. *Transitional SJS/TEN:* widespread purpuric macules with epidermal detachment between 10 and 30% BSA
   c. *TEN:* widespread purpuric macules with epidermal detachment >30% BSA

Associated Clinical Features

1. The exact incidence of SJS is unknown; it is an uncommon to a rare disease with a peak incidence in the second decade of life.
2. Leukocytosis and an elevated ESR may be present. Electrolytes and liver enzyme abnormalities and chest x-ray abnormalities may also be present (depending on multiorgan involvement).
3. The diagnosis is usually made clinically. H&E staining of a frozen sample of the exfoliating skin will show a full-thickness epidermis.
4. Complications of SJS include secondary bacterial infection, fluid and electrolyte imbalances, scarring of the skin, loss of the nails and hair, contractures, and strictures of the esophagus, vagina, bronchi, urethra, and anus. Ocular findings and sequelae include symblepharon, corneal ulceration, keratitis, uveitis, panophthalmitis and blindness (in 3 to 10%).
5. SJS runs a protracted course of 3 to 6 weeks with a mortality rate varying from 5 to 15%.

Consultations

Dermatology and ophthalmology consultations (usually obtained after hospitalization)

Emergency Department Treatment and Disposition

1. Hospitalize all patients with a clinical diagnosis of SJS, preferably in an ICU.
2. *Discontinue the offending drug (all drugs introduced within the past month).*
3. *No member* of a similar drug family should be reintroduced (unless the risk of abrupt discontinuation is too high). For example, phenobarbital, carbamazepine, and phenytoin

share a common metabolic pathway (cytochrome P450) and may induce a cross-reaction; thus, all three drugs are contraindicated after SJS/TEN resulting from any one of them.

4. Supportive care includes
   a. Management of fluid and electrolytes, pain, thermoregulation, and nutritional support
   b. For meticulous skin care (see TEN; page 281)
   c. Daily ophthalmologic examination
   d. Mouthwashes and glycerin swabs for oral lesions
   e. Saline compresses for eyelids, lips, or nose
   f. Prophylactic use of systemic antibiotics is not recommended; daily examination for infection and periodic cultures of skin, eyes, and mucosa (monitoring for infection) are carried out.
5. Systemic corticosteroids
   a. *Their use is controversial* (risk of increased morbidity and mortality; hence routine use is discouraged).
   b. If they are used, consider using them early (within the first 2 days of eruption), at high doses (equivalent of prednisone 2 mg/kg per day), and discontinue after 4 days if no response.

Clinical Pearls: Stevens-Johnson Syndrome

1. Most common etiology for SJS (EM major) is drugs; most common etiology for EM minor is herpes simplex virus.
2. Consider SJS in any patient presenting with a rapidly-spreading rash while receiving a drug that was started recently (within the last 7 to 30 days) (Fig. 7-7).

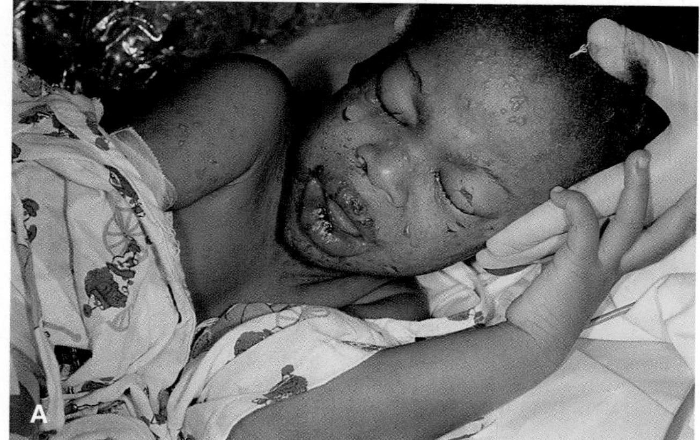

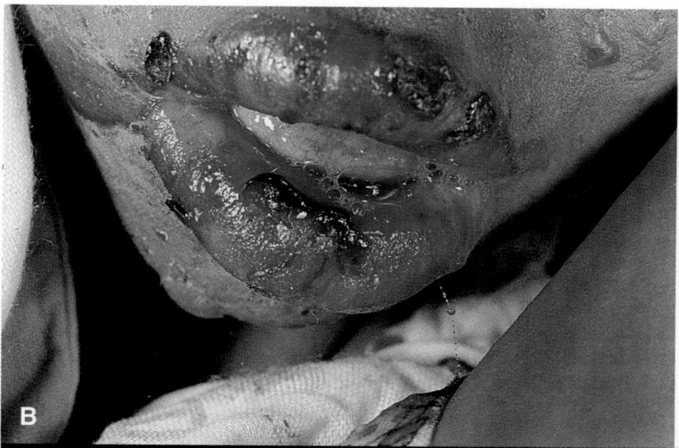

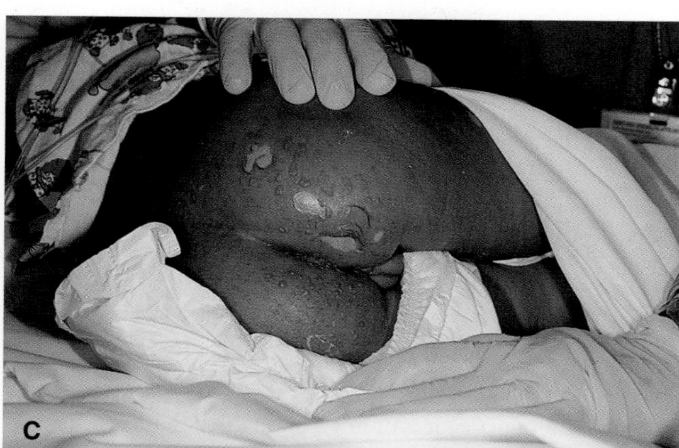

Figure 7-7. Stevens-Johnson Syndrome

A. A 7-year-old girl presented with this rash while receiving penicillin (on the eighth day) for pharyngitis. Nikolsky's sign was positive with peeling of the epidermis (seen on the face) with minimal pressure. The patient also had stomatitis and conjunctivitis. *B*. Close-up of erosive stomatitis with hemorrhagic-crusted erosions of lips. Lesions were also present on the buccal mucosa, palate, and posterior pharynx. *C*. Erythematous and purpuric macules are seen on the back with blistering leading to erosions on the buttocks. Less than 10% of the body surface area was involved.

BOX 7-9. ETIOLOGIES OF STEVENS-JOHNSON SYNDROME AND TOXIC EPIDERMAL NECROLYSIS

1. Drugs (most common etiology)

• ***Anticonvulsants***	• ***Antibiotics***
Barbiturates	Penicillins
Diphenylhydantoin	Sulfa drugs
Carbamazepine	Sulfadoxine, sulfadiazine
Valproic acid	Sulfasalazine, clotrimazole
	Quinolones
	Cephalosporins
• ***Nonsteroidal anti-inflammatory drugs***	• ***Other drugs***
Ibuprofen	Calcium channel blockers
Naprosyn	Allopurinol
Salicylates	Griseofulvin

2. Other etiologies

• ***Infections***	• ***Other***
Mycoplasma pneumoniae (most commonly identified infectious agent)	Foods (e.g., nuts, shellfish) Vaccines
Herpes simplex virus	Malignancy (leukemia, lymphoma)
Hepatitis B	
Epstein-Barr virus	

Clinical pearls

- The most common etiologies of SJS and TEN are drugs (anticonvulsants, antibiotics, NSAIDs).
- Typically rash is seen 7 to 21 days after introduction of a new medication.
- Rash may occur within 12 to 48 hours with a prior sensitization (e.g., prior EM due to drugs)
- It is uncommon to develop SJS or TEN if drug was started <7 days or >45 days ago.

BOX 7-10. CLINICAL FEATURES OF STEVENS-JOHNSON SYNDROME

- Abrupt onset
- Prodromal period 2 to 4 days that may include:
  (1) High fever, malaise
  (2) Cough, coryza, sore throat
  (3) Vomiting, diarrhea, dysuria
  (4) Headache, myalgias, arthralgia
- Skin lesions
  (1) Erythematous and/or purpuric macules
  (2) Papules
  (3) Blisters leading to erosions
  (4) *Target or iris lesions* (*unlike TEN*)
  (5) Erosions involve *<10% of body surface area*
  (6) Individual erosions *<3 cm in diameter*
  (7) Skin tenderness: *minimal to absent* (*unlike TEN*)
  (8) Positive Nikolsky's sign (with light stroking of the skin the epidermis peels off like wet tissue paper)
- Mucous membrane involvement (*two or more*)
  (1) Exudative or erosive stomatitis (most frequent)
  (2) Hemorrhagic-crusted erosions of lips, buccal mucosa, palate, posterior pharynx
  (3) Conjunctivitis (erythema or widespread blisters)
  (4) Vulvovaginitis
  (5) Tracheobronchial and esophageal mucosa (with severe disease)
  (6) Rectal and nasal mucosa (less common)
- Natural course
  (1) Active development of lesions usually lasts 4 to 6 days.
  (2) Blisters usually heal within 14 to 21 days.
- Other features
  (1) Pneumonitis
  (2) Polyarthritis
  (3) Hepatitis
  (4) Renal failure
  (5) Myocarditis
  (6) Enterocolitis

(Reproduced with permission from: Shah BR: Stevens-Johnson syndrome and toxic epidermal necrolysis. In: Perkin RM, Swift JD, Newton D (eds). *Pediatric Hospital Medicine*. Baltimore, Lippincott Williams & Wilkins, 2003, p. 833)

BOX 7-11. DIFFERENTIAL DIAGNOSIS OF STEVENS-JOHNSON SYNDROME

- Severe burn (see Fig. 18-2)
- Erythema multiforme minor (see Figs. 7-5 and 7-6)
- Drug eruptions
- Anticonvulsant hypersensitivity syndrome (see Figs. 7-10 to 7-12)
- Staphylococcal scalded skin syndrome (see Figs. 3-23 to 3-27)
- Toxic epidermal necrolysis (see Figs. 7-8 and 7-9)
- Kawasaki's disease (early in course; see Figs. 12-2 and 12-3)
- Scarlet fever (early in course; see Fig. 3-3)
- Toxic shock syndrome (early in course; see Figs. 3-21 and 3-22)
- Measles (see Fig. 3-53)
- Pemphigus vulgaris

DIAGNOSIS TOXIC EPIDERMAL NECROLYSIS

Definitions and Etiologies

1. Toxic epidermal necrolysis (TEN) is a severe life-threatening form of drug-induced hypersensitivity reaction characterized by widespread skin and mucous membrane involvement.
2. Stevens-Johnson syndrome (SJS; see Fig. 7-7) also is a severe life-threatening form of adverse drug reaction (most common etiology; rarely other etiologies) involving the skin and least two mucous membranes.
3. It is now believed that TEN is a disease spectrum beginning with SJS (*SJS is the least serious form of TEN*), and both diseases can be induced by the same drugs; thus, SJS and TEN represent the same drug-induced acute inflammatory process that varies in severity. A three-grade classification that has been proposed:
   a. *SJS:* mucosal erosions with widespread purpuric macules and epidermal detachment <10% body surface area (BSA)
   b. *Transitional SJS/TEN:* widespread purpuric macules with epidermal detachment between 10 and 30% BSA
   c. *TEN:* widespread purpuric macules with epidermal detachment >30% BSA

Associated Clinical Features

1. TEN is more common in adults than in children.
2. The incidence of TEN is increased in HIV-infected individuals.
3. Ocular findings and sequelae of TEN include symblepharon, corneal ulceration, keratitis, uveitis, panophthalmitis, and blindness (3 to 10%).
4. Leukocytosis, elevated ESR, fluid and electrolyte and liver enzyme abnormalities may occur. The chest radiograph may be abnormal, depending on the extent of multiorgan involvement.
5. The diagnosis of TEN is made clinically. Both staphylococcal scalded skin syndrome (SSSS, see Figs. 3-23 to 3-27) and TEN are exfoliating diseases and can be differentiated on histologic exam:
   a. In SSSS: cleavage occurs in the superficial upper layer of epidermis
   b. In TEN: full-thickness epidermis separation is seen (dermal-epidermal separation)
6. TEN runs a protracted course of 3 to 6 weeks. It is associated with significant morbidity (e.g., scarring of skin, loss of nails and hair, contractures, and strictures of the esophagus, vagina, bronchi, urethra, and anus) and a mortality rate of 30% (usually due to sepsis).

Consultations

Dermatology and ophthalmology (usually obtained after hospitalization)

Emergency Department Treatment and Disposition:

1. Hospitalize all patents with clinical diagnosis of TEN in a burn unit (preferred) or ICU.
2. *Discontinue the offending drug (all drugs introduced within the past month).*
3. *No member* of a similar drug family should be reintroduced (unless the risks of abrupt discontinuation outweigh the benefits). For example, phenobarbital, carbamazepine, and phenytoin share a common metabolic pathway, and may induce a cross-reaction; thus all three drugs are contraindicated after TEN resulting from any one of them.

4. Supportive care includes
   a. Management of fluid and electrolytes, pain, and thermoregulation, and nutritional support
   b. Daily ophthalmologic examination
   c. Mouthwashes and glycerin swabs for oral lesions
   d. Saline compresses for eyelids, lips, or nose
   e. Meticulous skin care
      1) Débridement of necrotic tissue
      2) Wash with normal saline or Burow solution compresses
      3) Remove loose skin and blisters.
      4) Apply petrolatum or paraffin gauze to provide a barrier over denuded areas.
      5) Do not use silver sulfadiazine in patients with sulfonamide-induced SJS or TEN.
      6) Warm water compresses and colloidal baths
      7) Sloughed skin should be covered with porcine xenograft (pig skin) until reepithelialization takes place.
5. Patients are put in reverse isolation to prevent secondary bacterial infection. Prophylactic use of systemic antibiotics is not recommended; daily examination for infection and periodic cultures of skin, eyes, and mucosa (to monitor for infection) are carried out.
6. Systemic corticosteroids
   a. *Their use is controversial* (due to risk of increased morbidity and mortality), *hence routine use is discouraged.*
   b. If they are used, consider using them early (within the first 2 days of eruption), at high doses (equivalent of prednisone 2 mg/kg per day), and discontinue after 4 days if no response.
7. Adjunct therapies reported in the literature for treating TEN (awaiting prospective studies) include use of plasmapheresis, gamma globulin, and immunosuppressive agents (azathioprine and cyclosporine).

Clinical Pearls: Toxic Epidermal Necrolysis

1. TEN is now considered part of a disease spectrum beginning with SJS (*SJS is the least serious form of TEN*), and both diseases can be induced by the same drugs.
2. The most common offending drugs for both SJS and TEN include anticonvulsants, nonsteroidal anti-inflammatory drugs, and sulfonamides.
3. Widespread skin and mucous membrane involvement leading to extensive exfoliation and exposure of the raw, tender skin are characteristic features of TEN (Figs. 7-8 and 7-9).
4. Consider SJS/TEN in any patient presenting with a rapidly spreading rash while receiving a drug that was started recently (within the last 7 to 30 days).
5. Both SJS and TEN are potentially life-threatening diseases due to multisystem involvement.

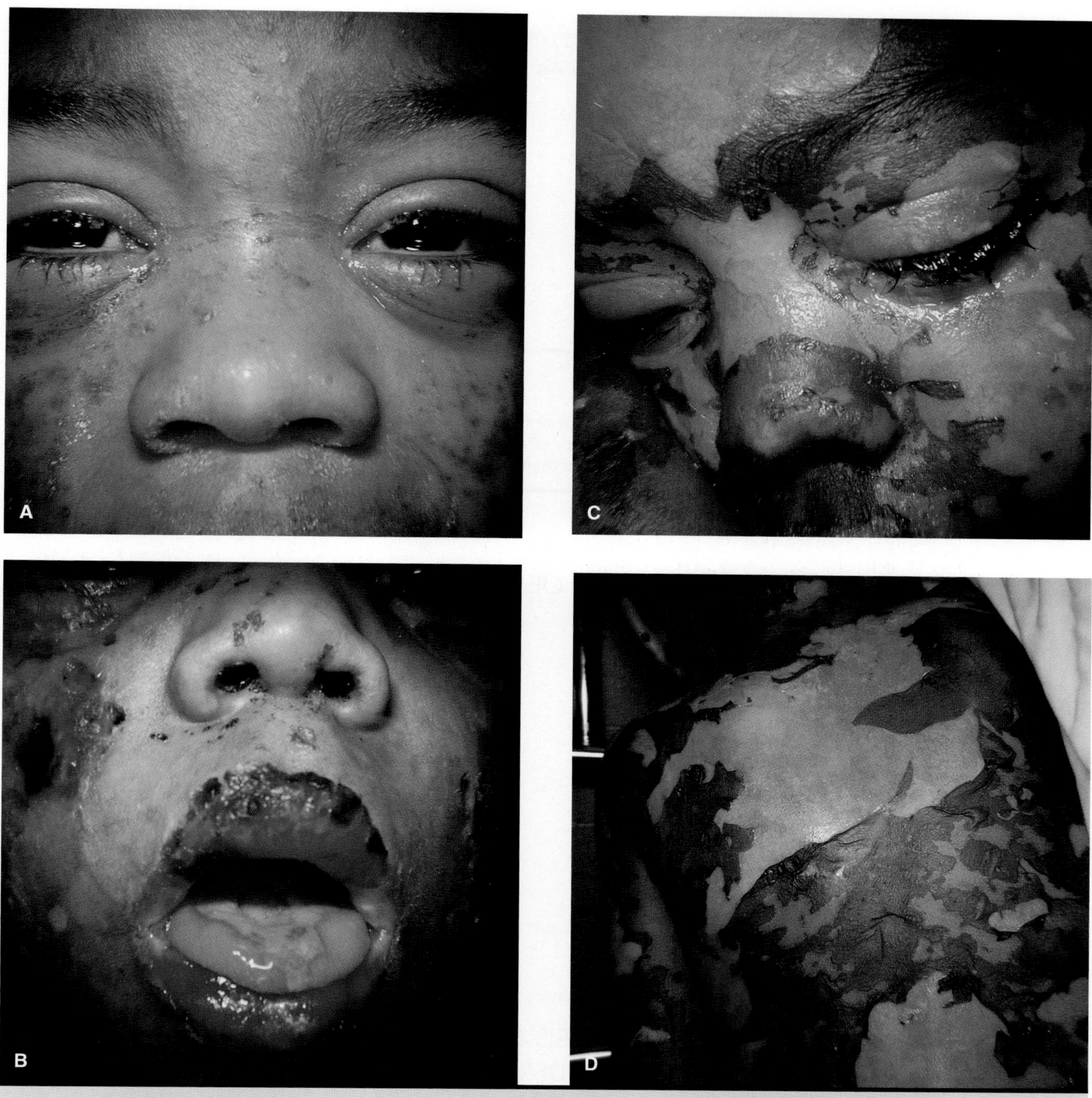

Figure 7-8. Toxic Epidermal Necrolysis

A 3-year-old boy with TEN (70% BSA involvement) presented with this rash a week after taking phenobarbital for a febrile seizure. *A*. Bilateral eye involvement with mucopurulent discharge (photograph taken on the second day of the illness). *B*. Erosive stomatitis and hemorrhagic crusted erosions of the lips (this photograph was taken on the second day of the illness). *C, D*. Abrupt onset and worsening within 24 hours after presentation, with dark necrotic skin peeling off, leaving a raw dermis (this photograph taken on the third day of the illness).

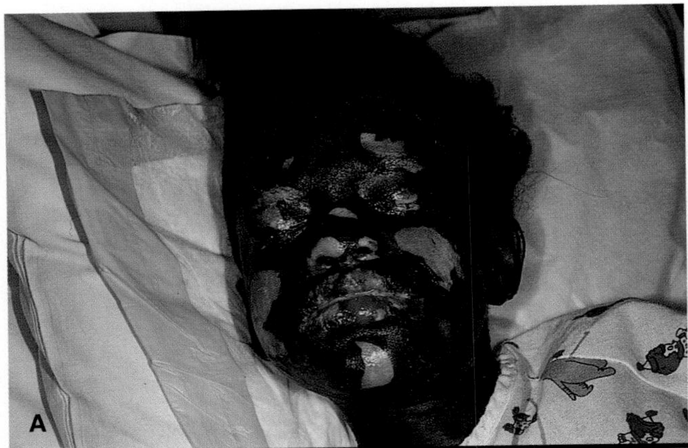

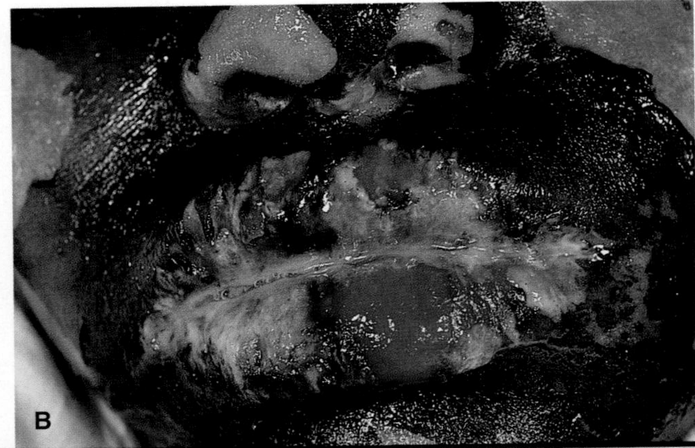

Figure 7-9. Toxic Epidermal Necrolysis

A 5-year-old girl presented with this rash while receiving trimethoprim-sulfamethoxazole (on the 10th day of therapy) for a urinary tract infection. She had 100% BSA involvement. *A*. Extensive involvement of the face with necrotic skin is seen (this photograph was taken on the seventh day after the onset of the rash). *B*. Close-up of mucosal involvement of the lips showing painful hemorrhagic erosions.

BOX 7-12. CLINICAL FEATURES OF TOXIC EPIDERMAL NECROLYSIS

- A prodrome of fever, myalgias, fatigue, arthralgia, nausea, vomiting, diarrhea, skin tenderness
- Abrupt onset
- Full-blown clinical picture within 24 hours
- Severe toxicity with fever and prostration
- Skin lesions
  (1) Necrotic
  (2) Dark skin peels off in sheets measuring >3 cm (*unlike SJS*)
  (3) Bullae and erosions involve >30% of body surface area (*unlike SJS*)
  (4) Target lesions absent (*unlike SJS*)
  (5) Skin tenderness present (*unlike SJS*)
  (6) The face and upper body parts are more prominently involved.
  (7) Positive Nikolsky's sign (same as in SJS)
- Mucous membrane involvement (same as SJS)
- Other features and natural course are the same as in SJS (see Box 7-10)

BOX 7-13. DIFFERENTIAL DIAGNOSIS OF STEVENS-JOHNSON SYNDROME VERSUS TOXIC EPIDERMAL NECROLYSIS

	SJS	*TEN*
Etiology	Drug-induced (most common), other (e.g., infection)	Drug-induced
Target lesions	May be present	Absent
Skin tenderness	Absent	Present
Skin erosion involvement	<10% of body surface area	>30% of body surface area
Individual erosions	<3 cm in diameter	>3 cm in diameter

DIAGNOSIS DRUG-INDUCED HYPERSENSITIVITY SYNDROME

SYNONYMS

Drug hypersensitivity syndrome
Antiepileptic hypersensitivity syndrome
Antiepileptic drug hypersensitivity syndrome
Hypersensitivity syndrome reaction
Drug reaction
DRESS (*d*rug *r*ash with *e*osinophilia and *s*ystemic *s*ymptoms)

Definition and Etiology

1. Drug-induced hypersensitivity syndrome (DIHS) is a subset of severe drug eruptions with a quite distinct triad of fever, rash, and systemic involvement (*of any internal organ*), that is seen in patients who are receiving a medication (either oral or parenteral) that is known to cause this reaction.
2. This syndrome was originally described in patients taking aromatic antiepileptic drugs (phenytoin, phenobarbital, carbamazepine, and primidone). However, it is also seen with other medications. A more informative, precise, and clinically relevant term has been proposed: the acronym DRESS, for *d*rug *r*ash (or *r*eaction) with *e*osinophilia and *s*ystemic *s*ymptoms.

Associated Clinical Features

1. DIHS is not a dose related, but an idiosyncratic, adverse drug reaction.
2. It has been reported to occur in all age groups.
3. If a patient has DIHS to one aromatic antiepileptic, exposure to another can cause an even more severe reaction.
4. Siblings of patients with DIHS may have an increased risk of a similar reaction.
5. A majority of patients present *within 2 months* of the start of the therapy.
6. Fever is usually the initial sign, often presenting for several days before other signs are apparent.
7. Internal organ involvement may predominantly involve one organ, or exclusively involve one organ, and may persist for weeks to months after the acute episode.
8. The diagnosis should be considered based on clinical findings in a patient receiving any of the medications known to cause DIHS. Laboratory evaluation should include CBC, liver enzymes, and urinalysis. Biopsy of the skin reveals a dense infiltrate of the papillary dermis, that is composed mostly of lymphocytes and occasionally of eosinophils.
9. The diagnosis of DIHS must be entertained even if the patient fails to recover promptly after discontinuation of the drug.

Consultations

Dermatology (if the diagnosis is unclear) and neurology (e.g., for continued management of seizures)

Emergency Department Treatment and Disposition

1. Discontinue the offending drug.
2. Hospitalize children with severe skin findings, evidence of systemic involvement, or inability to maintain hydration (e.g., during erythrodermic phase).
3. Treatment is mostly supportive and includes:
   a. Skin care (e.g., topical steroids to alleviate symptoms)
   b. Prevention of infection
   c. Treatment of ongoing seizures
4. Oral or IV steroids are sometimes used in patients with severe systemic involvement, but note that *no randomized, controlled studies have been published* to prove their efficacy in reducing the duration, morbidity, or mortality of DIHS.

Clinical Pearls: Drug-induced Hypersensitivity Syndrome

1. DIHS is a severe drug reaction most commonly seen with the use of antiepileptic medications (Fig. 7-10).
2. DIHS classically manifests as a triad of fever, rash, and multiorgan involvement (primarily hepatitis, lymphadenopathy and nephritis) and eosinophilia.
3. DIHS is often initially misdiagnosed as a viral infection, resulting in delay of the discontinuation of the responsible drug.
4. Prompt recognition and discontinuation of the drug is of *the utmost importance* in preventing or minimizing the severity and duration of internal organ involvement.

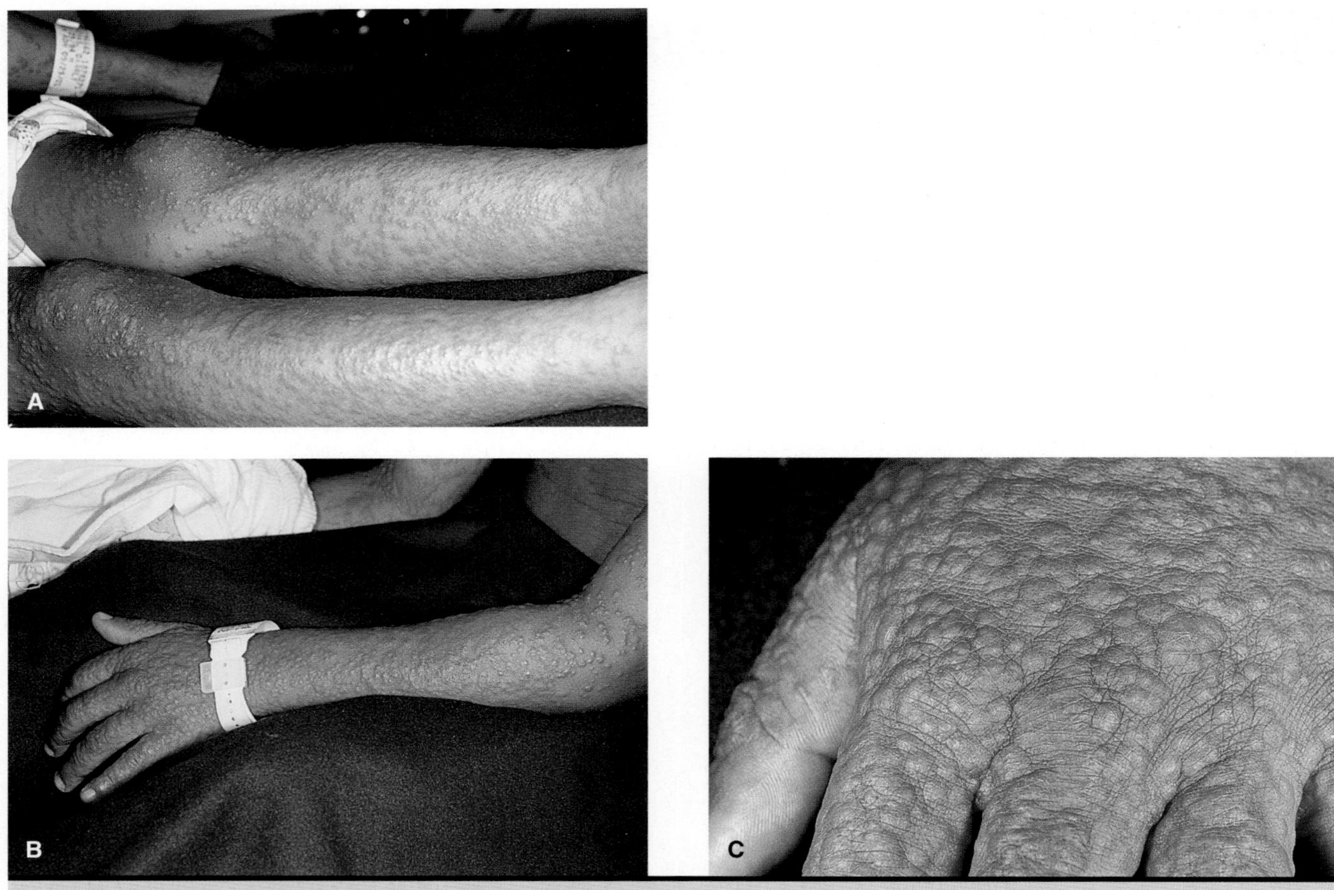

Figure 7-10. Drug-Induced Hypersensitivity Syndrome

A 7-year-old child presented with an extensive papular rash over his entire body 35 days after he was started on phenytoin for a seizure disorder. Papular lesions are seen on both legs (*A*), and arms (*B*), with a close-up showing the indurated nature of the rash (*C*).

BOX 7-14. ETIOLOGY OF DRUG-INDUCED HYPERSENSITIVITY SYNDROME

- *Anticonvulsants (most common etiology)*
  (1) Diphenhydantoin
  (2) Carbamazepine
  (3) Barbiturates
  (4) Primidone
  (5) Lamotrigine
  (6) Valproic acid
  (7) Ethosuximide
- *Other drugs*
  (1) Sulfa drugs (dapsone, sulfonamides, sulfasalazine)
  (2) Minocycline
  (3) Allopurinol

BOX 7-15. CLINICAL FEATURES OF DRUG-INDUCED HYPERSENSITIVITY SYNDROME

- Skin lesions
  (1) Begin on face, upper trunk, and proximal extremities
  (2) Begin as dusky red macules or papules that coalesce to become a generalized morbilliform eruption
  (3) Lesions become indurated and infiltrated
  (4) May progress to erythroderma
  (5) May progress to chronic exfoliative dermatitis
  (6) Vesicles or bullae may or may not be present
  (7) Petechiae or purpura may or may not be present
  (8) Absence of necrolysis (Nikolsky's sign negative [unlike SJS/TEN]; Fig. 7-11)
  (9) May have ichthyotic appearance in black patients
- Edema
  (1) Face (most striking)
  (2) Hands, legs, feet, penis, and scrotum
  (3) Usually symmetrical
- Mucous membrane involvement (either absent or minimal)
  (1) Mild conjunctivitis
  (2) Strawberry tongue, pharyngitis
  (3) Oral ulcerations absent (*the widespread ulcerations seen in SJS/TEN are not seen*; Fig. 7-12)
- Lymphadenopathy (localized or generalized)
  (1) Usually symmetrical
  (2) Cervical lymph nodes (most commonly involved)
  (3) Significant enlargement (pseudolymphoma)
  (4) Other: axillary, submandibular, inguinal, occipital, posterior auricular, submental
- Multiorgan involvement
  (1) Liver (most commonly affected): hepatomegaly, nonicteric hepatitis, liver failure
  (2) Hematologic: eosinophilia, leukocytosis, lymphocytosis, anemia, thrombocytopenia
  (3) Kidney: nephritis, hematuria, proteinuria
  (4) Pulmonary: pneumonitis, pulmonary edema, effusion
  (5) Cardiac: myocarditis
  (6) Splenomegaly
  (7) CNS: seizures, altered mental status
  (8) Myositis
  (9) Pancreatitis

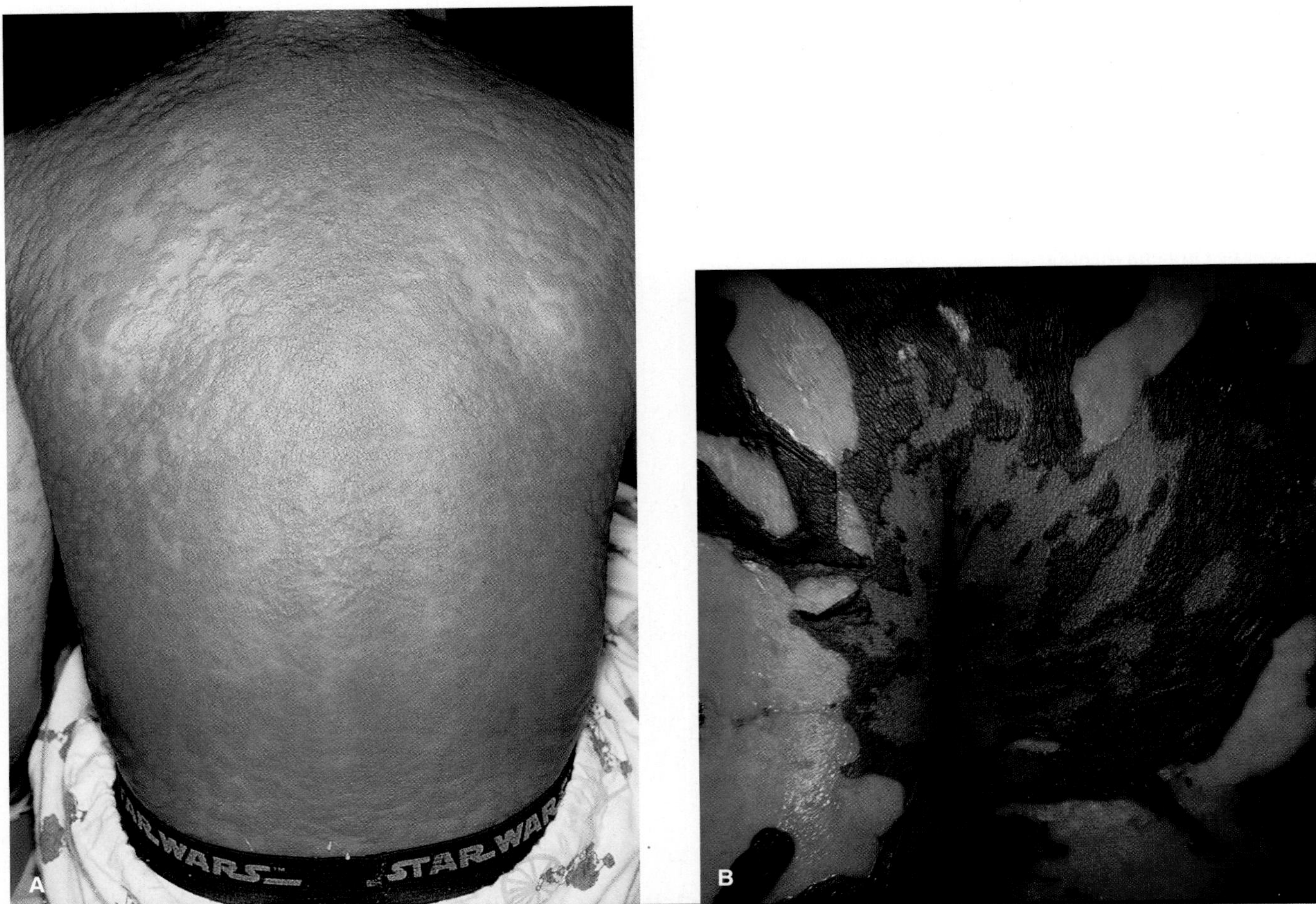

Figure 7-11. Drug-Induced Hypersensitivity Syndrome versus Stevens-Johnson Syndrome/Toxic Epidermal Necrolysis

A. Absence of necrolysis in spite of very extensive skin involvement is seen in DIHS. *B*. Vesicles, bullae, or purpuric lesions and necrolysis are typical findings in Stevens-Johnson Syndrome/Toxic Epidermal Necrolysis.

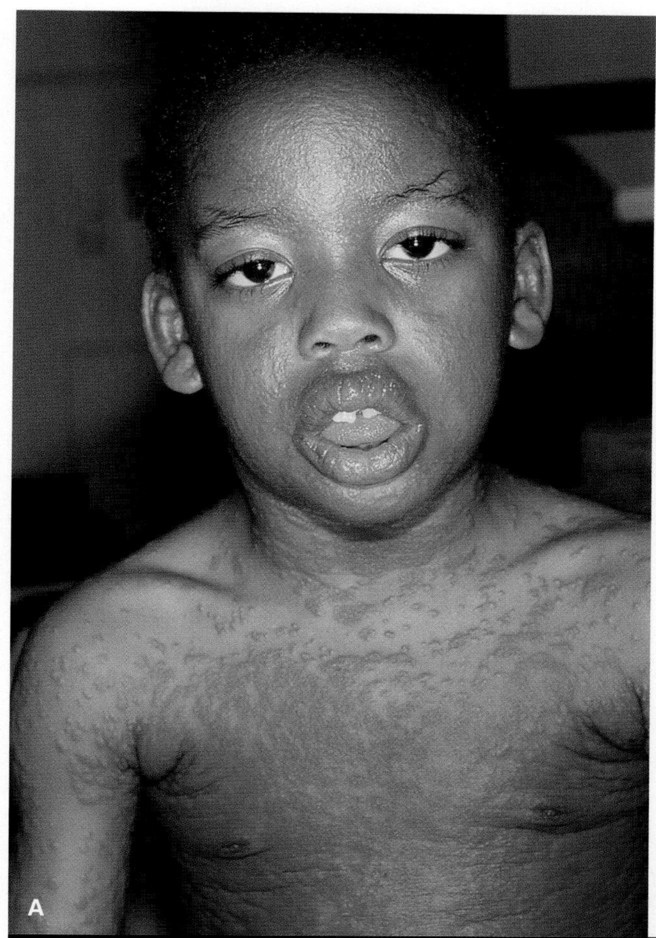

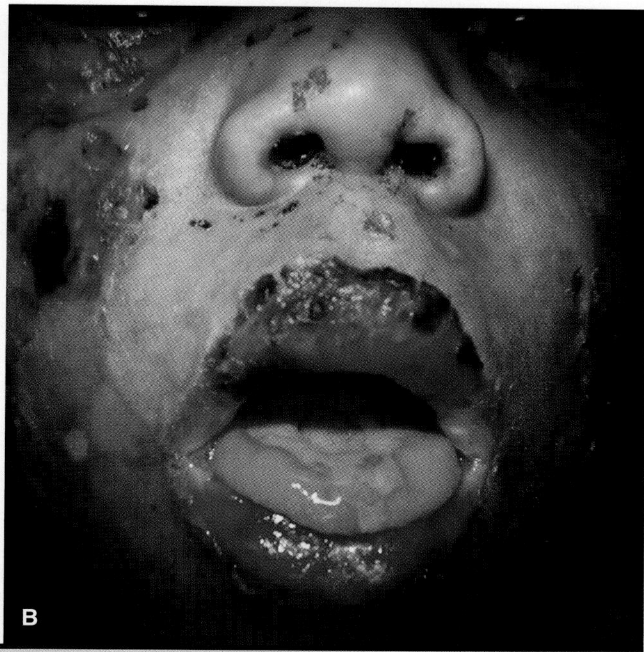

Figure 7-12. Mucous Membrane Involvement in Drug-Induced Hypersensitivity Syndrome versus Stevens-Johnson Syndrome/Toxic Epidermal Necrolysis

A. Mucous membrane involvement in patients with DIHS is either minimal or absent. *B*. Extensive mucous membrane involvement is seen in patients with Stevens-Johnson Syndrome/Toxic Epidermal Necrolysis.

BOX 7-16. DIFFERENTIAL DIAGNOSIS OF DRUG-INDUCED HYPERSENSITIVITY SYNDROME

- Bacterial infections
- Viral infections
- Serum sickness
- Kawasaki's disease
- Collagen vascular diseases
- Lymphoma
- Other drug eruptions
  (1) Stevens-Johnson Syndrome (SJS; see Fig. 7-7)
  (2) Toxic epidermal necrolysis (TEN; see Figs. 7-8 and 7-9)

BOX 7-17. DIFFERENTIAL DIAGNOSIS OF STEVENS-JOHNSON SYNDROME/TOXIC EPIDERMAL NECROLYSIS VERSUS DRUG-INDUCED HYPERSENSITIVITY SYNDROME

Involvement	***SJS/TEN***	***DIHS***
Etiologic drugs	Anticonvulsants, antibiotics	Anticonvulsants, antibiotics
Timing (usually)	Within 10–14 days	Within 30–40 days
Mucous membranes	Prominent	Seldom prominent
Skin	Necrolysis, flaccid bullae	Necrolysis absent, usually few bullae
Visceral	Limited to epithelium (tracheobronchial, GI)	Prominent involvement
	Liver rarely involved	Liver (~60%)
	Kidney rarely involved	Kidney (~15%)
Hematologic	Eosinophilia *not* present	Eosinophilia (~90%)
		Mononucleosis (~40%)

DIAGNOSIS

HENOCH-SCHÖNLEIN PURPURA

Synonym

Anaphylactoid purpura

Definition

Henoch-Schönlein purpura (HSP) is a syndrome resulting from widespread leukocytoclastic vasculitis due to IgA deposition in vessel walls, and is characterized by purpura, arthritis, and gastrointestinal and renal manifestations.

Etiology

1. The etiology of HSP remains unknown.
2. About 50% of children have preceding respiratory infection and as many as 75% of patients may have preceding group A beta hemolytic streptococcal infection. Other pathogens implicated in the etiology of HSP include hepatitis B virus, adenovirus, *Mycoplasma*, herpes simplex virus, parvovirus, and human immunodeficiency virus.
3. Certain foods, drugs, exposure to cold weather, and insect bites are other predisposing factors.

Associated Clinical Features

1. More common in children between 2 and 10 years of age (peak: 4 to 7 years)
2. HSP is rare in infants and uncommon in black children.
3. Diagnosis of HSP is usually made clinically with a typical distribution of the purpura.
4. There are no specific markers of HSP. Routine laboratory tests are neither specific nor diagnostic. Urinalysis should be performed to screen for renal involvement. Other tests are usually performed when the presentation is atypical or to exclude other diagnoses.
   a. CBC may show leukocytosis, thrombocytosis, and anemia (GI blood loss).
   b. Antinuclear antibody and coagulation studies are normal.
   c. ESR may be elevated and serum complement level may be depressed.
   d. Serum IgA and IgM concentrations may be elevated.
   e. Urinalysis may show hematuria (gross or microscopic), proteinuria, and white blood cells and casts.
   f. Gross or occult blood may be detected in the stool.
   g. Anticardiolipin or antiphospholipid antibodies may be present.
5. In doubtful cases skin biopsy helps in confirming leukocytoclastic vasculitis (acute vasculitis of arterioles and venules in the superficial dermis, capillary endothelial swelling, fibrin deposits, and perivascular neutrophilic fragments ("nuclear dust"). Immunofluorescence staining reveals presence of IgA in walls of arterioles and in renal glomeruli.
6. Ultrasound (US) study (as clinically indicated)
   a. Helpful for the intestinal complications (demonstrates presence of edematous hemorrhagic infiltration of the intestinal wall, e.g., duodenum, jejunum, ileal segments), detects ileoileal intussusception or perforation
   b. US with doppler flow studies helpful for evaluation of acute scrotum (demonstrates marked edema of scrotal skin and contents with intact vascular flow in testicles [these findings help prevent surgical exploration])
7. Complications of HSP include
   a. Gastrointestinal (bowel obstruction or perforation, intussusception)
   b. Renal (nephrotic syndrome, azotemia, oliguria, chronic glomerulonephritis [<1% develop persistent renal disease and <0.1% develop serious renal disease])
   c. Hypertensive encephalopathy
   d. Pulmonary hemorrhage, pulmonary interstitial disease
   e. Central nervous system (seizures, coma, paresis)
   f. Acute scrotum (mimicking acute testicular torsion)

Consultations

Nephrology or surgery for HSP-related complications, and dermatology for atypical cases

Emergency Department Treatment and Disposition

1. There is no specific treatment. The majority of cases are self-limiting, and symptoms resolve in a few weeks. Supportive, symptom-directed treatment includes bland diet and pain control with nonsteroidal anti-inflammatory drugs for the relief of arthritis, fever, or angioedema. Elevation of the scrotum helps in relieving scrotal edema.
2. Hospitalize any patient presenting with HSP-related complications (e.g., hypertension, oliguria, intestinal obstruction, or GI bleeding).
3. Remove the offending antigen, if identified (e.g., drugs).
4. Systemic corticosteroids (given intravenously or orally)
   a. For life-threatening complications (e.g., intestinal hemorrhage, obstruction, intussusception, or CNS complications) or for severe arthritis (may hasten resolution of arthritis)
   b. In usual doses does not have any effect on established nephritis
   c. Corticosteroid therapy does not prevent recurrences.
5. Other therapies that have been tried include plasmapheresis (removes IgA-immune complexes from circulation) and intravenous immunoglobulin.

6. Recurrences after an initial episode of HSP
   a. Usually seen in up to 50% of cases within the first few months
   b. Recurrences are usually milder and more common in patients with nephritis
   c. In <10% of children, recurrence of rash may continue up to a year, and rarely for several years.
7. Long-term morbidity and mortality is attributed almost exclusively to renal disease. Serial urinalyses and follow-up of renal functions are recommended, if the initial tests show any abnormalities.

Clinical Pearls: Henoch-Schönlein Purpura

1. HSP is the most common cause of nonthrombocytopenic purpura.
2. The sine qua non of HSP is palpable purpura seen most prominently on the lower extremity (Figs. 7-13, 7-14). The rash begins as an erythematous, maculopapular, blanching rash that later progresses to nonblanching petechiae or purpura.
3. HSP is usually benign and self-limiting; long-term morbidity and mortality is attributed almost exclusively to renal involvement.
4. Arthritis or gastrointestinal symptoms may precede the appearance of HSP rash by up to 2 weeks.
5. Testicular involvement occurs in up to 35% of patients with HSP. Acute scrotal swelling may be a presenting sign of HSP (*prior to the appearance of purpura*), and may mimic acute testicular torsion or incarcerated inguinal hernia.
6. Young infants with HSP often have atypical presentations consisting of urticaria and angioedema.

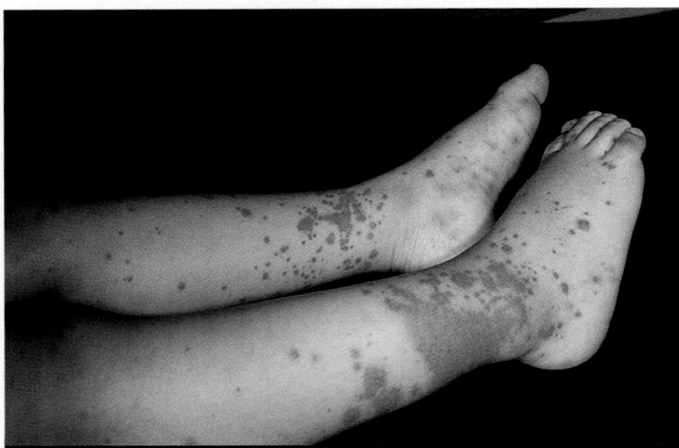

Figure 7-13. Henoch-Schönlein Purpura

Typical distributions of palpable purpuric lesions are on the lower extremities and buttocks (below the waistline). Lesions can appear on the arms, face, and ears, but the trunk is usually spared.

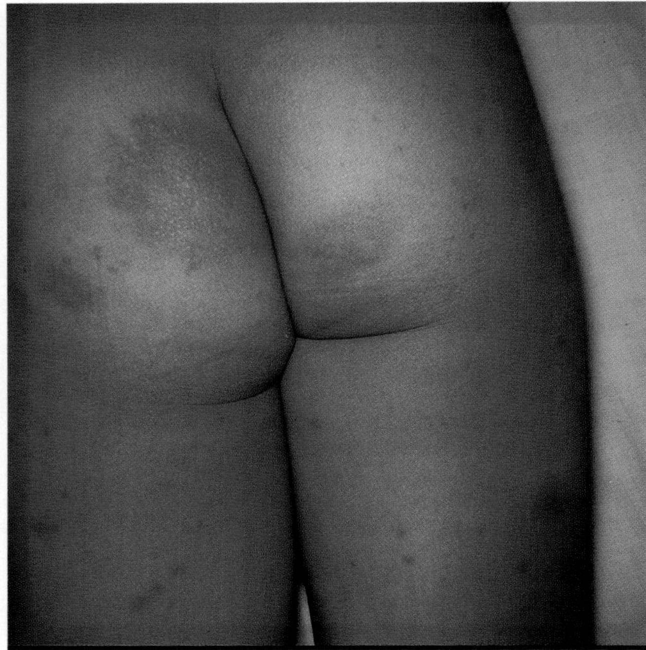

Figure 7-14. Henoch-Schönlein Purpura

Large area of ecchymosis on the buttocks with purpuric lesions are seen. This large ecchymotic lesion can be mistakenly attributed to child abuse (bruises on the buttocks are usually due to inflicted injuries from child abuse).

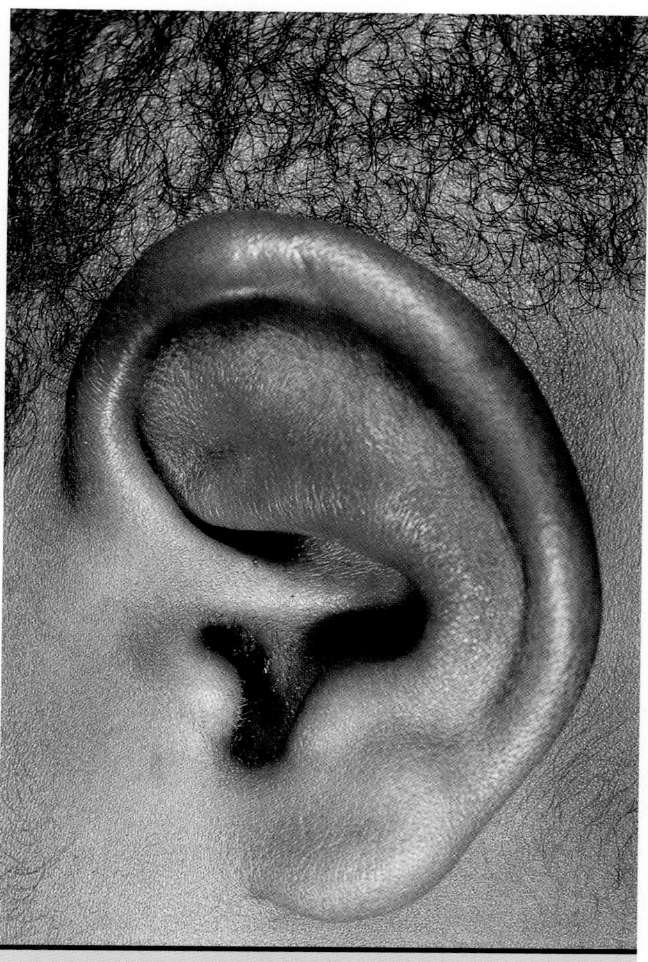

Figure 7-15. Henoch-Schönlein Purpura with Vasculitis

Purpuric lesion with edema affecting the ear in a patient with HSP. This finding can be mistakenly attributed to child abuse, especially when the patient presents with ear involvement that precedes the purpura (like buttocks, ears are not frequently injured in childhood accidents, and bruises at these sites are strong indicators of abuse).

BOX 7-18. CLINICAL FEATURES OF HENOCH-SCHÖNLEIN PURPURA

- Typical skin lesions
  (1) Lesions evolve from pinkish maculopapular or urticarial papules to palpable purpura.
  (2) Purpura appears to be gravity- and pressure-dependent.
  (3) Lesions occur in crops and last from 3 to 10 days.
  (4) Lesions appear at intervals varying from a few days to months.
  (5) Bullous or necrotic lesions may be present.
- Distribution of skin lesions
  (1) *From the buttocks down the lower extremities*
  (2) The upper extremities may be involved.
  (3) Primarily effects extensor surfaces
  (4) *The torso is usually spared.*
  (5) *The face, palms, and soles are usually spared.*
  (6) Brownish pigmentation may result from hemosiderin deposits in skin.
- Gastrointestinal symptoms (75% of cases)
  (1) Colicky abdominal pain (may precede the onset of purpura)
  (2) Vomiting, diarrhea
  (3) Gross or occult blood in stool (>50% of cases)
  (4) Hematemesis, hematochezia, or melena
- Joint symptoms (60%)
  (1) Arthritis or arthralgia
  (2) Most commonly involved joints: knees, ankles, dorsum of hands and feet
  (3) Often incapacitating
  (4) Self-limiting, nondeforming
  (5) May precede the onset of purpura
- Renal involvement (25 to 50% of cases)
  (1) Microscopic or macroscopic hematuria (most common renal feature)
  (2) Proteinuria
  (3) Hypertension
- Atypical presentations
  (1) Lesions may be urticarial
  (2) Angioedema

    May precede palpable purpura

    Sites (dependent areas or greater tissue distensibility): scalp, periorbital regions, hands/feet, chest wall, scrotum

  (3) Acute infantile hemorrhagic edema (Finkelstein's disease, Seidlmayer's syndrome)

    Variant of HSP in young infants (2 to 24 months)

    Systemic involvement extremely rare

    Erythematous, edematous, urticarial lesions of hands and feet

    Medallion-like purpura

BOX 7-19. DIFFERENTIAL DIAGNOSIS OF HENOCH-SCHÖNLEIN PURPURA

- *Other conditions with purpura/petechiae*
  (1) Meningococcemia
  (2) Rocky Mountain spotted fever
  (3) Enteroviral exanthema
  (4) Erythema multiforme
  (5) Drug eruptions
  (6) Gonococcemia
  (7) Child abuse
  (8) Protein S or protein C deficiency
  (9) Thrombocytopenia from any etiology (e.g., idiopathic thrombocytopenic purpura, leukemia)
- *Differential diagnosis of other features of HSP (renal, GI, joints, vasculitis)*
  (1) Acute abdomen from any etiology
  (2) Inflammatory bowel disease
  (3) Glomerulonephritis from other etiology (e.g., poststreptococcal)
  (4) Arthritis from other etiology (e.g., systemic juvenile rheumatoid arthritis, postinfectious reactive arthritis)
  (5) Kawasaki's disease
  (6) Familial Mediterranean fever
  (7) Polyarteritis nodosa

DIAGNOSIS SEBORRHEIC DERMATITIS

Synonyms

Cradle cap
Dandruff

Definition and Etiology

1. Seborrheic dermatitis is an inflammatory disorder occurring in the extremes of pediatric age groups (infancy and adolescence). This age group distribution parallels the distribution, size, and activity of the sebaceous glands; however, the etiology and contribution of sebaceous glands in this disorder are unknown.
2. *Malassezia furfur* or *Pityrosporum ovale* has been implicated as a causative agent, although its role in the etiology of infantile seborrheic dermatitis is unclear.
3. Genetic and environmental factors including stress, poor hygiene, and excessive perspiration are some of the contributory factors.

Associated Clinical Features

1. Seborrheic dermatitis is more commonly seen in early infancy and adolescence.
2. It is also a common cutaneous manifestation of AIDS among children and adolescents. Thick, greasy scales on the scalp and large hyperkeratotic erythematous plaques on the face, chest, and genitals are common presentations.
3. Complications include secondary monilial infection (due to colonization with *Candida albicans*) and secondary bacterial infections.

Emergency Department Treatment and Disposition

1. For infants
   a. Minor amounts of scale are easily removed by frequent shampooing with products containing sulfur and salicylic acid (e.g., Sebulex shampoo)
   b. Warm mineral or olive oil compresses followed by washing several hours later and lifting off the scale with a fine-toothed comb may be helpful for scales that are dense, thick, and adherent.
2. For older children and adolescents
   a. Any of the antiseborrheic shampoos containing selenium sulfide (e.g., Selsun Blue), zinc pyrithione (e.g., Head & Shoulders), coal tar (e.g., Neutrogena T/Gel), or ketoconazole (e.g., Nizoral) can be used intermittently (e.g., 2 to 3 times per week)
   b. Instruct the patient/parent to lather the shampoo and let it sit on the scalp for 5 to 10 minutes before rinsing.
3. Apply a topical low- to mid-potency corticosteroid solution to the scalp and cream to nonhairy inflamed areas. Caution patients that topical steroids should not be used as maintenance therapy.
4. Topical antifungal agents effective against *M. furfur* (e.g., ketoconazole cream) may be helpful in adolescents.
5. Reassure patients that seborrheic dermatitis does not cause permanent hair loss.

Clinical Pearls: Seborrheic Dermatitis

1. Seborrheic dermatitis is the most common rash in the first month of life (Figs. 7-16 and 7-17).
2. Lesions consist of greasy scales and erythematous papular dermatitis on the scalp, face, and other parts of body.
3. Suspect coexisting atopic dermatitis when lesions are weeping and associated with pruritus.
4. With pronounced scaling, seborrheic dermatitis may resemble psoriasis.
5. Seborrheic dermatitis is one of the most common cutaneous manifestations of AIDS in older children, adolescents, and adults, and onset usually occurs before the development of AIDS symptoms.

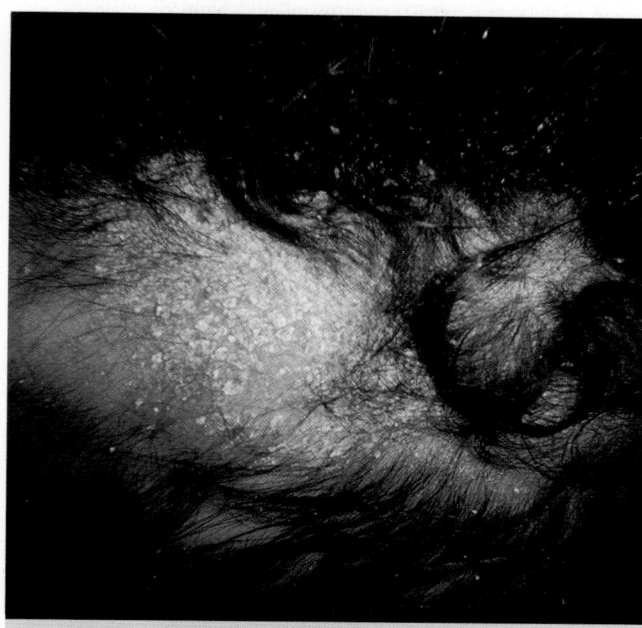

Figure 7-16. Seborrheic Dermatitis

Scalp of a 3-week-old newborn with scaly lesions. Tinea amiantacea refers to seborrheic dermatitis of the scalp with dense patches of yellow-white scale firmly adherent to the hair shafts.

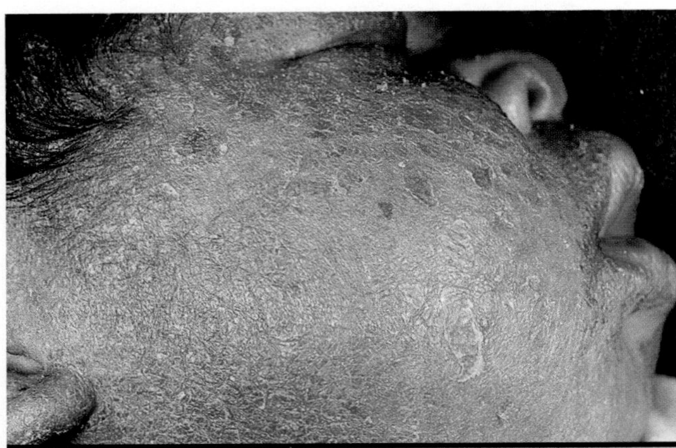

Figure 7-17. Seborrheic Dermatitis

Greasy papular eruption on the face of an infant. Scales may be scraped from the eyebrows. The ears were similarly involved in this infant.

BOX 7-20. CLINICAL FEATURES OF SEBORRHEIC DERMATITIS

- Onset: usually between 2 and 6 weeks of age
- Duration: until 6 months of age, then disappears until puberty
- Skin lesions in infancy

A. Scalp:

(1) Greasy, adherent, yellowish-red scales

(2) Involvement focal on the vertex of the scalp or diffuse

B. Other sites: central part of the face (medial parts of eyebrows, cheeks), ears, postauricular folds, neck, intertriginous areas, extremities, diaper region

(1) Greasy, scaly with erythematous or yellow-colored papular dermatitis

(2) Involvement either focal or may spread to involve almost entire body

C. Little or no pruritus

D. Postinflammatory pigmentary changes (either hypo- or hyperpigmentation)

- Skin lesions in adolescents

A. Scalp:

(1) Fine diffuse scales (dandruff) or focal areas of thick, oily, yellow crusts with underlying erythema

(2) Loss of hair

B. Other sites:

(1) Scaly papules in the central part of the face (medial aspects of eyebrows, nasolabial folds)

(2) Red, scaly plaques in intertriginous areas (axillae, inguinal region, gluteal cleft, umbilicus)

(3) Blepharitis

C. Pruritus: absent to marked

BOX 7-25. DIFFERENTIAL DIAGNOSIS OF ATOPIC DERMATITIS

- For all types of AD
  (1) Seborrheic dermatitis
  (2) Contact dermatitis
  (3) Fixed drug eruption
  (4) Fungal infections
  (5) Scabies
- For severe infantile AD
  (1) Histiocytosis X
  (2) Wiskott-Aldrich syndrome
  (3) Phenylketonuria
  (4) Bruton's X-linked agammaglobulinemia
  (5) Psoriasis
  (6) Job syndrome (hyperimmunoglobulin E syndrome)
  (7) Chronic granulomatous disease

DIAGNOSIS ECZEMA HERPETICUM

Synonym

Kaposi's varicelliform eruption

Definition/Etiology

1. Eczema herpeticum (EH) is a disseminated cutaneous herpes simplex virus (HSV) infection superimposed on a preexisting skin disorder (e.g., eczema).
2. EH is most commonly caused by HSV-1, and less commonly by HSV-2.

Associated Clinical Features

1. EH is seen in infants, children, and adults of any age.
2. EH is seen most commonly in patients with eczema (atopic dermatitis); however, it occurs with a number of other primary and acquired dermatologic disorders (e.g., seborrheic dermatitis, ichthyosis vulgaris, burns, skin grafts, irritant contact dermatitis, Darier's disease, pityriasis rubra pilaris).
3. Often there is a history of contact with a family member (usually a parent) with recurrent oral/facial HSV infection.
4. If indicated, CBC, blood culture, and bacterial cultures from the vesiculopustules may be done to exclude secondary bacterial superinfection.
5. The diagnosis of EH is usually made clinically. Diagnosis can be confirmed by Tzanck smear (see Fig. 3-49), HSV culture, or PCR.
6. Complications include secondary bacterial infection (*Streptococcus pyogenes* and *Staphylococcus aureus*), sepsis, and scarring.

Consultation

Dermatology (if diagnosis is unclear)

Emergency Department Treatment and Disposition

1. Mild cases of EH can be managed as an outpatient with acyclovir given orally.
   a. Dose for immunocompetent children: 1200 mg/24 hours divided every 8 hours for 7 to 10 days
   b. Max dose of oral acyclovir in children: 80 mg/kg per 24 hours
2. Topical penciclovir cream may be applied to affected areas every 2 hours.
3. Topical mupirocin applied bid or tid to affected areas or antibiotic given orally (e.g., dicloxacillin or cephalexin) for localized uncomplicated bacterial superinfection
4. Hospitalize patients with severe EH with systemic signs (e.g., fever, prostration)
   a. IV acyclovir dose for immunocompetent children: 15 mg/kg per 24 hours or 750 mg/m^2 per 24 hours divided every 8 hours for 5 to 7 days
   b. Topical penciclovir cream may be applied to affected areas every 2 hours.

c. Antibiotics (if indicated) given for bacterial superinfection (e.g., IV oxacillin)

Clinical Pearls: Eczema Herpeticum

1. "Punched out" ulcers superimposed on a preexisting skin disorder like eczema are important clues (Figs. 7-26, and 7-27).
2. Suspect EH when infected-appearing eczema does not respond to appropriate antibiotic therapy; this may indicate HSV infection.

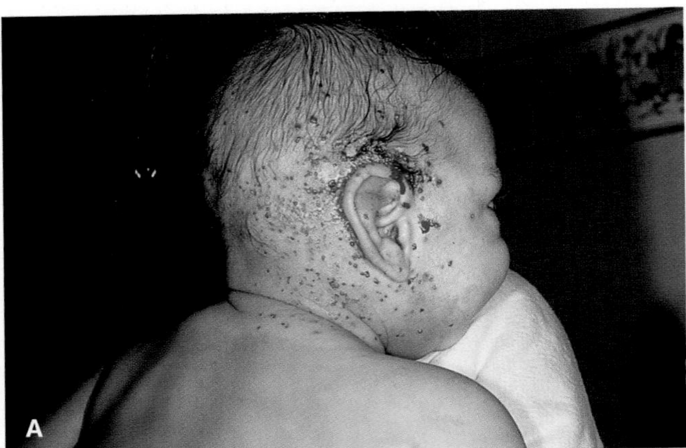

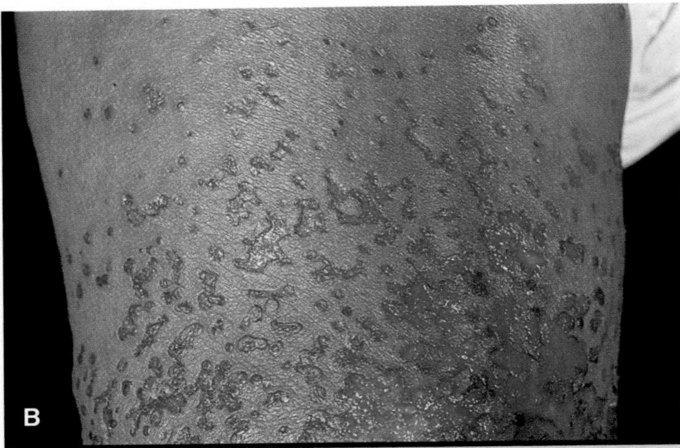

Figure 7-26. Eczema Herpeticum

A. Widespread "punched-out" lesions on upper trunk, neck, and extremities were seen in a highly febrile 4-month-old infant with infantile eczema. The mother suffered from recurrent cold sores (herpes simplex labialis), and had cold sores 5 days prior to the appearance of this infant's rash. *B*. Close-up of the "punched-out" lesions is shown here.

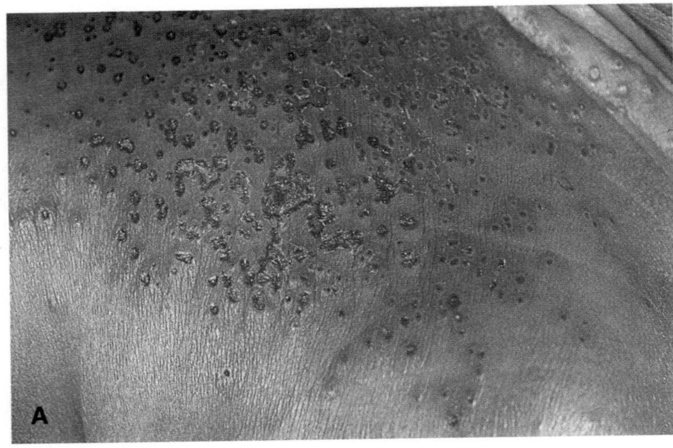

Figure 7-27. Eczema Herpeticum

(A) Close-up of the "punched-out" lesions seen over the trunk in a 3-month-old infant who was brought to the ED with a history of worsening rash, fever, and irritability. This infant's mother also had cold sores 4 days prior to the onset of this rash. (B) Schematic drawing illustrating a typical course of eczema herpeticum. (Reproduced with permission from: Katz SL et al (eds): *Krugman's Infectious Disease of Children*, 10th ed. St. Louis, Mosby-Year Book, 1998, p. 713)

BOX 7-26. CLINICAL FEATURES OF ECZEMA HERPETICUM

- Confined to areas of preexisting skin disorder (e.g., areas of atopic dermatitis)
- Rapid development of numerous umbilicated vesicles
- Vesicles evolve into "punched-out" ulcers
- Ulcers may become confluent, producing large denuded areas.
- Lesions painful
- Lesions may become hemorrhagic and crusted
- Lesions begin as clusters of vesicles, then rapidly become widespread over affected skin areas.
- Common sites: face, neck, trunk
- Lesions usually spread for 7 to 10 days.
- Primary infection resolves in 2 to 6 weeks.
- Systemic signs and symptoms: fever, malaise, sometimes irritability
- Lymphadenopathy in some cases
- Bacterial superinfection indicated by golden-yellow crusted lesions (*S. pyogenes* and *S. aureus*) or follicular pustules (*S. aureus*)
- Systemic dissemination can occur in immunocompromised patients
- Recurrent episodes of EH may occur.
- Recurrent episodes usually milder and without severe systemic symptoms
- Recurrent episodes resolve more quickly.

BOX 7-27. DIFFERENTIAL DIAGNOSIS OF ECZEMA HERPETICUM

- Disseminated (systemic) HSV infection
- Disseminated varicella zoster infection
- Staphylococcal folliculitis
- Widespread bullous impetigo
- *Candida* folliculitis
- Pseudomonal (hot-tub) folliculitis

DIAGNOSIS PSORIASIS

SYNONYM

Psoriasis vulgaris for plaque psoriasis

Definition/Etiology

1. Psoriasis is a chronic hereditary skin disorder of unknown etiology that is characterized by epidermal proliferation.
2. The process of cell maturation to shedding to replacement takes 3 to 4 weeks in normal skin. In psoriasis, there is a defective inhibitor of epidermal cell proliferation; thus, this cycle is shortened to 3 to 4 days. This leads to a rapid epidermal cell turnover with decreased shedding and subsequent accumulation of dead cells. Silvery white scales that are seen in psoriasis represent accumulated dead skin cells.

Associated Clinical Features

1. Psoriasis is more common in adults than in children.
2. About 10% of patients have their onset before the age of 10 years, and onset may be seen as early as the first months of life.
3. A positive family history is seen in 30% of patients and there is an association with certain histocompatibility leukocyte antigens.
4. Psoriasis vulgaris or plaque psoriasis is the most common variant of psoriasis.
5. Precipitating factors of psoriasis include:
   a. Minor trauma (psoriatic lesions seen mainly at sites of repeated trauma)
   b. Infection (e.g., upper respiratory tract infections leading to guttate psoriasis; see Fig. 7-29)
   c. Lack of sunlight exposure
   d. Cold weather
6. Generalized pustular psoriasis (Fig. 7-28)
   a. Patients often have fever, chills, diarrhea, and arthralgias.
   b. Leukocytosis and toxic appearance are also common.
   c. Most patients have an antecedent nonpustular psoriasis or a genetic predisposition for the disease.
   d. Episodes may be precipitated by medications such as tar and anthralin or by withdrawal of both topical and systemic steroids.
   e. Relapses are common.
7. The diagnosis of psoriasis is usually made clinically. In doubtful cases, skin biopsy will confirm the diagnosis.
8. Complications of psoriasis include generalized exfoliative dermatitis (erythroderma) and psoriatic arthritis.

Consultation

Dermatology for severe forms of psoriasis (e.g., generalized pustular psoriasis)

Emergency Department Treatment and Disposition

1. Hospitalize patients with severe forms of psoriasis (e.g., generalized pustular psoriasis, which can be a serious and at times a fatal disease). Other patients are treated as outpatients.
2. Establish realistic parental expectations.
   a. Psoriasis is characterized by relapses and remissions.
   b. Educate parents and older patients that psoriasis is a chronic disease that can be treated but not cured, and that goals of therapy are to control the flare-ups.
3. General instructions:
   a. Avoid trauma or scratching the lesions (Koebner's phenomenon [trauma-induced lesions]).
   b. Emollient to maintain skin hydration (e.g., Vaseline, petrolatum, mineral oil)
   c. Lukewarm brief baths (adding bath oil or coal tar may help).
   d. For thick scalp lesions use shampoo two or three times per week (coal tar, selenium sulfide, or zinc pyrithione).
   e. Sunlight exposure helps psoriasis (use sunscreens and avoid sunburn, as it aggravates psoriasis).
4. Topical corticosteroids creams
   a. Low-potency steroid creams on face and groin no more than bid for 2 weeks
   b. Medium-potency steroid creams on other body parts no more than bid for 2 weeks
   c. High-potency steroid creams are reserved for older children and adolescents with severely affected areas no more than bid for 2 weeks.
5. A course of antibiotics may be helpful (e.g., guttate psoriasis precipitated by streptococcal infection; see page 311). Antibiotics are also indicated for lesions that are crusted or open and weeping (e.g., penicillin, cefalexin, or erythromycin).
6. Refer the patient to a dermatologist for continuity of care. Other therapeutic options in refractory cases include topical vitamin D analogue creams or retinoids, UVB phototherapy, PUVA (psoralen plus UVA phototherapy), or oral therapies that include steroids, retinoids, methotrexate, or cyclosporine.

Clinical Pearls: Psoriasis

1. Psoriasis is characterized by erythematous plaques that are covered with thick silvery or yellow-white scales and irregular, sharply-demarcated borders.
2. Koebner's phenomenon (new lesions appearing at the site of trauma) is an important feature of psoriasis.
3. Involvement of nails is also an important feature of psoriasis.

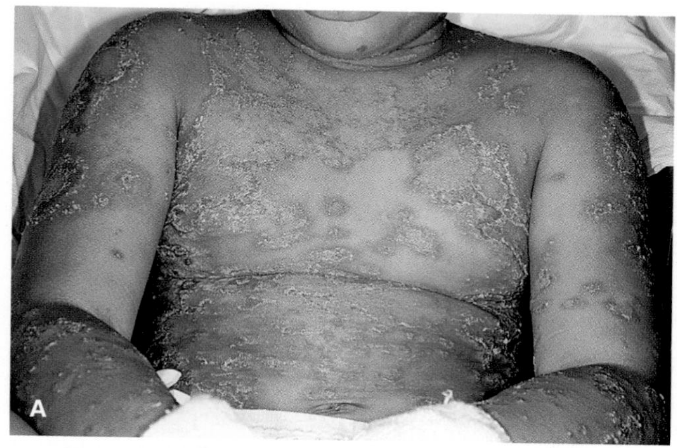

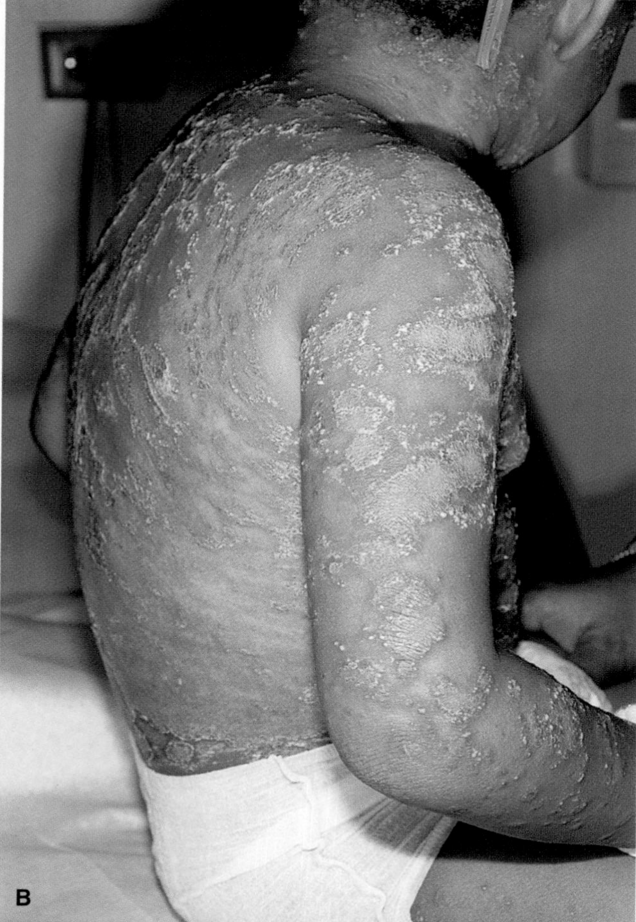

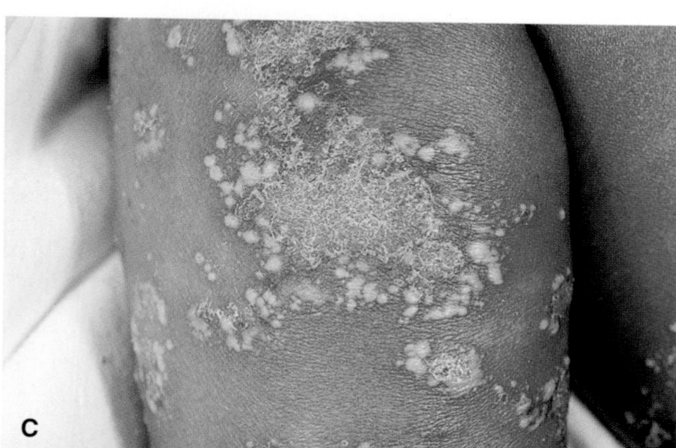

Figure 7-28. Generalized Pustular Psoriasis

Pustular psoriasis may occur in a localized (often seen on palms and soles) or generalized pattern. Generalized pustular psoriasis often occurs suddenly in patients who have a history of chronic plaque psoriasis. *A, B*. Numerous tiny, sterile pustules developed from an erythematous base in this child. Typically the patient develops large patches of erythema with sharply demarcated gyrate or serpiginous margins with small pustules. *C*. Close-up of pustular psoriasis is shown. Numerous tiny, sterile pustules evolve from an erythematous base and coalesce into lakes of pus. Pustules are superficial (upper epidermal) and are easily ruptured. Patients with pustular psoriasis are usually toxic-appearing and highly febrile. Burning and pruritus result in severe discomfort. Patients with pustular psoriasis may also have mucous membrane involvement, as well as fissuring and ulceration of the tongue and erythematous, scaly lips. Certain medications can trigger pustular psoriasis (e.g., prednisone withdrawal).

BOX 7-28. CLINICAL FEATURES OF PSORIASIS

- Well-delineated erythematous plaques
- Plaques are round, oval, or polymorphous.
- Plaques are covered with thick silvery-white scales.
- Removal of scales results in pinpoint bleeding (Auspitz sign).
- Pruritic to varying degrees
- Koebner's phenomenon (new lesions appear at the sites of trauma, often in a linear fashion).
- Location of plaques
  (1) Bilateral (rarely symmetrical) distributed on extensor surfaces of extremities (usually on unexposed or frequently traumatized areas, such as knees and elbows)
  (2) Scalp
  (3) Perianal
  (4) Umbilical
  (5) Intragluteal cleft
  (6) Lumbosacral
  (7) Genitals/diaper area (infants)
  (8) May be generalized (e.g., guttate psoriasis)
- Nail changes
  (1) Pitting of nail plates
  (2) Detachment of plates
  (3) Oil spot sign (yellow-brown discoloration)
  (4) Subungual hyperkeratosis
- Other presentations of psoriasis
  (1) Localized or generalized pustular psoriasis (see Fig. 7-28)
  (2) Napkin psoriasis (seen in the groin in a young infant; well-circumscribed erythematous plaque with minimal scaling [due to constant wetness of area])
  (3) Guttate psoriasis (see Fig. 7-29)
  (4) Psoriatic arthritis (more common in adults and may precede skin lesions)

BOX 7-29. DIFFERENTIAL DIAGNOSIS OF PSORIASIS

- Other conditions with scalp involvement
  (1) Seborrheic dermatitis
  (2) Tinea capitis
  (3) Atopic dermatitis
- Nummular eczema
- Tinea corporis
- Pityriasis rosea
- Pityriasis rubra pilaris
- Contact dermatitis
- Lichen simplex chronicus
- Reiter's syndrome
- Psoriasiform drug eruptions (e.g., beta-blockers, gold)
- Other conditions with Koebner's phenomenon (e.g., lichen planus)

DIAGNOSIS GUTTATE PSORIASIS

Definition

Guttate psoriasis is a variant of psoriasis characterized by an abrupt onset of profuse oval or round droplike lesions, most commonly following group A beta-hemolytic streptococcal infections (Fig. 7-29).

Etiology

1. Group A beta-hemolytic streptococcal infection (streptococcal pharyngitis, perianal streptococcal dermatitis, otitis, or sinusitis)
2. Viral infections (e.g., upper respiratory tract infections [URIs])
3. Withdrawal of systemic corticosteroid therapy
4. Sunburn

Associated Clinical Features

1. About a third of patients with psoriasis have their first episode before the age of 20. An episode of guttate psoriasis may be the first indication of the patient's propensity for the disease.
2. Streptococcal pharyngitis or a viral URI precedes the eruption of guttate psoriasis by 1 to 3 weeks.
3. *Guttate* in Latin means "spots that resemble drops." Guttate psoriasis lesions are small oval or round lesions that are morphologically identical to larger plaques of psoriasis.
4. Laboratory tests should include a throat culture and serological titer (e.g., antistreptolysin O titer) to confirm streptococcal infection.

Emergency Department Treatment and Disposition

1. Antibiotic therapy for guttate psoriasis associated with streptococcal infection
   a. Drug of choice: penicillin (see streptococcal pharyngitis, page 67)
   b. For patients allergic to penicillin: erythromycin or clindamycin
2. Guttate psoriasis usually resolves spontaneously in a few weeks or months (especially with antibiotic therapy).
3. Tonsillectomy or monthly injections of benzathine penicillin may be necessary if flares are precipitated by recurrent streptococcal infections.
4. Exposure to sunlight also helps in resolution of lesions.
5. For persistent lesions, the same therapy as that for psoriasis is recommended (see page 308).

Clinical Pearls: Guttate Psoriasis

1. Guttate psoriasis is a variant of psoriasis that is seen more commonly in children and adolescents.
2. Guttate psoriasis may herald the development of generalized plaque psoriasis.
3. Guttate psoriasis is characterized by an abrupt onset of droplike lesions, mainly on the trunk, buttocks, hips, and proximal extremities.

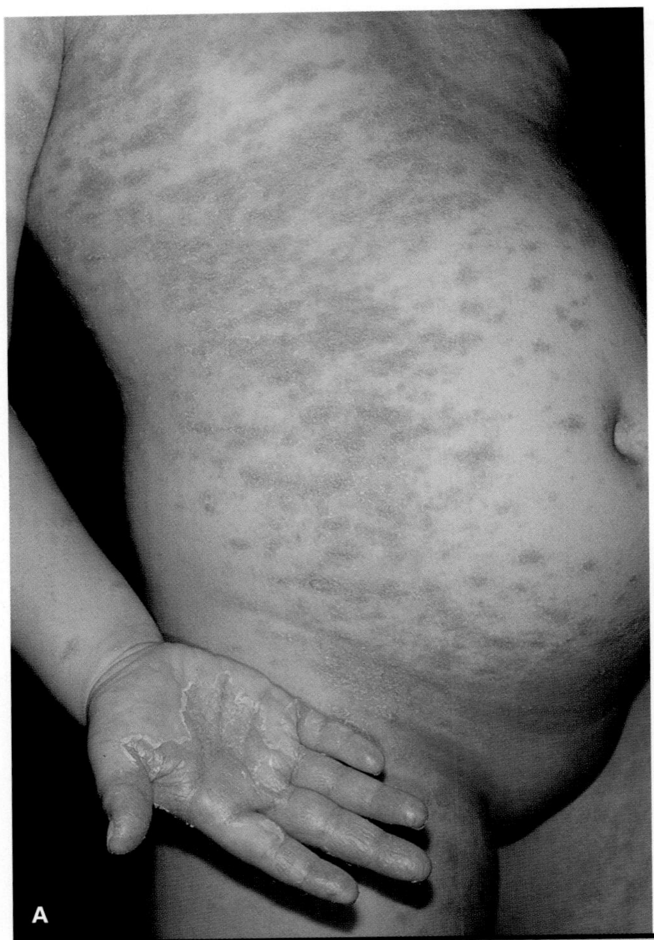

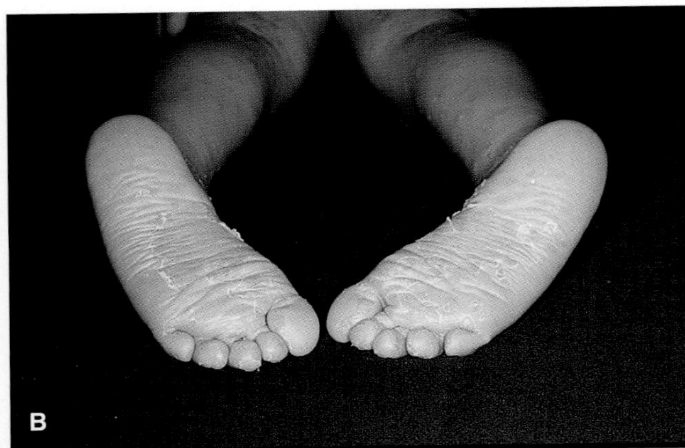

Figure 7-29. Guttate Psoriasis

An abrupt onset of erythematous, scaly, droplike plaques mainly concentrated on the trunk of a 6-year-old child following a streptococcal infection. About 8 days prior to this rash, the patient had a sore throat, low-grade fever, and "goose-bumps" on the skin (scarlet fever) by history. Her throat culture was positive for group A beta-hemolytic streptococci. Intense erythema and desquamation is also seen on the palms (*A*) and both feet (*B*) following streptococcal infection.

BOX 7-30. CLINICAL FEATURES OF GUTTATE PSORIASIS

- Abrupt onset
- Skin lesions
  (1) Small droplike round or oval scaly nonconfluent plaques
  (2) Number varies from few to hundreds
  (3) Size varies from pinpoint up to 1 cm (increases in diameter with time)
  (4) Salmon pink color
  (5) Location: trunk (highest concentration)
  (6) Other sites: proximal extremities, face, scalp, nails
  (7) Palms and soles usually spared
  (8) Varying degree of pruritus

BOX 7-31. DIFFERENTIAL DIAGNOSIS OF GUTTATE PSORIASIS

- Viral exanthemas
- Pityriasis rosea
- Drug eruptions
- Secondary syphilis
- Disseminated tinea corporis
- Mucha-Habermann disease

DIAGNOSIS PITYRIASIS ROSEA

Definition/Etiology

1. Pityriasis rosea (PR) is a benign, self-limiting eruption of unknown etiology with a distinct presentation of a solitary "herald patch" lesion followed by an exanthema.
2. It is presumed to be caused by a viral agent, but no single consistent virus has been identified to date.
3. The name pityriasis rosea is derived from Greek (pityriasis = scaly) and Latin (rosea = pink).

Associated Clinical Features

1. Common age at presentation
   a. Older children, adolescents, and young adults (age range: 10 to 35 years)
   b. About 50% of cases occur before age 20.
   c. Incidence highest among adolescents
   d. Rare in children <5 years
2. PR is commonly seen during fall, winter, and spring.
3. About 5% of patients have prodrome of fever, malaise, arthralgia, and pharyngitis preceding the PR eruption (usually seen in patients with florid PR).
4. Atypical clinical variants of PR that are seen less commonly (~25% of cases):
   a. Papular PR (especially in African-American children)
   b. PR with intensely irritated or inflamed edematous lesions
   c. "Inverse form of PR": lesions limited to face, scalp, distal extremities, groin, axillae
   d. PR with vesicular, pustular, urticarial, or hemorrhagic (purpuric) or large annular erythema multiforme-like lesions
   e. PR with oral lesions
5. The diagnosis of PR is made clinically. Very rarely a skin biopsy may be required for atypical cases. Histopathology findings in PR are nonspecific regarding the diagnosis, but allows other diseases to be excluded. It reveals extravasated erythrocytes within dermal papillae and dyskeratotic cells within the dermis.
6. Recurrences of PR are rare (about 2% of cases).

Consultation

Dermatology (for atypical PR variant cases)

Emergency Department Treatment and Disposition

1. Most patients are asymptomatic and do not need any specific treatment except reassurance about the *benign nature* of the rash and the *total duration* of the eruption.
2. Printed patient information is available from the American Academy of Dermatology.
3. Patients do not need any isolation and should not be considered contagious.

4. Symptomatic relief from pruritus may be obtained by any of the following:
   a. Soothing nonprescription lotions containing calamine, menthol, or pramoxine
   b. Lukewarm colloidal oatmeal bath (not hot, as this may intensify itching)
   c. Nonflurorinated topical corticosteroid (e.g., hydrocortisone lotion 1 or 2%)
   d. Antihistamine given orally, especially at night (when pruritus is more troublesome)
5. A rare patient with extensive disease with intense itching may respond to a short course of prednisone (dose: 0.5 to 1 mg/kg per day given orally for 7 days). This is rarely indicated in children and is best reserved for patients with intractable pruritus with severe disease.
6. Direct sun exposure hastens the resolution of individual lesions (but must avoid burning which can exacerbate the rash).
7. Ultraviolet B (UVB) administered in five consecutive daily erythemogenic exposures, results in decreased pruritus and hastens the involution of lesions. Therapy is most beneficial within the first week of eruption (rarely indicated in children).

Clinical Pearls: Pityriasis Rosea

1. PR is a self-limiting eruption lasting about 6 to 12 weeks and is characterized by pink oval papules or plaques on the trunk and proximal extremities.
2. Skin lesions are parallel to the ribs, forming a "Christmas tree" appearance on the trunk (Figs. 7-30 and 7-31).
3. A herald patch is seen in 80% of cases and heralds the onset of PR; however, its absence does not preclude the diagnosis of PR (Fig. 7-30).
4. Secondary syphilis may be indistinguishable from PR, especially if the herald patch is absent; thus, serology for syphilis must be obtained in all sexually active patients presenting with a rash of PR.

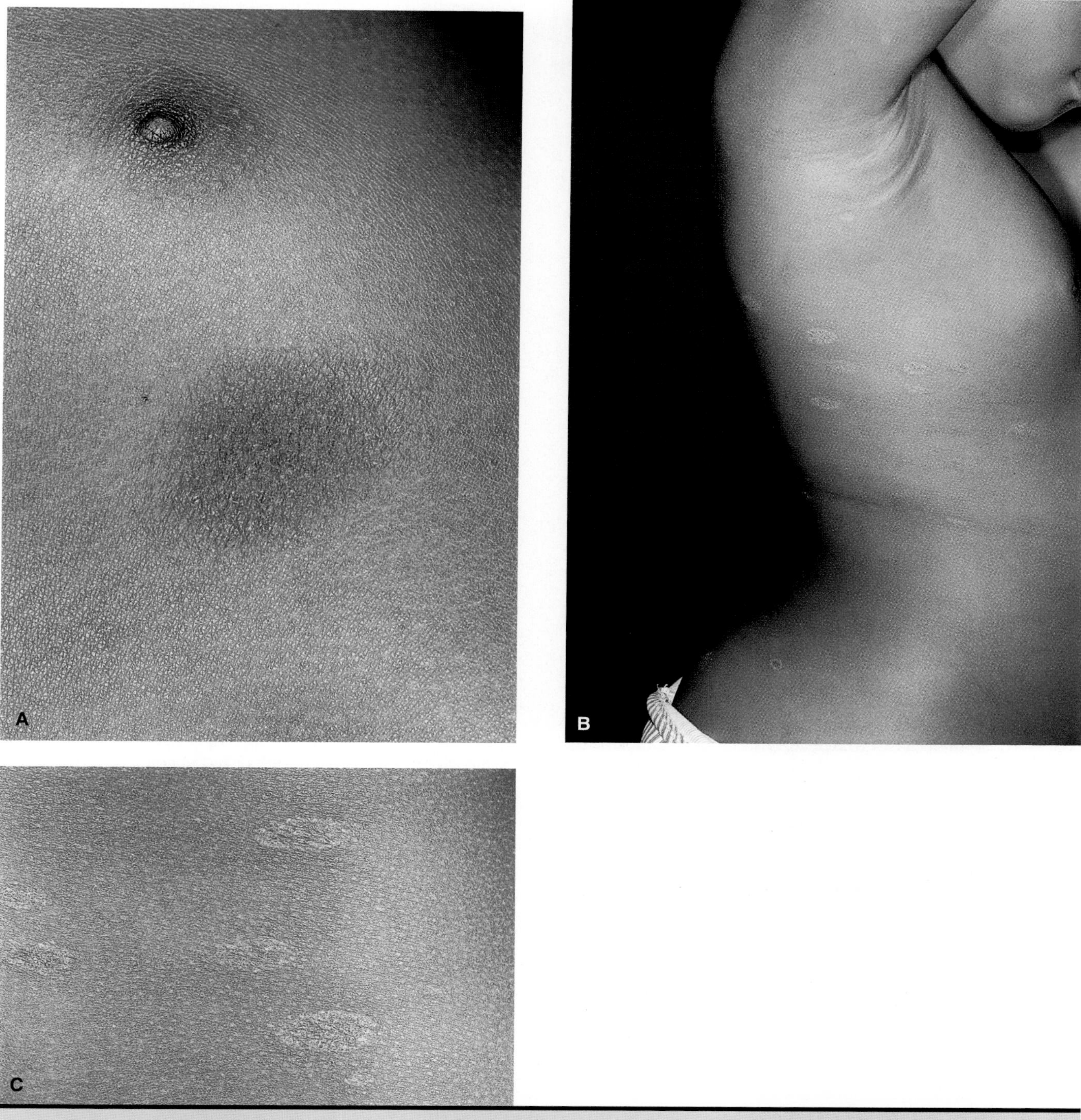

Figure 7-30. Pityriasis Rosea

This herald patch (*A*) preceded the PR eruption by about 10 days in this child. Oval-shaped papulosquamous lesions of PR are seen (*B*). Most of the eruptions are truncal in distribution. Conformation to skin lines is often more discernible in the anterior and posterior axillary folds and supraclavicular areas. A fine, wrinkled, tissuelike scale remains attached within the border of the plaque, giving the characteristic ring of scale, called collarette scale. The long axis of the oval plaques is oriented along skin lines. Numerous lesions on the back, oriented along the skin lines (parallel to the ribs), give the appearance of drooping pine-tree branches (Christmas-tree distribution). Close-up of the papulosquamous oval-shaped lesions is shown (*C*).

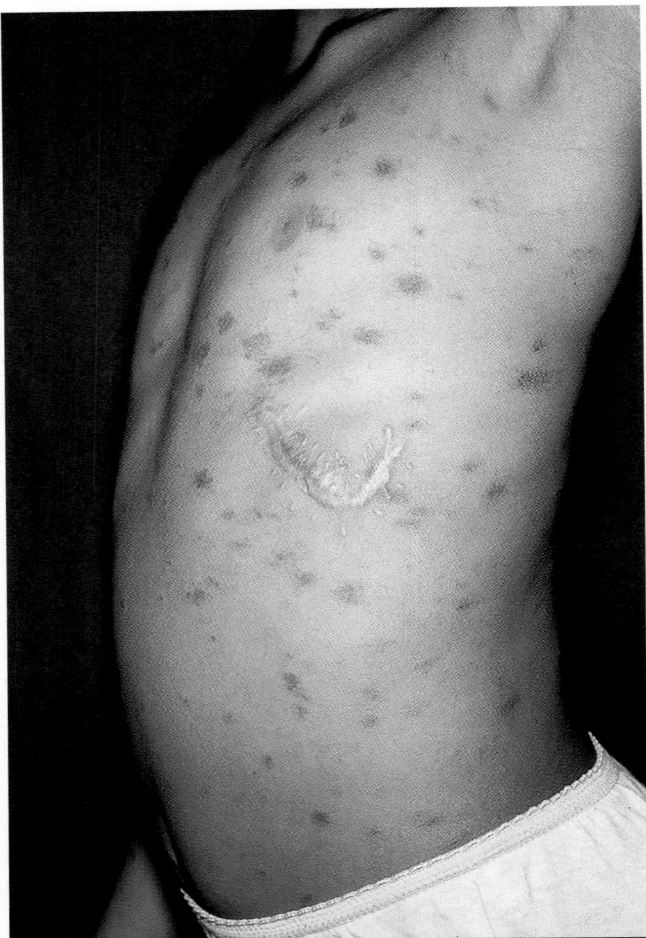

Figure 7-31. Pityriasis Rosea

Postinflammatory hyperpigmentation (or hypopigmentation) may be pronounced as seen here, particularly in black patients, after the PR eruption has resolved. These changes disappear during subsequent weeks to months.

BOX 7-32. CLINICAL FEATURES OF PITYRIASIS ROSEA

- *Herald patch*
  - (1) Heralds the onset of PR
  - (2) Precedes generalized eruption of PR by 1 to 2 weeks
  - (3) Seen in 80% of patients
  - (4) Usually a solitary lesion (rarely several lesions)
  - (5) Round-to-oval lesion varying from 1 to 10 cm in diameter
  - (6) Most common location: trunk or proximal extremities (can occur anywhere)
  - (7) Erythematous plaque with a raised border and marginal collarette of fine scale
  - (8) Retains the same features as subsequent oval lesions of PR
  - (9) Usually asymptomatic, but sometimes associated with mild pruritus
- *Eruptive phase*
  - (1) Widespread, symmetrical, multiple, discrete papular lesions
  - (2) Lesions oval to round in shape, ranging 1 to 3 cm in size
  - (3) Lesions dull pink or red in color
  - (4) Lesions covered with fine scale
  - (5) Some lesions clear centrally leaving a collarette of scale attached only at the periphery.
  - (6) Number of lesions varies from few to hundreds
  - (7) Lesions mostly on trunk, neck, and proximal parts of upper arms and legs
  - (8) Lesions may involve the face, scalp, distal extremities (in children or with extensive disease)
  - (9) *Palms and soles usually spared* (but *not always* spared)
  - (10) Long axes of lesions parallel to skin cleavage lines resulting in a "Christmas tree" pattern
  - (11) Highly variable pruritus (severe pruritus with extensive inflammatory eruption)
- *Natural course*
  - (1) New eruption continues in crops for 2 weeks
  - (2) Total duration of rash 6 to 12 weeks

BOX 7-33. DIFFERENTIAL DIAGNOSIS OF PITYRIASIS ROSEA

- *Differential diagnosis of herald patch*
  (1) Tinea corporis
  (2) Nummular eczema
- *Differential diagnosis of skin eruption*
  (1) Secondary syphilis
  (2) Viral exanthemas
  (3) Mucha-Habermann disease
  (4) Guttate psoriasis
  (5) Parapsoriasis
  (6) Tinea versicolor
  (7) Id reaction of fungal infection
  (8) PR-like drug eruption caused by many drugs (e.g., captopril, isotretinoin, metronidazole, clonidine, barbiturates, levamisole, vaccines [e.g., diphtheria toxoid])
  (9) Lichen planus
  (10) Eczema

DIAGNOSIS SCABIES

SYNONYM

Seven-year itch

Definition/Etiology

1. Scabies is a contagious skin infestation caused by the female mite *Sarcoptes scabiei* subsp. hominus (Fig. 7-32).
2. The female mite tunnels into the upper layer of the skin and produces a burrow. She deposits 2 eggs daily for 4 to 5 weeks (the life span of the mite) in the burrows. The larvae then hatch in a few days causing intense itching. Only 10% of the eggs develop into adult mites. An infested person has an average of 12 mites on the skin.
3. Signs and symptoms of scabies are a result of delayed hypersensitivity cell-mediated immune response to the proteins of the parasite. Nodules are a granulomatous response to the dead mite antigens and feces.

Associated Clinical Features

1. The incubation period is 4 to 6 weeks in persons without previous exposure. With a previous infestation, symptoms may develop in 1 to 4 days after repeated exposure to the mite.
2. It affects persons from all socioeconomic levels without regard to age, sex, or standards of personal hygiene; however, it is more common in crowded living quarters and nursing homes.
3. Dogs and cats may be infested by nearly identical organisms (*Sarcoptes scabiei* subsp. canis) and sometimes may serve as a source for human infestation.
4. The diagnosis of scabies is usually made clinically, based on distribution of the lesions, worsening pruritus at night, and a history of a similar rash in other family members.
5. When the diagnosis is not clear, light microscopic examination of a skin scraping from a burrow or a new unexcoriated lesion can be done with a #15 surgical blade, and it may

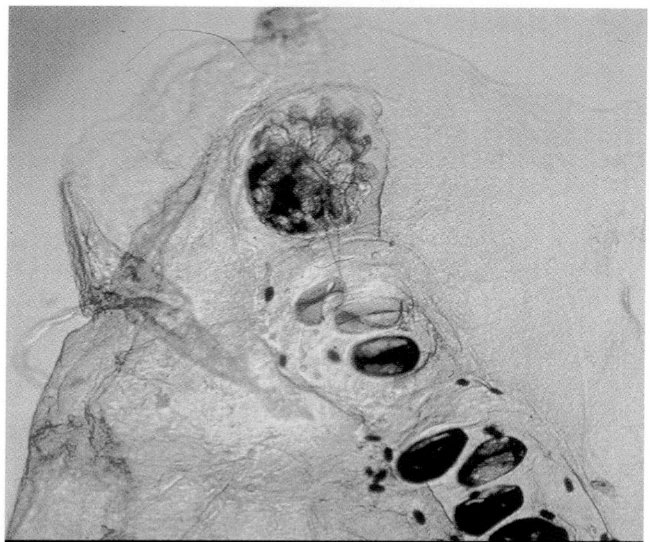

Figure 7-32. *Sarcoptes scabiei*

The causative mite, 400 μm in size, alongside ova (large black ovals) and feces (scattered smaller black dots). (Reproduced with permission from: Kane KS, Ryder JB, Johnson RA, Baden HP, Stratigos A: Scabies. In: *Color Atlas & Synopsis of Pediatric Dermatology*. New York, McGraw-Hill, 2002, p. 619.)

demonstrate a mite, egg, or feces (scybala). A negative scraping does not rule out scabies. A drop of mineral oil may be placed over the suspected lesion prior to scraping (skin scrapings adhere, feces are preserved, and the mite remains alive and motile in the clear oil). Mites are found in burrows and at the edges of vesicles, but rarely in papules.

6. Complications of scabies include secondary infection (*Staphylococcus aureus* or *Streptococcus pyogenes*). Scabies incognito is undiagnosed scabies resulting from the use of topical steroids.

Emergency Department Treatment and Disposition

1. Untreated scabies can last for months or years.
2. *Treat all the patient's contacts.*
3. Permethrin 5% cream (preferred treatment)
   a. Safe and effective
   b. Apply from the neck down (older children and adolescents) including intertriginous and genital areas, the intergluteal cleft, and under trimmed nails.
   c. Because scabies can affect the head, scalp, and neck in infants and young children, treatment of the entire head, neck, and body in this age group is required (avoid areas around the eyes and mouth).
   d. Leave the medication on overnight (about 8 hours).
   e. Change all the clothes and bed sheets the following morning.
   f. Repeat 1 week later for best results
   g. Side effects include mild, transient burning, stinging, redness, and rash.
4. Gamma benzene hexachloride (lindane 1%) cream or lotion
   a. Alternate preparations for school-aged children, adolescents, and adults
   b. *Caution: If improperly used and a significant amount is systemically absorbed, it may be neurotoxic.*
   c. *Do not use lindane under the following circumstances:*
      1) *Children <5 years of age* (infants have a larger surface area to body weight ratio and can absorb the drug through the skin, leading to neurotoxicity, and if the drug is applied to palms and soles in infants [common sites of scabies], they may lick the drug, also leading to toxicity).
      2) Premature infants
      3) Patients with crusted lesions
      4) Children with a prior history of seizure disorders
      5) Malnourished children (lindane seeks fat; lack of fat in a malnourished patient may lead to toxicity)
      6) Children with severe excoriations or inflamed or traumatized skin
      7) Children with chronic and preexisting dermatosis
      8) Use cautiously in women who are pregnant or breastfeeding
5. Alternative therapies include sulfur (5 to 10% precipitated sulfur in petrolatum) and crotamiton cream.
6. Educate the patient/parent about the following issues:
   a. Wash all clothing, towels, and bed linens that have touched the skin (use a normal washing machine cycle).
   b. Itching may continue for days to weeks (3 to 4 weeks) after treatment.
   c. Continued application of medication is unnecessary and worsens itching by causing irritation (overtreatment must be avoided).
   d. Bland lubricants or oral antihistamines may be used to relieve itching.
   e. Nodules can persist for weeks and even months after effective treatment.
   f. Children may return to school or child care after completing treatment.
7. Topical or systemic antibiotic therapy is indicated for secondary bacterial infections of the excoriated lesions.
8. The patient should be referred to their primary care physician for reexamination for treatment failures in 1 week and 4 weeks.
9. For crusted or Norwegian scabies:
   a. Isolate the patient.
   b. Several or sequential courses of topical permethrin or gamma benzene hexachloride
   c. Oral ivermectin at a single dose of 200 μg/kg

Clinical Pearls: Scabies

1. Scabies is an intensely pruritic, erythematous, generalized papular eruption (Figs. 7-33 and 7-34).
2. Scabies is a highly contagious disease transmitted by direct skin contact with an infected person. It usually infests the entire household and common contacts are household members, baby sitters, or playmates. *Treat all the contacts.*
3. The presence of a similar rash in other family members is an important clue.
4. Interdigital web lesions are less commonly seen in children.
5. Young infants may have hyperpigmented nodular lesions, especially along the axillary line.
6. Because scabietic lesions are the result of a hypersensitivity reaction to the mite, itching may not subside for several weeks despite successful treatment. Use of oral antihistamines and topical corticosteroids can help relieve this itching.
7. Treatment failures are usually due to failure to treat all the contacts (exposed individuals) simultaneously.

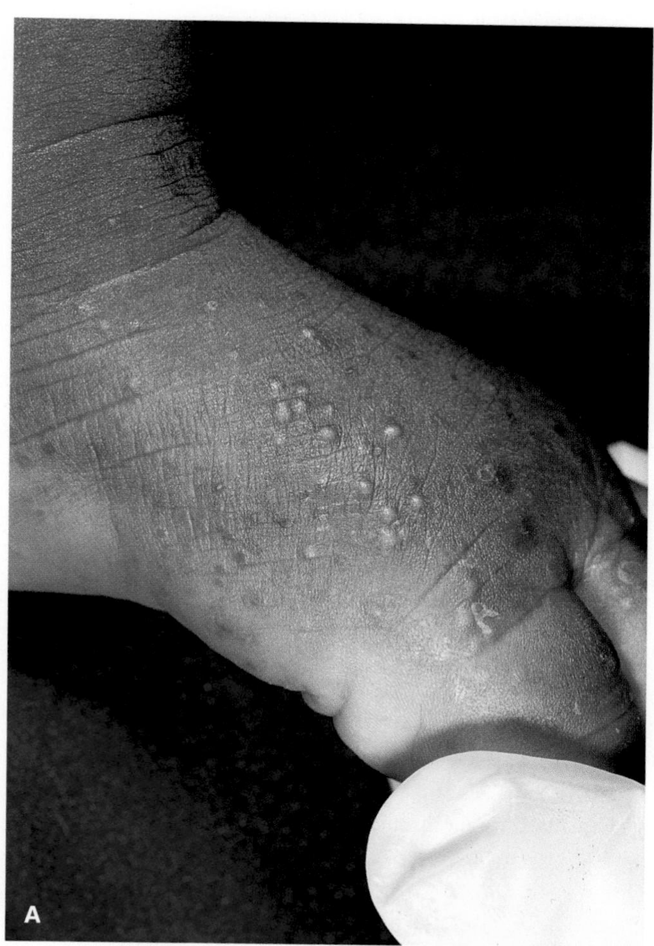

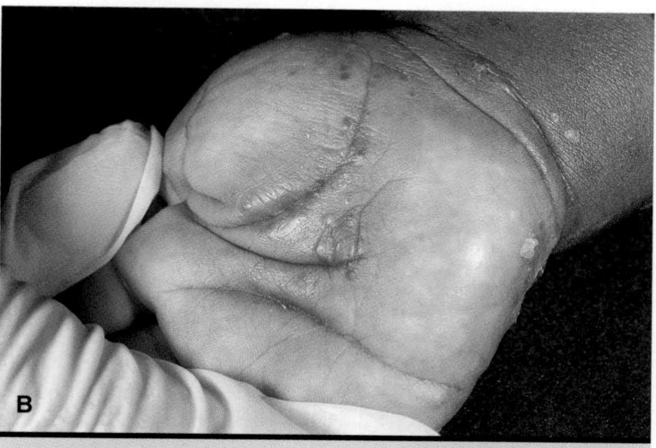

Figure 7-33. Scabies

An infant with papular and vesicular lesions on the foot and palm. The babysitter had a similar rash involving the wrist and interdigital spaces.

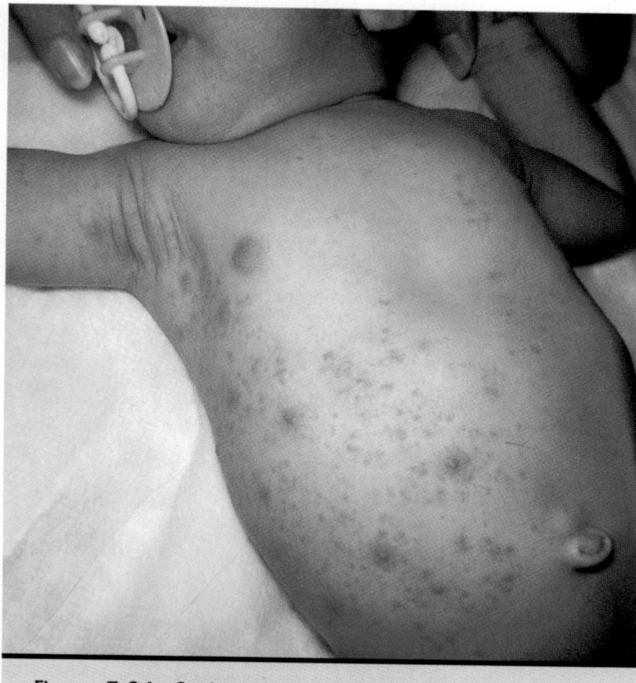

Figure 7-34. Scabies

A 2-month-old infant with lesions on the trunk and axillae. The mother also had an intensely pruritic rash on her hands and waistline.

BOX 7-34. CLINICAL FEATURES OF SCABIES

Primary lesions

- Intensely pruritic, papular lesions
- Excoriations common
- Pruritus worse at night
- Lesions show pleomorphism
- Distribution (older children/adults)
  (1) Generalized
  (2) Highest concentration: waist, male genitalia, interdigital webs, wrists, axillae, areolae of breasts
  (3) Face and scalp spared (except in infants and immunocompromised hosts)
- Burrows
  (1) Linear, serpiginous, or S-shaped
  (2) Tortuous, threadlike line
  (3) Gray-white
  (4) Common locations: finger webs, wrists, sides of hands and feet, penis, buttocks, scrotum, palms and soles of infants
  (5) Scratching destroys burrows.
  (6) May not always be demonstrated, especially in children (burrows seen in only 10% of cases)
- Nodular scabies (variant)
  (1) Red-brown lesions
  (2) Seen in covered areas (buttocks, groin, scrotum, penis, axillae)
  (3) Lesions do not represent inadequately treated scabies
  (4) Lesions are persistent and resolve spontaneously after weeks or months.
- Norwegian or crusted scabies (variant)
  (1) Seen in patients with Down's syndrome, immunocompromised hosts, or institutionalized individuals
  (2) Lesions consists of thick, psoriasiform crusted lesions
  (3) Involvement of hands and feet with asymptomatic crusting (rather than typical inflammatory papules and vesicles)
  (4) Gray scales and thick crusts may be present over the trunk and extremities.
  (5) Lesions teem with mites and are very contagious.

Secondary lesions (from scratching)

- Pinpoint erosions
- Scaling
- Erythema
- Eczematization (chronic scratching)

BOX 7-35. SCABIES IN INFANTS

- Often widespread involvement (as the diagnosis is not readily suspected)
- Palms, soles, face, and scalp often involved (unlike older children/adults)
- Lesions seen above the neck (unlike older children/adults)
- Vesicles or pustules on palms and soles (*highly characteristic sign of scabies in infants*)
- Burrows *not* common
- Secondary eczematization and impetiginization common
- Hyperpigmented nodules may be seen in axilla, diaper area, groin

BOX 7-36. DIFFERENTIAL DIAGNOSIS OF SCABIES

- Impetigo
- Papular urticaria
- Other arthropod bites
- Atopic dermatitis
- Seborrheic dermatitis
- Contact dermatitis
- Drug eruptions
- Crusted (Norwegian) scabies may be mistaken for psoriasis

DIAGNOSIS

TINEA VERSICOLOR

Synonym

Pityriasis versicolor

Definition/Etiology

Tinea versicolor is a superficial skin infection caused by the yeast *Malassezia furfur* (previously known as *Pityrosporum ovale* or *Pityrosporum orbiculare*).

Associated Clinical Features

1. Tinea versicolor is a common disease. It affects 1 to 2% of the general population in temperate zones and 30 to 40% in subtropical and tropical zones.
2. The organism is part of the normal skin flora and appears in highest numbers in areas with increased sebaceous gland activity.
3. Predisposing factors (that allow lowering the body's resistance and proliferation of the yeast) include malnutrition, burns, immunosuppressive or corticosteroid therapy, Cushing's syndrome, and pregnancy. Excess heat and humidity and oily skin or application of oils (e.g., cocoa butter, bath oil) on children leads to yeast overgrowth.
4. Tinea versicolor is more common in adolescents and young adults (years of higher sebaceous gland activity); however, it may occur in prepubertal children and infants.
5. The diagnosis is made clinically by the characteristic distribution and the appearance of the lesions.
6. The skin lesions may be inconspicuous in fair-skinned individuals during winter, and white hypopigmentation becomes more obvious as unaffected skin tans.
7. Scraping the lesions lightly with a surgical blade followed by potassium hydroxide examination of the scale shows numerous short, rod-shaped hyphae mixed with round spores in grapelike clusters ("chopped spaghetti-and-meatballs" appearance) (Fig. 7-37).
8. The yeast is transmitted by personal contact during periods of scaling. Fungal elements may be also be retained in frequently worn garments that are in contact with the skin. Thus, boiling such clothing might decrease the chance of recurrence.
9. The disease may vary in activity for years, but it diminishes or disappears with advancing age. In athletes, the rash may persist all year round.

Emergency Department Treatment and Disposition

1. Various topical treatment options (used for limited disease) include:
   a. Selenium sulfide 2.5% lotion or shampoo (treatment options include):
      1) Apply over affected areas and wash off after 30 minutes daily for 1 week; follow with monthly applications for 3 months (to help prevent recurrences).
      2) Apply over affected areas and wash off in 24 hours; repeat once a week for a total of 4 weeks.
   b. Terbinafine spray or cream twice daily for 1 week
   c. Sodium hyposulfite or thiosulfate in 15 to 25% concentrations; apply twice a day for 2 to 4 weeks.
   d. Antifungal antibiotics (e.g., miconazole, clotrimazole, ketoconazole) applied to entire affected area one to two times a day for 2 to 4 weeks

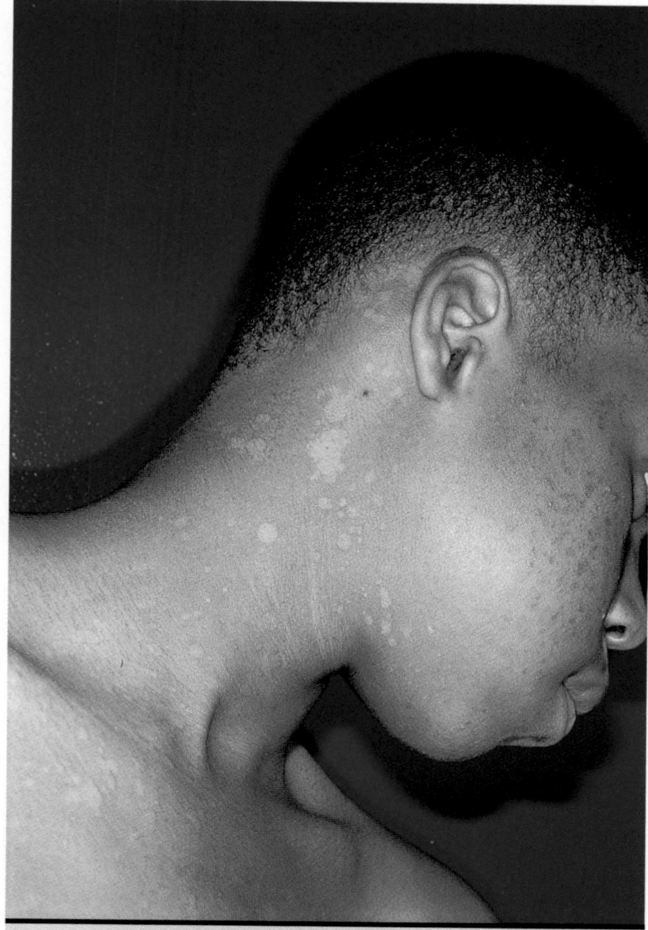

Figure 7-35. Tinea Versicolor

Numerous circular, scaly lesions on the neck and anterior chest. The lesions are slightly hypopigmented, confluent macules. This patient had liver failure from chronic active hepatitis.

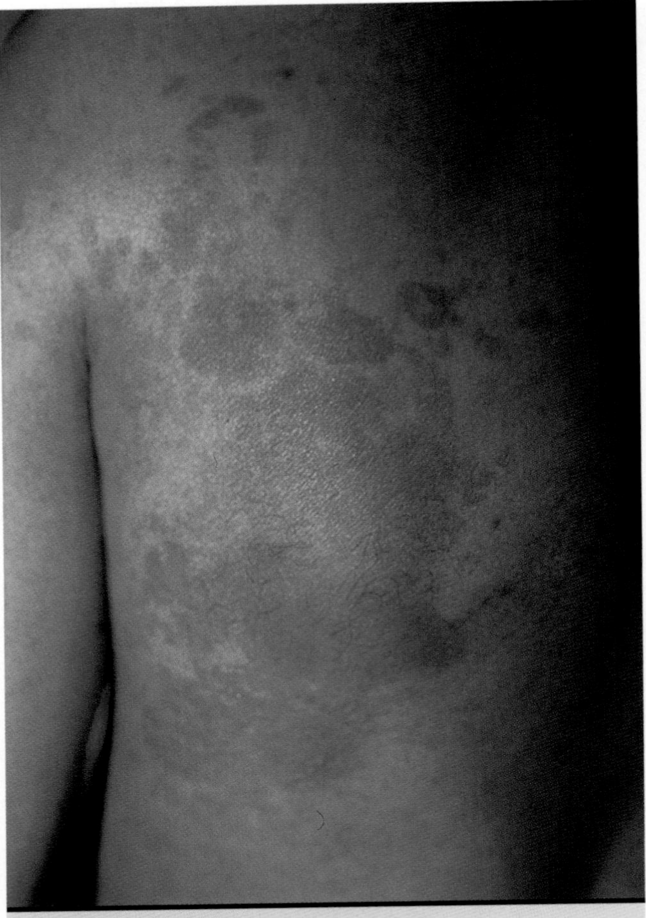

Figure 7-36. Tinea Versicolor

Lesions are hyperpigmented, confluent macules on the posterior chest. The blotchy pigmentation is what usually brings the patient to a physician.

2. Various treatment options that are given orally for either extensive disease or failure with conventional therapy or with recurrences include:
   a. Ketoconazole (dose: 200 mg once daily for 5 days; refraining from bathing for at least 12 hours after treatment allows the medication to accumulate in the skin)
   b. Itraconazole (dose: 200 mg once daily for 5 days)

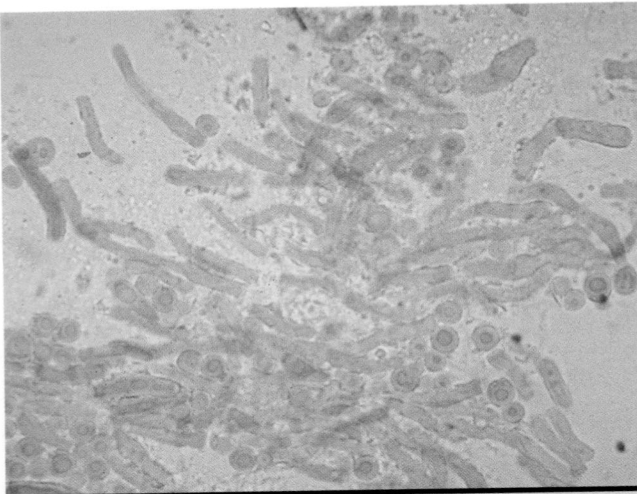

Figure 7-37. Tinea Versicolor; Potassium Hydroxide (KOH) Preparation

KOH preparation demonstrating filamentous hyphae and spores ("spaghetti-and-meatballs") appearance characteristic of tinea versicolor. (Reproduced with permission from: Mei Kane KS, Ryder JB, Jonson RA et al: Pityriasis versicolor. In: *Color Atlas & Synopsis of Pediatric Dermatology*. New York, McGraw-Hill, 2002, p. 529.)

3. Recurrence rates
   a. Vary from 15 to 60%
   b. Monthly prophylaxis with 50% propylene glycol in water, selenium shampoo, or azole creams can help prevent recurrences.

Clinical Pearls: Tinea Versicolor

1. As the name implies, lesions of tinea versicolor can be a *variety of colors* including pink, tan, or white (hypopigmented).
2. There is a high rate of recurrence in spite of adequate treatment; in fact, recurrences are considered the rule rather than the exception.
3. Warn patients that pigmentary changes may return to normal only after many months, even when the infection has been successfully treated.

BOX 7-37. CLINICAL FEATURES OF TINEA VERSICOLOR

- The rash begins insidiously and spreads over months to years.
- Multiple small, circular macules of *various colors* (white, pink, or brown) with scales
- Lesions are typically reddish-brown in white patients.
- Lesions are either hypopigmented (off-white to white or fawn) or hyperpigmented (brown) in blacks (Figs. 7-35 and 7-36).
- Color is uniform in each individual.
- *Lesions fail to tan during the summer.*
- Lesions enlarge radially and become confluent.
- Distribution of lesions is highly characteristic:
  (1) Upper chest (most common site)
  (2) Back
  (3) Shoulder
  (4) Neck
  (5) Upper arms
  (6) Abdomen
  (7) Forehead (children)
  (8) Dorsum of hands and feet
- No involvement of hair or nail plates
- Lesions usually asymptomatic
- Mild pruritus may be present in some patients
- Wood's light: pale, yellow-orange, or yellow-green fluorescence of some lesions

BOX 7-38. DIFFERENTIAL DIAGNOSIS OF TINEA VERSICOLOR

- Vitiligo
- Seborrheic dermatitis
- Postinflammatory hypopigmentation
- Pityriasis rosea
- Pityriasis alba
- Secondary syphilis
- Gutatte psoriasis
- Tinea corporis
- Nummular eczema

DIAGNOSIS TINEA CAPITIS

SYNONYM

Ringworm of the scalp

Definition

Tinea capitis is a highly contagious fungal infection of the scalp.

Etiology

1. The prevalent dermatophyte that causes this infection in the United States is *Trichophyton tonsurans*.
2. The other organisms are:
   a. *Microsporum canis*
   b. *Trichophyton violaceum*
   c. *Trichophyton verrucosum*
   d. *Microsporum audouinii*

Associated Clinical Features

1. Tinea capitis is more common among African-American children than among other racial groups (reasons unclear).
2. It occurs most commonly in areas of poverty and crowded living conditions.
3. Most common age
   a. Preschool children (2 to 6 years; most common age)
   b. Increasingly recognized in adults, infants, and neonates
4. Modes of transmission include
   a. *T. tonsurans, T. violaceum,* and *M. audouinii* are transmitted from person to person.
   b. *M. canis* and *T. verrucosum* are acquired from infected animals: cats, dogs, and cattle.
   c. Other sources of infection are inanimate objects such as combs, brushes, blankets, telephones, hats, pillowcases, and barber's shears. Asymptomatic classmates or household members also spread the infection (spores are shed in the air in the vicinity of the patient). Thus, tinea of the scalp may be contagious by direct contact or from contaminated fomites.
5. Hair loss occurs because hyphae grow within the shaft, rendering it fragile, so that the hair strands break off 1 to 2 mm above the scalp.
6. The diagnosis is usually made clinically. The following tests may help in the diagnosis:
   a. KOH preparation of a diseased hair
      1) *T. tonsurans* tinea capitis: endothrix (fungal spores are inside the hair shaft)
      2) *Microsporum* species: ectothrix (fungal spores are outside the hair shaft)
   b. Fungal culture on DTM (dermatophyte test media), Mycosel, or Sabouraud media
   c. Both KOH preparation and culture may be negative in kerion or pustular type tinea (Fig. 7-38).
   d. Consider bacterial culture in case of kerion to exclude superinfection.
   e. Wood's lamp examination
      1) *T. tonsurans* tinea capitis does not fluoresce
      2) *Microsporum* tinea (*M. canis* and *M. audouinii*): hair fluoresces with apple green or blue-green color (skin and scales do not fluoresce)

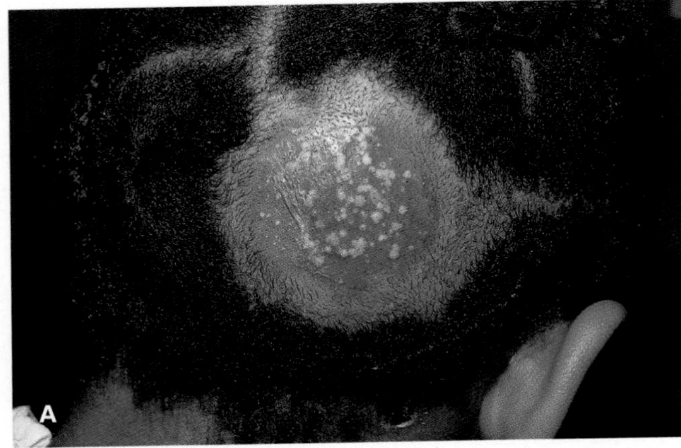

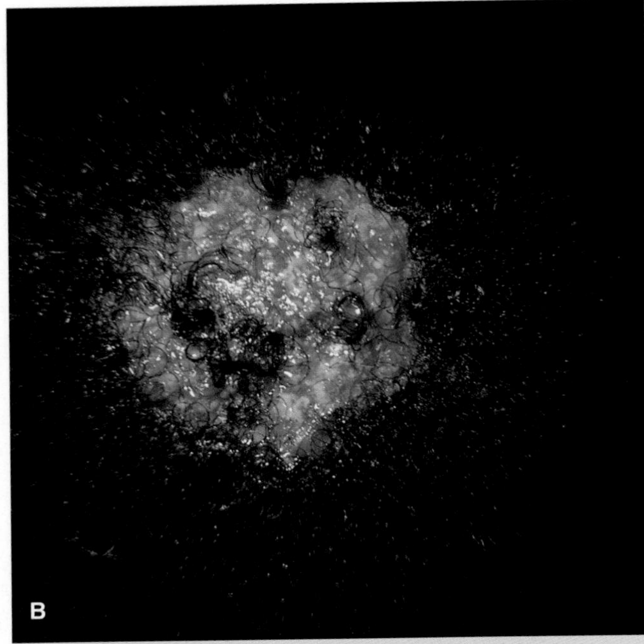

Figure 7-38. Kerion of Inflammatory Tinea Capitis

A. Indurated, boggy, painful mass with pustules on the scalp. *B.* Indurated, boggy, painful mass appearing as an abscess on the scalp.

7. Complications include lymphadenitis, bacterial pyoderma, and permanent scarring alopecia in severe untreated cases, tinea corporis and secondary bacterial infection.

Emergency Department Treatment and Disposition

1. Topical antifungal agents are ineffective and systemic therapy is required for tinea capitis.
2. Griseofulvin
    a. Dose: 15 to 20 mg/kg per day once or twice daily given with milk or a fatty meal
    b. Duration of therapy: 6 weeks minimum or 2 weeks after clinical resolution of inflammation (overall duration may vary from 6 to 12 weeks)
    c. Refractory cases may need higher doses (20 to 25 mg/kg per day).
    d. Laboratory monitoring is usually not necessary in a healthy child.
3. Newer antifungals that may be used include itraconazole, fluconazole, or terbinafine. These agents are used if the organism is resistant to griseofulvin.
4. Prednisone therapy can dramatically resolve the severe inflammation of a kerion.
    a. Dose: 1 mg/kg per day for 1 to 2 weeks
    b. If bacterial superinfection exists, oral cephalexin or dicloxacillin can be added for the first week of treatment.
5. Antifungal shampoo (e.g., selenium sulfide 2.5% or ketoconazole 2%) 2 to 3 times/week
    a. Decreasing shedding of spores decreases the spread of infection.
    b. Instruct the patient to lather the shampoo and keep it on the scalp for 5 to 10 minutes before rinsing.
6. Patients are referred to their primary care physician for reexamination in 4 weeks.
7. The patient can attend school once treatment is started. Patient should be advised to use his or her own towels, hairbrush, comb, and hats, and not to share such items with others.
8. *T. tonsurans* lesions may occur outside of the scalp in patients, their families, and their close friends. These lesions serve as a reservoir for reinfection. Therefore, advise evaluation of all siblings or close contacts in the family for tinea capitis and corporis.
9. Id reactions are treated by wet compresses and topical corticosteroids, and eradication of the primary source of infection.

Clinical Pearls: Tinea Capitis

1. Clinical variants of tinea capitis include noninflammatory, inflammatory (kerion), seborrheic, and pustular types.
2. Kerion is commonly confused with bacterial infections, the seborrheic form is commonly mistaken for dandruff, and the pustular type is commonly mistaken for bacterial infection (Figs. 7-39 and 7-40). Patients with kerion or pustular type tinea may receive several courses of antibiotics before the correct diagnosis is made.

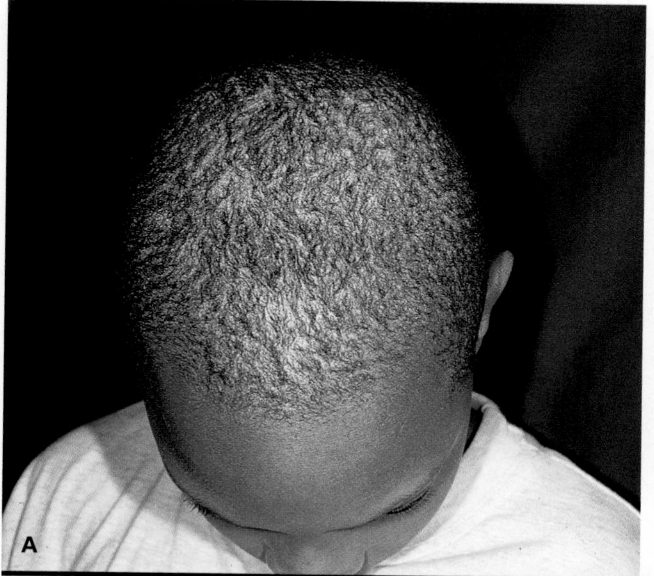

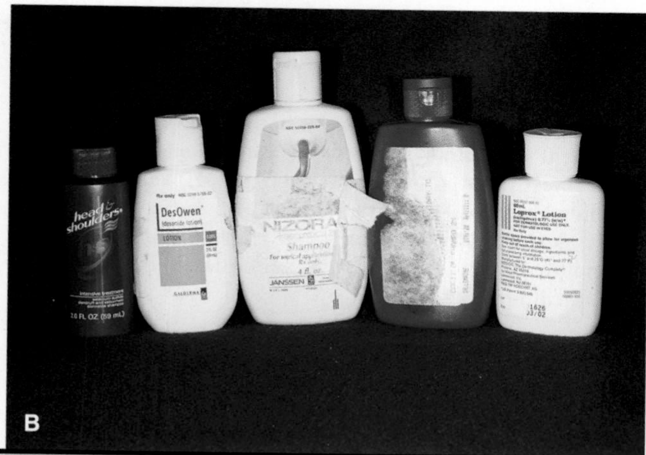

Figure 7-39. Seborrheic Tinea Capitis

A. Diffuse, fine, white adherent scaling on scalp resembling dandruff is seen in this child. Usually hair loss is minimal with this form of infection *B.* Antidandruff medications that were used to treat this child are shown. Patients with seborrheic tinea capitis are often misdiagnosed as having dandruff and often get several antidandruff medications (as shown here) prior to specific antifungal therapy.

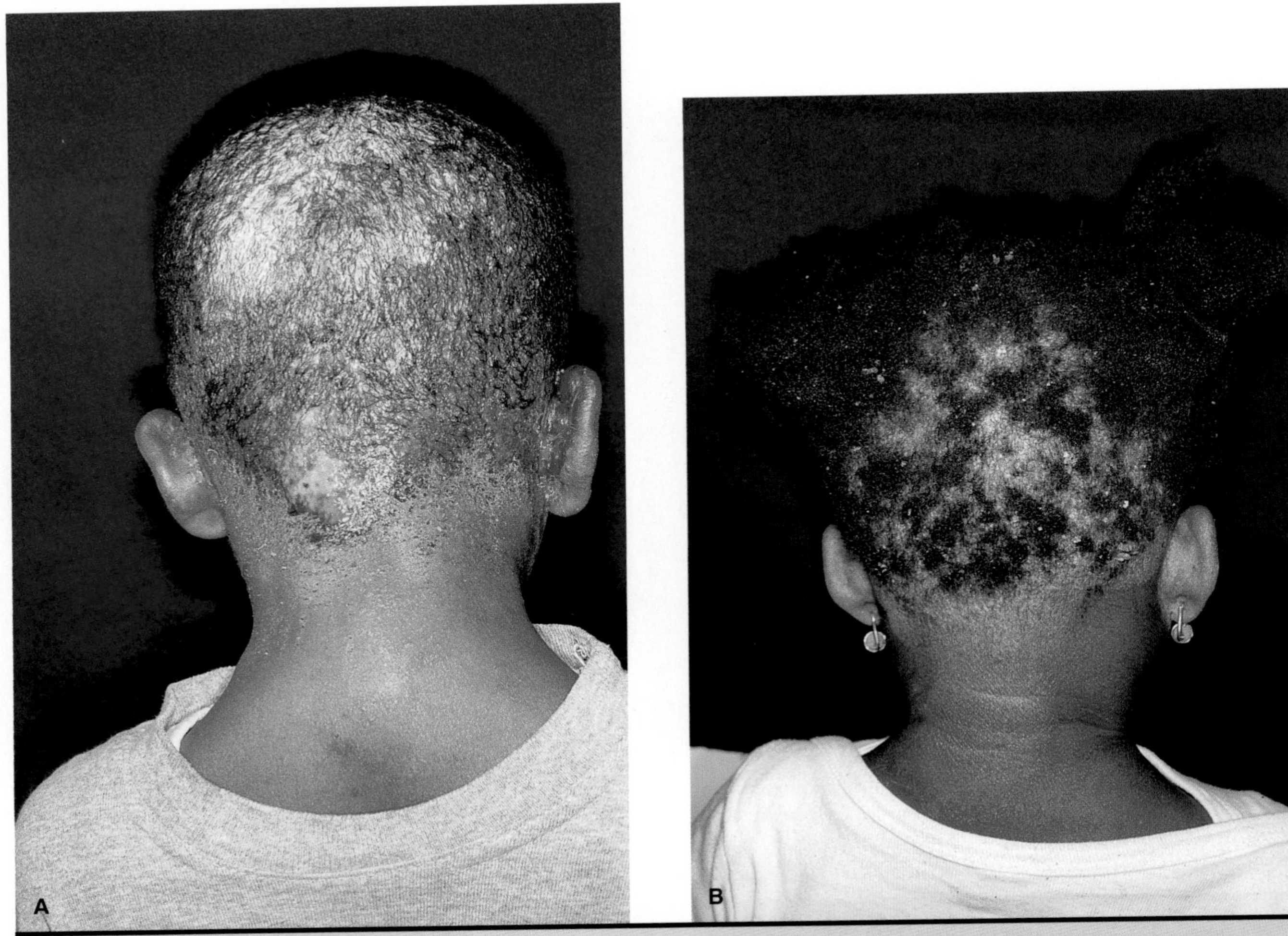

Figure 7-40. Tinea Capitis in Patients with AIDS

Extensive involvement of the scalp with scaling is seen in two different patients suffering from AIDS.

3. An intense inflammation seen in the kerion represents the patient's immune response (as suggested by a positive skin test to *Trichophyton* antigen). KOH wet mounts and fungal cultures are often negative in kerion because of the destruction of the fungal structures by inflammation, and treatment often has to be initiated based on the clinical appearance.

4. Diffuse, patchy, or discrete alopecia, scalp scaling, scalp pruritus, and lymphadenopathy (postauricular or occipital) are characteristic findings of tinea capitis.

5. Id reaction may be seen with kerion, and is commonly misdiagnosed as griseofulvin allergic reaction (the rash frequently coincides with the start of griseofulvin treatment).

BOX 7-39. CLINICAL FEATURES OF TINEA CAPITIS

- Noninflammatory tinea
  (1) Single or multiple lesions
  (2) Patchy or circular areas of hair loss
  (3) Absence of inflammation (*Trichophyton* antigen skin test negative)
  (4) Mild to moderate amount of scalp scale
  (5) "Black-dot" appearance (hairs broken off at surface of scalp; broken hairs typically <2 mm long) (Fig. 7-41)
  (6) Occipital or postauricular adenopathy (strong marker of tinea capitis)
- Inflammatory tinea

A. Kerion
  (1) Indurated, boggy, painful, single or multiple lesions
  (2) Inflammatory tumorlike mass studded with follicular pustules
  (3) Secondary regional lymphadenopathy sometimes present which represents a hypersensitivity reaction to the fungus (*Trichophyton* antigen skin test positive).
  (4) May heal with scarring and some hair loss

B. Id hypersensitivity reaction
  (1) May be seen in children with kerions
  (2) A true delayed hypersensitivity reaction (*Trichophyton* antigen skin test positive)
  (3) Presents as acute papular eruption on face, neck, trunk

- Seborrheic tinea
  (1) Diffuse or patchy, fine, white adherent scaling on scalp
  (2) *Resembles dandruff*
  (3) Minimal hair loss (less commonly patchy or diffuse hair loss)
  (4) More common among girls
  (5) Adenopathy sometimes present
- Pustular type
  (1) Discrete pustules or scabbed areas without scaling or significant hair loss
  (2) Pustules either sparse or numerous
  (3) Pustules often mistaken as bacterial infection

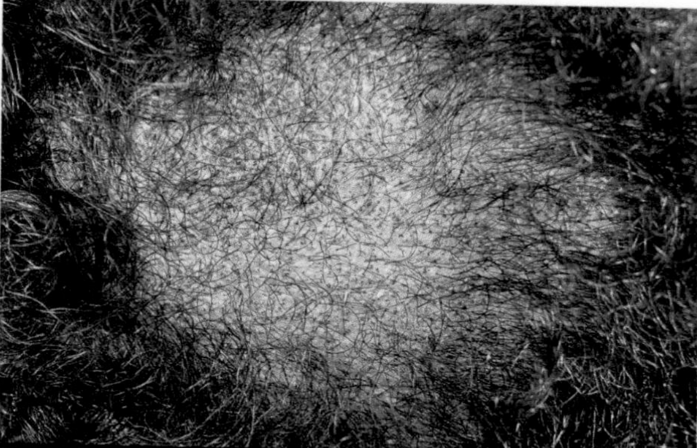

Figure 7-41. "Black-Dot" appearance of Tinea Capitis

This appearance is typically seen with infection from *Trichophyton tonsurans*. There is an area of alopecia with scale but no inflammation. Arthrospores inside the shafts of infected hairs weaken the hair and cause it to break off at or below the scalp surface, resulting in the "black dot" appearance of the surface.

BOX 7-40. DIFFERENTIAL DIAGNOSIS OF TINEA CAPITIS

- Alopecia areata (Fig. 7-42)
- Trichotillomania (hair pulling)
- Scalp furunculosis
- Psoriasis of scalp
- Seborrheic dermatitis (Fig. 7-16)
- Pityriasis rubra pilaris
- Langerhans cell histiocytosis
- Tinea amiantacea (a form of seborrheic dermatitis seen in children; a localized patch of large, brown, polygonal-shaped scales that adheres to the scalp and mats the hair with little or no inflammation)

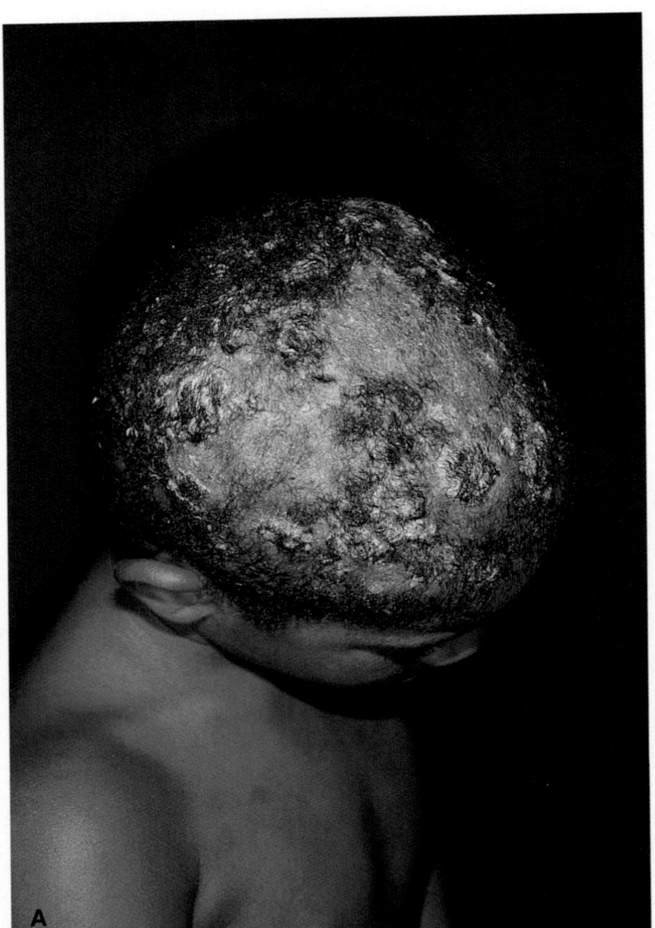

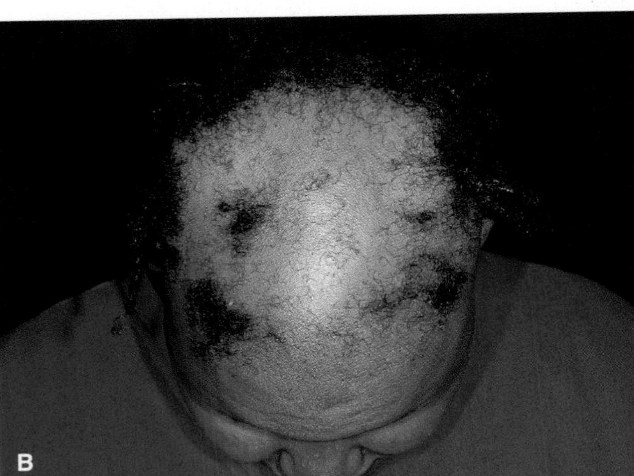

Figure 7-42. Differential Diagnosis: Tinea Capitis versus Alopecia Areata

Signs of inflammation (e.g., "black-dot" appearance, scaling, or pustules) are seen in tinea (*A*), while smooth, nonscarring areas of hair loss on the scalp without any signs of inflammation are seen in alopecia areata (*B*). The presence of lymphadenopathy (e.g., postoccipital) is a strong marker of *T. capitis*.

DIAGNOSIS

TINEA CORPORIS

Synonyms

Ringworm (of smooth or glabrous skin or ringworm of body)
Tinea corporis gladiatorum
Tinea circinata

Definition

1. Tinea corporis is a dermatophyte infection of the body involving the face (excluding the beard area in men), trunk (excluding the groin), or extremities (excluding palms and soles).
2. As the name ringworm implies, it is an annular lesion that spreads peripherally with an active papulovesicular border while clearing in the center (Figs. 7-43 and 7-44).

Etiology

1. *Trichophyton* species (*T. mentagrophytes, T. rubrum*)
2. *Microsporum* species (*M. canis, M. audouinii*)
3. *Epidermophyton floccosum*

Associated Clinical Features

1. Tinea corporis is seen in all age groups.
2. It may be present concurrently with tinea capitis.
3. It is more common in warm climates.
4. Infection is transmitted by infected scales from skin lesions of an infected person or contact with infected scales or hairs deposited on environmental surfaces. *M. canis* infections are usually acquired from infected pets (especially kittens and puppies).
5. Tinea from cats may appear suddenly as multiple round-to-oval plaques on the trunk and extremities.
6. Treatment with topical steroids (when mistaken for nummular eczema) suppresses inflammation but not infection and this entity is referred to as tinea incognito.
7. The diagnosis is made clinically and usually no tests are required.
8. Tests that help in arriving at the diagnosis in doubtful cases:
    a. Direct microscopic examination with KOH preparation from the scales of the advancing border demonstrates hyphae, budding yeasts, or arthrospores
    b. Fungal culture of skin scrapings from the affected area and inoculated on DTM (dermatophyte test media), Mycosel, or Sabouraud media identifies the specific dermatophyte.

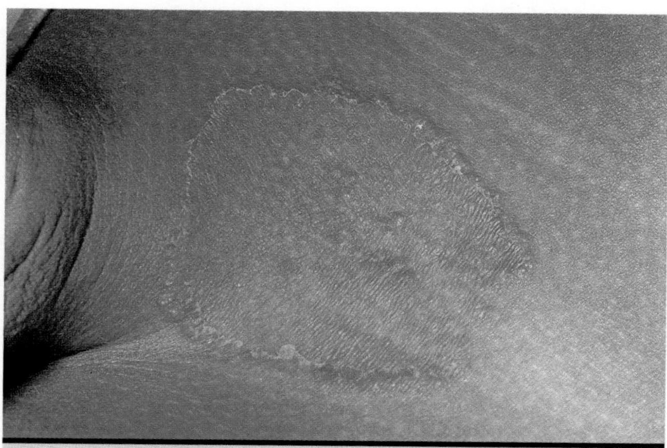

Figure 7-43. Tinea Corporis

As the name "ringworm" implies, the lesion is an annular lesion which spreads at the periphery with an active, erythematous, scaly, advancing border with a clearing in the center.

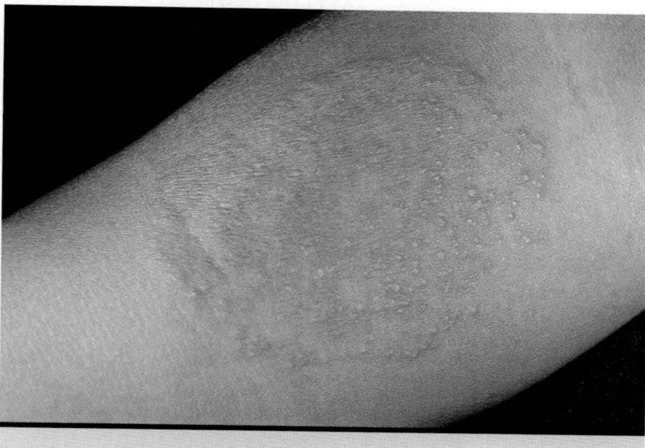

Figure 7-44. Tinea Corporis

A ring within a ring (one or two rings within a larger ring) may be seen.

Emergency Department Treatment and Disposition

1. Topical antifungals are effective for treatment:
    a. Apply twice daily for 10 to 14 days (or until lesions clear).
    b. Apply topically at least 2 cm beyond the advancing edge of the skin lesion.
    c. Continue topical application for 1 more week after clearing to ensure clinical cure.

d. Examples of topical antifungals:
   1) *Imidazoles:* clotrimazole (Mycelex, Lotrimin), miconazole (Micatin), ketoconazole (Nizoral), econazole (Spectazole)
   2) *Allylamines:* terbinafine (Lamisil), naftifine (Naftin)
   3) *Naphthiomates:* tolnaftate (Tinactin)

2. For extensive tinea corporis: Griseofulvin given orally with food (dose: 15 to 20 mg/kg per day for 1 week)

Clinical Pearls: Tinea Corporis

Tinea corporis consists of a scaly annular lesion with an active advancing border and a clearing in the center.

BOX 7-41. CLINICAL FEATURES OF TINEA CORPORIS

- Skin lesions
  (1) Solitary or multiple lesions
  (2) Varying size (1 to 10 cm)
  (3) Annular configuration
  (4) Active, scaly, raised, erythematous, papulovesicular border with central clearing
  (5) Central area becomes brown or hypopigmented and less scaly and inflamed as the active border progresses outward.
  (6) Some red papules may be seen in the central area.
  (7) Sharply marginated lesion with a distinct border
  (8) One or two rings within a larger ring may be seen.
  (9) *Does not* fluoresce with Wood's lamp
- Location (any exposed area, excluding palms, soles, and the beard area in men)
  (1) Body (tinea corporis)
  (2) Face (tinea faciei)
  (3) Extremities

BOX 7-42. DIFFERENTIAL DIAGNOSIS OF TINEA CORPORIS

- Herald patch of pityriasis rosea (see Fig. 7-30).
- Nummular eczema
- Granuloma annulare
- Contact dermatitis
- Psoriasis
- Seborrhea
- Erythema chronicum migrans
- Tinea versicolor
- Systemic lupus erythematosus

DIAGNOSIS

TINEA CRURIS

SYNONYMS

Jock itch
Tinea of the groin

Definition

Tinea cruris is a fungal infection of the groin and upper thigh.

Etiology

1. *Epidermophyton floccosum*
2. *Trichophyton rubrum* or *T. mentagrophytes*

Associated Clinical Features

1. It is commonly seen in adolescents, young adults, and athletes. It is rarely seen in children.
2. Men are affected much more frequently than women.
3. Predisposing factors include
   a. Concomitant tinea pedis
   b. Summer months: warm humid environment, sweating, tight (exercise outfits) or wet clothing (bathing suits) that often serve as an occlusive dressing
   c. Winter months: wearing several layers of clothing
   d. Obesity
4. The diagnosis is made clinically.
5. Tests that help in arriving at the diagnosis in doubtful cases:
   a. Direct microscopic examination with KOH preparation from the scales of the advancing border demonstrates hyphae, budding yeasts, or arthrospores.
   b. Fungal culture of skin scrapings from the affected area and inoculated on DTM (dermatophyte test media), Mycosel, or Sabouraud media identifies the specific dermatophyte.

Emergency Department Treatment and Disposition

1. Topical antifungal therapy (see page 329 for preparations)
   a. Imidazole cream twice daily for 2 to 4 weeks
   b. Do not use antifungal preparations combined with high-potency topical steroids.
2. For severe cases, consider use of a short course of griseofulvin.
3. Other measures that help include
   a. Wearing loose-fitting underwear
   b. Use of antifungal foot powder
   c. Treat tinea pedis simultaneously if present.
   d. Instruct patients to put on socks first *before* their underwear in order to avoid carrying the fungal elements from the infected feet up to the groin area.

Clinical Pearls: Tinea Cruris

1. Tinea cruris and tinea pedis are commonly seen together in the same patient.
2. Typically tinea pedis precedes the groin infection (due to spread of infection from the infected feet to the groin).
3. Tinea incognito (modified form of tinea) may not be recognized as tinea; the only clue may be a history of a typical, half moon–shaped plaque treated with cortisone cream (Fig. 7-45).

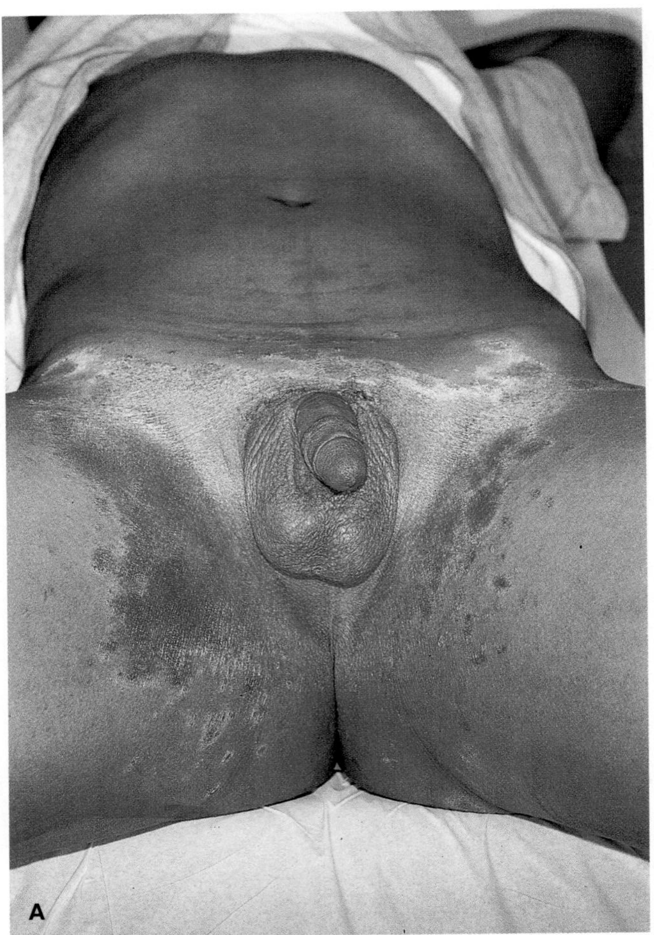

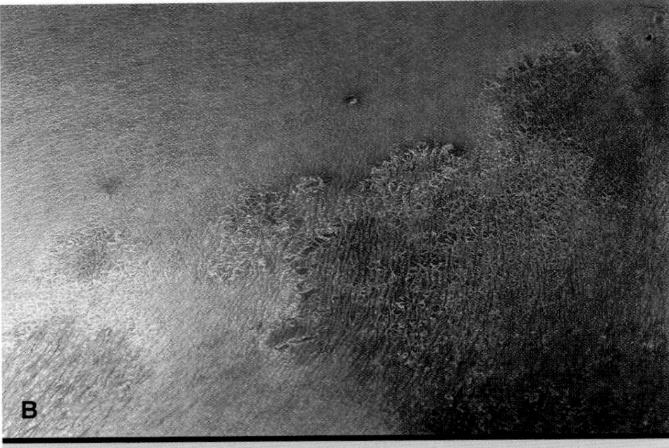

Figure 7-45. Tinea Corporis

A. Bilateral, irregular, half moon-shaped, sharply bordered patches with hyperpigmented, scaly centers are seen. Note the absence of involvement of the scrotum or penis (an important distinction from candidiasis). *B*. Close-up showing a well-defined advancing border with scaling. KOH preparation of the scale was positive for numerous hyphae.

BOX 7-43. CLINICAL FEATURES OF TINEA CRURIS

- Skin lesion
  (1) Erythema
  (2) Pruritus
  (3) Well-demarcated plaques with papules (occasional pustules or vesicles)
  (4) Lesion with active borders with well defined scaling and central clearing
  (5) Skin within border red-brown with papules
  (6) Does not fluoresce under Wood's light
- Location
  (1) Begins in crural folds, then advances on to the thigh, forming half moon-shaped plaques
  (2) Bilateral irregular plaques on upper thighs
  (3) May extend to buttock and gluteal cleft
  (4) No involvement of scrotum or penis (as opposed to candidiasis)
  (5) No satellite pustules beyond free margin of rash (as opposed to candidiasis)
- Tinea incognito
  (1) Modified form of tinea from prior use of topical steroid creams
  (2) Modified appearance (e.g., very extensive rash instead of a half moon-shaped plaque, lack of advancing, scaly border)

BOX 7-44. DIFFERENTIAL DIAGNOSIS OF TINEA CRURIS

- Intertrigo/candidiasis (Fig. 7-46)
  (1) *Involvement of scrotum or labia*
  (2) Satellite pustules beyond margin of rash
- Psoriasis
  (1) Rash with vivid red color and uniform scaling
  (2) Presence of typical psoriatic plaques at other sites
- Erythrasma
  (1) Noninflammatory lesion
  (2) Uniformly brown and scaly (no advancing edge like tinea cruris)
  (3) Fluoresces pink or coral-red under Wood's light
  (4) Rash covered with fine wrinkles
- Seborrheic dermatitis
- Allergic contact dermatitis

Clinical pearl:

Erythrasma or candidiasis may coexist with tinea cruris.

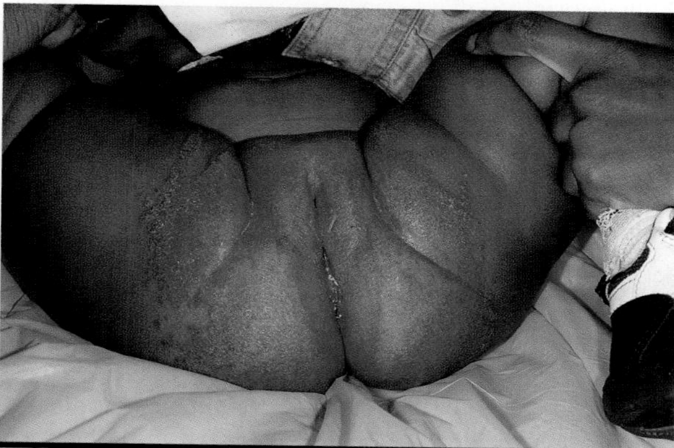

Figure 7-46. Intertrigo; Differential Diagnosis of Tinea Cruris

A red, half moon-shaped plaque, resembling tinea of the groin and extending to the groin and down the thigh, forms after moisture accumulates in the crural fold. The sharp borders touch where the opposed surfaces of the skin folds of the groin and thigh meet. Obesity contributes to this inflammatory process, which may be infected with a mixed flora of bacteria, fungi, and yeast. Groin intertrigo recurs after treatment unless weight and moisture are controlled.

DIAGNOSIS

TINEA PEDIS

Synonyms

Athlete's foot
Ringworm of the feet

Definition

Tinea pedis is a fungal infection of the feet.

Etiology

1. *Trichophyton rubrum*
2. *T. mentagrophytes* (interdigitale)
3. *Epidermophyton floccosum*

Associated Clinical Features

1. Tinea pedis is more common in adolescents and young adults and uncommon in young children.
2. Infection is acquired by contact with skin scales containing fungi or with fungi in damp areas (e.g., swimming pools, locker room floors, communal baths).
3. Infection in one family member tends to spread throughout the household (e.g., infection may occur in children whose parents are infected).
4. Communicability persists as long as the infection is present. Once infection is established, the individual becomes a carrier and is more susceptible to recurrences.
5. Predisposing factors include hot, humid weather (summer months) and occlusive footwear.
6. Infection may be associated with id reaction (erythematous papulovesicular eruption on legs and trunk, and vesicular eruptions on palms and sides of fingers).
7. Secondary bacterial infection may occur, as macerated skin serves as portal of entry for the bacteria.
8. The diagnosis is usually made clinically.

9. A potassium hydroxide wet mount demonstrates fungal elements and helps in differentiating tinea pedis from other conditions. Skin scrapings inoculated on fungal culture (e.g., dermatophyte test media) can also help in confirming the diagnosis.

Emergency Department Treatment and Disposition

1. Tinea pedis runs a chronic course. Exacerbations occur with hot, humid weather or with exercise.
2. General instructions for treatment and to prevent recurrences:
   a. Improve foot hygiene (keeping feet cool and dry, especially between toes; frequent airing of affected areas)
   b. Use absorbent antifungal foot powder on the feet.
   c. Avoid occlusive footwear (shoes promote warmth and sweating which encourage fungal growth) and wear wider shoes.
   d. Use cotton socks (avoid nylon or other fabric that interferes with dissipation of moisture) and change wet socks as soon as possible.
   e. Dry groin area before drying feet to avoid inoculating fungal scales into the groin.
3. Topical application of antifungal preparation
   a. Few examples: miconazole, haloprogin, clotrimazole, or terbinafine applied bid, or econazole, ketoconazole, or naftifine once a day
   b. Duration of treatment: 2 to 3 weeks
4. For hyperkeratotic diffuse involvement of soles
   a. Terbinafine given orally for 2 to 6 weeks
   b. Griseofulvin given orally for 6 to 8 weeks
5. Acute vesicular tinea pedis
   a. Burow's solution–soaked wet compresses applied for 30 minutes several times a day
   b. Griseofulvin given orally for 6 to 8 weeks
   c. Topical antifungal agents (as mentioned above) once macerated tissue is dried
   d. Antibiotics for secondary bacterial infection (Fig. 7-47)
   e. Treatment of id reaction includes wet dressings and low-potency topical steroids (rarely, a short course of prednisone therapy)
6. Inquire about other family members with a similar rash and recommend treatment of all infected family members.
7. Advise patients with active infection not to go to swimming pools to avoid spread of the infection.
8. Treat tinea cruris simultaneously, if present.
9. Consider and treat toenail involvement (onychomycosis; see page 337) when treating tinea pedis. Toenail infection can serve as a reservoir for the reinfection of the rest of the foot.

Clinical Pearls: Tinea Pedis

1. Tinea pedis is the most common fungal infection in adolescents and adults.
2. Tinea pedis is uncommon in children and most cases are actually eczema or contact or shoe dermatitis. Nonetheless, tinea pedis should be considered in the differential diagnosis of foot dermatitis in children.
3. Tinea pedis commonly occurs in association with tinea cruris.
4. Tinea pedis begins as interdigital scaling and fissuring and spreads to involve the plantar aspects of both feet (Fig. 7-48).

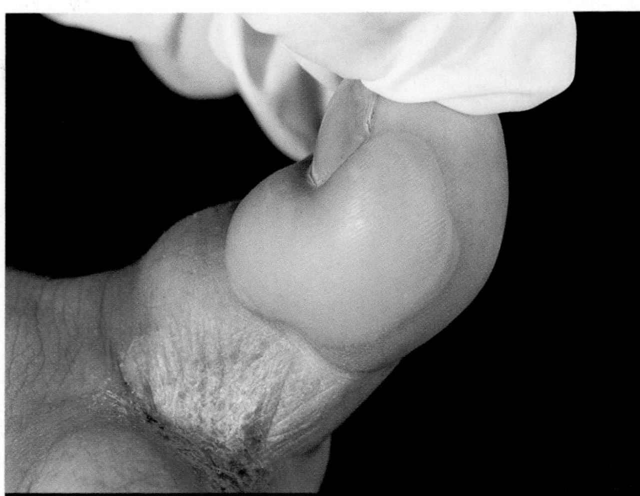

Figure 7-47. Tinea Pedis with Secondary Bacterial Infection

The toe web space with macerated scale is seen with a bullous impetigo secondary to *S. aureus* infection.

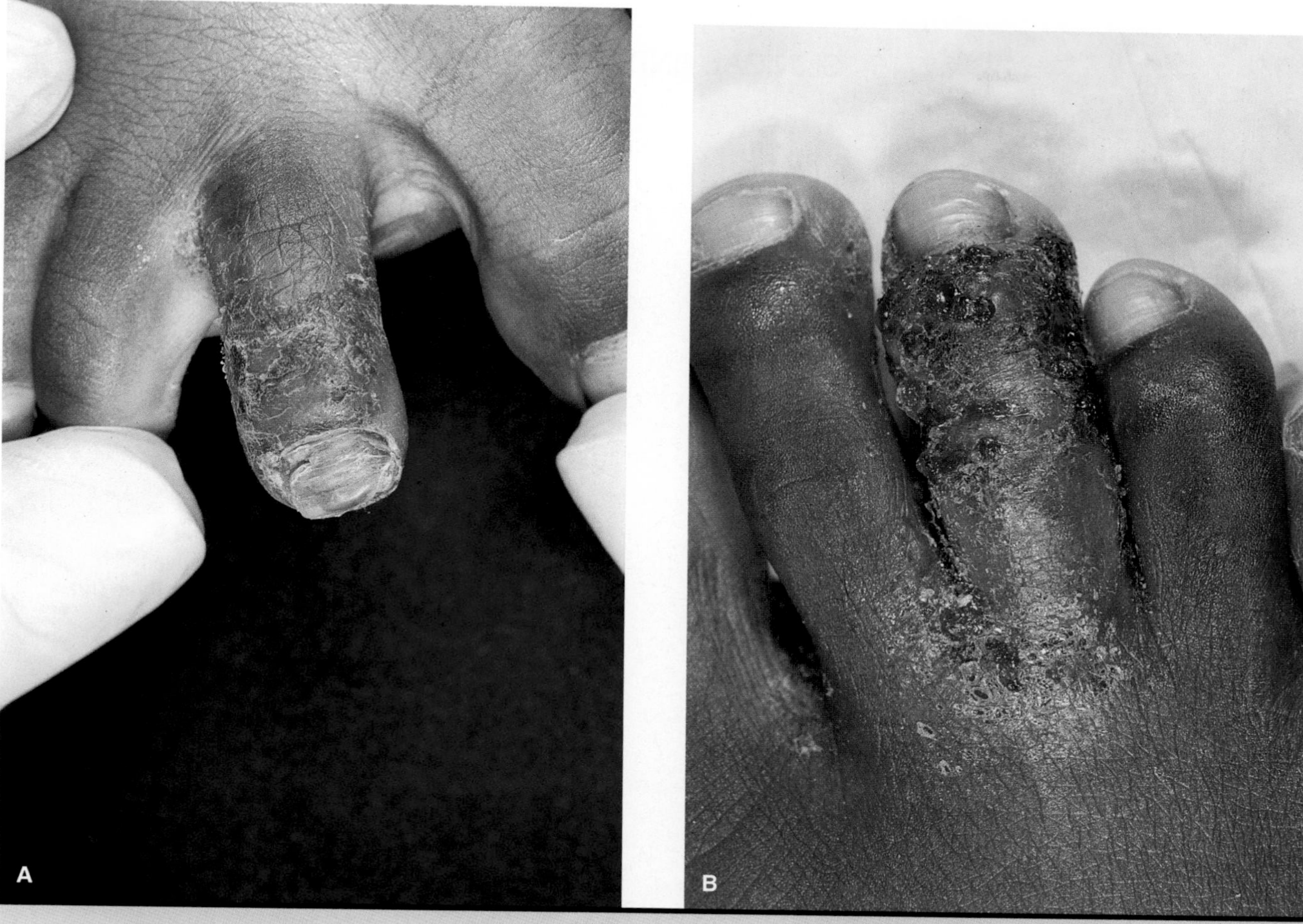

Figure 7-48. Tinea Pedis

The toe web space with macerated scale and inflammation that has extended from the web area onto the dorsum of the foot is seen in two different patients.

BOX 7-45. CLINICAL FINDINGS OF TINEA PEDIS

- Incubation period: unknown
- Skin lesions

A. *Interdigital infection (toe web infection)*
   (1) Foul odor
   (2) Pruritus
   (3) Dry and fissuring webs with white scaling, or white webs that are macerated and soggy
   (4) Fissuring on the plantar surface of foot

B. *Vesicular/pustular form (inflammatory)*
   (1) Least common type (severity resembles allergic contact dermatitis)
   (2) Usually originates from a chronic web infection
   (3) Rapid, acute development of vesicles on the sole or dorsum of the foot
   (4) Papules, then vesicles, then bullae, then pustules
   (5) Secondary bacterial infection (in eroded areas after bullae rupture)
   (6) May have associated *dermatophytid* or *id reaction*

C. *Chronic diffuse hyperkeratosis of sole ("moccasin-type" or "dry-type" tinea)*
   (1) Usually infection of the entire sole
   (2) Sole covered with fine, silvery white scales
   (3) Scaling more prominent along lateral borders of the sole
   (4) Skin of the sole pink and tender
   (5) Pruritus
   (6) Similar involvement of hands
   (7) Usually two feet and one hand involvement

- Sites
   (1) Web space (most common between the third, fourth, and fifth toes, but all webs may be infected)
   (2) Plantar aspects of both feet
   (3) Lesions usually patchy in distribution
   (4) Involvement of the entire sole (severe cases)
   (5) Rarely involves the dorsum of the foot
   (6) Rarely one or two palms may be involved
   (7) Associated infection of groin and upper thigh (tinea cruris)
   (8) May have associated infection of the toenails (tinea unguium)

BOX 7-46. DIFFERENTIAL DIAGNOSIS OF TINEA PEDIS

- Contact dermatitis or shoe dermatitis
- Atopic dermatitis
- Dyshidrotic eczema
- Juvenile plantar dermatosis ("wet foot, dry foot" syndrome or soggy sock dermatitis)
- Infection with *Candida albicans*
- Erythrasma
   (1) Bacterial infection caused by *Corynebacterium minutissimum*
   (2) Same appearance as interdigital tinea pedis
   (3) Wood's light shows a bright coral-red color

chemical or physical destruction of the infected epithelium and include any of the following:

a. Topical application of salicylic acid, as solution, patches, or plasters (e.g., Duofilm, Compound W, Mediplast, Occlusal-HP)
   1) Soak wart in warm water for 5 minutes, remove loose tissue, and dry.
   2) Apply a thin layer (avoiding normal skin) once or twice daily; allow to dry and apply a bandage.
   3) Therapy may be required for up to 12 weeks.
b. Cryotherapy with liquid nitrogen (5 to 10 seconds of liquid nitrogen applied to each wart with a cotton swab or cryotherapy gun)
c. Daily treatment with tretinoin gel or cream (applied nightly and washed off in the morning) for several weeks for widespread flat warts
d. Curettage with local anesthesia
e. Laser surgery

4. Oral cimetidine at moderately high doses (25 to 40 mg/kg per day for 2 to 3 months) has been used for treatment of refractory warts (the efficacy of cimetidine has not been established in controlled clinical trials).
5. For treatment of condyloma acuminata, see page 171.
6. Refer patients with warts on the face, periungual warts, large plantar warts, or warts resistant to conservative therapy to a dermatologist for other therapeutic considerations (e.g., cryotherapy or electrodesiccation or curettage).

Clinical Pearls: Warts

1. Cutaneous warts are benign infections of the skin and are self-limiting in a majority of cases.
2. Common warts occur most frequently in children and adolescents. Anogenital warts are most common in young sexually active patients.
3. Genital warts are the most common viral sexually transmitted disease in the United States.
4. Warts will often resolve spontaneously without treatment and watchful waiting may be done in asymptomatic patients (about two-thirds of warts disappear spontaneously within 2 years); however, failure to treat incurs a risk of spread to other sites.

BOX 7-49. CLINICAL FEATURES OF WARTS

- *Common wart (verruca vulgaris)*
  (1) Begins as flesh-colored single or multiple papules
  (2) Lesions evolve into dome-shaped, gray-brown growths with a roughened surface.
  (3) Black dots (thrombosed capillaries) may be seen on the surface.
  (4) Usually asymptomatic
  (5) Most common location: dorsal surface of hands, fingers
  (6) Can occur on any skin surface (e.g., paronychial areas, face, knees, elbows)
- *Flat wart ("juvenile wart" or verruca plana)*
  (1) Seen in children and adolescents
  (2) Common on the face (forehead, around mouth, and beard area in men), back of hands, neck
  (3) Soft, grouped, flat-topped papules
  (4) Flesh-colored to light brown-yellow
  (5) Contiguous lesions become confluent and form plaques.
  (6) Distribution of several lesions along a line of cutaneous trauma (important diagnostic clue)
- *Plantar wart (verruca plantaris)*
  (1) Seen on weight-bearing areas of the soles
  (2) Grows inward into the sole of the foot (with pressure of walking)
  (3) Painful
  (4) Flat, marked hyperkeratosis with black dots on the surface
  (5) Lesions may coalesce into a single plaque (mosaic wart)
- *Palmar wart*
  (1) Seen on palms
  (2) Sharply demarcated
  (3) Often with a ring of thick callus
- *Periungual wart*
  (1) Lesions around nail
  (2) History of nail biting
  (3) Often painful
  (4) May spread beneath the nail plate, separating it from the nailbed
- *Mucous membrane warts (Condylomata acuminata; see Figs. 4-1 and 4-2)*
  (1) Moist, fleshy, papillomatous lesions
  (2) Sites: perianal mucosa, labia, vaginal introitus, perineal raphe, penile shaft, corona, glans penis, lips, gingivae, tongue, conjunctivae
  (3) Condylomata (if untreated) may proliferate and become confluent, forming large cauliflower-like masses

BOX 7-50. DIFFERENTIAL DIAGNOSIS OF WARTS

- Molluscum contagiosum (differential diagnosis of common warts)
- Skin tags
- Differential diagnosis of plantar or palmar warts
  (1) Calluses
  (2) Corns
  (3) Punctate keratoses
  (4) Black heel
- Differential diagnosis of juvenile flat warts
  (1) Lichen planus
  (2) Lichen nitidus
  (3) Angiofibromas
  (4) Syringomas
  (5) Milia
  (6) Acne
- Condylomata lata (differential diagnosis of condylomata acuminata)
- Periungual fibroma of tuberous sclerosis (differential diagnosis of periungual warts)
- Epidermal nevi
- Varicella zoster virus in patients with AIDS
- Recurrent infantile digital fibroma
- Squamous cell carcinoma

DIAGNOSIS MOLLUSCUM CONTAGIOSUM

Definition/Etiology

Molluscum contagiosum is viral infection of the skin caused by the poxvirus molluscum contagiosum virus, and is characterized by discrete pearly white papules that are umbilicated (Fig. 7-53).

Associated Clinical Features

1. Molluscum contagiosum is more common in children and usually presents between the ages of 3 and 16 years. Swimming pools and bathing together are predisposing conditions for the development of molluscum contagiosum.
2. Humans are the only known source of the virus. The disease is acquired by direct contact with an infected person or from fomites (e.g., towels) and is spread by autoinoculation.
3. Predisposing conditions for disseminated lesions
   a. Children with atopic dermatitis (widespread involvement in areas of dermatitis)
   b. Human immunodeficiency virus (HIV) infection
   c. Other immunodeficiency states including leukemia
4. Unilateral conjunctivitis may develop with lesions located on or near the eyelids. Rarely, lesions may appear on the conjunctiva or cornea.
5. The diagnosis is usually made clinically.
6. If the diagnosis is in doubt, a papule can be removed and crushed between two microscope slides. Wright or Giemsa staining of the expressed material reveals characteristic intracytoplasmic inclusions. Skin biopsy reveals epithelial cells with large intracytoplasmic inclusions (molluscum bodies).

Emergency Department Treatment and Disposition

1. Molluscum contagiosum is a self-limited disease with an average duration of lesions lasting about 6 to 9 months.

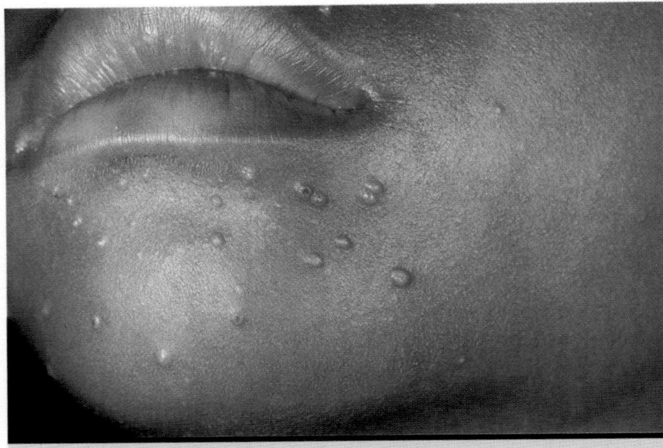

Figure 7-53. Molluscum Contagiosum

Mulitiple, dome-shaped papules with some lesions with central umbilication (umbilication from which a plug of cheesy material can be expressed) are seen in a child with AIDS.

However, lesions can persist for years, can spread to distant sites, and may be transmitted to others. Enlarging or spreading lesions are treated and genital lesions should be definitively treated to prevent spread through sexual contact.

2. Treatment depends on the number and size of lesions, age of the patient, and availability of treatment methods. Any of the following may be used (conservative nonscarring methods should be used for children who have many lesions):
   a. Conservative (e.g., no treatment for lesions around the eye)
   b. Mechanical removal of the central core of each lesion with a needle, a sharp curette, or a comedo extractor (lesions involute faster after they are irritated)
   c. Small papules can be removed with a curette with or without local anesthesia (EMLA cream applied 30 to 60 minutes before treatment effectively prevents pain of curettage). This technique in not chosen for cosmetically significant areas, as scar tissue may form.
   d. Salicylic acid applied each day without tape occlusion may cause irritation and encourage resolution.
   e. Tretinoin gel or cream applied once or twice daily to individual small lesions (weeks or months of treatment may be required)
   f. Cantharone (blistering beetle extract) applied to each lesion without occlusion and washed off after 2 to 6 hours (results in inflammation to facilitate spontaneous extrusion of the plug)
3. Patient can be referred to a dermatologist for other therapeutic modalities that include manual curettage of large lesions, cryotherapy with liquid nitrogen, electrocautery, or carbon dioxide laser therapy.
4. Advise affected patients to avoid shared baths and towels until the infection is clear.

Clinical Pearls: Molluscum Contagiosum

1. Molluscum lesions are benign and self-limited.
2. Patients with eczema and HIV infection tend to develop widespread eruptions.
3. Although lesions can regress spontaneously, treatment may prevent autoinoculation and spread to other persons.
4. Molluscum lesions may be associated with other venereal diseases in sexually active individuals.
5. Molluscum lesions are often misdiagnosed as warts or herpes simplex virus lesions.
6. Genital molluscum contagiosum in children may be a manifestation of sexual abuse.

BOX 7-51. CLINICAL FEATURES OF MOLLUSCUM CONTAGIOSUM

- Incubation period: 2 to 7 weeks (may be as long as 6 months)
- Absence of systemic manifestations
- Skin lesions
  (1) Usually asymptomatic nonpruritic papules
  (2) Size: 2 to 5 mm in size
  (3) Central umbilication in some lesions (absent in small lesions)
  (4) Umbilication often appears to contain tiny keratin plugs
  (5) Umbilication from which a plug of cheesy material can be expressed
  (6) Firm papules with a smooth surface (unlike irregular and velvety surface of warts)
  (7) Multiple (usual 2 to 20 lesions)
  (8) Lesions discrete or in small clusters
  (9) Round or oval dome-shaped papules
  (10) Flesh-colored to pearly white (waxy) papules
  (11) Erythema and scaling at the periphery of the papule
  (12) Papules may appear inflamed or secondarily infected during spontaneous involution
- Most common sites: face, eyelids, neck, axillae, trunk, thigh (lesions may appear anywhere except palms and soles)
- Other sites: genitals (vulva, labia majora, penile shaft, glans, buttocks [autoinoculation or from close sexual or nonsexual contact])
- Molluscum contagiosum in HIV-infected patients
  (1) Generalized distribution
  (2) Atypical facial lesions (either multiple small papules or giant nodular tumors)

BOX 7-52. DIFFERENTIAL DIAGNOSIS OF MOLLUSCUM CONTAGIOSUM

- Nevi
- Acne
- Milia
- Warts (see Figs. 7-50 to 7-52)
- Herpes simplex lesions
- Other infections in HIV patients (e.g., disseminated cryptococcosis, histoplasmosis, coccidioidomycosis)
- Basal cell carcinoma (adults)

DIAGNOSIS HEMANGIOMA

Definition and Etiology

Hemangiomas are benign, vascular hamartomas consisting of dilated vessels in the dermis surrounded by masses of proliferating endothelial cells. Superficial hemangiomas have a bright red appearance and are called strawberry hemangiomas (Fig. 7-54). Deeper purple lesions are referred to as cavernous hemangiomas.

Associated Clinical Features

1. Hemangiomas are more common in premature infants, and three to four times more common in girls than in boys.
2. Hemangiomas may occur as isolated tumors or be associated with syndromes:
   a. Diffuse neonatal hemangiomatosis (hemangiomas of GI tract, liver, CNS, and lungs)
   b. PHACE syndrome (*p*osterior fossa malformations [Dandy-Walker malformation], large facial *h*emangiomas, *a*rterial anomalies [aneurysmal carotid dilation, aplasia or hypoplastic carotid arteries], *c*ardiac defects [coarctation of the aorta], and *e*ye abnormalities [glaucoma, cataracts, microphthalmia, and optic nerve hypoplasia])
   c. Klippel-Trenaunay-Weber syndrome (port-wine stain, varicose veins, and hemangiomas over a limb associated with limb hypertrophy)
3. Hemangiomas with special regional involvement:
   a. Hemangiomas in beard distribution (mandibular region, lips, chin, neck): patients are at risk for airway involvement (e.g., associated hemangiomas in the subglottic region)
   b. Midline hemangiomas in the lumbosacral region: associated spinal malformations, tethered cord, and anomalies of the anorectal and urogenital regions
   c. A hemangioma around the urethra may interfere with urination.
4. Hemangiomas are diagnosed clinically.
5. CBC with platelet count and coagulation profile are done in very rapidly enlarging cavernous hemangiomas leading to Kasabach-Merritt syndrome.
6. Ultrasonography, MRI, or CT scan helps in differentiating hemangiomas from other vascular malformations and neoplastic diseases. Patients with large facial hemangiomas also need neuroimaging (CT or MRI) to exclude posterior fossa vascular malformations (see PHACE syndrome, above). These imaging techniques also help in evaluation for possible visceral involvement in a patient with numerous cutaneous hemangiomas.
7. Complications of hemangioma include:
   a. Ulceration (hemangioma in an area of friction) (Fig. 7-55)
   b. Secondary infection (ulcerated hemangioma); superinfection can lead to cellulitis, osteomyelitis, or septicemia
   c. Compromise of a vital function (e.g., a periorbital hemangioma may cause amblyopia from obstruction of the visual axis or astigmatism from compression of the globe or by extension into the retrobulbar space)
   d. High-output congestive heart failure (CHF; e.g., diffuse hemangiomatosis with hepatic lesions)

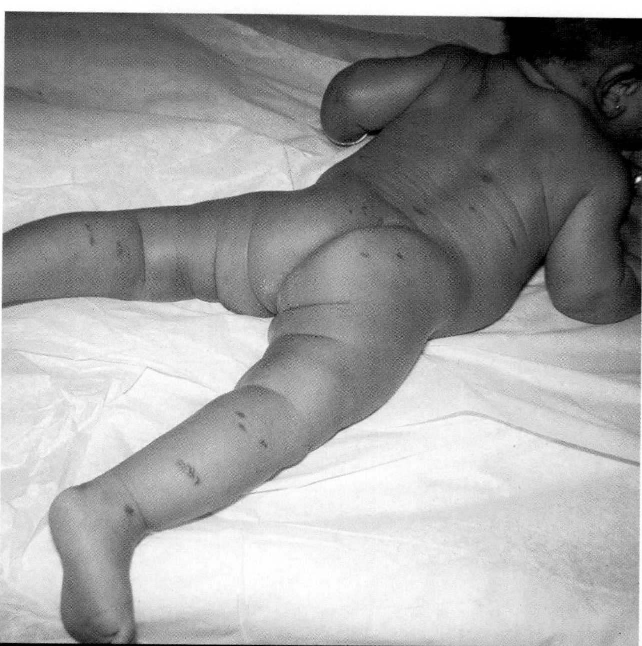

Figure 7-59. Urticaria Pigmentosa

Multiple hyperpigmented flat lesions on the back of a infant.

BOX 7-55. CLINICAL FEATURES OF MASTOCYTOSIS

- *Three clinical forms of mastocytosis are seen in childhood:*

A. Urticaria pigmentosa (generalized)

(1) Most common manifestation
(2) Seen in infants and children
(3) Onset of lesions: from a few weeks to 2 years after birth (usually lesions erupt in crops during the first 6 months of life)
(4) Lesions sparse or numerous
(5) Size varying from 0.5 to 3.5 cm in diameter
(6) Early lesions bullous, urticarial, or hyperpigmented
(7) Color ranges from yellow-tan to chocolate brown or reddish-brown
(8) Individual lesions can be macules, papules, or nodules.
(9) Vesiculation usually abates by 2 years of age.
(10) Generalized distribution (often symmetrically distributed) mainly involving trunk
(11) May spare the palms, soles, mucous membranes, and face

B. Solitary mastocytoma (individual lesions)

(1) Second most common manifestation
(2) Early lesion may present as recurrent, evanescent wheals or bullae
(3) Lesion becomes infiltrated, rubbery, pink, yellow (with a peau d'orange surface) or tan plaque (at site of whealing or blistering)
(4) Plaque usually measures 1 to 3 cm
(5) Present at birth or shortly thereafter
(6) May occur at any site (common sites: wrist, neck, trunk)
(7) Usually involute spontaneously during early childhood

C. Diffuse cutaneous or erythrodermic mastocytosis

(1) Diffuse involvement of skin
(2) Infant is usually normal at birth
(3) Onset usually after the first few months of life
(4) Diffusely erythrodermic infant with *a boggy or doughy appearance*
(5) Skin hard with reddish-brown or peau d'orange discoloration
(6) Recurrent bullae, intractable pruritus common
(7) Systemic symptoms include flushing, wheezing, headache, diarrhea, or syncope

- *Other features*

(1) Positive Darier's sign (stroking results in urtication of the lesion due to release of histamine)
(2) Pruritus
(3) Lesions may become bullous in young infant
(4) Dermographism

BOX 7-56. DIFFERENTIAL DIAGNOSIS OF MASTOCYTOSIS

- Differential diagnosis of urticaria pigmentosa
  (1) Postinflammatory hyperpigmentation
  (2) Drug eruptions
  (3) Bullous impetigo
  (4) Café au lait spots
  (5) Arthropod bite reaction
  (6) Juvenile xanthogranuloma
  (7) Chronic urticaria
  (8) Pigmented nevi
  (9) Lentigines
- Differential diagnosis of solitary mastocytoma
  (1) Nodular scabies
  (2) Recurrent bullous impetigo
  (3) Nevi
  (4) Juvenile xanthogranuloma

DIAGNOSIS CAFÉ AU LAIT SPOTS

SYNONYM

Coffee-with-cream hue spots

Definition and Etiology

Café au lait spots (CALS) are tan to dark brown macules seen on any cutaneous surface. Histologically, they are characterized by scattered giant melanin granules as well as increased melanocytic activity of melanocytes. There is an increase in melanin in both melanocytes and keratinocytes without melanocytic proliferation.

Associated Clinical Features

1. CALS are relatively common, with 10 to 20% of the general population having one or several lesions.
2. Solitary CALS are common and their prevalence varies with age; in contrast, multiple lesions are an uncommon finding at any age, and their presence, particularly in Caucasian patients, should encourage further investigation.
3. Wood's lamp examination may accentuate and reveal CALS inapparent in visible light.

Emergency Department Treatment and Disposition

1. Treatment of CALS is medically unnecessary. Most patients need only reassurance about the benign nature of these lesions.
2. CALS can be masked by cover-up makeup. Bleaching creams and laser treatment have also been used with variable success for cosmetically significant areas. Patients should be referred to a dermatologist for such interventions.
3. Patients with multiple CALS are at risk of having an underlying disorder. It is important to recognize whether the presence of multiple CALS in a particular patient is normal or indicates an association with a multisystem disorder.

Clinical Pearls: Café Au Lait Macules

1. Solitary CALS are common in the pediatric population and in most children represent a normal finding (Fig. 7-60). No investigation is needed for a normal child presenting with a solitary lesion, even with an unusual morphology or an exceptional size.
2. The most frequent disorder seen in association with multiple CALS is neurofibromatosis type 1 (NF1) (Fig. 7-61).
3. CALS are present in 90 to 100% of patients with NF1. Intertriginous freckling in the axillae, inframammary region, or groin is a pathognomonic sign of NF1.
4. CALS alone are not pathognomonic of NF1, regardless of their size and number.

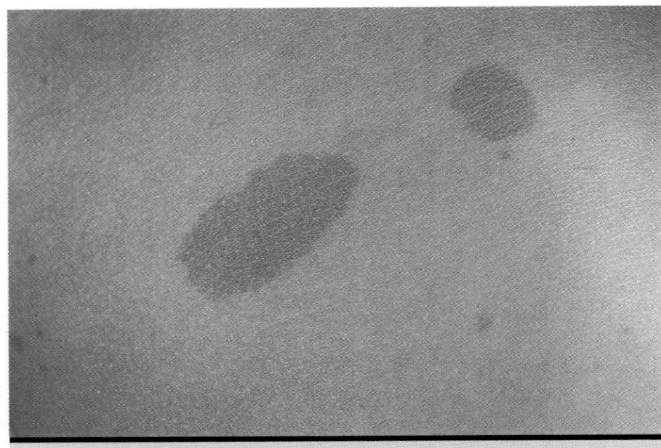

Figure 7-60. Café au Lait Spot

Irregular brown macules that are found in 10 to 20% of normal children. Number and size are increased in neurofibromatosis.

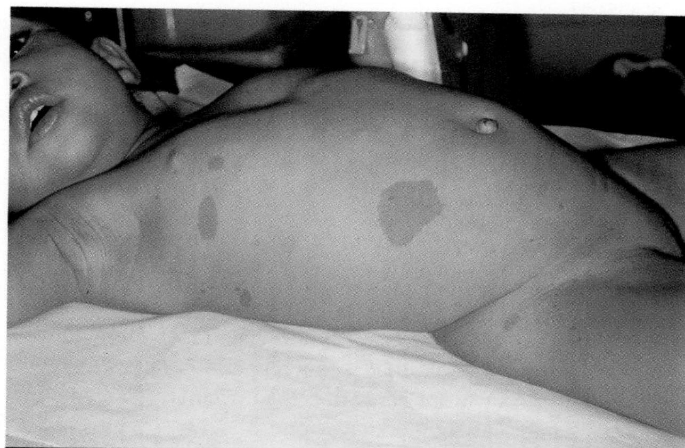

Figure 7-61. Café au Lait Spots in Neurofibromatosis

Uniform brown macules are seen on the trunk of this 3-year-old child who presented with an episode of afebrile seizure. There was a strong family history of mental retardation and epilepsy in two other siblings. Crowe's sign or axillary freckling (tiny freckle-like lesions in the axillae) are highly characteristic of neurofibromatosis.

BOX 7-57. CLINICAL FEATURES OF CAFÉ AU LAIT SPOTS

- Skin lesions
  (1) May be present at birth or develop during childhood
  (2) May increase in size and number with age
  (3) *Macular* lesion
  (4) Discrete, well circumscribed
  (5) Round or oval
  (6) Light or dark brown color (coffee-with-cream hue; hue varies with degree of pigmentation of the individual [tan or light brown in white children and dark brown in black children])
  (7) Uniform hyperpigmentation
  (8) Seen on any cutaneous surface
  (9) Lesions vary in size from 0.5 to 20 cm.
- Borders
  (1) Irregular, jagged, and shaggy borders (McCune-Albright syndrome, Fig. 7-62)
  (2) Smooth, regular borders (neurofibromatosis)

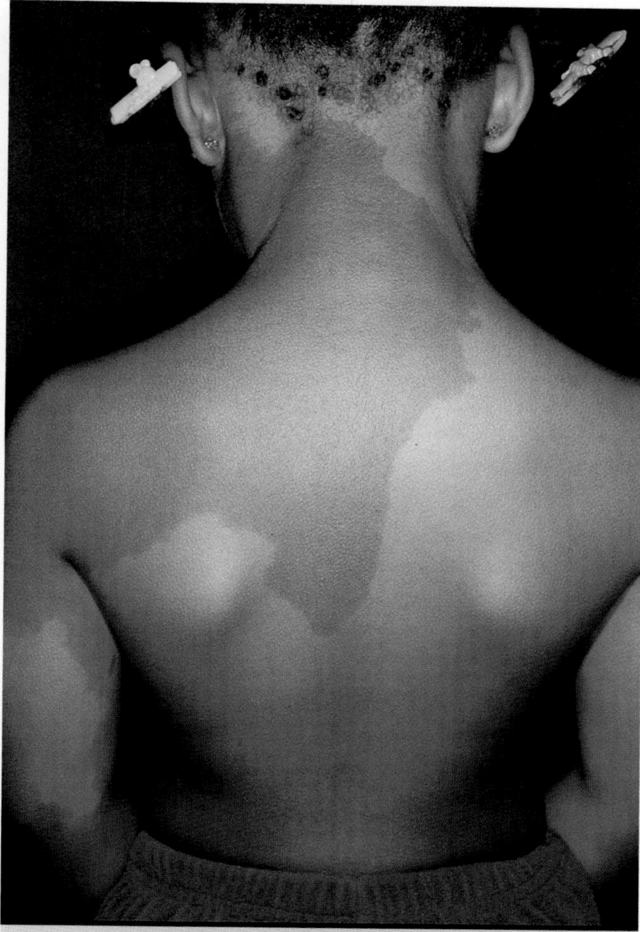

Figure 7-62. Café au Lait Spots in McCune-Albright Syndrome

CALS with irregular, jagged, and shaggy borders is seen on the back of a 4-year-old girl. She also had precocious puberty and polyostotic fibrous dysplasia.

BOX 7-58. DISORDERS WITH MULTIPLE CAFÉ AU LAIT SPOTS

- Neurofibromatosis (either type 1 or type 2)
- McCune-Albright syndrome (CALS may be single and large)
- Tuberous sclerosis
- Proteus syndrome
- Familial café au lait spots
- Fanconi's anemia
- Watson's syndrome (pulmonic stenosis, freckling, mental retardation)
- Ring chromosome syndromes (microcephaly, mental retardation, short stature, limb and cardiac anomalies)
- Ataxia-telangiectasia
- Silver-Russell syndrome
- LEOPARD syndrome
- Turner's syndrome

BOX 7-59. DIAGNOSIS OF NEUROFIBROMATOSIS

Neurofibromatosis type 1 (NF1)

- NIH consensus criteria for diagnosis includes two or more of the following:
  (1) Five or more CALS >5 mm in greatest diameter in prepubertal children and >1.5 cm in postpubertal adolescents and adults
  (2) Two or more neurofibromas of any type (dermal, subcutaneous) or one plexiform neurofibroma
  (3) Freckling in the axillae (Crowe's sign) or inguinal regions
  (4) Optic glioma
  (5) Two or more Lisch nodules (iris hamartomas; seen in >90% of patients >6 years of age)
  (6) Bone lesions (sphenoid dysplasia, scoliosis)
  (7) A first-degree relative with NF-1 (by the above criteria)

Neurofibromatosis type 2 (NF2)

- Diagnosis is made in presence of:
  (1) Bilateral eighth nerve masses (visualized with CT or MRI) *or*
  (2) First-degree relative with NF2 *and either*
    a) Unilateral eighth nerve deafness *or*
    b) Any two of the following: neurofibroma, meningioma, spinal glioma, schwannoma, juvenile posterior subcapsular lenticular opacity

BOX 7-60. DIFFERENTIAL DIAGNOSIS OF CAFÉ AU LAIT SPOTS

- Nevus spilus
- Lentigo
- Nevocellular nevus
- Becker's melanosis
- Segmental pigmentation disorder (hypopigmentation or hyperpigmentation)

DIAGNOSIS

ERYTHEMA NODOSUM

Definition and Etiology

Erythema nodosum (EN) represents a cell-mediated hypersensitivity reaction to a variety of antigenic stimuli. It occurs in association with several diseases (e.g., infections, malignancies) and during drug therapy.

Associated Clinical Features

1. EN occurs more commonly in adolescents and young adults (predominant age range: 20 to 30 years) and is seen more commonly in females (female:male ratio of 3:1).
2. Laboratory tests should be done depending on the suspected etiology. Usually initial evaluation should include throat culture, antistreptolysin O titer, tuberculin skin test, and ESR (usually elevated in patients with EN).
3. Chest radiograph may show bilateral hilar adenopathy. It is seen in EN produced by coccidioidomycosis, histoplasmosis, tuberculosis, streptococcal infections, lymphoma, and as a nonspecific reaction in many cases.
4. The diagnosis is made clinically based on a very characteristic presentation, and in most cases biopsy is not required. Skin biopsy shows septal panniculitis (lymphohistiocytic infiltrate, granulomatous inflammation, and fibrosis in the septa of subcutaneous fat).

Consultation

Dermatology (in doubtful cases)

Emergency Department Treatment and Disposition

1. In most instances EN is a self-limited disease and requires only symptomatic relief.
   a. Nonsteroidal anti-inflammatory agents (e.g., indomethacin or naproxen) given orally
   b. Bed rest, leg elevation, and elastic wraps or support stockings may help.
2. Identify and treat the precipitating factor:
   a. Discontinue offending drug
   b. Specific treatment of the underlying infection

Clinical Pearls: Erythema Nodosum

1. EN lesions are multiple, bilateral, tender nodules that undergo characteristic color changes ending in temporary bruise-like areas, and occurs most commonly on the extensor surfaces of the shins (Fig. 7-63).
2. The most common cause of EN is streptococcal infection and tuberculosis in children and streptococcal infection and sarcoidosis in adults.
3. EN may recur with recurrent infections (e.g., recurrent EN seen in children with recurrent streptococcal infections).

BOX 7-61. ETIOLOGY OF ERYTHEMA NODOSUM

- Idiopathic (up to 50% of cases)
- Infections
  (1) *Streptococcus pyogenes* infections
  (2) Tuberculosis
  (3) Psittacosis
  (4) *Yersinia enterocolitica* infection
  (5) Lymphogranuloma venereum
  (6) Cat-scratch disease
  (7) Coccidioidomycosis (most common cause in west and southwest United States)
  (8) Histoplasmosis
  (9) Blastomycosis
  (10) Leprosy
- Drugs
  (1) Sulfonamides
  (2) Oral contraceptives
  (3) Phenytoin
- Sarcoidosis
- Inflammatory bowel disease
- Malignancy (e.g., Hodgkin's disease, leukemia, sarcoma)
- Pregnancy

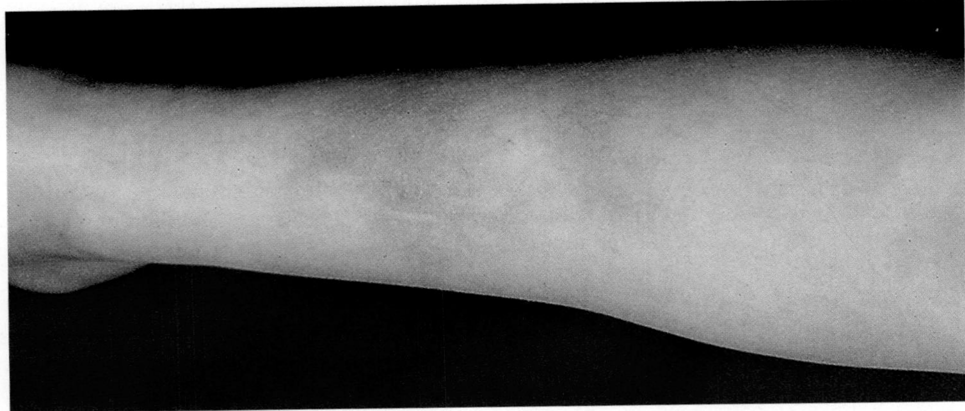

Figure 7-63. Erythema Nodosum

Erythema Nodosum Tender, red nodules on the pretibial area of an adolescent. (Reproduced with permission from: Kane KS, Ryder JB, Johnson RA et al. Erythema Nodosum. In: Color Atlas & Synopsis of Pediatric Dermatology, New York, McGraw-Hill, 2002, p. 345)

BOX 7-62. CLINICAL FEATURES OF ERYTHEMA NODOSUM

- *Skin lesions*
  (1) Subcutaneous nodules with poorly defined borders
  (2) Discrete lesions
  (3) Size: 2 to 6 cm
  (4) Shape: Oval
  (5) Nodules are erythematous, tender, tense, and hard during the first week.
  (6) Nodules become fluctuant but do not suppurate during the second week.
  (7) Overlying skin changes in color: bright red to blue to greenish to yellow, then they fade
  (8) Common location: extensor surfaces (shins; extensor aspects of forearms; thighs, trunk)
  (9) *Symmetrically* distributed
  (10) Individual lesions disappear in 1 or 2 weeks.
  (11) New lesions may appear for 3 to 6 weeks.
  (12) Nonulcerating and nonscarring lesions
  (13) Overlying skin desquamates
- *Other associated features*
  (1) Low-grade fever, malaise
  (2) Arthralgias/arthritis (seen in 50% of cases either during eruptive phase of EN, or preceding EN by 2 to 8 weeks)

BOX 7-63. DIFFERENTIAL DIAGNOSIS OF ERYTHEMA NODOSUM

- Cellulitis
- Erysipelas
- Ecchymoses
- Child abuse
- Arthropod bites
- Calcified hematoma
- Superficial and deep thrombophlebitis
- Weber-Christian panniculitis (localized subcutaneous inflammation [e.g., trunk, thighs])
- Lupus panniculitis
- Panniculitis secondary to pancreatic disease
- Erythema induratum (cold, ulcerating nodules on the calves)

DIAGNOSIS ACANTHOSIS NIGRICANS

Definition

Acanthosis nigricans (AN) is velvety thickening and hyperpigmentation of the skin with a characteristic distribution.

Associated Clinical Features

1. Acanthosis nigricans can occur at any age and is commonly seen in children.
2. It may be familial with autosomal dominant inheritance.
3. The diagnosis of AN is made clinically. Skin biopsy (not required for diagnosis) shows acanthosis, hyperkeratosis, papillomatosis, and increased melanin in the basal layer and upper dermis.
4. Laboratory tests as indicated by signs and symptoms should be performed to exclude any underlying syndromes.

Emergency Department Treatment and Disposition

1. Acanthosis nigricans lesions are usually asymptomatic and do not require treatment.
2. Refer the patient to a subspecialist depending on the underlying etiology of AN.
3. Usually correction of the underlying disorder (e.g., discontinuing the causative drug, weight reduction) improves AN.
4. For cosmetic concerns or to promote comfort in areas with thicker lesions, the following therapies may be tried.
   a. Topical tretinoin
   b. Topical hydroxyl acids (e.g., lactic acid, 10 to 20% urea).

Clinical Pearls: Acanthosis Nigricans

1. The majority of cases of AN are associated with obesity (pseudoacanthosis nigricans).
2. Acanthosis nigricans represents a cutaneous marker of tissue insulin resistance regardless of its cause.
3. Correction of the underlying etiology of AN (e.g., obesity, withdrawal of drugs) usually improves AN.
4. Acanthosis nigricans is rarely a sign of malignancy in children; however, a rapidly progressing and widespread AN is caused by malignancy until proved otherwise at any age.

BOX 7-64. ETIOLOGY OF ACANTHOSIS NIGRICANS

- Hereditary or idiopathic AN (without any underlying etiology)
- Obesity-associated AN (pseudoacanthosis nigricans)
  (1) Most common type of AN
  (2) Obesity produces insulin resistance.
  (3) Regresses with weight loss
- Syndrome-associated AN (various endocrine disorders associated with insulin resistance)
  (1) Insulin-resistant diabetes
  (2) Cushing's syndrome
  (3) Hyperandrogenic or hypogonadal syndromes
  (4) Acromegaly and gigantism
  (5) Addison's disease
  (6) Hypothyroidism or hyperthyroidism
  (7) Stein-Leventhal syndrome
  (8) HAIR-AN syndrome (*h*yper*a*ndrogenemia, *i*nsulin *r*esistance, *a*canthosis *n*igricans) (Fig. 7-64)
- Drug-induced AN
  (1) Corticosteroid therapy
  (2) Oral contraceptives
  (3) Niacin
  (4) Nicotinic acid
- Malignancy-associated AN (seen in adults)
  (1) Gastric adenocarcinoma [most common]
  (2) Carcinomas of colon, ovary, pancreas, rectum, and uterus
  (3) Lymphoma

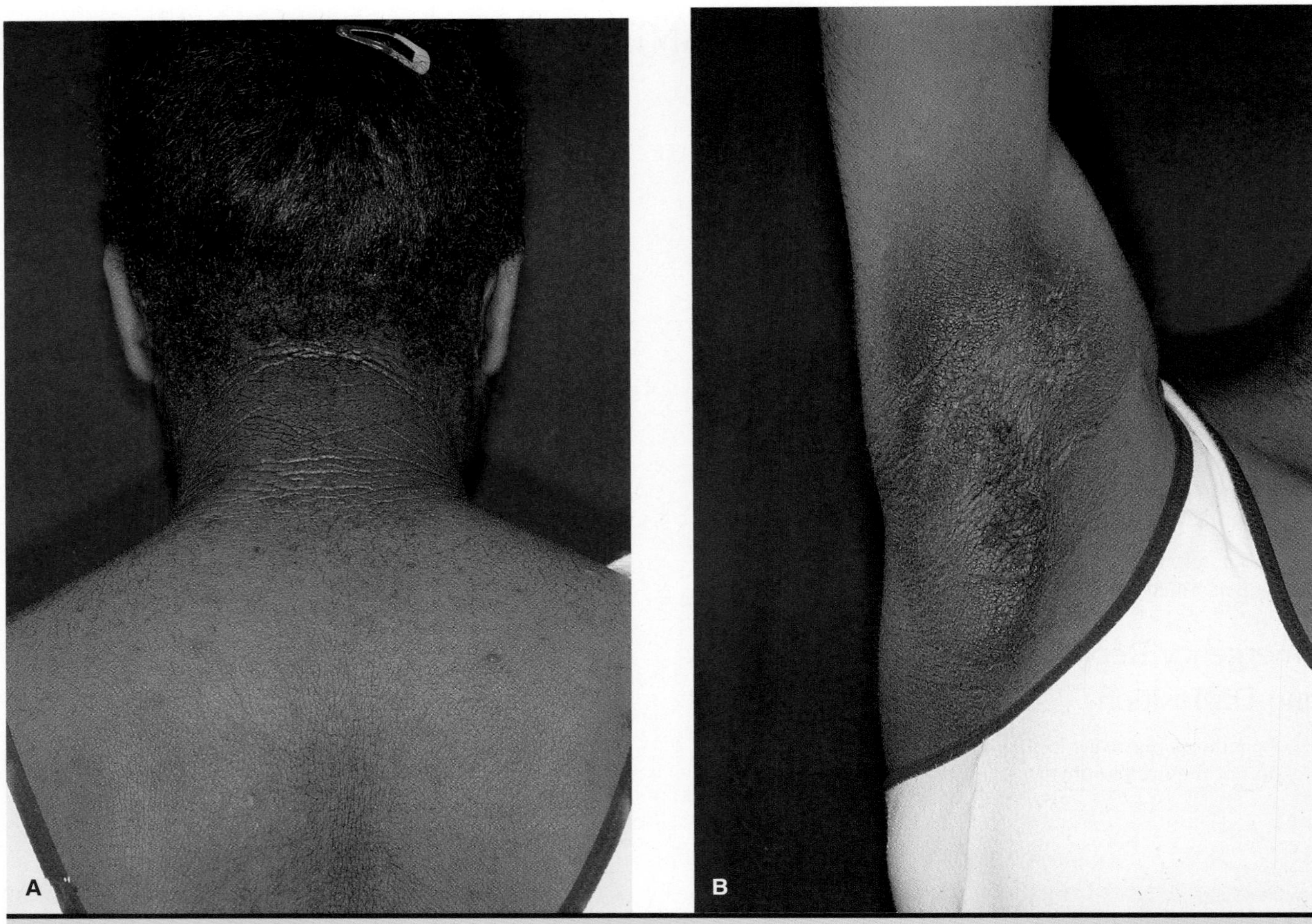

Figure 7-64. Acanthosis Nigricans

A 15-year-old girl with type II diabetes presented with these hyperpigmented, velvety, papillomatous (verrucous) plaques accompanied by accentuation of skin markings on the back of the neck (*A*) and both axillae (*B*). AN may be a marker for insulin resistance, hyperinsulinemia, and eventually type II diabetes. This patient had HAIR-AN syndrome, which is usually seen in young African-American women who present with virilization or accelerated growth, hirsutism, polycystic ovaries, clitoral hypertrophy, elevated testosterone levels, and onset of AN in infancy or childhood with subsequent rapid progression of AN during puberty.

BOX 7-65. CLINICAL FEATURES OF ACANTHOSIS NIGRICANS

- Symmetrical distribution
- Rarely unilateral or localized
- Dark brown to black in color
- Leathery, warty, or papillomatous surface
- Velvety texture as skin thickens
- Skin lines accentuated
- Most common location: body folds (axillae, back and sides of neck, groin, antecubital fossae)
- Other locations
  (1) Flexures of the knees
  (2) Knuckles
  (3) Submammary and around areolae of the breasts
  (4) Umbilicus
  (5) Beltline
  (6) Anogenital areas
  (7) Inner thighs
- Mucous membrane/mucocutaneous involvement (seen in malignancy-associated AN)
  (1) Oral mucosa
  (2) Vermilion borders of the lips
  (3) Warty papillomatous thickening periorbitally and periorally

BOX 7-66. DIFFERENTIAL DIAGNOSIS OF ACANTHOSIS NIGRICANS

- Other conditions associated with hyperpigmentation
  (1) Postinflammatory hyperpigmentation
  (2) Epidermal nevus
  (3) Tinea versicolor

DIAGNOSIS HIDRADENITIS SUPPURATIVA

SYNONYMS

Hidradenitis axillaris
Apocrinitis
Abscess of apocrine sweat glands

Definition

Hidradenitis suppurativa (HS) is a chronic, suppurative abscess of apocrine sweat glands in the axillary, genital, and perianal areas.

Etiology

1. Developmental sequence of HA: primary keratinous occlusion of apocrine duct, followed by dilatation of the duct and hair follicle, followed by secondary bacterial infection, then rupture of the apocrine gland with extension of infection/inflammation to adjacent areas, leading to ulceration and fibrosis, sinus tract formation, and scarring
2. Bacteria are *not* the underlying cause of hidradenitis, but they participate in the process, thus representing a secondary infection.
3. *Staphylococcus aureus*, nonhemolytic streptococci, *Streptococcus milleri*, *S. viridans*, *Escherichia coli*, *Proteus* spp., and *Pseudomonas* spp. are often isolated from the draining lesions. Anaerobes (*Bacteroides*, anaerobic gram-positive cocci) have also been reported from such lesions (presence of anaerobes often is suggested by foul odor of the discharge).

Associated Clinical Features

1. HS is more common in African-Americans (due to their larger number of apocrine sweat glands) than in whites.
2. Age at presentation (among the pediatric population)
   a. Most commonly seen during puberty (with development of apocrine glands)

b. Rarely seen in children before the onset of puberty

3. More common in females (female:male ratio of 3 to 4:1)

4. Axillary lesions are more common in females; groin lesions are more common in males.

5. Most cases of HS occur sporadically; familial occurrence with autosomal dominant inheritance (with a tendency towards follicular occlusion) has been seen.

6. HS may be associated with endocrinopathies (e.g., diabetes, Cushing's syndrome).

7. Several factors that predispose to the occurrence of HS include obesity, warm tropical climates, and hormonal (low estrogens or presence of androgenic progestins) and end-organ hypersensitivity to androgens.

8. Use of antiperspirants or deodorants may exacerbate the condition.

9. The diagnosis of HS is made clinically. Gram-stained smears, culture, and sensitivity results are helpful in guiding therapy in the initial phases of infection. Instruct the laboratory to look specifically for *S. milleri* and anaerobes and to assess sensitivity to erythromycin and tetracycline in particular.

10. Complications include cellulitis, ulceration, and burrowing abscesses that may perforate adjacent structures, forming fistulas to the urethra, bladder, rectum, or peritoneum; squamous cell carcinoma (in area affected for >10 years); and pyoderma gangrenosum.

Consultation

Dermatology (for recurrent difficult-to-treat patients) and surgery (for recalcitrant cases)

Emergency Department Treatment and Disposition

1. Early stages of disease
   a. Antibiotic therapy (mainstay of treatment)
      1) Topical (e.g., clindamycin)
      2) Empirical therapy may be initiated with tetracycline, doxycycline, or minocycline for patients 8 years or older (clindamycin or cephalosporins are alternative agents).
      3) Some patients require long-term oral therapy (e.g., erythromycin [dose: 1 g/day] *or* tetracycline [dose: 1 g/day] *or* minocycline [dose: 200 mg/day] for patients >8 years).
   b. Warm compresses encourage spontaneous rupture of abscesses and assists in incision and drainage of the bulging abscesses.
   c. Intralesional corticosteroids (e.g., triamcinolone acetonide) injected into inflamed areas may help reverse the process.
   d. Systemic corticosteroids (e.g., prednisone 40 to 60 mg/day for 7 to 10 days, tapering gradually as inflammation subsides) for patients who respond poorly to antibiotics may decrease fibrosis and scarring.
   e. Isotretinoin (dose: 1 mg/kg per day for 20 weeks) may be effective in early cases that present with inflammatory cystic lesions without undermining sinus tracts.

2. In recalcitrant cases
   a. Surgical extirpation of apocrine glands
   b. Total excision of the hair-bearing area, followed by split-thickness skin grafting may be the only curative option.

3. General measures include weight reduction, wearing loose-fitting clothes, improving local hygiene, and applying antiseptic compresses (e.g., povidone-iodine or chlorhexidine) or Burow's solution soaks.

Clinical Pearls: Hidradenitis Suppurativa

1. HS is a chronic, recurrent inflammatory disease of apocrine sweat glands.

2. HS presents as painful nodules and abscesses with chronically draining sinuses involving the axillae, groin, or perineum (Fig. 7-65). Restriction to areas of the body with more apocrine glands helps in arriving at the diagnosis.

3. HS runs a chronic course punctuated by relapses and partial remissions, and if severe leads to fistulae, dermal scarring with hypertrophic scars, lymphedema, and even restriction of arm or leg movement.

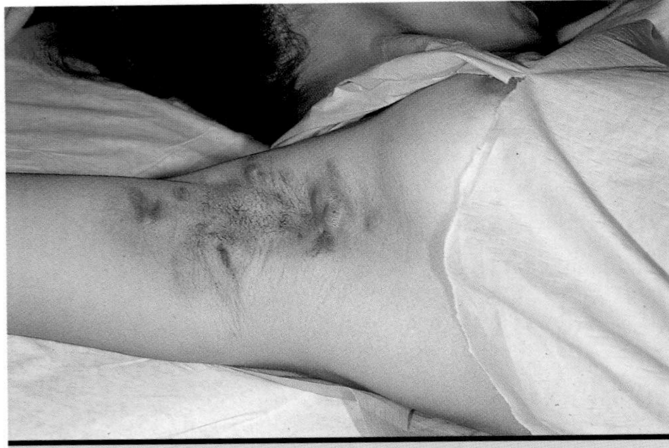

Figure 7-65. Hidradenitis Suppurativa

Nodules, abscess, and draining sinus tracts are seen. Both axillae were involved in this 18-year-old African-American girl. This was her fourth recurrence. A hallmark of HA is a double and triple comedone, a blackhead with two or more surface openings that communicate under the skin. The chronic, uncomfortable, malodorous, and unsightly nature of this patient's disease was causing significant social debilitation. She had failed many courses of antibiotic therapy and was referred for surgical extirpation of the apocrine glands.

BOX 7-67. CLINICAL FEATURES OF HIDRADENITIS SUPPURATIVA

- Skin lesions
  (1) Begin as deep-seated tender, erythematous inflammatory nodules that coalesce into a single large abscess
  (2) Malodorous discharge (thin/serous or frankly purulent)
  (3) Lesions moderately to exquisitely tender
  (4) Milder cases: resolve spontaneously or after incision and drainage of abscess
  (5) Severe cases: new crops of lesions suppurate, rupture and can become progressive and self-perpetuating
  (6) During healing: deep fibrosis with cicatricial scarring, sinus tracts, and fistulas admixed with new lesions
  (7) Involvement often bilateral
- Most common sites
  (1) Axilla
  (2) Anogenital areas
  (3) Inguinal creases
  (4) Buttocks
  (5) Upper inner thighs
- Less common sites
  (1) Areolae, periareolar, and submammary regions of the breasts
  (2) Periumbilical region
  (3) Scalp, face, posterior neck, shoulders

BOX 7-68. DIFFERENTIAL DIAGNOSIS OF HIDRADENITIS SUPPURATIVA

- *Axillary region*
  (1) Suppurative lymphadenitis (any cause)
  (2) Furuncles
  (3) Carbuncles
  (4) Nodulocystic acne
  (5) Cat-scratch disease
  (6) Tularemia
  (7) Scrofuloderma
  (8) Actinomycosis
- *Anogenital region*
  (1) Furunculosis
  (2) Crohn's disease with fistulae/sinus tracts
  (3) Ulcerative colitis with fistulae/sinus tracts
  (4) Bartholin's gland abscesses
  (5) Lymphogranuloma venereum
  (6) Donovanosis
  (7) Granuloma inguinale

Suggested Readings

Carroll MC, Yueng-Yue KA, Esterly NB, Drolet BA: Drug-induced hypersensitivity syndrome in pediatric patients. *Pediatrics* 2001;108:485.

Habif TP: The SJS/TEN spectrum of disease. *Clinical Dermatology*, 3rd ed. Philadelphia, Mosby-Year Book, 2004, page 630.

Hartley AH: Pityriasis rosea. *Pediatr Rev* 1999;20:266.

Haruda F: Phenytoin hypersensitivity: 38 cases. *Neurology* 1979;29: 1480.

Landau M, Krafchik BR: The diagnostic value of café-au-lait macules. *J Am Acad Dermatol* 1999;40:877.

Lapidus CS, Honig PJ: Atopic dermatitis. *Pediatr Rev* 1994;15:327.

Revuz J: Dermatology clinic. New Advances in Severe Adverse Drug Reactions. 2001.

Wolkenstein P, Revuz J: Toxic epidermal necrolysis. *Dermatol Clin* 2000;18:485.

Zacharisen MC: Pediatric urticaria and angioedema. *Immunol Allergy Clin North Am* 1999;19:363.

BOX 8-5. CLINICAL FEATURES OF VIRAL CONJUNCTIVITIS

- Diffuse mild conjunctival hyperemia
- Thin discharge
- Bilateral symptoms (often one side will predominate, especially early)
- Itching
- Tearing
- Foreign body sensation
- Diffuse lid edema may occur, mimicking periorbital cellulitis.
- Normal visual acuity (though blurred by secretions)
- Photophobia (minimal, if any)
- Preauricular adenopathy
- Often associated with upper respiratory tract infection
- Patients usually highly contagious (especially adenovirus conjunctivitis)

BOX 8-6. FEATURES OF BACTERIAL CONJUNCTIVITIS

- Generally of rapid onset in one eye; progresses to other eye in 2 to 5 days
- Conjunctival injection and inflammation
- Normal visual acuity
- *Photophobia is not a feature of bacterial conjunctivitis; its presence should raise the suspicion of iritis or herpes keratoconjunctivitis.*
- Thick purulent discharge (Fig. 8-4)
- Wet, sticky mucopurulent matting of lashes upon awakening
- May be either bilateral or unilateral
- Eyelid edema
- Conjunctivitis caused by chlamydia and gonorrhea must be considered in sexually active teens.
- Unusually copious purulent drainage, pronounced lid edema, and chemosis should raise the suspicion for gonococcal conjunctivitis.
- Management
  (1) Cultures and Gram's stain are not performed routinely for mild to moderate conjunctivitis.
  (2) Topical therapy that provides broad-spectrum coverage (e.g., a fluoroquinolone [ciprofloxacin, ofloxacin])
  (3) Ointment is preferred due to extended contact time with eye (3 to 5 hours).
  (4) Typically a self-limited condition with a duration of 8 to 10 days (consider another etiology if "red eye" lasts >10 days)
  (5) Ophthalmology referral for severe conjunctivitis or conjunctivitis that does not improve after 7 days of treatment

BOX 8-7. FEATURES OF VERNAL CONJUNCTIVITIS

- Onset from 3 to 13 years of age
- More common in spring and summer and in warm climates
- Represents type I and type IV hypersensitivity reactions
- Pronounced allergic conjunctivitis
  (1) Severe eye itching
  (2) Thick mucous, stringy discharge
  (3) Usually bilateral involvement
  (4) Photophobia may result
  (5) Cobblestone appearance due to large conjunctival papillae on the back of the upper lid
- Management
  (1) Topical antihistamines and mast cell stabilizers
  (2) *Do not* use oral antihistamines (eyes become drier and more irritated).
  (3) Cool compresses, refrigerated gel masks, or ice packs
  (4) Ophthalmologist may choose to prescribe steroids.
- Preventive measures: washing hair before going to sleep (allergens become trapped by hair during the course of the day and get into the eyes as children move about in bed).

BOX 8-8. DIFFERENTIAL DIAGNOSIS OF CONJUNCTIVITIS

- Bacterial conjunctivitis
- Vernal or allergic conjunctivitis
- Viral conjunctivitis
  (1) Acute hemorrhagic conjunctivitis (adenovirus)
  (2) Measles conjunctivitis
  (3) HSV keratoconjunctivitis
- Inclusion conjunctivitis
- Periorbital cellulitis
- Corneal abrasion
- Blepharitis
- Stye
- Internal hordeolum
- Foreign body
- Trauma
- Uveitis
- Acute angle closure glaucoma
- Systemic diseases (e.g., Kawasaki disease)

DIAGNOSIS HORDEOLUM AND CHALAZION

Synonym

Stye for hordeolum

Definition

1. A hordeolum is a focal painful inflammation of the sebaceous glands of the eyelid margin with abscess formation.
   a. Internal hordeolum: infection of the meibomian glands (sebaceous glands embedded in the tarsal plate)
   b. External hordeolum: infection of the glands of Zeis (sebaceous glands located in the eyelash follicles) (Fig. 8-7)
2. A chalazion is a chronic painless granulomatous reaction of the same region (Fig. 8-8).

Etiology

1. Infection is largely caused by *Staphylococcus aureus*.
2. A chalazion is a chronic granulomatous reaction to the lipid material secreted by the meibomian glands.
   a. While it is not, strictly speaking, caused by a bacterial infection, it is more likely to occur as a consequence of one.
   b. The edema of a blepharitis may mechanically block the meibomian glands and predispose a patient to the development of a chalazion.

Associated Clinical Features

1. While they may be difficult to distinguish visually, a patient with a chalazion will not report any pain or discharge, whereas these symptoms are typical of a hordeolum.
2. A hordeolum is erythematous and localized, though it may produce a more generalized lid edema as well as a discrete abscess with purulent discharge.
3. A chalazion is typically a firm, localized, swollen lump at the lid margin or in the midportion of the lid. It is slow-growing, nontender, and non-erythematous. Occasionally a chalazion will become secondarily infected.
4. Fever is not a feature of either diagnosis, and if present should alert the clinician to the possibility of cellulitis.

Emergency Department Treatment and Disposition

1. Hot, moist compresses applied for 15 minutes, four times daily will cure about half of patients with hordeola or acute chalazia.
2. In the case of a large discrete abscess that is not resolving, incision with an 18-gauge needle will speed resolution. Care

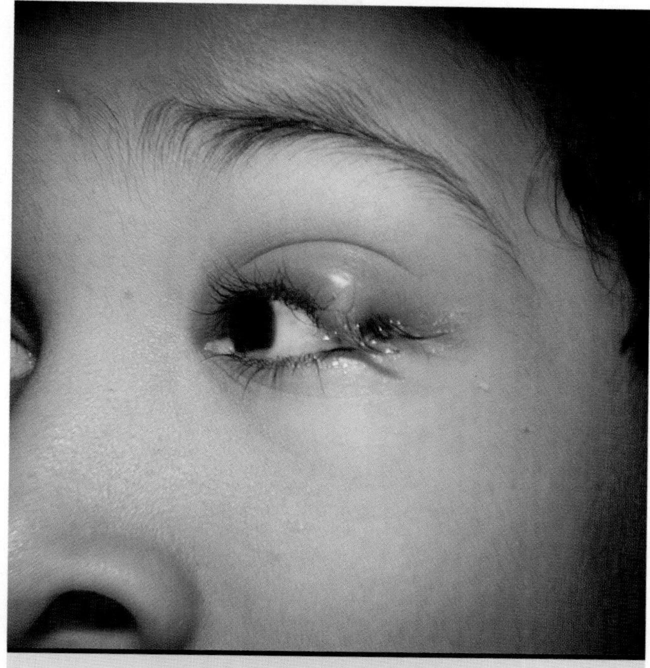

Figure 8-7. External Hordeolum

An erythematous tender swelling at the lid margin with purulent discharge is seen. There is also mild erythema and edema of the upper eyelid.

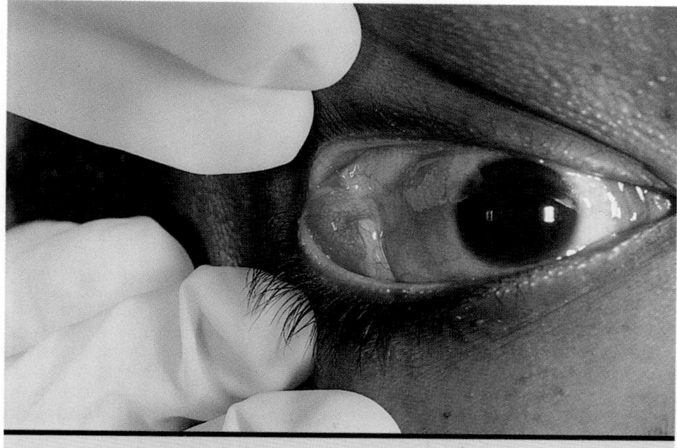

Figure 8-8. Chalazion

A pea-sized, mobile, painless, noninflamed nodule is seen within the body of the eyelid.

should be taken to avoid external incisions that may leave scars, as well as incisions that pierce the tarsal plate that may lead to anatomic distortion.

3. Granulomatous chalazia unresponsive to conservative therapy may require excision, or rarely, steroid injection by an ophthalmologist.
4. Topical antibiotics are of limited value in either of these diagnoses.

Clinical Pearls: Hordeolum and Chalazion

1. Hordeola are purulent staphylococcal infections of the eyelid sebaceous glands that generally resolve with conservative measures.
2. A chalazion is a lipogranulomatous reaction that causes focal, nonpurulent swelling of the eyelid.

BOX 8-9. CLINICAL FEATURES OF HORDEOLUM

- Tender
- Erythematous nodule at lid margin
- May have purulent drainage
- Associated lid edema may be present.
- Usually unilateral and single
- External hordeolum
  (1) Smaller, superficial abscess at lid margin
  (2) Tends to point to skin surface
- Internal hordeolum
  (1) Larger, located on subconjunctival surface of the lid
  (2) May point to the skin or to the palpebral conjunctival surface

BOX 8-10. CLINICAL FEATURES OF CHALAZION

- Typically a firm, localized, swollen nodule
- More common on upper lid
- Occurs in mid-portion of the lid more often than the lid margin
- Slow-growing
- Nontender
- Non-erythematous

BOX 8-11. DIFFERENTIAL DIAGNOSIS OF HORDEOLUM AND CHALAZION

- Pyogenic granuloma
- Periorbital cellulitis (see Figs. 8-9 and 8-11)
- Blepharitis
- Nevus
- Molluscum contagiosum
- Hydrocystoma (translucent cyst located at lid margin)

DIAGNOSIS

PRESEPTAL CELLULITIS

Synonym

Periorbital cellulitis

Definition

Preseptal cellulitis is an infection of the superficial eyelid and periorbital soft tissues anterior to the orbital septum (without involvement of the eye or orbital contents) (Fig. 8-9).

Etiology

1. Local infection from a portal of injury such as an insect bite or local trauma
2. Spread from a contiguous soft tissue infection (e.g., hordeolum, dacryocystitis, impetigo) (Fig. 8-10)
3. Spread from upper respiratory tract infections (e.g., paranasal sinusitis)
4. Bacteremic spread
5. The most commonly encountered organisms include:
   a. *Staphylococcus aureus*
   b. *Streptococcus pyogenes*
   c. *Streptococcus pneumoniae*
   d. *Haemophilus influenzae* (once a leading cause of this condition, it is much less common since the initiation of routine childhood vaccination)

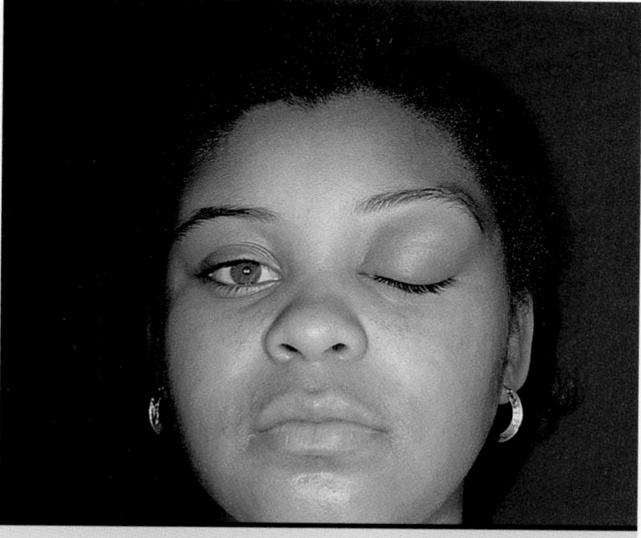

Figure 8-9. Preseptal Cellulitis

Intense erythema, eyelid edema, and tenderness with no clinical signs of orbital involvement were present in the left eye in this adolescent girl, CT scan showed left maxillary sinusitis and absence of proptosis or involvement of the orbital contents.

Associated Clinical Features

1. Preseptal cellulitis is commonly seen in younger children (average age: around 2 years), while patients with orbital cellulitis are older (average age: around 12 years).
2. Leukocytosis may be present (though this is neither reliable nor relevant). Blood culture and Gram's stain and culture (aerobic, anaerobic) of aspirated material from an abscess may be indicated. Corneal surface cultures are diagnostic approximately 50% of the time.
3. The following findings would warrant evaluation by orbital CT scan to rule out orbital involvement:
   a. Pain on eye movement or limitation of extraocular movements
   b. Diminishment of visual acuity
   c. An afferent pupillary defect or dilated pupil
   d. Proptosis
   e. Unreliable eye exam (e.g., difficult eye examination with swollen eyelids)

Consultations

Ophthalmology and otolaryngology (if orbital involvement cannot be excluded)

Emergency Department Treatment and Disposition

1. Hospitalization for intravenous antibiotics should be considered for children who are under 5 years of age or immunocompromised, those with signs of sepsis, or those who cannot be expected to follow-up reliably.

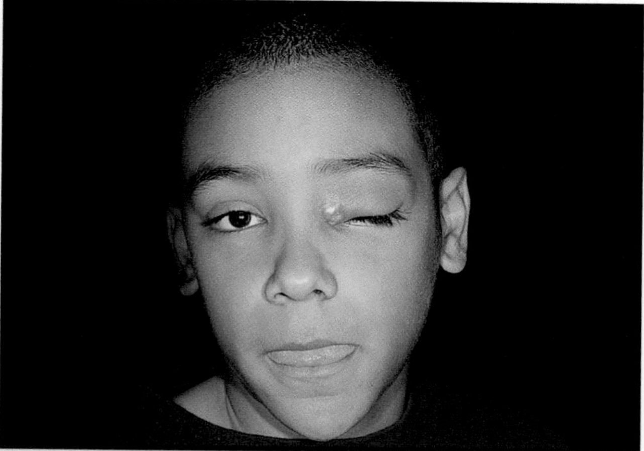

Figure 8-10. Hordeolum with Preseptal Cellulitis

Spreading from a contiguous infection can lead to preseptal cellulitis.

2. In the era of routine *H. influenzae* immunization, uncomplicated preseptal cellulitis in older children may be treated with oral antibiotics and close follow-up on an outpatient basis, provided the child is well appearing and every effort has been made to exclude the more concerning diagnosis of orbital cellulitis.
3. Antibiotic therapy
   a. Inpatient parenteral regimen:
      1) Ceftriaxone or cefotaxime (cefuroxime is another alternative if the possibility of meningitis has been excluded; it covers gram-positive bacteria including *S. aureus* and *H. influenzae*)
      2) If there is a clear cutaneous portal of entry (e.g., hordeolum, superficial laceration): cefazolin or nafcillin
      3) Parenteral antibiotic therapy is continued until clinical improvement is noted and the patient has remained afebrile for at least 24 to 48 hours.
      4) Oral antibiotic therapy (e.g., amoxicillin-clavulanate) is continued for an additional 7 to 10 days after discharge from the hospital.
   b. Outpatient regimen
      1) Amoxicillin-clavulanate (usual duration: 10 to 14 days)
      2) Close follow-up
      3) Hospitalize if patient is not improving after 48 hours of oral antibiotic therapy

Clinical Pearls: Preseptal Cellulitis

1. Preseptal cellulitis must be carefully distinguished from orbital cellulitis. CT scan of the orbits is indicated if there is any question of the diagnosis. Because they differ in severity and urgency of management, it is important early in a patient's course to distinguish the two.
2. Antibiotic therapy should commence in the ED and close follow-up must be ensured should the patient be discharged home.
3. Allergic reactions and insect bites resulting in swelling of the eyelid may be differentiated from preseptal cellulitis by usual absence of painful eyelid swelling.

BOX 8-12. CLINICAL FEATURES OF PRESEPTAL CELLULITIS

- Unilateral involvement much more common (about 95% of cases)
- Bilateral involvement seen in viral etiology (Fig. 8-11)
- Presence of significant pain, warmth, and swelling of lid
- Sometimes completely obscures eye and blocks vision
- The eye itself is not involved.
- No intrinsic difficulties with eyesight (provided lid may be opened and discharge cleared away)
- Chemosis or conjunctivitis with thin or purulent drainage may be present.
- Inflammation may spread over the superior orbital rim and onto the brow (in contrast to orbital cellulitis, in which superior spread is blocked by orbital septum).
- Local inflammation may cause lymphatic or venous obstruction, resulting in edema distant from site of infection.
- Absence of proptosis, resistance to globe retropulsion, or any restriction of spontaneous eye movement (these findings should alert the clinician to the possibility of orbital cellulitis)
- Patients febrile or afebrile (systemic signs unusual except in patients with bacteremia)

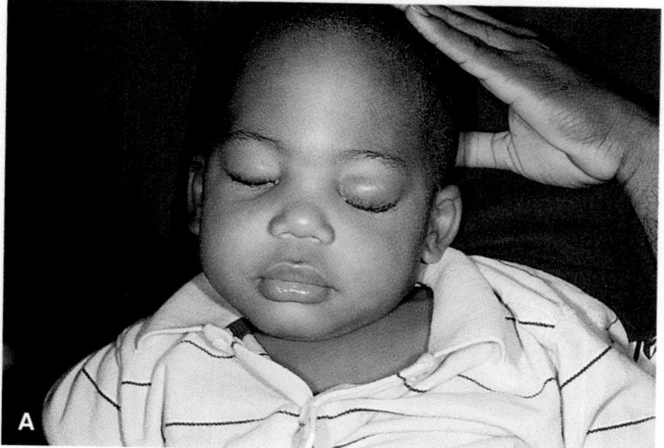

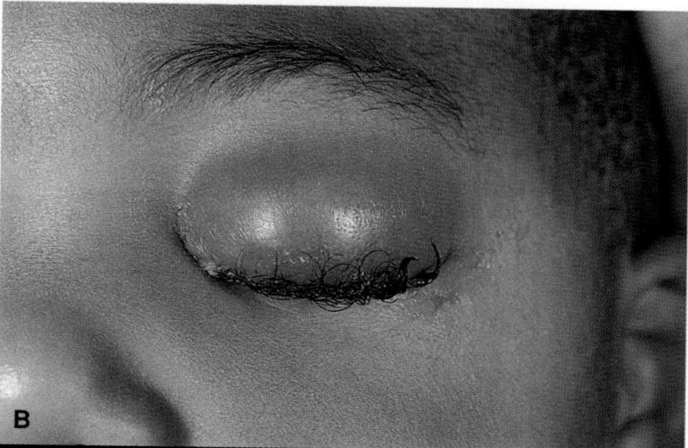

Figure 8-11. Bilateral Preseptal Cellulitis

A. Intense erythema and swelling associated with extreme tenderness were presenting complaints in this child. He had no clinical signs of orbital involvement. Preseptal cellulitis is unilateral in the majority (about 95% of cases). However, bilateral involvement may be seen. This patient had bilateral conjunctivitis with mucopurulent discharge. *B*. Close-up showing the left eye, which was more involved than the right eye.

BOX 8-13. DIFFERENTIAL DIAGNOSIS OF PRESEPTAL CELLULITIS

- Orbital cellulitis (Figs. 8-14 and 8-15)
- Hordeolum (Fig. 8-7)
- Conjunctivitis
- Allergic reaction
- HSV infection (Fig. 8-12)
- Herpes zoster
- Dacryoadenitis
- Dacryocystitis
- Contact dermatitis

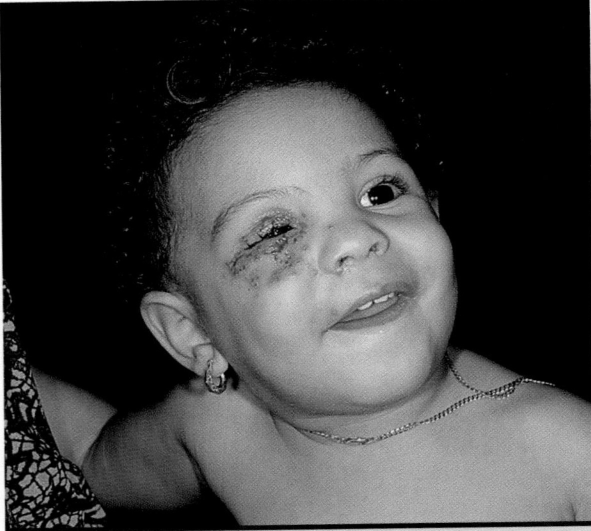

Figure 8-12. Herpes Simplex Virus Infection: Differential Diagnosis of Preseptal Cellulitis

Multiple vesicular lesions on an erythematous base were present that quickly progressed to pustular and scab formations in this 9-month-old infant with primary HSV infection. The cornea was not involved in this patient (the cornea is involved in 10 to 30% of patients with primary ocular type I HSV infection). Type 1 HSV was cultured from the vesicle. Ocular infections are usually caused by HSV-1 except in newborns, where HSV-2 predominates (see also Fig. 8-5).

DIAGNOSIS

ORBITAL CELLULITIS

SYNONYM

Postseptal cellulitis

Definition

Orbital cellulitis is an infection of the soft tissues of the orbit posterior to the orbital septum. Infection may involve all the orbital structures, including extraocular muscles, sensory and motor nerves, and the optic nerve.

Etiology

1. Orbital cellulitis may result from diverse causes:
   a. About 75 to 90% of cases of orbital cellulitis are associated with either preceding or concurrent acute paranasal sinusitis. The most commonly involved sinuses are the ethmoid, followed by the maxillary and frontal sinuses (Fig. 8-13).
   b. Extension of odontogenic infection
   c. Inoculation after penetrating ocular injury or intraorbital surgery
   d. Hematogenous spread from bacteremia (more likely in younger patients)
2. Pathogenesis of infection (extension from sinusitis) predicts causative pathogens. It may be polymicrobial.
   a. *Streptococcus pneumoniae*
   b. Nontypable *Haemophilus influenzae*
   c. *Moraxella catarrhalis*
   d. *Staphylococcus aureus*
   e. *Streptococcus pyogenes*
   f. Anaerobes: *Peptostreptococcus*, *Bacteroides*, *Fusobacterium*

Associated Clinical Features

1. Orbital cellulitis usually follows sinusitis; thus it is seen more often in older children than younger children (mean age: about 12 years). In contrast, preseptal cellulitis is commonly seen in younger children (average age: around 2 years).
2. Leukocytosis is usually present. Blood, nasal, and nasopharyngeal cultures are usually negative or noncontributory. Gram's stain and culture (aerobic, anaerobic) of aspirated material either from the sinuses or from the surgically drained abscess also helps in determining the cause.
3. Patients with suspected orbital cellulitis should receive an orbital contrast-enhanced CT scan.
   a. To confirm the diagnosis and assess the spread of infection, see the modified Chandler staging system (Box 8-15). CT scan identifies proptosis, soft tissue swelling, subperiosteal abscess, retrobulbar abscess, and sinusitis.
   b. Contrast-enhanced study is superior to a nonenhanced study in differentiating true abscess from phlegmon formation (which is not amenable to surgical drainage).
4. Other tests include blood cultures (though their utility is limited) and culture of purulent nasal drainage, if present. Lumbar puncture is indicated in the setting of meningeal signs.

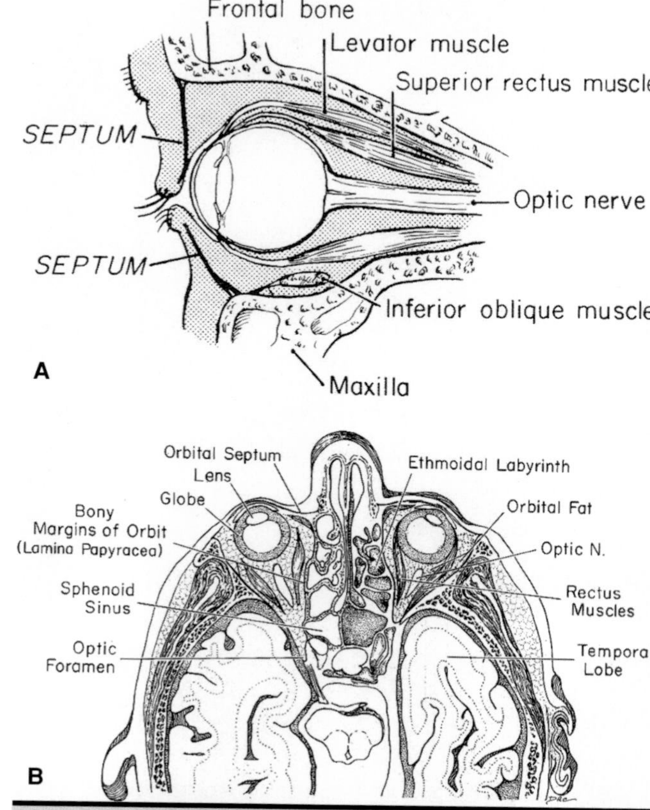

Figure 8-13. Orbital Anatomy

A. Sagittal view of the orbit, illustrating the position of the orbital septum. The orbital septum is an extension of the orbital periosteum to the tarsal plate in both upper and lower eyelids and acts as a physical barrier to preseptal infection, thus preventing spread of infection to the orbital contents. (Reproduced with permission from: Smith TF, O'Day D, Wright PF: Clinical implications of preseptal cellulitis in childhood. *Pediatrics* 1978;62:1007.) *B.* Schematic drawing of structures important in CT evaluation of preseptal and orbital cellulitis. The orbit is bordered on three sides by sinuses (floor of the frontal sinus, lateral wall of the ethmoid sinus, and roof of the maxillary sinus), and thus is susceptible to contiguous infection. The orbital cavity is separated from the ethmoid air cells by the orbital bone lamina papyracea (paperlike layer). Congenital bony dehiscence is commonly found in the lamina, through which sinus infection can easily spread into the orbit. (Reproduced and modified with permission from: Goldberg F, Berne AS, Oski FA: Differentiation of orbital cellulitis from preseptal cellulitis by computed tomography. *Pediatrics* 1978;62:1001.)

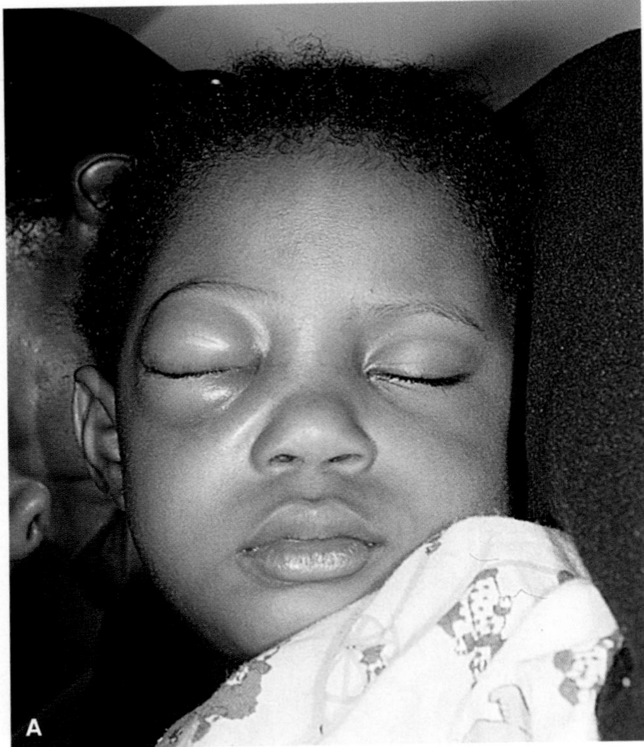

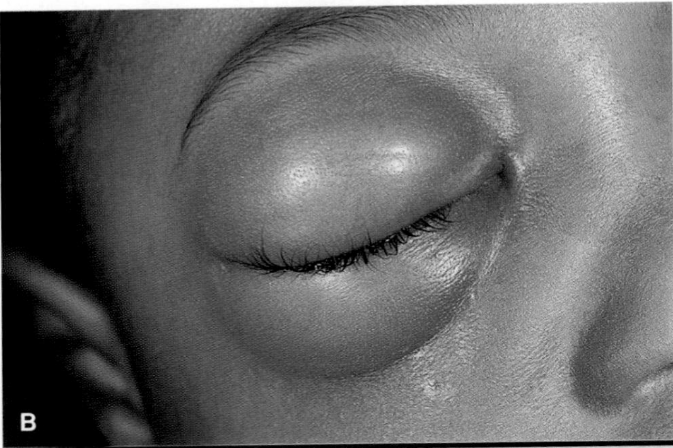

Figure 8-14. Orbital Cellulitis

A. Unilateral eye involvement with marked swelling of both upper and lower eyelids with intense erythema (*B*), and proptosis are seen in this highly febrile child. He required surgical drainage of a subperiosteal abscess that grew *S. aureus*. Axial CT scan at the level of the sinuses and orbit showed complete opacification of the maxillary and ethmoid sinuses on the right side.

5. Orbital complications from orbital cellulitis include subperiosteal and orbital abscess, endophthalmitis, septic uveitis, retinitis, exudative retinal detachment and optic neuropathy, and secondary glaucoma.
6. Intracranial complications of orbital cellulitis include meningitis, brain abscess, epidural or subdural empyema, and cavernous sinus thrombosis.

Consultations

Emergent ophthalmology evaluation, otolaryngology evaluation (if orbital cellulitis arises from sinus involvement), infectious disease, and neurosurgical evaluation (if intracranial involvement is suspected)

Emergency Department Treatment and Disposition

1. Patients with orbital cellulitis must be admitted to the hospital for intravenous antibiotics and close monitoring. Patients should receive broad-spectrum IV antibiotics as soon as possible to cover organisms implicated in sinusitis as well as superficial soft tissue infection:
   a. A third-generation cephalosporin (e.g., ceftriaxone sodium or cefotaxime) and oxacillin are good initial choices.
   b. Metronidazole or clindamycin is added when anaerobic infection is suspected.
   c. The antibiotic coverage may be narrowed following culture and sensitivity results from surgical specimen or blood.
   d. Patient is very closely reevaluated daily with assessments of visual acuity, pupillary reaction, extraocular motility, and color vision.
   e. Mean hospital stay is between 10 and 14 days. Depending on the clinical response, parenteral therapy is given for at least 7 to 10 days followed by oral therapy (usually two to three times the usual regimen) to complete a total of 3 weeks.
2. Nasal decongestant therapy and warm compresses may also help.
3. The decision to perform decompressive surgery depends on a number of factors. Selected patients with subperiosteal abscess may be followed very closely with IV antibiotic therapy. However, patients with diminishment of visual acuity, development of an afferent pupillary defect, frontal sinusitis, intracranial complications, or those showing a lack of response to IV antibiotics within 72 hours must undergo emergent drainage (Fig. 8-15).

Clinical Pearls: Orbital Cellulitis

1. Orbital cellulitis is a vision-threatening and life-threatening infection whose clinical course advances rapidly.
2. The cardinal symptoms are proptosis, decreased vision, and decreased ocular motility.
3. Malignancies like neuroblastoma, rhabdomyosarcoma, and retinoblastoma need to be distinguished from orbital cellulitis. Orbital imaging must be obtained in all patients with clinical suspicion of orbital cellulitis.
4. Uncomplicated sinusitis may result in periorbital edema, which is differentiated from cellulitis by absence of soft tissue induration or tenderness.

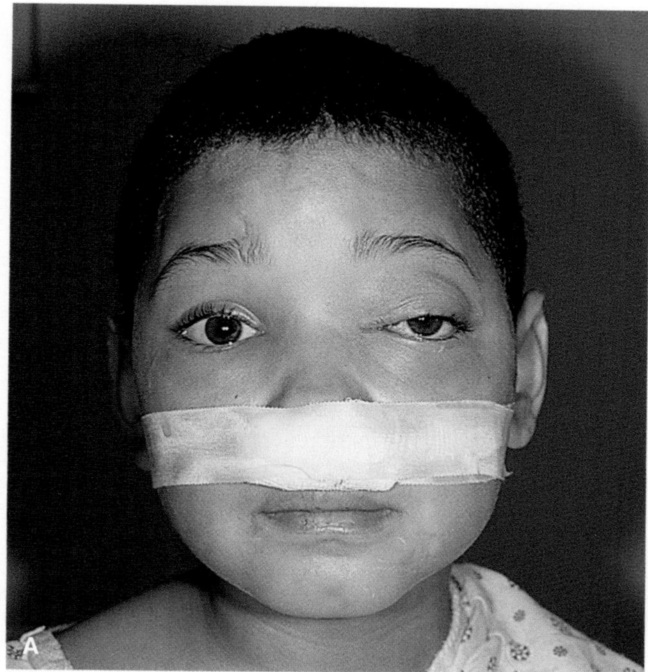

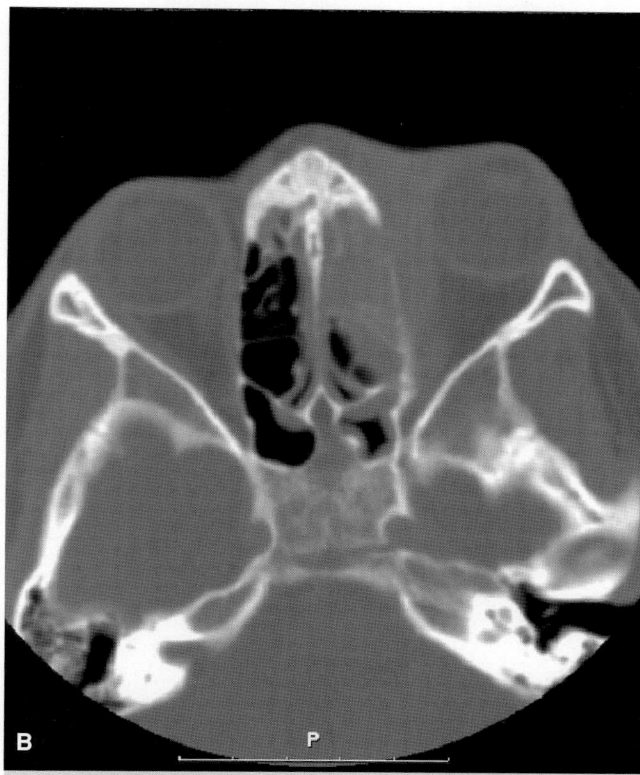

Figure 8-15. Orbital Cellulitis Secondary to Sinusitis

Unilateral eye involvement with proptosis (outward and inferior displacement of the globe) and impaired extraocular movements were seen this 8-year-old child. He also had exquisite tenderness over the ethmoid and maxillary sinuses. This picture was taken on the second day after he underwent surgical drainage. *B*. An axial CT scan of the orbit (bone windows) shows an erosion of the left lamina papyracea with soft tissue in the ethmoid sinus and orbit. A proptosis of the left orbit is also seen (see also Fig. 9-5).

BOX 8-14. CLINICAL FEATURES OF ORBITAL CELLULITIS

- Almost always unilateral
- Proptosis
- Tender and swollen eyelid
- Chemosis
- Ocular and retro-orbital pain or orbital discomfort
- Resistance to retropulsion of the globe
- Limitation of spontaneous extraocular movement or painful extraocular movements
- Systemic signs (fever, septic appearance, headache) more likely than with preseptal cellulitis
- Elevated intraocular pressure
- A dilated pupil or afferent pupillary defect (signals compression of the optic nerve)
- Complete or partial loss of vision or double vision
- Papilledema, vomiting, severe headache, or meningeal signs may signal intracranial spread to meninges or cavernous sinus.

BOX 8-15. MODIFIED CHANDLER STAGING SYSTEM FOR ORBITAL CELLULITIS

- Stage I: preseptal cellulitis
- Stage II: inflammatory orbital edema
- Stage III: subperiosteal abscess
- Stage IV: orbital abscess
- Stage V: cavernous sinus thrombosis

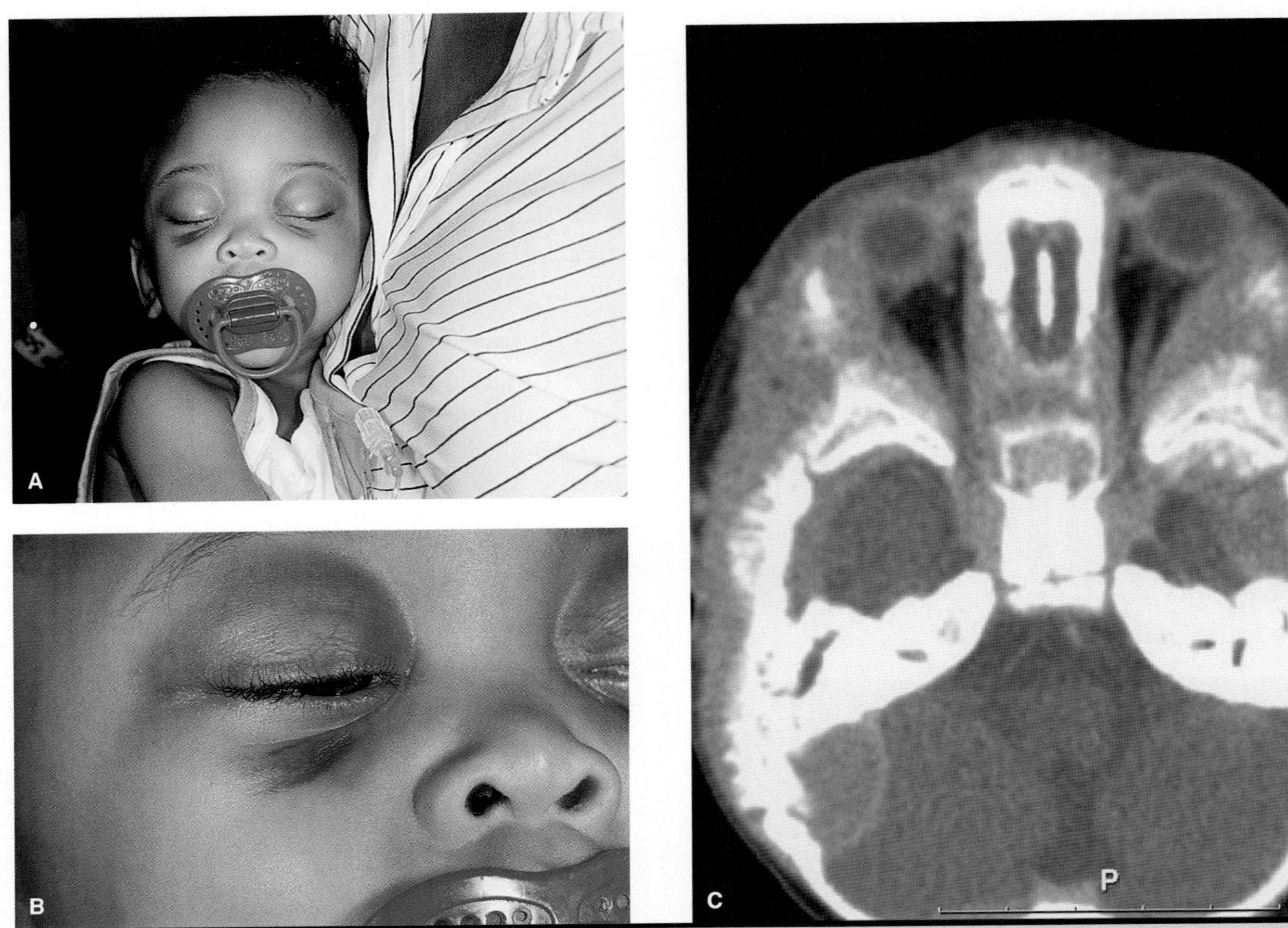

Figure 8-16. Metastatic Neuroblastoma: Differential Diagnosis of Proptosis

A. An 11-month-old infant presented with bilateral raccoon eyes and orbital proptosis. *B*. Close-up showing periorbital ecchymosis. Rapid onset of painless proptosis and periorbital ecchymosis in a young infant are common presenting signs of metastatic neuroblastoma. Neuroblastoma is the most common tumor to metastasize to the orbit in childhood. About 20% of patients with neuroblastoma develop orbital metastasis. Primary sites are either in the abdomen (e.g., adrenal medulla or paraspinal ganglia) or sympathetic chains at other sites (e.g., mediastinum). Other findings include Horner's syndrome and increased urinary vanillylmandelic acid (VMA) and homovanillic acid (HVA). *C*. Aggressive bony erosion and periosteal reaction are seen involving the orbits and temporal bone. Abnormally enhancing soft tissue masses in the extraconal spaces are also seen bilaterally with the epidural enhancing masses. These findings are consistent with metastatic neuroblastoma.

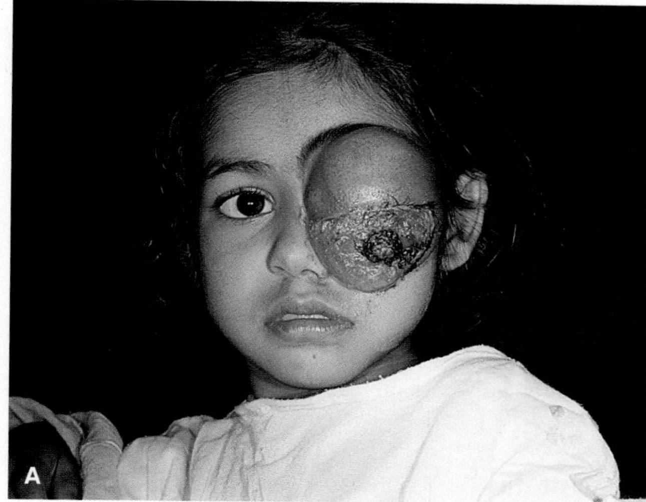

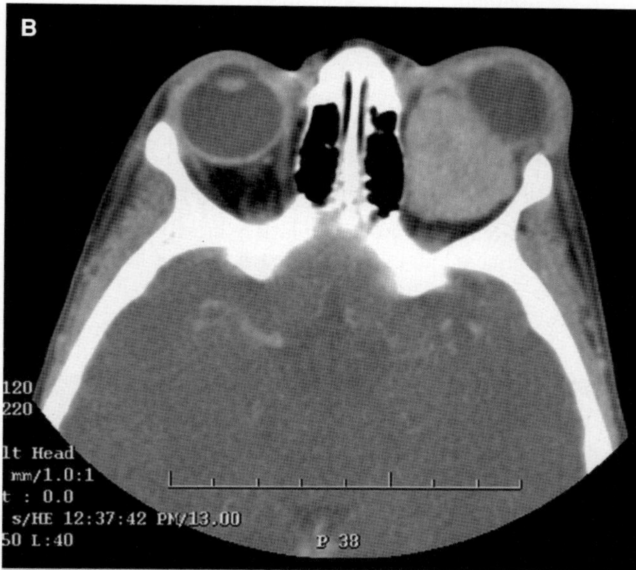

Figure 8-17. Rhabdomyosarcoma: Differential Diagnosis of Proptosis

A rapidly growing orbital mass was the complaint of this 7-year-old girl. Common physical findings of rhabdomyosarcoma are painless proptosis, inferior displacement of the globe, and edema and erythema of the lids. Median age at presentation is 7 to 8 years. *B*. Postcontrast CT through the orbits reveals a large enhancing intraconal soft tissue mass posterior to the left globe causing proptosis of the left eye. No evidence of extraorbital invasion is seen.

BOX 8-16. DIFFERENTIAL DIAGNOSIS OF ORBITAL CELLULITIS

- Preseptal cellulitis (Figs. 8-9 to 8-12)
- Allergic reaction
- Dysthyroid exophthalmos
- Intraocular tumor
- Metastatic tumor to orbit (e.g., neuroblastoma; Fig. 8-16)
- Sarcoidosis
- Cavernous sinus thrombosis
- Ruptured dermoid cyst
- Rhabdomyosarcoma (Fig. 8-17)
- Orbital vasculitis
- Dacryoadenitis
- Dacryocystitis
- Conjunctivitis

DIAGNOSIS LEUKOCORIA

Synonym

White pupillary reflex

Definition and Etiology

1. Leukocoria is a white discoloration of the pupil, typically noted during direct ophthalmoscopic examination in a darkened room.
2. It is an abnormal pupillary reflex and indicates an opacity at or behind the pupil. It may result from pathology anywhere in the eye, though typically it results from retinal or corneal pathology.

Associated Clinical Features

1. The presence of bilateral red reflexes suggests the absence of cataracts and intraocular pathology (Fig. 8-18).
2. Leukocoria is commonly brought to the attention of the physician by parents after a flash photograph reveals asymmetric pupillary color.
3. The most concerning suggested diagnosis in a pediatric patient is retinoblastoma, a malignancy thought to arise from retinal germ cells (Figs. 8-19 and 8-20).
4. Rapid pupillary constriction of a pupil that has not been chemically dilated may mask the diagnosis of leukocoria. For this reason, some pediatricians recommend routine exams with pupillary dilation in the first year of life.

Consultation

Emergent ophthalmology consultation

Emergency Department Treatment and Disposition

1. Patients noted to have leukocoria should receive emergent ophthalmologic consultation and hospital admission.
2. While untreated retinoblastoma is almost uniformly fatal, with treatment, cure rates can reach 90% or better.

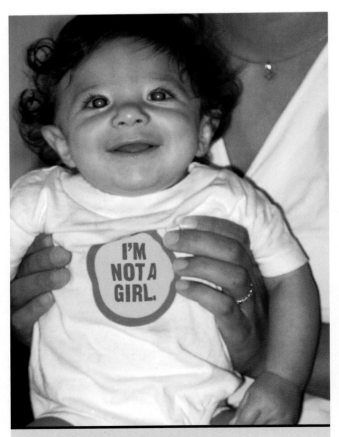

Figure 8-18. Normal Red Reflexes.

The presence of bilateral red reflexes suggests the absence of cataracts and intraocular pathology. Courtesy of Aden Benjamin Spektor and his parents.

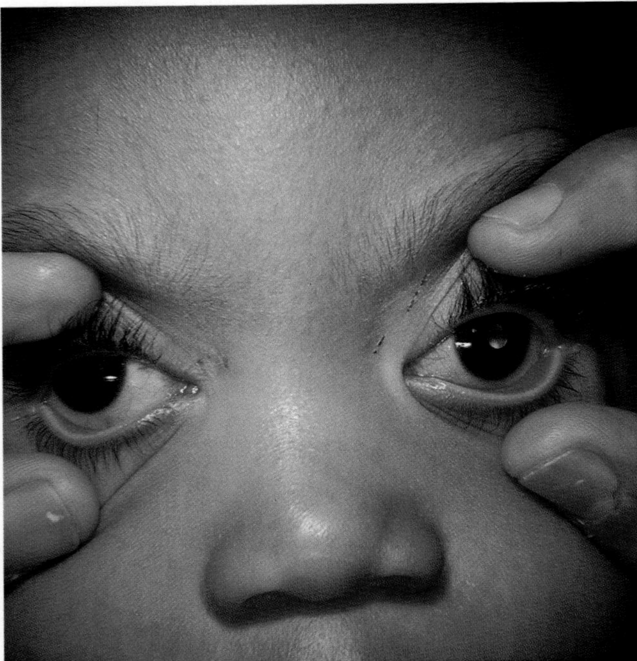

Figure 8-19. Leukocoria in Retinoblastoma

An 18-month-old child presenting with white pupil.

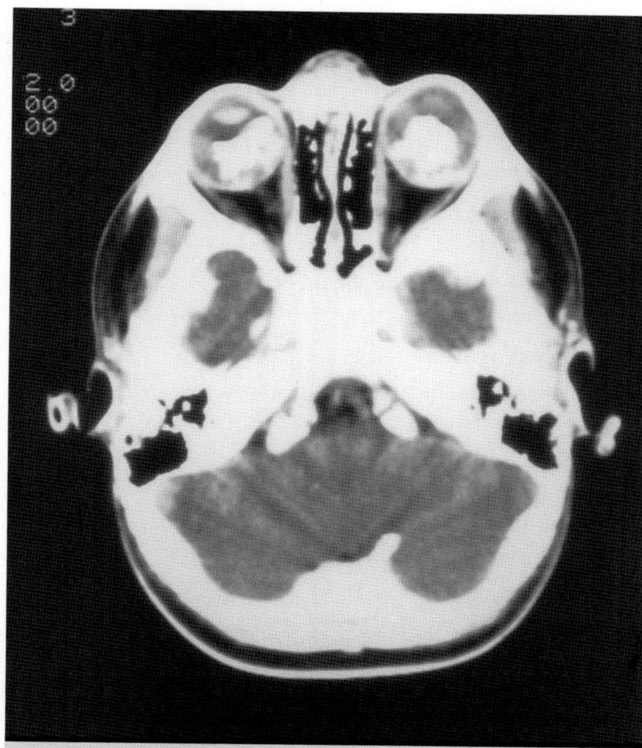

Figure 8-20. Bilateral Retinoblastoma

Axial CT scan of the head. Soft tissue window demonstrates bilateral large calcified intraorbital masses in a patient with bilateral retinoblastoma. (Reproduced with permission from: Shah BR, Laude TL: Retinoblastoma. In: *Atlas of Pediatric Clinical Diagnosis*. WB Saunders, Philadelphia, 2000, p. 146.)

Clinical Pearls: Leukocoria

1. Leukocoria is defined as white pupil and indicates an opacity at or behind the pupil.
2. Leukocoria is a marker of underlying pathology that should be evaluated promptly by an ophthalmologist.
3. The diagnosis of leukocoria might be obscured by rapid pupillary constriction with direct illumination of the eye.
4. The most common presenting signs of retinoblastoma are leukocoria and strabismus.

BOX 8-17. DIFFERENTIAL DIAGNOSIS OF LEUKOCORIA

- Retinoblastoma
- Coats' disease (exudative retinopathy)
- Cataract (Fig. 8-21)
- Corneal opacity
- Vitreous hemorrhage (e.g., leukemia)
- Endophthalmitis
- Ocular larva migrans (*Toxocara canis*)
- Toxoplasmosis
- Uveitis
- Phakomatosis
- Persistent hyperplastic primary vitreous
- Retinopathy of prematurity
- Congenital retinal folds
- Retinal coloboma
- Retinal detachment
- Retinal dysplasia
- Hematoma
- Hemangioma
- Medulloepithelioma

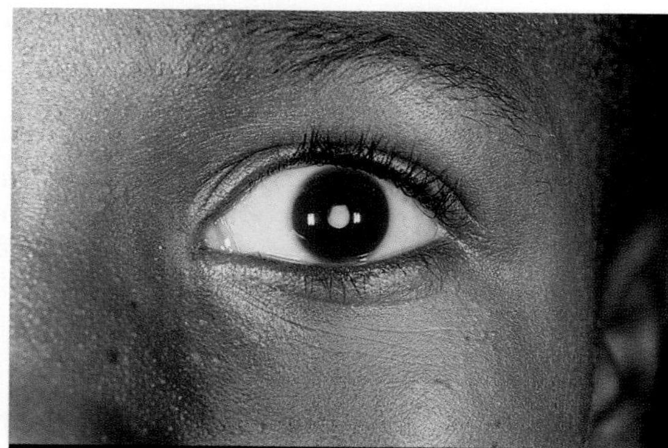

Figure 8-21. Cataract: Differential Diagnosis of Leukocoria

BOX 8-18. CLINICAL FEATURES OF RETINOBLASTOMA

- Most common ocular malignancy in children
- Average age at diagnosis: 18 months
- Arises from stem cells of retina
- Inheritance patterns
  (1) Hereditary (30 to 40%)
  Hereditary and bilateral (25%)
  Hereditary and unilateral (15%)
  (2) Nonhereditary (sporadic) and unilateral (60%)
  Chromosomal deletion (6%)
  95% of patients with retinoblastoma have no family history of ocular tumors.
- Clinical features at presentation include:
  (1) Leukocoria (60% of cases)
  (2) Strabismus (20% of cases)
  (3) Proptosis (a late finding)
  (4) Retinal detachment
- Other signs include, glaucoma, hyphema, hypopyon, vitreous hemorrhage, and preseptal cellulitis.
- Funduscopy and slitlamp examination with pupillary dilation should be done to exclude cataract.
- A complete blood count should be sent to exclude bone marrow involvement.
- Radiography: (detection of calcifications)
  (1) Computed tomography of the orbit
  (2) Ultrasonography
- Treatment options
  (1) Radiation
  (2) Chemotherapy
  (3) Surgery for refractory cases

DIAGNOSIS CORNEAL ABRASION

Definition

A superficial abrasion of the cornea or sclera that does not penetrate Bowman's membrane

Etiology

Corneal abrasions may result from mechanical disruption of the superficial cornea by a foreign body (FB) or other irritant such as dust, ultraviolet radiation, chemical caustic, or improper use of contact lenses.

Associated Clinical Features

1. The history usually suggests a mechanism, though occasionally patients will present without a clear inciting cause.
   a. Direct trauma by finger or other FB
   b. Contact lens trauma
   c. Ultraviolet light exposure (e.g., snow blindness)
   d. Wind injury (generally caused by dust or other fine particulate matter)
   e. Atraumatic recurrence of an old corneal abrasion
2. Diagnosis rests on demonstrating fluorescein uptake.
   a. Fluorescein should be instilled in the inferior fornix and the patient's eye examined with blue light, ideally with a slitlamp or magnifying loupe.
   b. A corneal epithelial defect will fluoresce under blue light. The size, shape, and location of the abrasion must be documented (Fig. 8-22).
   c. A dendritic pattern of fluorescence is suggestive of herpes simplex virus keratoconjunctivitis.
   d. Suspect the presence of a retained FB under the upper or lower lid with a staining pattern with one or more vertical linear abrasions.
   e. Fluid flowing out of an area of fluorescein uptake (Seidel's sign) should alert one to the possibility of globe rupture and leaking aqueous humor.
3. The lid must be everted to rule out FB (especially if fluorescein staining demonstrates a linear vertical pattern).

Consultation

Emergency ophthalmology consultation if there is concern for globe rupture or concern for penetration into deeper corneal tissues

Emergency Department Treatment and Disposition

1. A topical ocular anesthetic may help in both diagnosis and therapy. Pain limited to a corneal abrasion should resolve

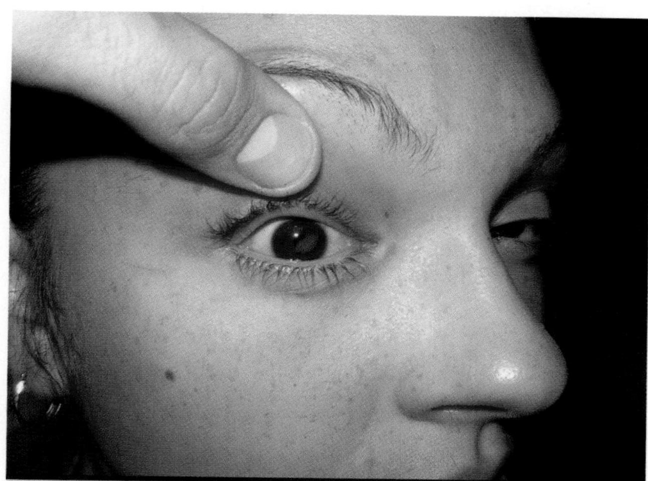

Figure 8-22. Corneal Abrasion

Fluorescein is instilled in the inferior fornix and the patient's eye is examined with blue light, ideally with a slitlamp or magnifying loupe. A corneal epithelial defect fluoresces under blue light. (*Important:* When using impregnated strips, wet the strip before instillation; otherwise the strip itself may cause corneal abrasion.)

with a topical ocular anesthetic. If pain persists, consider other etiologies such as traumatic iritis or uveitis.

2. While a topical anesthetic is effective, prolonged use delays epithelial healing and should be avoided outside the acute setting (i.e., ED or physician's office).
3. Use of an eye patch
   a. Patching is *not* recommended routinely for corneal abrasions.
   b. *Do not use a patch in a patient who wears contact lenses.*
   c. Patching does not promote re-epithelialization, and there is no significant difference in rate of healing or reduction of pain in patients treated with or without patching.
   d. Patching prevents blinking and keeps children from putting their fingers into their eyes (thus patching may provide comfort). However, use of a patch should be limited (do not use for longer than 24 hours to avoid developing infection), and all such cases need evaluation by an ophthalmologist.
   e. In patients with considerable photophobia, a patch (pressure patch) and topical cycloplegics may minimize discomfort from ciliary spasm.
4. Patients may be safely discharged home with topical antibiotic ointment (e.g., bacitracin or erythromycin). Do not use ointments containing steroids or neomycin.
5. The practice of using routine tetanus prophylaxis for uncomplicated corneal abrasions has been challenged (a tetanus booster may be given as necessary).
6. Significant oral analgesia is often required.
7. Cool compresses will minimize corneal edema.
8. Any patient with a prior history of ocular herpes presenting with a staining corneal defect should be seen by an ophthalmologist emergently.
9. Any patient with a history of contact lens wear presenting with a staining corneal defect should be seen by an ophthalmologist emergently and the contact lens should be removed. Bacterial corneal infection needs to be excluded in such patients.
10. Routine corneal abrasions may be referred to an ophthalmologist for outpatient evaluation.
    a. Patients need to be re-examined in 24 hours and restained with fluorescein to ensure that the epithelial defect is improving.
    b. Corneal abrasions generally heal well after 24 to 48 hours, but may progress to form an ulcer (see Fig. 8-23) or abscess.
    c. Healing time is longer for larger abrasions, but there should be daily improvement of symptoms (e.g., decreasing redness and pain, improving vision). If symptoms do not improve daily, an infection must be ruled out.
    d. Deep injuries may leave permanent scars.
    e. Abrasions caused by vegetable matter may cause fungal keratitis.
    f. Abrasions resulting from contact lens trauma may develop pseudomonal keratitis.
11. A retained foreign body must be aggressively excluded (e.g., by rechecking beneath the upper eyelid), especially if the abrasion does not appear to be healing.

Clinical Pearls: Corneal Abrasion

1. Pain and FB sensation are the cardinal symptoms of corneal abrasion.
2. Infants with corneal abrasions present with excessive crying.
3. *Topical anesthetic should never be dispensed to any patient for continued use.*
4. Corneal abrasion is a relatively minor eye injury that can lead to more serious consequences if mistreated. All patients with corneal abrasions need topical antibiotics and close follow-up.
5. Exclude other injuries such as globe rupture or traumatic iritis.
6. Symptoms of corneal abrasion (pain, tearing, and photophobia) mimic uveitis. Topical anesthetic will cause immediate relief of pain in corneal abrasion, while pain due to uveitis will persist. Such patients need immediate referral to an ophthalmologist.
7. Pseudomonal infections occur commonly following patching of corneal abrasions in patients who wear contact lenses. *Do not use patches in patients who wear contact lenses.*

BOX 8-19. CLINICAL FEATURES OF CORNEAL ABRASION

- Severe pain
- Excessive crying in infants
- Tearing
- Photophobia
- Foreign body sensation (even in the absence of a FB)
- Blepharospasm
- Blurred vision (if corneal defect large or lies in the visual axis)
- Fluorescein uptake

BOX 8-20. DIFFERENTIAL DIAGNOSIS OF CORNEAL ABRASION

- Uveitis
- Ultraviolet keratitis
- Iritis
- Corneal foreign body
- Conjunctivitis
- Corneal ulcer
- Herpetic keratoconjunctivitis
- Penetrating globe injury
- Trichiasis
  (1) Misdirection of eyelashes toward the globe
  (2) Frequently caused by epiblepharon in children

BOX 8-24. CLINICAL FEATURES OF SUBCONJUNCTIVAL HEMORRHAGE

- Subconjunctival hemorrhage in patients with minor trauma (without severe globe injury) or Valsalva maneuvers
  - (1) Bright or dark red patch of scleral blood
  - (2) Does not obscure iris
  - (3) May be patchy or continuous
  - (4) May be associated with chemosis
  - (5) Distinctive and somewhat alarming appearance to patients
  - (6) Patch may spread and change color over time (as blood pigments break down)
  - (7) Usually spontaneously resolves in 2 weeks
- Exclude severe injury to the globe in patients presenting with subconjunctival hemorrhage associated with any of the following
  - (1) Severe eye pain
  - (2) Photophobia
  - (3) Decreased visual acuity
  - (4) Extension of the hemorrhage beyond the limbus

BOX 8-25. ETIOLOGY AND DIFFERENTIAL DIAGNOSIS OF SUBCONJUNCTIVAL HEMORRHAGE

- Trauma to the eye
- Conjunctivitis (e.g., adenovirus, *Haemophilus influenzae*)
- Chemical irritation
- Bleeding disorders/coagulopathy
- Anticoagulant medications
- Hypertension
- Diabetes mellitus
- Conditions that increase venous pressure
  - (1) Chest trauma (increased intrathoracic pressure)
  - (2) Forceful vomiting
  - (3) Coughing
  - (4) Valsalva
  - (5) Strangulation

DIAGNOSIS HYPHEMA

Definition and Etiology

A hyphema is a layering meniscus of blood in the anterior chamber of the eye between the cornea and iris (Figs. 8-26 and 8-27). A hyphema is generally caused by trauma (blunt or penetrating injury) to the globe with subsequent hemorrhage from the vessels of the anterior chamber structures.

Associated Clinical Features

1. Penlight examination will show larger hyphemas, while smaller hyphemas and microhyphemas will require slitlamp examination.
2. A diffuse hyphema occurs when blood cells are still suspended in the anterior chamber and have not yet settled to form a meniscus.
3. Blood clot in the anterior chamber may occlude the trabecular meshwork and lead to glaucoma. This is more common after a complete hyphema or after a rebleed.
4. Hyphema-related optic neuropathy is seen in patients with sickle cell hemoglobinopathy (SS, S-thalassemia, or SC disease). Thus, a sickle cell preparation or hemoglobin electrophoresis should be performed in all patients who are at risk for having sickle cell hemoglobinopathy (e.g., African-Americans or those of Mediterranean descent).
5. Complete blood count, platelet count, bleeding time, prothrombin time, and partial thromboplastin time should be done for patients with nontraumatic hyphema.
6. Non-Caucasian patients should be screened for sickle cell hemoglobinopathy. Sickle cell disease is an uncommon cause of hyphema, and its presence may lead to more complications or alter the treatment plan.
7. Rebleeding occurs as a complication of hyphema:
   a. Typically seen within 3 to 5 days after the initial hemorrhage
   b. Seen in approximately 30% of patients
   c. It is believed to result from clot degradation and retraction
   d. Rebleeds are usually more severe than the initial bleed and generally leave the patient with a permanent degradation of visual acuity.
8. Patients with small hyphemas generally do well. The chance of recovering visual acuity of 20/50 or better is 75 to 90% with grade I hyphemas, 65 to 70% with grade II hyphemas, and 25 to 50% with grade III and IV hyphemas.

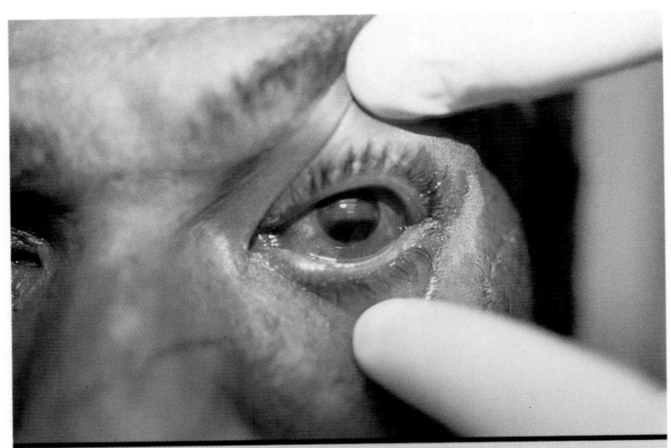

Figure 8-26. Hyphema

Blood filling almost one-half of the anterior chamber following blunt trauma.

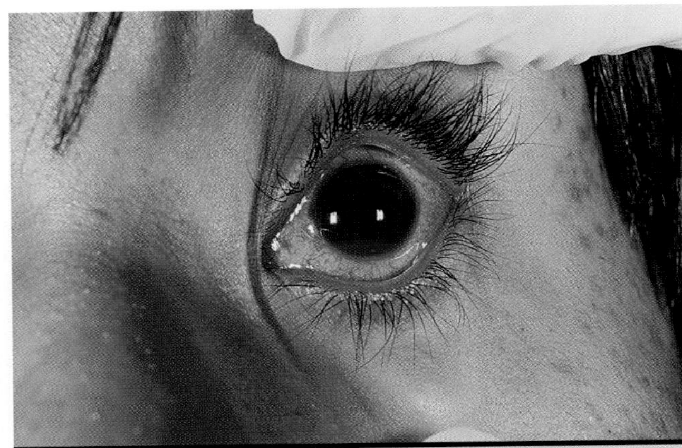

Figure 8-27. Hyphema

Blood filling less than one-third of the anterior chamber following blunt trauma.

Consultation

Emergent ophthalmology consultation

Emergency Department Treatment and Disposition

1. Patients with hyphema have undergone a significant globe injury and should be evaluated for other eye injuries such as corneal abrasions and globe rupture. This evaluation should be carried out promptly by a consultant in the ED.
2. There is considerable controversy regarding management of hyphemas, including hospitalization, bed rest, topical and systemic medications, and surgical intervention. The goals of management include rapid resolution of hyphemas, patient comfort, and prevention of secondary complications.
3. Elevate the head of the bed to promote settling and reabsorption of the clot.
4. Prevention of posttraumatic glaucoma is of paramount concern; patients should have their intraocular pressure (IOP) measured, and every effort should be made to protect the eye from further trauma. In children this may entail rigid shielding.
5. In patients with normal IOP, activity should be limited for 72 hours to prevent rebleeding. In children, hospital admission is the best method to ensure this in most cases. Rapid eye movements should be discouraged, such as those that occur when reading or playing video games.
6. Patients with elevated IOP should be treated with ocular antihypertensives:
    a. Topical beta-blockers
    b. Topical cycloplegics (e.g., homatropine) dilate the pupil and relax the injured ciliary body.
    c. Topical steroids decrease intraocular inflammation and prevent the formation of synechiae in the angle of the anterior chamber.
    d. Avoid carbonic anhydrase inhibitors (e.g., acetazolamide) in patients with sickle cell disease.
7. Aminocaproic acid is an antifibrinolytic agent that reduces rebleeding by preventing lysis of the initial clot until the injured vessels heal.
8. Patients who do not respond to topical measures may require surgical drainage.
9. Avoid aspirin and NSAIDs that may inhibit platelet activity.

Clinical Pearls: Hyphema

1. Hyphema is a layering of blood in the anterior chamber generally caused by trauma.
2. Since a hyphema indicates severe eye trauma, concurrent injuries to the retina or other ocular tissues must be excluded. Thus, all patients who present with hyphema *must be seen* by an ophthalmologist.
3. The most important complications of hyphema include late rebleeding into the anterior chamber, increased IOP, and corneal blood staining.
4. The presence of hyphema in the absence of trauma should prompt an investigation for underlying disease (e.g., leukemia or coagulopathy).
5. Hyphema can lead to posttraumatic glaucoma.

BOX 8-26. CLINICAL FEATURES OF HYPHEMA

- Varying degrees of pain
- Red meniscus layering in anterior chamber
- Blurred vision
- History of trauma
- Microhyphema
  (1) No blood seen on gross examination
  (2) Suspended RBCs seen on slitlamp examination
- Grades of hyphema
  (1) Grade 1: blood filling less than one-third of the anterior chamber
  (2) Grade 2: blood filling one-third to less than one-half of the anterior chamber
  (3) Grade 3: blood filling one-half to less than the total space of the anterior chamber
  (4) Grade 4: Total hyphema ("eight-ball" or "blackball" hyphema) blood filling the entire anterior chamber

BOX 8-27. ETIOLOGY AND DIFFERENTIAL DIAGNOSIS OF HYPHEMA

- Trauma (either blunt or penetrating)
- Nontraumatic (spontaneous hyphemas)
  (1) Sickle cell disease
  (2) Leukemia
  (3) Retinoblastoma (rarely may be a presenting symptom)
  (4) Hemophilia/bleeding disorder
  (5) Iris tumors (e.g., juvenile xanthogranuloma)
  (6) Severe iritis
  (7) Iris neovascularization (e.g., intraocular tumors, diabetes)

DIAGNOSIS CORNEAL FOREIGN BODY

Definition

A foreign object embedded in the eye, generally in the cornea

Etiology

1. Metal (frequently from grinding or welding without adequate eye protection)
2. Glass
   a. Proximity to breaking glass
   b. Glass foreign bodies are particularly difficult to detect.
3. Organic material (e.g., wood)
4. Dust or other inorganic matter blown by the wind

Associated Clinical Features

1. A foreign body (FB) may be visible on direct examination or slitlamp examination. The corneal epithelial defect will stain yellow with fluorescein.
2. Foreign bodies propelled with some velocity may penetrate the cornea and lodge in deeper structures. These may damage the iris, lens, or retina, and may lead to endophthalmitis.
3. Penetrating globe injury should be suspected with a suggestive history or the following findings:
   a. Irregular pupil
   b. Prolapsed iris
   c. Reduced intraocular pressure
   d. Hyphema
   e. Lens opacification
4. Suspicion of intraocular FBs requires imaging and ophthalmologic consultation.
   a. Plain films may localize metallic FBs.
   b. CT of the orbits is a superior test and may also demonstrate radiolucent FBs such as wood and glass.
   c. Ultrasound (B-mode ultrasound, ultrasound biomicroscopy) may also be used to localize a FB in the globe or sclera and may aid in detecting retinal and choroidal detachments.

d. MRI is potentially useful, though strictly contraindicated if there is any suspicion of a metallic FB.

5. Corneal FBs may lead to infection or scarring. Metal FBs may develop a rust ring within hours. This may be removed acutely or on follow-up (Fig. 8-28).

Consultation

Emergent ophthalmology consultation if there is any suspicion of globe rupture

Emergency Department Treatment and Disposition

1. Simple FBs may be treated by nonophthalmologists.
2. Locating the FB may be challenging if none is immediately apparent.
   a. The corneal epithelial defect will stain yellow with fluorescein.
   b. The upper lid must be everted to find a FB located underneath the lid.
   c. A moist cotton swab should be wiped over the complete undersurface of the upper lid to localize FBs in the fornix that may be beyond the area exposed by lid eversion. Care should be taken to avoid swabbing the cornea itself, since this will cause an abrasion and compound the problem.
   d. Multiple FBs may be present.
3. Once located, corneal FBs may be removed by a number of methods, provided the patient is cooperative.
   a. Topical anesthetic is instilled on the lower palpebral conjunctiva.
   b. Superficial FBs may be irrigated off the conjunctival surface with a syringe and then picked off the inferior fornix or palpebral conjunctiva with the dab of a moistened cotton swab.
   c. A narrow-gauge needle (held tangentially across the globe) or a rotary spud may be used to remove embedded objects
      1) This should be done with magnifying loupes or under slitlamp examination.
      2) The supervening corneal epithelium is gently picked off and the FB exposed and then irrigated off.
      3) Care must be taken to avoid creating unnecessarily large epithelial defects or penetrating the anterior chamber.
   d. Rust ring removal
      1) Metal FBs will oxidize to produce a rust ring within hours.
      2) This ring may be removed en bloc by gently shaving it off the cornea with a rotary spud or a fine needle.
4. In young children or uncooperative patients, an ophthalmologist should be consulted.
5. Tetanus immunization should be updated.
6. Topical antibiotic drops should be used as prophylaxis to prevent infectious keratitis.
7. Pain medicine: these patients have significant requirements for analgesia.
8. Follow-up should be arranged with an ophthalmologist to ensure proper corneal healing.

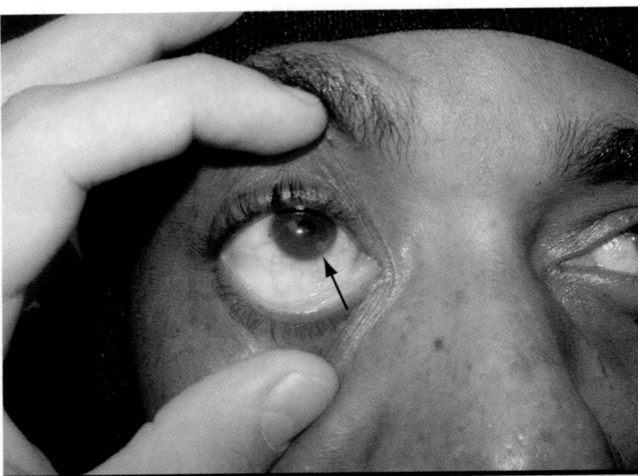

Figure 8-28. Rust Ring; Corneal Foreign Body

This patient, who was working as welder, accidentally got a piece of metal in his eye a few days ago. He had a FB sensation and burning pain but figured it would go away. When it did not, he came to the ED. The piece of metal had already fallen out, but a little "pit", where the metal was imbedded, is seen. A rust colored ring surrounding it and a white ring of edema around it is also seen.

Clinical Pearls: Corneal Foreign Body

1. Evaluation of ocular FBs must ensure that the deeper structures of the eye are unaffected.
2. If there is an appropriate mechanism or clinical findings suggestive of deeper penetration, the patient should be evaluated with imaging modalities and evaluated by an ophthalmologist.

BOX 8-28. CLINICAL FEATURES OF CORNEAL FOREIGN BODY

- Pain
- Photophobia
- Tearing
- Foreign body sensation
- Blurred vision (variable; depending on location of foreign body and the depth of penetration)
- Visible foreign body
- Irregular pupil
  (1) Represents a deeper injury with distortion of the normal ocular architecture
  (2) An apparent FB in this setting may actually be a prolapsed iris

BOX 8-29. DIFFERENTIAL DIAGNOSIS OF CORNEAL FOREIGN BODY

- Corneal abrasion
- Corneal ulceration
- Glaucoma
- HSV keratitis
- Other infection

DIAGNOSIS TRAUMATIC GLOBE RUPTURE

Definition

Traumatic globe rupture is a disruption of the ocular architecture from blunt or penetrating forces that creates a fissure or tear in the cornea and/or sclera, allowing potential communication of the globe contents with the environment.

Etiology

1. Even though the globe is protected by the bony orbit, direct trauma to the eye may cause rupture.
2. In blunt trauma, compressive forces may tear the sclera at its weak points (usually the corneoscleral junction or insertion of extraocular muscles).
3. In penetrating trauma, perforation of the cornea by a missile or foreign body (FB) such as glass may invade deeper structures.

Associated Clinical Features

1. Injuries can be divided into anterior segment trauma (injuries to the cornea, anterior chamber, iris, and lens) and posterior segment trauma (perforation of the sclera, retina, and vitreous).
2. Orbital fractures
   a. Extraocular movements may be compromised in the setting of orbital wall fracture and subsequent entrapment of extraocular muscles.
   b. Bony fragments may penetrate the globe in severe injuries.
3. Diagnosis is generally made clinically from examination findings, but may be facilitated with imaging techniques if indicated.
   a. A CT scan with fine cuts through the orbits may detect occult rupture.
   b. In the setting of penetrating trauma, a retained FB should be suspected and CT scan is useful.

Consultation

Emergent ophthalmology consult (must see these patients in the ED)

Emergency Department Treatment and Disposition

1. Suspicion of globe rupture requires the immediate attention of an ophthalmologist.
2. The patient with globe rupture will need urgent operative repair, and should be kept NPO.
3. Once the diagnosis is suspected, further ocular examination should be stopped immediately.
4. *Do not* use an eye patch. The eye should be protected with a plastic shield such that the edges of the shield touch the bony prominences above and below the eyeball. Further

manipulation of the area must be kept to an absolute minimum.

5. *Do not* instill any topical analgesics.
6. No attempt should be made to measure the intraocular pressure.
7. Changes in intraocular pressure (through coughing, vomiting, or agitation) should be prevented pharmacologically if necessary.
8. The patient's activity should be kept to a minimum and every attempt should be made to keep the child calm.
9. Tetanus immunization should be updated as required.
10. Broad-spectrum IV antibiotics should be given as prophylaxis (e.g., ceftazidime and vancomycin) that provide coverage against gram-positive and gram-negative organisms including *Bacillus* species (contamination with organic FB).

Clinical Pearls: Traumatic Globe Rupture

1. Check the "ocular vital signs" (red reflex, pupil, visual acuity and motility) in any child presenting with ocular trauma.
2. *Once the diagnosis of ruptured globe is suspected, the eye should be protected with a shield and further manipulation of the area kept to an absolute minimum.*
3. Ruptured globe is an ophthalmologic emergency that may not be immediately apparent on initial exam. An ophthalmologist should see the patient in the ED.
4. Following blunt trauma to the eye, a 360° subconjunctival hemorrhage may obscure underlying ruptured globe.
5. Liberal use of antiemetics, analgesics, and sedation may minimize expulsion of intraocular contents.

BOX 8-30. CLINICAL FEATURES OF TRAUMATIC GLOBE RUPTURE

Symptoms

- Eye pain
- Usually marked visual disturbances including blurred vision or diplopia (normal visual acuity is sometimes present and does not exclude the diagnosis)
- Redness
- Swelling

Eye findings

- Gross extrusion of globe contents
- Chemosis (conjunctival edema and swelling; Fig. 8-29)
- Peaked (teardrop) or irregular pupil or eccentric pupil (Fig. 8-30)
- Hyphema
- Subconjunctival hemorrhage
- Poor red reflex
- Decreased intraocular pressure (*though measurements of intraocular pressure should be avoided in patients suspected of harboring a globe injury*)
- Exophthalmos (with retrobulbar hemorrhage) or enophthalmos
- Conjunctival abrasion/laceration (Fig. 8-31)
- Limitation of extraocular movement
- Scleral buckling
- Bubbles in the anterior chamber
- Shallow anterior chamber (anterior perforating injury)
- Deep anterior chamber (posterior perforating injury)
- Iris prolapse or incarceration (may simulate a foreign body)
- Seidel's sign (aqueous humor leaking through the wound; this may be facilitated with instillation of fluorescein and examination through a slitlamp)

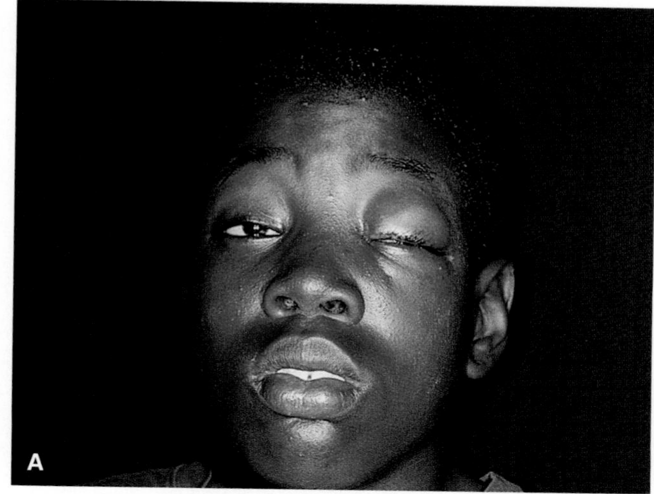

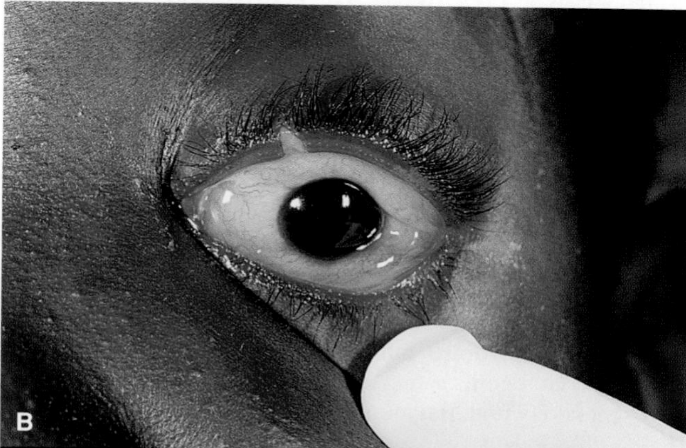

Figure 8-29. Traumatic Ruptured Globe

A. Swelling, redness, eye pain, and blurred vision were the presenting complaints following blunt trauma in this patient. *B*. Close-up showing severe chemosis. Patients presenting with severe 360° subconjunctival chemosis without hemorrhage following trauma should be treated as if they have a ruptured globe.

BOX 8-31. DIFFERENTIAL DIAGNOSIS OF TRAUMATIC GLOBE RUPTURE

- Hyphema
- Ocular foreign body
- Traumatic iritis
- Retinal detachment
- Subconjunctival hemorrhage (from another etiology)
- Vitreous hemorrhage

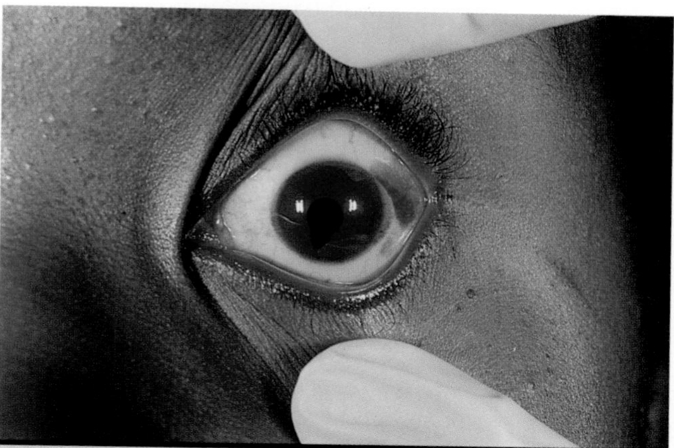

Figure 8-30. Teardrop Pupil with Subconjunctival Hemorrhage: Traumatic Ruptured Globe

Immediately after laceration, the iris or choroid will plug the corneal wound. Because of this, the pupil may appear as a teardrop shape with the narrowest segment pointing toward the rupture.

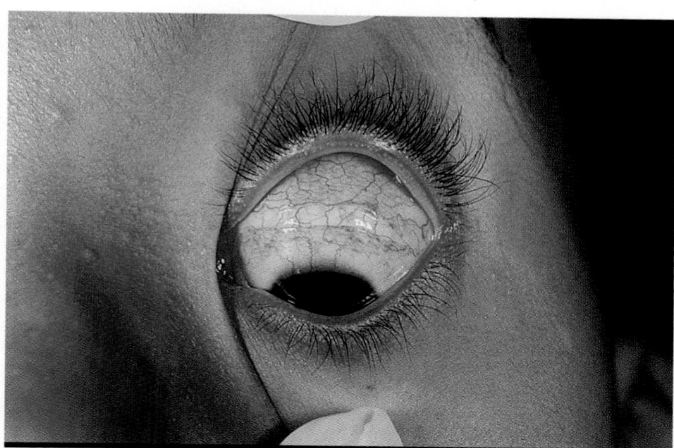

Figure 8-31. Conjunctival Laceration

This can be one of the signs of ruptured globe. This patient presented with redness and eye pain following accidental injury by a pencil point that poked his eye. The rest of the examination was normal.

DIAGNOSIS INFANTILE GLAUCOMA

SYNONYM

Primary congenital glaucoma

Definitions

1. Glaucoma is a condition marked by increased intraocular pressure that causes pathologic changes in the optic disc.
2. Infantile glaucoma is a congenital disorder that may be present at birth or may manifest before the third year of life.
3. Primary congenital glaucoma refers to a developmental disorder of the trabecular meshwork leading to a reduction of aqueous outflow from the anterior chamber. It should be differentiated from the myriad secondary causes of glaucoma due to ocular malformation or systemic illness.
4. Juvenile glaucoma refers to glaucoma that occurs after 2 to 3 years of age.
5. Traumatic glaucoma is an increase in intraocular pressure following traumatic disruption of the aqueous drainage systems.

Etiology

1. The problem is a malformation of the structures responsible for draining aqueous humor from the anterior chamber. As aqueous humor accumulates, intraocular pressure rises and compresses the blood supply to the optic disc. Prolonged optic nerve ischemia can lead to blindness.
2. There are numerous causes of infantile glaucoma, most of which have their roots in heterogeneous congenital abnormalities.
3. Glaucoma is associated with a number of named syndromes (Box 8-34).

Associated Clinical Features

1. Symptoms may be present at birth or may develop gradually during infancy.
2. Acute symptoms occur when pupillary constriction in response to bright light causes the iris to pull on the trabecular meshwork and abruptly block the aqueous outflow from the eye, leading to a sudden increase in intraocular pressure. Typically, the child cries when exposed to bright light and tries to close his or her eyes.
3. Over time, increased intraocular pressure causes structural changes in the eye related to expansion of the anterior chamber and stretching and edema of the cornea.
4. Visual field loss is initially peripheral and is related to optic nerve ischemia. With time the deficit becomes global.
5. Corneal opacities and scarring along with myopia and astigmatism from an elongated globe lead to further visual defects. Deprivation amblyopia also diminishes visual acuity if there is unilateral involvement.
6. Prognosis is worse for early onset.
   a. If glaucoma is present at birth, over 50% of affected eyes will be legally blind.
   b. If glaucoma occurs later, 20% of affected eyes will be blind.

Consultation

Emergent referral to an ophthalmologist

Emergency Department Treatment and Disposition

1. Principles of management of congenital glaucoma include lowering the intraocular pressure to prevent optic nerve damage and progressive enlargement of the eye and to reduce corneal edema.
2. Medical treatment of increased intraocular pressure can be temporizing before surgery. Various medications that are used include beta-blockers (e.g., timolol), pilocarpine, carbonic anhydrase inhibitors (e.g., acetazolamide), α_2-adrenergic agonists (e.g., brimonidine), and prostaglandin $F_{2\alpha}$ analogs (e.g., latanoprost).
3. Surgery is considered definitive therapy, though it is not always curative.
   a. The goal is to improve drainage of aqueous humor from the anterior chamber.
   b. Goniotomy is the first-line treatment. It involves excision of abnormal tissue with the aid of a microscopic lens.
   c. Trabeculotomy ab externum involves passage of a probe through the canal of Schlemm and then sweeping through the trabecular meshwork and into the anterior chamber to open up the angle.

Clinical Pearls: Infantile Glaucoma

1. Infantile glaucoma is a vision-threatening disorder marked by increased intraocular pressure that presents before the age of 3.
2. The classic triad of excessive tearing, blepharospasm, and photophobia is absent in the majority of cases (they are seen in a third of affected patients at the time of diagnosis).
3. Tearing is one of the most common presenting signs of infantile glaucoma.
4. Infantile glaucoma should be considered in the differential of the fussy infant.

BOX 8-32. CLINICAL FEATURES OF INFANTILE GLAUCOMA

- Usually bilateral (about 70% of cases)
- Photophobia
- Tearing (epiphora; secondary to eye irritation resulting from stretch trauma to the cornea)
- Buphthalmos
  - (1) Distention of the globe caused by increased intraocular pressure
  - (2) "Ox-eye"
  - (3) Unilateral large, bulging eyeball (eye wall is elastic and stretches)
- Corneal edema/clouding (Fig. 8-32)
- Megalocornea (corneal diameter of >10 mm in a term infant or >12 mm in an infant at 1 year of age strongly suggests glaucoma)
- Red eye (secondary to injected conjunctival vessels)
- Blue sclera (expansion and thinning of the sclera unmasks the underlying choroids, giving the sclera a blue appearance)
- Increased intraocular pressure (>25 mmHg)
- Globe may feel subjectively firm
- Haab's striae
  - (1) Horizontal "stretch lines" crossing the central cornea
  - (2) Caused by tears in Descemet's membrane
- Amblyopia (visual impairment of affected eye)
- Eyelid spasm

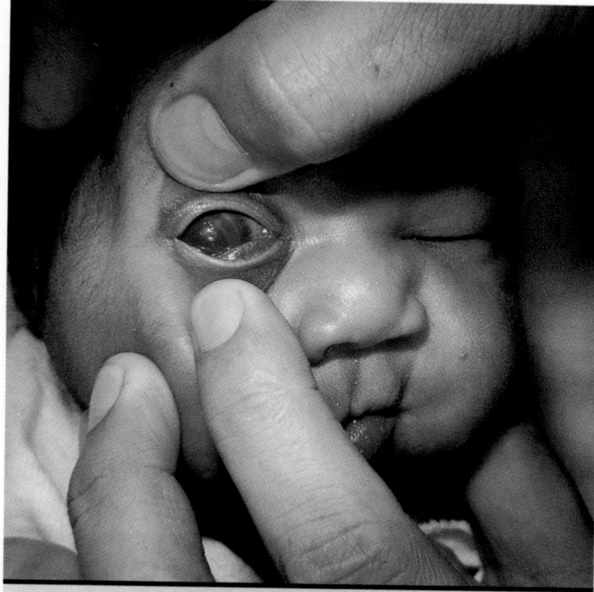

Figure 8-32. Infantile Glaucoma

Congenital glaucoma in a patient with congenital rubella syndrome. Congenital glaucoma occurs in about 10% of patients with congenital rubella. Glaucoma develops because of abnormal angle development. When this is present at birth, it causes an enlarged, hazy cornea as seen in this patient.

BOX 8-33. DIFFERENTIAL DIAGNOSIS OF INFANTILE GLAUCOMA

- Conjunctivitis
- Iritis
- Corneal abrasion (excessive tearing)
- Foreign body (excessive tearing)
- Nasolacrimal duct obstruction (excessive tearing)
- Keratomalacia
- Birth trauma (leading to corneal haziness [e.g., forceps injury])
- Congenital infections (leading to corneal haziness [e.g., herpes simplex virus])
- Congenital megalocornea

BOX 8-34. SYNDROMES ASSOCIATED WITH GLAUCOMA

- Prader-Willi syndrome
- Cystinosis
- Sturge-Weber syndrome
- Neurofibromatosis (NF-1)
- Stickler's syndrome
- Oculocerebrorenal (Lowell) syndrome
- Rieger's syndrome
- Fetal alcohol syndrome
- Short syndrome
- Hepatocerebrorenal syndrome
- Pierre Robin syndrome
- Marfan's syndrome
- Rubinstein-Taybi syndrome
- Infantile glaucoma associated with mental retardation and paralysis
- Oculodentodigital dysplasia
- Open angle glaucoma associated with microcornea and absence of frontal sinuses
- Mucopolysaccharidosis
- Trisomy 13
- Congenital rubella
- Duplication 3q syndrome
- Trisomy 21 (Down syndrome)
- Cutis marmorata telangiectasia congenita
- Warburg's syndrome
- Kniest syndrome (skeletal dysplasia)
- Michel syndrome
- Nonprogressive hemiatrophy

DIAGNOSIS

CHEMICAL EYE INJURIES

SYNONYM

Ocular burn

Definition

Injury to the eye caused by exposure to chemical irritants (Fig. 8-33). The majority of ocular exposures in children result from household (as opposed to industrial) preparations.

Etiology

1. Acids
   a. Coagulative necrosis: proteins in the corneal epithelium are denatured, leading to the formation of a barrier to further penetration.
   b. These burns are more likely to be superficial than alkali burns.
2. Alkalis
   a. Liquefactive necrosis: alkalis are lipophilic substances that cause saponification of lipid membranes and penetrate deeply into ocular tissues.
   b. They can cause persistent and delayed injury if the eye is not properly decontaminated.
3. Hydrofluoric acid
   a. Present in commercial cleaners such as Armor-All, rust removers, and aluminum cleaners
   b. Penetrates deeply into tissues and causes catastrophic, often delayed injury
   c. Ocular injury may occur from direct splash or from contact with vapors.
4. Bleach
   a. Household bleach (e.g., Clorox) is generally a 3 to 6% solution of sodium hypochlorite.
   b. Dry bleach ("all fabric" bleach): either sodium carbonate/perborate or sodium carbonate/percarbonate
   c. Mildly alkaline
5. Hydrogen peroxide
   a. Household hydrogen peroxide solution is generally a 3% solution.
   b. Some hair bleaches contain 10% peroxide, which is more corrosive.
   c. Industrial sources of peroxide may exceed concentrations of 30%.
6. Cyanoacrylate adhesives (e.g., "Superglue")

Associated Clinical Features

1. Alkali injuries occur more frequently than acid injuries due to their presence in various household cleaning agents and home construction materials.
2. The extent of caustic injury is dependent on the pH, quantity, and time elapsed between exposure and irrigation.
3. Acid burns are more often self-limited given the barrier function of coagulation necrosis. Alkali burns are more likely to progress to deeper structures.
4. After the acute burn, damage and corneal breakdown continue. Collagenase is released from the regenerating tissue, producing even more destruction.
5. Hydrofluoric acid burns may be asymptomatic initially. Complications of eye exposure include corneal opacification,

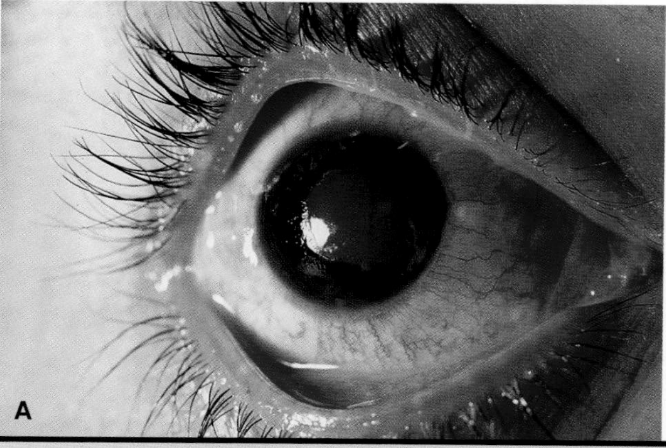

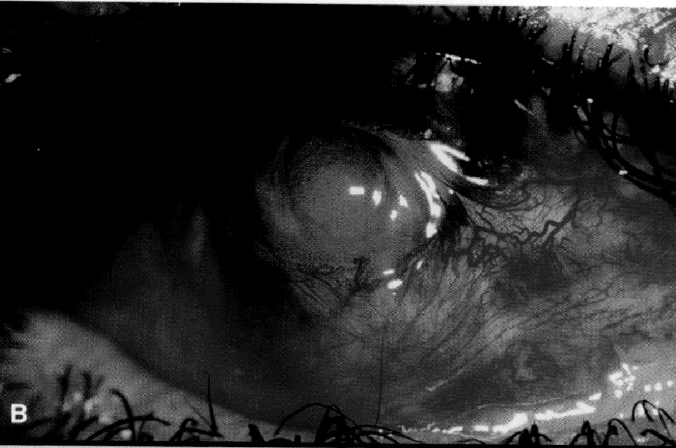

Figure 8-33. Chemical Burns

Corneal burns (*A*) and subacute alkali burn to the conjunctiva and cornea (*B*) are seen. The use of fluorescein confirms injury to the corneas in addition to the conjunctiva. (Reproduced with permission from: Christian CW, Lane WG: Ophthalmic involvement in nonaccidental trauma. In: Hertle RW, Schaffer DB, Foster JA (eds). *Pediatric Eye Disease. Color Atlas and Synopsis*. New York, McGraw-Hill, 2002, p. 107.)

corneal sloughing, keratoconjunctivitis, and necrosis of the anterior chamber.

6. Contamination with household bleach is generally a benign exposure, provided adequate irrigation is instituted.

Consultations

Ophthalmology (for any hydrofluoric acid exposure as well as for nontrivial acid and alkali exposures to ensure that deeper ocular structures are not involved) and toxicology or poison control center (for chemical ocular exposures)

Emergency Department Treatment and Disposition

1. Any ocular exposure should be immediately irrigated with generous amounts of water as soon as possible after the incident (begin irrigation in the prehospital setting).
2. Patients who arrive in the ED
   a. Patients should have their conjunctival pH measured immediately with litmus paper (or the pH indicator of a urine dipstick) before undergoing repeat ocular irrigation using a Morgan lens or similar device.
   b. Irrigation with a minimum of 1 liter of fluid is recommended. Retract the lids during irrigation and the stream of irrigating fluid should be directed onto the globe and conjunctival fornices.
   c. There is no therapeutic difference between ocular irrigation with normal saline, sterile water, lactated Ringer's, or normal saline with bicarbonate.
   d. Ocular local anesthetic (or if required, sedation with a parenteral agent) may reduce the discomfort associated with this process.
   e. Any particulate matter should be removed from the fornices using a cotton swab.
   f. After an initial liter of irrigation, the ocular pH should be rechecked to determine the need for further irrigation. It may be difficult to precisely return to a neutral pH, but continue irrigation until a general trend toward a neutral pH is documented.
   g. After stopping the irrigation, recheck the pH again after about 10 minutes to ensure a persistently stable reading.
3. Both eyes should be assessed given the likelihood of migration of the contaminant from one eye to the other via the nasolacrimal apparatus.
4. After irrigation is complete, a thorough ocular examination, including visual acuity and fluorescein testing, is required to assess the extent of injury.
5. Patients with mild injuries (e.g., absent corneal opacification) can be followed daily by an ophthalmologist as outpatients to document healing. Such patients are usually sent home on a topical antibiotic, a cycloplegic, and pain medication.
6. Patients with moderate to severe injuries (e.g., hazy cornea or total loss of corneal epithelium, or opaque cornea without any visualization of the iris or pupil) usually are admitted for close monitoring of intraocular pressure, adhesions, and infection.
7. Hydrofluoric acid exposures
   a. May require irrigation with 1% calcium gluconate (a 1:10 dilution of the generally available solution) if pain persists after irrigation
   b. Physicians should have a high suspicion for any inhalational exposure.
   c. Dermal exposures should reveal themselves with the presence of pain, and should be treated accordingly.
   d. Consult a poison control center for recommendations.
8. Cyanoacrylate exposures should be managed conservatively.
   a. They do not appear to cause significant long-term morbidity.
   b. The adhesive may dry quickly after it encounters the cornea, but will be absorbed over time by the body's own mechanisms.
   c. Attempts to forcefully peel away the adhesive may cause further epithelial trauma and should be kept to a minimum.

Clinical Pearls: Chemical Eye Injuries

1. A chemical burn is a true ophthalmic emergency.
2. Caustic injury to the eye is one of the few conditions in which treatment must occur *prior to* additional history and eye examination. Copious irrigation *as early as possible* is the most important treatment intervention.
3. In general alkali burns are more severe than acid burns.
4. *Do not* attempt to neutralize acids with alkalis or vice versa.
5. Alkali and hydrofluoric acid burns are likely to cause delayed injury and corneal perforation.
6. Complications of caustic injuries include perforation, blindness, corneal neovascularization, secondary glaucoma, cataract formation, and retinal damage.

BOX 8-35. TYPICAL ACID AND ALKALI EXPOSURES

- *Acids*
  (1) Sulfuric acid: typically from a car battery, liquid drain cleaner, or rust removers
  (2) Hydrofluoric acid: aluminum cleaners, Armor-All, industrial exposure
  (3) Hydrochloric acid: various tile and ceramic cleaners, toilet bowl cleaners
  (4) Nitric acid
  (5) Acetic acid
- *Alkali*
  (1) Ammonia: household cleaners
  (2) Sodium hydroxide: airbag injury
  (3) Potassium hydroxide
  (4) Magnesium hydroxide: sparklers, fireworks

BOX 8-36. CLINICAL FEATURES OF CHEMICAL EYE INJURIES

- Depending on offending agent, symptoms may include:
  (1) Eye pain
  (2) Photophobia
  (3) Foreign body sensation
  (4) Conjunctival injection
  (5) Lacrimation
  (6) Blepharospasm
  (7) Disturbances in visual acuity
- Variable degrees of corneal injury manifested by:
  (1) Fluorescein uptake
  (2) Corneal opacification
  (3) Epithelial sloughing
  (4) Anterior chamber and globe perforation (if injury is profound or is allowed to progress without intervention)

Suggested Readings

Arnold LD, Eppich WJ: A clear-sighted approach to conjunctivitis: State of the art clinical practice. *Pediatr Emerg Med Rep* 2003;8:99.

Bertolini J, Pelucio M: The red eye. *Emerg Med Clin North Am* 1995;13:561.

Givner LB: Periorbital versus orbital cellulitis. Concise reviews of pediatric infectious diseases. *Pediatr Infect Dis J* 2002;21:1157.

Greenberg MF: The red eye in childhood. *Pediatr Clin North Am* 2003;50:105.

Kipp MA: Childhood glaucoma. *Pediatr Clin North Am* 2003;50:89.

Mahadevan SV, Savitsky E: Emergency management of traumatic eye injuries. *Trauma Rep* 2001;VOL 2, No. 4, Page 1.

Mester V: Intraocular foreign bodies. *Ophthalmol Clin North Am* 2002;15:235.

Sheikh A, Hurwitz B, Cave J: Antibiotics for acute bacterial conjunctivitis. *The Cochrane Database of Systematic Reviews* 2000, Issue 1. Art. No.: CD001211. DOI:10.1002/14651858. CD001211.

Starkey CR, Steele RW: Medical management of orbital cellulitis. *Pediatr Infect Dis J* 2001;20:1002.

Tingley DH: Eye trauma: Corneal abrasions. *Pediatr Rev* 1999;20:320.

Weiss AH: Conjunctivitis in the neonatal period (ophthalmia neonatorum). Long SS (ed). In: *Principles and Practice of Pediatric Infectious Diseases*, 2nd ed. Elsevier, Philadelphia 2003, page 488.

CHAPTER 9

OTOLARYNGOLOGY

Peter Peacock / Mark Spektor / Binita R. Shah
Edited by Binita R. Shah

DIAGNOSIS ACUTE OTITIS MEDIA

Definition

Acute otitis media (AOM) is an infection of the middle ear. It does not affect the ear canal; however, infectious material may be present if tympanic perforation has occurred.

Etiology and Pathophysiology

1. Most episodes begin with viral upper respiratory tract infection (URI). Mucous membrane edema results in occlusion of the eustachian tube, causing fluid accumulation in the middle ear. This fluid may then become superinfected with bacteria.
2. The most common bacterial pathogens include:
   a. *Streptococcus pneumoniae*
   b. *Moraxella catarrhalis*
   c. *Haemophilus influenzae*
   d. Group A beta-hemolytic streptococci

Associated Clinical Features

1. Vertigo and hearing impairment are uncommon but result from vestibulocochlear involvement.
2. Other findings may include those associated with primary viral infection (e.g., fever, lymphadenopathy, rhinorrhea).
3. The diagnosis is clinical (although there are several diagnostic adjuncts, such as reflex tympanography, which may be used).

Complications

1. Mastoiditis
2. Bacteremia
3. Sepsis
4. Tympanic membrane perforation
5. Cholesteatoma
6. Facial paralysis
7. Intracranial suppurative complications (e.g., meningitis, brain abscess, encephalitis)

Consultation

Otolaryngology (emergently in cases complicated by mastoiditis and perhaps in cases with sepsis in an immunocompromised host when tympanocentesis for culture may be helpful)

Emergency Department Treatment and Disposition

1. Analgesia should be considered to reduce the pain, especially during the first 24 hours of an episode of AOM. Both systemic (e.g., acetaminophen or ibuprofen) and topical analgesics (e.g., benzocaine preparations) may have utility.
2. The American Academy of Pediatrics clinical practice guidelines on diagnosis and management of acute otitis media in patients *2 months through 12 years of age* with *uncomplicated AOM* were published in 2004. Observation without the use of antibacterial agents in a child with uncomplicated AOM is an option. The "observation option" for AOM refers to deferring antibacterial treatment of selected children (based on diagnostic certainty, age, illness severity, and assurance of follow-up) for 48 to 72 hours and limiting management to symptomatic relief (please refer to Clinical Practice Guidelines, 2004 for details).
3. Antibacterial agents
   a. If the decision is made to treat AOM with an antibacterial agent, it should cover *S. pneumoniae*, nontypable *H. influenzae*, and *Moraxella catarrhalis*.
   b. Amoxicillin is the first-line drug for most children (dose: 80 to 90 mg/kg per day).
   c. In patients presenting with severe illness (moderate to severe otalgia or fever of 39°C or higher) and in those for whom additional coverage for beta-lactamase–positive *H. influenzae* and *M. catarrhalis* is desired, begin

therapy with high-dose amoxicillin-clavulanate (dose: 90 mg/kg per day of the amoxicillin component with 6.4 mg/kg per day of clavulanate in two divided doses).

d. Between 30 and 60% of isolates of *S. pneumoniae* are resistant to penicillin and standard-dose amoxicillin.
e. Risk factors for the presence of bacterial species likely to be resistant to amoxicillin include attendance at child care, recent receipt (<30 days) of antibacterial treatment, and age <2 years.
f. The course of antibiotics should be for 10 days for younger children and for children with severe disease. For children 6 years and older with mild to moderate disease, a 5- to 7-day course is acceptable.
g. For patients allergic to penicillin (type I reactions [urticaria or anaphylaxis]), azithromycin or clarithromycin is recommended.
h. In patients who are vomiting or those who for other reasons cannot tolerate oral medication, a single dose of parenteral ceftriaxone can be used for the initial treatment of AOM.
i. Treatment with a 3-day course of parenteral ceftriaxone is recommended in a patient who fails amoxicillin-clavulanate therapy

4. Patients should be followed-up by their primary care clinicians after the course of antibiotics is complete to ensure clearance of the infection. They should also be instructed to be reevaluated more quickly if pain and fever persist for 48 hours, as this suggests resistance to the prescribed antibiotic.

Clinical Pearls: Acute Otitis Media

1. Otitis media is a localized abscess; systemic toxicity cannot be attributed to this infection. A primary cause should be sought when disease more significant than a viral URI is suggested by the overall clinical picture.
2. *S. pneumoniae*, nontypable *H. influenzae*, and *Moraxella catarrhalis* account for 95% of bacterial cases of AOM. However, the microbiology of AOM may be changing as a result of routine use of the pneumococcal vaccine.
3. Topical antibiotics can be considered in cases in whom there is rupture of the tympanic membrane.
4. As indicated, pain management must be addressed during an episode of AOM regardless of the use of antibacterial agents.

BOX 9-1. CLINICAL FEATURES OF ACUTE OTITIS MEDIA

- Symptoms include:
  (1) Distinct otalgia (pain that interferes with sleep or normal daily activities)
  (2) Fever
  (3) Associated URI symptoms (e.g., cough, coryza)
- Signs of middle ear inflammation as indicated by otoscopic abnormalities of the tympanic membrane (TM) as suggested by:
  (1) Distinct erythema (a pink erythematous flush caused by crying or high fever usually is less intense and subsides as the child quiets down)
  (2) Presence of middle ear effusion (MEE) is indicated by
    a. Otorrhea (Fig. 9-1)
    b. Fullness or bulging of TM (highest predictive value for the presence of MEE)
    c. Reduced or absent mobility on insufflation (a finding of immobility is significantly more accurate than any of the other findings)
    d. Air-fluid level behind TM
  (3) Opacification or cloudiness
  (4) Loss of visible landmarks
  (5) Retraction

Clinical pearls

- A diagnosis of AOM requires:
  (1) A history of acute onset of signs and symptoms
  (2) Presence of MEE
  (3) Signs and symptoms of middle-ear inflammation

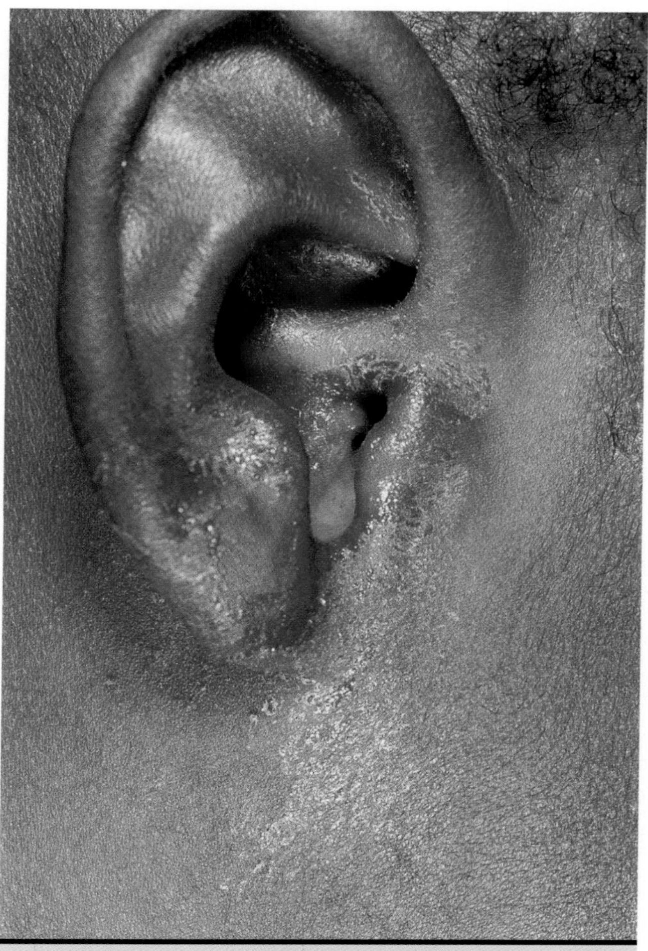

Figure 9-1. Acute Otitis Media Presenting with Otorrhea

Purulent drainage from the external auditory canal (EAC) was seen in this otherwise healthy patient who presented with a history of fever and severe earache of 3 days' duration, followed by drainage from the right ear. Otorrhea is defined as a discharge from the ear. The common etiologies of otorrhea include otitis externa, acute otitis media with perforation, or drainage through an indwelling tympanostomy tube. Less common causes of otorrhea include foreign body in the EAC, cholesteatoma, chronic suppurative otitis media or basilar skull fracture.

BOX 9-2. DIFFERENTIAL DIAGNOSIS OF ACUTE OTITIS MEDIA

- Viral infection
- Otitis externa
- Barotrauma
- Foreign body
- Referred pain from lymphadenitis or pharyngitis
- Cholesteatoma

DIAGNOSIS OTITIS EXTERNA

SYNONYM

Swimmer's ear

Definition

Otitis externa is inflammation or infection of the external auditory canal (EAC).

Etiology and Pathophysiology

1. Most episodes begin with dampness and maceration of the skin of the EAC. Thus, it is most commonly seen in the summertime due to swimming (Fig. 9-2).
2. Diabetes plays an important role in progression of the initial infection to temporal osteomyelitis or malignant otitis externa.
3. Otitis externa usually results from a mixed infection
   a. Bacteria (*Pseudomonas aeruginosa, Klebsiella, Enterobacter, Staphylococcus aureus, Streptococcus pyogenes*)
   b. Fungi (*Aspergillus* and *Candida*)

Clinical Features

1. The diagnosis is made clinically.
2. There is a role for CBC, ESR, and CT scanning of the temporal bones when temporal osteomyelitis is suspected.

Complications

1. Temporal osteomyelitis/malignant otitis media
2. Meningitis, bacteremia, and sepsis may occur.

Consultation

Otolaryngology consultation for cases complicated by osteomyelitis

Emergency Department Treatment and Disposition

1. Analgesia should be considered. Both systemic (e.g., acetaminophen) and topical analgesics may have utility. The pain from this disorder may be intense.
2. Topical broad-spectrum antibiotics with coverage of *Staphylococcus* and *Streptococcus* species and gram-negative pathogens should suffice in most cases (e.g., polymyxin B-neomycin combination).
3. Topical steroids may also have efficacy in reducing the inflammation. Preparations of antibiotics and steroids are available (e.g., Cortisporin).
4. The addition of antipseudomonal coverage should be considered in diabetic patients, and this should be administered intravenously in patients thought to have malignant otitis externa.
5. Use of a suspension rather than a solution may be appropriate when there is concern that tympanic rupture may be present, as the latter agents are more caustic to the middle ear or may cause pain. Instill the drops either directly or with the help of a cotton ear wick so as to cover the entire EAC.
6. Patients must be instructed to refrain from swimming to keep the ears dry (or use ear plugs).
7. Complete resolution usually takes about a week in the majority of patients. Cases that do not respond quickly to topical therapy should be referred to an otolaryngologist.
8. Cases complicated by osteomyelitis warrant admission for IV antibiotics and emergent otolaryngologic consultation, as surgery may be indicated for débridement of necrotic temporal bone.

Clinical Pearls: Otitis Externa

1. Discharge from the EAC can be seen in both otitis media with perforation and otitis externa. Extreme pain or discomfort when pulling the pinna or tragus is seen with otitis externa; this helps in distinguishing the two disease processes.
2. Most cases of otitis externa respond quickly to topical therapy.
3. Malignant otitis externa is a disorder of immunocompromised hosts and diabetics.
4. Screening for malignant otitis externa is a primary clinical goal. Some clinicians evaluate the serum glucose in all patients presenting with otitis externa, as this is the primary risk factor for malignant disease.

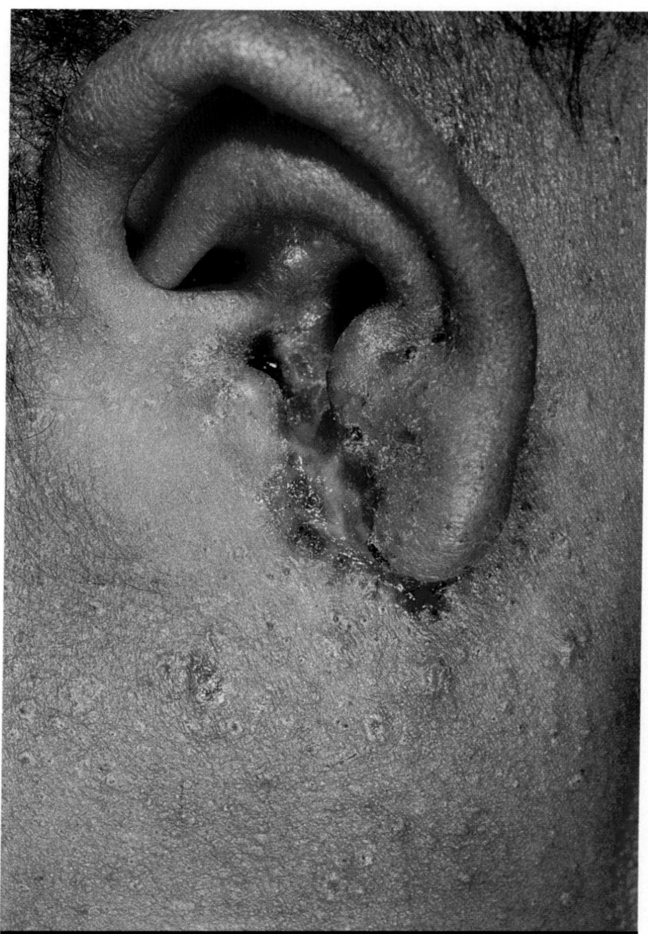

Figure 9-2. Otitis Externa (Swimmer's Ear)

White-yellow discharge from the EAC associated with excoriation of the surrounding skin were seen in a 8-year-old patient who gave a history of swimming every day during summer camp. Otorrhea from the EAC can be seen in both otitis media with perforation and otitis externa. Extreme pain when pulling the pinna and tragus were present (these findings are consistent with otitis externa and help in differentiating it from otitis media with perforation). This patient's EAC was also very edematous and filled with dried debris. Other less common etiologies of otorrhea from otitis externa include fungal otitis externa, eczematous otitis externa, and furunculosis (hair follicle infection usually due to *S. aureus*).

BOX 9-3. CLINICAL FEATURES OF OTITIS EXTERNA

- Recent history of swimming
- Otalgia (most common complaint)
- Discharge from the ear (common complaint)
- Itching
- Patients usually afebrile; constitutional symptoms suggest complications
- Physical examination
  (1) Edema and thick discharge from the EAC
  (2) Discharge may be substantial and the EAC may be occluded with debris (in this setting the tympanic membrane will be obscured)
  (3) Discharge usually white, yellow, or green
  (4) Exquisite tragus tenderness (characteristic of this infection)
  (5) Pain on movement of the pinna

BOX 9-4. DIFFERENTIAL DIAGNOSIS OF OTITIS EXTERNA

- Cellulitis
- Otitis media with perforation
- Malignant otitis externa (temporal osteitis)
- Foreign body in EAC

DIAGNOSIS PERITONSILLAR ABSCESS

SYNONYM

Quinsy

Definition

The palatine tonsils are surrounded by a capsule. Peritonsillar abscess (PTA) is a localized accumulation of pus between the faucial pillars and the tonsillar capsule. Inflammation progresses from peritonsillar cellulitis to the phlegmon stage and abscess formation.

Etiology

1. The etiology of PTA is usually polymicrobial.
2. Group A beta-hemolytic streptococci (GABHS or *Streptococcus pyogenes*) is the most common aerobic pathogen along with anaerobes like *Fusobacterium* spp., *Peptostreptococcus*, *Peptococcus*, *Bacteroides*, *Streptococcus viridans*, and *Streptococcus sanguis*.
3. Less common pathogens include *Staphylococcus aureus*, *Haemophilus influenzae*, and *Neisseria* spp.

Associated Clinical Features

1. Predisposing factors include chronic tonsillitis and a prior history of multiple trials of antibiotics to cure acute tonsillitis. However, it can occur de novo without any prior history of recurrent or chronic tonsillitis.
2. Peritonsillar cellulitis (PTC) and PTA have similar presentations (i.e., histories and time course) and differentiation may be difficult, especially during the early stages. In PTC, trismus is uncommon and fluctuance is absent.
3. The diagnosis is usually made by history and clinical examination and confirmed by collection of pus from the abscess via needle aspiration.
4. A CBC does not help in diagnosis or management. Throat culture, blood culture, and culture of the aspirate may help in identification of the pathogens and in directing subsequent antibiotic therapy (if the patient is not responding to the initial empiric therapy).
5. Intraoral or transcutaneous sonography (placing the transducer over the submandibular gland) has been used in differentiating PTC from PTA (abscess is seen as an echo-free cavity with a well-defined circumference).
6. A CT scan with contrast of the neck and head should be considered if extension from the peritonsillar space is suspected or when the patient fails to respond to the initial empiric therapy.

Complications

1. In untreated patients, the abscess becomes fluctuant and may spontaneously rupture.
2. Complications of PTA include extension to the peripharyngeal space, and submandibular and sublingual spaces within the floor of the mouth (Ludwig's angina); airway obstruction; aspiration pneumonia; mediastinitis; sepsis; meningitis; cerebral abscess; and recurrent PTA.

Consultation

Otolaryngology

Emergency Department Treatment and Disposition

1. Hospitalize patients who are unable to maintain good oral intake, and those who are dehydrated, toxic appearing, and those with suspected complications. However, the majority of patients can be managed as outpatients. Patients may need IV hydration as fluid deficits are not uncommon because of decreased to absent oral intake.
2. Needle aspiration versus incision and drainage (I&D) of PTA:
   a. Controversy exists over needle aspiration alone versus I&D.
   b. Treatment decisions should be made in consultation with an otolaryngologist.
   c. *Either procedure should be performed only by a trained physician,* and only in a cooperative patient without severe trismus (very young or uncooperative patients or abscess in an unusual location may require general anesthesia).
   d. No significant difference (e.g., duration of signs and symptoms or treatment failure) was found between needle aspiration alone versus needle aspiration followed by I&D in some studies.
   e. A majority of patients can be treated with needle aspiration of pus alone followed by antibiotic therapy.
   f. Antibiotic therapy alone, without drainage, may suffice for certain patients with early peritonsillar cellulitis.
   g. Complications of either procedure include external carotid artery laceration (carotid artery is located 2.5 cm behind and lateral to the tonsil).
3. Needle aspiration
   a. Gold standard for confirming the diagnosis (aspiration of pus is diagnostic of PTA), as well as therapeutic (relief of pain)

b. Negative needle aspiration does not rule out PTA (abscess may be located posteriorly, which is not accessible to aspiration).
c. Allows accurate location of the abscess cavity in patients who may need I&D

4. Empiric antibiotic therapy
   a. Clindamycin or ampicillin-sulbactam is usually given, initially intravenously.
   b. Oral antibiotic therapy once oral intake is tolerated (either clindamycin or amoxicillin-clavulanate)
   c. Usual duration 10 days
   d. Some physicians still use penicillin alone and follow the patient very closely (due to the recent emergence of beta-lactamase-producing organisms, treatment failure may be seen).
5. Following the procedure, warm saline gargles, analgesics, and antipyretics are used as indicated.
6. Arrange close follow-up (within 24 hours) if the patient is discharged home. The patient is evaluated for reaccumulation of pus and response to antibiotic therapy (e.g., defervescence, ability to maintain good oral intake, improvement in tonsillar inflammation, resolution of cervical adenopathy).
7. The recurrence rate in the absence of a history of chronic tonsillitis is low (~10%), and patients do not require routine tonsillectomy. Most recurrences occur shortly after the initial PTA episode (often from ongoing infection rather than recurrence) and about 90% of recurrences occur within a year. Tonsillectomy may be considered with a prior history of recurrent PTA or recurrent tonsillitis.

Clinical Pearls: Peritonsillar Abscess

1. PTA occurs as a complication of an acute tonsillitis, and is the most common deep infection of the head and neck in adolescents and young adults.
2. The classic triad of PTA consists of trismus, fullness or frank bulging of the superior pole of the palatine tonsil, and deviation of the uvula toward the contralateral tonsil (Fig. 9-3).
3. Trismus is a cardinal sign of PTA and results from spasm of the pterygoid muscle.
4. Speech quality in PTA is often characterized as a "hot potato" voice.
5. Treatment decisions about PTA in the ED should be made in consultation with an otolaryngologist. Needle aspiration confirming the presence of pus remains the gold standard for the diagnosis, followed by appropriate antibiotic therapy to cover both aerobic and anaerobic pathogens.

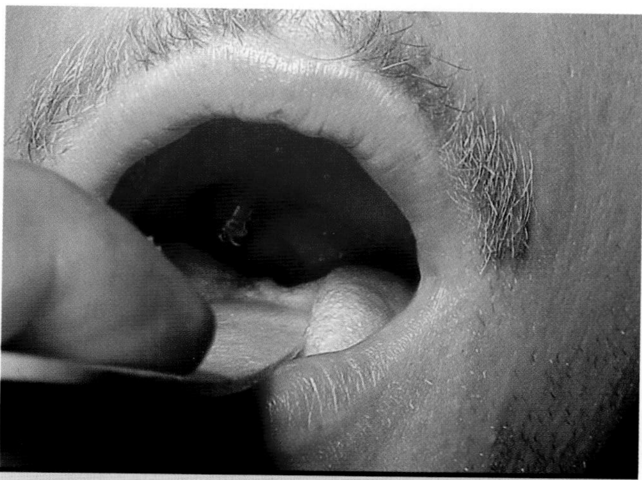

Figure 9-3. Peritonsillar Abscess

An adolescent patient presented with a severe sore throat and a fever of 39°C. Clinically he had the classic triad of PTA, consisting of trismus, fullness and bulging of the left tonsil, with deviation of the uvula toward the contralateral side. He also had difficulty swallowing. A diffuse white coating on the tongue is also seen.

BOX 9-5. CLINICAL FEATURES OF PERITONSILLAR ABSCESS

- Age at presentation
  (1) Adolescence and young adults
  (2) Most common age: 15 to 35 years
  (3) Rare in children <12 years of age (unless immunocompromised)
- Acute tonsillopharyngitis leads to increasing discomfort
- Fever (history of an afebrile interval of several days following acute tonsillopharyngitis, or persistent fever [up to 40°C])
- Severe sore throat ("worst sore throat" the patient ever had)
- Other constitutional symptoms like malaise, headache, and fatigue
- Trismus (difficulty or inability to open the mouth due to spasm of pterygoid muscles)
- Difficulty swallowing (first with solids, followed by liquids, and finally saliva)
- Drooling
- Difficult speech ("hot potato" quality)
- Torticollis (spasm of ipsilateral muscles of the neck)
- Limitation of neck mobility
- Odynophagia
- Otalgia (ipsilateral)
- Throat exam
  (1) Tonsillopharyngitis
  (2) Exudates may be present
  (3) *Unilateral* peritonsillar edema and marked inflammation (most common location of abscess is at the superior pole of the tonsil, leading to fullness or frank bulging of the superior pole of the palatine tonsil)
  (4) *Asymmetry* of the soft palate
  (5) *Uvula displaced* to opposite side of abscess
  (6) Inferior or medial displacement of the tonsil
- *Ten percent of cases of PTAs are bilateral* (diagnosis in these patients is difficult).
- Upper cervical lymphadenopathy (ipsilateral; single or multiple nodes)

BOX 9-6. DIFFERENTIAL DIAGNOSIS OF PERITONSILLAR ABSCESS

- Peritonsillar cellulitis
- Uncomplicated tonsillitis
- Retropharyngeal abscess
- Parapharyngeal abscess
- Infectious mononucleosis
- Dental infections
- Pharyngitis (from other etiology; e.g., diphtheria)
- Cervical adenitis/abscess
- Salivary gland infection
- Foreign body aspiration
- Malignancy (leukemia, lymphoma)
- Aneurysm of internal carotid artery

DIAGNOSIS RETROPHARYNGEAL ABSCESS

Diagnosis

1. Retropharyngeal abscess (RPA) is an accumulation of pus in the retropharyngeal space (a pocket of connective tissue that extends from the base of the skull to the tracheal carina [T1 level] between the posterior pharyngeal wall and the prevertebral fascia).
2. The retropharyngeal space contains lymph nodes that drain the nasopharynx, adenoids, and posterior paranasal sinuses. Bacterial infections of these areas may lead to suppuration of lymph nodes resulting in abscess formation. These lymph nodes usually begin to atrophy during the third to fourth years of life and usually regress completely by 6 years of age.

Etiology

1. RPA usually results as a complication of nasopharyngitis, tonsillitis, otitis, sinusitis, adenitis, or dental infections.
2. Rarely, it results from penetrating trauma to the posterior oropharynx (e.g., a child running and falling down with an object [e.g., a pencil] in their mouth), trauma from a retained foreign body (e.g., a fish bone in an older child), an extension of vertebral osteomyelitis, or following instrumentation (e.g., laryngoscopy, endotracheal intubation, endoscopy).
3. Bacterial pathogens include *Streptococcus pyogenes*, *Staphylococcus aureus*, anaerobes (e.g., *Peptostreptococcus*, *Fusobacterium* spp., *Bacteroides*), *Eikenella* species, *Haemophilus influenzae*, and *Haemophilus parainfluenzae*.

Associated Clinical Features

1. The infection progresses through three stages, beginning with cellulitis, then proceeding to phlegmon, and then to abscess.
2. A simple examination of the throat may not show RPA. Attempting to visualize the oropharynx/posterior pharyngeal wall in an uncooperative child may result in agitation and worsening of airway compromise and must be avoided.
3. CBC may show leukocytosis with a shift to the left. Blood culture, and culture and Gram stain of the purulent material after incision and drainage will help in identifying the pathogen.
4. Radiological studies that help in confirming the diagnosis:
   a. A lateral radiograph of the nasopharynx and neck in hyperextension (Fig. 9-4)
      1) May show a swollen prevertebral soft tissue space (retropharyngeal mass) with or without air within the mass
      2) Normal spinal lordosis may be absent or reversed
      3) This view also helps in excluding epiglottitis (normal epiglottis and aryepiglottic folds) and radiopaque foreign body.

   b. A chest x-ray is usually done to exclude any pathology (e.g., aspiration pneumonia or mediastinitis).
   c. Color flow doppler ultrasonography is a new modality that may improve diagnostic accuracy in differentiating phlegmon from abscess.
   d. CT scan of neck with contrast (*imaging modality of choice*; Fig. 9-4)
      1) Helps in differentiating retropharyngeal cellulitis from mature abscess (central areas of lucency)
      2) Helps in determining the location and extent of the abscess
      3) Helps in locating a foreign body
      4) Helps in detecting complications (e.g., dissection of infection into the mediastinum)
      5) Overall accuracy ~75%

Complications

1. Airway obstruction
2. Rupture of abscess with asphyxiation or aspiration of pus into the lungs (pneumonia, empyema, pyopneumothorax), mediastinitis, and purulent pericarditis/tamponade.
3. Vascular complications (septic thrombophlebitis of the internal jugular vein [Lemierre's syndrome] or erosion through the carotid artery sheath).

Consultations

Radiology and otolaryngology

Emergency Department Treatment and Disposition

1. Management includes stabilization of the airway depending on the degree of airway compromise, O_2 therapy, continuous pulse oximetry monitoring, IV hydration, and keeping the child from eating or drinking.
2. Very close monitoring is required for the onset of airway compromise or increased severity of the illness.
3. Allow the patient to remain in a position of comfort. Most patients prefer the supine position with their necks extended (to relieve obstruction). Neck flexion (which often happens while sitting) occludes the airway.
4. Younger patients may not cooperate for CT and may need sedation. *Use extra care when sedating a patient with a compromised airway* (sedation may lead to relaxation of the airway muscles, resulting in complete obstruction).
5. Intravenous antibiotic therapy to cover penicillinase-producing *S. aureus* and anaerobes
   a. Clindamycin (dose: 40 mg/kg per day divided every 6 hours) *and* ceftriaxone (dose: 100 mg/kg per day divided

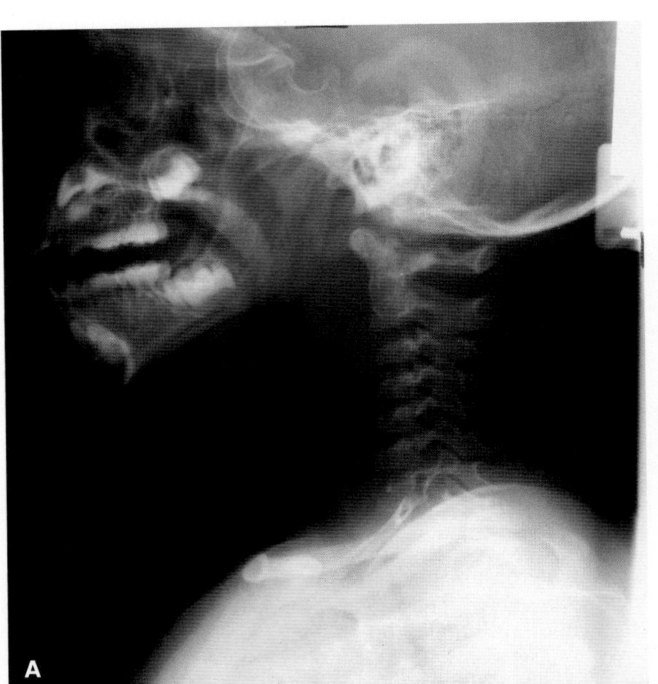

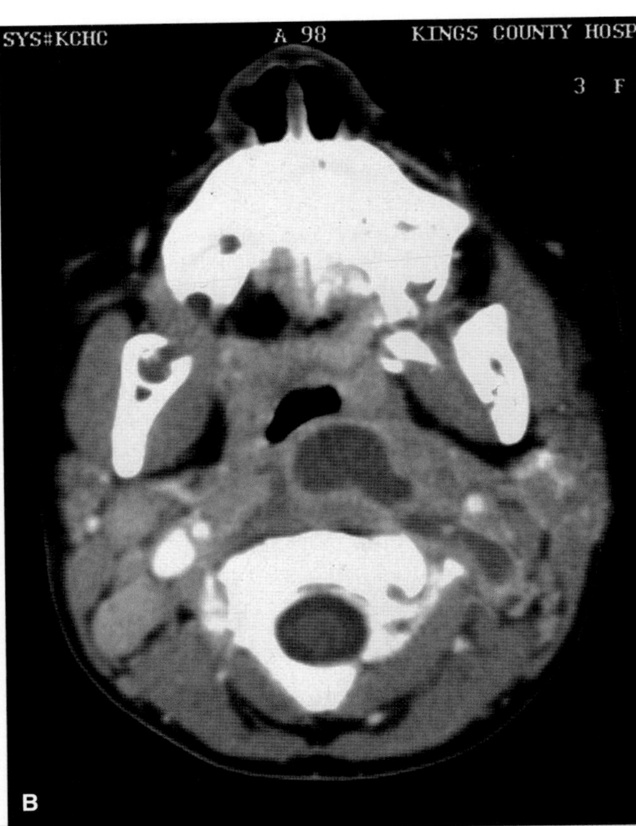

Figure 9-4. Retropharyngeal Abscess.

A. A 3 year of child presented with high fever, drooling and inspiratory stridor of 2 days duration. A lateral radiograph of the neck reveals a loss of normal axial lordosis with a widening of the prevertebral soft tissue extending from C1-C4 with a bulging of the nasopharyngeal airway. *B*. Post-contrast CT of the neck in the same patient reveals a well-defined peripherally enhancing and centrally low-density lesion in the nasopharyngeal region causing a mass effect on the adjacent airspace. These findings are consistent with a retropharyngeal abscess.

every 12 hours) *or* cefotaxime (dose: 150 mg/kg per day divided every 8 hours)

b. Alternative therapy includes oxacillin (dose: 150 mg/kg per day divided every 6 hours) *and* ceftriaxone or cefotaxime.

6. If the infection is diagnosed in the prefluctuant stage (cellulitis or phlegmon), patients require hospitalization, preferably in the ICU for continuous monitoring for possible airway compromise, parenteral antibiotics, and observation for development of an abscess.
7. After securing the airway by endotracheal intubation, incision and drainage under general anesthesia is performed in the operating room in patients with frank RPA. Postoperative monitoring is continued in the ICU.

Clinical Pearls: Retropharyngeal Abscess

1. RPA is a life-threatening surgical emergency with potential for airway compromise and catastrophic complications. If left untreated, the abscess may rupture spontaneously into the pharynx, resulting in aspiration of pus into the lungs and mediastinum.
2. RPA is a disease almost exclusively seen in pre–school-age children (as opposed to peritonsillar abscess, which is a disease of school-age older children and adolescents).
3. Suspect RPA in any sick-appearing infant or young child presenting with stridor, neck stiffness, and/or torticollis, who refuses to eat, with or without drooling.
4. *RPA can mimic meningitis (stiff neck/meningismus) or epiglottitis (toxic appearance, high fever, stridor).*
5. *Do not try to feel for fluctuance in the bulging mass in the posterior pharyngeal wall (especially in an uncooperative child); this can lead to rupture of the abscess with subsequent aspiration of the pus.*

BOX 9-7. CLINICAL FEATURES OF RETROPHARYNGEAL ABSCESS

- Age at presentation
  (1) Most common in children <4 years of age (about 96% of cases are <6 years of age)
  (2) About 50% of cases are between 6 and 12 months old
- Signs and symptoms:
  (1) Recent or current history of acute nasopharyngitis or pharyngitis
  (2) Abrupt onset of high fever
  (3) Toxic appearance
  (4) Inspiratory stridor or gurgling respirations
  (5) Varying degree of respiratory distress (depending on the severity of obstruction)
  (6) Refusal to eat
  (7) Drooling
  (8) Dysphagia (difficulty swallowing)
  (9) Odynophagia (pain on swallowing)
  (10) Sore throat
  (11) Neck pain
  (12) Torticollis
  (13) Neck stiffness/meningismus (irritation of the paravertebral ligaments)
  (14) Voice change ("hot potato" or muffled voice)
  (15) Trismus
  (16) Anterior bulge in the posterior pharyngeal wall or a forward bulge of the soft palate (depending on the location of abscess)
  (17) Opisthotonic posture (hyperextension of the neck and head to relieve the obstruction)
  (18) Neck swelling (cervical adenopathy [usually unilateral] or parapharyngeal abscess)

BOX 9-8. DIFFERENTIAL DIAGNOSIS OF RETROPHARYNGEAL ABSCESS

- Other conditions presenting with airway obstruction:
  (1) Viral croup
  (2) Epiglottitis
  (3) Bacterial tracheitis
  (4) Foreign body aspiration
  (5) Peritonsillar abscess
  (6) Infectious mononucleosis
- Meningitis
- Penetrating pharyngeal foreign body
- Caustic burns of the posterior pharynx
- Vertebral osteomyelitis
- Angioedema of epiglottis
- Hematoma (e.g., hemophilia or inflicted injuries)
- Lymphoma, lymphangioma (cystic hygroma), or hemangioma

BOX 9-9. PREVERTEBRAL SPACE ON A LATERAL NECK RADIOGRAPH

- For proper interpretation, the x-ray should be made with the patient in a sitting position with neck hyperextended and during inspiration (if possible).
- Normal buckling of the upper cervical prevertebral soft tissues that occurs during flexion or extension may mimic RPA (false-positive result)
- Soft tissue space normally seen between the posterior border of the radiolucent airway and the anterior surface of the vertebrae:
  (1) Normal distance <7 mm at the level of C2
  (2) Normal distance <4 mm at the level of C3 and C4
  (3) Normal distance <14 mm in children <15 years old at level of C6 (normal distance in adults is 22 mm)
- A rough (but less precise) guide:
  (1) Normal soft tissue space should be *less than one half the width of the adjacent vertebral body*
  (2) Increased soft tissue space would be *retropharyngeal soft tissue greater than one half the width of the adjacent vertebral body*

DIAGNOSIS ACUTE SINUSITIS

Definition

Sinusitis is inflammation or infection of the lining of any sinus. Sinuses include maxillary, ethmoid, frontal, and sphenoid. The inflammatory process may lead to or be precipitated by collection of fluid within the sinuses. Sinusitis is arbitrarily categorized by duration of symptoms as:

1. Acute sinusitis: symptoms lasting 10 to 30 days
2. Subacute sinusitis: symptoms lasting 30 to 90 days
3. Chronic sinusitis: symptoms lasting over 3 months

Etiology and Pathophysiology

1. The ethmoid and maxillary sinuses are the first to develop, and are present at birth. Sphenoid and frontal sinuses develop between age 4 and 7 years. The sphenoid sinuses are rarely infected alone. They are usually involved as a part of pansinusitis.
2. Sinusitis can be viral (e.g., adenovirus, rhinovirus, or parainfluenza virus), bacterial, or allergic in origin.
3. Most episodes begin with viral upper respiratory tract infection. Mucous membrane edema and ciliary paralysis result in mucosal stasis and occlusion of the sinus ostia with resultant fluid accumulation.
4. As with other ENT infections, while the initial infection is usually viral, bacterial superinfection may supervene, in which case the offending agents are usually *Streptococcus pneumoniae*, nontypable *Haemophilus influenzae*, *Moraxella catarrhalis*, group A streptococci, and anaerobes.

Associated Clinical Features

1. The proximity of the frontal sinus to the inner table of the skull results in relatively frequent complication of frontal sinusitis by cerebral abscess.
2. The American College of Radiology has recommended that diagnosis of sinusitis be made on clinical grounds, and recommends the use of imaging studies only after the patient does not respond or worsens after antibiotic treatment.
   a. A plain "sinus series" includes Waters' view (occipitomental) for maxillary sinuses, Caldwell's view (anteroposterior) for ethmoid and frontal sinuses, and submentovertex and lateral views for sphenoid sinuses. Normal findings make a diagnosis of sinusitis highly unlikely, but abnormal findings are only moderately helpful because an uncomplicated viral URI also results in abnormal radiographic signs.
   b. A CT scan should be considered for those patients in whom sinus surgery is being considered or in the set-

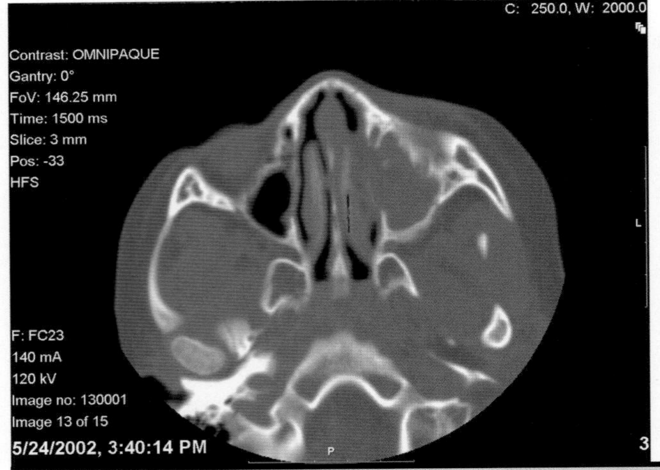

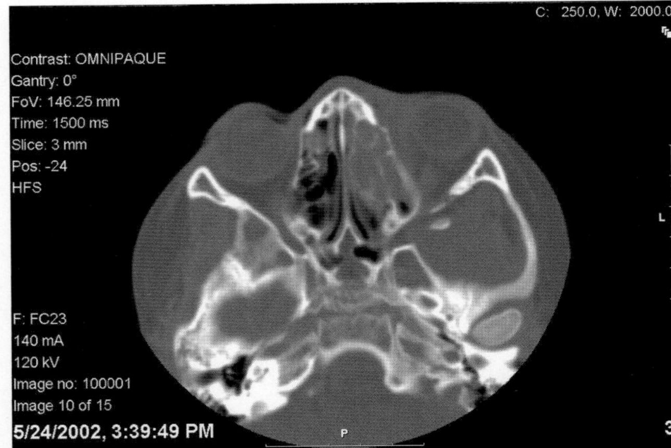

Figure 9-5. Acute Bacterial Sinusitis

A CT scan of the orbit showed a near complete opacification of the left ethmoid, left maxillary, and left frontal sinus associated with a subperiosteal collection along the medial wall of the left orbit. An elevation of the left medial rectus muscle was also seen. This image is of a 12-year-old boy who presented with sudden onset of high fever with "eye swelling." On physical examination, he had orbital cellulitis (unilateral periorbital swelling of the left eye associated with proptosis, pain on eye movement, and decreased vision). He had a persistent cold (yellow-green nasal discharge) without improvement lasting for about 14 days. He required surgical drainage (endonasal endoscopic surgery).

ting of complications of sinusitis (e.g., orbital cellulitis or intracranial complications associated with frontal sinusitis; Fig. 9-5).

Complications

1. Cerebral abscess
2. Cavernous sinus thrombosis
3. Periorbital cellulitis
4. Orbital cellulitis
5. Bacteremia, sepsis, and meningitis

Consultation

Otolaryngology (e.g., for patients presenting with suppurative complications such as orbital cellulitis or intracranial abscess, for patients with underlying immunodeficiency in whom aspiration for culture may be helpful, or for patients with recurrent or chronic infection)

Emergency Department Treatment and Disposition

1. Hospitalize any patient presenting with suppurative or intracranial complications associated with acute sinusitis. These patients need parenteral antibiotics, subspecialty consultation, and if indicated surgical drainage.
2. Antimicrobial therapy is given usually for 10 to 14 days (for at least 7 days past the point of substantial improvement or resolution of signs and symptoms).
   a. Amoxicillin in conventional doses (usually initial drug of choice in absence of risk factors for penicillin-resistant *S. pneumoniae* [PRSP] such as day care attendance, antibiotic therapy <90 days previously, or age <2 years)
   b. High-dose amoxicillin (90 mg/kg per day in two divided doses) *or* amoxicillin-clavulanate or a second- or third-generation cephalosporin (cefaclor, cefuroxime) for patients at high risk for PRSP or for treatment failures.
3. Analgesia should be considered.
4. Patients should be followed-up by their primary care clinicians after the course of antibiotics to ensure clearance of the infection. They should also be instructed to revisit more quickly if pain and fever persist for 48 hours, as this suggests resistance to the prescribed antibiotic or complications.

Clinical Pearls: Acute Sinusitis

1. The initial symptoms of sinusitis are generally indistinguishable from viral URI. Symptoms of more than 10 days' duration or high fever lasting more than 3 days should suggest the diagnosis of sinusitis.
2. Nasal foreign body should be considered in a patient presenting with persisting nasal discharge (especially unilateral).
3. Orbital cellulitis is the most frequent serious complication of acute sinusitis. Intracranial extension of the infection can also occur from acute sinusitis.
4. Classic signs and symptoms of sinusitis that are seen in older children and adults are not usually not seen in young children.
5. Acute sinusitis is diagnosed clinically and usually diagnostic imaging is not necessary to confirm the diagnosis (unless complications are suspected).

BOX 9-10. CLINICAL FEATURES OF ACUTE SINUSITIS

- Common cold (rhinosinusitis and/or cough) persisting without improvement for more than 10 to 14 days:
  (1) Nasal discharge of any color (yellow, green, or white)
  (2) Nasal discharge of any quality (clear or thick)
  (3) Daytime cough (dry or wet, may be worse at night); cough occurring only at night is a common residual symptom of uncomplicated URI.
- Classic signs and symptoms that are usually seen in older children and adults include:
  (1) Periorbital edema (edema may involve the upper or lower lid, and usually develops gradually over hours to days; it is most obvious in early morning after awakening and may decrease and actually disappear during the day)
  (2) Facial pain (facial pain that changes with head position and nose blowing may be more specific)
  (3) Fever (usually high >39°C)
  (4) Tooth pain
  (5) Tenderness to percussion over affected sinuses or facial swelling overlying the maxillary, ethmoid, or frontal sinus
  (6) Headache (feeling of fullness, dull ache in either supraorbital or retro-orbital area)
  (7) Halitosis (especially in the absence of pharyngitis, tooth decay, or a nasal foreign body)
  (8) Opacity on transillumination
- Other clinical findings may include those associated with primary viral infection (e.g., fever, lymphadenopathy, pharyngeal erythema)

BOX 9-11. DIFFERENTIAL DIAGNOSIS OF ACUTE SINUSITIS

- Nasal foreign body
- Viral URI
- Nasal polyps
- Periorbital cellulitis

DIAGNOSIS ACUTE MASTOIDITIS

Definition

Mastoiditis is inflammation or infection of any part of the mastoid process. It is classified as acute or chronic mastoiditis.

Etiology

1. Middle ear infection is the inciting event, which progresses through temporal osteitis to involve the mastoid air cells.
2. The most common causative organisms in acute mastoiditis are *S. pneumoniae*, *Streptococcus pyogenes*, and *Staphylococcus aureus*. Other pathogens include *Haemophilus influenzae*, *Pseudomonas aeruginosa*, and other gram-negative bacilli.

Associated Clinical Features

1. Symptoms include otalgia (often manifesting as irritability in a young infant), headache, fever, and systemic toxicity.
2. Physical and otoscopic examination findings include those associated with the primary otitis media (in most cases otorrhea or a bulging, immobile, opaque tympanic membrane; for other signs and symptoms see acute otitis media, Box 9-1).
3. Torticollis may also be a presenting sign.
4. The diagnosis should be suggested by the physical examination, although laboratory markers of inflammation are useful adjuncts.
5. When mastoiditis is suspected clinically, CT scan of the temporal bone should be performed to further clarify the nature and extent of the disease. Bony destruction of the mastoid must be differentiated from the simple clouding of mastoid air cells that is often found in uncomplicated cases of otitis media.

Complications

1. Bacteremia and sepsis
2. Because of close anatomical proximity, this inflammatory process may result in thrombosis of the sigmoid cerebral sinus.
3. Mastoiditis may also result in meningitis through contiguous spread. Other intracranial complications include temporal lobe or cerebellar abscess, epidural empyema, and subdural empyema.

Consultation

Otolaryngology

Emergency Department Treatment and Disposition

1. Hospitalization and otolaryngology consultation are required for all patients presenting with acute mastoiditis.
2. Critical care may be appropriate when mastoiditis is complicated by sepsis, meningitis, or cerebral venous sinus thrombosis.
3. Parenteral antibiotics (pending culture results) to cover the most common pathogens is chosen:
   a. Cefuroxime or ampicillin-sulbactam
   b. Clindamycin (in a penicillin-allergic patient)
   c. IV antibiotics are given for at least 7 to 10 days.
   d. If the clinical response to treatment has been satisfactory, oral antimicrobial therapy can be substituted for 3 weeks longer to complete a 4-week course.
3. Myringotomy with or without insertion of a tympanostomy tube is usually performed for drainage. If the patient does

not show improvement in 24 to 48 hours, a simple mastoidectomy may be required.

Clinical Pearls: Acute Mastoiditis

1. This diagnosis should be considered in patients with otitis media and systemic toxicity.
2. Diagnosis of acute mastoiditis is usually made by clinical findings.
3. Parenteral antibiotics and surgical consultation should be initiated as quickly as possible. Intracranial complications (e.g., meningitis, cerebral venous sinus thrombosis) may occur.

BOX 9-12. CLINICAL FEATURES OF ACUTE MASTOIDITIS

- Findings indicative of mastoiditis (Fig. 9-6):
  - (1) Retroauricular pain and swelling
  - (2) Erythema and tenderness to palpation over the mastoid air cells
  - (3) The pinna may be displaced inferiorly and anteriorly (outward)
  - (4) A fluctuant, erythematous, and tender mass overlying the mastoid bone (accumulation of subperiosteal pus)
  - (5) Findings of otitis media (in most cases otorrhea or a bulging, immobile, opaque tympanic membrane)

BOX 9-13. DIFFERENTIAL DIAGNOSIS OF MASTOIDITIS

- Otitis media
- Herpes zoster oticus
- Otitis externa
- Trauma
- Acute barotrauma
- Intracranial infection
- Trigeminal neuralgias
- Venous sinus thrombosis

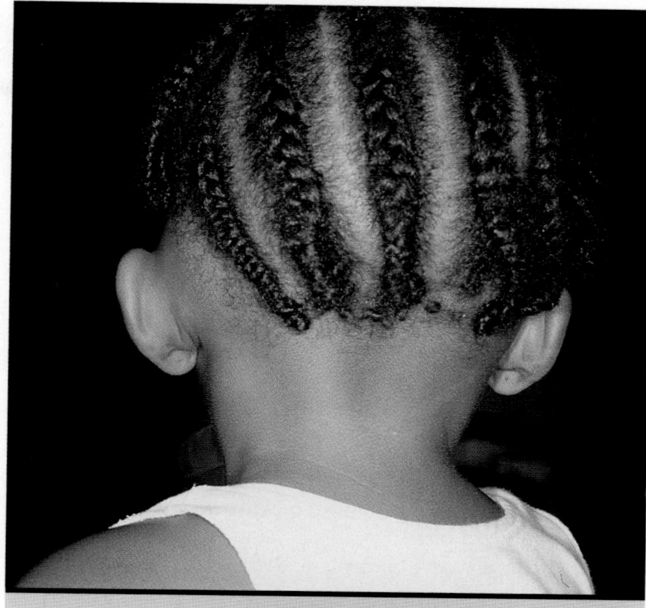

Figure 9-6. Acute Mastoiditis

A downward and lateral (outward) displacement of the auricle associated with erythema and swelling over the mastoid bone were seen in this 14-month-old infant. She also had purulent otorrhea and tenderness to palpation over the mastoid air cells (postauricular area). She was prescribed antibiotic therapy for acute otitis media 1 week prior to this photograph; however, the antibiotic prescription was not filled by the mother. (Reproduced with permission from: Shah BR, Laude TA: *Atlas of Pediatric Clinical Diagnosis.* WB Saunders, Philadelphia, 2000, p. 158.)

DIAGNOSIS EPISTAXIS

Definition

Epistaxis is bleeding from the nose. It can either be anterior or posterior.

Etiology

1. Most episodes of epistaxis originate from the anterior nasal septum in a vascular bed known as Kiesselbach's plexus.
2. Less commonly hemorrhage may originate from branches of the sphenopalatine arteries.
3. The primary initiating factors for anterior epistaxis:
    a. Local trauma due to nose picking (epistaxis digitorum) or a direct blow
    b. URI, a dry environment, or allergies may also contribute

Associated Clinical Features

1. The key clinical discrimination is between anterior and posterior hemorrhage. With brisk bleeding this may be a difficult determination.
2. Look carefully for the presence of a nasal foreign body as an etiological factor leading to epistaxis.
3. Also look carefully for the presence of septal hematoma that can occur following blunt trauma. Untreated septal hematoma can lead to septal perforation or abscess formation.
4. A complete blood count including hemoglobin value and type and cross-match are indicated in a patient presenting with signs of hypovolemia (e.g., a patient with significant blood loss due to a posterior bleed, or patients with bleeding disorders).
5. Laboratory screening for coagulopathy is not indicated in uncomplicated anterior epistaxis, but is mandated by a posterior bleed or by clinical findings (e.g., history of recurrent mucosal hemorrhage or anticoagulant use or the presence of petechiae or easy bruising).
6. While anterior epistaxis is usually not life-threatening, posterior bleeds may be and are difficult to control, usually requiring surgical intervention.

Consultation

Emergent otolaryngologic consultation in cases of suspected posterior epistaxis

Complications

1. Exsanguination
2. Infection complicating nasal packing

Emergency Department Treatment and Disposition

1. Direct compression of the soft bulb of the nose should be maintained for several minutes while necessary equipment is brought to the bedside.
2. After having the patient blow their nose to evacuate any clot, pledgets moistened with solutions of anesthetic and vasoconstrictive agents should be placed in the nares.
3. After several minutes, the pledgets should be removed and the nasal passage examined with the use of a nasal speculum and head lamp.
4. If the bleeding has stopped, emollient antibiotic ointment may be an appropriate intervention.
5. Expandable thrombogenic anterior packing can be used for anterior hemorrhage that persists.
6. Posterior hemorrhage can be managed in the short term with commercially-available devices, gauze packing with petroleum jelly, or Foley catheter tamponade.
7. Adjunctive therapies for pediatric epistaxis, which most often occurs due to nose picking or dry nasal mucosa, include use of a humidifier and rubbing petroleum jelly onto the anterior nasal septum. Educating both patient (if appropriate) and family in order to avoid the trauma caused by nose picking include trimming the fingernails and covering the hands with mittens or socks during sleep.

Clinical Pearls: Epistaxis

1. Most cases of epistaxis can be easily managed with local care.
2. It is uncommon for childhood epistaxis to require nasal packing. Nasal packing should be done in consultation with an otolaryngologist.
3. Posterior hemorrhage is a challenging clinical entity mandating surgical consultation and admission.
4. A history of prolonged bleeding or a history of easy bruisability in a patient or a family member suggests a possible bleeding disorder (Fig. 9-7).

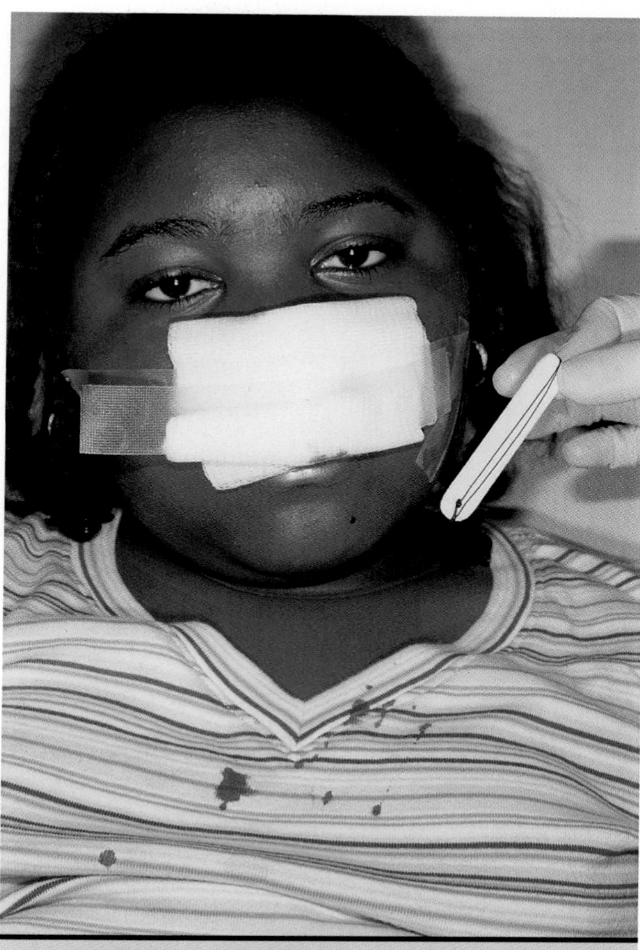

Figure 9-7. Epistaxis in a Patient with Immune Thrombocytopenic Purpura (ITP)

Repeated episodes of epistaxis with prolonged bleeding were the presenting compliant of this patient with a diagnosis of chronic ITP. Her platelet count during this episode of epistaxis was 5000. Nasal packing was applied to control her bleeding and she was hospitalized for close monitoring. A history of prolonged bleeding or a history of easy bruisability in a patient or a family member suggests a systemic disorder and such patients require a thorough history and physical examination and laboratory tests.

BOX 9-14. DIFFERENTIAL DIAGNOSIS OF EPISTAXIS

- Trauma
- Local inflammation including viral or bacterial URI
- Nasal foreign body
- Allergic rhinitis
- Nasal polyps
- Telangiectasias and tumors
- Hematologic disorders (e.g., platelet disorders)
- Drugs (e.g., aspirin, warfarin, NSAIDs)

DIAGNOSIS AURICULAR HEMATOMA

Definition

Auricular hematoma is a collection of blood within the tissue layers of the pinna, most frequently between the cartilage and the perichondrium.

Etiology

Direct trauma to the pinna may result in accumulation of blood between the cartilage and perichondrium. The perichondrium is the only blood supply to the structural cartilage and hematoma accumulation can thus result in necrosis and destruction of the auricular cartilage with resultant cosmetic deformity.

Associated Clinical Features

1. A history of auricular trauma should prompt concern. A common accidental injury in contact sports is auricular hematoma.
2. Auricular hematoma can also occur due to inflicted injury (e.g., child abuse; Fig. 9-8).

Complications

Auricular cartilage necrosis (deformity such as "cauliflower ear")

Consultation

Otolaryngology (if needed for emergent drainage and compressive dressing)

Emergency Department Treatment and Disposition

1. Auricular block will provide appropriate procedural analgesia.
2. Many different therapeutic approaches have been proposed. Hematoma evacuation is the first priority. Most methods depend on evacuation of hematoma and replacing the perichondrium on the cartilage. Various methods include repeated aspiration, incision and drainage with pressure dressing, and suction drainage. Packing sufficient to prevent reaccumulation is also necessary.

Clinical Pearls: Auricular Hematoma

1. Recognition of this condition is essential because of the long-term cosmetic morbidity-associated with improper management.
2. Drainage and prevention of recurrence are the key principles of management.

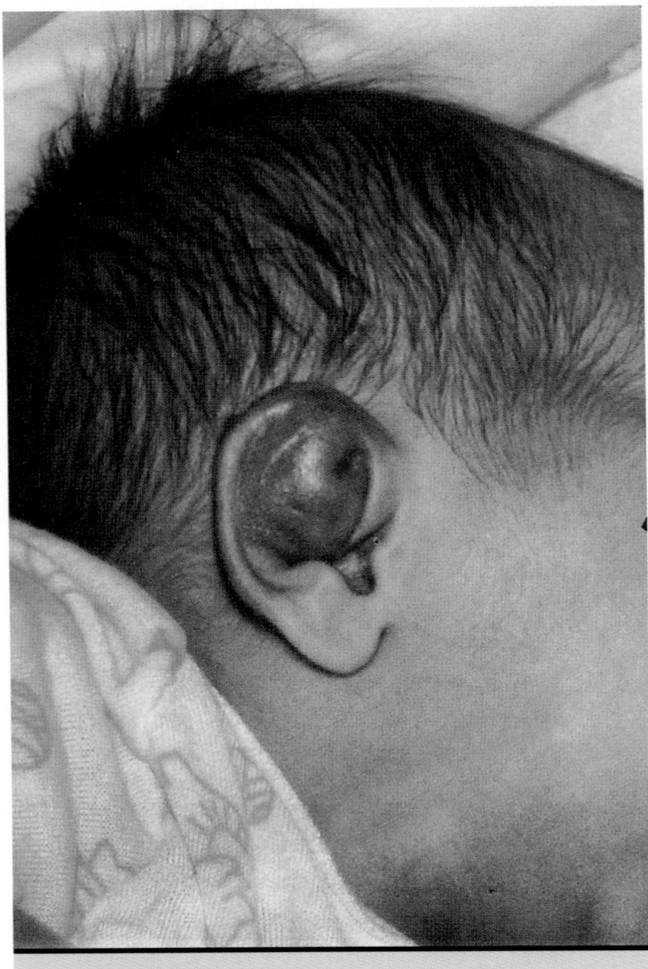

Figure 9-8. Auricular Hematoma due to Child Abuse.

A five-week-old infant presented with 1-week history of cough, vomiting and recent ear swelling. Physical examination revealed a large hematoma of the left pinna. This may lead to the later formation of a cauliflower, or boxer's ear. Physical examination also revealed a torn labial frenulum and multiple healing rib fractures confirming a diagnosis of child abuse.

Reproduced with Permission. Giardino AP, Christial CW and Giardino ER. A Practical Guide to the Evaluation of Child Physical Abuse and Neglect. Sage Publications, Inc; 1997.

BOX 9-15. CLINICAL FEATURES OF AURICULAR HEMATOMA

- Usually within hours after the injury, the skin covering the anterior surface of the auricle is raised by a hematoma (or seroma) which forms in a plane between the cartilage and perichondrium.
- Clinical findings include:
  (1) Distortion of the helix and antihelix
  (2) Tenderness
  (3) Erythema
  (4) Soft tissue swelling

BOX 9-16. DIFFERENTIAL DIAGNOSIS OF AURICULAR HEMATOMA

- Cellulitis
- Abscess

DIAGNOSIS NASAL FOREIGN BODY

Definition

A multitude of objects are commonly inserted into the nasal cavity. Some examples include toys, beads, earrings, marbles, buttons, and vegetable materials (Fig. 9-9).

Clinical Features

1. As with other ENT foreign body (FB) syndromes, risk is determined by behavioral development. Children between 6 months and 6 years of age are generally at risk, as are those with developmental delay.
2. Direct visualization can usually be accomplished with an otoscope, though fiberoptic rhinoscopy may occasionally be a necessary adjunct.
3. Plain radiographs will not detect the majority of FBs, which are not radiopaque. Computed tomography may occasionally be indicated to evaluate infectious or inflammatory complications.

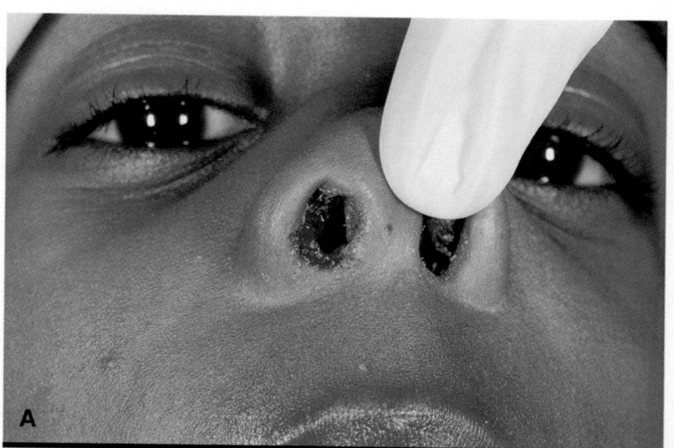

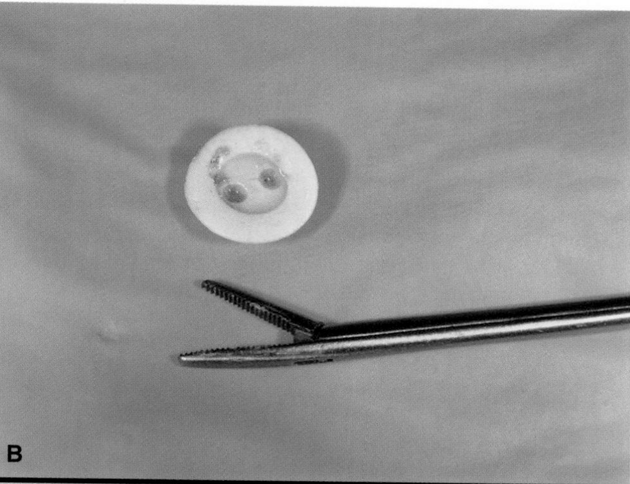

Figure 9-9. Nasal Foreign Body

A. A 6-year-old child was brought to the ED with a complaint of a foul-smelling serosanguineous discharge from the right nostril. He confessed to putting a button in his nostril about 1 week prior to this visit. The button that was removed is shown in *B*.

Complications

1. Airway occlusion
2. Rhinosinusitis

Consultation

Otolaryngology (with unsuccessful attempts at the removal of a FB; while this need not be emergent, mucosal edema and infection may complicate delayed management)

Emergency Department Treatment and Disposition

1. Many of these FBs can be managed by having the parent assist the child in blowing the nose. The parent gives the child a "kiss", blowing into the mouth while occluding the unaffected nare. The insufflated air follows the path of least resistance, usually dislodging the offending object.
2. If the above method is unsuccessful, the following method can be tried:
   a. Restrain the child with immobilization of the head.
   b. For better visualization of a FB, anesthetize the nasal mucosa with lidocaine spray and reduce the edema with phenylephrine nose drops followed by suctioning the nasal discharge.
   c. The FB can often be removed with the help of an alligator forceps or a curette.
3. Otolaryngological consultation is indicated where the emergency physician is unable to remove the object.

Clinical Pearls: Nasal Foreign Body

1. Unilateral, foul-smelling nasal discharge is due to a FB until proven otherwise.
2. Antibiotics are not necessary once the FB has been dislodged, unless sinusitis has developed.
3. Both sides of the nose and both ears must be examined, as patients presenting with one FB are at greater risk for FBs at other sites.
4. Removal attempts under suboptimal conditions may lead to bleeding and movement of the FB to a less accessible location. FBs that are pushed into the nasopharynx during such attempts can be swallowed or aspirated.
5. Signs and symptoms of a FB may be subtle and history of insertion of a FB may be lacking.
6. Nasal FBs can mimic chronic infections or tumors.

BOX 9-17. CLINICAL FEATURES OF NASAL FOREIGN BODY

- Foreign bodies are most often self-inserted (usually as a part of play).
- The nose is the most common site for insertion of a FB in children <3 years of age (as opposed to the ear, which is the most common site in children between 3 and 8 years of age).
- Most cases will present with a complaint of an FB in the nose.
- Chronic or foul-smelling nasal discharge, usually unilateral
- Unilateral nasal obstruction
- Usually the FB can be readily seen (however, mucosal edema may obscure its visualization).
- Recurrent epistaxis (undiscovered FBs may lead to mucosal erosions, leading to recurrent epistaxis)

BOX 9-18. DIFFERENTIAL DIAGNOSIS OF NASAL FOREIGN BODY

- Sinusitis
- Viral URI
- Nasal polyps
- Tumor

BOX 10-1. CLINICAL FEATURES OF PYLORIC STENOSIS

- Infant is usually normal at birth without vomiting for the first few weeks of life.
- *Onset of symptoms:*
  (1) Mean age: 2 to 3 weeks after birth
  (2) Range: birth to 5 months of age
  (3) Rare before first week or after third month of life
- Prominent gastric peristaltic waves crossing from left to right across the abdomen may be seen after feeding.
- *Characteristics of vomitus:*
  (1) First begins as regurgitation of feedings; eventually becomes forceful or projectile
  (2) Vomiting occurs shortly after feeding or near the end of feeding
  (3) Nonbilious and nonbloody (rarely may contain streaks of blood)
  (4) Contains milk feeding that infant had just taken earlier
  (5) Infant appears hungry after vomiting and wants to feed again.
- *Pyloric "olive":*
  (1) A firm, fusible, ballotable mass with size and shape of an olive (~2 cm in length)
  (2) Best palpated when stomach is empty or immediately after the infant has vomited (the abdominal musculature is more relaxed after vomiting)
  (3) Best palpated from the left side
  (4) Palpated in 60 to 80% of patients
  (5) Usually palpated in midepigastric area beneath liver edge
  (6) *If palpated, pathognomonic for pyloric stenosis*
  (7) *Absence of the "olive" does not exclude the diagnosis.*
- *Metabolic derangements:*
  (1) Hypochloremia
  (2) Hypokalemia
  (3) Metabolic alkalosis
  (4) Serum sodium *normal*
  (5) Blood urea nitrogen elevated (with dehydration)
  (6) Urine pH acidic (*paradoxical aciduria* in the face of metabolic alkalosis)
- *Late signs of PS include:*
  (1) Signs of wasting or poor weight gain
  (2) Signs of dehydration (e.g., sunken eyes, poor skin turgor, dry mucous membranes, and lethargy)
  (3) Decrease in stool number or constipation

BOX 10-2. DIFFERENTIAL DIAGNOSIS OF PYLORIC STENOSIS

- Nonbilious vomiting and/or regurgitation from other etiologies
  (1) Normal regurgitation
  (2) Gastroesophageal reflux
  (3) Milk intolerance
  (4) Acute gastroenteritis
  (5) Acute abdomen (e.g., intestinal obstruction)
  (6) Other gastric malformations (e.g., pyloric atresia, antral webs, gastric duplication, gastric volvulus)
  (7) Peptic ulcer disease
  (8) Salt-wasting adrenogenital syndrome
  (9) Bezoars
- Hypochloremic, hypokalemic metabolic alkalosis from other etiologies
  (1) Gastric outlet obstruction from other etiologies (e.g., pyloric atresia, antral webs, gastric duplication, gastric volvulus, choledochal cyst)
  (2) Bartter's syndrome

DIAGNOSIS

INTUSSUSCEPTION

Definition

Intussusception occurs when the proximal part of the intestine invaginates into the lumen of the distal adjoining bowel segment.

Etiology and Pathogenesis

1. Infants
   a. Idiopathic (about 90 to 95% of cases)
   b. Lead point is hypertrophied Peyer's patches and lymph nodes following a viral infection (e.g., adenoviral gastroenteritis)
   c. An association between rotavirus vaccine and intussusception led to the voluntary withdrawal of the vaccine from the market.
2. Older children
   a. Recognizable anatomical lead point is the rule (about 75% of cases)
   b. Some examples include Meckel's diverticulum (most common), Peutz-Jeghers' syndrome, tumors (lymphoma, hemangioma), duplication cysts, appendix, and Henoch-Schönlein purpura (HSP) with intramural hematoma (Fig. 10-3) and *Ascaris lumbricoides* worm infestation.
   c. Intussusception also occurs in dehydrated patients with cystic fibrosis.
4. Intussusception usually starts with a lead point just proximal to the ileocecal valve leading to an ileocolic invagination. During telescoping, the mesentery is dragged along with the *intussusceptum* (proximal invaginating portion of the bowel) into the *intussuscipiens* (the adjacent distal recipient portion of the bowel). As the process continues and intensifies, the mesentery of the intussusceptum becomes compressed leading to venous engorgement, edema, and bleeding from the mucosa (clinically, bloody stools mixed with mucus). Further pressure of entrapment may lead to obstruction of the mesenteric arteries leading to gangrene perforation of the bowel and peritonitis.

Associated Clinical Features

1. Intussusception may occur at any point along the GI tract.
   a. The most common site of intussusception is ileocolic (90% of cases) and ileoileocolic.
   b. Less common sites are cecocolic, and rarely just ileoileal.
   c. Ileoileal intussusceptions may occur in children with HSP.
3. The intussusceptum along with its mesentery may continue through the colon a variable distance, occasionally as far as the rectum, where it can be palpated on rectal exam (Fig. 10-4).
4. Ileoileal intussusception (e.g., typically seen with HSP) may have a less typical clinical picture, the symptoms and signs being chiefly those of small intestinal obstruction.
5. Signs of systemic toxicity (due to gangrenous bowel or peritonitis) may be present and include fever and marked abdominal distention and leukocytosis.

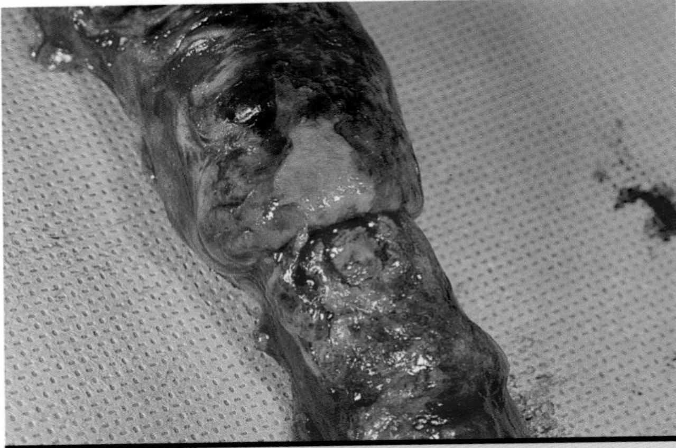

Figure 10-3. Intussusception in Henoch-Schönlein Purpura

A magnified view of ileoileal colic intussusception after bowel resection in a patient with Henoch-Schönlein purpura in whom the intussusception could not be reduced by barium enema. The proximal portion of the ileum (intussusceptum) telescopes into the more distal ileum and cecum (intussuscipiens). This image also illustrates necrosis of both the intussusceptum and intussuscipiens.

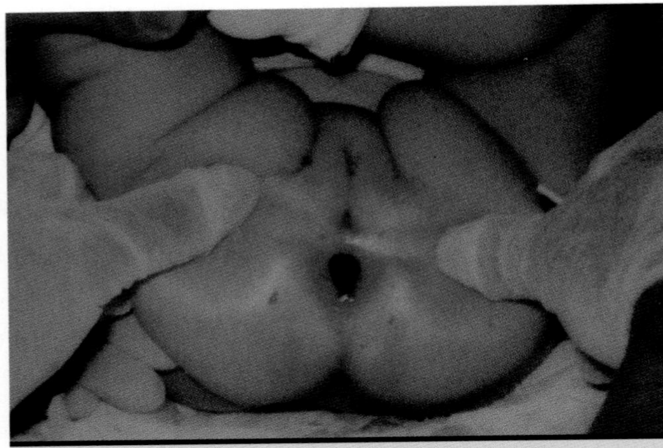

Figure 10-4. Intussusception

The apex of the intussusception may extend into the transverse, descending, or sigmoid colon—even to and through the anus. This presentation must be distinguished from rectal prolapse. This type of intussusception can be distinguished from prolapse of the rectum by the separation between the protruding intestine and the rectal wall, which does not exist in rectal prolapse.

6. Laboratory tests include CBC, serum electrolytes, glucose, and blood type and cross-match.
7. Acute abdomen series (upright chest and a supine and upright abdomen)
   a. Radiographs are usually nonspecific in the diagnosis of intussusception, but help in identification of free air in the abdomen.
   b. Radiologic findings that suggest a diagnosis of intussusception include minimal intestinal gas, minimal fecal contents in colon, mass lesion, and air-fluid levels in dilated small bowel loops (particularly if the large bowel appears empty; or signs of obstruction (usually appear later in the course).
   c. *Normal radiographs do not rule out intussusception and should not deter one from administering an enema in a infant with a strong suspicion of intussusception.*
8. Abdominal ultrasound (US)
   a. A sensitive and specific noninvasive test that can be used for the diagnosis of intussusception
   b. US can be reliably used as an initial screening test to exclude intussusception (US has been shown to correlate well with the negative findings of contrast enemas).
   c. US use is limited by the therapeutic implications of using barium or air contrast enemas for diagnosis.
   d. Findings of intussusception include:
      1) Concentric loops of intestine within intussusception are seen as a tubular or kidney-shaped mass in longitudinal views and a doughnut or target-shaped mass in transverse images.
      2) US images may also show the presence of lymph nodes in the intussusception (attesting to the fact that most lead points result from hyperplasia of lymph nodes associated with infections).
9. Complications include intestinal hemorrhage, necrosis secondary to local ischemia, bowel perforation, peritonitis, sepsis, and shock.

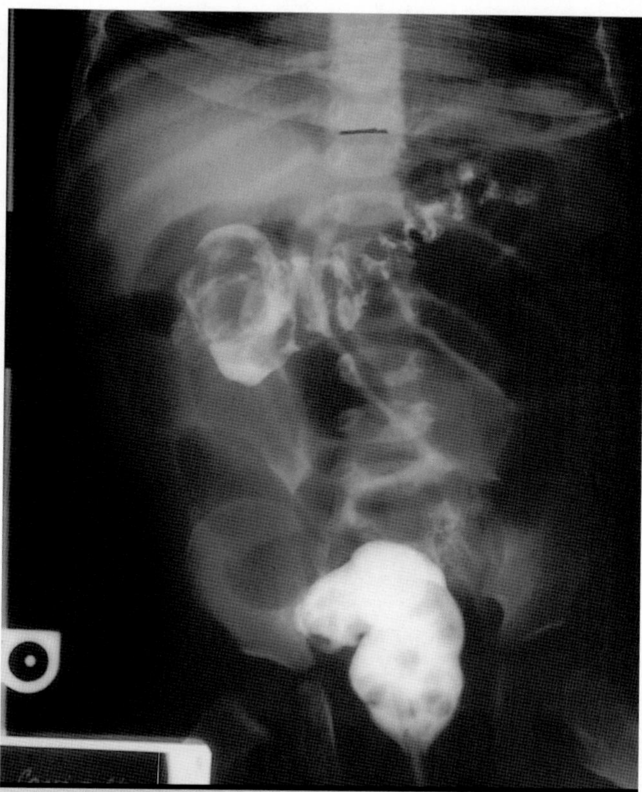

Figure 10-5. Intussusception

Post-evacuation film of barium enema shows a large filling defect (coil-spring appearance) in the hepatic flexure, an unresolved ileocolic intussusception. Contrast material between the intussusceptum and the intussuscipiens is responsible for the coil-spring appearance.

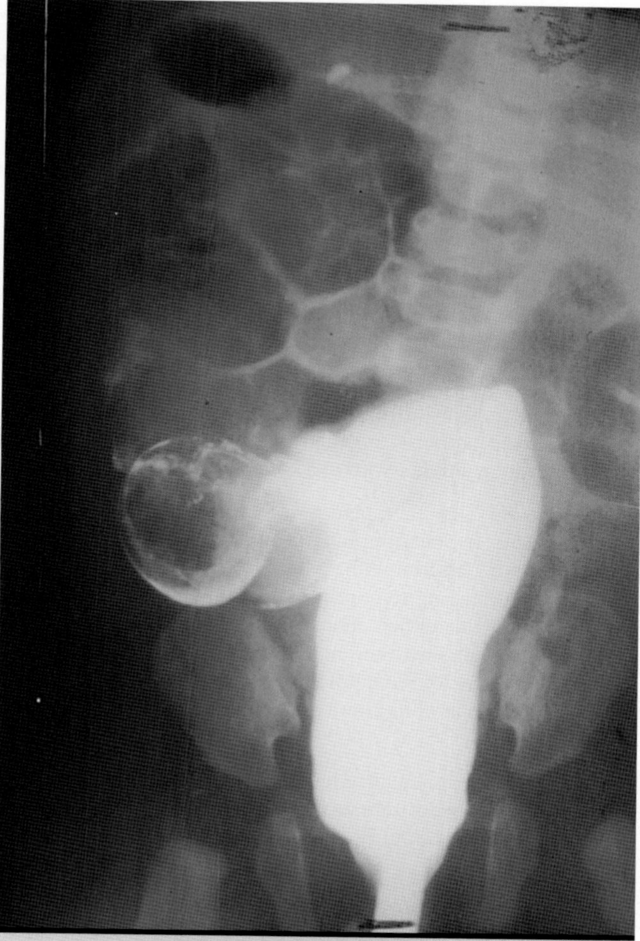

Figure 10-6. Intussusception Extending into the Sigmoid Colon

Consultations

Emergent surgical and radiologist consultations

Emergency Department Treatment and Disposition

1. Stabilization of the patient based on abnormal vital signs (e.g., patient presenting with shock or peritonitis) including continuous cardiac and pulse oximetry monitoring
   a. Fluid resuscitation is carried out, as clinically indicated, by IV fluid boluses of 20 mL/kg of crystalloid until adequate vascular volume is achieved.
   b. For febrile or ill-appearing patients with shock, broad-spectrum triple antibiotic coverage is given (e.g., ampicillin and gentamicin, and either clindamycin or metronidazole).
2. Keep the patient off of oral intake and insert a nasogastric tube to decompress any gaseous distention or to prevent aspiration in infants who are vomiting.
3. Diagnostic and therapeutic interventions are somewhat dependent on location and resources available in a given institution. Children with suspected intussusception require definitive imaging to confirm the diagnosis and subsequent reduction with either enema (hydrostatic reduction using barium) or air insufflation. The surgical staff should be in attendance for the attempted reduction, with an anesthesiologist and operating room staff alerted should reduction be unsuccessful.
4. Intraoperative manual reduction is required for cases with unsuccessful hydrostatic reduction, and if indicated, resection of gangrenous bowel or a recognizable lead point is done.
5. Hospitalization is recommended for all patients after reduction because of the possible risk of recurrence. Recurrent intussusception is seen in about 5 to 8% of cases. It is more common after hydrostatic than surgical reduction. Recurrence is also more common in an older child and an anatomical lead point must be suspected.

Clinical Pearls: Intussusception

1. Intussusception is the second most common cause of acute intestinal obstruction between 3 months and 2 years of age (the first being an incarcerated inguinal hernia).
2. Up to 60% of cases of intussusception are initially misdiagnosed; gastroenteritis most commonly is confused with intussusception.
3. Currant-jelly stool is a late finding of intussusception; its absence does *not* exclude the diagnosis (Fig. 10-7).
4. *Profound lethargy without a preceding history of abdominal pain* may be the only presenting sign of intussusception (up to 10% of cases). Such neurologic signs of intussusception often get misdiagnosed as sepsis or as a postictal state, delaying the correct diagnosis and management.
5. Intussusception rarely reduces spontaneously; if left untreated it would result in death in most cases.

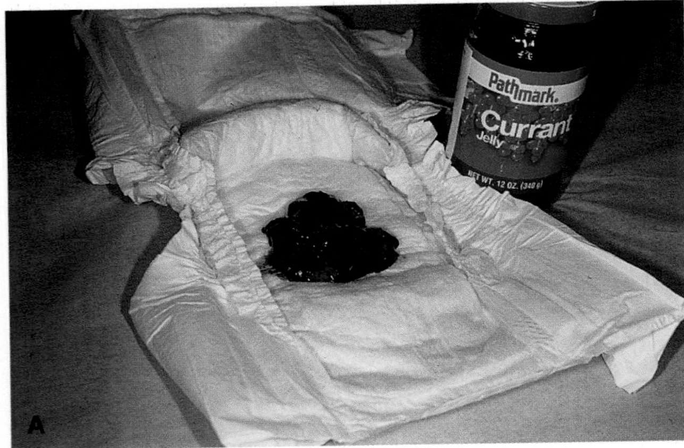

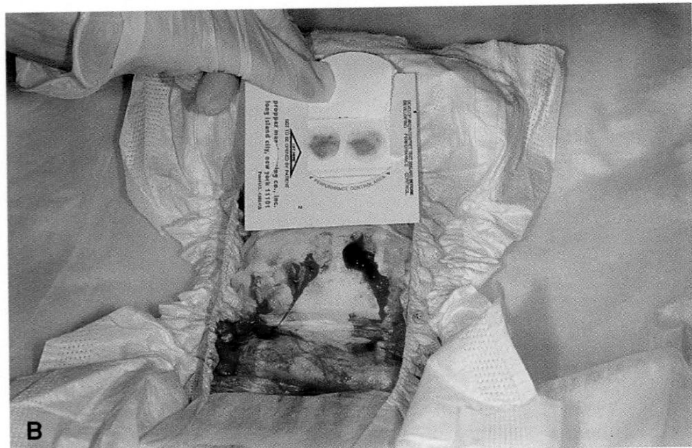

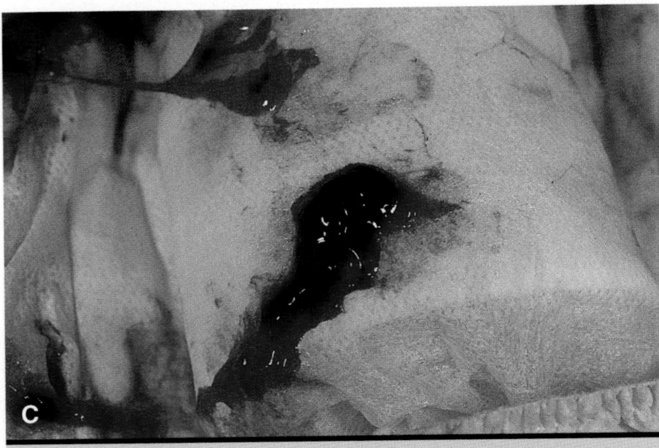

Figure 10-7. Currant-Jelly Stool

A. Commercially available currant jelly. *B*., *C*. Diarrhea containing mucus and blood constitutes the classic currant-jelly stool most often associated with intussusception, although it occurs relatively infrequently. This stool was passed by an 8-month-old infant who presented with inconsolable crying episodes and bilious vomiting.

BOX 10-3. CLINICAL FEATURES OF INTUSSUSCEPTION

- Age at presentation
  - (1) Peak incidence: 7 to 9 months (range: 2 months to 5 years)
  - (2) About 60% of patients: <1 year
  - (3) About 80% of patients: <2 years
- Abdominal pain (80 to 95% of cases)
  - (1) Pattern of pain fairly characteristic
  - (2) Episodic severe colicky pain (often infants rock back and forth) often leading to episodic bouts of crying or moaning with pain
  - (3) Guarded position with knees and legs pulled up onto the abdomen
  - (4) The infant may sleep or may appear listless, lethargic, or playful between episodes of pain.
- Abdominal mass (65% of cases)
  - (1) An ill-defined variably tender sausage-shaped mass
  - (2) Mass palpable in right upper quadrant or mid-abdomen
  - (3) Absence of bowel in the right lower quadrant (Dance's sign)
- Vomitus (75% of cases)
  - (1) Initially nonbilious but may progress to bilious
  - (2) Vomitus may be feculent
- Stool (currant-jelly stools; 60% of cases)
  - (1) Diarrheal stool with gross blood and mucus (either passed spontaneously or following rectal exam)
  - (2) A normal-appearing stool positive for occult blood
- Rectal exam (rectal exam may reveal the first evidence of bleeding)
  - (1) Presence of blood mixed with stool
  - (2) Occasionally intussusception can be felt on rectal examination (Fig. 10-4.)
- Neurologic signs of intussusception
  - (1) Lack of interaction
  - (2) Extreme lethargy or coma or shock-like state (out of proportion to abdominal signs)
  - (3) Irritability and alternating or progressive lethargy
  - (4) Seizures or seizure-like activity
  - (5) Weak cry
  - (6) Apnea
  - (7) Hypotonia
  - (8) Opisthotonic posturing
- Classic triad of intussusception (classic triad seen in *only 21% of cases*; 75% of cases have two findings, and 13% have none or only one finding)
  - (1) Intermittent colicky abdominal pain (85% of cases)
  - (2) Bilious vomiting (75% of cases)
  - (3) Currant-jelly stool (60% of cases)

BOX 10-4. DIFFERENTIAL DIAGNOSIS OF INTUSSUSCEPTION

- Gastroenteritis
- Enterocolitis (abdominal pain with bloody mucoid diarrhea)
- Meckel's diverticulum (painless rectal bleeding)
- Henoch-Schönlein purpura (abdominal pain and bleeding due to vasculitis)
- Trauma (e.g., child abuse)
- Incarcerated inguinal hernia
- Infantile colic
- Appendicitis
- Inflammatory bowel disease
- Polyps

BOX 10-5. INTUSSUSCEPTION AND ENEMA

- Gold standard for diagnosis and treatment of intussusception is barium enema (Figs. 10-5 and 10-6) or air contrast enema.
- Sedation is often helpful for relaxing the infant during the study.
- Contraindications for enema
  - (1) Evidence of peritonitis
  - (2) Intestinal perforation or pneumatosis intestinalis
  - (3) Shock or very ill-appearing patient
- Barium enema
  - (1) Reduction confirmed *only* with adequate reflux of barium into the ileum
  - (2) Successful reduction is done in 50 to 75% of cases.
  - (3) Ileoileal intussusception is usually not demonstrable by barium enema and reduction using hydrostatic technique may not be possible (it is suspected because of gaseous distention of the intestine above the lesion).
  - (4) Complications include chemical peritonitis and perforation (risk ~2.5 to 5% of attempted barium reductions)
- Air enema
  - (1) Reflux of air into the terminal ileum and disappearance of the mass at the ileocecal valve document successful reduction.
  - (2) Air contrast obviates the risk of barium peritonitis should a perforation be present.
  - (3) Less radiation than a barium enema
  - (4) Complications include tension pneumoperitoneum and perforation (risk ~0.1 to 0.2%)

DIAGNOSIS ACUTE APPENDICITIS

Definition and Etiology

1. The appendix is a diverticulum that extends from the inferior tip of cecum. The lining of the appendix is interspersed with lymphoid follicles. Common locations of the appendix are anterior or retrocecal. Uncommon locations include subcecal, within the hernial sac, and in the right and left upper and lower quadrants.
2. Obstruction of the appendiceal lumen due to various etiologies (e.g., fecalith, viral infections leading to lymphoid follicle hyperplasia, foreign body) leads to inflammation of the appendix. Distension due to mucus secretion leads to secondary infection of the appendix.
3. Ulceration of the inflamed mucosa may result in necrosis and rupture of the appendix. Peritonitis with or without abscess formation occurs due to spillage of the appendiceal contents into the peritoneal cavity.

Associated Clinical Features

1. Appendicitis is most commonly seen in the second and third decade of life (peak incidence is between 10 and 30 years of age); however, it can occur at any age.
2. Appendicitis is more common in males than in females (male:female ratio 2:1).
3. A typical sequence of acute appendicitis:
   a. The first symptom is periumbilical pain (distension of the appendix) followed by anorexia, nausea, right lower quadrant pain (involvement of visceral and parietal peritoneum), vomiting, and fever.
   b. This sequence of events is seen less commonly in children.
4. Nonspecific symptoms and signs that often lead to a delay in the diagnosis in neonates, infants, and young children include fever, irritability or lethargy, abdominal distension, vomiting and diarrhea, refusal to walk or limping, a palpable mass, abdominal wall cellulitis, respiratory distress or grunting respirations, and signs of shock.
5. A genitourinary examination (examination of the testes in males and examination of the perineum including a rectal-abdominal or pelvic exam, as indicated) must be performed while evaluating patients for appendicitis, as many genitourinary disorders present with right lower quadrant pain.
6. Rectal examination:
   a. Controversy exists about whether a rectal exam is mandatory for diagnosis of appendicitis in children, as it is a nonspecific and insensitive test for appendicitis.
   b. It may show tenderness or bogginess (a mass consistent with a growing pelvic abscess) on the right with the appendix directed toward the pelvis.
   c. A rectal exam does not add data that cannot be obtained with an anterior abdominal exam; however, it helps in patients for whom the diagnosis of appendicitis is not straightforward.

7. Laboratory evaluation includes:
   a. Complete blood cell count
      1) White blood cell count (WBC) can be normal in early appendicitis. *Do not rely entirely on a normal WBC to exclude appendicitis.*
      2) Significant elevation with a left shift is usually seen with perforated appendicitis.
      3) An elevated WBC count can be seen in other conditions that often mimic appendicitis (e.g., pelvic inflammatory disease [PID], gastroenteritis).
   b. Urinalysis to exclude urinary tract infection; microscopic pyuria or hematuria may be found in patients with an inflamed appendix near the bladder.
   c. Serum electrolytes, glucose, creatinine, and blood urea nitrogen values to assess the status of hydration
   d. Pregnancy test in all postmenarchal adolescent females
8. Acute abdomen series:
   a. Include upright chest film (to exclude pneumonia that may present with acute abdominal symptoms); supine and upright abdomen films may help when the diagnosis is uncertain
   b. Some findings that are suggestive of appendicitis but not pathognomonic include:
      1) Fecalith or appendicolith (the lumen of the appendix may contain fecal material, and if calcified may be seen radiographically; radiographic evidence of a fecalith is seen in 20% of cases)
      2) A few localized loops (sentinel loops) of small intestine and/or dilated cecum containing an air-fluid level in the right lower quadrant (RLQ) associated with scoliosis with concave curvature of the lumbar spine to the right due to muscle spasm (even though nonspecific, this is one of the most common findings of nonperforated AP)
      3) Loss of the psoas shadow on the right
      4) Obliteration of the right properitoneal fat line
      5) Gas in the appendix
      6) Haziness over the right sacroiliac joint
      7) Signs of perforated appendix include a paucity of air in the RLQ (due to development of an inflammatory process [abscess or phlegmon]) with functional obstruction of the small bowel (absence of gas in the ascending colon due to spasm of the cecum and ascending colon due to perforation and a subsequent inflammatory process).
9. Ultrasound (US) of abdomen may be used as an initial screening test
   a. Specificity usually in excess of 90%; thus, a positive US helps rule in the diagnosis of AP.
   b. A negative US examination by an inexperienced examiner does not exclude AP. *Appendicitis is ruled out reliably only if an experienced examiner confidently visualizes a normal appendix.*
   c. Advantages of US: it is noninvasive, there is no ionizing radiation exposure, and it requires only minimal patient preparation.
   d. US is extremely helpful in identifying gynecological disorders that are commonly considered in the differential diagnosis of AP.
   e. Limitations of US include: it is operator dependent, technically limited in certain situations (e.g., obesity, abdominal guarding), and visualization of the appendix in an atypical location is difficult. US is also more likely to miss perforated appendicitis.
10. Computed tomography (CT) of abdomen:
    a. Contrast protocols vary among institutions (e.g., CT done with oral, intravenous, and rectal contrast, or limited CT of the abdomen with rectal contrast).
    b. CT serves as a useful adjunct in the diagnosis of ,appendicitis with sensitivity ranging from 87 to 100% and specificity ranging from 89 to 98% (CT is sensitive enough to virtually rule out appendicitis with a negative test).
    c. Excellent for showing the presence of appendicitis (both nonperforated and perforated)
    d. Findings of nonperforated CT: fluid-filled dilated appendix with stranding of surrounding fat (Fig. 10-8)

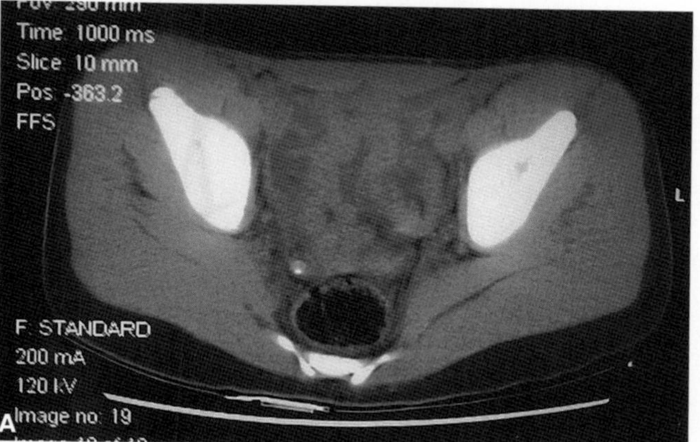

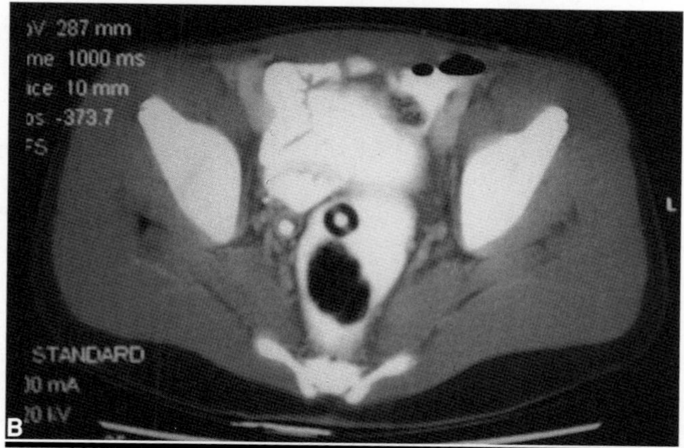

Figure 10-8. Acute Appendicitis

A. A non–contrast enhanced axial CT scan through the pelvis reveals a calcific appendicolith in a pelvic appendix. Inspissated, sometimes calcified fecal material leads to obstruction followed by secondary bacterial invasion. Radiographic evidence of a fecalith is seen in 20% of cases. The presence of an appendicolith along with inflammation is indicative either of acute appendicitis or of impending appendicitis. *B*. Contrast enhanced CT scan of the pelvis reveals the previously described appendicolith in a dilated fluid-filled and thick-walled appendix. Enhancement of the appendiceal wall is also noted.

e. Findings of perforated appendicitis: phlegmon and/or abscess formation

Consultation

1. Surgery consultation for the operative management of straightforward cases
2. Surgery consultation for patients for whom the diagnosis is uncertain (keep a low threshold for early consultation for such cases).

Emergency Department Treatment and Disposition

1. Appendectomy is the treatment for appendicitis. Patients can be taken directly to the operating room (OR) in the absence of metabolic derangements or fluid deficits.
2. Patients with significant fluid losses (due to vomiting, diarrhea, or third spacing [sequestration of intraluminal or intraperitoneal fluid]) should be fluid resuscitated *prior* to surgery (as indicated, crystalloid boluses of 20 mL/kg given to restore intravascular volume).
3. Patients with a perforated appendix are given antibiotics to cover both anaerobic and aerobic pathogens (e.g., ampicillin, gentamicin, and clindamycin) prior to surgery. In the OR, peritoneal fluid is cultured (for both anaerobic and aerobic pathogens), and subsequent therapy may be modified accordingly.
4. If appendicitis is suspected but not definite, observe the patient in the ED or as an inpatient for serial abdominal examinations (*remember the value of repeated frequent examinations*).

Clinical Pearls: Acute Appendicitis

1. Acute abdomen is not a diagnosis; its a term used to define the area of concern.
2. Appendicitis is the most common acute atraumatic surgical condition of the abdomen in children aged 2 years and older.
3. Appendicitis is very difficult to diagnose in younger children; the perforation rate in children younger than 8 years is twice that in those older than 8 years.
4. Appendicitis remains primarily a clinical diagnosis; however, imaging is strongly recommended in clinically equivocal cases.
5. *No* laboratory test is diagnostic for appendicitis. *Do not* rely entirely on a normal white blood cell count to exclude appendicitis. Confirmation of the clinical diagnosis of appendicitis by plain radiography, US, or CT should be pursued only after surgical consultation, if the diagnosis is in doubt.
6. About 15% of patients with appendicitis present with diarrhea. Diarrhea is the most confusing symptom leading to a delay in diagnosis, as patients often get misdiagnosed with gastroenteritis.
7. The lower abdominal pain described by the patient with AP is virtually always crescendo, building without any periods of relief. If the pain suddenly but only temporarily recedes, it signals perforation of the appendix and release of intraluminal pressure.
8. Missed appendicitis is one of the most common diagnoses resulting in malpractice claims. Initial misdiagnosis rates range from 28 to 57% for children 12 years old or younger, to nearly 100% for those 2 years or younger.

BOX 10-6. CLINICAL SIGNS OF ACUTE APPENDICITIS

- McBurney's point tenderness
  (1) With classic location of the appendix, the area of maximum pain and tenderness is at McBurney's point, which is located one-third of the distance from the right anterior superior iliac spine to the umbilicus.
  (2) About 75% of normal appendices lie inferior and medial to McBurney's point.
  (3) About 50% of appendices are located 5 to 10 cm from McBurney's point.
  (4) About 15% of appendices are located more than 10 cm from McBurney's point.
- Right lower quadrant tenderness
- Rovsing's sign: percussion or deep palpation of the left lower quadrant causes pain referred to the right lower quadrant.
- Positive psoas sign: extension of the right hip to stretch the psoas muscle will produce pain if an inflamed appendix is lying near the psoas muscle.
- Obturator sign: pain on passive internal rotation of the flexed right hip
- Signs suggestive of peritonitis (seen with a perforated appendix; Box 10-7)

BOX 10-7. SIGNS OF PERFORATED APPENDICITIS

- Progression of appendicitis to necrosis and perforation are seen:
  (1) In 10% of patients by 24 hours
  (2) In 50% of patients by 48 hours
- Patients with a perforated appendix appear ill with signs of toxicity/prostration:
  (1) Higher temperature
  (2) Significant tachycardia (e.g., out of proportion to fever)
  (3) Dyspnea, grunting
  (4) Pallor
  (5) Signs of septic shock
  (6) Leukocytosis (leukopenia with overwhelming sepsis/septic shock)
  (7) *Patients do not like to move* and feel most comfortable lying on their sides with the hips and knees flexed.
  (8) Patients walk very slowly in a bent-over position with a shuffling gait while holding the right side of the abdomen.
  (9) Patients will refuse to hop or jump due to extreme pain.
  (10) *Remember: Patients with obstruction are restless, and move around the bed, while patients with peritonitis are quiet, without movement.*
- Abdominal mass
- Patients with a perforated appendix show signs of peritonitis:
  (1) Rigidity
  (2) Involuntary guarding
  (3) Rebound tenderness
  (4) Percussion tenderness (best method for eliciting peritonitis, beginning in the area that you suspect will not be tender)
  (5) Cough sign (abdominal pain while coughing)
  (6) Abdominal distension
  (7) Absent or decreased bowel sounds
  (8) Striking the right heel while the patient is lying supine causes pain in the RLQ.
- Most common bacterial pathogens seen with perforated appendicitis:
  (1) Aerobes: *Escherichia coli*, *Klebsiella* spp., *Pseudomonas* spp.
  (2) Anaerobes: *Bacteroides fragilis*, *Peptostreptococcus* spp.

BOX 10-8. ATYPICAL PRESENTATIONS OF ACUTE APPENDICITIS

- Prominent flank or back pain with less anterior abdominal pain (extraperitoneal or retrocecal appendix)
- Genitourinary symptoms (irritation of ureter or bladder by inflamed appendix):
  (1) Pain on urination
  (2) Testicular pain
  (3) Penile pain
- Appendicitis and diarrhea (seen in about 15% of patients):
  (1) Seen with a pelvic appendix that is lying in proximity to the sigmoid colon and rectum (extension of the inflammatory process to the muscular wall of the sigmoid colon)
  (2) Diarrhea is the most confusing symptom leading to delay in diagnosis (patients often are misdiagnosed with gastroenteritis)
  (3) Two features that may help in differentiating gastroenteritis from appendicitis:
    A. Rectal exam: tenderness present with pelvic appendicitis while patients with gastroenteritis do not have tenderness
    B. Stool volume/character: a child with appendicitis passes small amount of stool and gas followed by relief of symptoms until the sigmoid colon becomes distended again with fluid or gas; child with gastroenteritis typically passes voluminous liquid stools

BOX 10-9. COMPONENTS OF THE MANTRELS SCORE USED FOR DIAGNOSING ACUTE APPENDICITIS

	Score
Symptoms:	
*M*igration of abdominal pain from the epigastrium to the RLQ	1
*A*norexia	1
*N*ausea or vomiting	1
Signs:	
*T*enderness in the RLQ	2
*R*ebound tenderness	1
*E*levation of temperature	1
Laboratory tests:	
*L*eukocytosis	2
*S*hift to left of WBC count	1
Total possible score	10

Recommendations

Score <5: appendicitis unlikely

Score 5 or 6: appendicitis possible

Score >6: appendicitis likely

- The eight variables described above that are associated with appendicitis have been tested in children presenting with abdominal pain:
  (1) With a cutoff value of 7, its sensitivity and specificity improve as the age of the child increases.
  (2) In patients 16 or 17 years old with a score of 7: 100% sensitivity and 93% specificity for having appendicitis
  (3) In other age groups, the value of the score is limited.
  (4) The score is not as accurate in women as in men (due to gynecological problems mimicking appendicitis)
  (5) Despite its limitations, this scoring system serves as a useful checklist of signs and symptoms in evaluating patients for possible appendicitis.

(Reproduced with permission from: Alvarado A: A practical score for the early diagnosis of appendicitis. *Ann Emerg Med* 1986;15:557.)

BOX 10-10. DIFFERENTIAL DIAGNOSIS OF ACUTE ABDOMEN/ACUTE APPENDICITIS

- Intussusception
- Midgut volvulus
- Testicular torsion
- Pelvic inflammatory disease
- Ectopic pregnancy
- Ovarian torsion
- Ruptured ovarian cyst or *mittelschmerz* (mid–menstrual cycle ovulatory pain)
- Ovarian tumors (e.g., teratoma)
- Incarcerated hernia
- Constipation with fecal impaction
- Trauma
- Mesenteric adenitis
- Meckel's diverticulum
- Henoch-Schönlein purpura
- Right lower lobe pneumonia
- Bacterial enterocolitis (e.g., pseudoappendicitis due to *Yersinia eneterocolitica* or *Campylobacter jejuni* infection)
- Diabetic ketoacidosis
- Gastroenteritis
- Acute pyelonephritis

DIAGNOSIS

INCARCERATED INGUINAL HERNIA

Definition and Etiology

1. The majority of inguinal hernias in children are indirect hernias (i.e., they occur as a result of incomplete or abnormal obliteration of the processus vaginalis).
2. The processus vaginalis is a diverticulum of the peritoneal cavity and accompanies the testicle as it descends into the scrotum. Layers of the processus fuse after the testicle is in the scrotum; however, the timing of this closure varies among different individuals. In the majority, it fuses by 2 years of age (up to 30% of adults may have a patent processus vaginalis).
3. An indirect inguinal hernia exists when abdominal or pelvic viscera enter the patent processus and travel through the internal ring into the inguinal canal. The bowel is the most commonly found organ within the hernia sac in the boys, while ovaries or fallopian tubes are commonly seen within hernia sacs in girls.
4. Incarceration is defined as an inability to reduce the hernia (hernial sac contents) into the abdominal cavity.

Associated Clinical Features

1. The incidence of inguinal hernias is 1 to 5%.
2. Boys are 3 to 10 times more likely to have hernias than girls.
3. Premature and low birth-weight infants have a higher risk of developing an inguinal hernia.
4. Inguinal hernias usually present with an asymptomatic bulge in the groin that becomes more prominent with crying, straining, or laughing.
5. Inguinal hernias may be either unilateral or bilateral, especially in premature and low birth-weight infants.
6. About two-thirds of hernias are seen on the right side, one-third are seen on the left side and few are seen bilaterally.
7. Parents may describe a mass that is noticed when the child cries or strains.
8. Hernias are commonly seen in conditions that are associated with increased intra-abdominal pressure (e.g., ascites, presence of ventriculoperitoneal shunts).
9. Incidence of incarceration:
   a. More than 60% of incarcerated hernias occur before 2 years of age.
   b. Greatest risk of incarceration is before 6 months of age (about 30% of hernias at <2 months of age incarcerate)
   c. The rate of incarceration decreases with age and it becomes rare later in life.
10. An incarcerated hernia may remain asymptomatic; however, a significant number will lead to intestinal strangulation and testicular ischemia. Both testicular atrophy and subsequent infertility have been reported following incarcerated hernias.
11. Incarcerated hernia is usually diagnosed by history and physical examination. If it is difficult to differentiate an acute hydrocele from an incarcerated hernia:
    a. Plain radiographs may show gas-filled loops of bowel in the scrotum in addition to other signs of obstruction in hernia.
    b. A scrotal ultrasound can also differentiate an inguinal hernia from a hydrocele.

Consultation

Emergent surgical consultation for incarcerated or strangulated hernia or when reduction is not possible

Emergency Department Treatment and Disposition

1. Elective repair of inguinal hernias is done in children to prevent complications such as incarceration and strangulation. The complication rate is high if hernia repair is done in patients with incarceration.
2. There is some controversy about whether patients undergoing hernia repair should undergo exploration of the contralateral groin at the time of surgery (because of high incidence of a persistent patent processus vaginalis and the associated risk of a subsequent inguinal hernia and potential incarceration).
3. Regardless of whether a hernia is symptomatic or not, every attempt should be made to reduce it when it is first recognized.
   a. Attempts should be made to reduce the hernia manually as long as the child appears well, without any evidence of bowel ischemia or peritonitis.
   b. Attempts to calm the crying child help in reduction.
   c. Analgesia and sedation is recommended if reduction is difficult or if it causes pain or crying (sedation is given only after the patient is seen by the surgeon).
   d. Placing a child in the Trendelenburg position for some time may also help (gravity helps in reduction).
   e. Once the patient is quiet, gently squeeze the most dependent part of the hernia in the direction of the inguinal canal with one hand while providing gentle pressure on the external ring with the thumb and the index finger of the other hand.
   f. If hernia is not reduced by the above method, consult the surgeon.

g. *Do not try to reduce the hernia if there is evidence of peritonitis or the child appears toxic.*

4. For incarcerated hernias that fail reduction or incarcerated hernias with strangulation, emergent repair is required. Prior to surgery, take the following preparations:
   a. Intravascular access and volume resuscitation as indicated
   b. Placement of a nasogastric tube
   c. Administer intravenous antibiotics.
5. Even though surgical repair as an outpatient is possible after manual reduction, parents must be educated and must understand that recurrence is possible and the patient must be brought back to the ED. The patient must be seen by the surgeon before discharge.
6. Admit any patient if you are uncertain about either the follow-up or the reducibility of the hernia.

Clinical Pearls: Incarcerated Inguinal Hernia

1. Incarcerated hernia is a surgical emergency.
2. Look for evidence of an incarcerated hernia in any infant who presents with inconsolable crying or irritability (other entities that cause inconsolable crying in an infant include corneal abrasion, fracture [e.g., inflicted trauma from abuse], and hair-tourniquet syndrome).
3. Incarceration may be the presenting sign of a previously undiagnosed inguinal hernia.
4. Incarceration with or without strangulation is one of the most common complications of an inguinal hernia.
5. An infant with a previously reducible inguinal hernia who presents with irritability or inconsolable crying, vomiting, or poor feeding has a surgical emergency with an incarcerated hernia unless and until proven otherwise.

BOX 10-11. CLINICAL FEATURES OF INCARCERATED INGUINAL HERNIA

- Abrupt onset of symptoms
  (1) Irritability
  (2) Poor feeding
  (3) Vomiting (may become bilious and sometimes feculent with obstruction)
  (4) Lack of bowel movements
  (5) Abdominal distension
- Swelling in the groin (inguinal mass; Fig. 10-9)
  (1) Firm
  (2) Immobile
  (3) Tender
  (4) Irreducible
  (5) Erythematous or indurated over time (if not reduced)

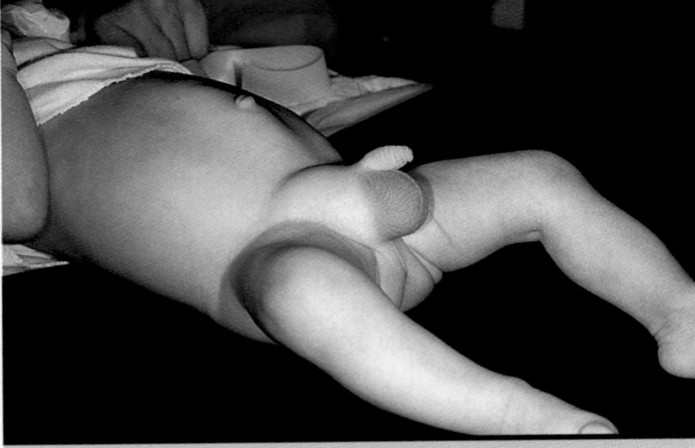

Figure 10-9. Incarcerated Inguinal Hernia

This infant presented with inconsolable crying and a few episodes of vomiting. Inguinal hernia may be either unilateral or bilateral. This patient's hernia (hernial sac contents) could not be reduced into the abdominal cavity and the patient required surgical repair.

BOX 10-12. DIFFERENTIAL DIAGNOSIS OF INCARCERATED INGUINAL HERNIA

- Hydrocele
  (1) Most commonly confused with hernia
  (2) Hydrocele cannot be reduced
  (3) Hydrocele lacks a mass at the inguinal ring
  (4) Seen more often bilaterally
  (5) The majority resolve by the second year of life
  (6) Transillumination positive (unreliable, as a hernia sac containing bowel filled with fluid will also transilluminate)
- Testicular torsion
- Undescended testis
- Retractile testis
- Inguinal lymphadenopathy

DIAGNOSIS

TESTICULAR TORSION

Synonym

Spermatic cord torsion

Definition

Testicular torsion is defined as twisting of the testis leading to venous engorgement, edema, progressive arterial compromise, and subsequent infarction if not relieved in a timely fashion.

Etiology

1. Each testicle is 4 to 6 cm in length and 3 to 4 cm in width. The epididymis is attached directly to the posterolateral aspect of the testis. The testes are anchored posteriorly to the scrotal wall by the tunica vaginalis and inferiorly by the scrotal ligament (gubernaculum).
2. Two types of torsion are seen:
   a. Intravaginal testicular torsion ("bell-clapper deformity"; Figs. 10-10 and 10-11)
      1) Most common form of testicular torsion
      2) The tunica vaginalis completely surrounds the testicle, epididymis, and distal part of the spermatic cord (normally it anchors the testis only to the posterior wall of the scrotum).
      3) The testis rotates freely inside the processus vaginalis like a clapper in a bell. Twisting of the testis and spermatic cord on a vertical axis leads to venous engorgement, obstruction, and secondary edema of the spermatic cord with progressive arterial compromise and subsequent infarction.
      4) Present in 12% of asymptomatic men
      5) Anomaly *almost always* bilateral
   b. Extravaginal
      1) Testis not fixed in the scrotum
      2) Entire cord, tunica vaginalis, and testis rotate within the lax subcutaneous tissue of the scrotum, producing torsion
      3) Seen in neonates or in infants with cryptorchidism

Associated Clinical Features

1. Torsion affects the left testis twice as often as the right (most likely due to the longer length of the left spermatic cord).
2. Although unilateral testicular torsion is more common, bilateral torsion has been reported in the newborn period.
3. A thickened cord and an anterior location of the epididymis may be palpated earlier in the course of the torsion. With intense swelling and edema, the testis and epididymis are indistinguishable by palpation as distinct structures (Figs. 10-11, 10-12, and 10-13).

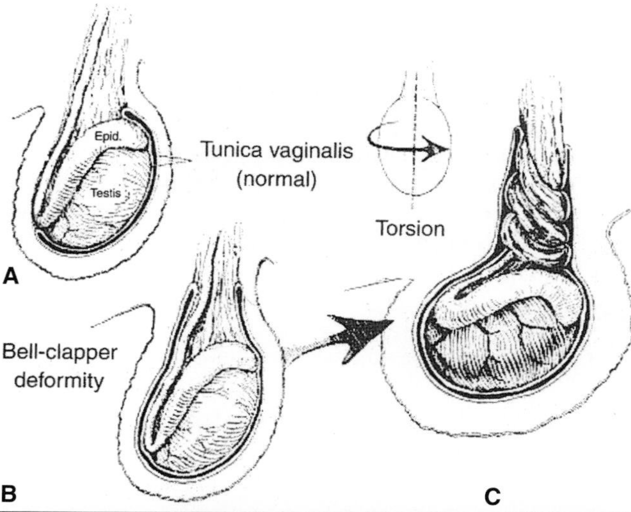

Figure 10-10. Bell-Clapper Deformity

The mechanism of testicular torsion associated with bell-clapper deformity. *A*. The normal position of the testicle in relation to the tunica vaginalis. As shown, the tunica vaginalis does not extend fully around the testicle, thus anchoring it to the opposite side. *B., C.* Bell-clapper deformity. Abnormally high placement of the tunica on the spermatic cord; thus the tunica vaginalis surrounds the testicle and it is free to rotate. (Reproduced with permission from: Fleisher GR, Ludwig S: *Textbook of Pediatric Emergency Medicine*, 3rd ed. Williams & Wilkins, Baltimore, 1993, p. 382.)

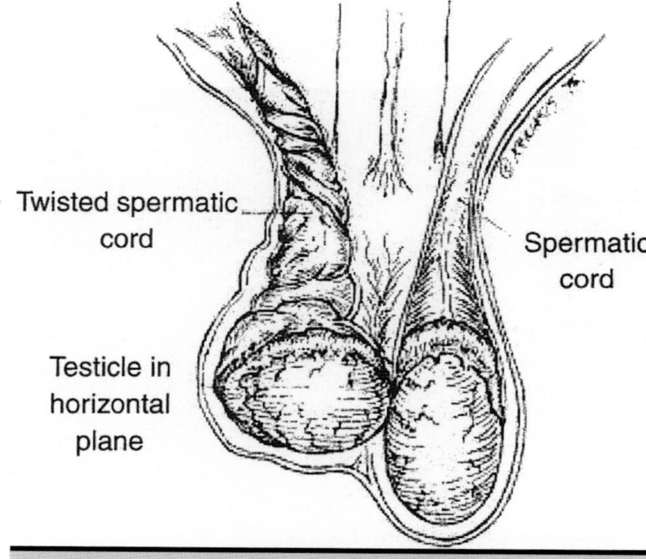

Figure 10-11. Bell-Clapper Deformity; Testicular Torsion

The horizontal lie seen in testicular torsion. Note the abnormal position of the epididymis of the torsed testicle compared to the other side. (Reproduced with permission from: Knoop K: *Atlas of Emergency Medicine*, 2nd ed. McGraw-Hill, New York, 2002, p. 218.)

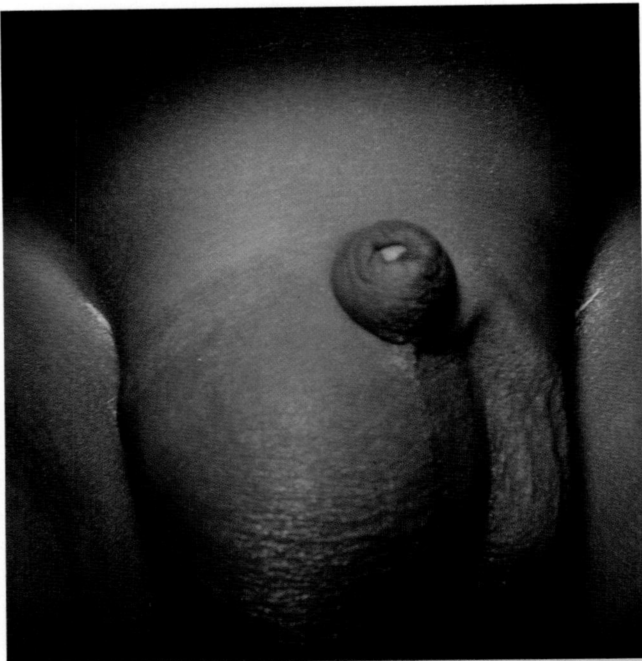

Figure 10-12. Testicular Torsion

An erythematous scrotal swelling in this neonate, noted shortly after birth, with a right-sided testicular torsion. He was found to have an infarcted testis.

4. Special varieties of torsion:
   a. Neonatal torsion
      1) Usually occurs as a prenatal event
      2) Usually the testis is salvaged only if torsion has occurred after delivery.

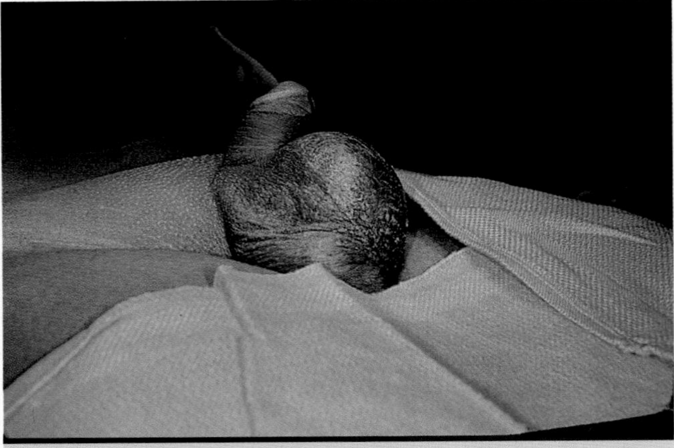

Figure 10-13. Testicular Torsion

Acute onset of scrotal pain and swelling of the left hemiscrotum of 24 hours' duration were the presenting complaints in this 14-year-old adolescent male. His left testis was retracted high into the scrotum with a horizontal lie. His cremasteric reflex was also absent on the left side. (Reproduced with permission from Shah BR, Laude TL: *Atlas of Pediatric Clinical Diagnosis*. WB Saunders, Philadelphia, 2000, p. 330.)

      3) Presents as a hard, painless nontransilluminating mass
      4) Edema and discoloration of scrotal skin may be present.
   b. Torsion of an undescended testis
      1) Tender mass is noted high in the groin in association with an empty scrotum
      2) May be confused with lymphadenitis or an inguinal hernia
   c. Henoch-Schönlein purpura (Fig. 10-14)
      1) Pain and swelling of the spermatic cord and testicle is seen in 2 to 38% of patients.
      2) Purpura usually precedes scrotal swelling by a few days; however, acute scrotal swelling may be an initial presentation *before* the onset of purpura.

5. Laboratory studies (*saving time is crucial*):
   a. CBC is not helpful.
   b. Markedly elevated serum values of interleukin-6 and C-reactive protein are seen more often in epididymitis than in torsion.
   c. Urinalysis is usually negative for pyuria or bacteriuria (negative urine microscopy is suggestive but not diagnostic of torsion).

6. Testicular torsion is a clinical diagnosis. When the diagnosis cannot be made on clinical grounds alone, an imaging study may be considered. The most commonly used imaging studies include:
   a. Testicular real-time color-flow doppler ultrasonography (Fig. 10-16)
      1) This is the diagnostic study of choice.
      2) It may be helpful to differentiate between torsion and epididymo-orchitis.
      3) A decrease or absent blood flow is seen with torsion, while blood flow is increased in epididymo-orchitis.
   b. Testicular scintigraphy
      1) This study analyzes testicular perfusion.
      2) Testicular torsion shows a "cold spot" (decrease or absence of blood flow), while there is an increased flow in epididymo-orchitis.

Consultation

Emergent urological or surgical consultation

Emergency Department Treatment and Disposition

1. Emergent surgical exploration is indicated for detorsion and evaluation of testicular viability. Scrotal orchiopexy (fixing the testis to the scrotal wall) is performed for a viable testis. If infracted, the testis is removed. Fixation orchiopexy of the contralateral testis is also done (contralateral testis with the "bell-clapper" deformity is seen in >50% of cases).

2. Testicular salvage
   a. Time is the critical factor that determines salvageability.
   b. Damage to the gonad varies with the degree of torsion (360 degrees versus 720 degrees; one turn = 360 degrees), its tightness, and its duration.

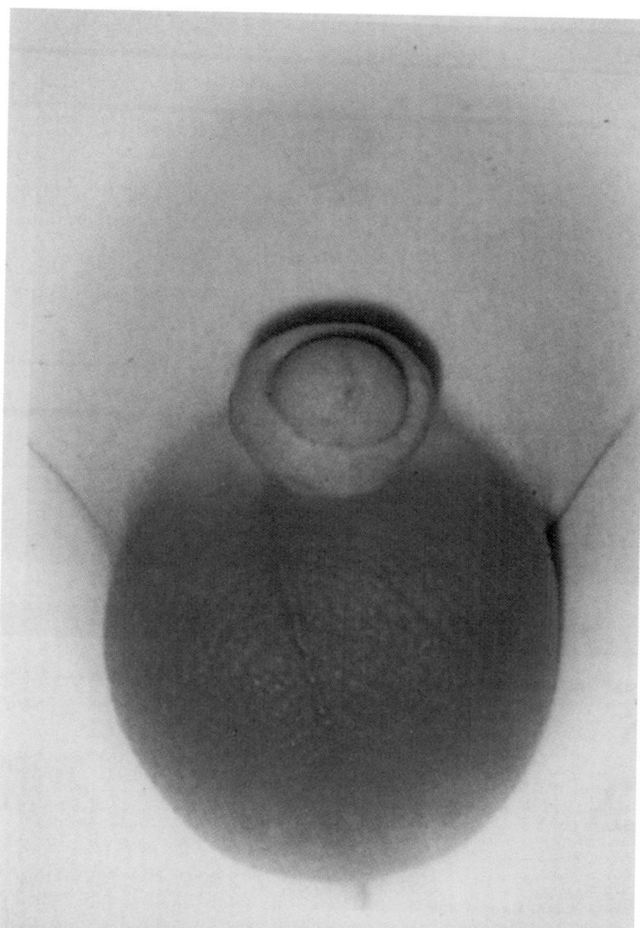

Figure 10-14. Henoch-Schönlein Purpura with Swollen Scarlet Scrotum; Differential Diagnosis of Acute Scrotum/Testicular Torsion

Painless swelling and redness of the scrotum (with minimally tender testes) in an 8-year-old boy with HSP. This patient presented with severe intermittent abdominal pain of 4 days' duration. These scrotal changes developed 12 hours prior to development of a red rash over the legs, buttocks, and ankles. The sudden onset of scrotal swelling with redness seen in HSP mimics acute testicular torsion. Making a diagnosis of HSP in a patient prior to the appearance of the typical rash could be challenging. Scrotal ultrasound with doppler flow study or radionuclear imaging will show hyperemia of the testis in HSP, as opposed to an absence of blood flow in testicular torsion. Patients have been taken for surgical exploration to exclude testicular torsion (prior to appearance of the typical rash of HSP), and subsequently been diagnosed with HSP. (Reproduced with permission from: Gunasekaran TS, Hassall E: The swollen, scarlet scrotum: An uncommon manifestation of a common disorder. *J Pediatr* 1999;134:97.)

c. If the blood supply is totally obstructed for >6 hours, than surgical detorsion is unlikely to salvage the testis.
d. Patients with testicular torsion should undergo scrotal exploration even when symptoms have been present for >12 hours, because individual variation in blood supply and degree of torsion may allow for salvage.

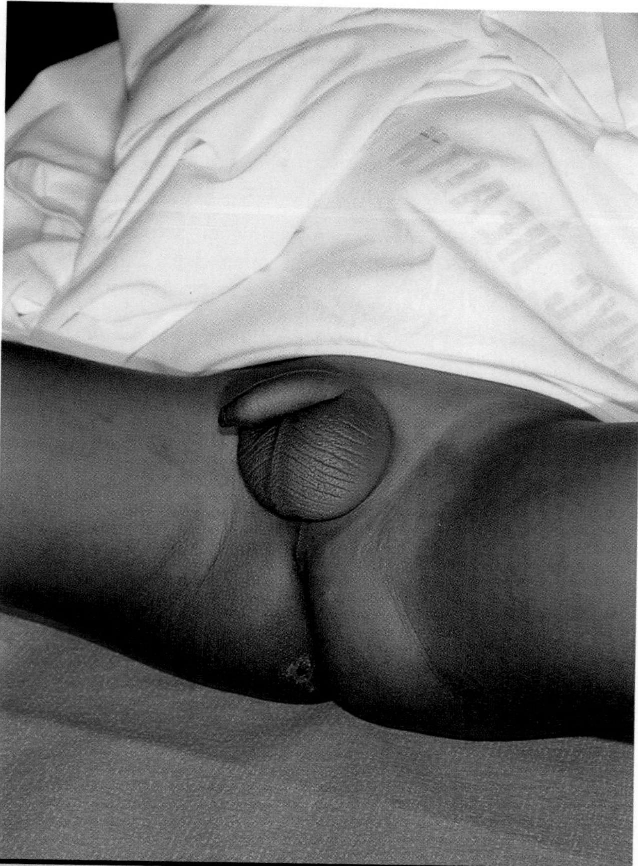

Figure 10-15. Cellulitis with Acute Scrotal Swelling; Differential Diagnosis of Acute Scrotum/Testicular Torsion

Acute onset of scrotal swelling, extreme pain, and fever were the presenting complaints of this child. The patient had impetigo over the perineum and scratching the skin led to the spread of the infection.

3. Manual detorsion
   a. A temporizing procedure and *not* a definitive treatment (*perform while awaiting surgical exploration*)
   b. Indicated if surgical intervention is not available in a timely fashion
   c. Torsion usually occurs from a lateral to medial direction (from outward to inward). Detorsion should be done in the opposite direction. Detorsion can be tried by lifting the scrotum and rotating the testis (on its vascular pedicle) outward toward the thigh (*from a medial to a lateral orientation*).
   d. Perform only if symptoms are present for <4 to 6 hours.
   e. Sedation is required prior to detorsion.
   f. Successful detorsion is indicated by relief of the pain and attainment of a lower testicular position (from a prior high-riding position).
   g. Surgical fixation must be performed following successful detorsion to prevent recurrence.

Clinical Pearls: Testicular Torsion

1. The most common cause of acute painful scrotal swelling in boys 12 years of age and older is testicular torsion.
2. A true surgical emergency; for testicular salvage, prompt diagnosis and treatment are required.
3. Boys with acute scrotal pain should be presumed to have testicular torsion until proven otherwise. Exploration is harmless in epididymo-orchitis but critical in torsion.
4. Any male child presenting with abdominal pain *must* have a testicular exam to exclude torsion.
5. Preceding history of testicular trauma is often misleading.
6. Clinical distinction between testicular torsion and epididymo-orchitis is often difficult.
7. An imaging study should be performed only after surgical consultation, and only when the tentative clinical diagnosis is unlikely to be testicular torsion.
8. Scrotal exploration should not be inappropriately delayed while awaiting a diagnostic study or attempt at manual detorsion.
9. No radiologic tests are 100% accurate or pathognomonic for testicular torsion.
10. In testicular torsion, *saving time is crucial* (testicular salvage is inversely proportional to the duration of ischemia).

BOX 10-13. CLINICAL FEATURES OF TESTICULAR TORSION

- Most common age at presentation
  - (1) Between 10 and 20 years of age
  - (2) About 66% of cases occur between 12 and 18 years of age.
  - (3) Peak incidence: around 13 years of age (coincides with onset of puberty)
  - (4) Second most frequent peak: neonatal period
  - (5) Torsion can occur at any age.
- Scrotal or testicular pain
  - (1) Most common symptom (>80% of patients)
  - (2) Usually sudden onset or gradual onset *with increasing severity* (excruciating character)
  - (3) Pain may awaken patient from sleep.
  - (4) Pain can follow exercise or sex.
  - (5) Pain may radiate to the ipsilateral inner thigh or abdomen, groin, or flank.
  - (6) Pain unaffected by position
  - (7) Preceding history of trauma (20% of patients)
  - (8) History of prior short-lived episodes of testicular pain with spontaneous resolution (~30 to 50% of patients)
  - (9) Associated abdominal pain, nausea, vomiting (*often mimics acute appendicitis*)
  - (10) Absence of urinary symptoms such as dysuria, frequency, urgency, or fever
- Scrotal/testicular examination (affected side Figs. 10-12 and 10-13);
  - (1) A red, swollen, and tender hemiscrotum
  - (2) Testis swollen, exquisitely tender
  - (3) Testis riding high in scrotum; *horizontal lie* (*instead of normal vertical lie*)
  - (4) Epididymis may be difficult to palpate with intense edema (normal position of epididymis: posterolateral to testis; with torsion it is in abnormal position and axis)
  - (5) Absent cremasteric reflex
  - (6) Negative Prehn's sign (elevation of affected testis above pubic symphysis does not relieve pain, and may even cause a sharp increase in pain)
  - (7) Contralateral testis is normal on examination (should be examined first for comparison)

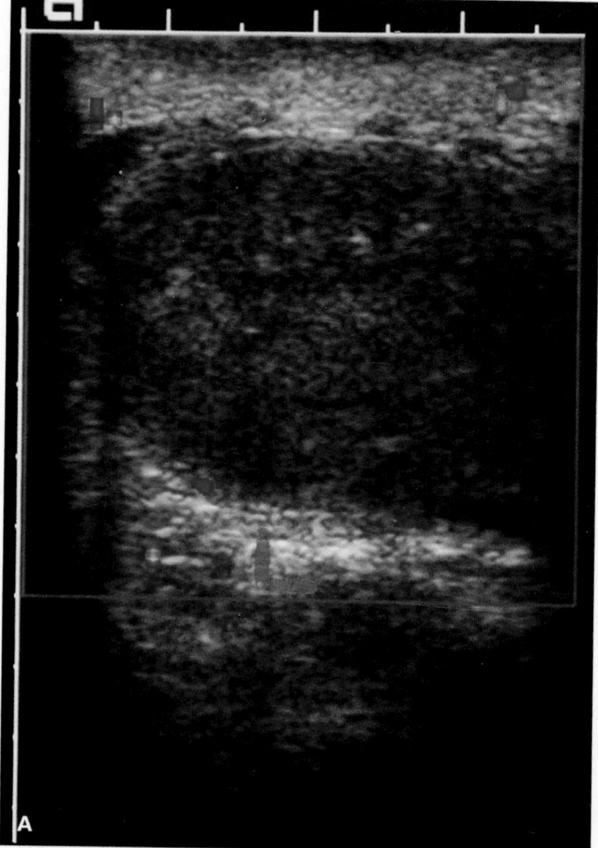

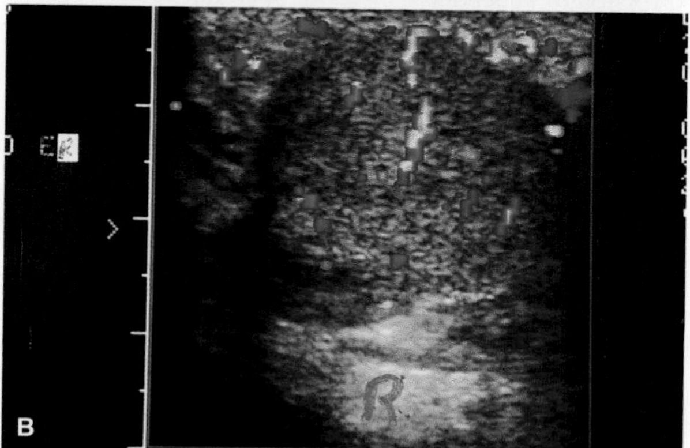

Figure 10-16. Grayscale and Color Doppler Images of the Testes in Testicular Torsion

These images were obtained in a 15-year-old patient with a 2-hour history of left scrotal pain. The left testis (*A*) is heterogeneous and hypoechoic and slightly enlarged compared to the right. The left epididymis is enlarged and heterogeneous. There is thickening of the overlying scrotal skin and soft tissues, along with a reactive left hydrocele. There is an absence of vascular flow in the parenchyma of the left testis with flow in the surrounding soft tissues. The right testis (*B*) demonstrates normal perfusion.

BOX 10-14. TESTICULAR TORSION AND THE CREMASTERIC REFLEX

- Cremesteric reflex
  (1) Superficial skin reflex mediated by L1 and L2 nerves
  (2) Stroking skin of upper medial thigh results in contraction of the ipsilateral cremaster muscle, leading to homolateral elevation of testis and the scrotal contents (*not just scrotal skin*)
  (3) Best elicited with patient lying down
  (4) Normally present in all boys >30 months old
  (5) Seen in 48% of boys <1 month old and in 45% of boys between 1 and 30 months old
- How reliable is the cremesteric reflex?
  (1) Earlier reports: 100% correlation between presence of cremasteric reflex and nontorsion of testis
  (2) Recent case reports: testicular torsion seen with *preserved* cremasteric reflex
  (3) Absence of cremasteric reflex raises suspicion of torsion, *but its presence should not be considered to exclude torsion*

BOX 10-15. DIFFERENTIAL DIAGNOSIS OF ACUTE PEDIATRIC SCROTUM

Painful and swollen

- Testicular torsion
- Acute epididymitis (with or without orchitis)
- Orchitis (e.g., mumps)
- Torsion of appendix testis
- Torsion of appendix epididymis
- Trauma
  (1) Testicular hematoma
  (2) Fracture/rupture of testis
- Testicular tumor (hemorrhage within tumor)
- Incarcerated inguinal hernia
- "Blue balls"
- Acute hydrocele
- Vasculitis
  (1) Henoch-Schönlein purpura
  (2) Kawasaki's disease

Nonpainful and swollen

- Acute idiopathic scrotal edema
- Hydrocele (Fig. 10-17)
- Reducible inguinal hernia
- Varicocele
- Spermatocele
- Testicular tumor

Differential diagnosis of acute scrotum: A diagnostic dilemma

- The three most common etiologies, comprising about 90% of cases of acute scrotal pain:
  (1) Testicular torsion (early surgical intervention)
  (2) Acute epididymitis (medical therapy)
  (3) Torsion of appendage (medical therapy)

  (In one study of 3021 patients of all ages with acute scrotum, the diagnoses were divided roughly evenly between the above three etiologies.)

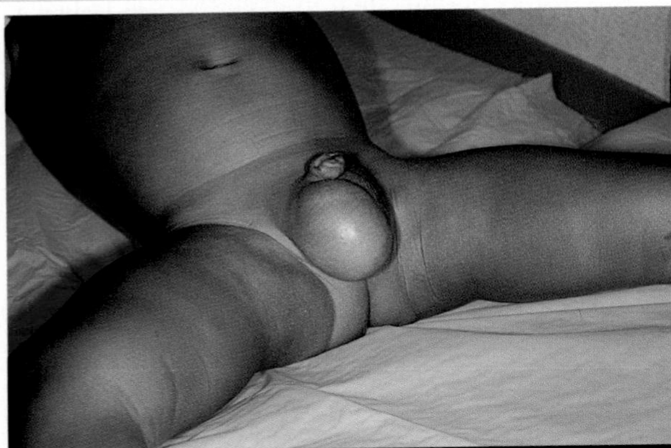

Figure 10-17. Hydrocele; Nonpainful Scrotal Swelling; Differential Diagnosis of Acute Scrotum

A swelling of the right hemiscrotum due to a hydrocele is seen in this infant. A change in size indicates a communicating hydrocele with a patent processus vaginalis.

BOX 10-16. DIFFERENTIAL DIAGNOSIS: TESTICULAR TORSION VERSUS ACUTE EPIDIDYMITIS

	Testicular torsion	*Acute Epididymitis*
Average age	12–15 years	25 years
Rare	<8 or >35 years	
Pain	Usually sudden	Gradual
Severity	Peaks in hours	Peaks in days
Fever	Uncommon	Common
Vomiting	Common	Uncommon
Dysuria	Rare	Common
Discharge	Rare	Common
Laterality	Unilateral	Usually unilateral (~10% bilateral)
Testis	Riding high in scrotum	Normal position
Long axis of testis	Horizontal lie	Normal vertical lie
Cremasteric reflex (affected side)	Absent (usually)	Present
Prehn's sign	Negative	Positive
Prostate	Nontender	Tender
Pyuria/ bacteriuria	Rare	~50%
Color doppler flow	Decreased	Increased

- An enlarged epididymis can be felt distinctly on the testis early in the course of acute epididymitis. With time, as edema spreads to the testis as well as to the scrotal wall, it may become difficult to differentiate torsion from epididymo-orchitis.
- Testicular torsion and epididymitis together comprise up to 75% of final diagnoses in patients presenting with acute scrotum.
- *Acute epididymitis is the most common entity confused with testicular torsion (a study of malpractice claims found that in 61% of cases, torsion was misdiagnosed as epididymitis).*

BOX 10-17. DURATION OF TORSION AND TESTICULAR SALVAGE

Duration of torsion (hours)	*Testicular salvage (%)*
Less than 6	85–97
6–12	55–85
12–24	20–80
>24	<10

(Reproduced with permission from: Smith-Harrison LI, Knoontz WW Jr: Torsion of the testis. Changing concepts. In: Ball TP Jr et al (eds). *American Urological Association Update Series*, Vol. IX, lesson 32. American Urological Association Office of Education, Houston, 1990.)

DIAGNOSIS ACUTE EPIDIDYMITIS (EPIDIDYMO-ORCHITIS)

Definitions

1. Acute epididymitis is an infection/inflammatory process involving the epididymis.
2. If the inflammatory process also involves the testis, it is referred to as epididymo-orchitis.
3. Orchitis is an inflammatory process involving the testis; orchitis as an isolated infection is uncommon.

Etiology

1. Acute epididymitis in adults results from a urethral infection that passes in a retrograde fashion through the vas deferens to the epididymis. In children it is usually due to refluxed urine secondary to an underlying anatomic abnormality.
2. In rare instances, acute epididymitis may result from hematogenous spread.
3. Acute epididymitis is divided into sexually transmitted and non–sexually transmitted epididymitis, based on the etiology.
4. Sexually transmitted epididymitis
   a. Seen in sexually active adolescents and young adults; various etiologies in adolescents to persons 35 years old include:
      1) *Chlamydia trachomatis* (nearly two-thirds of all cases)
      2) *Neisseria gonorrhoeae*
      3) *Mycoplasma* spp.
      4) Coliforms (most common) in homosexual men; other rare etiologies include fungal and syphilis
   b. Patients older than 35 years develop epididymitis due to *Escherichia coli* or other gram-negative uropathogens such as *Klebsiella* and *Pseudomonas* spp. (usually associated with urinary tract infection [UTI]).
5. Non–sexually transmitted epididymitis
   a. Seen in younger children
   b. *Escherichia coli* or other gram-negative uropathogens (usually associated with UTI)
   c. Predisposing conditions in younger children include
      1) Anatomical abnormality of the genitourinary tract (e.g., congenital anomaly of the wolffian duct such as an ectopic ureter entering the vas, or ectopic vas deferens), neurogenic bladder, hypospadias, or urethral stricture
      2) Recent UTI
      3) Recent urinary surgery or instrumentation (e.g., catheterization)
      4) Anatomical abnormality of the gastrointestinal tract (e.g., imperforate anus, rectourethral fistula)

Associated Clinical Features

1. Most patients infected with *Chlamydia* do not complain of urethral discharge but have a demonstrable discharge characteristic of nongonococcal urethritis.
2. Of patients with gonococcal epididymitis, 21 to 30% have no history of urethral discharge and no demonstrable discharge 50% of the time.
3. Complications of acute epididymitis include
   a. Scrotal and testicular abscess (seen with gonococcal epididymitis)
   b. Sterility or impaired fertility
4. Laboratory tests include
   a. Urinalysis typically in patients with epididymitis show pyuria with or without bacteriuria (all prepubertal boys with epididymitis may not have an abnormal urinalysis).
      1) Examination of first-void urine sample for leukocytes
      2) Presence of bacteriuria (Gram-stained smear of uncentrifuged urine)
   b. Urine culture
   c. Urethral discharge or intraurethral swab specimen for Gram-stained smear, culture, and sensitivity
   d. In patients with sexually transmitted epididymitis, syphilis serology and HIV testing should be done.
5. To differentiate between testicular torsion and epididymo-orchitis (if the diagnosis is in doubt), the following studies may be helpful:
   a. Testicular real-time color-flow doppler ultrasonography
      1) Diagnostic study of choice
      2) A decreased or absent blood flow is seen with torsion.
      3) Blood flow is increased in epididymo-orchitis (Fig. 10-18).
   b. Testicular scintigraphy
      1) Analyzes testicular perfusion
      2) Testicular torsion: "cold spot" (decrease or absence of blood flow)
      3) Epididymo-orchitis: increased flow

Consultation

Emergent urology consultation (if the diagnosis of testicular torsion cannot be excluded and for non–sexually transmitted epididymitis to exclude anatomic abnormality)

Emergency Department Treatment and Disposition

1. Most patients can be managed as outpatients with supportive measures as long as fever and local inflammation subside. Patients must be followed closely to ensure efficacy of therapy and referred to urologist for follow-up.
   a. Bed rest
   b. Scrotal support and testicular elevation
   c. Sitz baths or ice pack
   d. Nonsteroidal anti-inflammatory medications for pain
2. Hospitalization is recommended for patients with complications (e.g., abscess) or for patients with systemic toxicity (e.g., high fever, vomiting).

3. For sexually-acquired epididymitis in adolescents
   a. Begin antibiotic therapy pending culture results.
      1) For *C. trachomatis* and *N. gonorrhoeae* coverage: ceftriaxone 250 mg IM in a single dose *and* doxycycline 100 mg orally bid for 10 days
      2) For enteric organisms or for patients allergic to cephalosporins and/or tetracycline: ofloxacin 300 mg orally bid for 10 days *or* levofloxacin 500 mg orally once daily for 10 days
   b. Sex partners should be evaluated and treated when sexually-transmitted epididymitis is either suspected or confirmed.
   c. Counseling about refraining from sexual intercourse until the patient and his sexual partners are treated and cured (completion of therapy and absence of symptoms)
   d. Encourage practicing safe sex to prevent recurrences.
4. For non–sexually transmitted epididymitis associated with UTI in prepubertal children
   a. Trimethoprim-sulfamethoxazole
   b. Urology consultation

Clinical Pearls: Acute Epididymitis (Epididymo-orchitis)

1. Acute epididymitis is the most common intrascrotal inflammatory disease.
2. Acute epididymitis is the most common entity confused with testicular torsion. If infection spreads to the testis (epididymo-orchitis), it is often indistinguishable from testicular torsion on examination. (A study of malpractice claims found that in 61% of cases, torsion was misdiagnosed as epididymitis.)
3. *The presence of pyuria, bacteriuria, dysuria, or fever does not exclude a diagnosis of torsion.* Any patient with an equivocal examination requires perfusion imaging by color doppler US or nuclear scintigraphy (the diagnosis of acute epididymitis is confirmed by normal to increased testicular blood flow; Fig. 10-18).
4. Acute epididymitis is the most common cause of acute painful scrotal swelling in young adults >18 years of age.
5. All young children with acute epididymitis must be investigated (e.g., renal ultrasound, voiding cystourethrogram) for an underlying urinary tract anomaly.
6. The two most common causes of sexually transmitted bacterial epididymitis in young men are *Chlamydia trachomatis* and *Neisseria gonorrhoeae*.

BOX 10-18. CLINICAL FEATURES OF ACUTE EPIDIDYMITIS

- Bimodal presentation (corresponds to peaks in genitourinary infections)
  (1) Most common age: postpubertal sexually active adolescents and young adults (19 to 35 years old [average age: 25 years])
  (2) Smaller peak: around age 2 years (rare in younger preadolescent children)
- Symptoms
  (1) Usually unilateral
  (2) About 10% bilateral
  (3) Pain and swelling *typically grow more gradually* than in testicular torsion
  (4) Peak pain is felt over days rather than hours (*unlike torsion*)
  (5) Adolescents: urethral discharge, urinary frequency, urgency, dysuria
  (6) Preadolescent boys: urinary symptoms (dysuria or pyuria)
  (7) Initially symptoms of abdominal, groin, and/or flank pain (due to vasitis [inflammation begins in the vas deferens and descends to the lower pole of the epididymis in the initial stages])
  (8) Fever common (*unlike torsion*)
  (9) Vomiting rare (*common with torsion*)
  (10) Young infants may cry with diaper changes and toddlers may refuse to walk because of the pain.
- Genitourinary examination
  (1) Tenderness and firm swelling initially localized to the epididymis
  (2) May involve the testis after a few hours (epididymo-orchitis)
  (3) Scrotal erythema and tenderness may be present.
  (4) Testis in normal vertical position
  (5) Long axis of testis usually matches the long axis of the body
  (6) *Cremasteric reflex present* (unlike torsion; however, *this is not a 100% reliable sign to differentiate the two*)
  (7) Prehn's sign positive (elevation of scrotum results in relief of pain [as opposed to torsion in which there is no relief]; however, *this is not a 100% reliable sign to differentiate the two*)
  (8) There may be tenderness over the groin and lower abdomen.
  (9) A tender, boggy prostate may be present.

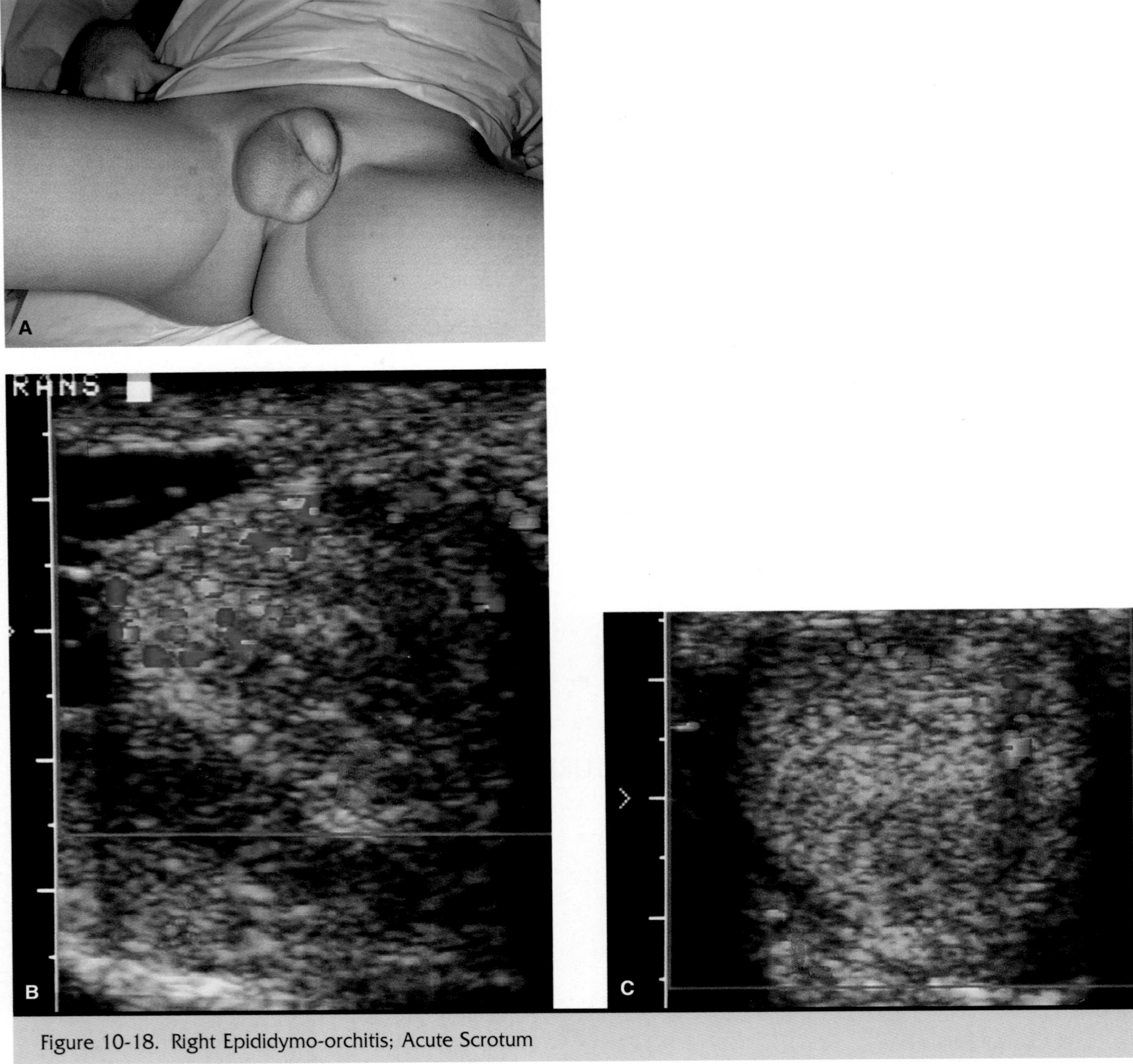

Figure 10-18. Right Epididymo-orchitis; Acute Scrotum

A. An erythematous right-sided scrotal swelling of 3 days' duration is seen in this 6-year-old child. The orientation of the testis was in the normal position, with its long axis parallel to the long axis of the body. *B*., *C*. Transverse color doppler images of the right and left testes in the same patient are shown. There is increased vascular flow in the right testis (*B*) as compared to the left (*C*). The right testes is hypoechoic and heterogeneous and slightly enlarged relative to the left; also, there is a complex hydrocele.

BOX 10-19. CLINICAL FEATURES OF MUMPS ORCHITIS OR EPIDIDYMO-ORCHITIS

- Mumps virus is the most common cause of isolated orchitis.
- Most common age: adolescents and adults
- Seen in about 10 to 30% of postpubertal boys with mumps (oophoritis occurs in 5 to 10% of postpubertal girls with mumps)
- Testes often affected with or without epididymis
- Epididymitis may occur alone.
- Usually unilateral testicular involvement
- Bilateral orchitis uncommon (about 15 to 30% of patients)
- Typically orchitis develops 5 to 7 days after the onset of parotitis.
- Rarely orchitis may precede parotitis or occur as an isolated manifestation of mumps without clinical parotitis.
- Usually resolves in 7 to 10 days with symptomatic treatment
- Sterility due to secondary atrophy of testicle rare (orchitis usually unilateral)
- Mumps vaccine is highly effective in preventing mumps and mumps orchitis.
- Other rare viral etiologies causing orchitis include
  (1) Enteroviruses (e.g., coxsackieviruses, echoviruses)
  (2) Epstein-Barr virus
  (3) Varicella-zoster virus
  (4) Influenza virus
  (5) Lymphocytic choriomeningitis virus
  (6) Dengue virus

BOX 10-20. DIFFERENTIAL DIAGNOSIS OF ACUTE EPIDIDYMITIS OR EPIDIDYMO-ORCHITIS

(See also Box 10-16)

- Sexually-transmitted epididymitis
- Non–sexually transmitted epididymitis
- Other etiologies of acute scrotum (Box 10-15)

Clinical pearls

- The three most common etiologies, accounting for about 90% of cases of acute scrotal pain:
  (1) Testicular torsion
  (2) Acute epididymitis
  (3) Torsion of the appendix testis/epididymis

DIAGNOSIS TORSION OF THE APPENDIX TESTIS

Definition

Torsion of the appendix testis (a testicular appendage or hydatid of Morgagni)

Etiology

1. In a normal scrotum, several vestigial appendages exist that may undergo torsion and cause an acute, painful scrotal mass. The testicular and epididymal appendages are two vestigial remnants that commonly are involved (Fig. 10-19).
2. The appendix of the testis is a vestigial embryonic remnant representing a degenerated müllerian (mesonephric) duct. It is located on the superior pole of the testis or between the testis and epididymis.
3. The cause of torsion of the appendage is unclear. The effect of estrogen before puberty leading to enlargement and subsequent strangulation has been considered as one of the causes. When pedunculated, it may twist around its base, producing venous engorgement, edema, and subsequent infarction.

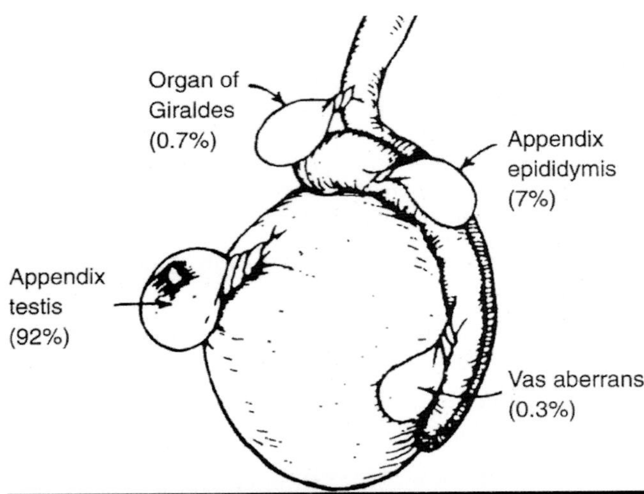

Figure 10-19. Location and Incidence of Intrascrotal Appendages

The appendix testis is present in almost all boys, the appendix epididymis is present in approximately 7% of boys, and the other appendages are rarely present. (Reproduced with permission from: Sheldon CA: Undescended testis and testicular torsion. *Surg Clin North Am* 1985;65:1303.)

Associated Clinical Features

1. Even though early on there are some differences in the presentation of torsion of the appendix and torsion of the testis, signs and symptoms can be very similar in both, and the scrotum can be inflamed and tender in patients presenting later in the course of torsion of the appendix (thus the distinction between the two can be very difficult).
2. Torsion of the appendix testis occurs more often (or at least as often) than testicular torsion.
3. Torsion of the appendix testis is a clinical diagnosis.
4. Urinalysis may be normal or show the presence of pyuria with or without bacteriuria in patients with epididymo-orchitis, while it is usually normal in patients with torsion of the appendix testis or testicular torsion.
5. If a diagnosis of testicular torsion cannot be excluded, a testicular real-time color-flow doppler ultrasonogram may help in differentiating between torsion, epididymo-orchitis, and torsion of the appendix testis.
   a. A decrease or absence of blood flow is seen with testicular torsion.
   b. Blood flow is increased in epididymo-orchitis.
   c. Blood flow to testis is normal or increased with torsion of the appendix testis.
   d. *Important: Ultrasound results are often similar in both torsion of the appendix and epididymo-orchitis* (look for other signs and symptoms that may help to differentiate the two; see Box 10-16).

Consultation

Urology (especially when testicular torsion cannot be excluded by examination)

Emergency Department Treatment and Disposition

1. Surgical excision is not required if the diagnosis of torsion of the appendix is entertained *and* the examiner is confident about the diagnosis. However, surgical exploration is required if a diagnosis of the testicular torsion cannot be excluded.
2. Once the testicular torsion can be ruled out with certainty, generally supportive therapy is offered and includes:
   a. Scrotal support
   b. Bed rest
   c. Analgesia with nonsteroidal anti-inflammatory medications
3. Resolution of symptoms can be expected within 7 to 10 days.
4. Patients can be discharged home and followed closely in 48 to 72 hours.

Clinical Pearls: Torsion of the Appendix Testis

1. The most common cause of testicular pain in boys between 3 and 13 years of age is torsion of the appendix testis.
2. Among all embryonic remnants, the appendix testis is the most commonly involved appendage in torsion.
3. Torsion of the appendix testis is rare in adolescents.
4. Torsion of the appendix is very likely if tenderness is present at the upper pole of the testis with the remainder of the testis being nontender.
5. The "blue dot" sign, a pathognomonic sign of an infarcted appendage, is often not seen because of the overlying scrotal wall edema. This sign is seen in only 20% of cases.
6. Distinguishing torsion of the appendix from testicular torsion can be difficult in some patients. A testicular flow scan or color doppler US may be helpful in such cases.

BOX 10-21. CLINICAL FEATURES OF TORSION OF THE APPENDIX TESTIS

- Common age at presentation
  (1) Average: 10 years (range, 3 to 13 years)
  (2) Preadolescents (rare in adolescents)
- Both the right and left testes are equally affected (unlike testicular torsion in which left testis is involved more often than the right testis)
- Symptoms
  (1) *Gradual onset* of scrotal pain and swelling (*unlike testicular torsion*)
  (2) History of previous episodes is uncommon (*unlike testicular torsion*)
  (3) Nausea and vomiting rare (*unlike testicular torsion*)
  (4) Fever rare (*unlike epididymo-orchitis*)
  (5) Urinary symptoms of dysuria and pyuria rare (*unlike epididymo-orchitis*)
  (6) History of penile discharge uncommon (*unlike epididymo-orchitis*)
- Genitourinary examination (affected side)
  (1) Tenderness and swelling localized to the superior lateral aspect of the testis (where the appendage is located)
  (2) Firm swelling distinct from the epididymis
  (3) Testis normal or enlarged
  (4) Testis with a normal lie (vertical lie)
  (5) Erythema and edema of the scrotal wall
  (6) Cremasteric reflex present
  (7) "Blue dot" sign (a localized area of bluish discoloration secondary to infarction of the appendage; this sign is rarely seen because of overlying scrotal edema)
- Natural course
  (1) Inflammation resolves gradually following infarction.
  (2) Usually resolves completely within 7 to 10 days from the onset of symptoms (the involved appendage undergoes autoamputation within 1 week)

BOX 10-22. DIFFERENTIAL DIAGNOSIS OF TORSION OF THE APPENDIX TESTIS

- Testicular torsion
- Acute epididymo-orchitis
- Other causes of acute scrotum (see Box 10-15)

Clinical pearls

- The three most common etiologies of acute scrotal pain (about 90% of cases)
  1) Testicular torsion
  2) Acute epididymitis
  3) Torsion of the appendix testis/epididymis

DIAGNOSIS CONGENITAL IMPERFORATE HYMEN WITH HEMATOMETROCOLPOS

Definition and Etiology

1. A layer of epithelialized connective tissue that forms the hymen has no opening, leading to vaginal obstruction. This is referred to as an imperforate hymen.
2. Imperforate hymen is usually an isolated anomaly and patency of the cervix and uterus is maintained.
3. Imperforate hymen leads to hydrocolpos or one of its variants (Box 10-23).

Associated Clinical Features

1. Female newborns should have a through examination of the genitalia rather than the usual cursory look for gender identification.
    a. A normal perforate hymen can be seen on careful examination of the newborn.
    b. Vaginal length can be determined by inserting a moistened cotton-tipped applicator into the vagina.
    c. A normal vagina in the full-term infant is approximately 4 cm in length.
2. Familial occurrences of imperforate hymen have been described.
3. Children with imperforate hymens may be brought in for evaluation of sexual abuse. Trauma to the hymen as a result of sexual abuse can lead to scarring and subsequently an imperforate hymen (*acquired*).
4. The diagnosis of an imperforate hymen is made clinically.
5. An imperforate hymen is usually an isolated anomaly. Rare associated anomalies described with it include imperforate anus, multicystic dysplastic kidney, and bifid clitoris. Pelvic

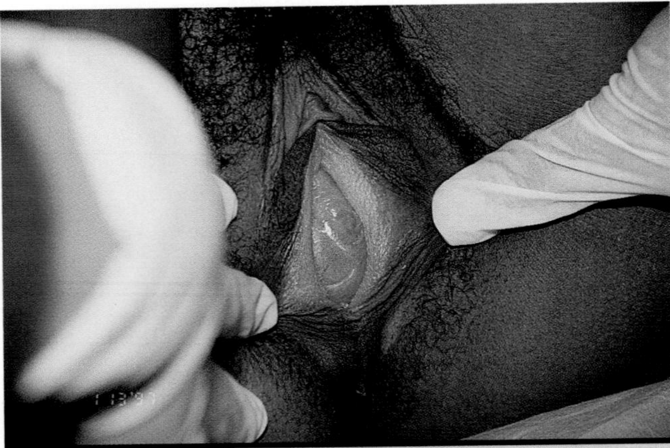

Figure 10-20. Congenital Imperforate Hymen with Hematometrocolpos

A 12-year-old girl presented with intermittent crampy abdominal pain of 24 hours' duration. She had similar pain about 4 weeks prior to this episode, was seen by her physician, and sent home on antacids for her abdominal pain. Because of persistent pain, she decided to come to the ER. She denied any prior menstruation. Her examination showed an imperforate hymen with a bulging mass at the introitus.

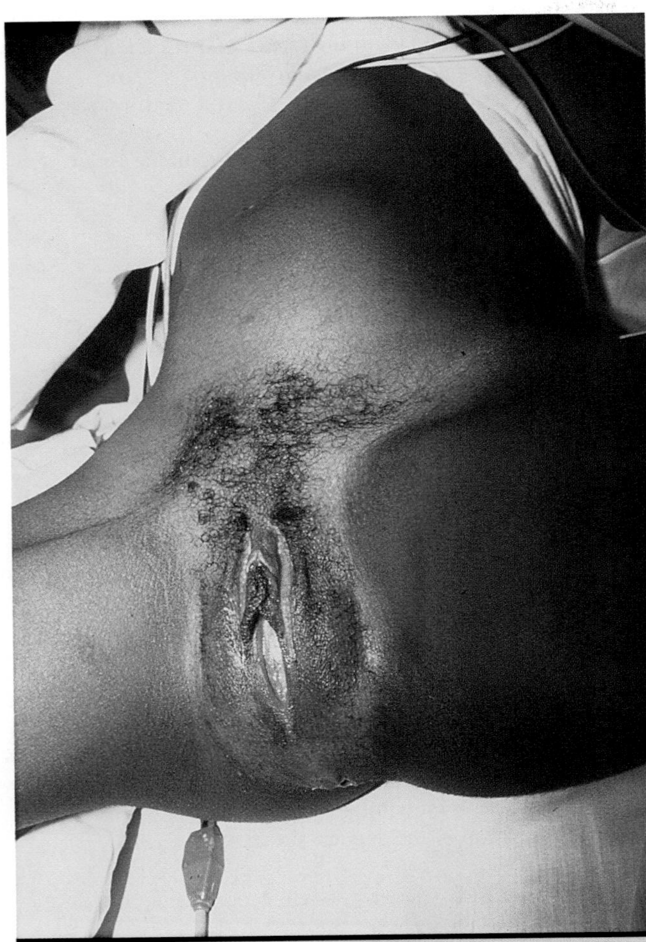

Figure 10-21. Congenital Imperforate Hymen with Hematometrocolpos

A 13-year-old girl presented with abdominal pain. She had similar pain about 5 weeks prior to this episode. She also had difficulty voiding. She had Tanner IV sexual development level, but denied having prior menstruation. An abdominal mass (distended uterus) was palpable in the mid-abdomen. An imperforate hymen with a bulging mass was also visualized at the introitus. Hymenectomy was performed leading to drainage of about 1.0 liter of blood, fluid, and menstrual debris.

ultrasonography may be used for confirmation and to exclude the presence of any other associated anomalies.

Consultation

Surgery

Emergency Department Treatment and Disposition

1. An asymptomatic neonate with imperforate hymen (without hydrocolpos or hydrometrocolpos) can be followed conservatively, as spontaneous opening can occur.
2. In a symptomatic patient hymenotomy (stellate incisions at the 2, 4, 8 and 10 o'clock positions) with excision of excessive hymenal tissue is performed. The margins are then approximated using a fine absorbable suture. Caution must be exercised to avoid urethral and rectal injuries.
3. Following the drainage of menstrual blood and debris with the relief of the symptoms, the patient can be discharged home with follow-up with the primary care physician. Patients need to be monitored for possible recurrence of symptoms with the development of adhesions.
4. Puncturing the imperforate hymen in the ED setting without a full surgical resection is not recommended, as complete drainage may not be obtained and a small perforation may allow ascension of bacteria with a possibility of extension of infection to intra-abdominal organs.
5. Carbon dioxide laser therapy also has been used as an alternative to surgical repair of imperforate hymen.
6. The patient needs to be reassured about the normal nature of her female genitalia. In many cultures integrity of the hymen is considered symbolic of virginity, and the patient and her family need to be reassured that the surgical intervention carried out to treat imperforate hymen should not alter this symbolic value.
7. If imperforate hymen is detected during infancy and the patient is asymptomatic, hymenotomy is delayed until adolescence because approximation is best facilitated by estrogenized tissue.

BOX 10-23. TYPES OF FEMALE PEDIATRIC GENITAL DISORDERS

- Hydrocolpos or mucocolpos
  (1) Vaginal distention with mucus secretions
  (2) Secondary to excessive intrauterine stimulation of an infant's cervical mucus glands by maternal estrogens
- Hydrometrocolpos
  (1) Distention of the uterus and vagina with mucus secretions
  (2) Secondary to excessive intrauterine stimulation of an infant's mucus glands by maternal estrogens
- Hematocolpos
  (1) Vaginal distension with menstrual products
  (2) Seen at menarche
- Hematometrocolpos
  (1) Distention of the uterus and vagina with menstrual products
  (2) Seen at menarche

BOX 10-24. CLINICAL FEATURES OF IMPERFORATE HYMEN

- *In infancy: (any of the following)*
  (1) Asymptomatic
  (2) Difficulty in micturition
  (3) Hydrocolpos or hydrometrocolpos presenting as
    A. Palpable lower midline abdominal mass or mass extending superiorly to the umbilicus *and/or*
    B. Visible bulging mass or membrane at the introitus
- In adolescents: (any of the following)
  (1) Abdominal pain (which may be cyclic)
  (2) Normal pubertal changes with "primary amenorrhea" or cryptomenorrhea if a small opening is present
  (3) Urinary retention or symptoms of urgency, dysuria, or frequency
  (4) Hematocolpos or hematometrocolopos presenting as
    lower abdominal mass *and/or*
    B. Visible bulging mass at the introitus (mass may appear blue from hematocolpos)
  (5) Persistent low back pain (sacral plexus/nerve root irritation secondary to a large hematocolpos)
- *Complications of imperforate hymen:*
  (1) Acute urinary retention
  (2) Hydronephrosis or hydroureter (secondary to chronic extrinsic pressure)
  (3) Constipation (secondary to extrinsic pressure on the colon)
  (4) Hematosalpinx with rupture (acute abdomen)

Clinical Pearls: Imperforate Hymen

1. Congenital imperforate hymen is the most common obstructive anomaly of the female reproductive tract (seen in 0.1% of female newborns).
2. If an imperforate hymen is asymptomatic in the neonatal period, it often remains undetected until adolescence.
3. Inspect the hymen in any pubescent girl who has never menstruated and presents with an abdominal mass.
4. Cyclic abdominal pain in a girl with normal pubertal changes and "primary amenorrhea" are important diagnostic clues.

BOX 10-25. DIFFERENTIAL DIAGNOSIS OF CONGENITAL IMPERFORATE HYMEN

- Labial agglutination (see Fig. 2-24)
- Congenital absence of the vagina
  (1) Often associated with major genitourinary (GU) or gastrointestinal (GI) anomalies
  (2) Some examples: imperforate anus, bicornuate uterus, renal hypoplasia, fistulas, polydactyly
- Transverse imperforate vaginal septum
  (1) Often associated with major GU or GI anomalies
  (2) Some examples: imperforate anus, bicornuate uterus, renal hypoplasia
- Acquired imperforate hymen from sexual abuse
  (1) Genital trauma of sexual abuse
  (2) Trauma leading to scarring that leads to an imperforate hymen

DIAGNOSIS VAGINAL FOREIGN BODY IN A PREPUBERTAL CHILD

Definition

Young girls may put foreign objects in their vaginas (e.g., toilet tissue being the most common, though sometimes it is a crayon or bead) during normal exploration of the body. Insertion of a foreign body (FB) into the vagina leads to either vaginal bleeding or blood-stained and foul-smelling vaginal discharge.

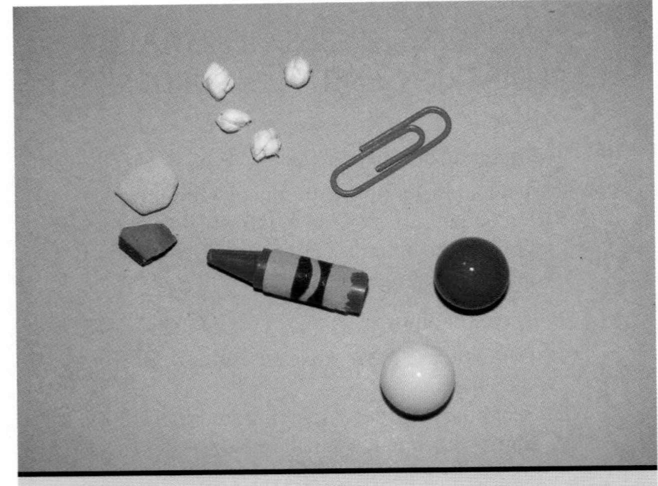

Figure 10-22. Examples of Vaginal Foreign Bodies.

Few examples of objects found in the vagina of prepubertal children by accident or intention are shown and include wades of toilet paper, crayon, pieces of rubber or clay, paper clip and marbles. Other items include food items, bottle caps or toys. In adults, objects found in vagina include objects like oranges, bottles, dringking glasses and sexual stimulants such as vibrators, leaves, ginger root, chili pepper or gun powder. Foreign objects in a child's vagina may also indicate child sexual abuse.

Associated Clinical Features

1. In the majority of patients (especially younger ones), the history is not helpful because the parent has usually not witnessed, nor does the child remember, putting an FB into the vagina. Older patients may recall insertion of an FB. Usually FBs are inserted by the girl herself.
2. Children can be examined in either the frog leg position, with the parent holding the child's legs flexed, or the knee-chest position, with the patient prone and kneeling with the buttocks and perineum exposed. The knee-chest position allows the vestibule to open, resulting in better visualization of the distal vaginal mucosa and introitus. Use of a speculum or attempts to visualize the cervix are usually not necessary.
3. External genital examination of a child with a vaginal FB may appear normal or may show evidence of an irritative vulvitis leading to erythematous, hyperpigmented changes secondary to chronic vaginal discharge.

4. Commonly seen FBs in an adolescent patient include retained tampons, diaphragms, or contraceptive sponges. These retained objects lead to chronic irritation and bleeding, usually accompanied by a foul discharge.
5. Radiographic and ultrasonographic studies are not recommended because they fail to detect most vaginal foreign objects. Magnetic resonance imaging has been used to confirm presence of vaginal FBs when plain radiographs are negative (e.g., for plastic FBs).
6. Vaginal foreign bodies in young girls may be a previously unrecognized indicator of sexual abuse. Thus, girls with vaginal FBs should be evaluated for possible sexual abuse.

Consultation

Surgery (with unsuccessful attempts at removal in the ED)

Emergency Department Treatment and Disposition

1. All suspected or confirmed vaginal FBs must be removed. Vulvovaginitis will only resolve after the removal of the FB.
2. A foreign body may become embedded in the atrophic mucosa of the vaginal walls. This requires great care to remove, and damage to the adjacent organs must be avoided. Procedures that may help in removal include:
   a. Irrigation of the vagina using an angiocatheter (without the needle) filled with lukewarm water; this may allow extrusion of small wads of toilet paper.
   b. Rectal examination in the lithotomy position with a bimanual examination (recto-abdominal exam) may allow palpation of a FB in the vagina. Gentle milking may help in extrusion of the FB or expression of vaginal blood or discharge.
3. Indications for examination under general anesthesia for vaginoscopy for direct visualization and removal of a FB include:
   a. Suspected perforation or significant internal injury
   b. Patient extremely agitated or too young to undergo the procedure without the use of a deep sedative or general anesthetic
   c. With suspected child abuse when forensic examination and documentation is required
   d. The size and configuration of the FB may pose a risk of serious injury if attempts are made for its removal without proper sedation and a cooperative patient.
4. Topical estrogen cream may be used to hasten healing of any residual mucosal lesions.
5. To prevent future occurrences, young girls should be taught to pat their vulva dry after going to the bathroom rather than rubbing it with tissue. Rubbing causes balls of tissue to break off and become lodged in the vagina.

Clinical Pearls: Vaginal Foreign Body

1. The classic symptom of a vaginal FB is a foul-smelling, bloody vaginal discharge.
2. Persistent or recurrent foul-smelling, bloody vaginal discharge in a child should alert the clinician to the possibility of a retained vaginal FB.
3. Wads of toilet paper are the most frequent FBs found in prepubertal children and forgotten tampons in postpubertal adolescents.

BOX 10-26. CLINICAL FEATURES OF A VAGINAL FOREIGN BODY IN A PREPUBERTAL CHILD

- The most common type of FB seen in vagina is wads of toilet paper.
- Other types of FBs seen in the vagina include a wide variety of objects (e.g., crayons, safety pins, plastic toys, glass beads)
- The vast majority of FBs are found in girls between 3 and 9 years of age
- Most common symptom: vaginal bleeding or blood-stained vaginal discharge (>90% of cases) or foul-smelling vaginal discharge (recurrent or persistent)
- Other symptoms may include pain in the abdomen or groin or painful urination.
- Physical signs may include skin redness and swelling due to irritation from vaginal discharge.
- The duration of symptoms may vary from days to months to years.

BOX 10-27. DIFFERENTIAL DIAGNOSIS OF GENITAL BLEEDING IN PREPUBERTAL CHILD

- Foreign body (vaginal)
- Vulvovaginitis from various etiologies
  (1) Nonspecific (e.g., poor perineal hygiene)
  (2) *Streptococcus pyogenes*
  (3) *Shigella flexneri, S. sonnei*
  (4) *Neisseria gonorrhoeae*
  (5) *Chlamydia trachomatis*
  (6) *Haemophilus influenzae, H. parainfluenzae*
  (7) *Staphylococcus aureus*
  (8) *Neisseria meningitidis*
  (9) *Escherichia coli*
  (10) Pinworms
- Trauma
  (1) Accidental (straddle injury; see Fig. 2-28)
  (2) Sexual abuse (see Fig. 4-4)
- Lichen sclerosis et atrophicus (see Fig. 2-22)
- Urethral prolapse (often mistaken for vaginal bleeding; see Figs. 2-26 and 2-27)
- Labial adhesions (see Fig. 2-24)
- Condyloma acuminata (see Fig. 4-2)
- Urinary tract infections
- Neonatal maternal estrogen withdrawal
- Exposure to estrogen-containing medications
- Precocious puberty
- Blood dyscrasias
- Sarcoma botryoides (vaginal rhabdomyosarcoma)
- Hemangiomas
- Polyps of the genital tract
- Periurethral cysts

DIAGNOSIS PARAPHIMOSIS

Definition

Paraphimosis occurs when the foreskin is retracted behind the coronal sulcus and cannot be replaced in its normal position. Phimosis is stenosis of the preputial ring, such that the foreskin cannot be retracted back over the glans penis. Unlike phimosis, paraphimosis is always pathological and needs to be treated emergently.

Etiology and Pathogenesis

1. Etiologies of paraphimosis include:
   a. Iatrogenic causes:
      1) Failure to reduce the foreskin after it has been retracted for cleaning by a child or caretaker
      2) Failure to reduce the foreskin after it has been forcibly retracted by a health professional during cleansing prior to bladder catheterization or medical examination
   b. Infection (e.g., usually seen in men with chronic balanoposthitis [chronic infection leading to contracture of the foreskin, forming a tight ring that constricts the glans when retracted])
   c. Hair or thread tourniquets (Fig. 10-23)
   d. Trauma
   e. Masturbation

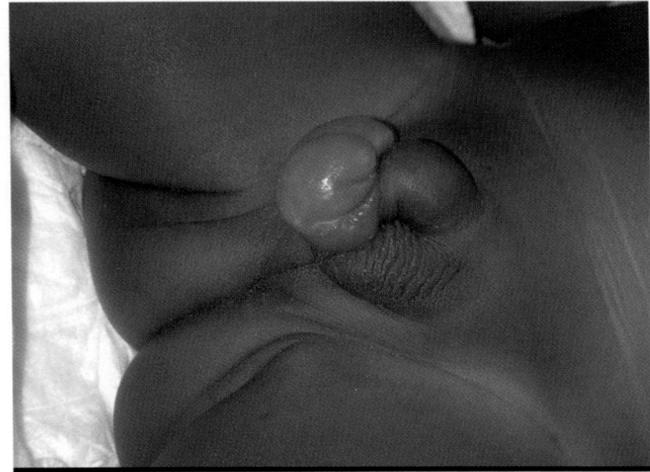

Figure 10-23. Paraphimosis-like Presentation Due to Hair-Tourniquet Syndrome

The hair-tourniquet syndrome is a surgical emergency similar to paraphimosis. Penile constriction may result in swelling and ischemic injury distal to the constrictive process. Careful examination is required to identify the tourniquet (e.g hair) which is mobilized gently, divided, and removed (see Fig. 2-16).

2. A tight foreskin retracted behind the glans and left in that position forms a constricting ring leading to impairment of lymphatic and venous return from the glans. This leads to edema of the prepuce, penile shaft, and glans distal to the incarcerated foreskin (Fig. 10-24). If not reduced promptly, arterial insufficiency, ischemia, and gangrene of the glans penis will follow. When constriction is relieved, normal blood flow into and out of the foreskin and glans penis will return.

Associated Clinical Features

1. The diagnosis of paraphimosis is made clinically.
2. *Verify by history* that the patient is uncircumcised, as a paraphimosis-like condition may occur in the circumcised male due to a constricting band of hair (hair-tourniquet) or fiber just proximal to the glans.

Consultation

Urology or surgery (if attempts at reduction are unsuccessful)

Emergency Department Treatment and Disposition

1. Treatment of paraphimosis is emergent reduction of the foreskin. For the reduction procedure, see Fig. 10-25.
2. In rare cases of paraphimosis, emergency circumcision under general anesthesia is necessary.
3. Elective circumcision is advisable to avoid recurrence.
4. Educate the caretaker that inability to retract the foreskin completely is normal in young children (up to 4 to 5 years of age); attempting to retract it may cause paraphimosis.

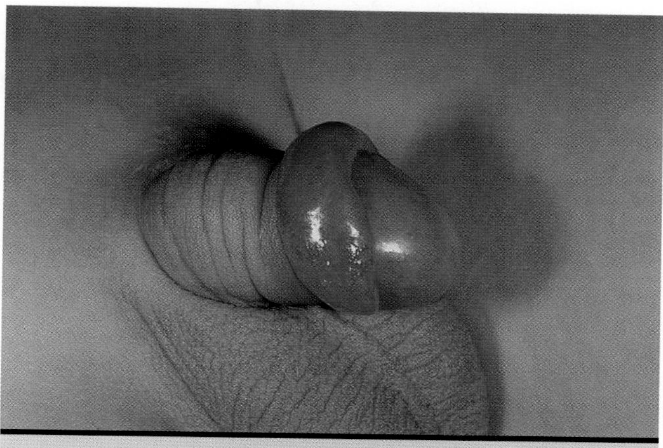

Figure 10-24. Paraphimosis

A 10-month-old uncircumsized male infant presented with inconsolable crying. Edematous foreskin trapped proximal to the glans penis is seen.

5. Educate parents that no special care is required for an uncircumcised penis. The external surface of the foreskin requires gentle cleaning like other parts of the body, and the foreskin should not be forcibly retracted for cleansing.

Clinical Pearls: Paraphimosis

1. Paraphimosis is a surgical emergency and can result in arterial compression, penile necrosis, and gangrene if not promptly reduced.
2. Advise parents, or older boys who are uncircumcised with a retractable foreskin, to return the foreskin to its unretracted (normal) position after cleaning.

BOX 10-28. CLINICAL FEATURES OF PARAPHIMOSIS

- Most common age: uncircumcised young infants and children
- Most common presentation
  (1) Pain and swelling of the glans penis
  (2) Rarely difficulty voiding and urinary retention (urethral obstruction due to edema)
- Young infants
  (1) Swelling usually noticed by a caretaker during a diaper change
  (2) May present with inconsolable crying (because of pain)
- Older children
  (1) Very anxious
  (2) Severe pain as swelling increases, leading to ischemia of the glans penis
- Examination
  (1) A flaccid proximal penis
  (2) Erythema and engorgement distal to the obstruction
  (3) Foreskin retracted

BOX 10-29. DIFFERENTIAL DIAGNOSIS OF PARAPHIMOSIS

- Hair-tourniquet syndrome (penile strangulation by a constrictive band of hair just proximal to the glans)
- Allergic reactions (angioedema) of the genitalia (e.g., due to insect bite)
- Contact dermatitis of the penis
- Penile trauma
- Acute soft tissue infection

BOX 10-30. DIFFERENTIAL DIAGNOSIS OF INCONSOLABLE CRYING IN INFANTS

- Paraphimosis
- Hair-tourniquet syndrome (accidental or inflicted [child abuse])
- Intussusception
- Child abuse (e.g., fractures or shaken impact syndrome)
- Corneal abrasion
- Incarcerated/strangulated hernia
- Testicular torsion

PROCEDURE REDUCTION OF PARAPHIMOSIS

Indication

Emergent reduction of paraphimosis is indicated in all cases.

Contraindication

None

Equipment

1. Surgical gloves
2. 4 × 4 gauze
3. Ice packs or crushed ice
4. Anesthetic lubricant jelly (e.g., 1% lidocaine)
5. 25- and 23-gauge needles and 3-ml and 5-ml syringes
6. Sedative agent (e.g., midazolam)
7. Local anesthetic (e.g., lidocaine without epinephrine) for dorsal nerve block
8. Babcock clamps (4 to 6)

Anesthesia

1. Apply 1% lidocaine jelly to the glans penis and undersurface of edematous foreskin (not to the shaft of the penis) to lubricate as well as to anesthetize the area.
2. Sedation (e.g., midazolam) or a dorsal penile nerve block may be required to reduce the pain of the procedure if the paraphimosis is not quickly and easily reduced.

Technique

1. Treatment of paraphimosis involves moving the foreskin back into its normal position. Explain the need for the procedure to the caretaker.
2. Paraphimosis is usually reduced by nonsurgical techniques. Surgical reduction is indicated when nonsurgical techniques are unsuccessful.
3. Nonsurgical/noninvasive reduction techniques include:
   a. Gentle manual reduction technique (Fig. 10-25):
      1) Hold one gauze sponge in each hand, and place the index and third fingers of each hand in apposition proximal to the phimotic ring (with the gauze covering the fingers for traction) and both thumbs are aligned on the urethral meatus.
      2) Thumb pressure is used to push the glans back through the prepuce against the counter pressure on the shaft generated by four fingers, which are behind this ring and are supporting it.
      3) It is critical to attempt to advance the most distal foreskin ring (the foreskin closer to the coronal margin). If this tight ring can be reduced, then the remainder of the foreskin will follow. The key to success is application of slow, steady pressure.

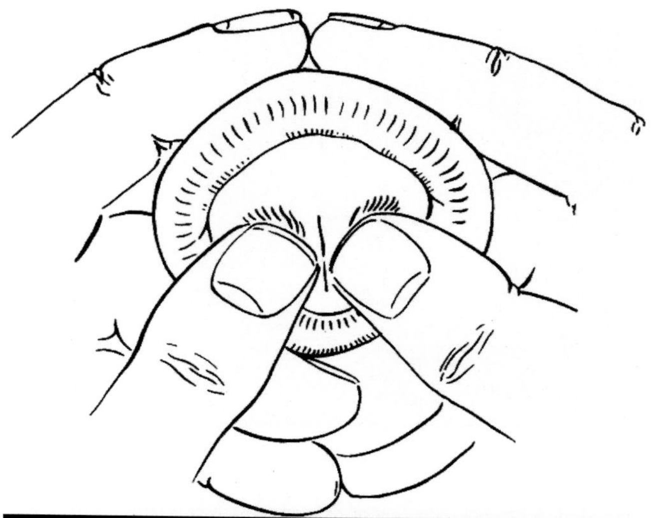

Figure 10-25. Manual Reduction of Paraphimosis

With the thumbs on the glans penis and fingertips on the tight band of foreskin, the glans is pushed as the foreskin is pulled over the glans penis. The foreskin can be reduced by pressure on the glans, like that used to turn a sock inside out. (Reproduced with permission from: Kelalis PP, King LR, Belman AB: *Clinical Pediatric Urology,* 2nd ed. Philadelphia, WB Saunders, 1985).

b. Attempt an assisted manual reduction technique (if the above method is unsuccessful). Reduction is attempted by either reducing the swelling or by using Babcock clamps.
   1) Apply gentle, continuous manual compression using the clinician's hand (for 3 to 5 minutes) *and/or*
   2) Apply the iced-gloved method to induce vasoconstriction (the patient requires close monitoring to prevent pressure or cold injury): A large rubber glove is half filled with a mixture of crushed ice and water and the cuff end is tied. The thumb of the glove is invaginated and held securely in place over the lubricated penis for brief periods (3 minutes at a time). With reduction of the swelling, manual reduction is attempted.
   3) Reduction using Babcock clamps (noncrushing clamps): Clamps are placed on the constricting ring in each quadrant followed by a gentle, slow, continuous equal traction pulling the foreskin over the glans.

c. Successful reduction results in the appearance of an uncircumcised penis with a phimotic foreskin.

d. Postreduction bleeding, if it occurs, is slight and generally responds to compression.

4. Surgical reduction techniques include (urologic/surgical consultation is usually requested):
   a. Puncture technique: After application of antiseptic to the foreskin, the edematous foreskin is punctured with a 25- or 23-gauge needle. Either a single shallow puncture or punctures at multiple sites may be required. This is followed by application of gentle compression between the thumb and forefingers to express the fluid and relieve the edema. Paraphimosis is then reduced by manual reduction.
   b. A dorsal incision in the foreskin ring is made when any of the above techniques fail or when skin ulceration, gangrene, or infection is present. Though this may be done in the ED, it is optimally done in the operating room.
   c. Perform an emergency circumcision if all other measures fail.

Complications

1. Complications related to manual reduction include ischemia of the glans due to excessive compression, laceration of the foreskin due to overly zealous attempts at manual reduction, and cold injury related to application of ice.

2. Complications from surgical reduction include infection, contusion, or laceration to the penile shaft, glans, or urethra.

Follow-Up

1. Patients can be discharged home after a successful reduction after they have voided with a follow-up with a pediatric surgeon (or urologist) for possible elective circumcision.

2. Considerable postreduction edema is the rule in these cases, and it may take hours to days to fully resolve (Fig. 10-26). Instruct the caretaker and/or patient to avoid retracting the foreskin for several days.

Clinical Pearls: Reduction of Paraphimosis

1. Paraphimosis is a surgical emergency and can result in arterial compression, penile necrosis, and gangrene if not promptly reduced.

2. Prompt reduction of paraphimosis obviates the need for later, more difficult reduction of an extremely swollen foreskin and glans penis.

3. Prolonged and painful attempts by manual reduction must be avoided.

4. Nonsurgical reduction techniques are successful in the majority of cases.

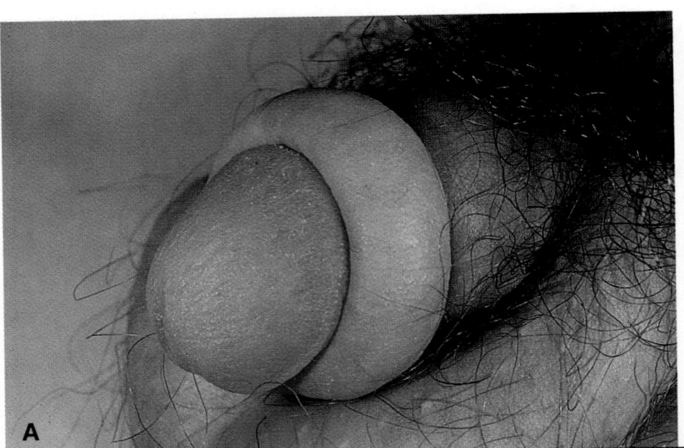

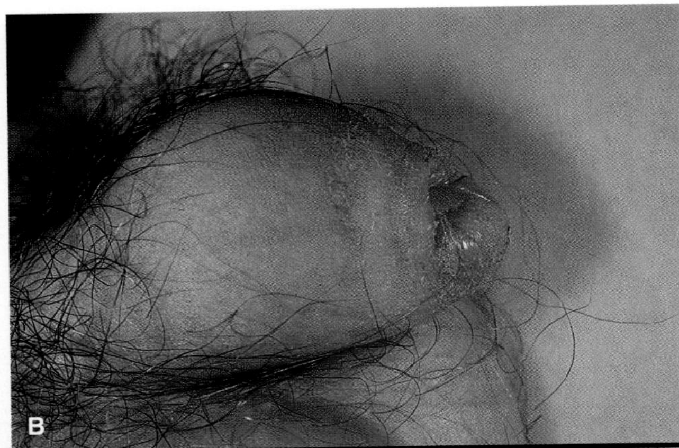

Figure 10-26. Reduction of Paraphimosis

A. A mentally retarded adolescent patient presented with paraphimosis of 3 days' duration. A manual reduction of paraphimosis was performed. *B*. Penile edema after manual reduction of paraphimosis. Postreduction residual edema may take hours to days to fully resolve.

Suggested Readings

Hughes ME, Currier SJ, Della-Guistina D. Normal cremasteric reflex in a case of testicular torsion. *Am J Emerg Med* 2001;19:241–242.

Berkowitz CD, Elvik SL, Logan M: A simulated acquired imperforate hymen following the genital trauma of sexual abuse. *Clin Pedaitr* 1987;26:307.

Botash AS: Imperforate hymen: congenital or acquired from sexual abuse? *Pediatrics* 2001;108:E53.

Green M, Strange GR: Paraphimosis reduction. In: Henretig FM, King C (eds). *Textbook of Pediatric Emergency Procedures*. Williams & Wilkins, Baltimore, 1997, p. 1007.

Kahn R, Duncan B, Bowes W: Spontaneous opening of congenital imperforate hymen. *J Pediatr* 1975;87:768.

Kanegaye JT: Reduction of paraphimosis. In: Walsh-Sukys MC, Krug SE (eds). *Procedures in Infants and Children*. Philadelphia, WB Saunders, 1997, p. 386.

Sanfilippo JS: Gynecologic problems of childhood. In: Behrman RE, Kliegman RM, Jenson HB (eds). *Nelson Textbook of Pediatrics*, 16th ed. WB Saunders, 2000, p. 1669.

Schneider K, Hong J, Fong J, Sanders CG: Hematocolpos as an easily overlooked diagnosis. *Curr Opin Pediatr* 1999;11:249.

Shah BR: Hydrometrocolpos with imperforate hymen. In: Shah BR, Laude TL: *Atlas of Pediatric Clinical Diagnosis*. WB Saunders, Philadelphia, 2000, p. 320.

Shah BR, Laude TL: Paraphimosis. In: *Atlas of Pediatric Clinical Diagnosis*. WB Saunders, Philadelphia, 2000, p. 336.

DIAGNOSIS SICKLE CELL ANEMIA WITH ACUTE CHEST SYNDROME

Synonym

Pneumonia in a patient with Sickle cell disease

Definition

Acute chest syndrome (ACS) is defined as acute pulmonary findings in a child with sickle cell disease (SCD). These findings may include tachypnea, which is sometimes subtle; retractions; diminished (often asymmetrical) breath sounds; and rales, vesicular sounds, or other signs of consolidation. Hypoxemia is often present and new pulmonary findings may be seen on chest radiograph. However, many patients present with clinical findings of ACS that precede abnormal radiographic findings by 24 to 72 hours.

Associated Clinical Features

1. Patients with chest pain should be examined carefully for clinical findings of consolidation.
2. Abdominal pain and/or distension may be a presenting symptom of ACS or sometimes a complication. Any patient with abdominal pain should have careful monitoring of pulmonary status and oxygen saturation.

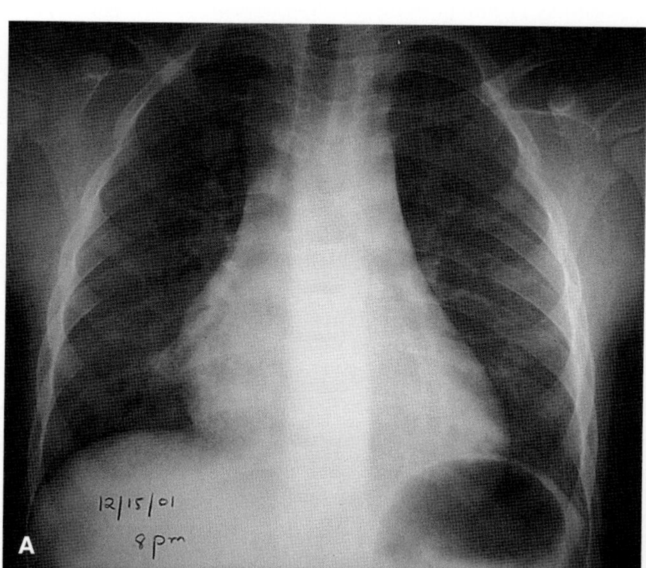

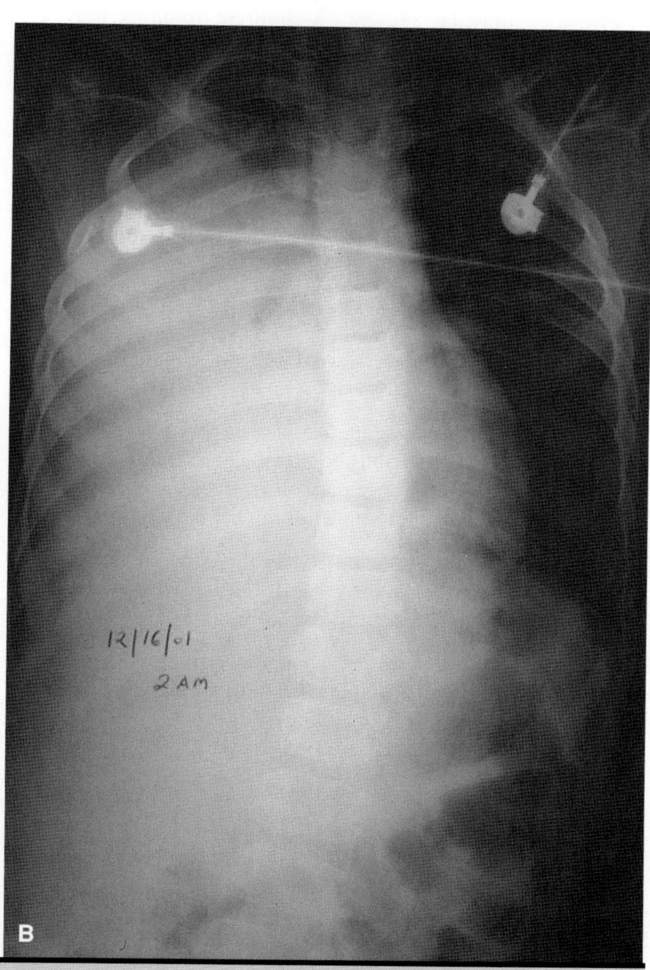

Figure 11-4. Acute Chest Syndrome

A. Frontal view in a patient with sickle cell anemia showing cardiomegaly with a minimal ill-defined parenchymal infiltrate seen in the right lower lobe. This patient presented with chest pain associated with fever and cough. *B*. Six hours later, the radiograph shows near complete opacification of the right hemithorax with a mediastinal shift to the contralateral side. This may represent a large consolidation with or without pleural effusion. This patient developed severe respiratory distress associated with hypoxemia. Patients with ACS can have a fulminant clinical course, including progressive respiratory failure, acute respiratory distress syndrome, and 2% mortality. Recurrent episodes of ACS are associated with chronic sickle cell lung disease in adults (associated with a 25% mortality rate and significant morbidity).

3. Neurological problems may be seen in ACS. This may be due to embolization of bone marrow fat from the lungs to the brain or ischemia/infarction due to systemic hypoxemia and underlying cerebrovascular disease (see SCD with cerebrovascular disease). There is a temporal association of ACS and stroke.

4. Complete blood count often shows a significant drop in hemoglobin value from baseline, a decrease in platelet count, and an elevated number of nucleated RBCs. Other tests include arterial blood gases (monitoring of acid-base status and hypoxemia), type and cross-match for blood transfusion, baseline values of serum electrolytes, blood urea nitrogen, lactic dehydrogenase, and liver function tests.

5. Chest radiograph shows pulmonary infiltrates that may be present unilaterally or bilaterally. Infiltrates are either confined to a single lobe or diffusely spread. Pleural effusions may be present. Radiologic findings may lag behind clinical findings; a repeat chest radiograph may be required to confirm the diagnosis.

Consultation

A pediatric hematologist should assist in management of a patient with ACS and assist in deciding about the need for blood transfusion.

Emergency Department Treatment and Disposition

1. Due to its variable and often severe clinical course, all patients with ACS should be hospitalized, preferably in an intensive care unit. These patients need oxygen therapy and continuous cardiac and pulse oximetry monitoring.

2. Close monitoring of analgesic therapy is needed to prevent hypoventilation secondary to splinting (hypoventilation may lead to atelectasis and hypoxemia).

3. Maintain hydration by offering maintenance fluids with close monitoring of intake and output (avoid pulmonary edema and worsening of ACS).

4. Blood transfusion
   a. Simple transfusion with packed RBCs is usually given for a moderately severe episode, especially when associated with a drop in hemoglobin concentration.
   b. Exchange transfusion is usually reserved for patients who do not respond to simple transfusion.

5. Sickle cell patients with fever as a presenting finding should have urgent administration of antibiotics after blood culture is obtained (see sickle cell anemia with fever, Box 11-1).
   a. All patients with ACS ultimately should be treated with a macrolide or other antibiotic to treat infection by atypical bacteria.
   b. Cefuroxime or ceftriaxone is often used to cover common bacterial pathogens such as *Streptococcus pneumoniae*, and erythromycin to cover *Mycoplasma pneumoniae* and *Chlamydia pneumoniae*.

6. Incentive spirometry is used as an adjunctive therapy.

7. Patients presenting with recurrent episodes should be referred to a hematologist for consideration of hydroxyurea therapy, which clearly reduces the frequency of this serious complication.

Clinical Pearls: Acute Chest Syndrome

1. Due to the fact that fever may be the only early manifestation of ACS, all febrile sickle cell patients should have a chest radiograph as part of their evaluation.

2. Maintain a high index of suspicion for ACS in any patient with SCD who presents with chest, back, or abdominal pain or respiratory symptoms.

3. Acute chest syndrome not only has significant acute morbidity and mortality, but may predispose to chronic sickle cell lung disease and pulmonary hypertension.

4. Clinical or radiological diagnosis of ACS mandates hospitalization.

5. Many patients present with clinical findings of ACS that precede abnormal radiographic findings by 24 to 72 hours. Thus, a chest radiograph may be negative during the early course; repeat radiographs 24 to 72 hours later may show evidence of pulmonary infiltrates (Fig. 11-4).

BOX 11-4. CLINICAL FEATURES OF ACUTE CHEST SYNDROME IN SICKLE CELL DISEASE

- ACS means acute pulmonary findings in a child with sickle cell disease.
- Presenting complaints of ACS may include any of the following:
  (1) Only fever
  (2) Chest pain
  (3) Abdominal pain
  (4) Back pain
  (5) Cough
- Pulmonary findings may include any of the following:
  (1) Tachypnea (which is sometimes subtle)
  (2) Retractions
  (3) Diminished (often asymmetrical) breath sounds
  (4) Rales
  (5) Vesicular sounds
  (6) Other signs of consolidation
- Hypoxemia often present
- New pulmonary findings may be seen on chest radiograph.
- Many patients present with clinical findings of ACS that precede abnormal radiographic findings by 24 to 72 hours.
- Neurological problems that may be seen in ACS and require assessment include:
  (1) Seizures
  (2) Confusion, obtundation
  (3) Focal neurologic deficits

BOX 11-5. ETIOLOGY AND DIFFERENTIAL DIAGNOSIS OF ACUTE CHEST SYNDROME IN SICKLE CELL DISEASE

- The term *acute chest syndrome* underlines the difficulty of establishing the etiology of acute pulmonary findings in children with SCD.
- Infection may be a predominant factor in many patients.
  (1) Common pathogens include *Chlamydia pneumoniae* and *Mycoplasma pneumoniae* (often associated with a severe clinical course).
  (2) Bacterial infection with *Streptococcus* spp. (especially *S. pneumoniae*), *Staphylococcus*, and gram-negative organisms can occur (fewer than 10% of cases).
  (3) Various viruses may also cause ACS (e.g., respiratory syncytial virus, influenza)
  (4) Parvovirus B19 (associated with transient aplastic crises in sickle cell patients) is also associated with ACS.
- Noninfectious etiologies include:
  (1) At least some cases may be due to acute bone marrow infarction and subsequent pulmonary fat embolization (even in patients without parvovirus infection, pulmonary fat embolism is a common cause of ACS, often severe).
  (2) ACS is often diagnosed after hospitalization for other causes, particularly pain episodes.
  (3) Notably associated with nosocomial ACS is thoracic pain (chest or back), resulting in splinting and hypoventilation and use of opioid analgesia (may induce hypoventilation and pulmonary sickling). Incentive spirometry reduces this risk.

DIAGNOSIS SICKLE CELL ANEMIA WITH PRIAPISM

Definition

Priapism is defined as an unwanted painful penile erection. Clinically it can be a prolonged episode or shorter, often recurrent "stuttering" episodes. The word *priapism* is derived from Priapus, the Greek god of fertility, who was depicted in statues as having an erect phallus of exaggerated proportions.

Etiology

1. Priapism can be classed as low-flow or high-flow.
   a. Low-flow ischemic priapism is presumably due to sludging and stasis of blood in the corporal spaces. Ischemia and infarction will injure cavernosal smooth muscle and ultimately may result in fibrosis and impotence.

b. The etiology of high-flow priapism is not clear, but may be related to vascular disease and autonomic dysfunction.

2. The glans and corpus spongiosum are generally spared in sickle cell-related priapism. Tricorporal priapism is associated with a more prolonged, difficult course and more severe systemic disease.

Associated Clinical Features

1. Stuttering episodes are more commonly seen in prepubertal males and the prognosis is probably better than in older patients with low-flow episodes; however, in a large series from Jamaica, all patients with stuttering ultimately did have a prolonged episode lasting longer than 24 hours.
2. The diagnosis of priapism is made clinically in a patient with a history of sickle cell disease.
3. Noninvasive methods used to assess penile perfusion include radionuclide penile scan and doppler ultrasonography.

Consultations

Emergent consultation with urology and pediatric hematology for patients who have a priapism episode lasting >2 hours; many of these episodes will extend to 24 hours and beyond without intervention.

Emergency Department Treatment and Disposition

1. Patients should be treated with fluids at 1.5 times maintenance and given adequate analgesia (i.e., morphine sulfate 0.1 to 0.15 mg/kg per dose every 2 to 3 hours).
2. If priapism is not resolved in 2 to 3 hours, patients should generally be admitted to the hospital.
3. Aspiration and irrigation of the corpora cavernosum
   a. Especially for older, cooperative patients, consultation by urology may be obtained in the ED prior to admission for an attempt at aspiration and irrigation of the corpora cavernosum with 1:1,000,000 dilution of epinephrine (Fig. 11-5).
   b. With local and/or regional anesthesia, approximately 10 mL of dilute epinephrine is slowly injected into the base of the corpora cavernosum after aspiration; this will often result in detumescence.
   c. Younger children may require mild to moderate sedation or admission to the hospital for deep sedation/general anesthesia.
   d. If detumescence occurs, patients may be discharged.
   e. If aspiration fails or priapism recurs, hospitalization is required.
4. Transfusion therapy (especially exchange transfusion) for treatment of priapism
   a. It may be associated with the appearance of neurological events within 2 weeks. Patients often have severe headache as a prodrome (ASPEN syndrome; *a*ssociation of *s*ickle cell disease, *p*riapism, *e*xchange transfusion, and *n*eurological events).
   b. Those with ischemic priapism, even with exchange transfusion, often have minimal passage of normal blood into the congested corpora cavernosum. However, transfusion may be required in patients who fail aspiration/irrigation, and it may be especially effective in high-flow patients.
   c. Patients with persistent priapism should have another attempt at aspiration after transfusion; if retumescence occurs, perfusion of the corpora cavernosum with some

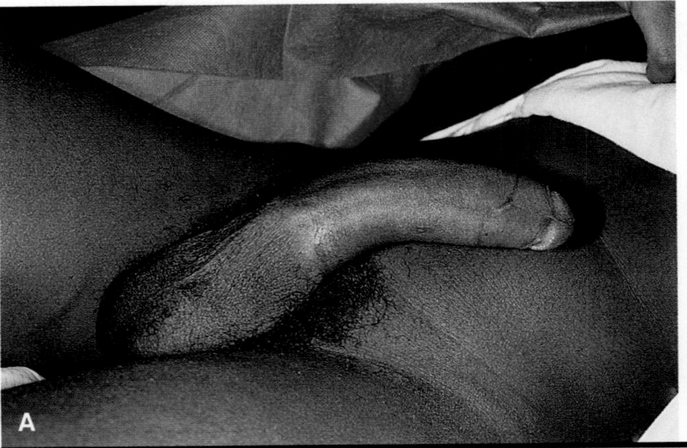

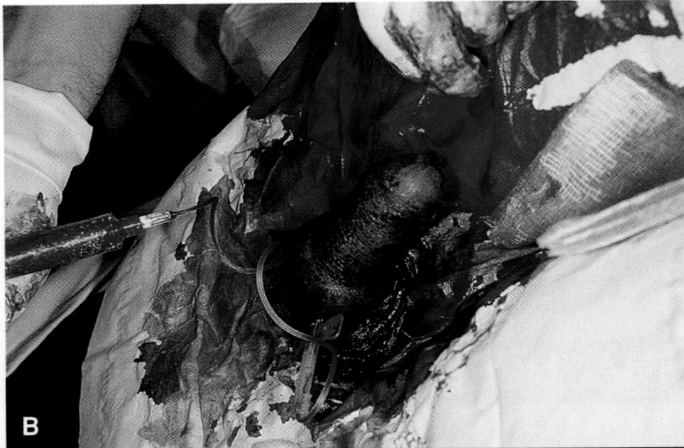

Figure 11-5. Priapism in Sickle Cell Disease

A. An adolescent male patient with sickle cell anemia presented with a swollen, edematous, and very tender penile erection of 5 hours' duration. He awoke from the sleep around 5 o'clock in the morning with penile pain. The diagnosis of priapism is usually made by clinical examination. Both corporal bodies are turgid and tender, while the glans penis and spongiosum are usually spared. *B*. A 21-gauge butterfly needle was placed in the corpora cavernosum after lidocaine injection, aspiration and irrigation with saline and phenylephrine was performed, with subsequent resolution of the priapism.

DIAGNOSIS ACUTE IMMUNE THROMBOCYTOPENIC PURPURA

SYNONYM

Acute idiopathic thrombocytopenic purpura

Definition

1. Immune thrombocytopenic purpura (ITP) in children is an *acquired thrombocytopenia* due to excessive destruction of autoantibody-coated platelets by phagocytic cells, predominantly in the spleen.
2. It is classified into:
   a. Acute ITP
   b. Chronic ITP (thrombocytopenia persisting >6 months)

Etiology and Pathophysiology

1. The autoantibodies are directed against some of the platelet membrane glycoproteins.
2. About 70% of patients have a history of an antecedent viral infection which is implicated in the production of the antibodies.
3. Immune thrombocytopenic purpura has been associated with common childhood illnesses (e.g., varicella, rubella, rubeola, mumps, upper respiratory tract infection, infectious mononucleosis) and immunizations.

Associated Clinical Features

1. Complete blood count findings include:
   a. Platelet count is generally less than 20,000/mm^3 (although severity of thrombocytopenia is variable)
   b. The blood smear shows many large platelets indicative of increased platelet turnover.
   c. Hemoglobin may be low due to bleeding.
   d. White blood cell count and differential are usually normal.
2. Prothrombin time, partial thromboplastin time, fibrinogen, and fibrin split products, while generally not done, are all normal.
3. Bleeding time, although not a recommended test, is generally prolonged.
4. Bone marrow aspiration is not needed for diagnosis in most patients. It shows:
   a. Normal erythroid and granulocytic series
   b. Normal or increased numbers of megakaryocytes
5. Antinuclear antibody and HIV tests, especially in an adolescent or as indicated should be done.
6. The most serious complication is intracranial bleeding. It is usually seen with a platelet count <10,000 to 20,000/mm^3, and when signs of significant hemorrhage are present (e.g., oral mucosal bleeding, hematuria, or hematochezia). It occurs in 0.1 to 0.5% of patients.
7. Acute ITP is a self-limited disorder in 90% of children. Complete recovery is seen in 75% of patients within 12 weeks and in 90% by 9 to 12 months after onset. Most patients recover in about 8 weeks.
8. Chronic ITP develops in 10% of children. It is usually not possible at diagnosis to predict which patients will have acute ITP and which patients will go on to develop chronic ITP.

Consultation

Hematology

Emergency Department Treatment and Disposition

1. Mild ITP (platelet count between 20,000 and 50,000/mm^3):
   a. In the absence of mucosal hemorrhages, patients can be observed without specific therapy.
   b. Follow patients as outpatients with once or twice weekly CBCs.
2. Hospitalization and hematology consultation are recommended, especially for:
   a. Patients with mucosal or retinal hemorrhages
   b. Patients at high risk for bleeding (platelet count <20,000/mm^3)
3. Treatment modalities (any of the following modalities for patients with platelet counts<20,000/mm^3 and/or mucosal bleeding):
   a. Intravenous immune globulin (IVIG)
      1) Advantages include rapid onset of action and highly effective (~90%)
      2) It can be given *without* bone marrow examination.
      3) Usual dose is 1 g/kg for 1 to 2 days.
      4) May not be suitable for ED administration since IV infusion takes 4 to 6 hours
   b. Intravenous methylprednisolone (30 mg/kg per day for 3 days) *or*
   c. Prednisone: 2 to 4 mg/kg for 5 to 7 days followed by 2 mg/kg for 2 to 3 weeks
      1) Advantages include: inexpensive therapy, given orally, and effective in 75 to 80% of patients
      2) A bone marrow exam is recommended by most pediatric hematologists prior to starting corticosteroids.
   d. Intravenous anti-D immune globulin
      1) Immune globulin against D-antigen of the Rh blood group system, when given to Rh-positive children with ITP, produces a rapid rise in platelet count.

2) Advantages are that it can be given in an ambulatory setting (ED or office) by IV infusion over 3 minutes. The recommended dose is 50 to 75 µg/kg.
3) Premedication with prednisone and acetaminophen prior to anti-D is known to result in a higher platelet count with fewer side effects.
4) The most common adverse effect is a fall in Hb concentration by 1 to 2 g/dL.

4. Life-threatening hemorrhages (e.g., intracranial bleeding or retroperitoneal bleeding):
   a. Patient needs to be hospitalized and managed in an ICU setting.
   b. The treatment may be started in the ED. The patient should receive a dose of methylprednisolone and started on IVIG infusion if Rh blood group status is unknown.
   c. If the patient is Rh-positive, slow IV push of anti-D immune globulin (50 to 75 µg/kg) can be given in the ED.
   d. Methylprednisolone IV 30 mg/kg per day to be given for 3 days
   e. IVIG 1 g/kg per day for 2 days
   f. Platelet transfusions every 6 to 8 hours; while platelet survival following platelet transfusion is poor, it is better when combined with corticosteroids and IVIG or anti-D immune globulin.
5. *Education of the family and patient at the time of discharge includes:*
   a. Activities that increase the risk of head injury, falls, or trauma should be restricted (e.g., rollerblading, skating, contact sports).
   b. Strictly enforce use of helmets and seat belts.
   c. Avoid taking the temperature rectally and avoid intramuscular injections.
   d. Avoid aspirin, aspirin-containing drugs, and ibuprofen.
   e. Avoid direct exposure to sunlight for prolonged periods (this produces petechiae and purpura in a child with thrombocytopenia).
   f. Educate the patient and family about signs and symptoms of increased intracranial pressure.
   g. A rule of thumb for a child with a low platelet count: *avoid any activity where one foot is not on the ground at all times.*

Clinical Pearls: Immune Thrombocytopenic Purpura

1. ITP is the most common cause of acquired thrombocytopenia in childhood.
2. Acute ITP is a clinical diagnosis reached by exclusion of other causes of thrombocytopenia (e.g., leukemia and aplastic anemia), usually by careful physical examination and evaluation of blood count and blood smear.
3. Typical presentation of acute ITP is that of an otherwise healthy child who presents with an acute onset of easy bruising and purpuric rash (Fig. 11-7).
4. Treat the child and not the platelet count.

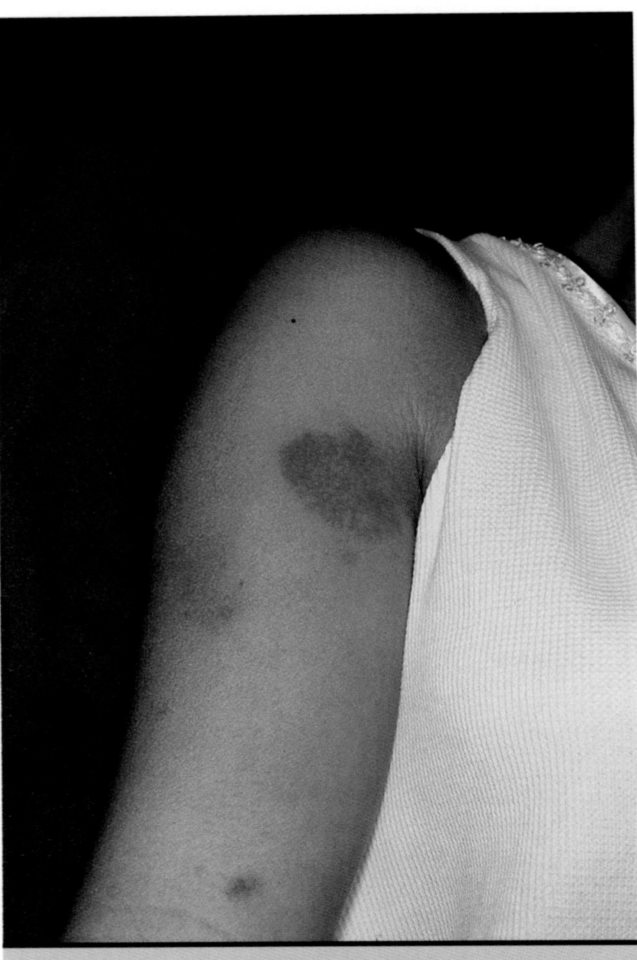

Figure 11-7. Immune Thrombocytopenic Purpura

Sudden onset of petechiae and ecchymoses over the hands and lower extremities were the presenting complaints in this otherwise healthy 5-year-old girl. Her WBC, differential, and hemoglobin values were normal. Her platelet count was <11,000/mm^3. She had an upper respiratory tract infection 4 days prior to the appearance of these skin lesions. Her examination was otherwise negative. Purpura is most prominent over the legs and typically it is asymmetrical in acute ITP.

BOX 11-10. CLINICAL FEATURES OF IMMUNE THROMBOCYTOPENIC PURPURA

- Peak age of presentation: between 2 and 6 years
- Gender prevalence equal in prepubertal children
- Female preponderance in adolescents and adults
- The illness is characterized by sudden onset of skin and/or mucosal bleeding in otherwise healthy children.
- Sites of hemorrhages:
  (1) Skin: petechiae (pinpoint hemorrhages), ecchymosis (large areas of hemorrhage; Fig. 11-7)
  (2) Oral mucosal bleeding, gum bleeding, epistaxis
  (3) Hematuria
  (4) Melena
  (5) Menorrhagia may be seen in adolescent females.
- Physical examination may be normal except for skin and mucosal bleeding.
- Absence of lymphadenopathy and hepatosplenomegaly (except when ITP is associated with mononucleosis)

BOX 11-11. DIFFERENTIAL DIAGNOSIS OF IMMUNE THROMBOCYTOPENIC PURPURA

- Differential diagnosis of ITP:
  (1) Acute ITP is a clinical diagnosis reached by exclusion of other causes of thrombocytopenia such as leukemia and aplastic anemia.
  (2) Acute leukemia almost never presents with isolated thrombocytopenia.
  (3) Immune thrombocytopenia from another etiology
    a. Systemic lupus erythematosus (can be a presenting manifestation)
    b. Evans' syndrome
    c. AIDS (specially in adolescents)
- Differential diagnosis of purpura/petechiae:
  (1) Bruising due to child abuse (platelet count normal)
  (2) Accidental trauma (e.g., bruising in a normal, active, healthy child [bruising seen in exposed areas, especially over hard bony surfaces like the shins])
  (3) Bacterial infection (e.g., meningococcemia, endocarditis)
  (4) Viral infections (e.g., Epstein-Barr virus, measles)
  (5) Rickettsial infections (e.g., Rocky Mountain spotted fever)
  (6) Henoch-Schönlein purpura (Fig. 11-8)
  (7) Factor deficiencies (e.g., hemophilia)
  (8) Drugs (e.g., sulfonamides, penicillins)
  (9) Letterer-Siwe disease
  (10) Ehlers-Danlos syndrome
  (11) Scurvy

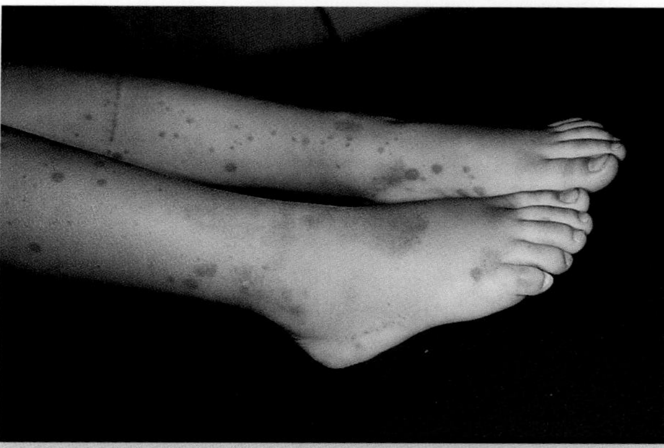

Figure 11-8. Differential Diagnosis of Immune Thrombocytopenic Purpura: Henoch-Schönlein Purpura

Purpuric lesions are symmetrically distributed over the lower extremities in HSP. Skin lesions in HSP are characteristically palpable purpura in dependent parts of the body. This patient also had angioedema of both feet. Patients with HSP may also have other systemic involvement including joints (e.g., arthritis or arthralgias), renal (e.g., hematuria), and GI (e.g., abdominal pain or bleeding). Unlike ITP, platelet counts in patients with HSP are either normal or elevated.

DIAGNOSIS HEMOPHILIA

Synonyms

Hemophilia A (classical hemophilia)
Hemophilia B (Christmas disease)

Definitions

1. Hemophilia is an inherited bleeding disorder of variable severity due to decreased amount or abnormal function of plasma coagulation protein.
2. Hemophilia A is due to deficiency of coagulation factor VIII and hemophilia B is due to deficiency of coagulation factor IX. Both are X-linked recessive disorders with very similar clinical features.
3. Hemophilia C, factor XI deficiency, is an autosomal recessive disorder of mild severity and is more common in Ashkenazi Jews.

Associated Clinical Features

1. Patients with mild and moderate hemophilia usually bleed after trauma. Those with severe hemophilia bleed either spontaneously or after minor injury.
2. Initially after trauma, bleeding stops promptly but recurs after 30 to 60 minutes. Other manifestations include oral bleeding, hematuria, and gastrointestinal or central nervous system bleeding.
3. Only a third of hemophilia patients bleed after circumcision.
4. Specific coagulation factor assay is needed for definitive diagnosis.
5. It is essential to know:
   a. Type of hemophilia (i.e., factor VIII, IX, or XI deficiency)
   b. Usual plasma level of deficient coagulation factor
   c. History of inhibitors to coagulation factor
   d. Usual replacement coagulation product used for treatment of prior bleeding episodes

Consultation

Hematology (urgent consultation for all children with hemophilia who present with bleeding)

Emergency Department Treatment and Disposition

1. The unconscious patient with a history of hemophilia poses a challenge unless the patient has a MedicAlert bracelet or similar device.
2. Severe or life-threatening bleeding
   a. Intracranial or retroperitoneal bleeding may be life-threatening in patients with hemophilia.
   b. *A history of head injury should be taken seriously.*
      1) Even in the absence of external bleeding, the patient should be given appropriate clotting factor in a dose of 50 units/kg.
      2) Obtain a head CT scan soon after factor infusion.
   c. Any patient with significant head injury (e.g., loss of memory, hematoma, or laceration) should be hospitalized after factor replacement in the ER and receive factor replacement for 3 to 5 days even if head CT is negative.
   d. Monitoring the levels of coagulation factor is mandatory in patients receiving factor replacement for serious and life-threatening bleeding.
3. DDAVP
   a. Intravenous DDAVP or nasal desmopressin (Stimate) is recommended to treat hemarthrosis in mild to moderate hemophilia A.
   b. The dose of IV DDAVP is 0.3 μg/kg given as an IV infusion over 15 minutes.
   c. This dose may be repeated at 24-hour intervals for 2 or 3 days.
   d. Stimate nasal spray requires 1 spray in 1 nostril (150 μg) for children less than 50 kg or 1 spray in each nostril (total dose 300 μg) for children over 50 kg.
   e. IV and nasal administration had similar increases in factor VIII level in one study.
4. Severe hemophilia A or B: Recombinant technology–derived coagulation factor VIII or IX is available and is used most frequently to treat bleeding episodes.
5. Hemarthrosis (Fig. 11-9)
   a. Factor VIII: 20 to 40 units/kg IV
   b. Factor IX: 25 to 50 units/kg IV
   c. Above dose may need to be repeated in 12 to 24 hours if pain persists.
   d. Prednisone: 1mg/kg per day in two divided doses for 3 to 5 days to prevent inflammation in the joint.
   e. Adjuvant therapy
      1) Physical therapy, splints, and crutches as required for abnormalities in gait or joint function after resolution of acute hemorrhage
      2) During acute phase: immobilization as required by bed rest, ice, compression, and elevation
6. Muscle bleeding
   a. Similar dosing as in hemarthrosis
   b. Prednisone is not recommended.
7. Oral bleeding
   a. Factor VIII or IX: 30 to 50 units/kg IV
   b. Aminocaproic acid is an important adjunct to factor replacement in the management of oral bleeding.

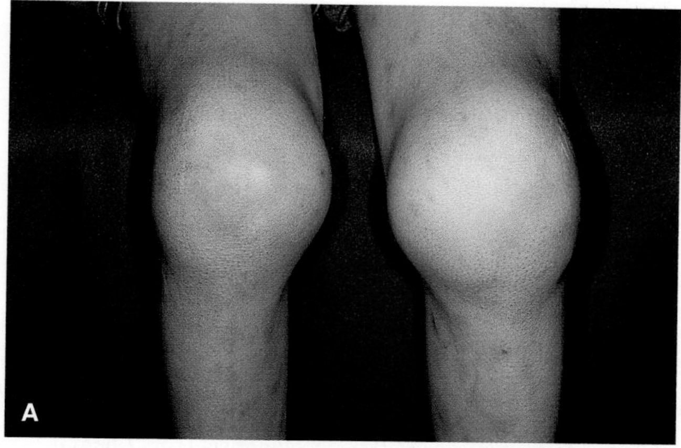

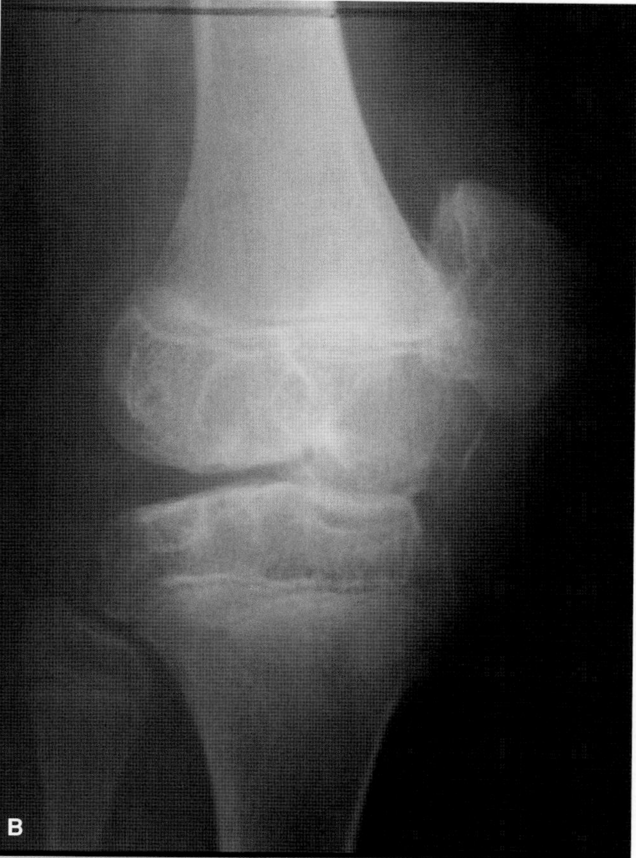

Figure 11-9. Hemarthrosis

A. A 9-year-old male child with hemophilia A presented with swelling of both knees (left > right) with significant pain in the left knee and limitation of movement. Markedly swollen knees seen here represent an acute bleeding in a hemophilia patient with hemophilic arthropathy or synovitis. *B.* Lateral view of the knee shows diffuse osteopenia, widening of the intercondylar notch, cortical irregularity, and a suprapatellar effusion. There is a subcortical cyst, and increased synovial density secondary to hemosiderin deposition.

1) It is an antifibrinolytic agent that prevents clot lysis and promotes healing.
2) Given in a dose of 75 to 100 mg/kg per dose every 6 hours (usually orally) for 5 to 7 days

Clinical Pearls: Hemophilia

1. Accurate diagnosis of the type of hemophilia is required for the proper management of the patient.
2. Deep hematomas and bleeding into joints are the most common findings in patients with hemophilia.
3. For patients with mild to moderate hemophilia A, do not prescribe DDAVP spray (used to treat patients with diabetes insipidus); instead prescribe Stimate nasal spray.
4. Monitor levels of plasma clotting factor (VIII or IX) when treating life-threatening bleeding.
5. Aminocaproic acid is an important medication when treating oral bleeding in any type of hemophilia.
6. CT scan or MRI of head must be done if there is any suggestion of head trauma, even if symptoms are minimal.
7. All head injuries should be treated very aggressively with factor infusion, even if there are no signs of intracranial bleeding.

BOX 11-12. CLINICAL FEATURES OF HEMOPHILIA

- Presenting signs and symptoms depend on the concentration of deficient plasma coagulation protein.
  - (1) Severe: Coagulation factor level <1%
  - (2) Moderate: 1 to 5%
  - (3) Mild: >5%
- Hemarthrosis
  - (1) Hallmark of hemophilia
  - (2) May occur spontaneously or following trauma
  - (3) Typically presents during toddler years
  - (4) Most commonly involved joints: elbows, knees, ankles
  - (5) Less frequently involved joints: shoulders, wrist, hips
  - (6) Clinically: acute joint swelling, erythema, or discoloration may be present, with pain, warmth, and limitation of movement
- Deep hematomas
- Oral bleeding
- Hematuria
- Laboratory findings
  - (1) CBC usually normal (anemia may be due to bleeding)
  - (2) Platelet count normal
  - (3) Partial thromboplastin time (PTT) prolonged
  - (4) Prothrombin time (PT) normal
  - (5) Decrease concentration of factor VIII, IX, or XI

BOX 11-13. DIFFERENTIAL DIAGNOSIS OF HEMOPHILIA

- Other clotting factor deficiencies
- Platelet function disorders
- Vitamin K deficiency
- Von Willebrand's disease
  - (1) A congenital disorder of hemostasis characterized by defective or deficient von Willebrand factor (vWF)
  - (2) Primary symptoms: ecchymosis (small hematomas in areas of trauma) and epistaxis
  - (3) Other sites of mucocutaneous bleeding: gingival bleeding, bruising, menorrhagia, bleeding after dental extraction, severe postoperative bleeding (e.g., after tonsillectomy)
  - (4) Hemarthrosis rare
  - (5) Prolonged bleeding time in some patients
  - (6) Prolonged PTT in some patients
  - (7) Factor VIII and vWF levels are decreased in type 1 disease.

SYMPTOM ABDOMINAL MASS

Background

1. Any abdominal mass in a child requires urgent medical attention since it may be a presenting manifestation of malignancy (Figs. 11-10 and 11-11).
2. Abdominal masses tend to be retroperitoneal in origin.
3. In infants most abdominal masses tend to be due to benign conditions.
4. It is not always easy to palpate the abdomen in infants. One should make a serious attempt to feel the abdomen.
5. Any mass detected during a routine well child visit may increase the chance of early diagnosis and treatment of a malignancy and a favorable outcome.

Clinical Evaluation

1. Obtain detailed history including:
   - a. Duration of the mass and rapidity of increase in the size of the mass
   - b. Pain
   - c. Constipation (suggests either a tumor compressing the bowel or that the mass is stool)
   - d. Diarrhea
   - e. Fever
   - f. Weight loss
2. Thorough physical exam that may show:
   - a. General appearance irritable or cachectic (may suggest malignancy)

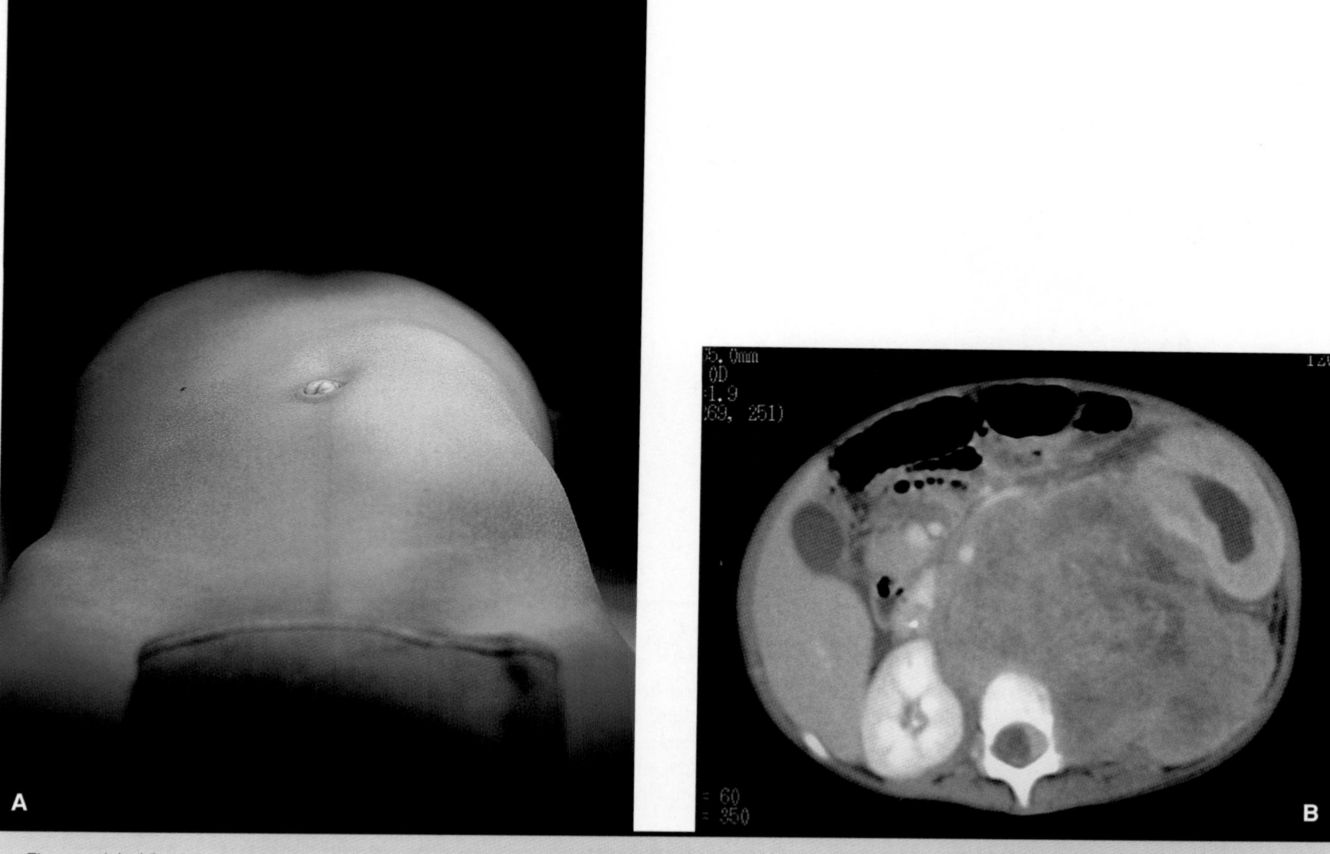

Figure 11-10. Neuroblastoma Presenting as an Abdominal Mass

A. A left-sided abdominal mass was the presenting complaint in this 3-year-old girl who also had a history of weight loss. She was anemic (Hgb/Hct 10/32) with an elevated LDH value (826 U/L [normal 80 to 200]). The rest of her examination and laboratory tests were normal. Excessive catecholamine secretion by the tumor may result in tachycardia, hypertension, diarrhea, and skin flushing. Other findings of neuroblastoma include exophthalmos, ecchymoses ("raccoon eyes"; see Fig. 8-16), hepatomegaly, constipation, abdominal pain, localized back pain, weakness, scoliosis, bladder dysfunction, and palpable nontender subcutaneous nodules. *B*. Complex predominantly left-sided heterogenous mass with necrotic areas and calcifications arising from the retroperitoneum is seen on the CT scan. The left kidney is seen displaced anteriorly with hydronephosis. Histology confirmed the diagnosis of neuroblastoma.

b. Presence of proptosis and ecchymosis (suggests metastatic malignancy such as neuroblastoma; see Fig. 8-16)
c. High blood pressure (suggests Wilms' tumor, neuroblastoma, hydronephrosis, multicystic kidney)
d. Sporadic aniridia or hemihypertrophy (may be associated with Wilms' tumor)
e. Marked pallor and petechiae (suggest marrow infiltration by the tumor, typically neuroblastoma)
f. Fecal masses are usually mobile, multiple, and palpable in the left lower quadrant (see Fig. 15-14) or on the entire left side corresponding to the course of the descending colon. Rectal examination confirming rectum filled with stool suggests that the abdominal mass may be a stool mass. Fecal masses disappear after a cleansing enema.
g. Uncommon masses include intussusception (mass in right lower or upper quadrant) or incarcerated hernia (see page 439).
h. Imperforate hymen with an abdominal mass suggests hydrocolpos, hydrometrocolpos, hematocolpos, or hematometrocolopos (see Fig. 10-21).

3. In differential diagnosis of abdominal masses in children, the age of the child should be considered.
    a. Greater than 50% of masses are of renal origin in neonates (and of these, most are caused by multicystic kidney disease or congenital hydronephrosis) (Fig. 11-12).
    b. Abdominal masses in infants and children are either retroperitoneal tumors (e.g., Wilms' tumor or neuroblastoma) or enlarged liver and spleen (often from diseases like leukemia or lymphoma).

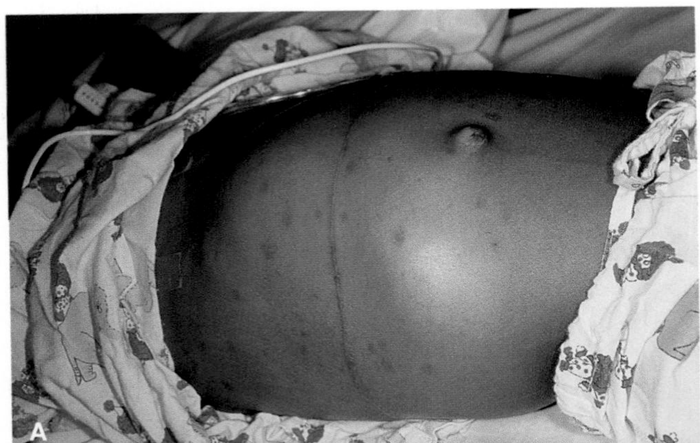

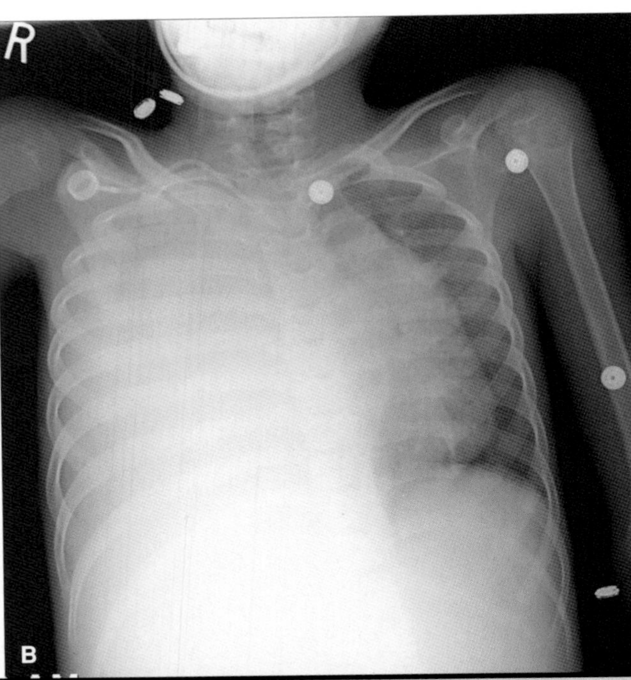

Figure 11-11. Wilms' Tumor Presenting as an Abdominal Mass

A. A 7-year-old child presented with a huge abdominal mass and respiratory distress. Pelvic CT scan followed by laparotomy confirmed the mass as Wilms' tumor. Wilms' tumor most often presents as an asymptomatic mass in the flank. Because of the retroperitoneal location of the kidney, these tumors can be quite large at diagnosis without significant impingement of other vital structures. *B*. Right-sided pleural effusion. Almost complete opacification of the right hemithorax with mediastinal shift to the left is seen. Approximately 10 to 15% of patients with Wilms' tumor will have hematogenous metastatic disease at presentation. The most common site is the lungs (80 to 85% of cases), then the liver with or without the lungs (15% of cases). A large abdominal mass with a large pleural effusion led to respiratory failure in this patient.

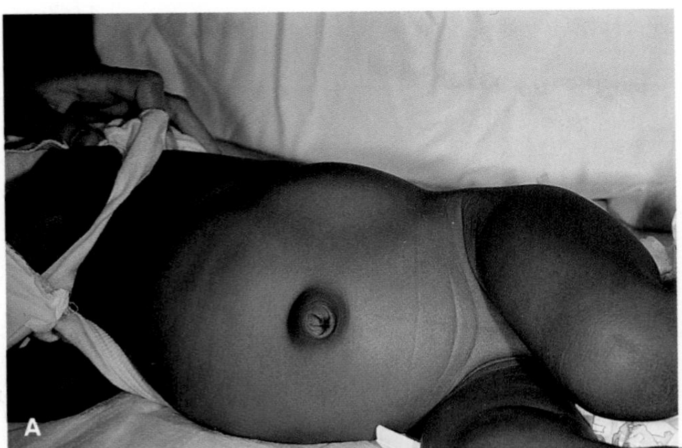

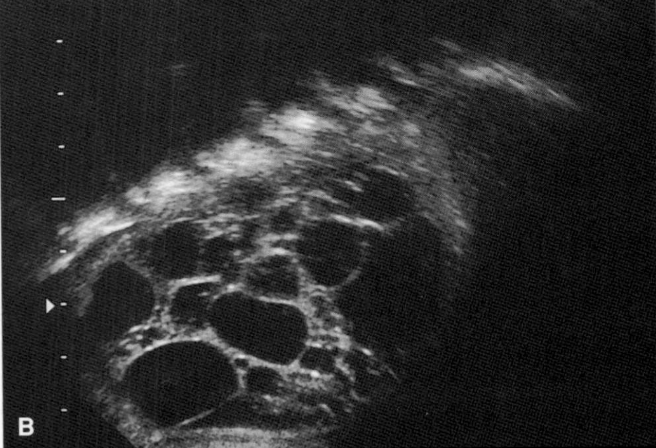

Figure 11-12. Multicystic Kidney with Dysplasia Presenting as an Abdominal Mass

A. A left-sided abdominal mass was accidentally detected in this 10-month-old infant who presented to the ED with complaints of fever and rhinorrhea. *B*. Pelvic ultrasound showing a large mass consisting of multiple noncommunicating cysts of varying sizes occupying the left renal fossa. No normal renal parenchyma is identified and the mass has no solid structure. A renal scan subsequently confirmed an enlarged distorted left kidney with poor uptake of radiotracer.

BOX 12-1. CLINICAL FEATURES OF KAWASAKI DISEASE

The diagnosis is established clinically by:

a. Presence of fever and at least four of the five criteria listed below, *or*

b. Presence of fever and at least three of the five criteria listed below, and evidence of coronary artery abnormalities (Figs. 12-2 and 12-3)

(1) *Fever:* high and unremitting; lasting 5 days or more; unresponsive to antipyretics and antibiotics

(2) *Skin rash:* polymorphic (morbilliform, maculopapular, scarlatiniform, or erythema multiforme–like); nonvesicular; commonly seen on trunk and extremities

(3) *Mucous membrane changes* (at least one of the following): erythematous or fissured lips; erythema of the buccal mucosa and pharynx; "strawberry" tongue

(4) *Conjunctivitis:* bilateral bulbar involvement; nonexudative

(5) *Changes in distal extremities* (at least one of the following): erythema of the palms or soles; indurative edema of the hands or feet; periungual desquamation of fingers and toes (1 to 3 weeks after the onset of illness)

(6) *Cervical lymphadenopathy:* unilateral; at least one node 1.5 cm or larger in diameter; nonpurulent; this is the least constant finding

Clinical phases (after onset of illness):

- *Acute febrile phase:* up to 1 to 2 weeks (fever and other acute signs)
- *Subacute phase:* up to 2 to 4 weeks (fever abated, desquamation, thrombocytosis, development of coronary aneurysms)
- *Convalescent phase:* up to 6 to 8 weeks (illness disappears, ESR returns to normal)

Clinical pearl

- *Perineal desquamation seen within the first week of illness is an important early diagnostic clue.*
- The diagnosis of KD requires exclusion of other illnesses that might mimic its clinical features (e.g., acute adenoviral infection).

BOX 12-2. OTHER LESS COMMON FINDINGS IN KAWASAKI DISEASE

- Extreme irritability
- Aseptic meningitis (50%)
- Urethritis (sterile pyuria, 70%)
- Hepatic dysfunction (40%)
- Hydrops of the gallbladder (<10%)
- Diarrhea, vomiting, abdominal pain
- Arthritis or arthralgia (10 to 20%; knees, ankles, hips)
- Uveitis
- Pneumonitis
- Testicular swelling
- Peripheral gangrene
- Erythema or induration at bacille Calmette-Guérin inoculation site

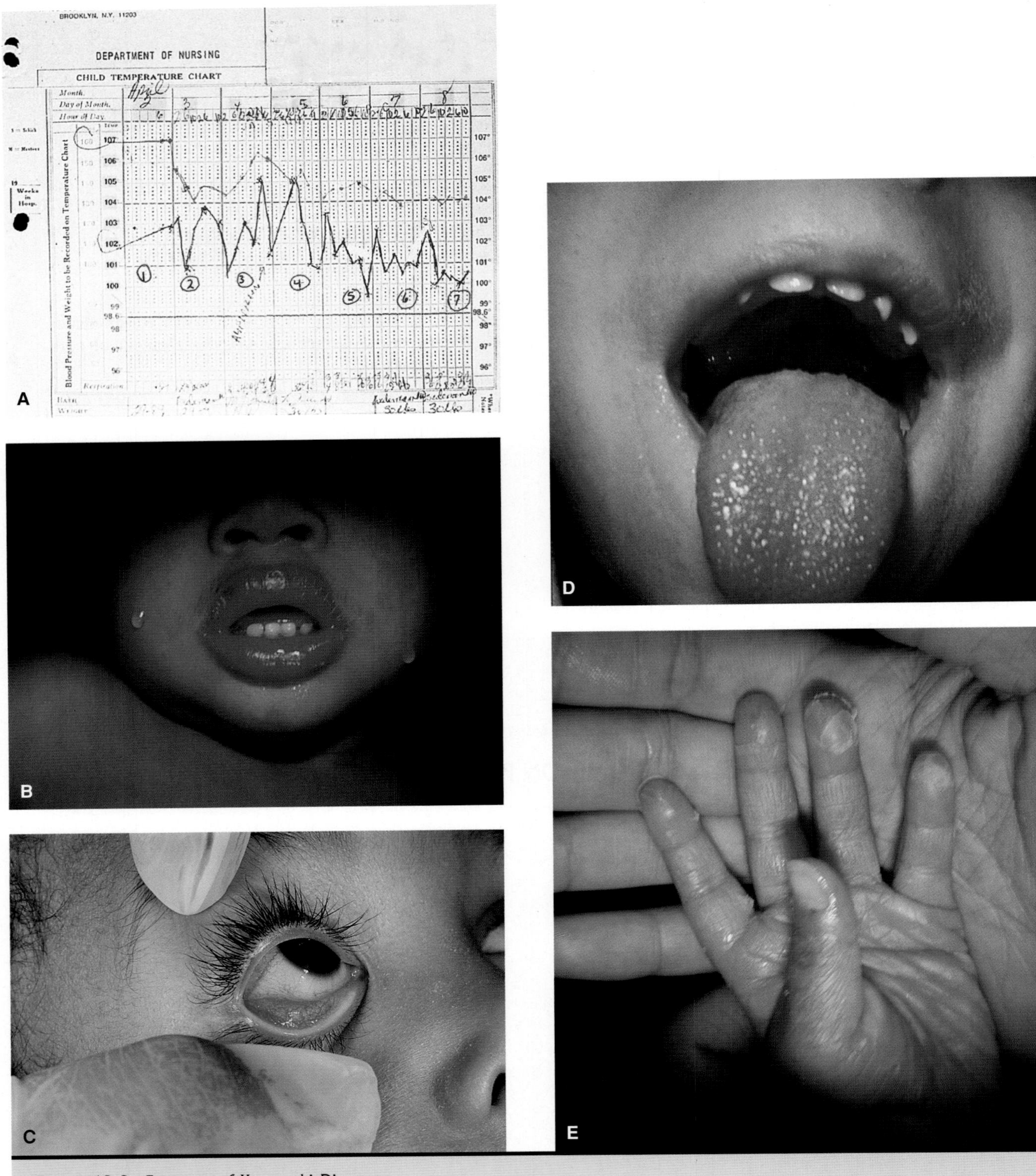

Figure 12-3. Features of Kawasaki Disease

A. Temperature curve in a typical untreated case of KD. With the administration of IVIG on the seventh day of hospitalization (when the diagnosis of KD was entertained), temperature returned to normal. *B*. Red lips with fissuring, giving the appearance of red lipstick. *C*. Nonexudative conjunctivitis. *D*. Red strawberry tongue. *E*. Erythema of the palm with desquamation of the fingers, seen on the eighth day of illness (the patient's hand is against the mother's hand). *F*. Erythema of the soles. *G*. Perineal desquamation seen in this 18-month-old infant with KD on the fourth day of illness. *H*. Cervical adenopathy. *I*. Desquamation of the fingers on the 12th day of illness.

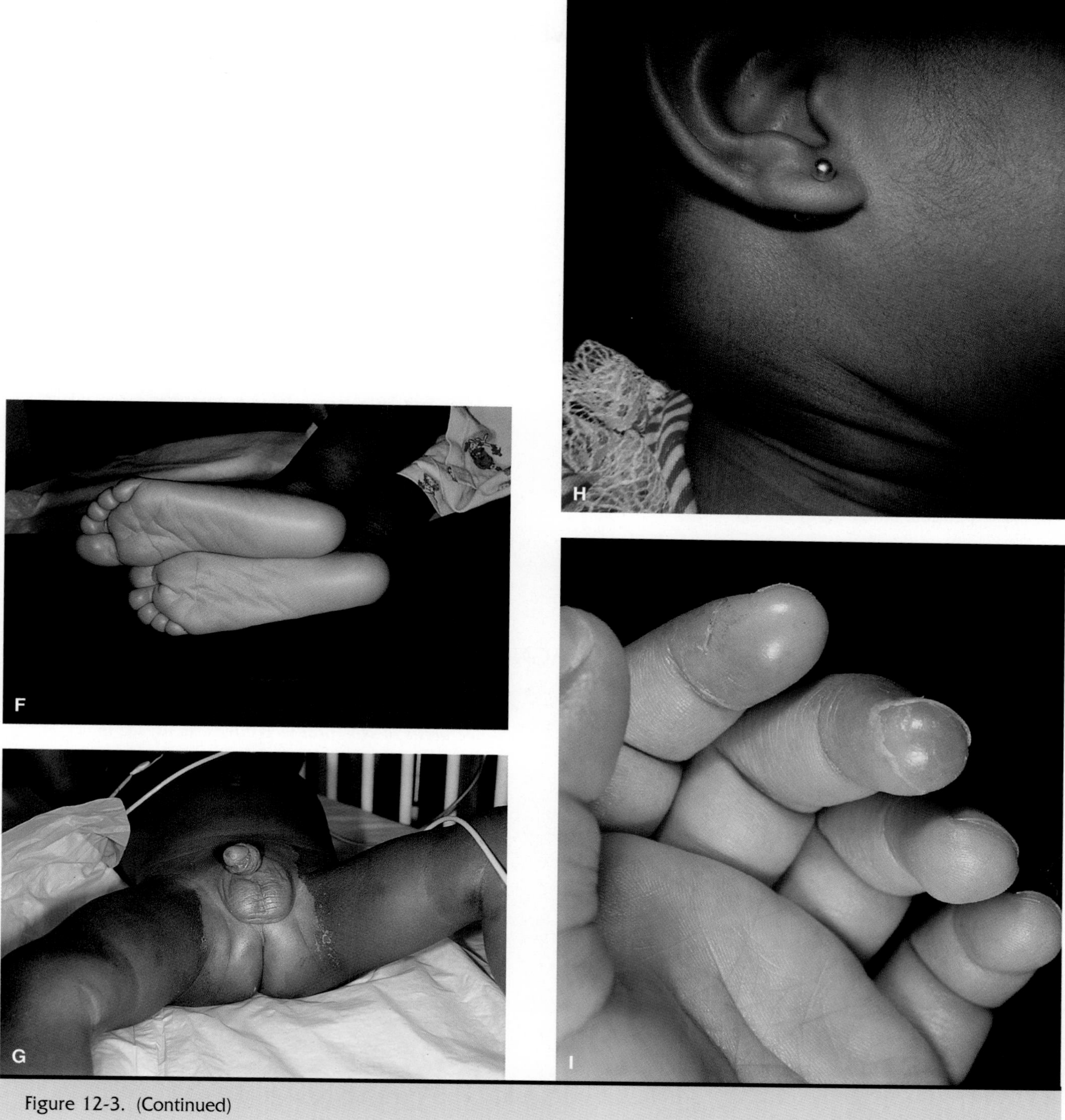

Figure 12-3. (Continued)

6. Measles can be differentiated from KD by the presence of exudative conjunctivitis, Koplik's spots, and severe cough. Measles rash starts on the face behind the ears, becomes confluent, and fades with a brownish hue (Fig. 3-53). Leukopenia and low ESR are other findings in measles. KD rash is most prominent on the trunk and extremities and fades abruptly without residua. *Perineal desquamation is also typical of KD and not of measles.*

BOX 12-3. CARDIAC INVOLVEMENT IN KAWASAKI DISEASE

- Myocarditis (tachycardia, decreased ventricular function, arrhythmias, CHF) seen during acute illness in about 50% of patients
- Pericarditis (pericardial effusion) seen during acute illness in about 30% of cases
- Coronary aneurysm (during second and third weeks of illness; seen in 20 to 25% of untreated patients)
- Giant coronary aneurysms (diameter >8 mm) with risk of rupture, thrombosis, or stenosis
- Myocardial infarction (coronary thrombosis or stenosis; principal cause of death)
- Patients at higher risk for coronary aneurysm:
  (1) Male gender
  (2) Infants <12 months of age
  (3) Prolonged fever (>14 days)
  (4) Presence of cardiac involvement (e.g., pericardial effusion, mitral regurgitation)
  (5) Thrombocytosis (platelet count >1 million)
  (6) WBC count >30,000/mm^3, higher absolute band count
  (7) ESR >101 mm/h (Westergren method)
  (8) Persistent elevation of ESR or CRP >4 weeks
  (9) Elevated LDH
  (10) Decreased albumin
  (11) Hgb <10 g/dL
  (12) Palpable axillary arterial aneurysms
  (13) Recurrence of fever after an afebrile period of at least 24 hours

Clinical pearl

- Prevalence of coronary artery abnormalities is highly dependent on gamma globulin dose, but independent of salicylate dose (IVIG 2 g/kg combined with at least 30 to 50 mg/kg per day of aspirin provides maximum protection against development of coronary abnormalities [meta-analysis from U.S. and Japanese multicenter studies])

BOX 12-4. DIFFERENTIAL DIAGNOSIS OF KAWASAKI DISEASE

- Scarlet fever (*lack of conjunctivitis, response to antibiotics in 24 to 48 hours;* see Fig. 3-3)
- Measles (see Clinical Pearls: Kawasaki Disease)
- Viral infections (e.g., EBV, enterovirus, adenovirus; see Clinical Pearls: Kawasaki Disease)
- Staphylococcal or streptococcal toxic shock syndrome (*hypotension [very rare in KD unless patient is in cardiogenic shock], renal involvement, elevations of CPK, focus of infection*; see Figs. 3-19 to 3-22)
- Stevens-Johnson syndrome (*Nikolsky's sign positive, necrolysis of skin, oral ulcerative lesions*; see Fig. 7-7)
- Hypersensitivity drug reactions
- Systemic juvenile rheumatoid arthritis
- Staphylococcal scalded skin syndrome (see Fig. 3-23 and 3-24)
- Rocky Mountain spotted fever (see Fig. 3-34)
- Mercury poisoning
- Leptospirosis

DIAGNOSIS INCOMPLETE KAWASAKI DISEASE

SYNONYMS

Kawasaki syndrome
Mucocutaneous lymph node syndrome

Definition

1. Kawasaki disease (KD) is an acute febrile illness of unknown etiology characterized by an acute generalized vasculitis. Diagnosis of KD is based on clinical criteria summarized by the American Heart Association (Box 12-1).
2. Incomplete KD refers to KD with incomplete clinical manifestations. Even though patients with incomplete KD do not have all the classic signs that are required to make a clinical diagnosis of KD, they do not present with any atypical signs normally not seen in patients with classic KD. Thus, incomplete KD is the preferred term over atypical KD.

Associated Clinical Features

1. Incomplete KD is seen more commonly in young infants than in older children.
2. Laboratory findings are similar in both classic and incomplete KD (see Box 12-1 for classic features of KD). Leukocytosis or a normal WBC count with a left shift, elevated acute phase reactants (ESR and C-reactive protein), and sterile pyuria are common findings. Thrombocytosis is typically seen during the second week of illness. Additional findings may include CSF pleocytosis, elevations of serum transaminases, anemia, and hypoalbuminemia. Thrombocytosis and elevated ESR also persist for weeks in incomplete KD (Figs. 12-4, 12-5 and 12-6).
3. Even though laboratory findings in KD (both classic and incomplete) are nondiagnostic, they are characteristic and

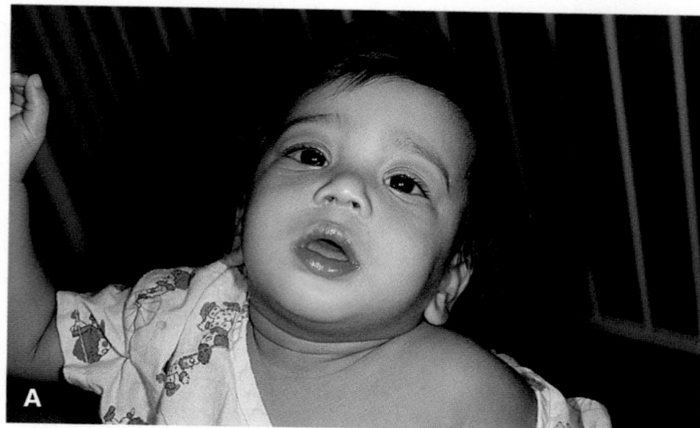

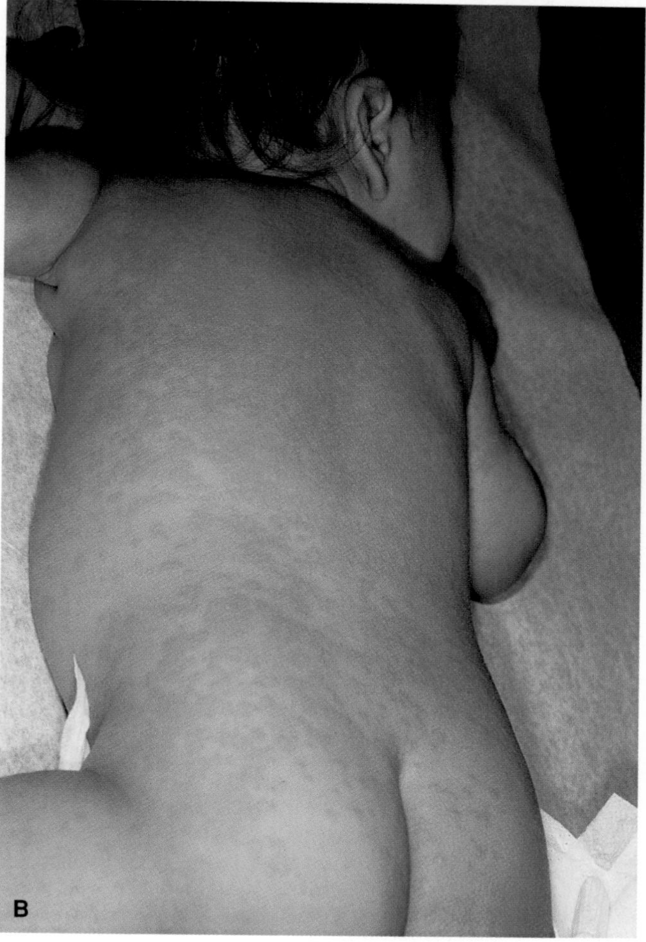

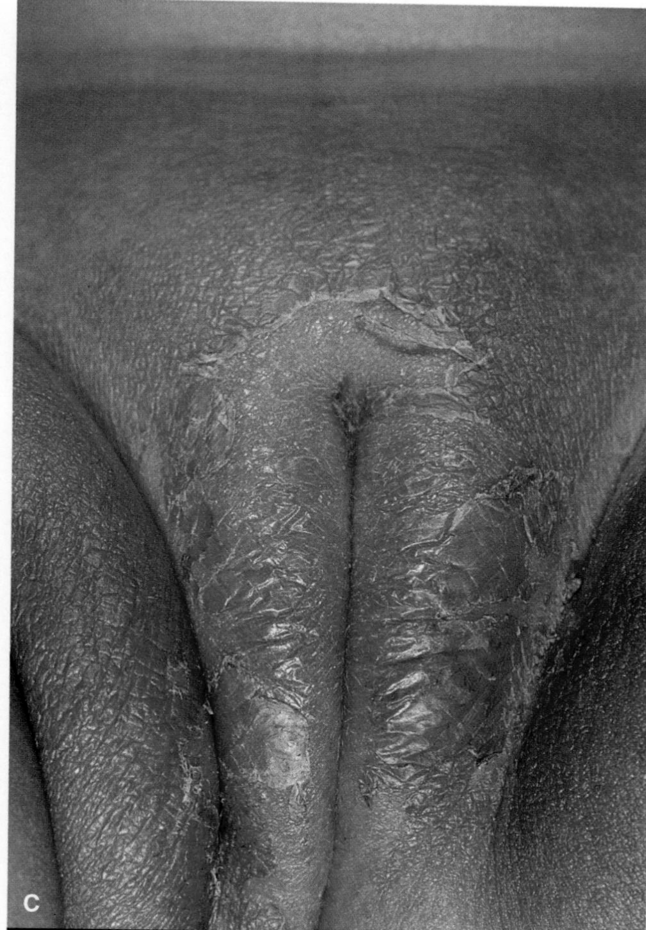

Figure 12-4. Incomplete Kawasaki Disease

Red lips (*A*), erythematous maculopapular rash (*B*), and perineal desquamation (*C*), present since the third day of illness in a 7-month-old infant who presented with persistent fever (9 days' duration) that did not respond to either antibiotic therapy (given for a clinical diagnosis of otitis media) or antipyretic therapy. This infant did not have any eye or extremity changes or cervical adenopathy (findings that are typically seen in a patient with classic KD). Her echocardiogram showed coronary dilation.

may help in including or excluding incomplete KD. The presence of leukopenia and a normal ESR in an infant or child with fever, rash, and red eyes does not suggest a laboratory profile compatible with KD (and usually suggests a viral infection, such as adenovirus).

Etiology, Consultation, Differential Diagnosis, Emergency Department Treatment and Disposition

See Kawasaki disease, page 492

Clinical Pearls: Incomplete Kawasaki Disease

1. The presentation of KD is often incomplete in young infants with *fever and fewer than four of the other features*; thus recognition of such cases is difficult. Infants are at greatest risk for developing coronary artery aneurysms. The

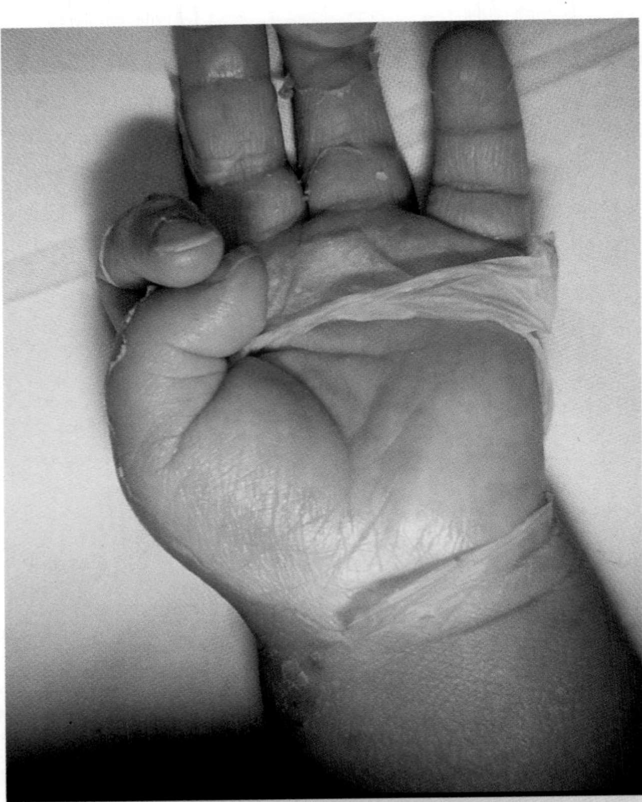

Figure 12-5. Incomplete Kawasaki Disease

Desquamation of the hand seen in a highly febrile 4-month-old infant. This infant was not suspected of having KD until this desquamation was seen on the 11th day of the illness. He remained extremely irritable and highly febrile and did not respond to IV antibiotic therapy that was given for a clinical diagnosis of sepsis (all cultures were negative). Prolonged fever followed by peripheral desquamation are among the most common signs of incomplete KD. His echocardiogram showed the presence of coronary artery dilation.

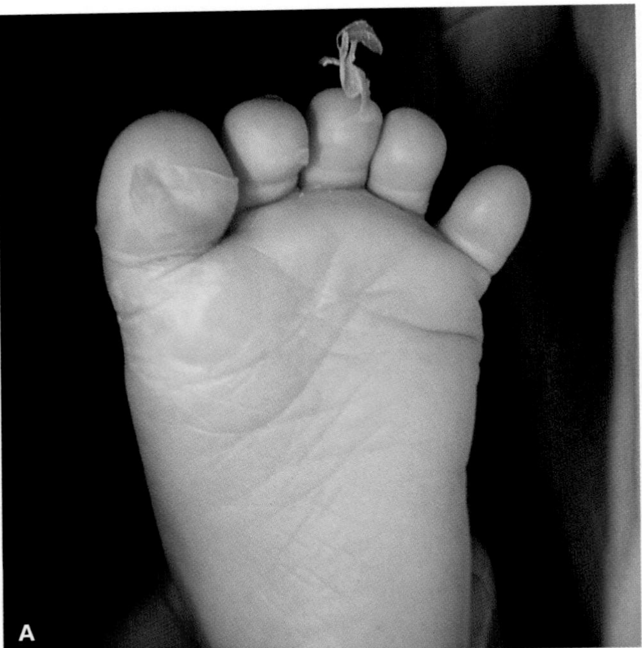

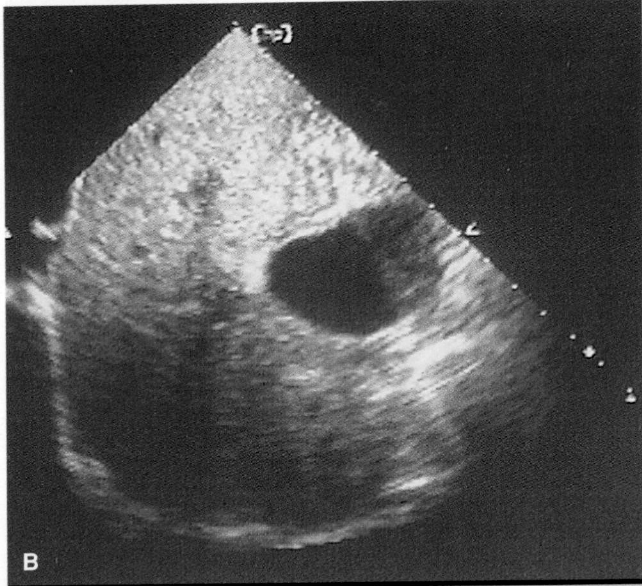

Figure 12-6. Incomplete Kawasaki Disease

An 11-month-old male infant presented with persistent fever of 7 days' duration, erythematous maculopapular rash, red lips, perineal desquamation, and hypotension. He was admitted with a clinical diagnosis of toxic shock syndrome. All of the cultures including blood, CSF, and urine were negative except for scant growth of group A beta-hemolytic streptococci from the throat. He developed peripheral desquamation on the 11th day of illness (*A*). His initial echocardiogram was negative except for hydrops of the gallbladder that was found incidentally (*B*). He did not respond to IV antibiotic therapy and remained persistently febrile for 20 days, and a diagnosis of KD was entertained. He received IV immune globulin, after which he became afebrile. He had persistent leukocytosis (with a WBC count up to 31,000), markedly elevated ESR, and marked thrombocytosis. His repeat echocardiogram on the 21st day of illness showed giant coronary artery aneurysm. This infant had several risk factors for the development of coronary artery abnormalities (see Box 12-3).

diagnosis of incomplete KD is often based on finding a coronary artery aneurysm on echocardiography.

2. Like classic KD, fever is a characteristic finding in incomplete KD. Occasionally prolonged fever is *the sole manifestation* of KD in infants.

3. Incomplete KD should be considered in any infant who has prolonged and unexplained fever lasting for >5 days even in the absence of other clinical criteria; maintain a high index of suspicion for the possible diagnosis.

BOX 12-5. CLINICAL AND LABORATORY FINDINGS THAT SHOULD PROMPT CONSIDERATION OF INCOMPLETE (ATYPICAL) KAWASAKI DISEASE

(For typical features of Kawasaki disease see Box 12-1).

Clinical findings:

- Daily high spiking fevers, especially >5 days, and particularly in infants, without evidence of bacterial infection

with or without

1. One or more other diagnostic criteria for KD, especially conjunctival injection, oral mucosal changes, and/or rash
2. Anterior uveitis on slitlamp examination

and

Laboratory findings:

- Markedly elevated ESR and/or C-reactive protein
- Elevated peripheral WBC or normal WBC with neutrophil predominance and immature forms on differential
- Thrombocytosis after the 7th day of fever

with or without

- Sterile pyuria
- Elevated alanine aminotransferase
- Aseptic meningitis
- Anemia
- Hypoalbuminemia
- Echocardiogram showing pericardial effusion

(Reproduced with permission from: Rowley AH: Incomplete (atypical) Kawasaki disease. *Pediatr Infect Dis J* 2002;21:21(6):page 563).

DIAGNOSIS SYSTEMIC LUPUS ERYTHEMATOSUS

Synonym

Lupus

Definition

Systemic lupus erythematosus (SLE) is a multisystem autoimmune disease of unknown etiology, characterized by production of autoantibodies and protean clinical manifestations. In Latin, "lupus" means wolf, and here it refers to the rash that extends across the bridge of the nose and upper cheekbones and was thought to resemble a wolf's bite (Fig. 12-7). Erythematosus is from the Greek word meaning "red" and refers to the color of the rash.

Etiology

1. SLE is an autoimmune disorder. Predisposing factors for lupus are many, including genetic (e.g., more common and more severe in African Americans, Latinos, and Asian Americans than in European Americans), environmental (e.g., ultraviolet light), and hormonal (e.g., female predominance and onset of SLE usually after puberty). Exposure to exogenous estrogens (e.g., oral contraceptive pills or hormone replacement therapy) increases the risk of developing lupus.
2. Certain drugs can lead to drug-induced SLE (e.g., isoniazid, hydralazine, and procainamide), and SLE remits when the drug is stopped. Sulfonamide antibiotics are a well known precipitant of idiopathic SLE.

Associated Clinical Features

1. About 15 to 25% of cases of SLE occur in patients <20 years old. SLE is less common in children <10 years old and rare in children <5 years old. Peak incidence in childhood is at age 11 to 13 years.

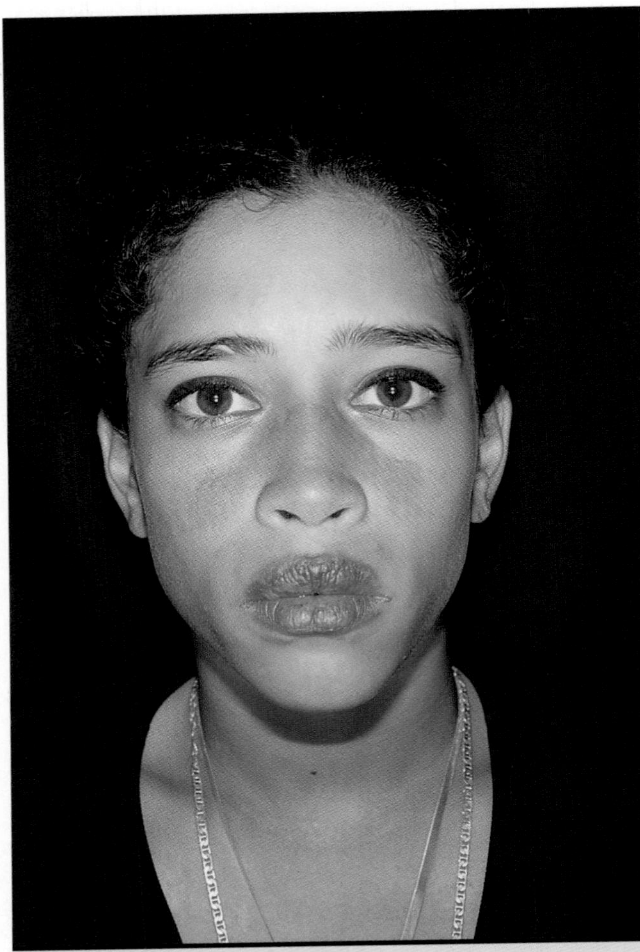

Figure 12-7. Butterfly Rash of Systemic Lupus Erythematosus

The butterfly rash is an erythematous macular blush or erythematous papules with fine scaling. It is usually quite well demarcated, and may be slightly raised and pruritic or painful. It is characteristically symmetrical, over both malar eminences, over the bridge of the nose, and sometimes on the forehead and ears. It spares the nasolabial folds. Malar rash is seen in one-third of SLE patients at onset of disease. This rash is highly suggestive of SLE but not pathognomonic. The rash is photosensitive and may be precipitated by exposure to sunlight. It usually does not leave scaring.

2. SLE is a predominantly a disease of women. The female: male ratio is 3:1 in children under 10 years of age, and 9:1 in those over 10 years.
3. Pericarditis is the most common cardiac manifestation of SLE (affects ~20 to 30% of patients).
4. Laboratory tests should include complete blood cell count with differential, platelet count, ESR (often elevated but not correlated with disease activity), urinalysis, a comprehensive metabolic panel (elevated creatinine with renal involvement and elevated liver function tests are seen in about 30% of patients). Serum complements C3 and C4 (commonly reduced, especially with renal lupus) and Coombs' test (if anemia is detected) are also useful.
5. The ECG may show evidence of pericarditis and a chest radiograph may show the presence of cardiomegaly (pericardial effusion) or pleural effusion.
6. Immunologic tests include:
   a. A majority of patients with SLE have a positive ANA test (often with a high titer >640). However, the specificity of this test is low, as about 20% of normal women can have a positive ANA.
   b. Antibodies that are specific for lupus include antibodies to double-stranded DNA (anti-dsDNA) and antibodies to Sm nuclear antigen (anti-Sm).
   c. Anti-Ro (SS-A), anti-La (SS-B), and anti-RNP are commonly seen in SLE (about 60% of patients), but are also found in other autoimmune diseases.
   d. Antiphospholipid antibodies (e.g., anticardiolipin antibodies, lupus anticoagulant) are seen in about 50% of SLE patients, and are associated with hypercoagulability.
7. The morbidity of SLE is related to nephritis, antiphospholipid antibody syndrome, infections, and complications related to corticosteroid therapy.

Consultations

Rheumatology and as indicated nephrology and hematology

Emergency Department Treatment and Disposition

1. Hospitalize all patients presenting with severe disease (e.g., nephritis, pericarditis, CNS-lupus) or patients presenting with complications of therapy (e.g., infection in a patient with neutropenia from cyclophosphamide therapy).
2. Treatment of SLE depends on organ system involvement and disease severity. Refer the patient to a pediatric rheumatologist for long-term management. Patients are treated to support clinical well being, using serologic markers of disease activity as guidelines.
3. Cutaneous lupus is treated by avoiding sun and using sunscreens that block both UV-A and UV-B. Treatment options include antimalarials (e.g., hydroxychloroquine), topical corticosteroids, and intradermal corticosteroids (discoid lesions).
4. Systemic therapeutic options to treat other manifestations include nonsteroidal anti-inflammatory drugs for musculoskeletal manifestations, serositis, and constitutional signs (e.g., fever), antimalarial drugs (e.g., hydroxychloroquine) and immunosuppressive agents (e.g., cyclophosphamide or azathioprine), and systemic corticosteroids.

Clinical Pearls: Systemic Lupus Erythematosus

1. SLE is an episodic disease. A history of intermittent symptoms such as arthritis, dermatitis, or nephritis may precede the diagnosis.

2. The most common clinical presentations of SLE are cutaneous, renal, and joint. SLE must be considered in the differential diagnosis of many signs and symptoms ranging from fevers of unknown origin to arthralgia, anemia, and nephritis.
3. CNS involvement occurs in 20 to 35% patients with SLE, and psychosis and seizures are the most common manifestations.
4. Lupus cerebritis must be considered in any patient with SLE and a change in behavior or mental status.

BOX 12-6. CLINICAL FEATURES OF SYSTEMIC LUPUS ERYTHEMATOSUS

The American College of Rheumatology classification of SLE requires *presence of four of the following eleven criteria* (a person is said to have SLE if any four or more of the eleven criteria are present, *serially or simultaneously,* during an interval of observation).

1. Photosensitivity (skin rash as a result of an unusual reaction to sunlight)
2. Malar rash (affects ~60% of patients; butterfly distribution on the face, spares the nasolabial folds; macular erythematous blush or erythematous papules)
3. Oral or nasopharyngeal ulcers (affects ~85% of patients; painless, often noted incidentally)
4. Discoid lupus (uncommon in children; deeper lesions showing atrophy, adherent scales, hyper- and hypopigmentation, erythema, scarring; most common on the face and scalp)
5. Arthritis (affects ~15% of patients; nonerosive arthritis involving the small joints of the hands or the large joints, characterized by tenderness, swelling, or effusion; Fig. 12-8)
6. Serositis (pleurisy, pericarditis, ascites)
7. Renal lupus (affects ~50 to 90% of children; diagnosed by persistent proteinuria >0.5 g/day or 3+ if quantitation not performed, RBCs and cellular casts in urine)
8. CNS lupus (e.g., psychosis, seizures, encephalopathy, myelitis, coma, stroke, peripheral neuropathy, migraines)
9. Hematologic lupus (anemia [hemolytic with positive direct Coombs' test or anemia of chronic disease], leukopenia, lymphopenia, thrombocytopenia)
10. Positive antinuclear antibody
11. Immunologic tests (anti-dsDNA, anti-Sm, antiphospholipid antibodies)

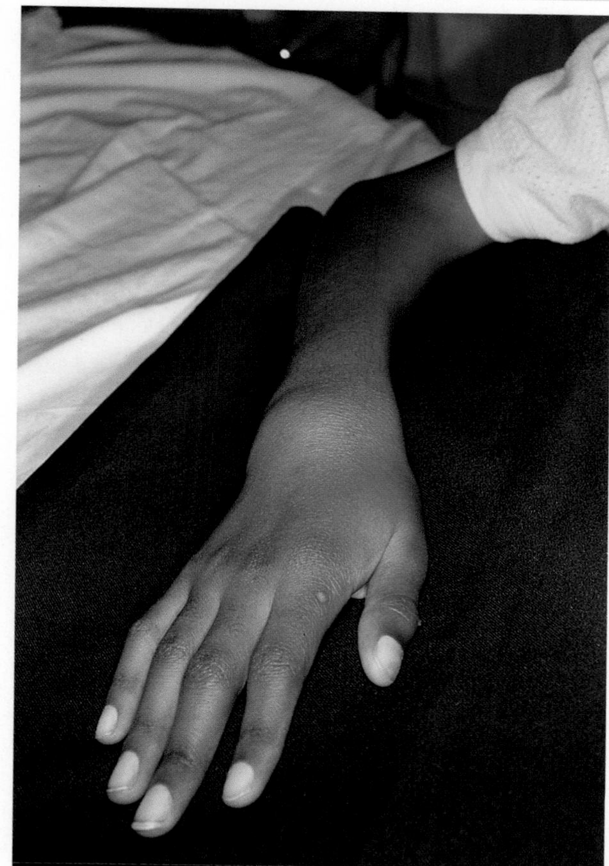

Figure 12-8. Arthritis of Systemic Lupus Erythematosus

Arthralgias and arthritis are frequent presenting manifestations of SLE. Arthritis is polyarticular and frequently affects proximal interphalangeal joints of the hands. Pain is intense and out of proportion to physical findings and may be migratory (thus mimicking postinfectious or reactive arthritis).

BOX 12-7. OTHER CLINICAL FEATURES OF SYSTEMIC LUPUS ERYTHEMATOSUS

- Alopecia (usually diffuse thinning)
- Raynaud's phenomenon (affects ~20% or more of SLE patients and may precede other signs and symptoms of SLE by months or years)
- Periungual telangiectasias
- Livedo reticularis (nonpalpable reticular rash)
- Vasculitis with palpable purpura (Fig. 12-9)
- Urticaria, angioedema
- Petechiae (Fig. 12-9)
- Embolic episodes
- Deep vein thrombosis
- Cerebrovascular accidents
- Digital ulceration
- Vesicobullous SLE (lesions consist of vesicles and bullae [may be hemorrhagic], common sites have a photosensitive distribution [e.g., face, neck, backs of hands])
- Nonspecific symptoms such as fever (~90% of patients), myalgia, arthritis/arthralgia, poor weight gain, depression
- Hepatosplenomegaly (~50 to 75% of patients)
- Lymphadenopathy (~50% of patients)
- Positive lupus erythematosus–cell preparation
- False-positive Venereal Disease Research Laboratory (VDRL) test
- Circulating autoantibodies (e.g., Anti-Ro, anti-La and anti-RNP antibodies)

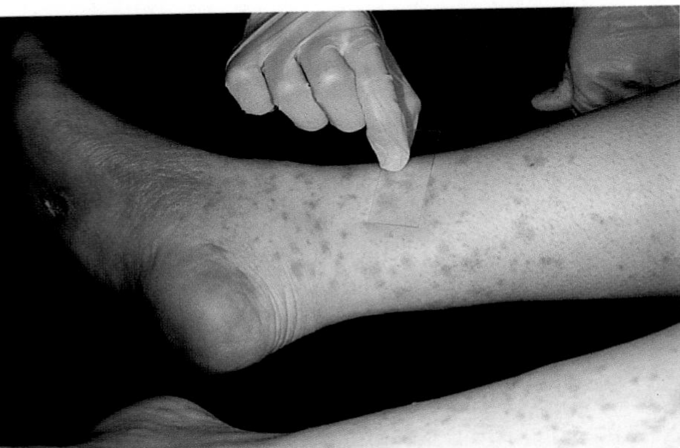

Figure 12-9. Vasculitis with Petechiae and Purpura of Systemic Lupus Erythematosus

BOX 12-8. DIFFERENTIAL DIAGNOSIS OF SYSTEMIC LUPUS ERYTHEMATOSUS

- Polymorphous light eruption
- Phototoxic and photoallergic drug eruptions
- Contact or allergic dermatoses
- Erysipelas (Fig. 12-10)
- Dermatomyositis
- Other collagen vascular diseases (e.g., Sjögren's syndrome, juvenile rheumatoid arthritis)
- Nephritis from another etiology (e.g., acute poststreptococcal glomerulonephritis)
- Malignancy (e.g., leukemia)
- Infections (e.g., infectious mononucleosis, acute rheumatic fever)
- Thrombocytopenia from other etiology (e.g., idiopathic thrombocytopenic purpura)
- Anemia from another etiology (e.g., idiopathic hemolytic anemia)

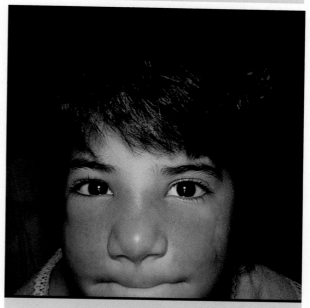

Figure 12-10. Butterfly Rash of Erysipelas

A rapidly spreading (<12 hours' duration), tender, fiery red, indurated rash on the face was seen in this 8-year-old girl. She had a temperature of 40°C with leukocytosis. The sharp demarcation between the salmon-red erythema and the normal surrounding skin is evident. Erysipelas may create a butterfly-like pattern on the face with involvement of both cheeks and the bridge of nose. An erysipelas rash spreads very rapidly like fire (hence the name "St. Anthony's fire") and is caused by group A beta-hemolytic streptococci.

DIAGNOSIS NEONATAL LUPUS ERYTHEMATOSUS

Definition

Neonatal lupus erythematosus (NLE) is an immune-mediated disease characterized by cutaneous lesions or congenital heart block or both in a neonate born to a mother who may have either overt or latent systemic lupus erythematosus (SLE) or other connective tissue disease.

Etiology

1. NLE is caused by the passively acquired transplacental passage of maternal Sjögren's syndrome A antibodies (also called anti-Ro/SS-A) and/or Sjögren's syndrome B antibodies (also called anti-La/SSB) or uridine-rich ribonucleoprotein antibody (anti-U1 RNP).
2. Predominant autoantibodies found in about 95% of cases of NLE are anti-Ro/SSA. These antibodies bind with an autoantigen in the heart, leading to an inflammatory process and resulting in fibrotic replacement and destruction of the sinoatrial bundle, the atrioventricular bundle, or the bundle of His. Transplacentally transmitted maternal antibodies may also cause immunomyocarditis and severe prenatal or postnatal dilated cardiomyopathy.
3. About 50% of mothers with babies with NLE have clinical features of either Sjögren's syndrome or SLE, while 50% of women are asymptomatic. However, more than 85% of mothers who have given birth to babies with NLE will demonstrate onset of sicca symptoms (e.g., dry eyes, dry mouth) and/or arthralgias or arthritis with time. Conversely,

most babies born to mothers with anti-Ro/SSA or anti-La/SSB or anti-U1 RNP do not develop NLE. It is also not possible to predict which neonates will be affected. Only about 1 to 2% of women with anti-Ro/SSA antibodies will have babies born with NLE. A prior history of giving birth to a baby with NLE or a diagnosis of SLE in the mother are risk factors that increase this percentage (the risk of a similarly affected infant in subsequent pregnancies is about 25%).

Associated Clinical Features

1. Congenital complete heart block (CHB) may lead to congestive heart failure (CHF).
2. Neonatal carditis and late-onset dilated cardiomyopathy (DCM) may also develop in these infants (cardiac muscle affected by an inflammatory process due to a prolonged exposure to anti-Ro/SSa antibodies).
3. Laboratory evaluation of the neonate includes complete blood count with differential and platelet count. Additional tests include anti-Ro/SS-A (seen in about 95% of cases of NLE), anti-La/SS-B (seen in 70% of NLE), and anti-U1 RNP (seen in 5% of NLE). These autoantibodies disappear with the rash. Antinuclear antibody may be also positive.
4. Chest radiograph, electrocardiogram, and echocardiogram are indicated to exclude DCM and associated heart defects (a higher incidence of atrial septal defect and patent ductus arteriosus is seen in these infants).
5. Scarring may result from the discoid lupus erythematosus (DLE)-like skin lesions.
6. Patients who had NLE may develop other autoimmune or connective tissue diseases (e.g., Hashimoto's thyroiditis, systemic-onset juvenile rheumatoid arthritis) later in life.
7. Despite early pacing, CHB carries a high mortality rate during the first 12 months of life.

Consultation

Cardiology (cardiac evaluation and pacemaker) and dermatology (if unclear diagnosis)

Emergency Department Treatment and Disposition

1. Hospitalize all symptomatic infants (e.g., those with CHB or with signs of CHF or significant thrombocytopenia).
2. Early pacing is indicated for most infants with CHB. Primary indications for placement of a pacemaker are CHF and a low ventricular rate averaging <60 bpm.
3. Cardiology consultation and follow-up must be obtained for all patients who are asymptomatic (possible development of DCM).
4. Refer the patient to a dermatologist for skin biopsy if the diagnosis is unclear.
5. For cutaneous lesions, sunscreen, protective clothing, and mild topical corticosteroids may be used. Systemic treatment is not indicated.
6. Refer the mother to a rheumatologist, as work-up is needed for SLE or other connective tissue disease.

Clinical Pearls: Neonatal Lupus Erythematosus

1. NLE is associated with cutaneous lesions and/or CHB (Fig. 12-11). Hepatic disease and thrombocytopenia may be present.
2. Periorbital "owl-eye" appearance of the facial rash is an important clue to the diagnosis of NLE (Fig. 12-12).
3. NLE is caused by transplacental autoantibodies transmitted from the mother to the fetus. IgG antibodies to Ro and/or La cross the placenta and induce the development of the clinical manifestations of NLE. The presence of anti-Ro/SSA antibodies in the infant and mother confirms the diagnosis of NLE.
4. Mothers of babies with NLE are likely to develop collagen vascular diseases with time. Infants with NLE are at risk of developing other autoimmune diseases during childhood or adolescence.
5. The heart block seen in NLE is permanent and irreversible; the skin lesions are benign and self-resolve, usually over a period of a few weeks to months.

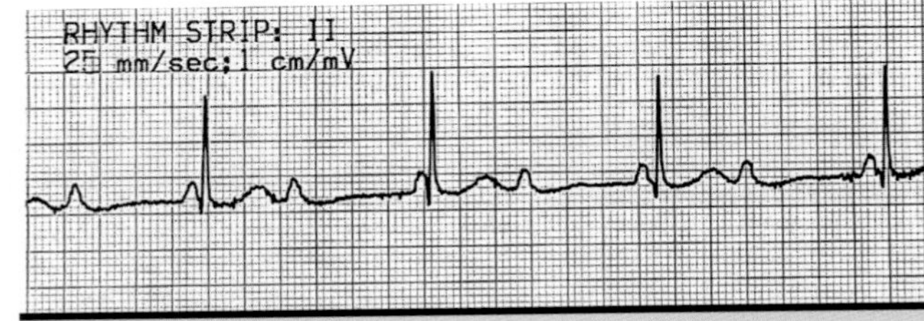

Figure 12-11. Congenital Complete Heart Block in Neonatal Lupus

In patients with CHB, a heart rate <55 bpm is associated with a greater likelihood of poor outcome. Early infancy is the time of greatest risk of death for those with CHB.

BOX 12-13. DIFFERENTIAL DIAGNOSIS OF RAYNAUD'S PHENOMENON

- Acrocyanosis
  (1) Represents exaggerated vasomotor response
  (2) Frequently seen in neonates
  (3) May occur at any age
  (4) Usually painless, persistent cyanosis of distal extremities
  (5) Typically poorly defined borders
  (6) Typically waxes and wanes with cold and emotional stress
  (7) Benign prognosis
- Chilblains
  (1) Represents spasm-induced vessel and tissue damage
  (2) Episodic color changes after exposure to cold
  (3) Typically patients present with nodules
- Frostbite (see Figs. 18-7 to 18-9)

DIAGNOSIS

LYME DISEASE

Synonyms

Borreliosis or Lyme borreliosis
Neuroborreliosis (Lyme disease with neurological manifestations)
Erythema chronicum migrans (for erythema migrans [EM])

Definition and Etiology

Lyme disease is a vector-borne disease caused by the spirochete *Borrelia burgdorferi* (Fig. 12-14). It is transmitted by a deer tick, *Ixodes scapularis* (also known previously as *Ixodes dammini*). It was first reported in Lyme, Connecticut in a group of children presenting with unexplained arthritis, hence the name Lyme disease.

Associated Clinical Features

1. Lyme disease occurs throughout the world. In Europe, it is seen mostly in Scandinavian countries, Germany, Austria, and Switzerland. In the United States it is most commonly seen in southern New England, New Jersey, southeastern New York, eastern Pennsylvania, as well as in Maryland, Delaware, Minnesota, and Wisconsin.
2. A diagnosis of Lyme disease is made clinically. Centers for Disease Control criteria include:
   a. Physician-diagnosed EM (>5 cm; Fig. 12-15)
   b. One or more clinical manifestations of early disseminated or of late Lyme disease plus positive serology
3. Routine laboratory tests are rarely useful in making the diagnosis of Lyme disease.
   a. CBC may show normal or elevated white blood cell count.
   b. ESR is usually elevated.
   c. In patients presenting with meningitis, CSF examination shows mild pleocytosis with predominance of lymphocytes (consistent with aseptic meningitis).
   d. In patients presenting with arthritis, joint fluid aspiration may show cells ranging from 25,000 to 125,000/mL, often with polymorphonuclear preponderance.
4. Tests for antibodies for Lyme disease:
   a. Use a two-step procedure when ordering antibody tests.
      1) Screening test: Either immunofluorescent antibody (IFA) or enzyme-linked immunosorbent assay (ELISA)
      2) Confirmation test (if screening test is positive or equivocal): Western immunoblot
      3) Immunoblot *not* necessary if screening test was negative.
   b. ELISA provides a quantitative measure of antibodies against *B. burgdorferi.*
   c. Immunoblot provides information about the specificity of the antibodies (antibodies against specific protein antigen of spirochete).
   d. Antibody tests are usually negative in the majority of patients with early localized Lyme disease.
   e. Antibodies to *B. burgdorferi* persist for many years despite adequate treatment and clinical cure.
5. Skin biopsy may demonstrate spirochetes in up to 40% of specimens.

Consultation

Rheumatology and as indicated, cardiology, neurology, or dermatology

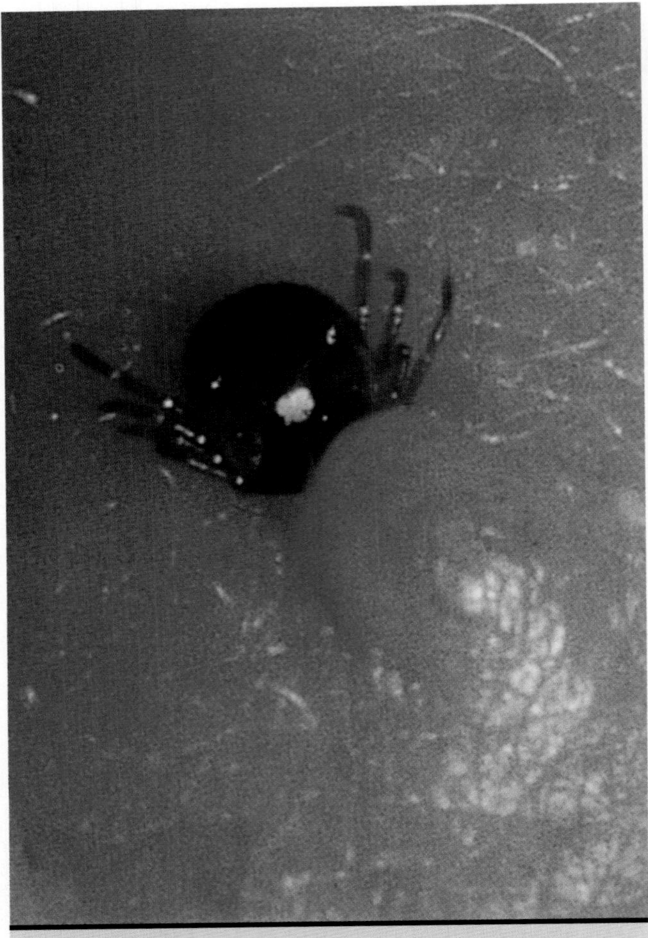

Figure 12-14. Lyme Borreliosis

A blood-distended *Ixodes scapularis* nymph (also known as the black-legged or deer tick) feeding on human skin. *Borrelia* transmission usually occurs after prolonged attachment and feeding (>48 hours). These tics are found in wooded areas, high grasses, gardens, marshes, and beach areas. (Reproduced with permission from: Kane KS, Ryder JB, Johnson RA, Baden HP, Stratigos A: Lyme borreliosis. In: *Color Atlas & Synopsis of Pediatric Dermatology*. McGraw-Hill, New York, 2002, p. 497.)

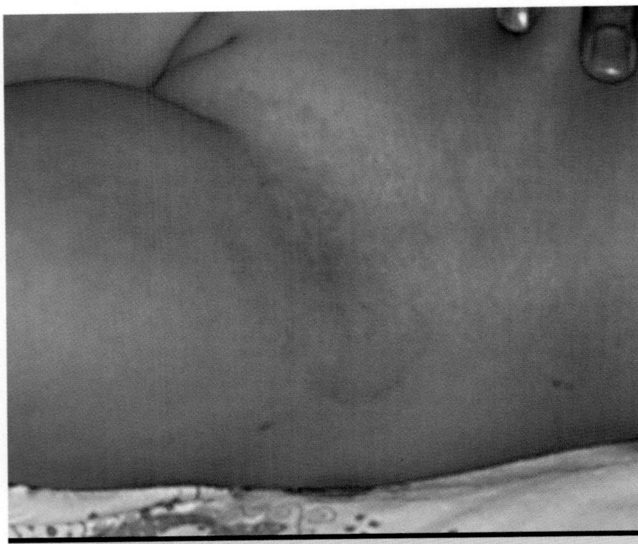

Figure 12-15. Erythema Migrans in Lyme Disease

Solitary target-shaped erythematous lesion with central clearing. If untreated, the erythema migrans lesion gradually expands and may reach a large size, sometimes >12 inches in diameter.

Emergency Department Treatment and Disposition

1. Hospitalize patients presenting with meningitis, encephalitis, carditis, or arthritis. Other patients can be followed closely by the PCP as an outpatient.
2. Patients with early localized (EM) or early disseminated disease, or those with first- or second-degree AV heart block:
   a. Amoxicillin 50 mg/kg per day divided tid (for patients <9 years of age; maximum dose 2 g/d) *or*
   b. Doxycycline 100 mg bid
   c. Total duration: 14 to 21 days
   d. For patients allergic to penicillin: erythromycin, azithromycin, or clarithromycin
3. Facial nerve palsy (Fig. 12-16):
   a. *Do not use corticosteroids.*
   b. Treat with antibiotics as above for 21 to 30 days. Although antibiotic therapy does not hasten the resolution of seventh nerve palsy; they are given to prevent further sequelae.
4. Treatment of carditis, third-degree AV heart block, meningitis, radiculopathy, or late neurologic disease:
   a. Ceftriaxone 75 to 100 mg/kg per day in a single dose (maximum 2 g) given IV or IM *or*
   b. Penicillin G 200,000 to 400,000 units/kg per day divided every 4 hours (maximum 20 million units/d) given IV
   c. Total duration: 14 to 21 days
5. Treatment of arthritis:
   a. Treatment same as EM for 30 days
   b. If recurrence or symptoms fail to resolve after 2 months: same treatment as late neurologic disease as mentioned above
6. Patients with Wenckebach or complete heart block may require a temporary pacemaker.
7. Removal of the tick:
   a. Ticks should be removed promptly, before transmission of *B. burgdorferi* occurs (transmission requires attachment for >48 hours).
   b. *Do not squeeze* the body of the tick during removal.
   c. Grasp the tick preferably with a pair of fine tweezers as close to the skin as possible and remove the tick by

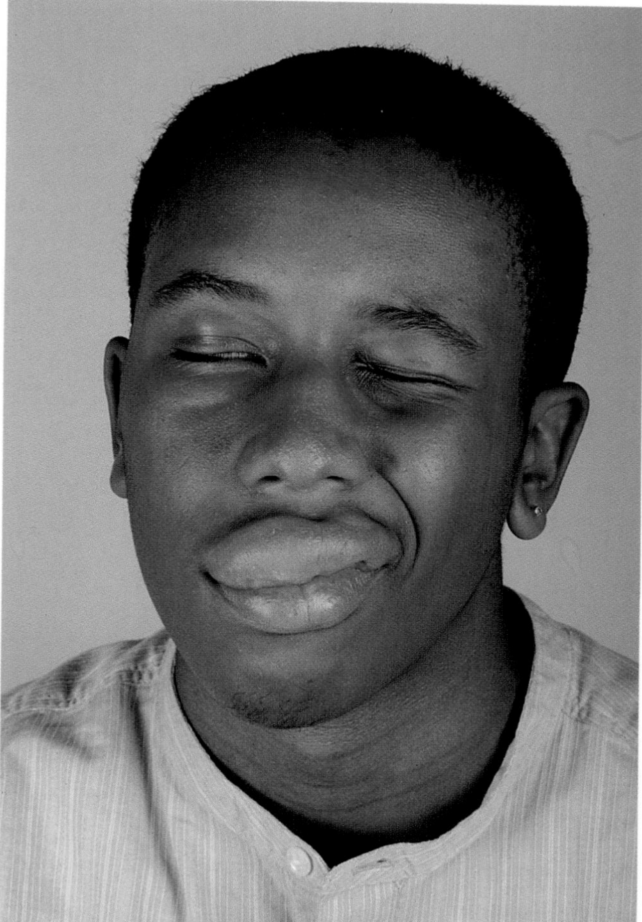

Figure 12-16. Peripheral Seventh Nerve Palsy

Acute peripheral facial palsy is the most frequent manifestation of neuroborreliosis in childhood (55% of cases). Seventh nerve palsy is seen in about 3% of children with Lyme disease (in highly endemic areas, Lyme borreliosis may be responsible for 25% of cases of seventh nerve palsy). Clinically it is indistinguishable from Bell's palsy. It may be the presenting as well as the only manifestation of Lyme disease. Usually it lasts from 2 to 8 weeks, is unaffected by treatment, and resolves completely. Rarely it may resolve only partially or not at all. Also note the markedly swollen upper lip (angioedema) in this patient following an arthropod bite.

gently pulling straight out, and *not* with a twisting motion.

d. Wear gloves or protect the fingers with facial tissue if fingers are used to remove ticks and wash thoroughly after tick removal.

8. Prevention of Lyme disease:
   a. Wear protective clothing (e.g., long sleeves and long pants that are tight at the wrists and waist; the pants should be tucked into light colored socks; wear a hat) when entering tick-infested areas.
   b. Use tick repellent for additional protection.

BOX 12-14. CLINICAL FEATURES OF LYME DISEASE

- The highest number of reported cases occur in children 2 to 15 years and persons 30 to 55 years of age and older.
- Clinical manifestations: three stages (these stages can overlap or occur alone):
  (1) Stage 1: early disease localized to the skin (erythema migrans [EM])
  (2) Stage 2: early disseminated disease with spirochetes spreading via the blood or lymph (multiple EM, seventh nerve palsy, cardiac disorders)
  (3) Stage 3: late disease with persistence of manifestations of infection (arthritis and chronic neurologic syndromes)
- Early localized disease:
  (1) EM (Box 12-15)
  (2) Nonspecific symptoms (fever, headache, myalgia, arthralgia, fatigue, lymphadenopathy
- Early disseminated disease:
  (1) Flulike illness with nonspecific symptoms (fever, headache, myalgia, arthralgia, fatigue, conjunctivitis)
  (2) Multiple EM (seen in about 25% of children)
  (3) Aseptic meningitis (uncommon)
  (4) Cranial neuritis (seventh nerve palsy relatively common)
  (5) Carditis (usually various degrees [first-, second-, or third-degree] of heart block, myopericarditis, left ventricular dysfunction)
  (6) Peripheral radiculoneuritis
  (7) Lymphadenopathy (regional or generalized)
- Late disease: arthritis (seen in about 7% of children):
  (1) Seen weeks to months (usually 4 to 6 weeks [range, 1 week to 22 months] after tick bite
  (2) Arthritis may occur without a history of earlier stages of illness (including EM)
  (3) Usually mono- or pauciarticular
  (4) Usually involves the large joints (knee, shoulder, hip, ankle, elbow; may also involve small joints)
  (5) Most commonly involved joint: knee (>90%)
  (6) Affected joint swollen and tender
  (7) Duration of arthritis variable (usually resolves in 1 to 2 weeks)
  (8) Usually resolves with treatment (if untreated, may last for months)
  (9) Arthritis may recur

c. Inspect the entire body and all clothing after spending time in an infested area.
d. Routine prophylactic antibiotics are not indicated following a deer tick bite.
e. Lyme vaccine (see CDC guidelines for recommendations)

Clinical Pearls: Lyme Disease

1. Lyme disease is the most common vector-borne disease in the United States.
2. Erythema migrans is the most characteristic manifestation of Lyme disease. It is seen in about 90% of children with Lyme disease. Multiple EM-like lesions are seen as a result of hematogenous spread and are the cutaneous markers of disseminated disease.
3. Acute peripheral facial palsy is the most frequent manifestation of neuroborreliosis in childhood.
4. Varying degrees of AV block are the most frequent manifestation of Lyme carditis.
5. The risk of developing Lyme disease following a deer tick bite is very low (1 to 2%), and if Lyme disease develops, it is an easily treatable disease. Thus, prophylactic antibiotics are not indicated routinely following a deer tick bite. Analysis of ticks to determine whether they are infected is not indicated because the predictive value of such tests for human disease is unknown.

BOX 12-15. CLINICAL FEATURES OF LYME DISEASE

- Erythema migrans (EM):
  (1) Usually seen 7 to 14 days after tick bite (range: 3 days to 4 weeks)
  (2) Location: initial rash at site of tick bite in 80% of patients (common locations: head or neck in younger children and extremities in older children)
  (3) Lesion begins as red macule or papule at bite site, then expands into slowly enlarging ring over days to weeks (thus is named "migrans")
  (4) Lesion forms into either annular uniform erythema or a target-shaped lesion with variable degrees of central clearing (very rarely central area may be vesicular or necrotic)
  (5) Annular lesion remains flat (border may be slightly raised), blanches with pressure, and does not desquamate, vesiculate, or have scale at the periphery (unlike ringworm)
  (6) Size: varies from 5 cm to more than 12 inches in diameter (median size: 15 cm)
  (7) Lesion asymptomatic or pruritic and painful
  (8) Lesion solitary or multiple (multiple smaller, secondary annular lesions may appear within days at other sites due to hematogenous spread of spirochetes)
  (9) About 75% of children with Lyme disease will have a single EM lesion.
  (10) EM lesions usually fade within 3 to 4 weeks, even in untreated patients.

BOX 12-16. DIFFERENTIAL DIAGNOSIS OF LYME DISEASE

Differential diagnosis of erythema migrans:

- Tinea corporis
- Herald patch of pityriasis rosea
- Cellulitis
- Erysipelas
- Nummular eczema
- Granuloma annulare
- Erythema multiforme
- Other arthropod or spider bite
- Fixed drug eruption
- Urticaria

Differential diagnosis of arthritis:

- Rheumatoid arthritis
- Systemic lupus erythematosus
- Acute rheumatic fever
- Septic arthritis

Differential diagnosis of other manifestations:

- Aseptic meningitis due to another etiology (e.g., enterovirus)
- AV heart block from another etiology (see Fig. 12-11)
- Peripheral seventh nerve palsy from another etiology (e.g., Bell's palsy)

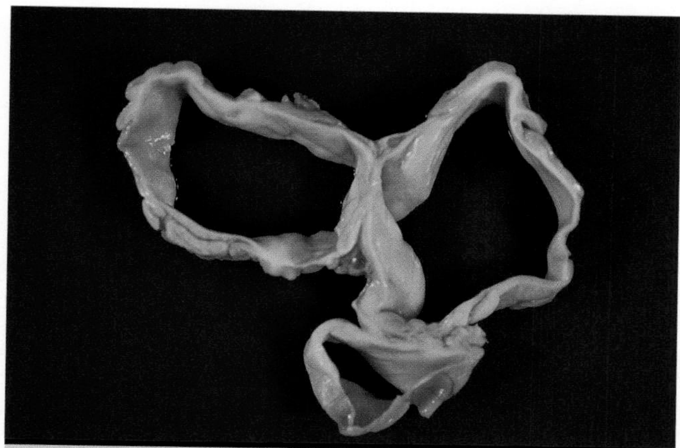

Figure 13-5. Severe Hydrocephalus as a Complication of Bacterial Meningitis

This autopsy photograph shows marked dilation of the ventricular system and prominent thinning of the cerebral mantle. This 3-year-old child who died from sepsis had a history of GBS neonatal meningitis complicated by the development of hydrocephalus that required a ventriculoperitoneal shunt at the age of 4 months.

8. Place a 5 TU PPD tuberculin test on the forearm of all patients with meningitis in areas where tuberculosis is endemic.
9. Radiographic tests
   a. Head CT scan *need not* be routinely performed in patients with a clinical diagnosis of uncomplicated meningitis (e.g., absence of focal neurological signs) prior to performing an LP.
   b. A head CT scan should be obtained prior to LP if elevated ICP or mass lesion is suspected (e.g., to exclude abscess, subdural empyema, brain tumor, or intracranial hemorrhage).
   c. A head CT scan or MRI is performed in patients with meningitis with focal neurological findings (e.g., suspected focal complications such as subdural effusion or empyema), prolonged obtundation or irritability, seizures, worsening ICP, persistent fever, persistently abnormal CSF indices, and neonates (who are prone to abscess formation).
10. Complications of meningitis include seizures, subdural effusion, hydrocephalus, cerebral infarction, hearing loss, and developmental delay (Figs. 13-3 to 13-5).

Emergency Department Treatment and Disposition

1. The keys to reducing morbidity and mortality in meningitis are high index of suspicion, prompt recognition, stabilization, and immediate initiation of antibiotic therapy.
2. The patient may need stabilization based on abnormal vital signs, continuous cardiac and pulse oximetry monitoring, and fluid resuscitation with crystalloids for septic shock.
3. If patient is not in shock, restrict IV fluid to basal requirement (800 to 1000 mL/m^2 per day) with 0.33% NaCl solution (sodium concentration of 40 mEq/L) because of possible SIADH.
4. Radiographic studies (e.g., CT scan in a patient with focal neurologic signs) should never delay prompt initiation of antibiotic therapy for suspected meningitis.
5. Empiric treatment of bacterial meningitis in patients <4 weeks of age:
   a. Provide coverage for GBS, *E. coli*, and *Listeria*.
   b. Ampicillin (100-200 mg/kg per day divided every 6 hours) *and* cefotaxime (300 mg/kg per day divided every 8 hours) *or* ampicillin and an aminoglycoside (e.g., gentamicin)
   c. Consider antiviral therapy if herpes is suspected (while awaiting confirmation of bacterial meningitis).
6. Empiric treatment of bacterial meningitis in patients 4 weeks to 12 weeks of age:
   a. Provide coverage for *H. influenzae*, pneumococci, and meningococci.
   b. Vancomycin (60 mg/kg per day divided every 6 hours) *and* cefotaxime (225 to 300 mg/kg per day divided every 8 hours) *or* ceftriaxone (100 mg/kg per day divided every 12 to 24 hours)
7. Empiric treatment of bacterial meningitis in patients >12 weeks of age:
   a. Provide coverage for pneumococci and meningococci.
   b. Vancomycin *and* cefotaxime *or* ceftriaxone
8. Offer antibiotic prophylaxis for exposure to *H. influenzae* type b and *N. meningitidis* (see page 106)
9. Administration of dexamethasone may be beneficial for treatment of infants and children with *H. influenzae* type b meningitis to decrease the hearing loss associated with meningitis, and its use may be considered for *H. influenzae* type b meningitis in infants older than 6 weeks.
10. Hospitalize all patients with a clinical diagnosis of meningitis.
    a. Patients presenting with septic shock requiring resuscitation (e.g., meningococcemia) will need ICU monitoring.
    b. Patients also need standard and droplet precautions for the first 24 hours after institution of appropriate antibiotics.

Clinical Pearls: Bacterial Meningitis

1. Meningitis is a life-threatening medical emergency; maintain a high index of suspicion in a patient presenting with any signs and symptoms shown in Box 13-1.
2. Neonates and young infants may present with nonspecific findings (e.g., paradoxical irritability or lethargy, hypothermia rather than high fever, and absence of neck stiffness).
3. The diagnosis of meningitis must not be excluded in young children based on an absence of signs of meningeal irritation (these signs are usually not seen in young children

[<18 months of age], and when present, usually represent a very late finding).

4. Stiff neck is a pathognomonic sign of meningeal irritation resulting from a purulent exudate or hemorrhage in the subarachnoid space.
5. CSF examination is the gold standard for the diagnosis; if there is any suspicion of meningitis, *perform a lumbar puncture*.
6. Classic signs of meningococcal infection (fever with petechiae or purpura) are seen in only 70% of cases. Patients with meningococcal meningitis may lack CSF abnormalities on initial LP even with a positive CSF culture. Thus, infections caused by *N. meningitidis* (including meningitis) must be considered even in the absence of skin lesions or CSF abnormalities (see meningococcemia, page 105).
7. Overall, seizures are seen in about 20 to 30% of patients with bacterial meningitis, and seizures are the presenting sign of meningitis in about 13 to 16% of children. Thus, meningitis must be considered in children presenting with febrile seizures (see page 537).
8. Delays in initiating antibiotic therapy while awaiting completion of diagnostic studies (e.g., LP in a patient with septic shock) must be avoided. Stabilization including antibiotic administration must be done in an unstable patient prior to LP.
9. Radiographic tests (e.g., CT scan in a patient with focal neurologic signs) should never delay prompt initiation of antibiotic therapy for suspected meningitis.
10. Failure to diagnose meningitis early is one of the leading causes of malpractice litigation in pediatrics.

BOX 13-1. TYPICAL SIGNS AND SYMPTOMS OF MENINGITIS

Neonate (signs and symptoms are often subtle and non-specific)

- Fever or hypothermia
- Poor suck/poor feeding
- Lethargy or irritability
- Weak or high-pitched cry
- Seizures
- Apnea or respiratory distress
- Septic shock

Infants

- Fever
- Lethargy or irritability
- Vomiting
- Bulging anterior fontanelle (Fig. 13-2)
- Seizures
- Coma
- Septic shock

Older child

- Fever
- Lethargy/mental status changes (confusion/coma)
- Petechiae or purpura (especially meningococcal infections; see Fig. 13-7, and Figs. 3-28-31)
- Headache
- Photophobia
- Seizures
- Septic shock
- Focal neurological findings
- Ataxia (labyrinthine dysfunction or vestibular neuronitis)
- Signs of meningeal irritation
  (1) Nuchal rigidity or meningismus (neck resists passive flexion)
  (2) Kernig's sign (attempt to passively extend the knee while patient is seated is met with resistance in the presence of meningitis)
  (3) Brudzinski's sign (passive flexion of the neck with the patient in a supine position results in spontaneous flexion of the hips and knees)

BOX 13-2. DIFFERENTIAL DIAGNOSIS OF MENINGITIS

- Bacterial meningitis of various etiologies
- Aseptic meningitis or meningoencephalitis
  (1) Enteroviruses (echovirus, poliovirus, coxsackievirus; occurs late summer and early fall)
  (2) Herpes simplex virus (typically associated with encephalitis)
  (3) Arboviruses
  (4) Mumps (rare due to routine immunization)
  (5) Measles (rare due to routine immunization)
  (6) Rubella (rare due to routine immunization)
- Tuberculous meningitis
- Fungal meningitis (e.g., *Cryptococcus neoformans*, *Coccidioides immitis*)
- Brain abscess, tuberculoma
- Parameningeal/paraspinal infection (e.g., subdural or epidural abscess)
- Sepsis
- Seizures from other etiologies and postitcal state
- Retropharyngeal abscess
- Cervical adenitis
- Trauma (e.g., shaken impact syndrome/child abuse, subdural or epidural hematoma, concussion)
- Subarachnoid hemorrhage (ruptured AVM/aneurysm)
- Focal intracranial mass lesions (e.g., intracranial or brainstem tumor)
- *Rickettsia* (e.g., Rocky mountain spotted fever, Q fever; seen in summer to late fall)
- Spirochetes (e.g., *Borrelia burgdorferi* [Lyme disease], *Treponema pallidum* [syphilis])
- Metabolic disturbances (e.g., electrolyte imbalance, hypoglycemia, uremia)
- Bacterial endocarditis with embolism
- Toxic ingestions (e.g., organophosphates, heavy metals [e.g., lead, mercury], phenothiazines)
- Collagen vascular diseases (e.g., systemic lupus erythematosus)
- Malaria
- Typhoid fever

BOX 13-3. CEREBROSPINAL FLUID FINDINGS IN MENINGITIS

Type of meningitis	*Leukocytes (number)*	*Glucose*	*Protein*	*Gram's stain*
Bacterial	Neutrophils (hundreds to thousands)	Low	High	Often positive
Viral	Lymphocytes (hundreds)	Normal	Slightly high	Negative
Tuberculous	Lymphocytes (hundreds)	Low	High	Negative
Cryptococcal	Lymphocytes (few to hundreds)	Low	Normal or high	Negative
Parameningeal (brain abscess, subdural abscess)	Lymphocytes (few)	Normal	High	Negative

(Reproduced with permission from: Bergelson J: Meningitis. In: Finberg L, Kleinman RE (eds). *Saunders Manual of Pediatric Practice*, 2nd ed. Philadelphia, WB Saunders, 2002, p. 389.)

DIAGNOSIS ALTERED LEVEL OF CONSCIOUSNESS

Definition

1. Consciousness is the state of awareness of self and environment. Consciousness requires intact function of both cerebral hemispheres and the brainstem ascending reticular activating system (ARAS) that traverses the diencephalon, midbrain, and upper pons.
2. Stupor or coma results from injury to or dysfunction of either the brainstem ARAS or both cerebral hemispheres (Fig. 13-6).
3. Injury or dysfunction of one cerebral hemisphere does not cause coma unless the contralateral hemisphere is affected by secondary effects of the primary injury (raised intracranial pressure [ICP] by tumor, trauma, abscess).
4. The spectrum of altered level of consciousness is described by:
   a. Lethargy: reduced wakefulness and lack of interest in the environment, but patient is easily arousable and can communicate
   b. Confusion: inattentiveness, mental slowness, dulled perception of the environment, incoherence in thinking
   c. Obtundation: severe blunting of alertness with a decreased response to stimuli and increased sleep
   d. Delirium: confusion with hallucinations and motor abnormalities (tremors/myoclonus); agitation may alternate with drowsiness.
   e. Stupor: unresponsiveness from which patient can be aroused only by vigorous and repeated stimuli, and patient lapses back into unresponsive state when the stimulus is withdrawn
   f. Coma: unresponsiveness from which patient cannot be aroused by verbal, sensory, or even vigorous physical stimuli

Etiology/Associated Clinical Features

1. Toxic metabolic encephalopathies that diffusely affect the brain (e.g., hypoglycemia, poisoning, meningitis)
   a. Most common causes in children (70 to 80% of cases)
   b. Progressive mental changes: comatose state, symmetric motor signs, brainstem reflex pathways spared, acid-base disturbances, seizures, tremors, myoclonus
   c. "Dissociation of findings": abnormal respiratory rate (e.g., apnea) with preserved pupillary reflexes
2. Structural abnormalities of the brain (20 to 30% of cases)
   a. Supratentorial lesion compressing or displacing diencephalon and brainstem (e.g., trauma, tumor)
      1) Focal asymmetric motor signs (hemiparesis, papilledema, reflex asymmetry)
      2) Pupillary reflexes: abnormal
   b. Infratentorial destructive or expanding lesions that damage or compress the ARAS (e.g., posterior fossa tumor, cerebrovascular disease)
      1) Sudden-onset coma, cranial nerve palsies
      2) Abnormal respiratory patterns, brainstem abnormalities
3. Vital signs: fever (e.g., infection, overdose), hypothermia (e.g., overdose, hypoglycemia), bradycardia (e.g., overdose,

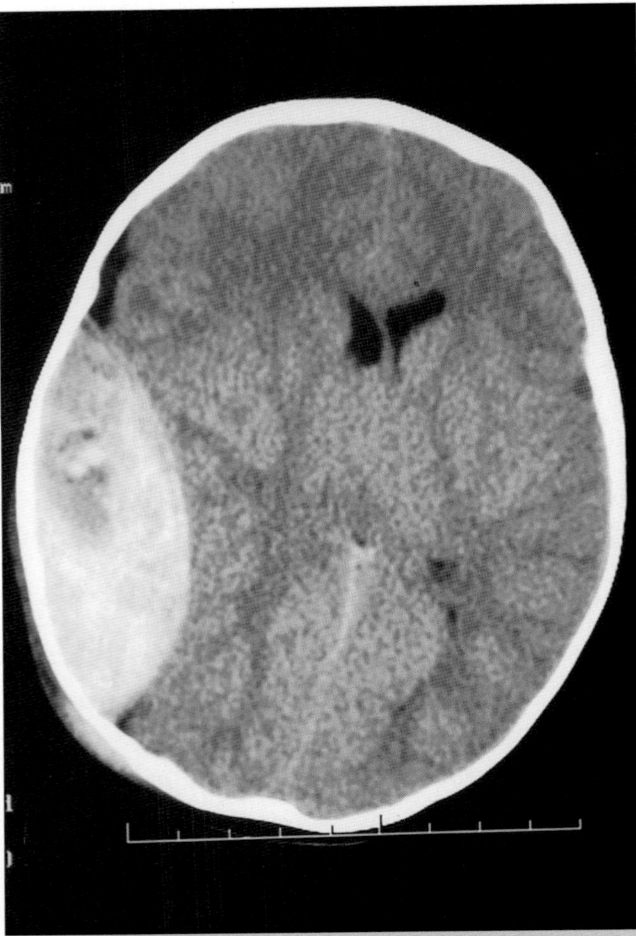

Figure 13-6. Epidural Hematoma with Herniation in Inflicted Head Trauma (Child Abuse) Presenting with Coma

A noncontrast CT axial image of the head shows a large right temporoparietal lenticular extradural hematoma with heterogenous density. There is a mass effect on the adjacent occipital lobe with evidence of subfalcine herniation, and a midline shift from right to left. This 4-month-old infant was brought to the ED with a history of vomiting and inability to arouse. His vital signs showed bradycardia, hypertension, and agonal respiration (Cushing's triad). His Hgb/Hct were 6.5/19.4. His skeletal survey showed the presence of a right parietal skull fracture with overlying soft tissue swelling. His mother subsequently confessed to shaking the infant violently and throwing him against the wall because he would not stop crying. He required neurosurgical intervention (intraoperative evacuation).

DIAGNOSIS

BELL'S PALSY

SYNONYMS

Idiopathic facial palsy
Acute peripheral facial paralysis
Lower motor neuron facial palsy

Definition

Bell's palsy is an acute, idiopathic, unilateral (in the vast majority) facial weakness affecting the muscles supplied by the seventh cranial nerve (Figs. 13-9 and 13-10).

Etiology

1. Bell's palsy results from a lesion of the cranial nerve VII nucleus or emergent facial nerve. The most commonly affected portion of the facial nerve is within the temporal bone.
2. The exact etiology of Bell's palsy is unknown, although serologic and DNA evidence suggests that herpes virus infection may be responsible for some cases. Reactivation of latent viruses (e.g., herpes simplex virus and varicella-zoster

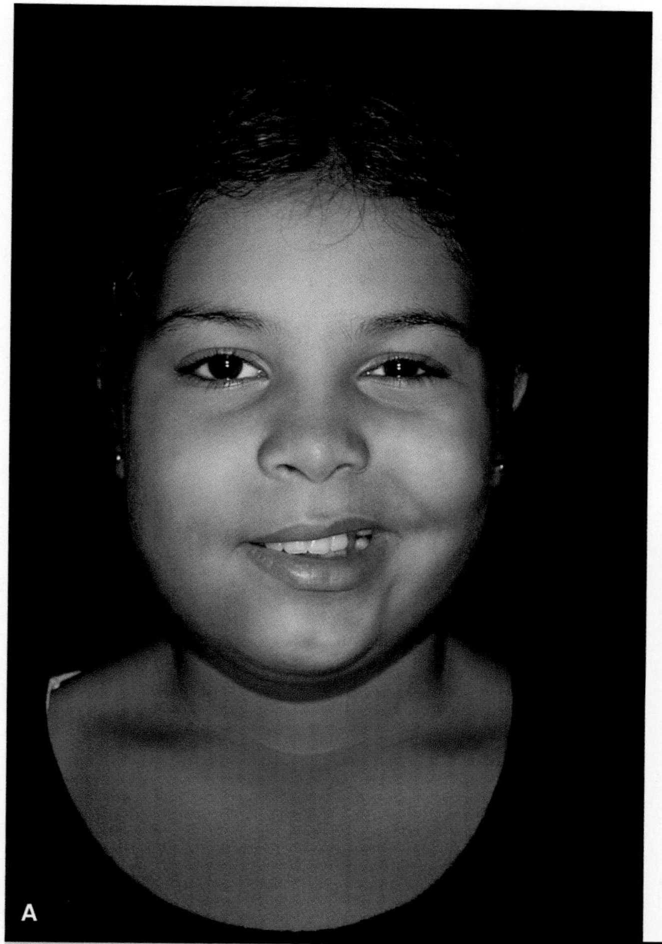

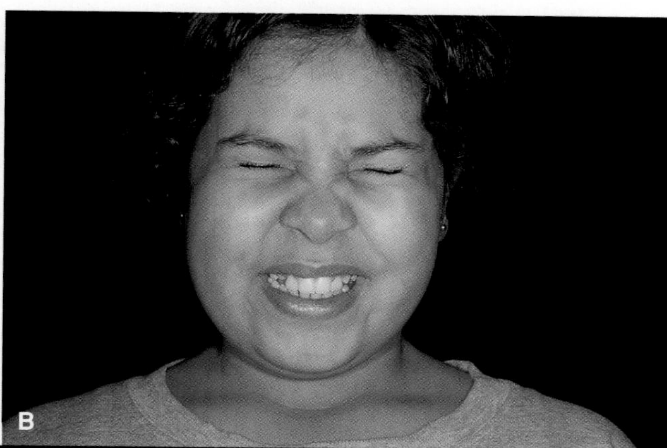

Figure 13-9. Right-Sided Bell's Palsy

A. Bell's palsy is a clinical diagnosis; there are no tests diagnostic of Bell's palsy. Ask the patient to smile, close eyes, raise eyebrows, and whistle or puff out the cheeks. Facial muscle paresis, facial asymmetry, drooling, widened palpebral fissure, smooth forehead, and flattened nasolabial fold are characteristic findings. *B*. Complete recovery from facial palsy confirms the diagnosis of Bell's palsy. These two photographs were taken 8 weeks apart in this otherwise healthy adolescent girl with Bell's palsy.

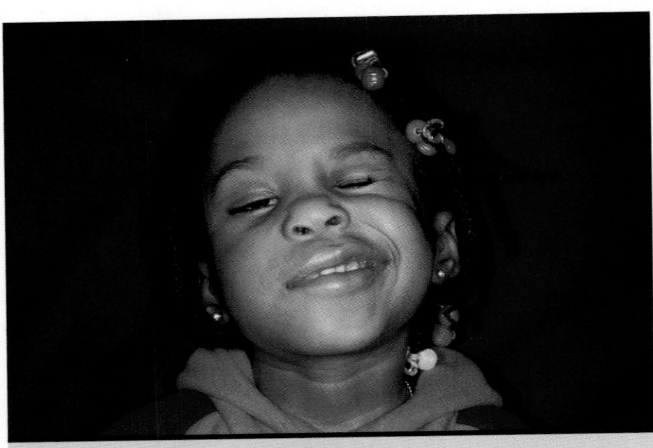

Figure 13-10. Right-Sided Facial Palsy Secondary to Rhabdomyosarcoma

Sudden onset of right lower motor neuron facial palsy was a presenting compliant in this 3-year-old girl who also had a history of intermittent bloody otorrhea from her right ear of 5 days' duration. She denied any history of fever, earache, headache, or vertigo. Her right tympanic membrane showed perforation with bloody discharge. A noncontrast CT scan of her temporal bone was obtained, and showed presence of external canal soft tissue mass on the right side extending in the middle ear cavity and mastoid cells associated with bony erosion of the mastoid cells.

virus) in the cranial nerves and sensory ganglia leading to dysfunction and neuropathy has been one suggested pathogenesis.

3. Other theories include immune-mediated demyelination and entrapment (edema and compression of the facial nerve within the bony facial canal, leading to ischemia).

Associated Clinical Features

1. Bell's palsy is uncommon in the first decade of life. Incidence increases with age after 10 years with a peak incidence in adulthood.
2. Preceding upper respiratory tract infection is present in greater than 50% of patients.
3. The first sign of Bell's palsy is usually pain or tingling in the ear ipsilateral to subsequent facial palsy followed by *rapid progression* over the next 48 hours. The severity of Bell's palsy can vary from mild weakness to complete paralysis.
4. Otoscopic exam and the remainder of the neurological exam is normal in patients with Bell's palsy.
5. Laboratory tests are usually *not* necessary in the absence of any sign or symptom suggestive of an underlying pathology (i.e., a patient with a normal history and physical examination except for evidence of Bell's palsy). Laboratory tests that may be useful include CBC (e.g., to exclude leukemia) and Lyme titers (in endemic areas).
6. Radiological evaluation is *not* necessary in Bell's palsy. Contrast-enhanced CT or MRI is done in patients with additional abnormal neurological findings (besides evidence of facial palsy) or if malignancy is suspected either from the history or physical examination.
7. Electromyography (EMG) may be used to predict recovery, but it is not needed for diagnosis. It is most informative until at least 3 weeks have elapsed after the onset of facial paralysis.
8. Recurrence is experienced in 5% of cases of Bell's palsy.

Consultation

Neurology (especially if the diagnosis is unclear or physical examination is abnormal in addition to peripheral facial palsy)

Emergency Department Treatment and Disposition

1. Nearly 85% of all patients spontaneously recover normal to near-normal facial function. About 85% of patients show the first signs of recovery within 3 weeks after the onset, and the remaining 15% of patients show recovery within 3 to 6 months.
2. Most patients recover from Bell's palsy without treatment. Treatment of Bell's palsy is controversial.
3. Some authorities recommend institution of antiviral therapy (e.g., acyclovir) at the onset of symptoms of Bell's palsy (on the basis of serologic and DNA evidence that herpes virus infection may be the cause of many cases of facial palsy).
4. A meta-analysis of randomized control trials performed in adults has supported the view that steroids given early in the course (most effective when given within 24 hours of onset) reduce the duration of paralysis and risk of long-term impairment.
   a. Oral prednisone 1 mg/kg per day in three divided doses given for 7 to 10 days followed by a 10-day taper is one suggested regimen.
   b. The efficacy of starting treatment with steroids more than two weeks after the onset of Bell's palsy is questionable.
5. Recommendations of the report of the Quality Standards Subcommittee of the American Academy of Neurology are as follows:
   a. Early treatment with oral steroids is recommended as *probably* effective to improve facial functional outcomes.
   b. Early treatment with acyclovir in combination with prednisone is recommended as *possibly* effective to improve facial functional outcomes.
   c. There is insufficient evidence to make recommendations regarding the use of facial nerve decompression to improve facial functional outcomes.
6. Corneal protection is required to prevent corneal exposure and ulceration until full recovery of tearing and lid closure has occurred. Measures include application of artificial tears during the daytime, wearing eyeglasses when outdoors, and using ophthalmic ointment at bedtime with an eye patch (to reduce the risk of scratching the cornea).

7. A follow-up appointment with the neurologist is recommended to follow the clinical course of the patient and for additional tests as indicated (e.g., EMG to follow the progress of recovery from the nerve injury).
8. Persistent redness or irritation of the eye requires referral to an ophthalmologist.

Clinical Pearls: Bell's Palsy

1. Bell's palsy is a lower motor neuron facial palsy.
2. Bell's palsy is the most common type of facial palsy, accounting for 80% of all facial palsies, and causes unilateral weakness of the entire face.
3. Patients presenting with acute lower motor neuron facial palsy require a thorough history and physical examination including a full neurological examination to exclude other causes of facial palsy. Diagnosis of Bell's palsy is made largely by excluding infectious or noninfectious diseases, trauma, and tumors.
4. Both the upper and lower parts of the face are affected in Bell's palsy. This feature distinguishes Bell's palsy from a central supranuclear lesion (upper motor neuron facial palsy), in which the ability to close the eye and to wrinkle the forehead is preserved.
5. Bilateral Bell's palsy is differentiated from Guillain-Barré syndrome on the basis that tendon reflexes are preserved in Bell's palsy, while they are absent in Guillain-Barré syndrome.
6. A weak cry or voice, pooling of oral secretions, nasal twang, and nasal regurgitation are signs of bulbar dysfunction and suggest Guillain-Barré syndrome, poliomyelitis, or malignancy (e.g. brain stem glioma).

BOX 13-7. CLINICAL FEATURES OF BELL'S PALSY

- *Typical features:*
  (1) 99% of patients have unilateral involvement
  (2) 1% of patients show clinical evidence of bilateral involvement
  (3) All muscles on affected side of face are involved
  (4) Flattening of nasolabial fold
  (5) Drooping of corner of mouth
  (6) Inability to close eye ipsilaterally (widened palpebral fissure)
  (7) Inability to wrinkle forehead ipsilaterally (smooth forehead)
  (8) Facial weakness when patient is asked to puff out cheeks against resistance
- *Other features (may be present depending on the site of injury):*
  (1) Impairment of ipsilateral lacrimation
  (2) Decreased corneal reflex on the involved side
  (3) Hyperacusis (painful sensitivity to loud sounds) in affected ear (if the stapedial nerve is affected)
  (4) A complaint of heaviness or numbness in the face (sensory loss is rarely demonstrable)
  (5) Loss of taste on anterior two-thirds of tongue
  (6) Difficulty in eating and drinking with dribbling of liquids from the weak corner of mouth

BOX 13-8. DIFFERENTIAL DIAGNOSIS OF BELL'S PALSY

- *Central facial palsy (upper motor neuron palsy)*
  (1) Results from lesion above the level of the facial nerve nucleus (e.g., brainstem tumor; frequently associated with hemiparesis)
  (2) Weakness of lower half or two-thirds of the face on contralateral side (of the lesion)
  (3) Sparing of the upper part of the face on contralateral side (of the lesion)
  (4) Ability to wrinkle forehead preserved
  (5) Ability to close eyes on both sides preserved
  (6) Flattening of nasolabial fold on contralateral side (of the lesion)
  (7) Inability to retract (drooping) corner of mouth on contralateral side (of the lesion)
  (8) Usually results in permanent deficit
  (9) Associated neurological signs and cranial neuropathies present

BOX 13-9. SYMPTOMS AND SIGNS INDICATIVE OF ADDITIONAL PATHOLOGY IN PATIENTS WITH FACIAL PALSY REQUIRING URGENT SPECIALIST REFERRAL

- Earache
- Hearing loss
- Pain or paresthesia
- Any abnormality on otoscopy (including otitis media)
- Associated cranial neuropathies or other neurological signs
- Hypertension
- Lymphadenopathy, pallor or bruising
- Vesicles in external meatus or on soft palate
- Single branch involvement
- Gradual progression of paralysis beyond 3 weeks
- Recurrence
- Mastoid swelling

(Reproduced with permission from the BMJ Publishing group: Riordan M: Investigation and treatment of facial paralysis. *Arch Dis Child* 2001;84: 286.)

BOX 13-10. DIFFERENTIAL DIAGNOSIS OF BELL'S PALSY

- Central facial palsy (see Box 13-8)
- Infections leading to facial palsy
  - (1) Lyme disease (in areas of Lyme endemicity: 30% of all facial palsies and bilateral facial palsy)
  - (2) Herpes simplex viral infection
  - (3) AIDS
  - (4) Acute or chronic otitis media
  - (5) Mastoiditis
  - (6) Temporal lobe abscess
  - (7) Chickenpox
  - (8) Infectious mononucleosis
  - (9) Mumps
  - (10) *Mycoplasma* infection
  - (11) Meningitis/encephalitis
  - (12) Cat-scratch disease
  - (13) Infant botulism (*bilateral facial muscle weakness due to neuromuscular junction disorder*)
  - (14) Ramsay-Hunt Syndrome
    - a. Herpes zoster infection of geniculate ganglia
    - b. Presents with facial palsy, vesicles on pinna or in external auditory canal
- Noninfectious diseases leading to facial nerve paralysis
  - (1) Stroke
  - (2) Guillain-Barré syndrome (*bilateral facial palsy*)
  - (3) Diabetes
  - (4) Sarcoidosis (*bilateral facial palsy*)
  - (5) Myasthenia gravis (*bilateral facial muscle weakness due to neuromuscular junction involvement*)
- Traumatic causes leading to facial palsy
  - (1) Blunt or penetrating temporal bone or facial trauma
  - (2) Basilar skull fracture
- Neoplastic diseases leading to facial palsy
  - (1) Parotid gland (e.g., rhabdomyosarcoma)
  - (2) Tumor in inner ear, middle ear, or adjacent brain (acoustic neuroma, pontine glioma, neurofibroma, cholesteatoma, meningeal carcinomatosis)
  - (3) Leukemia (leukemic meningitis)
  - (4) Cerebello pontine angle tumor (e.g., neurofibroma)
- Congenital facial palsy
  - (1) Birth trauma
  - (2) Congenital abnormality of the seventh cranial nerve (mobius syndrome)

DIAGNOSIS NEUROCYSTICERCOSIS

Definition and Etiology

Cysticercosis is a disease occurring after ingestion of larvae of the pork tapeworm (*Taenia solium*). Neurocysticercosis is an infection of central nervous system (CNS) with larval stages (cysticerci) of *T. solium* (Fig. 13-11).

Associated Clinical Features

1. *T. solium* is endemic in Mexico, South and Central America, many African countries, Korea, Cambodia, Laos, Asia, and Europe.
2. In the United States, neurocysticercosis cases have been reported from many states with the most cases occurring in the western states. Most cases are seen among immigrants arriving from areas endemic for cysticercosis; however, occasionally locally acquired cases have been seen. Thus, clinical suspicion is based on the travel history or a history of household contact with an individual with *Taenia solium* infection.
3. The brain is affected in 60 to 90% of cases of cysticercosis. Larvae undergo hematogenous dissemination forming cysts in the parenchyma, ventricles, and subarachnoid space. Ring-enhancing granulomas regress into end-stage calcified granulomas or totally disappear. This regression may take up to 2 years.
4. Diagnosis of neurocysticercosis is difficult because of the nonspecific clinical manifestations and nonpathognomonic findings on neuroimaging studies. Diagnostic criteria have been proposed (see Brutto Del, 2001).
5. Peripheral eosinophilia and presence of ova or proglottids in the stool may suggest the diagnosis. The cerebrospinal fluid (CSF) examination may show lymphocytic pleocytosis,

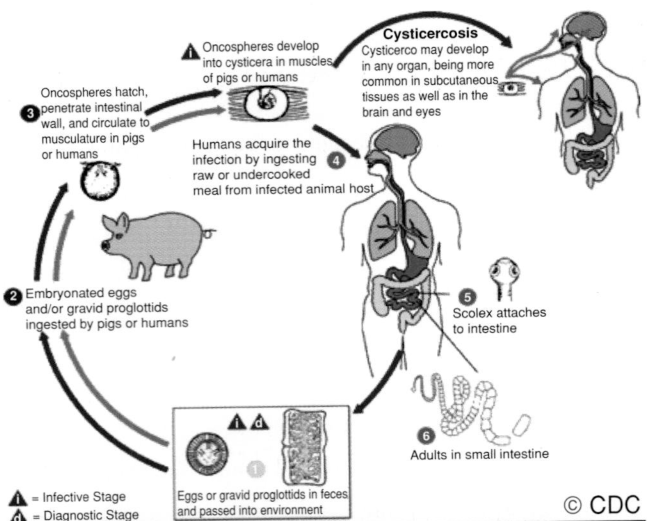

Figure 13-11. Life Cycle of Tapeworms (Taeniasis and Cysticercosis)

Cysticercosis is an infection of both humans and pigs with the larval stages of the parasitic cestode *Taenia solium*. This infection is caused by ingestion of eggs shed in the feces of a human tapeworm carrier (1). Pigs and humans become infected by ingesting eggs or gravid proglottids (2). Humans are infected either by ingestion of food contaminated with feces or by autoinfection. In the latter case, a human infected with adult *T. solium* can ingest eggs produced by the tapeworm, either through fecal contamination, or possibly from proglottids carried into the stomach by reverse peristalsis. Once eggs are ingested, oncospheres hatch in the intestine (3), invade the intestinal wall, and migrate to striated muscles, as well as the brain, liver, and other tissues, where they develop into cysticerci. In humans, cysts can cause serious sequelae if they localize in the brain, resulting in neurocysticercosis. The parasite life cycle is completed, resulting in human tapeworm infection, when humans ingest undercooked pork containing cysticerci (4). (Reproduced with permission from: Tapeworm diseases. Red Book Online. American Academy of Pediatrics, 2003.)

eosinophilia, and elevation of protein. The CSF enzyme-linked immunosorbent assay (ELISA) for anticysticercal antibodies or cysticercal antigens may be positive.

6. Plain radiographs may show cigar-shaped calcifications in the thigh and calf muscles or punctuate soft-tissue or intracranial calcifications.
7. Diagnosis can be confirmed by enzyme-linked immunotransfer blot assay for the detection of serum anticysticercal antibodies to *T. solium* glycoprotein antigen (available through the Centers for Disease Control and Prevention).
   a. High specificity (~100%) and sensitivity (~94 to 98%) in patients with two or more cystic or ring-enhancing lesions (Fig. 13-12)
   b. False-negative test possible in patients with solitary lesion or old calcified lesions.
   c. Test positive with cysticercosis in any tissue (brain, subcutaneous, muscle)
8. Diagnosis can also be confirmed by demonstration of the parasite from biopsy of a brain or spinal cord lesion.

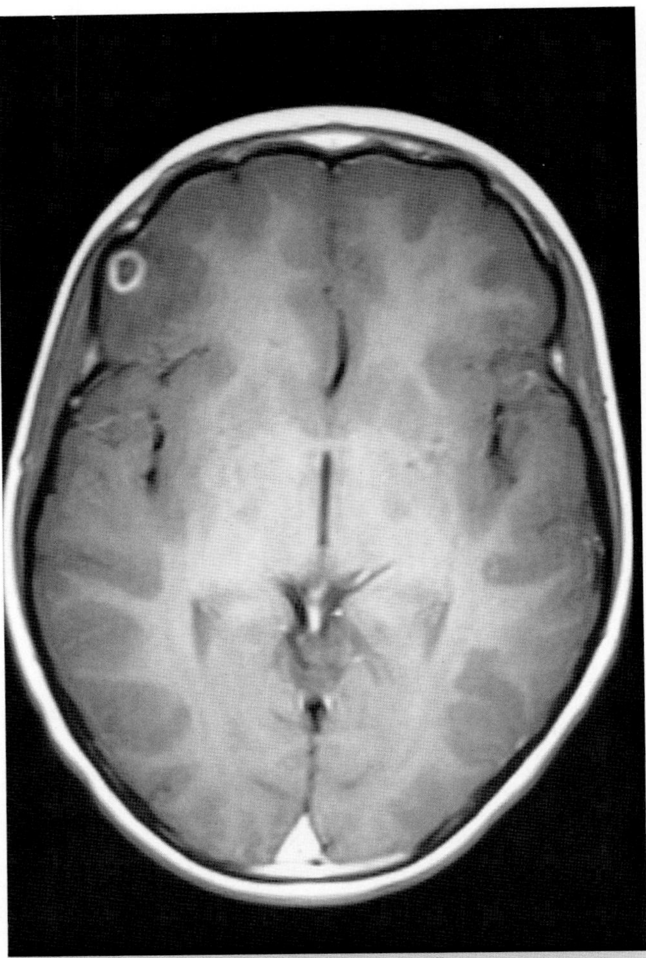

Figure 13-12. Ring-Enhancing Cortical Lesion of Neurocysticercosis

Axial T1 weighted gallium enhanced MRI image of the brain shows a solitary ring-enhancing lesion in the right frontal cortex (noncontrast CT scan of the head showed focal subcortical hypodensity in right frontal lobe). Differential diagnosis of ring-enhancing lesions is detailed in Box 13-13. This 11-year-old child presented with new-onset partial complex seizures. His CSF examination was negative for bacteria, mycobacteria, and fungi. His CSF neurocysticercosis antibody was positive.

Consultations

Neuroradiologist, neurology, neurosurgery, infectious disease

Emergency Department Treatment and Disposition

1. Stabilization of the patient based on abnormal vital signs, control of seizures, and increased ICP as indicated.
2. All patients with suspected neurocysticercosis require hospitalization for further evaluation and management (intensive care setting in patients with increased ICP or in patients with obstructive hydrocephalus requiring close monitoring)

3. Treatment of neurocysticercosis is individualized based on whether cysts are active or nonviable (assessed by neuroimaging studies [CT scan or MRI]) and their location.
   a. Patients with calcified lesions (nonviable cysts) need supportive therapy as indicated (e.g., anticonvulsants for seizures or shunt placement for intraventricular lesions presenting with hydrocephalus).
   b. There is controversy over the role of antiparasitic drugs in patients with active lesions (e.g., cysts or ring-enhancing lesions). Antiparasitic drugs hasten destruction and disappearance of intracranial cystic lesions or their transformation into calcified granulomas. However, as symptoms result from host inflammatory response, they may be exacerbated with treatment (especially ocular inflammation).
   c. Antiparasitic drugs are usually not recommended by most experts for patients with single inflamed cyst within brain parenchyma, as these patients do well without therapy.
   d. Antiparasitic drugs are recommended by many experts for patients with multiple cysticerci or nonenhancing lesions.
   e. Funduscopic examination *must be* performed before treatment to rule out intraocular cysts (ocular cysts are treated with surgical excision and usually are not treated with antiparasitic drugs, which can exacerbate inflammation).
   f. Antiparasitic drugs that are used include either praziquantel or albendazole.
4. Prophylactic anticonvulsant therapy is recommended for patients presenting with seizures. Therapy is usually continued until neuroradiologic resolution of active lesions, and the patient is seizure-free for 1 to 2 years.
5. Calcified lesions are inactive and not epileptogenic. Usually no therapy is required in an asymptomatic patient in whom a calcified lesion is picked-up incidentally (e.g., CT or MRI performed for other reasons).
6. Corticosteroids may be used for the first 2 to 3 days to reduce the adverse effects associated with antiparasitic therapy. They are usually used for patients with multiple cysts and increased ICP, or lesions near intraventricular foramina or the cerebral aqueduct with possible progression to obstructive hydrocephalus.

Clinical Pearls: Neurocysticercosis

1. Cysticercosis is the most prevalent parasitic disease of the CNS.
2. Neurocysticercosis is one of the most common causes of acquired (or adult-onset) epilepsy in endemic areas.
3. Seizures, focal neurological deficits, increased ICP, and intellectual deterioration are the most common clinical manifestations of neurocysticercosis.
4. Intracranial lesions in different reproductive stages (e.g., cystic, ring, or nodular-enhancing lesions, calcifications) on CT or MRI study are highly suggestive of neurocysticercosis.

BOX 13-11. CLINICAL FEATURES OF NEUROCYSTICERCOSIS

- Incubation period: months to years
- Seizures (afebrile; most common presentation)
- Focal neurological deficits
- Headache
- Signs and symptoms of increased intracranial pressure (ICP)
- Behavioral changes
- Intellectual deterioration
- Signs and symptoms of obstructive hydrocephalus (ventricular cysts)
- Signs and symptoms of meningitis (inflammation of basilar meninges)
- Gait disturbances, pain or transverse myelitis (cysts in spinal column)
- Notable *absence* of fever
- Extraneural evidence of cysticercosis may be present in patients with neurocysticercosis.
  (1) Ocular involvement with visual impairment (cysticerci seen in anterior chamber by funduscopic examination [subretinal cysticerci])
  (2) Subcutaneous or muscular cysticercosis (felt on palpation as nodules)
  (3) Radiographic evidence of soft-tissue calcification

BOX 13-12. NEUROIMAGING FEATURES OF NEUROCYSTICERCOSIS

- CT and/or MRI with contrast media (*any of the following findings depending on location and reproductive stages of disease*)
  (1) Solitary or multiple cystic lesions in brain parenchyma (near cerebral gray-white matter junction), subarachnoid space, or ventricular system
  (2) Lesions with or without contrast enhancement (ring or nodular enhancement = active granuloma stage)
  (3) Vasogenic edema around the cyst, contrast enhancement of the cyst wall, and transformation of the cyst wall into a granuloma (findings suggestive of larval death)
  (4) Cystic lesions showing scolex (pathognomonic sign; seen as a bright nodule within a cyst producing "hole-with-dot" appearance)
  (5) Parenchymal brain calcifications
  (6) Intraventricular cysts leading to hydrocephalus
  (7) Enhancement of leptomeninges

BOX 13-13. DIFFERENTIAL DIAGNOSIS OF NEUROCYSTICERCOSIS

- *Differential diagnosis of cysticerci-related cystic lesions on CT or MRI:*
  - (1) Low-grade astrocytomas
  - (2) Cystic cerebral metastasis
  - (3) Congenital arachnoid cysts
- *Differential diagnosis of cysticerci-related ring or nodular-enhancing lesions on CT or MRI:*
  - (1) Tuberculomas (Fig. 13-13)
  - (2) Toxoplasmosis
  - (3) Pyogenic brain abscess
  - (4) Mycotic granulomas
  - (5) Primary or metastatic brain tumors
- *Differential diagnosis of cysticerci-related calcification on CT or MRI:*
  - (1) Metabolic disorders (e.g., hypoparathyroidism, pseudo-hypoparathyroidism)
  - (2) Vascular malformations
  - (3) Tumors (e.g., craniopharyngioma)
  - (4) Infections (e.g., congenial toxoplasmosis or cytomegalovirus [TORCH syndrome], tuberculoma)
- *Differential diagnosis of cysticerci-related enhancement of leptomeninges on CT or MRI:*
  - (1) Chronic meningitis from tuberculosis
  - (2) Chronic meningitis from fungal etiology

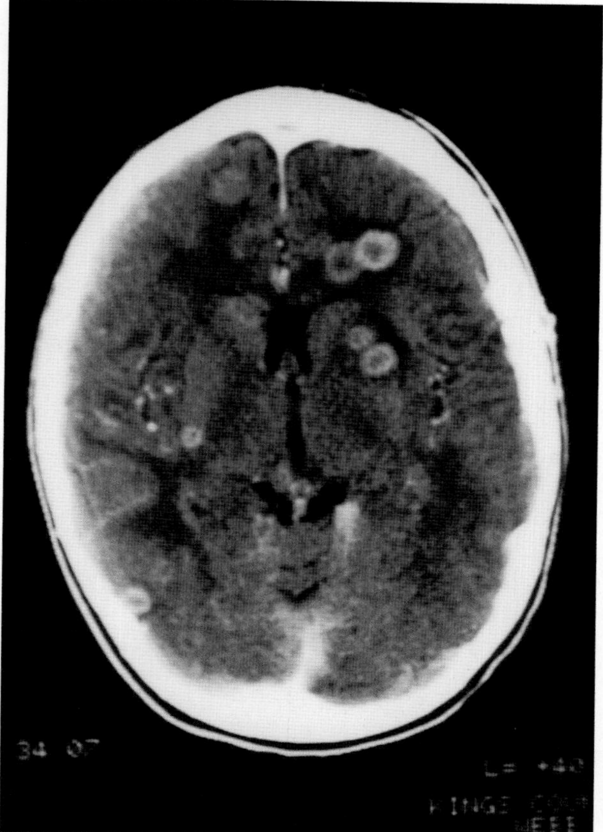

Figure 13-13. Multiple Ring-Enhancing Lesions of Tuberculoma (Differential Diagnosis of Neurocysticercosis)

A contrast-enhanced axial CT image of the brain shows multiple ring-enhancing lesions bilaterally with surrounding edema. This 5-year-old girl presented with afebrile seizure. Her chest radiograph was negative, but PPD was positive. Tuberculoma (CNS infection from *M. tuberculosis*) usually presents clinically as a space-occupying lesion ("brain tumor"). They occur most often in children $<$10 years of age. The most common location is infratentorial at the base of the brain near the cerebellum. Tuberculomas most often are singular but may be multiple. Common presenting symptoms are headache, fever, and convulsions. Most tuberculomas resolve with medical therapy, but these lesions may persist for months or even years.

DIAGNOSIS SUBARACHNOID HEMORRHAGE

Definition

Subarachnoid hemorrhage (SAH) is extravasation of blood into the subarachnoid space of the central nervous system (CNS).

Etiology

1. Nontraumatic SAH (spontaneous)
   a. Ruptured cerebral artery aneurysm
      1) Rupture of congenital berry aneurysm (most common etiology; 75% of cases)
      2) Aneurysms arise from intracranial arteries forming the circle of Willis (Fig. 13-14)
      3) Developmental weakness of the vessel wall at the sites of branching
      4) May be multiple (about 20 to 25% of cases)
      5) Sickle cell disease predisposes to formation of aneurysms due to weakening of vessel walls from ischemia.

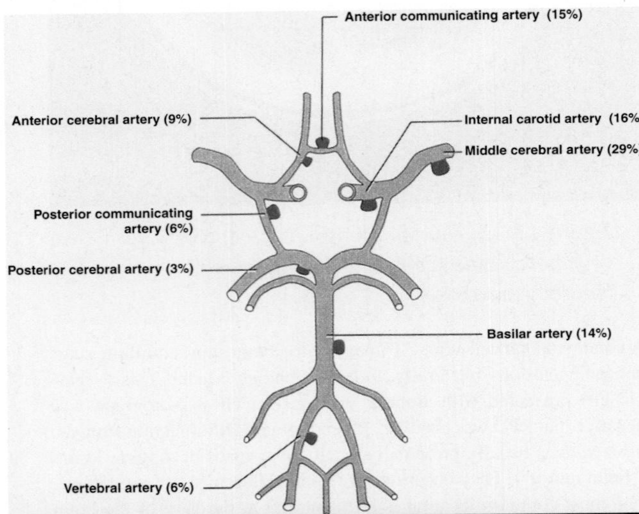

Figure 13-14. Frequency Distribution of Intracranial Aneurysms

Most aneurysms arise from arteries of the circle of Willis and their branches at the base of the brain. About 85% of aneurysms occur in the anterior circulation, usually at the site of vessel bifurcation. The most common sites are the junction of the internal carotid artery (ICA) and posterior communicating artery (PCoA), the anterior cerebral-anterior communicating complex, and the bifurcation of the middle cerebral artery (MCA). Aneurysms from the posterior circulation usually occur at the bifurcation of the basilar artery, and at the junctions of the basilar artery with the vertebral and posterior inferior cerebellar vessels. (Reproduced with permission from: Headache and facial pain. In: Aminoff MJ, Greenberg DA, Simon RP. *Clinical Neurology*, 3rd ed. Stamford, CT, Appleton & Lange, 1996, p. 77.)

   b. Ruptured arteriovenous malformation (AVM; 10% of cases)
      1) Abnormal vascular communication permitting arterial blood to enter the venous system (*without passing through a capillary bed*), leading to expansion of vein and rupture
      2) Most commonly located in the cerebral hemisphere (middle cerebral artery distribution)
      3) Other locations include cerebellum, brainstem, and spinal cord,
2. Trauma
   a. Seen in severe blunt trauma to the head or significant shear forces
   b. Results from tearing of small vessels of the pia mater
   c. Often seen with other intracranial injuries such as subdural hematoma, intraparenchymal bleeding or cerebral contusion
   d. Shaken impact syndrome/child abuse
3. Venous infarcts (thrombotic stroke)
4. Bleeding dyscrasias
5. Moyamoya disease
6. Mycotic aneurysms in subacute bacterial endocarditis
7. Substance abuse (e.g., cocaine, methamphetamine)
8. Tumors (rare)
9. Infections (rare)

Associated Clinical Features

1. SAH due to intracranial aneurysm
   a. Age at presentation: mean age around 30 to 40 years (can occur at any age, but rare in children)
   b. A fourfold increased risk of developing SAH compared to the general population in first-degree relatives of patients with SAH
   c. Patients with prior SAH are six times more likely to have a second hemorrhage later in life.
   d. "Warning bleed" occurs in 20 to 60% of patients about 14 days before the major bleed (range: 1 day to 4 months)
   e. An increased risk of aneurysm formation is seen in patients with sickle cell disease, Marfan's syndrome, coarctation of aorta, neurofibromatosis type 1, and autosomal dominant polycystic kidney disease.
2. SAH due to AVM
   a. AVM may remain asymptomatic throughout life or rupture and bleeding can occur at any age.
   b. Children often have a history of migraine-like headaches or seizures.
3. Depending on the etiology and severity of SAH, patients present with signs and symptoms ranging from severe

headache with signs of meningeal irritation to coma with signs of cerebral herniation.

4. Bleeding may cause injury to adjacent brain tissue leading to focal neurologic deficits.

5. ECG may show prolonged QTc, T-wave flattening and inversion to brady- or tachyarrhythmias.

6. *A noncontrast head CT* is the first test to be ordered in the evaluation (Fig. 13-15)
   a. May show a collection of hyperdense fluid in the CSF spaces (subarachnoid space overlying the cerebral convexity or basal cisterns)
   b. Sensitivity of about 98% for detecting SAH within the first 12 hours, about 93 to 95% within the first 24 hours (less sensitivity in patients presenting >24 hours after SAH)
   c. Helps in identifying other abnormalities if present (e.g., intraventricular or intracerebral hemorrhage)
   d. False-negative CT: small amount of blood or hemoglobin value of <10 g/dL
   e. False-positive CT: calcification of dural and vascular structures at the base of the brain

7. CSF examination
   a. CSF exam may show frank blood (Fig. 13-16) or xanthochromia (yellow-golden discoloration of the CSF that takes up to about 12 hours to become visible).
   b. Even though CSF exam may confirm bleeding, it is usually not performed because of the risk of cerebral herniation in the presence of brain edema or a focal intracranial lesion.

8. Angiography or magnetic resonance angiography for suspected SAH from ruptured aneurysm or AVM

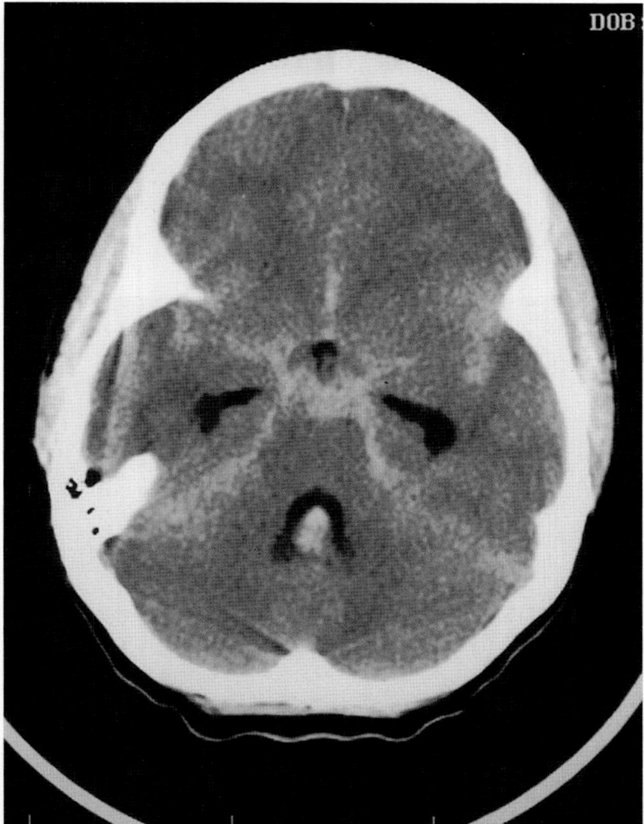

Figure 13-15. Subarachnoid Hemorrhage with Communicating Hydrocephalus

A noncontrast CT scan of the brain shows SAH in the basal cisterns, sylvian fissures, and intraventricular blood in the fourth ventricle with associated hydrocephalus (the ventricles are uniformly dilated out of proportion to the sulci, a finding consistent with a communicating hydrocephalus). This 10-year-old girl complained of severe headache that were followed by vomiting and unresponsiveness on the school playground. Cerebral angiography could not be completed due to the acute deterioration of the patient during the study, but the incomplete study showed an abnormal tangle of arterial vessels in the left vermian region arising from the left vertebral artery with anomalous anatomy (an aneurysm of the posterior inferior cerebellar artery could not be ruled out due to the incomplete study).

Consultation

Emergent consultation with neurologist and neurosurgeon

Emergency Department Treatment and Disposition

1. Resuscitation and stabilization (ABCs) of the patient based on the abnormal vital signs before any diagnostic work-up is performed

2. For emergent management of raised ICP with impending herniation, see page ??. Care should be taken not to reduce the ICP too rapidly, as this will increase the pressure gradient across the aneurysmal wall and increase the likelihood of rebleeding.

3. Anticonvulsant therapy (for patients at very high risk for seizures, and seizures may provoke rebleeding)

4. Hospitalize patients in ICU for continuous monitoring and further management.

5. Definitive surgery for SAH due to aneurysmal rupture requires isolating the aneurysm from the general circulation by surgical clipping. Alternative approaches include endovascular placement of balloons or coils obliterating the lumen of the aneurysm or decreasing the flow to the parent vessel.

Clinical Pearls: Subarachnoid Hemorrhage

1. Most common cause of nontraumatic SAH is a rupture of an intracranial aneurysm.

2. Presence of blood in the subarachnoid space causes meningeal irritation and clinically mimics signs and symptoms of meningitis.

3. *A truly bloody CSF sample may be mistaken for a traumatic tap, masking the SAH.*

4. Neck stiffness caused by SAH is often misdiagnosed as meningitis, and neck pain caused by SAH is often misdiagnosed as musculoskeletal neck pain.
5. Headaches associated with AVM classically remain on the same side (as the lesion), in contrast to a typical migraine that alternates from one side of the head to the other.

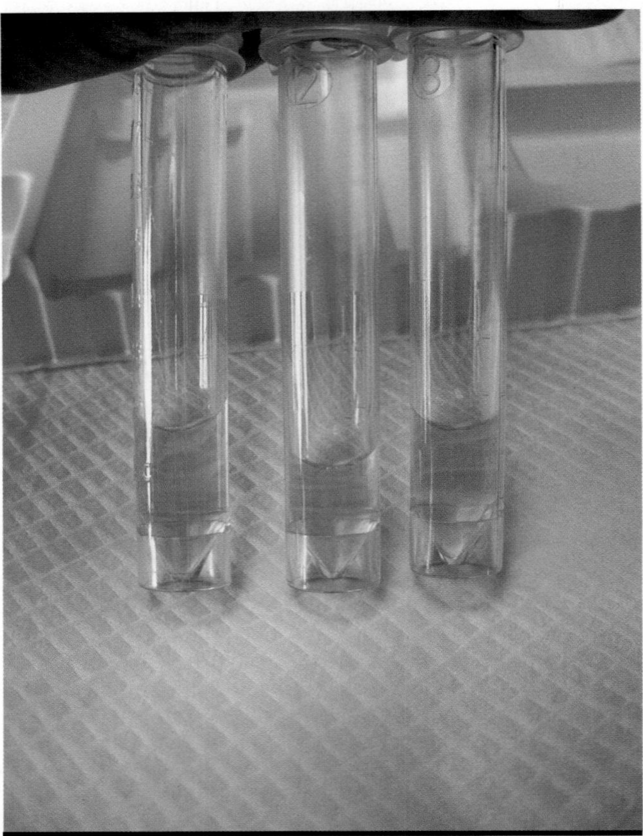

Figure 13-16. Cerebrospinal Fluid Examination in Subarachnoid Hemorrhage

A lumbar puncture is performed if the CT scan fails to confirm the clinical diagnosis. CSF exam usually reveals markedly elevated pressure. It is grossly bloody and contains from 100,000 to >1 million RBCs/cm^3. The supernatant of the centrifuged CSF becomes xanthochromic within several hours (usually by 12 hours) due to the breakdown of hemoglobin from RBCs. The number of WBCs in the CSF are in the same proportion to RBCs as in the peripheral blood. Presence of blood may produce chemical meningitis leading to pleocytosis (several thousand WBCs) during the first 48 hours, and a reduction of CSF glucose (usually between the fourth and eighth day posthemorrhage). CSF glucose is normal in the absence of pleocytosis.

BOX 13-14. CLINICAL FEATURES OF SUBARACHNOID HEMORRHAGE

SAH due to ruptured aneurysm

- Headache (raised intracranial pressure [ICP] with distortion of pain-sensitive structures)
  (1) New-onset headache or distinct change in a pattern of headache
  (2) Sudden onset
  (3) Generalized
  (4) Unusually severe ("the worst headache I ever had in my life")
  (5) *Absence of headache precludes the diagnosis of nontraumatic SAH*
  (6) Intensity of headache may remain unchanged for several days
  (7) History of milder (but similar) headaches in weeks prior to the acute event may be present ("warning bleeds")
  (8) Headache may improve spontaneously or with analgesics
- Loss of consciousness (confusion, stupor, or coma)
  (1) Raised ICP with decreased cerebral blood flow
  (2) Concussive effect of rupture
- Abnormal vital signs (precipitous raise in BP, temperature elevation)
- Signs of meningeal irritation (neck stiffness, Kerning's and Brudzinski's signs)
- Nausea and vomiting (common)
- Neck pain
- Notable absence of prominent focal neurological signs (bleeding into the subarachnoid space)
- Seizures (seen in about 10 to 25% of cases)

SAH due to rupture of AVM

- Previous history of migraine-like headaches and seizures
- Severe headache, vomiting, and signs of meningeal irritation (due to ruptured aneurysm)
- Generalized or focal seizures
- Progressive hemiparesis
- High-pitched bruit on auscultation of skull (~50% of cases)

BOX 13-15. DIFFERENTIAL DIAGNOSIS OF SUBARACHNOID HEMORRHAGE

- Headache from other etiology
  (1) Migraine
  (2) Tension headache
  (3) Sinus headache
  (4) Cluster headache
- Signs of meningeal irritation from other etiology
  (1) Meningitis
  (2) Meningoencephalitis
- Hemorrhage overlying cerebral hemisphere from other etiology (e.g., subdural hematoma [SDH])
  (1) SAH: subarachnoid blood may flow into the depths of brain sulci, fissures, or cisterns with no mass effect
  (2) SDH: limited by subdural space and does not penetrate into sulci, fissures, or cisterns and exerts mass effect

DIAGNOSIS FEBRILE SEIZURES

Definition and Etiology

1. A febrile seizure is an age-related phenomenon, characterized by generalized seizures occurring in young infants and children with fever, not associated with central nervous system infection and any other definable cause or previous history of afebrile seizures.
2. An NIH Consensus Conference (1980) defined febrile seizures as follows:
   a. A febrile seizure is an event in infancy or childhood, usually occurring between 3 months and 5 years of age, associated with fever but without evidence of intracranial infection or defined cause.
   b. Seizures with fever in children who have suffered a previous nonfebrile seizure are excluded.

Associated Clinical Features

1. Febrile seizures tend to run in the family. There is a history of febrile seizures in immediate family members in 25 to 40% of cases.
2. Viral infections are frequently associated with febrile seizures. Some examples of viral infections include infections caused by human herpes virus 6 and 7 (roseola infantum) and influenza A and B.
3. The rates of serious bacterial infections in patients with febrile seizures are similar to those in age-matched febrile control patients without seizures.
4. Risk factors for recurrent febrile seizures include the following:
   a. Early age at onset
   b. Epilepsy in a first-degree relative
   c. Febrile seizure in a first-degree relative
   d. Day nursery (increased frequency of febrile episodes)
   e. A first complex febrile seizure
5. The risk of having recurrent simple febrile seizures varies depending on the age of the child.
   a. There is a 30% risk of a second febrile seizure if a child's age is <12 months at the time of the first seizure. Of these patients 50% have additional risk of a third seizure.
   b. If there are no risk factors and age is >15 months at the time of the first seizure, the chances of recurrence are 10% in 18 months.
   c. In any child with a febrile convulsion, if one or two risk factors are present, the risk of recurrence is intermediate, with 25 to 50% recurrence. If three or more risk factors are present, the risk of recurrence is high, with 50 to 100% recurrence.
6. Evaluation of a child with a first febrile seizure is as follows (AAP Provisional Committee on Quality Improvement, 1996):
   a. Lumbar puncture (LP):
      1) Infants <12 months old: *LP must be strongly considered* (clinical signs and symptoms associated with meningitis may be minimal or absent in this age group)
      2) Children between 12 and 18 months old: *LP should be considered* (clinical signs and symptoms of meningitis may be subtle)
      3) Children >18 months old: LP is not routinely warranted, but should be done if meningeal signs and symptoms are present (e.g., neck stiffness and Kernig's and Brudzinski's signs) or for any child whose history or examination suggests the presence of intracranial infection.
      4) *In infants and children who have had febrile seizures and have received prior antibiotic treatment,*

treatment can mask the signs and symptoms of meningitis. In such children a lumbar puncture should be strongly considered.

b. Blood tests (serum electrolytes, calcium, phosphorus, magnesium, glucose, and CBC):
   1) These tests are not performed routinely (especially in children with a noncontributory history with a normal physical examination)
   2) A blood glucose determination, although not routinely needed, should be obtained if the child has a prolonged period of postictal obtundation.
   3) When fever is present, the decision regarding the need for laboratory testing should be directed toward identifying the source of the fever (based on history and physical examination, as indicated) rather than as part of routine evaluation of the seizure.

c. Neuroimaging (skull film, CT scan, or MRI) is not recommended routinely after the first febrile seizure.

d. EEG is *not* routinely recommended after the first febrile seizure. There is no published study that shows that an EEG can predict future epilepsy.

Consultation

Neurology for complex febrile seizures and febrile status epilepticus

Emergency Department Treatment and Disposition

1. Stabilize airway, breathing, and circulation and perform continuous cardiac and pulse oximetry monitoring and glucose dipstick testing in an actively seizing child before any diagnostic work-up.

2. For an actively seizing child, the aim is to stop the ongoing seizure activity.
   a. The drug of choice is a benzodiazepine.
   b. If IV access is present, then IV benzodiazepines (diazepam or lorazepam) may be administered.
   c. Rectal diazepam is a safe alternative, which is easy to use and effective in stopping the seizure. The rectal preparation comes in a premeasured syringe (2.5-, 5-, 10-, 15-, and 20-mg syringes), making it easy to deliver. Absorption is rapid, which helps to interrupt the seizure clusters or repetitive seizures.

3. Antipyretics help to make the child more comfortable by bringing down the temperature (*however, they will not prevent febrile seizures*).

4. Short-term intermittent prophylaxis
   a. This is done by administering intermittent diazepam during the febrile episode.
   b. This can reduce recurrence by one-third (provided doses are optimal and compliance is ensured).
   c. The suggested dose is 0.5 mg/kg given orally or rectally every 12 hours, if rectal temperature is >38.5°C. A maximum of four consecutive doses is allowed to avoid accumulation and development of side effects.

5. Continuous daily prophylaxis
   a. It is universally agreed that *this is not to be used routinely*.
   b. If it is used at all, it should only be used in carefully selected cases.
   c. The effective anticonvulsant medications are phenobarbital and valproate.
   d. Studies have shown that the following anticonvulsants are ineffective: phenytoin, carbamazepine, oxcarbazepine, and vigabatrin.

6. Long-term treatment of the child with simple febrile seizure (AAP Committee on Quality Improvement, 1999):
   a. No study has demonstrated that treatment for simple febrile seizures can prevent the later development of epilepsy.
   b. The consensus is that neither continuous nor intermittent anticonvulsant therapy is recommended for children with one or more simple febrile seizures.
   c. In situations in which parental anxiety is severe, intermittent oral diazepam at the onset of a febrile illness may be effective in preventing recurrence.

7. Educate parents about the possibility of recurrence of febrile seizures. Most of the seizures occur away from a medical center, and appropriate initial first aid management is essential. Some of the guidelines provided by the Epilepsy Foundation of America are mentioned below and are useful for teaching parents:
   a. Do not panic! These seizures might appear frightening but are generally harmless.
   b. Protect the child from nearby hazards.
   c. Protect the head from injury.
   d. Loosen clothes (including ties or shirt collars).
   e. Turn the child on his side to keep the airway clear.
   f. Do not put any hard implement into the mouth.
   g. Do not try to hold the tongue. It cannot be swallowed.
   h. Do not restrain the child.
   i. Do not use artificial respiration unless breathing is absent after muscle jerks subside or water has been inhaled.
   j. Reassure when consciousness returns.
   k. Febrile seizures generally last <1 minute but can last up to 15 minutes.
   l. With multiple seizures, or if one seizure lasts longer than 5 minutes, call an ambulance.

Clinical Pearls: Febrile Seizures

1. A simple febrile seizure is defined as a brief (<15 minutes) generalized seizure that occurs only once during a 24-hour period in a febrile child who does not have an intracranial infection or severe metabolic disturbance.

2. A simple febrile seizure is a benign and common event in children between the ages of 6 months and 5 years and most children have an excellent prognosis (Fig. 13-17).

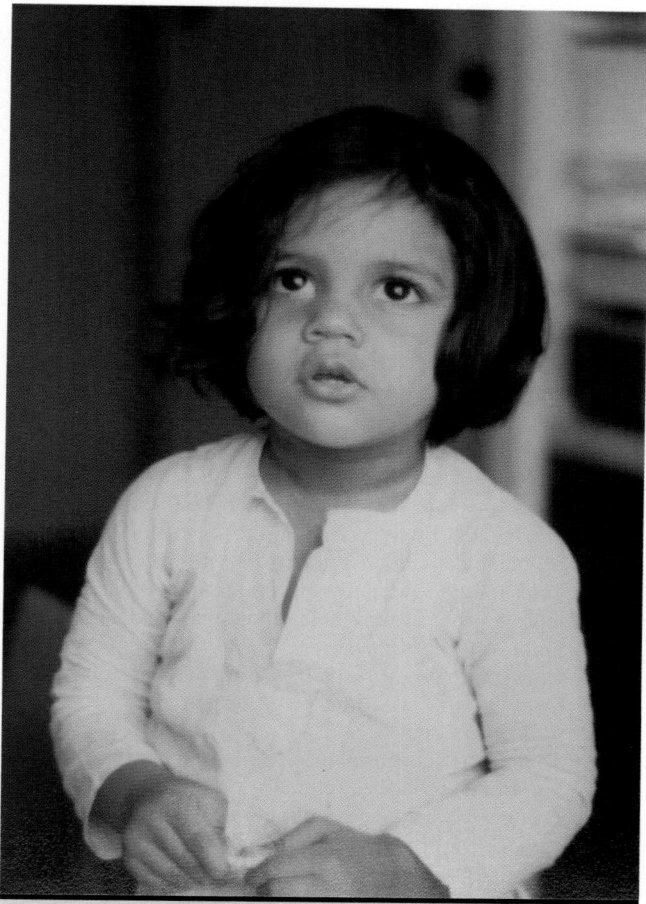

Figure 13-17. A Toddler Presenting to the ED with a Recent History of a Simple Febrile Seizure

As seen in this toddler, most patients present with a history of a brief febrile convulsion without any postictal neurological deficits (the overwhelming majority of febrile seizures will have terminated before presentation to the ED). In the absence of clinical signs or symptoms suggestive of CNS infection, such patients can be safely discharged home (once the etiology of fever has been determined). Discharge instructions include fever management, education about the possibility of recurrence of febrile seizures, and first aid management of seizures.

3. ED physicians evaluating an infant or a young child presenting with a first simple febrile seizure should direct their evaluation toward the diagnosis of the cause of the fever.
4. Seizures are the presenting sign of meningitis in about 13 to 16% of children, and in about 30 to 35% of these children (primarily children <18 months), meningeal signs and symptoms may be lacking. Thus, an LP should be strongly considered in such children.

BOX 13-16. CLINICAL FEATURES OF FEBRILE SEIZURES

- Incidence of febrile seizures: 2 to 5% of all children
- Types of febrile seizures

a. Simple febrile seizures
   (1) Seizures are generalized (tonic, clonic, tonic-clonic, rarely atonic).
   (2) Duration <15 minutes
   (3) Seizures *do not* recur within 24 hours.
   (4) Seizures *do not* exhibit any postictal neurologic abnormalities (including Todd's paralysis)

b. Complex febrile seizures (if one or more of the following features are present, the seizure is called a complex febrile seizure)
   (1) Partial onset or focal features during the seizure
   (2) Prolonged duration (>10 or 15 minutes)
   (3) Recurrent febrile seizures within 24 hours of the first episode

c. Febrile status epilepticus
   (1) Febrile seizures with duration 30 minutes or longer *or*
   (2) A series of short seizures without regaining consciousness in between the episodes

BOX 13-17. DIFFERENTIAL DIAGNOSIS OF SEIZURES ASSOCIATED WITH FEVER

- Meningitis
- Other central nervous system infection (e.g., encephalitis)
- Electrolyte imbalance associated with acute infection (e.g., acute gastroenteritis with hypo- or hypernatremia, hypoglycemia)
- Epilepsy with acute infection from any etiology
- Shigellosis (dehydration and related complications such as hyponatremia, hypoglycemia, or hypocalcemia)

DIAGNOSIS SEIZURES AND EPILEPSY

Definitions

1. *Seizure:* A seizure is a manifestation of an abnormal and excessive synchronized discharge of a set of neurons, with intermittent stereotypical, usually unprovoked, disturbance of consciousness, behavior, emotion, motor function, or sensation as a result of the cortical neuronal discharge.
2. *Convulsion:* A lay term used to describe an episode of excessive abnormal muscle contractions, usually bilateral, which may be sustained or interrupted.
3. *Epilepsy:* A condition in which a patient is prone to recurrent unprovoked seizures.
4. *Aura:* An aura is that portion of the seizure experienced before loss of consciousness occurs and for which memory is retained. It is a subjective ictal phenomenon that may precede an observable seizure. When it occurs alone, it constitutes a simple partial seizure.
5. *Automatism:* A more or less coordinated, repetitive, motor activity usually occurring when cognition is impaired and for which the subject is usually amnesic afterward. This may often resemble a voluntary movement and may consist of an inappropriate continuation of ongoing preictal motor activity.
6. *Status epilepticus* (see page 545): An ongoing condition in which seizures continue, or are repeated without regaining consciousness, for a period of 30 minutes. Recent definitions have shortened the duration to 5 to 10 minutes.
7. *Todd's phenomenon:* Transient focal neurologic deficit following a focal or secondarily generalized seizure.

Etiology

1. Seizures may be provoked by an acute event, when they are known as symptomatic seizures. The acute event may be fever, head trauma, electrolyte imbalance, hypo- or hyperglycemia, meningitis, encephalitis, etc.
2. Epilepsy (recurrent unprovoked seizures) may be cryptogenic, idiopathic, or genetic. Epilepsy may also result from a congenital malformation of the brain or a known etiology resulting in a focal injury, which becomes epileptogenic leading to unprovoked seizures.

Associated Clinical Features

1. Epidemiology of seizures
   a. The overall incidence of epilepsy between birth to 16 years is 40 per 100,000 births.
   b. In general, 1% of all children have at least one seizure by the age of 5 years.
   c. About 0.4 to 0.8% of all children have epilepsy by the age of 11 years.
   d. Generalized tonic-clonic seizures and partial seizures constitute 75% of all the seizure types in childhood. Absence epilepsy comprises 15%, and other generalized epilepsies (including catastrophic syndromes) make up the remaining 10%.
2. Generalized seizures are of the following types:
   a. Generalized tonic-clonic: Loss of consciousness, with tonic increase in muscle tone; followed by rhythmic (clonic) jerks, which subside slowly; the patient is unconscious after the seizure and recovers slowly; tongue biting or incontinence or both may occur.
   b. Absence: Rapid onset, with brief period of unresponsiveness (average 10 seconds) and rapid recovery; there may be increased or decreased muscle tone, automatisms or mild clonic movements. The seizure may be precipitated by hyperventilation.
   c. Myoclonic: Sudden brief (<100 milliseconds) involuntary single or multiple contractions of muscles or muscle groups of variable topography (axial, proximal limb, distal)
   d. Clonic: Regularly repetitive involuntary movements involving the same muscle groups, at a frequency of 2 to 3 per second.
   e. Tonic: A sustained increase in muscle contraction lasting a few seconds to minutes.
   f. Dystonic: Sustained contraction of both agonist and antagonist muscles producing athetoid or twisting movements, which when prolonged may produce abnormal postures.
   g. Epileptic spasm: A sudden flexion, extension, or mixed flexion-extension of predominantly proximal and truncal muscles that is usually more sustained than a myoclonic, but not as sustained as a tonic seizure (i.e., ~1 second).
3. Partial seizures have features depending on the lobe of origin:
   a. Temporal lobe:
      1) Seizures arising from this region are commonly preceded by an aura, which may be autonomic and/or psychic, and some sensory phenomena (e.g., rising epigastric sensation). This is followed by motor arrest, followed by oral automatisms (chewing, mouth movements), then reactive automatisms.
      2) Postictal confusion is common.
   b. Frontal lobe:
      1) Frequent short attacks with impairment of consciousness
      2) Rapid secondary generalization with prominent motor manifestations; automatisms are complex, stereotyped, and gestural at onset.
      3) Urinary incontinence common
      4) Minimal or no postictal confusion
      5) Drop attacks may occur.
   c. Occipital lobe:
      1) Fleeting visual symptoms include positive phenomena (sparks, flashes, phosphenes), negative phenomena (scotoma, hemianopsia, amaurosis),

perceptive illusions (macropsia, micropsia, metamorphopsia), and complex visual perceptions.
   2) At times, initial signs may also be clonic and/or tonic deviation of the eyes and head to the opposite side, palpebral jerks and forced closure of the eyelids, a sensation of ocular oscillations, headache, or migraine.
  d. Partial seizures involving the parietal lobe, supplementary motor area, or motor cortex are uncommon and present with varied manifestations.

4. Seizure recurrence risk:
   a. After a single unprovoked seizure, the risk of a second seizure is approximately 40%. This rises to 80% after a second unprovoked seizure.
   b. 75% of all recurrences occur within the first 6 months, and very few recurrences occur after 2 years.

5. Approximately 70% of children are able to discontinue medication after a 2-year seizure-free period. Of the remaining children, when medications are restarted, about 50% are seizure-free for 2 years, and a 70% success rate is seen with a second attempt of medication withdrawal.

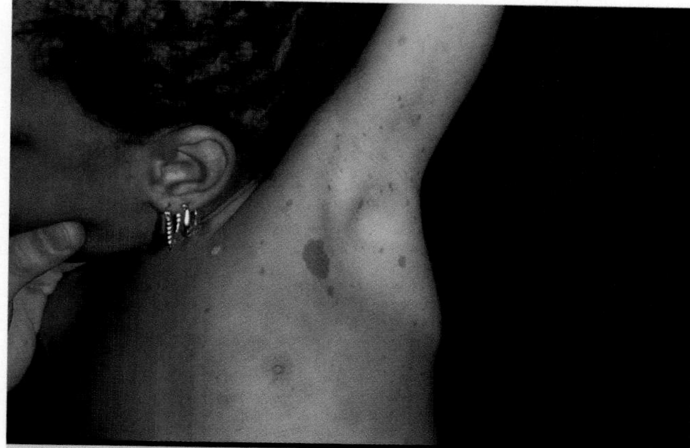

Figure 13-18. Crowe's Sign and Café au Lait Spots in Neurofibromatosis

Tiny freckle-like lesions in the axillae are highly characteristic of neurofibromatosis. These lesions were seen in a 6-year-old girl who presented with one episode of afebrile seizure.

Consultation

Neurology

Emergency Department Treatment and Disposition

1. Approach to a child with a seizure
   a. History: A detailed history of the event is necessary. In addition, the history should be taken to look for the probable cause of epilepsy. Important points include birth and developmental history, history of head trauma, CNS infections, alcohol or drug abuse, and family history of epilepsy.
   b. Physical examination: A thorough general physical and neurologic examination should be performed.
      1) On the general exam, one must look for neurocutaneous stigmata (café-au-lait spots, hypopigmented macules, port-wine stain) and other congenital anomalies (Fig. 13-18).
      2) On neurologic examination, focal deficits and asymmetry of findings should be sought.
      3) If absence epilepsy is suspected, hyperventilation should be performed for 3 minutes in the outpatient setting to trigger one of the typical seizures.

2. Practice parameter: Evaluating a first nonfebrile seizure in children:
   a. Goals of immediate evaluation:
      1) A careful history and neurologic examination should be done to determine if a seizure has occurred, and if so, if it is the child's first episode.
      2) The next step is to determine the cause of the seizure.
   b. Laboratory studies:
      1) Lab tests should be ordered based on individual clinical circumstances that include suggestive historic or clinical findings such as vomiting, diarrhea, dehydration, or failure to return to baseline alertness.
      2) Toxicology screening should be considered if there is any question of drug exposure or substance abuse.
      3) Lumbar puncture: In a child with a first nonfebrile seizure, LP is of limited value and should be considered primarily when there is concern about possible meningitis or encephalitis.
   c. An EEG is recommended as part of the neurodiagnostic evaluation of the child with an apparent first unprovoked seizure (an EEG will help to identify interictal abnormalities and provide information about the location of the seizure focus).
   d. Neuroimaging studies:
      1) Emergent neuroimaging should be performed in a child of any age who exhibits a postictal focal deficit (Todd's paresis) that does not quickly resolve, or who has not returned to baseline within several hours after the seizure.
      2) If a neuroimaging study is obtained, MRI is the preferred modality (since small lesions are better delineated due to higher resolution).

3. In the emergency room setting, when patients come in with a first episode of seizure, a CT scan of the head is performed only if a serious structural lesion is suspected (in all other circumstances, an MRI of the brain is preferably done on a nonemergent basis). Indications for CT include patients with any of the following:
   a. New-onset focal/partial seizures
   b. New focal neurologic deficits
   c. Persistent altered mental status
   d. Recent trauma

e. Fever (e.g. suspected CNS infection)
f. Persistent headache
g. History of malignancy
h. Immune deficiency states
i. Patients on anticoagulants

4. Practice parameter: Treatment of the child with a first unprovoked seizure:
   a. The majority of children who experience a first unprovoked seizure will have few or no recurrences.
   b. Only approximately 10% will go on to have many (≥10) seizures regardless of therapy.
   c. Treatment with an antiepileptic drug (AED) after a first seizure as opposed to after a second seizure has not shown to improve prognosis for long-term seizure remission.
   d. Treatment with an AED is not indicated for the prevention of the development of epilepsy.
   e. Treatment with an AED may be considered in circumstances in which the benefits of reducing the risk of a second seizure outweigh the risks of pharmacologic and psychosocial side effects.

5. First-line antiepileptic drugs in partial seizures:
   a. Simple: carbamazepine, phenytoin, valproic acid
   b. Complex: carbamazepine, phenytoin, valproic acid

6. First-line antiepileptic drugs in generalized seizures:
   a. Generalized tonic-clonic: carbamazepine, phenytoin, valproic acid
   b. Absence: ethosuximide, valproic acid
   c. Myoclonic: valproic acid
   d. Clonic: valproic acid

7. First aid: Most seizures occur away from a medical center, and appropriate initial first aid management is essential. The guidelines provided by the Epilepsy Foundation of America are useful for teaching parents (see febrile seizures, page 538)

Clinical Pearls: Seizures and Epilepsy

1. A majority of children who experience a first unprovoked seizure will have few or no recurrences.

2. An EEG is recommended as part of the neurodiagnostic evaluation of the child with an apparent first unprovoked seizure, to predict the risk of recurrence and to classify the seizure type and epilepsy syndrome.

3. The decision to perform other studies including laboratory tests, LP, and neuroimaging, for the purpose of determining the cause of the seizure and detecting potentially treatable abnormalities, will depend on age of the patient and the specific clinical circumstances.

BOX 13-18. CAUSES OF SEIZURES

- Inherited genetic (juvenile myoclonic epilepsy, absence)
- Acquired
  - (1) Trauma (immediate and posttraumatic)
  - (2) Infection (e.g., meningitis, encephalitis, abscess, toxoplasmosis)
  - (3) Vascular disease (e.g., stroke, intracranial hemorrhage)
  - (4) Hippocampal sclerosis
  - (5) Tumors (e.g., meningioma [Fig. 13-19], glioma, metastatic disease)
  - (6) Neurodegenerative disorders (e.g., neuronal storage diseases)
  - (7) Metabolic disorders (e.g., hypoglycemia, hyperglycemia, hypoxia, electrolyte disturbance [Na^+, Ca^{2+}, Mg^{2+})]
  - (8) Toxic (e.g., alcohol, drugs)
- Congenital
  - (1) Cortical dysplasia/dysgenesis (heterotopias, microgyria, pachygyria)
  - (2) Vascular malformations (e.g., Sturge-Weber syndrome)
  - (3) Prenatal injury (e.g., antenatal stroke, TORCH infections)
- Precipitating factors for seizures
  - (1) Stress
  - (2) Sleep deprivation and fatigue
  - (3) Metabolic disturbances
  - (4) Toxins and drugs
  - (5) Alcohol and alcohol withdrawal
  - (6) Menstrual cycle

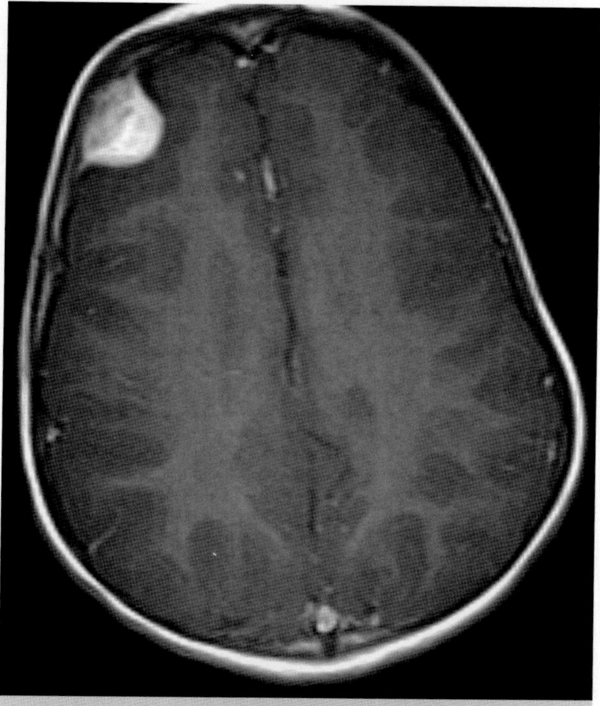

Figure 13-19. Meningioma Presenting with New-Onset Focal Seizure

A 22-month-old toddler presented with a left sided focal seizure with generalization lasting for about 3 to 5 minutes. While waiting in the ED, he had another left sided focal seizure with generalization. A noncontrast CT scan of the brain showed a right frontal extra-axial mass with peripheral curvilinear calcification. His contrast-enhanced axial T1 weighted MRI showed an enhancing extra-axial right frontal mass with "dural tail" anteriorly and posteriorly. Based on these imaging findings, meningioma was considered (even though this is an unlikely age for meningioma to present).

Modified and Reproduced with permission from: Shorvon SD. In: Handbook of Epilepsy Treatment. London Blackwell Science. 2000, p. 19.

BOX 13-19. CLASSIFICATION OF SEIZURES

The International League Against Epilepsy classifies seizures into the following types:

I. Partial or focal
   a. Simple partial, where there is no change in consciousness
      i. With motor symptoms
      ii. With somatosensory or special sensory symptoms
      iii. With autonomic symptoms
      iv. With psychic symptoms
   b. Complex partial, where there is alteration in consciousness
      i. With motor symptoms
      ii. With somatosensory or special sensory symptoms
      iii. With autonomic symptoms
      iv. With psychic symptoms
      v. With automatisms
   c. Partial with secondarily generalized seizure

II. Generalized
   a. Absence
   b. Myoclonic
   c. Clonic
   d. Tonic
   e. Tonic-clonic
   f. Atonic

III. Unclassified

Modified and Reproduced with permission from: Dreiffuss FE and Nordli DR Jr. Classification of Epilepsies in childhood. In: Pediatric Epilepsy. Diagnosis and Therapy. Pellock JM, Dodson WE and Bourgeois BF (eds). 2nd Edition. New York, Demos Med Publishing, Inc. 2001, p. 71.

BOX 13-20. DIFFERENTIAL DIAGNOSIS OF SEIZURES

- Other paroxysmal disorders that occur commonly in children, including:

a. Episodes without alteration in consciousness:
   (1) Tics
   (2) Rhythmic motor habits
   (3) Mannerisms
   (4) Shuddering spells
   (5) Rigors (with any febrile illness)
   (6) Jitteriness (newborn period)
   (7) Hypnagogic jerks (sleep myoclonus)
   (8) Benign myoclonus of infancy
   (9) Benign paroxysmal vertigo
   (10) Gastroesophageal reflux
   (11) Cardiac dysrhythmias
   (12) Munchausen's syndrome by proxy
   (13) Nonepileptic (pseudo) seizures

b. Episodes associated with change in consciousness may be mistaken for complex partial seizures.
   (1) Delirium (with any febrile illness)
   (2) Syncope (simple faint)
   (3) Cyanotic breath-holding attacks
   (4) Pallid syncopal attacks
   (5) Night terrors
   (6) Migraine (the aura, or confusional and basilar artery variants),
   (7) Narcolepsy
   (8) Munchausen's syndrome by proxy

DIAGNOSIS STATUS EPILEPTICUS AND ACUTE REPETITIVE SEIZURES

Definitions

1. Status epilepticus is defined as:
   a. An epileptic seizure that is so frequently repeated or so prolonged as to create a fixed and lasting condition (current definition set forth by the International League Against Epilepsy and the World Health Organization)
   b. Status epilepticus is functionally defined as a seizure lasting >30 minutes or recurrent seizures lasting >30 minutes from which the patient does not regain consciousness.
   c. A more practical definition of status epilepticus: Any seizure lasting >5 to 10 minutes, since the vast majority of self-limiting generalized convulsive seizures stop within 2 to 3 minutes of onset, almost all ceasing within 5 minutes.
2. Acute repetitive seizures (also termed serial seizures): Seizures recurring at frequent intervals, with full recovery between seizures
3. Seizure clusters: Clusters of seizures occurring regularly at certain times in some patients (e.g., around menstruation)

Associated Clinical Features

1. Status epilepticus
   a. One-third of cases of status epilepticus present as the initial manifestation of epilepsy.
   b. One-third of cases occur in previously diagnosed epilepsy.
   c. One-third of cases occur as a result of an acute isolated brain insult.
2. In patients with epilepsy, status epilepticus occurs in 0.5 to 6.6%.
3. Status epilepticus is more common in infants and young toddlers, and >50% of cases occur below the age of 3 years.
4. The overall mortality used to be 10 to 30%, but it is much less in children, as low as 3%. The morbidity of status epilepticus ranges from 11 to 15%.

Consultation

Neurology

Emergency Department Treatment and Disposition

1. Goals of treating status epilepticus include stopping the seizure safely and in a timely manner and minimizing treatment-related morbidity.
2. The systemic effects of status epilepticus should be understood and side effects of treatment anticipated (sedation, cardiovascular and respiratory compromise).
3. Airway, breathing, and circulatory support must be the first steps in management. Vital signs, pulse oximetry, and ECG should be closely monitored. Ensure adequate brain oxygenation and cardiorespiratory function.
4. Fingerstick assessment of glucose should be done as soon as possible to detect hypoglycemia. If hypoglycemia is found or suspected, IV glucose is administered (see page 521). In adolescents, IV thiamine 100 mg should be administered first.
5. Emergency antiepileptic drug therapy is needed if the convulsions persist for more than 10 minutes or longer than is usual for the individual patient.
   a. Fast-acting benzodiazepines are the traditional choice.
   b. Medication may be given either IV or rectally when IV access is not available.
   c. Give adequate doses of an effective drug, and watch carefully for hypoventilation and apnea.
      1) Diazepam: IV dosage is 0.3 mg/kg
      2) Lorazepam: IV dosage is 0.1 mg/kg
      3) Rectal diazepam gel: dose 0.5 mg/kg (rectal preparation comes in a premeasured syringe [2.5-, 5-, 10-, 15-, and 20-mg syringes] making it easy to deliver and absorption is rapid, which helps to interrupt the seizure clusters or repetitive seizures)
6. Hyperthermia can occur in 28 to 79% of patients, and should be recognized.
7. Laboratory tests should include CBC, chemistries, and as indicated toxicology screening and anticonvulsant levels.
8. If acute trauma is suspected, an emergent CT scan of the head should be performed.
9. Admit the patient to the ICU for further management and monitoring.
10. If the seizures continue or the patient continues to show an altered mental state for 30 to 60 minutes, a bedside EEG should be obtained, and if available, continuous bedside EEG monitoring is ideal. If the child's mental status is improving, an EEG may still be necessary, but not urgent.
11. Maintain patient on IV anticonvulsant medications during the initial evaluation. Further decisions about long-term therapy will depend on the results of the evaluation.

Clinical Pearls: Status Epilepticus

1. Status epilepticus is a medical emergency.

2. Identify precipitating factors such as hypoglycemia, electrolyte imbalance, lowered drug levels, infection, and fever (Figs. 13-20 and 13-21).
3. Consider giving a specific antidote if status epilepticus is due to toxicity from drugs (e.g., pyridoxine for acute isoniazid-induced status epilepticus or refractory seizures; see Fig. 17-21).
4. Terminate clinical and electrical seizure activity in status epilepticus as rapidly as possible.

BOX 13-21. CLASSIFICATION OF STATUS EPILEPTICUS

- Generalized
  (1) Convulsive: Tonic, tonic-clonic, clonic, or myoclonic
  (2) Nonconvulsive: absence
- Partial
  (1) Convulsive: Tonic or clonic
  (2) Nonconvulsive: simple or complex partial

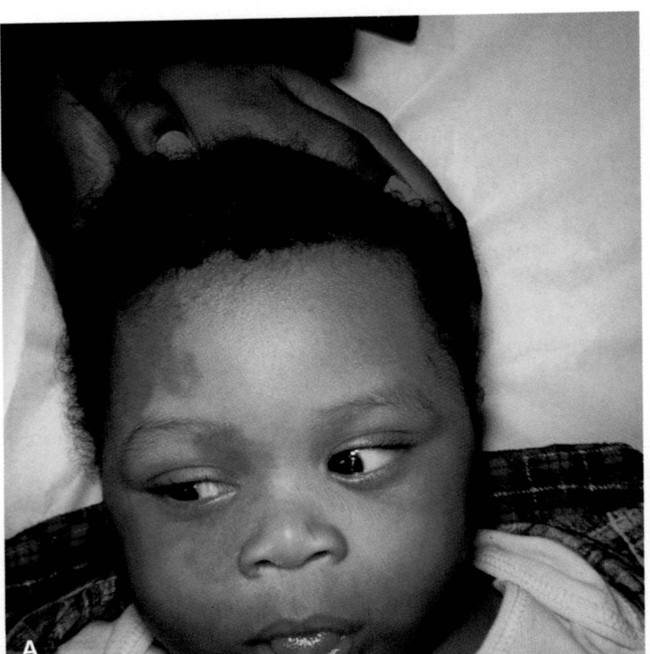

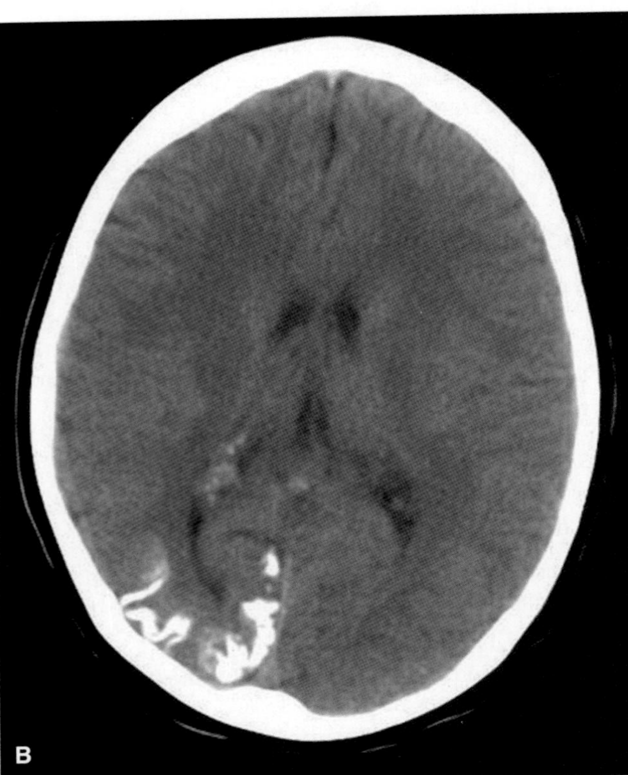

Figure 13-20. Port-Wine Stain and Intracranial Calcification in Sturge-Weber Syndrome

A. Port-wine stain in a patient who was brought to the ED with status epilepticus. As seen here, the most common location of a port-wine stain is the face. (PWS may also get confused with a red or purple bruise of inflicted injury or abuse, especially when it is very extensive as in this case). When a PWS is localized to the trigeminal area of the face (especially around the eyelids), a diagnosis of Sturge-Weber syndrome must be considered. *B*. Noncontrast CT of the head showing "tram-track" calcifications of the right occipital cortex with atrophy. An enlarged right-sided choroid plexus is also noted which may be secondary to an angioma.

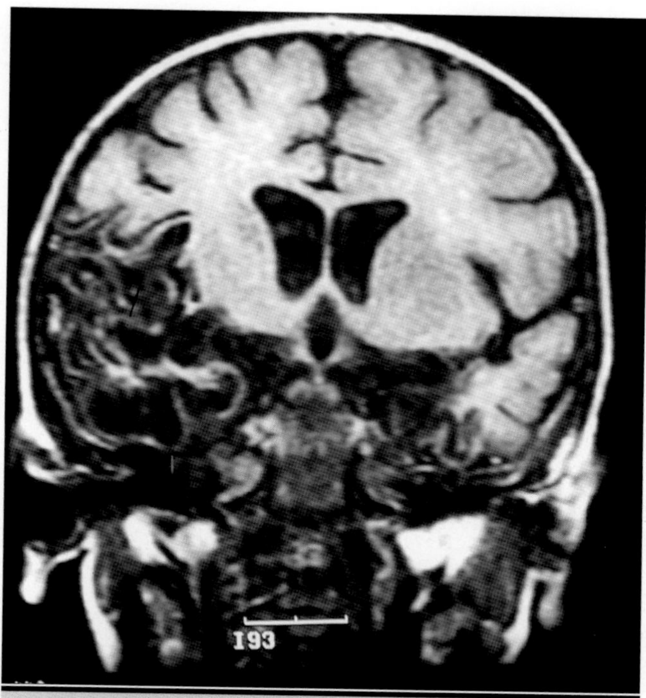

Figure 13-21. Herpes Encephalitis

An 18-month-old child was brought in status epilepticus to the ED. Past history was positive for HSV encephalitis at the age of 6 months in Puerto Rico. This patient cannot talk or sit and has developed choreoathetoid movements and seizures with extension of the legs and flexion of the arms. MRI showed encephalomalacia of the right temporoparietal lobe.

BOX 13-22. STATUS EPILEPTICUS: PRECIPITATING EVENTS

- Antiepileptic drug alterations
  (1) Withdrawal
  (2) Noncompliance
  (3) Drug interactions
  (4) Toxicity (e.g. carbamazepine toxicity)
- Infections
  (1) Central nervous system (e.g. meningitis)
  (2) Systemic
- Toxins
  (1) Alcohol
  (2) Drugs (e.g., isoniazid, bupropion)
  (3) Poisons (see mnemonic "CAMPHOR BALLS," Box 17-2)
  (4) Convulsive agents (e.g., high dose of penicillin)
- Structural
  (1) Trauma
  (2) Ischemic stroke
  (3) Hemorrhagic stroke
  (4) Acute hydrocephalus
- Hormonal change
- Electrolyte imbalance
- Diagnostic procedures and medications
- Emotional stress
- Progressive-degenerative disease
- Sleep deprivation
- Primary apnea
- Cardiac arrhythmias
- Fever

Modified and Reproduced with permission from: Leszczyszyn DJ and Pellock JM. Status Epilepticus. In: Pellock JM, Dodson WE and Bourgeois BF. Pediatric Epilepsy. Diagnosis and Therapy. 2nd ed. Demos Medical Publishing, Inc. 2001, p. 276.

BOX 13-23. PHYSIOLOGIC CHANGES IN TONIC-CLONIC STATUS EPILEPTICUS

Phase 1: Compensation

Cerebral changes

Increased blood flow
Increased metabolism
Increased glucose and O_2 utilization
Increased lactate concentration
Increased glucose concentration

Systemic and metabolic changes

Hyperglycemia
Lactic acidosis

Autonomic and cardiovascular changes

Hypertension (initial)
Increased cardiac output
Increased central venous pressure
Massive catecholamine release
Tachycardia
Cardiac dysrhythmia
Salivation
Hyperpyrexia
Vomiting
Incontinence

Phase 2: Decompensation

Cerebral changes

Failure of cerebral autoregulation (thus cerebral blood flow becomes dependent on systemic blood pressure)
Hypoxia
Hypoglycemia
Falling lactate concentrations
Falling energy state
Rise in intracranial pressure and cerebral edema

Systemic and metabolic changes

Hypoglycemia
Hyponatremia
Hypokalemia/hyperkalemia
Metabolic and respiratory acidosis
Hepatic and renal dysfunction
Consumptive coagulopathy, disseminated intravascular coagulation
Multiorgan failure
Rhabdomyolysis
Myoglobinuria
Leukocytosis

Autonomic and cardiovascular changes

Systemic hypoxia
Falling blood pressure
Falling cardiac output
Pulmonary edema
Pulmonary embolism
Respiratory collapse
Cardiac failure
Cardiac dysrhythmia
Hyperpyrexia

Modified and Reproduced with permission from: Shorvon SD. In: Handbook of Epilepsy Treatment. Blackwell Science, 2000, p. 176.

BOX 13-24. PROTOCOL FOR STATUS EPILEPTICUS

Time from start of intervention	*Procedure*
• 0–5 min	Monitor heart rate, respiratory rate, blood pressure, pulse oximetry, temperature, ECG ABCs of life support Insert IV line Collect blood for glucose, CBC, chemistry, anticonvulsant levels (if indicated)
• 6–9 min	IV fluids IV bolus 2 mL/kg of 50% glucose
• 10–30 min	IV Lorazepam 0.1 mg/kg, at rate of 1–2 mg/min (maximal dose: 2 mg/dose) IV Fosphenytoin 20 mg PE/kg (PE = phenytoin equivalent), at rate of 150 mg PE/min (monitor ECG and blood pressure) Repeat IV fosphenytoin 5–10 mg PE/kg if seizures persist
• 31–59 min	If seizures persist, IV phenobarbital 20 mg/kg, at a rate not to exceed 50 mg/min (anticipate intubation)
• 60 min	Stage of refractory status; choices include: (1) IV Midazolam 0.2 mg/kg, followed by 1–10 μg/kg per min IV infusion (2) IV Pentobarbital 5–15 mg/kg, followed by 0.5–5 mg/kg per hour IV infusion (3) IV Propofol 1–2 mg/kg, followed by 2–10 mg/kg per hour IV infusion (4) EEG monitoring should be performed to look for burst suppression pattern (5) Maintenance of IV infusions should continue for 12–24 hours and then tapered, while checking the EEG for reappearance of seizure activity; if clinical seizures or generalized discharges persist on EEG, then the infusion is increased until burst suppression; if not, then the infusion is gradually tapered over 12–24 hours
• 61–80 min	If seizures are still not controlled, anesthesia should be called to give general anesthesia with inhaled anesthetics and neuromuscular blockade

DIAGNOSIS

STROKE

Definition

1. Stroke is defined as the sudden occlusion or rupture of cerebral blood vessels resulting in focal cerebral damage causing clinical neurological deficits.
2. Types of strokes
   a. Arterial ischemic stroke (AIS)
      1) Embolic
      2) Thrombotic
   b. Sinovenous thrombosis (SVT)
   c. Hemorrhagic stroke

Associated Clinical Features

1. The incidence of pediatric stroke is 2.5 to 2.7 per 100,000 per year.
2. There are fundamental differences in stroke in children compared to adults.
3. Strokes in children are relatively rare and frequently result in lack of recognition and delay in diagnosis.
4. Radiographic imaging of the pediatric patient with stroke has dramatically improved in the past decade. Radiographic evaluation has significantly improved the assessment and treatment of stroke (Fig. 13-22 and 13-23).
   a. CT scan
      1) A noncontrast CT scan remains the modality of choice in acute stroke and is the preferred mode to look for fresh blood and subarachnoid hemorrhage.
      2) A CT scan is often normal within the first 12 hours after an ischemic stroke. In children, CT findings of ischemic stroke are similar to those in adults.

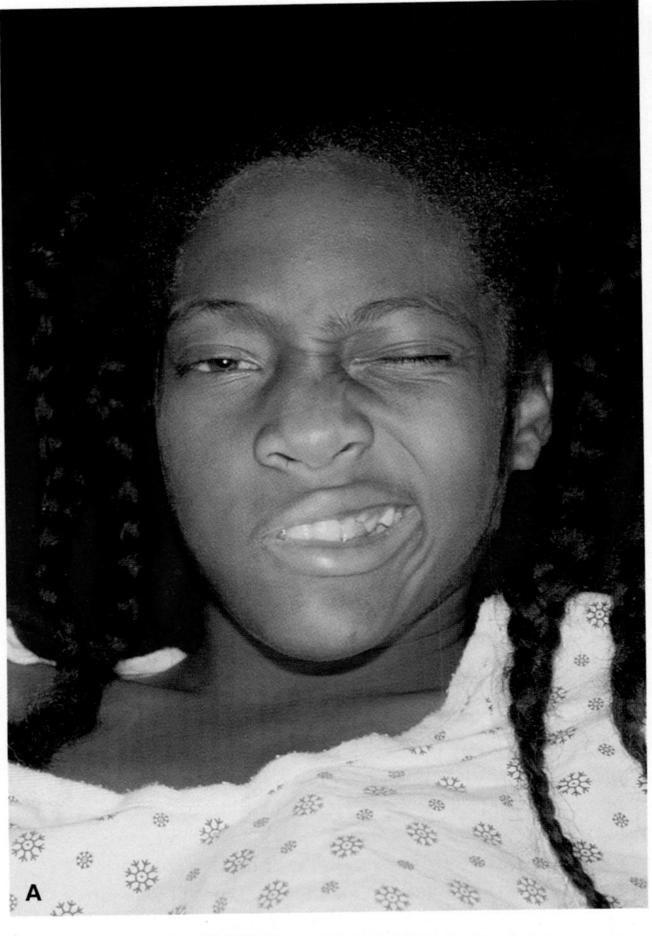

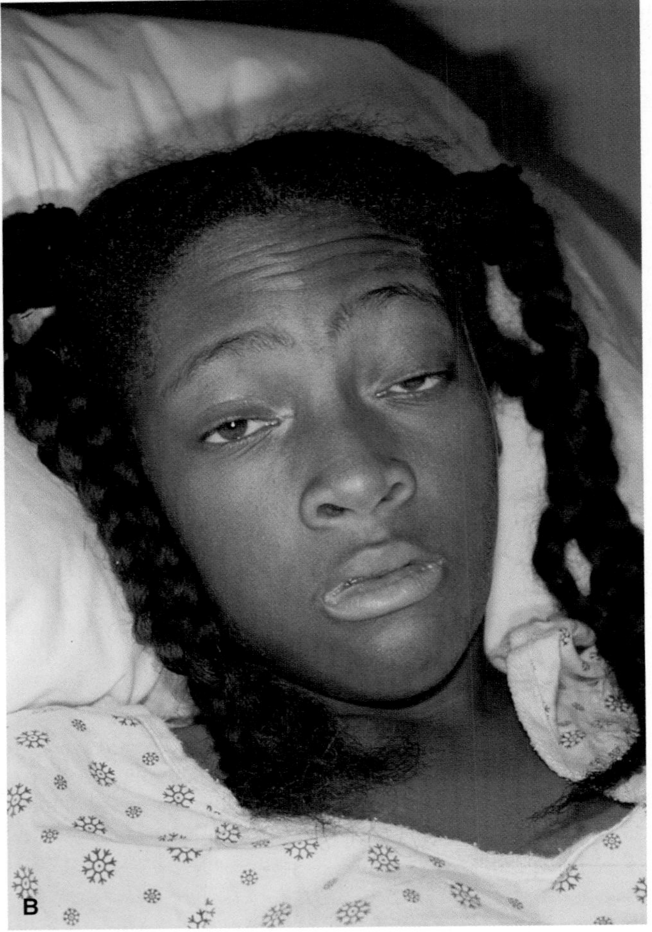

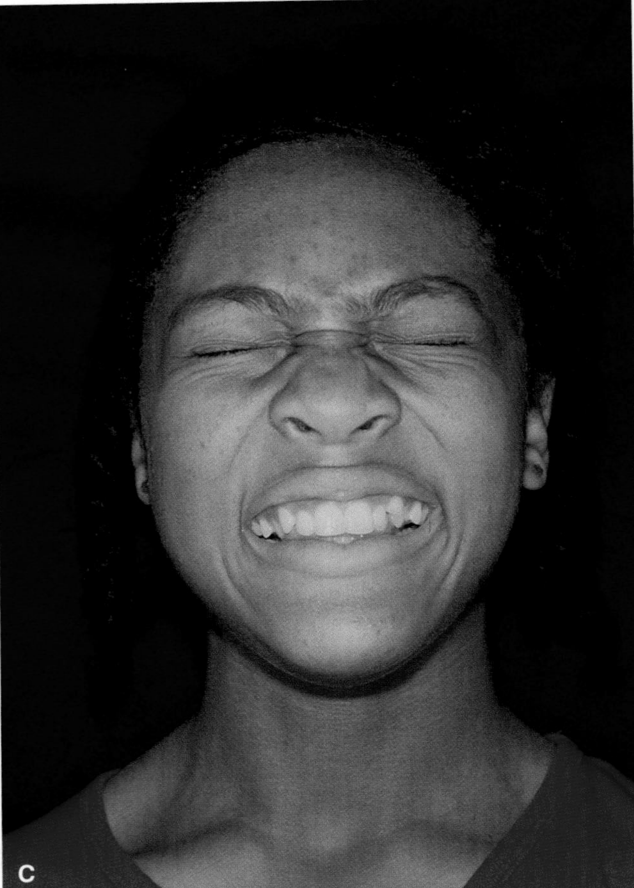

Figure 13-22. Right Facial Palsy (Central Facial Palsy or Upper Motor Neuron Palsy) Presenting with Stroke (Ischemic Stroke; Middle Cerebral Artery [MCA] Infarct)

A. Asymmetric movements of the facial muscles, inability to close the right eye (but ability to close the left eye), the angle of the mouth is deviated to the left (absence of movement of the right angle of the mouth), and flattening of the right nasolabial folds are seen. *B*. Ability to wrinkle the forehead equally on both sides and to raise the eyebrows symmetrically is preserved. Right-sided facial weakness involving the lower part of the face with sparing of the upper part (forehead) are classic findings for upper motor neuron facial palsy (in lower motor neuron facial palsy, the ability to wrinkle the forehead on the same side as the palsy is absent). *C*. Full recovery (after 6 months) from the right facial palsy is seen. Her smile is symmetrical and she is able to close her eyes well bilaterally. While in the gymnasium this 12-year-old-girl complained of nausea, vomiting, and headache. After coming home, she did not feel well, was agitated, and went to sleep. An hour later, she woke up with right-sided weakness (right facial palsy, right hemiparesis and aphasia). This history is suggestive of a thrombotic ischemic stroke (unlike acute history for an embolic stroke). Her diagnostic work-up including screening for protein C and S deficiency and collagen diseases was negative.

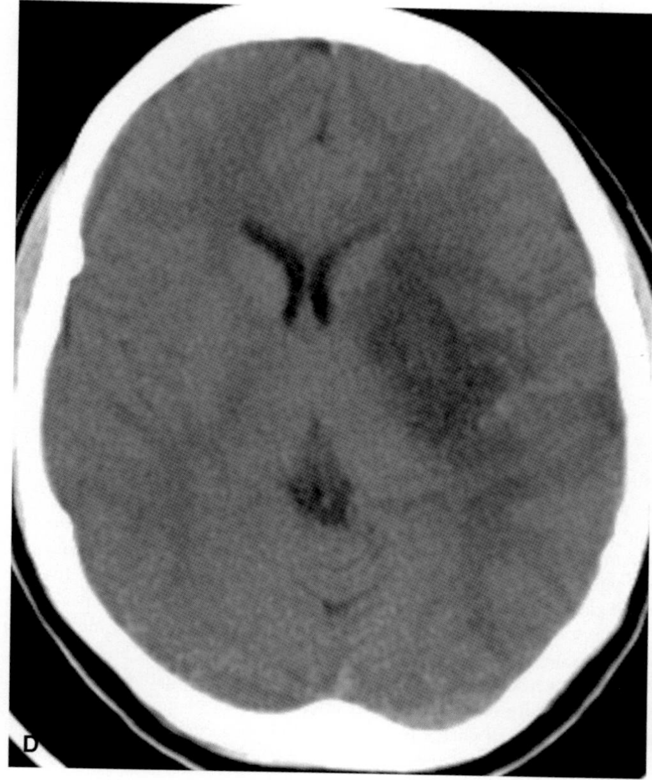

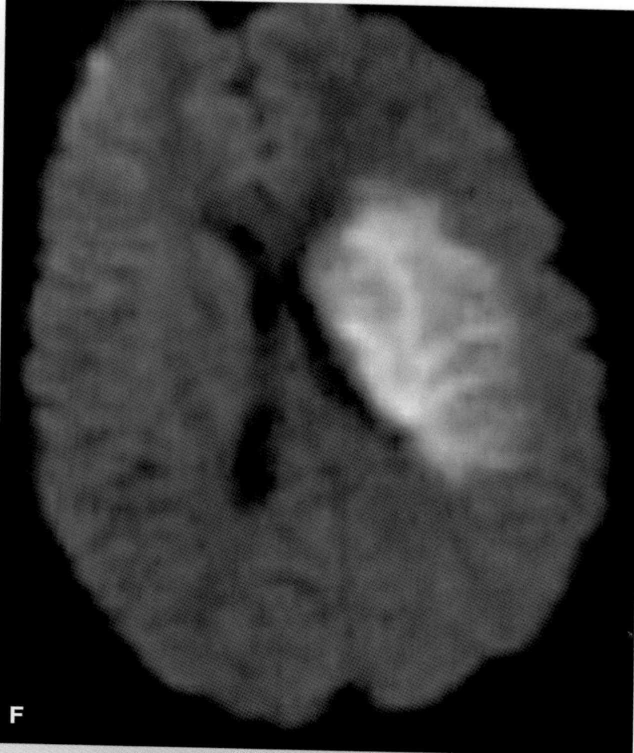

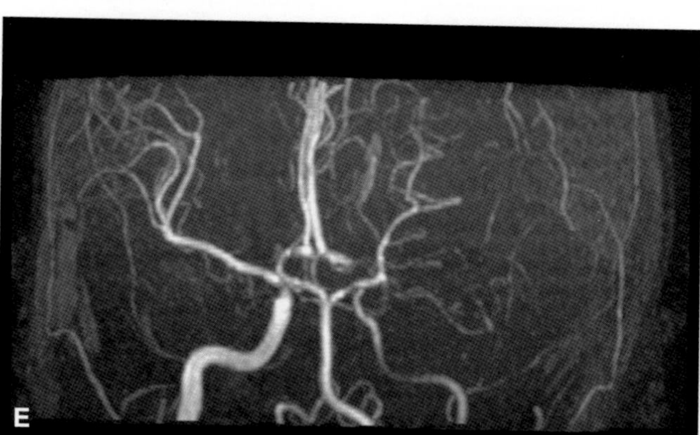

Figure 13-22. Ischemic Stroke; Middle Cerebral Artery [MCA] Infarct (Continued)

D. A non-contrast axial CT image of the head shows a left MCA infarct (an area of low attenuation) involving the left lentiform nucleus and parietal cortex. There is a evidence of a mass effect with a mild midline shift towards the right and mild compression of the left lateral ventricle. Other CT findings included left MCA hyperdense and areas of infarct involving left frontal temporal lobes including left basal ganglia. *E*. MRI and MRA with Gadolinium Images. 3 D time of flight MRA of the circle of Willis reveals decreased flow in the left internal carotid artery (along its entire course) and MCA with non visualization of sylvian branches. *F*. Diffusion weighted image of the brain reveals a large acute MCA infarct in the left basal ganglia and parietal lobe.

Ischemic infarcts appear as low-density lesion in a vascular area. Hemorrhagic infarcts have additional high-density components.

b. MRI is undoubtedly more sensitive than CT in detecting small and multiple infarcts. Diffusion weighted and perfusion weighted imaging have improved early detection and specifically ischemic injury.
c. Magnetic resonance angiography (MRA)
    1) MRA can be performed at the same time as MRI and adds valuable information regarding the cerebral arteries and angiomatous malformations.
    2) MRA is becoming a realistic noninvasive alternative to conventional angiography, particularly in children.
    3) MRA has been found to correlate well with conventional angiography in children with ischemic stroke.
d. Magnetic resonance venography (MRV) is the diagnostic study of choice in sinovenous thrombosis.

Consultations

Neurology (essential, as strokes in children may have many causes, are difficult to diagnose, and may have therapeutic implications), neurosurgery (hemorrhagic stroke), hematology (for transfusion in patients with sickle cell disease) and cardiology (if patient has congenital heart disease or cardiac disease is suspected)

Emergency Department Treatment and Disposition

1. Stabilize vital signs and intubate if the patient has increased intracranial pressure.

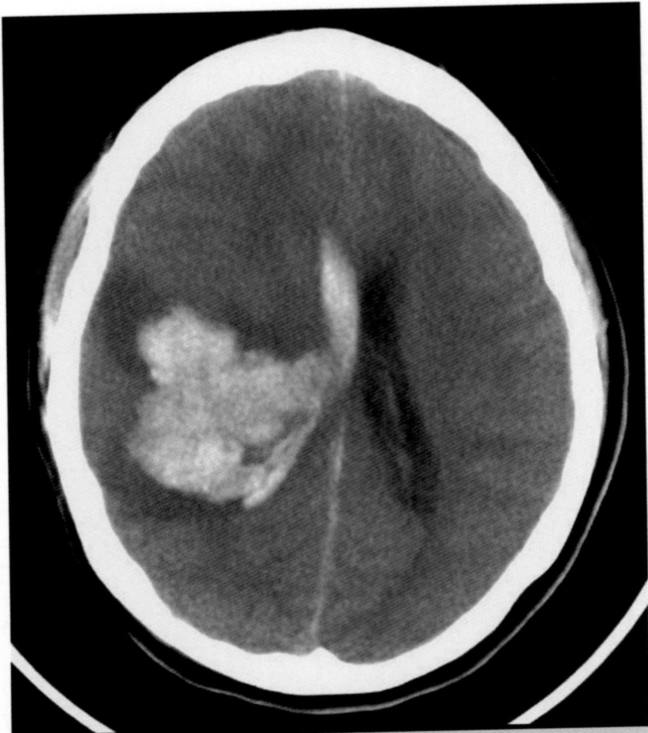

Figure 13-23. Hemorrhagic Stroke due to Intraparenchymal Hemorrhage

A noncontrast axial CT image of the head shows a large area of hyperdensity (hematoma) involving the right parietal area with surrounding hypodensity (representing associated edema) and intraventricular extension to the right lateral ventricle (the third and fourth ventricles and the right temporal and frontal regions were also involved). A significant mass effect with a significant right-to-left midline shift is also seen. This 13-year-old girl presented to the ED with a complaint of headache, stiff neck, and a history of fever. She was clinically suspected to have aseptic meningitis (CSF examination showed RBCs 720/mm^3, WBC 11/mm^3, protein 60 mg/dL, and glucose 65 mg/dL). All her cultures were negative, and she improved markedly to be discharged after 48 hours of hospitalization. Within 8 hours after discharge from the hospital, she complained of severe headache followed by seizures. On arrival to the ED, she was comatose with these CT findings.

BOX 13-25. COMMON ETIOLOGIES AND RISK FACTORS FOR STROKE IN CHILDREN

- *Cardiac abnormalities*
  - (1) Congenital heart disease
    - a. Atrial septal defect
    - b. Ventricular septal defect
    - c. Cyanotic heart disease
  - (2) Acquired heart disease
    - a. Myocarditis
    - b. Endocarditis
    - c. Arrhythmias
- *Vascular abnormalities*
  - (1) Vasculitis
    - a. Systemic lupus erythematosus
    - b. Primary cerebral angiitis
    - c. Meningitis
    - d. Varicella
  - (2) Vasculopathy
    - a. Moyamoya
    - b. Neurofibromatosis
    - c. Ehler-Danlos syndrome
  - (3) Vasospastic disorders
    - a. Migraine
    - b. Alternating hemiplegia
  - (4) Vascular anomalies
    - a. Fibromuscular dysplasia
    - b. Arteriovenous malformations
    - c. Cavernous angiomas
    - d. Sturge-Weber syndrome
- *Hematological disorders*
  - (1) Hemoglobinopathies
    - a. Sickle cell disease
    - b. Hemoglobin SC disease
  - (2) Coagulopathies
    - a. Protein C or S deficiency
    - b. Antithrombin III deficiency
  - (3) Platelet disorders
    - a. Thrombocytopenia
    - b. Thrombocytosis

BOX 13-26. UNCOMMON ETIOLOGIES AND RISK FACTORS FOR STROKE IN CHILDREN

- *Metabolic disorders*
  - (1) Homocystinuria
  - (2) Mitochondrial disorders (e.g., mitochondrial encephalopathy-lactic acidosis and stroke-like symptoms [MELAS])
  - (3) Organic acidurias
- *Trauma*
  - (1) Blunt cervical arterial trauma
  - (2) Child abuse
  - (3) Arterial dissection
  - (4) Intraoral trauma
- *Iatrogenic*
  - (1) Anticoagulation
  - (2) Arteriography/catheterization
  - (3) Carotid ligation (extracorporeal membrane oxygenation [ECMO])
  - (4) Chiropractic manipulation
- *Systemic diseases*
  - (1) Diabetes mellitus
  - (2) Hypertension
  - (3) Familial hypercholesterolemia

2. Patient needs to be hospitalized in a PICU for continuous monitoring.
3. Stroke treatment is a rapidly evolving field. There is ample reason to seek new acute treatments for children with ischemic cerebral infarction, because more than 50% of children have serious sequelae.
4. Thrombolytic agents (e.g., tissue plasminogen activator [t-PA]) have been effective in adults when administered within 3 hours of onset of stroke symptoms. Use of thrombolytic agents in children with arterial ischemic stroke has been rare.
5. Accumulating experience with antithrombotic and anticoagulant treatment (e.g., heparinization in patients with hypercoagulable states after consultation with a hematologist) in children suggests that these agents can safely be used in children.
6. For patients with sickle cell disease with stroke see Fig. 11-6.

Clinical Pearls: Stroke

1. Recognized stroke means "Brain attack."
2. Make immediate arrangements to obtain a noncontrast CT scan of the head.
3. Differentiate ischemic from hemorrhagic stroke.
4. Assess if the patient is a candidate for thrombolytic therapy (time is of the essence; administer within 3 hours).
5. Consider antithrombotic, anticoagulant, or anticonvulsant therapy, as clinically indicated.

BOX 13-27. CLINICAL FEATURES OF STROKE

- Typically, stroke is an acute neurologic event.
- Stroke manifests as hemiparesis with or without seizures.
- Seizures at onset of stroke (relatively frequent in children as compared to adults)
- Seizures, fever, headache, and lethargy occur more commonly in younger children.
- Dystonia is more common in children with basal ganglia infarction.
- Neonatal strokes manifest with persistent acute focal seizures.

BOX 13-28. DIFFERENTIAL DIAGNOSIS OF HEMIPARESIS

- Stroke
- Todd's paralysis (postictal following seizures)
- Tumor
- Trauma (subdural hemorrhage)
- Cerebral palsy (chronic history)
- Cerebral dysgenesis (schizencephaly; chronic history)

BOX 13-29. DIFFERENTIAL DIAGNOSIS: ISCHEMIC VERSUS HEMORRHAGIC STROKE

	Ischemic	*Hemorrhagic*
Clinical signs	Normal vital signs, minimal or no altered mental status	Signs of increased ICP, coma
CT findings	Low-density wedge-shaped lesion	Hemorrhage with or without midline shift
Management	Consider t-PA	Neurosurgical intervention

DIAGNOSIS RAISED INTRACRANIAL PRESSURE

SYNONYM

Intracranial hypertension

Definition

Raised intracranial pressure (ICP) is defined as ICP above 20 mm Hg in children and 11 mm Hg in neonates.

Etiology and Pathophysiology

1. The three components of the intracranial volume include:
   a. The brain, comprising 80% of intracranial volume
   b. CSF, 10% of intracranial volume
   c. Blood, 10% of intracranial volume
2. Monro-Kellie doctrine
   a. The compensation for an expanding mass lesion occurs via displacement/compression of the other compartments in the intracranial volume, as the brain is relatively incompressible. This is usually the CSF and venous volume of the brain, which allows a compensated normal ICP.
   b. However, at a critical mass, these compensatory mechanisms become exhausted and a sharp rise in ICP occurs.
3. Protean causes (many are interrelated)
   a. Traumatic brain injury (TBI; e.g., motor vehicle accidents, falls)
   b. Seizures (this as a cause of raised ICP would be after a minimum of 30 minutes of continuous seizures). Idiopathic epilepsy and seizures, alone or as a result of TBI, are among the other well known causes of raised ICP.
   c. Space-occupying lesions (benign and malignant pediatric tumors)
   d. Decreased reabsorption of CSF (arachnoid villi damage due to blood in the ventricles or infection)
   e. Increased production of CSF (e.g., choroid plexus tumor)
   f. Congenital causes (e.g., aqueductal stenosis)
   g. Metabolic causes (e.g., severe diabetic ketoacidosis)
   h. Infection (e.g., meningitis, brain abscess)
4. Types of cerebral edema: cerebral edema is a major cause of raised ICP and occurs in infections, tumors, head injury, Reye's syndrome, asphyxia, and a wide variety of other diseases in pediatrics.
   a. Vasogenic edema
      1) Due to increased permeability of brain capillary endothelial cells
      2) Neurons are not primarily injured and edema does not primarily reflect neuronal injury.
      3) Seen in tumors, abscesses, intracerebral hematomas, meningitis, and encephalitis
      4) Usually reversible and perfusion may be restored with therapy
   b. Cytotoxic edema
      1) As a result of cellular swelling secondary to cell injury
      2) It is due to failure of ATPase-dependent sodium exchange and may involve all cells within the brain, including neurons, astrocytes, and oligodendroglia.
      3) Water intoxication (a reversible cause) and diffuse axonal injury (DAI) secondary to TBI are other causes.
      4) Not usually reversible, as it is usually a manifestation of cell death
   c. Interstitial edema
      1) As a result of increased CSF hydrostatic pressure
      2) Hydrocephalus and decreased CSF reabsorption at the arachnoid villi are among the causes.
5. Therapy is directed at the cause and can be successful.

Associated Clinical Features

1. Symptoms of raised ICP range from asymptomatic to intense headache and vomiting, confusion, or other manifestations of altered mental status and seizures.
2. Perform a focused neurologic exam in all patients with suspected raised ICP.

3. Signs may range from asymptomatic to include Glasgow Coma Scale scores less than 15, unequal pupils, systolic hypertension, bradycardia, and irregular respirations (all three parts of Cushing's triad need not be present in severe raised ICP or impending herniation) (Fig. 13-24), and posturing or seizures.
4. CT scan of the head (contrast usually is not needed)
   a. Fastest and most efficient way of assessing severity of raised ICP
   b. It is noninvasive and does not require special equipment.
   c. CT scanning can assess the following:
      1) Ventricular size and compression
      2) If the basal cisterns are open (if compressed, herniation is imminent)
      3) Midline shift
      4) Edema
      5) Presence of hematomas, infarcts, or tumors
5. MRI takes too long and requires special nonmagnetic equipment.

Consultation

Emergent neurosurgery consultation

Emergency Department Treatment and Disposition

1. All patients with clinical/radiographic evidence of raised ICP require admission to the ICU for continuous monitoring after initial stabilization.
2. Patients may be brought to the operating room after initial stabilization for surgical evacuation of the hematoma, if present and/or decompressive craniotomy.
3. Management principles of first-line therapy:
   a. Stabilization of airway, breathing, and circulation, if clinically indicated
   b. Neurologic exam, and if necessary, emergency treatment for herniation (for signs and symptoms, see Box 13-30). When airway is secure, hyperventilate ($Paco_2$ 32 to 38 mm Hg), followed by sedation and pharmacological neuromuscular paralysis as needed, then CT scan
      (1) Controlled neuro intubation (use thiopental 4 mg/kg if blood pressure is stable, or fentanyl 1 to 2 μg/kg if hemodynamically unstable, lidocaine 1.5 mg/kg to blunt ICP spike and to facilitate laryngoscopy), followed by hyperventilation on the ventilator or via ambubag
      (2) Mannitol push 0.25 to 1 g/kg and/or hypertonic 3% saline 3 mL/kg
   c. Raise the head of the bed to 30° to optimize cerebral perfusion pressure (CPP).
      1) Mean arterial pressure (MAP) to the brain is highest in the supine position and ICP is lowest when the head is elevated.
      2) CPP is the difference between MAP and ICP. It is usually between 70 and 90 mm Hg in adults and lower in children. In treating raised ICP, the goal is to keep CPP between 40 and 50 mm Hg for infants and toddlers, 50 to 60 mm Hg for young children, and 60 to 70 mm Hg for older children, adolescents, and adults with vasopressor therapy if necessary till euvolemia has been achieved
   d. ICP monitoring (maintain ICP <20 mm Hg); for inadequate CPP, perform CSF drainage and reassess neurologic and cardiorespiratory status
      1) The ICP monitor type used depends on the neurosurgeon's preference (no objective data exist for this in children). Ventricular catheters are the most accurate, most reliable, and least expensive, and allow for therapeutic drainage of CSF, especially in herniation emergencies, but risks and consequences of infection may be higher. Parenchymal fiberoptic catheters are less accurate, with potential for drifting, and they cannot drain CSF. Subarachnoid, subdural, and epidural catheters are less invasive but also are less accurate.

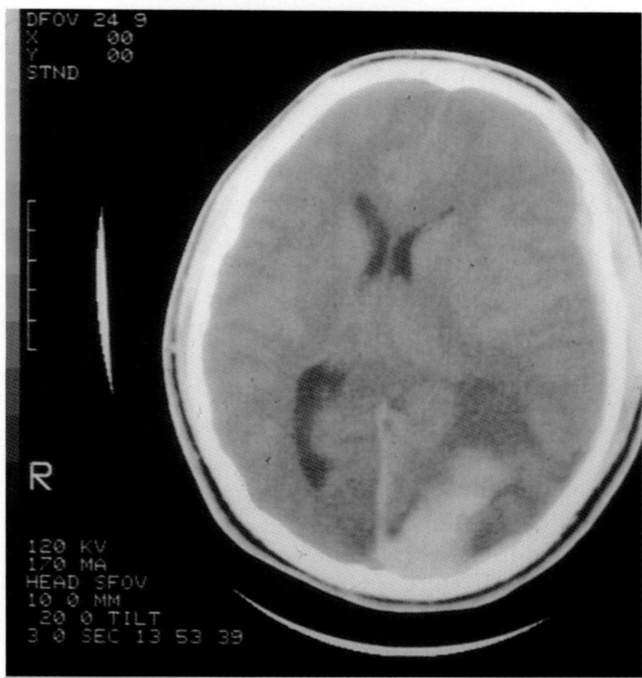

Figure 13-24. Intraparenchymal Bleed with Transtentorial and Subfalcine Herniation

A 16-year-old adolescent patient was brought to the ED with bradycardia, irregular respirations, and hypertension (Cushing's triad). He was found unresponsive in his bed with frothing at the mouth and urinary incontinence by his mother. About 12 hours prior to this, he complained of a bad headache and then went to sleep. A noncontrast CT scan of the head shows left parieto-occipital intraparenchymal bleeding with left frontoparietal subdural hematoma. The basal cisterns are obscured with a significant mass effect with evidence of transtentorial and subfalcine herniation. In the ED, he was intubated followed by hyperventilation and given a dose of mannitol prior to this CT scan (see also Fig. 13-6).

BOX 13-30. SIGNS OF HERNIATION OR IMPENDING HERNIATION

- Headache
- Vomiting
- Altered mental status
- Systolic hypertension
- Bradycardia
- Bradypnea
- Unequal pupils
- Seizures

2) Routine CSF drainage is associated with the least mortality and best outcome in adults.
3) Increased ICP above 20 mm Hg is strongly associated with poor outcome after severe TBI in children and adults. ICP must be kept below 20 mm Hg with an adequate CPP.

e. As indicated, treat fever.
f. Maintain normoglycemia.

4. Refractory intracranial hypertension
   a. Strongly consider osmotherapy (mannitol, hypertonic 3% saline).
   b. Barbiturates (e.g., pentobarbital bolus and drip); no response of raised ICP to pentobarbital is associated with poor outcome.
   c. Induced mild hypothermia to 34°C (treat fever aggressively)
   d. Vasopressor agents such as dopamine or norepinephrine via central venous catheter to increase MAP and improve CPP to at least 50 to 60 mm Hg
   e. Continuous exhaled carbon dioxide monitoring to ensure chronic mild hyperventilation to keep $Paco_2$ around 32 to 36 mm Hg
   f. Surgical evacuation of hematoma if present and/or decompressive craniectomy
5. Treatment of raised ICP should also include therapy to treat the underlying cause.
6. Potentially contraindicated therapeutic agents
   a. Nitroglycerin/nitroprusside have direct cerebral vasodilatory effects.
   b. Ketamine increases cerebral blood volume.
   c. Avoid free water administration, which causes hypo-osmolality.
   d. Steroids are contraindicated in raised ICP except in cases of vasogenic edema as may occur in tumors.
   e. Avoid propofol drips for sedation in children, which may give rise to propofol syndrome, which is associated with fatal intractable metabolic acidosis in children.

Clinical Pearls: Raised Intracranial Pressure

All three parts of Cushing's triad (systolic hypertension, bradycardia, and irregular respiration) need not be present in severe raised ICP with impending herniation.

Suggested Readings

AAP Committee on Quality Improvement, Subcommittee on Febrile Seizures: Practice parameter. Long-term treatment of the child with simple febrile seizures. *Pediatrics* 1999;103:1307.

AAP Provisional Committee on Quality Improvement, Subcommittee on Febrile Seizures: Practice parameter: The neurodiagnostic evaluation of the child with a first simple febrile seizure. *Pediatrics* 1996;97:769.

Baumann RJ, Duffner PK: Treatment of children with simple febrile seizures: The AAP Practice Parameter. *Pediatr Neurol* 2000;23:11.

Del Brutto OH: Proposed diagnostic criteria for neurocysticercosis. *Neurology* 2001;57:177.

Edlow JA: Subarachnoid hemorrhage. In: Bosker G (ed). *The Emergency Medicine Reports. Textbook of Adult and Pediatric Emergency Medicine*, 2nd ed. American Health Consultants, Atlanta, 2002, p. 537.

Greenes DS, Madsen JR: Neurotrauma. In: Fleisher GR, Ludwig S. (eds). *Textbook of Pediatric Emergency Medicine*, 4th ed. Lippincott Williams & Wilkins, Philadelphia, 2000, p. 1271.

Grogan PM, Gronseth GS: Practice parameter: Steroids, acyclovir, and surgery for Bell's palsy (an evidence-based review). Report of the Quality Standards Subcommittee of the American Academy of Neurology. *Neurology* 2001;56:830.

Haslem RH: Acute stroke syndromes. In: Behrman RE, Kliegman RM, Jenson HB (eds). *Nelson Textbook of Pediatrics*, 16th ed. WB Saunders, Philadelphia, 2000, p. 1856.

Knudsen FU: Febrile seizures: Treatment and prognosis. *Epilepsia* 2000;41:2.

Maria BL: *Current Management in Child* Neurology, 2nd ed. BC Decker, Hamilton, Ontario, 2002.

Pellock JM, Dodson WE, Bourgeois BF: *Pediatric Epilepsy—Diagnosis and Therapy*, 2nd ed. Demos Medical Publishing, New York, 2001, p. 276.

Riordan M: Investigation and treatment of facial palsy. *Arch Dis Child*, 2001;84:286.

Rogers MC and Nichols DG (ed). *Textbook of Pediatric Intensive Care*, 3rd ed. Lippincott Williams & Wilkins, Philadelphia, 1996, p. 645.

Shorvon S: *Handbook of Epilepsy Treatment*. Blackwell Science, London, 2000, p. 176.

Neuroimaging in the emergency patient presenting with seizure. *Neurology* 1996;47:26.

Practice parameter: Evaluating a first non-febrile seizure in children. *Neurology* 2000;55:616.

Practice parameter: Treatment of the child with a first unprovoked seizure. *Neurology* 2003;60:166.

CHAPTER 14

ENDOCRINOLOGY

Glenn D. Harris / Irma Fiordalisi / Binita R. Shah

DIAGNOSIS — DIABETIC KETOACIDOSIS

Definition and Etiology

1. Diabetic ketoacidosis/ketoacidemia (DKA) is a potentially life-threatening metabolic disturbance caused by an absolute or relative insulin deficiency with resultant ketone body production and concomitant decrease in the measured total carbon dioxide concentration (TCO_2) in serum. Initially, compensatory hyperventilation preserves a normal blood pH (ketoacidosis); without provision of sufficient insulin, ketonemia progresses, and a subnormal blood pH (ketoacidemia) ensues. The presence of even low concentrations of insulin in the portal circulation will usually inhibit the hepatic fatty acyl carnitine cycle, preventing DKA. In the absence of sufficient insulin this cycle is uninhibited, resulting in the production of ketone bodies.
2. Absolute or relative insulin deficiency causes impaired transport of glucose into cells resulting in hyperglycemia, glycosuria, and intracellular starvation. This condition leads to release of counterregulatory hormones (glucagon, epinephrine, cortisol, and growth hormone), which in turn results in lipolysis, proteolysis, glycogenolysis, gluconeogenesis, and insulin resistance.
3. Glycogenolysis and gluconeogenesis exacerbate the already-present hyperglycemia.
4. A negative cycle of progressive ketoacidemia and insulin resistance, accompanied by the surge of counterregulatory hormones, leads to increasing insulin resistance, hyperglycemia, dehydration, electrolyte losses, potential brain swelling, and metabolic death if untreated (and sometimes death even when treated).

Associated Clinical Features

1. DKA occurs most commonly among type 1 diabetics but is being more frequently recognized in association with type 2 diabetes mellitus.
2. DKA is an apparent paradoxical state of systemic dehydration with either subclinical or symptomatic brain swelling.
3. The most common cause of morbidity and mortality in pediatric DKA is raised intracranial pressure (ICP) that develops after treatment has begun (Fig. 14-1).
4. The degree of dehydration varies in DKA. The mean degree of dehydration among 97 episodes of pediatric DKA is reported to be 7.4% with a range of 1 to 22.7%; in another smaller study, similar findings were observed. This demonstrates that the traditional, arbitrary assumption of 10 to 15% dehydration in all patients with DKA overestimates the degree of dehydration in a majority of patients.
5. Overestimation of the degree of dehydration leads to excessive volume administration which may exacerbate brain swelling.
6. Severe DKA (i.e., severe ketoacidemia) does not necessarily mean that severe dehydration is present.

Consultation

Experts in the management of pediatric DKA should include emergency medicine physicians, pediatric critical care specialists, diabetologists, and/or endocrinologists.

Emergency Department Treatment and Disposition

1. Emergency management is directed toward assessment for and establishment of adequacy of airway, breathing and circulation, and the institution of insulin therapy.
2. Tracheal intubation is rarely required. However, when tracheal intubation is indicated, it should be accomplished using techniques that are protective for patients at risk for raised ICP.
3. Assessment for shock:
   a. If peripheral pulses, capillary refill time, skin temperature, and blood pressure are normal, shock is not present and rapid emergency volume resuscitation is not indicated (Figure 14-2).

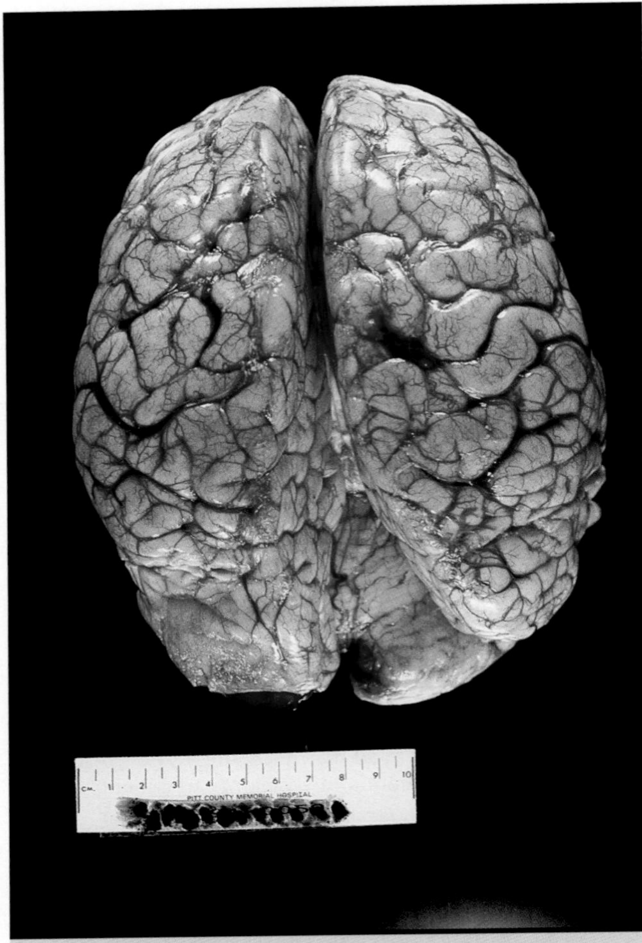

Figure 14-1. Brain Swelling Seen at Autopsy in a Patient with Diabetic Ketoacidosis

A dorsal view of the brain shows severe brain swelling. The gyri were flattened, the sulci were effaced, and the brain was markedly softened. On the ventral surface, there was evidence of brain swelling with herniation. The patient was a 17-year-old known type 1 diabetic with a history of polydipsia, lethargy, and vomiting. He collapsed at home and developed hypertension, bradycardia, and agonal respirations when first responders arrived. His hemoglobin A1c was 12.4%. Brain death was secondary to raised ICP with brain herniation prior to medical treatment.

b. If peripheral perfusion is poor, with or without hypotension, shock is present and requires emergency resuscitation. Follow pathway for shock (Figure 14-2).

c. *Notes on "adequate perfusion":*
   1) Severe ketonemia causes vasoconstriction.
   2) Cool, sometimes mottled skin may be attributable to a very low blood pH rather than hypovolemia. For this reason, if foot pulses are strong and blood pressure is appropriate but skin remains cool and/or mottled despite 10 to 20 ml/kg of resuscitation fluid in the presence of severe acidemia, further bolus volume resuscitation may not be warranted. In these cases, insulin and rehydration therapy is recommended with serial reassessments. The impaired perfusion should resolve as ketonemia is corrected with insulin and gradual rehydration.

4. Monitor closely for signs of raised ICP.
5. Start insulin as soon as possible by continuous intravenous infusion of regular human insulin at a rate of 0.1 unit/kg actual body weight per hour.
6. Rehydration (Box 14-1)
   a. Estimate the degree of dehydration based on physical examination and laboratory data.
   b. Subtract emergency volumes already given from the estimated volume deficit.
   c. Use rehydration solutions as described below.
   d. Give deficit plus maintenance allotments.
7. Once serum glucose is $<$300 mg/dL, glucose should be added to the electrolyte solutions described.
   a. For example, a 6-year-old child with uncomplicated DKA whose glucose is 280 mg/dL should receive 5% dextrose in lactated Ringer's with potassium, usually 40 mEq/L (*or* 5% dextrose in NaCl 100 mEq/L + $NaHCO_3$ 25 mEq/L + K^+ 40 mEq/L).
   b. Lower infusion rates of IV fluid (used in the physiologic management of DKA recommended here) may require that potassium concentrations be increased further in selected patients; up to 80 mEq/L K^+ can be given peripherally.
   c. Some patients may require solutions containing 10% or 12.5% dextrose (peripherally), or a greater dextrose concentration (via central venous access) plus appropriate electrolytes to maintain glucose in a safe range (usually 150 to 250 mg/dL) while delivering adequate insulin.
8. Identify any associated illnesses. These may be triggers or complications of DKA and may require additional, sometimes urgent, interventions.
   a. It is uncommon to require more than 30 ml/kg of isotonic saline resuscitation fluid, even when severe dehydration occurs in DKA.
   b. A need for emergency volumes in excess of 30 ml/kg of ideal body weight should raise suspicion for the possibility of the presence of a significant complicating illness such as septic shock, pancreatitis, or severe enteritis.
   c. In known pediatric diabetics, DKA is most commonly triggered by noncompliance with the prescribed insulin regimen.
9. Treat signs of raised ICP with mannitol 0.5 to 1 g/kg IV over 20 minutes and evaluate the patient for a concomitant decrease in rate of fluid administration. Tracheal intubation and hyperventilation may also be required.
10. Pediatric patients with moderate to severe DKA should be hospitalized. Initial resuscitation should be followed by contact with a PICU, where vital signs, neurologic examination, and metabolic progress can be appropriately monitored.

11. Although rehydration is planned over 48 hours, the vast majority of patients are fully recovered from DKA, no longer require IV fluids, and are receiving subcutaneous insulin within 12 to 24 hours.

12. After stabilization, a diabetes nurse educator and nutritionist should be involved with each patient who presents with DKA. Consider the following additional services, especially for patients with repeated episodes of DKA: child psychology or psychiatry if depression is suspected; social services.

13. Long-term management plans should be made in conjunction with a diabetologist or endocrinologist as well as with the primary care physician.

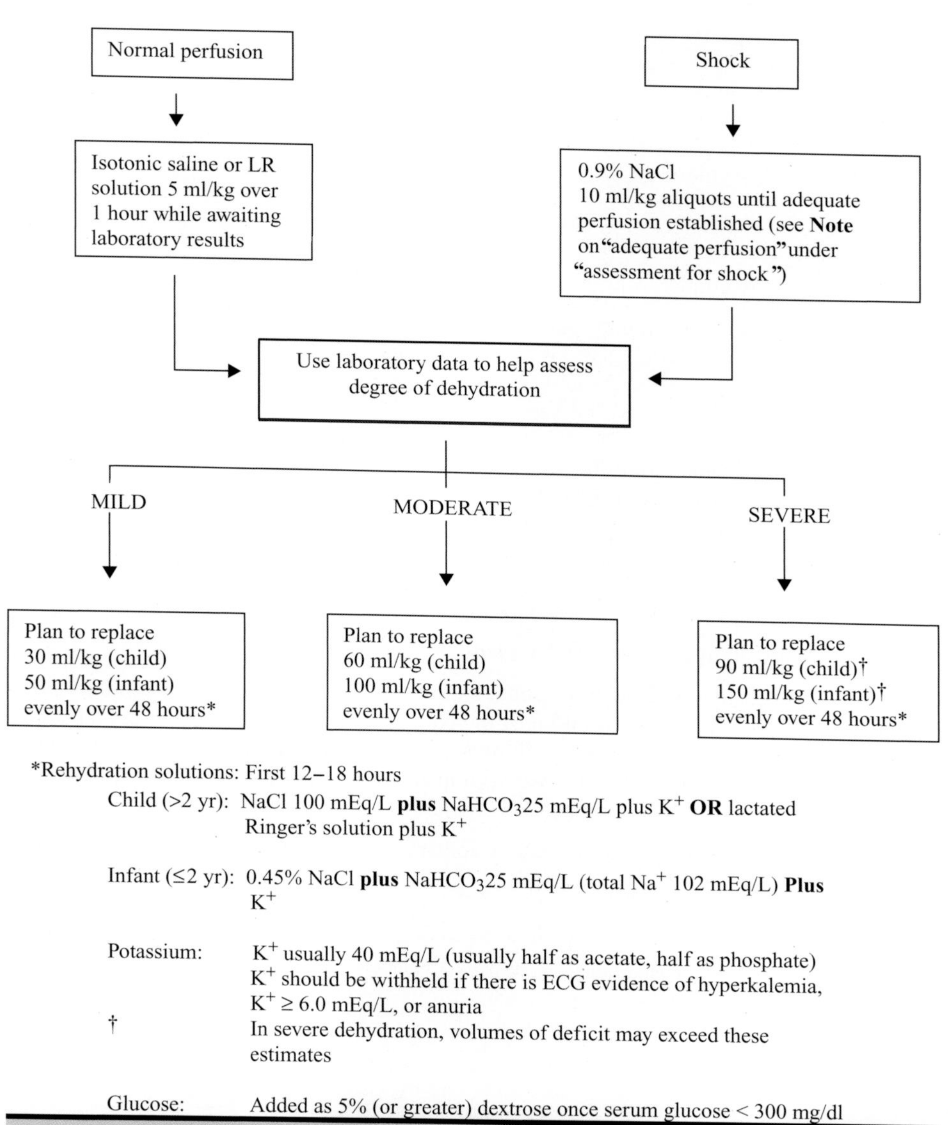

Figure 14-2. Rehydration in the Normally Nourished Infant or Child with DKA.

BOX 14-1. GUIDELINES FOR ESTIMATING THE VOLUME OF DEFICIT (DEGREE OF DEHYDRATION) IN DIABETIC KETOACIDOSIS

	Degree of Dehydration		
Guidelines	*Mild*	*Moderate*	*Severe*
Volume of deficit (ml/kg)*			
>2 years	30	60	≥90
≤2 years	50	100	≥150
Clinical measures			
Peripheral perfusion†			
Palpation of peripheral pulses (pulse volume)	Normal	Normal to decreased	Decreased to absent
Capillary refill time (s)‡	<2	2 to 3	≥3
Skin temperature (tactile)	Normal	Normal to cool	Cool to cold
Heart rate	Normal to mildly increased	Moderately increased	Moderately to severely increased
Blood pressure	Normal	Normal to mildly increased	Decreased to moderately increased
Blood urea nitrogen (mg/dL)	Normal to mildly increased, e.g., <20	Mildly increased, e.g., 20 to 25	Moderately to severely increased, e.g., 30
Predicted Na^+ (mEq/L)	Usually normal	Usually normal	Normal to increased
Glucose (mg/dL)	Mildly increased, e.g., 400	Moderately increased, e.g., 600	Severely increased, e.g., 800

*Use actual weight for normally nourished patients; for obese patients, use ideal body weight.

†If peripheral (foot) pulses are easily palpable on presentation but skin is cool to cold and capillary refill time is delayed, we give 0.9% NaCl (or lactated Ringer's) 10 ml/kg. If the patient has easily palpable peripheral (foot) pulses with cool to cold skin and delayed capillary refill *after* 10 to 20 ml/kg resuscitation fluid have been given, these findings are most likely due to severe ketonemia and should be treated with insulin and serial reassessments, not necessarily more resuscitation fluid.

‡Capillary refill time is modified by the hypertonic state. Capillary refill time between 2 and 3 seconds suggests moderate to severe dehydration.

(Modified from Harris GD, Fiordalisi I, Harris WL, et al: Minimizing the risk of brain herniation during treatment of diabetic ketoacidemia: a retrospective and prospective study. *J Pediatr* 1990;117:28.)

BOX 14-2. KEY FINDINGS IN DIABETIC KETOACIDOSIS

- *Clinical:*
  (1) Polyuria, polydipsia
  (2) Polyphagia, decreased appetite or no apparent change
  (3) Dehydration
  (4) Weight loss
  (5) Abdominal pain
  (6) Vomiting
  (7) Hyperventilation/Kussmaul breathing
  (8) Mental status changes/lethargy
  (9) Fruity odor of ketones on the breath
  (10) *Candida* infections (e.g., candidal vaginitis)
- *Laboratory:*

  Always present:
  (1) Hyperglycemia: may only be modest (blood glucose <300 mg/dL)
  (2) Glycosuria
  (3) Ketonemia, ketonuria
  (4) Metabolic acidosis/acidemia
  (5) Hypocarbia (compensatory)
- Sometimes present:
  (1) Apparent or actual hyponatremia
  (2) Hypernatremia
  (3) Hyperkalemia or hypokalemia
  (4) Hypophosphatemia
  (5) Increased blood urea nitrogen
  (6) Increased serum creatinine (may be anomalous due to presence of ketone bodies)
  (7) Hypertriglyceridemia
  (8) Increased serum amylase (primarily salivary in origin)

BOX 14-3. FACTORS THAT COMMONLY LEAD TO OVERESTIMATION OF THE DEGREE OF DEHYDRATION AND MAY LEAD TO ADMINISTRATION OF EXCESS RESUSCITATIVE FLUIDS

- An erroneous assumption that severe dehydration is present in all patients with DKA
- Severe ketonemia (e.g., $TCO_2 < 8$ mmol/L): this causes vasoconstriction, cool, mottled skin, and delayed capillary refill time
- Kussmaul breathing: This causes parched mucosa giving the patient a dehydrated appearance.
- Subnormal body temperature: common in severe DKA; may also be environmental or associated with sepsis

BOX 14-4. TRIGGERING FACTORS AND COMPLICATIONS OF DIABETIC KETOACIDOSIS

- *Triggering factors in DKA:*
  (1) Insulin noncompliance is the most common cause.
  (2) Depression leading to noncompliance
  (3) Behavioral disorders
  (4) Illicit drug use
  (5) Pregnancy
  (6) Infections: These may be minor (e.g., upper respiratory infection [URI], urinary tract infection [UTI]) or life-threatening, such as sepsis, necrotizing fasciitis, or mucormycosis (CNS, pulmonary, GI).
  (7) Acute appendicitis may trigger, complicate, or be confused with DKA.
  (8) Psychosocial disturbances, including physical and sexual abuse
- *Complications of DKA:*
  (1) Altered mental status
  (2) Brain swelling with or without raised ICP
  (3) Brain herniation
  (4) Central nervous system hemorrhage/infarction
  (5) Central nervous system acidosis
  (6) Acute hydrocephalus
  (7) Pancreatitis
  (8) Cardiac dysrhythmias due to electrolyte imbalance, especially hypo- or hyperkalemia
  (9) Hypoglycemia
  (10) Severe hypertriglyceridemia
  (11) Thromboses/thromboembolic disease
  (12) Hyperviscosity syndromes
  (13) Pulmonary edema; acute respiratory distress syndrome [ARDS]
  (14) Pulmonary air leak syndromes (e.g., pneumomediastinum)

BOX 14-5. DIFFERENTIAL DIAGNOSIS OF DIABETIC KETOACIDOSIS

- Nonketotic hyperosmolar coma (sometimes a misnomer since patients often have a mild degree of ketonemia and not all patients are in comas)
- Hypernatremic dehydration with associated hyperglycemia
- Stress hyperglycemia with lactic or hyperchloremic acidosis
- Starvation ketoacidosis
- Alcoholic ketoacidosis
- Salicylate intoxication
- Inborn errors of metabolism:
  (1) Methylmalonic acidemia
  (2) Proprionic acidemia
  (3) Isovaleric acidemia

BOX 14-6. DO'S OF DIABETIC KETOACIDOSIS

- Treat each episode as unique and tailor therapy to the individual patient.
- Assess and reassess airway, breathing, circulation, and neurologic status.
- Identify shock by diminished peripheral pulses and/or low blood pressure and administer aggressive fluid resuscitation.
- Give 10-ml/kg aliquots of an isotonic saline solution as quickly as warranted by the clinical situation until peripheral pulses are full (and blood pressure, if low, has normalized).
- Suspect complications such as sepsis or pancreatitis if more than 20 to 30 ml/kg of resuscitation fluid is required.
- Calculate fluids and electrolytes based on ideal body weight in the obese patient, but use actual body weight to calculate the insulin requirement (this is because fat cells contain little water, but do have insulin receptors).
- Provide continuous cardiorespiratory monitoring.
- At a minimum, record hourly vital signs, peripheral perfusion, mental status, and perform key laboratory tests.
- Start insulin by continuous IV infusion by the end of the first treatment hour and adjust the dose to effect a decrease in the base deficit by approximately 1 mEq/L per hour.
- Give continuous IV insulin and appropriate isotonic saline solutions to treat vomiting instead of antiemetics antiemetics.
- If continuous IV insulin is not possible or impractical (e.g., during transport), treat temporarily with hourly regular human insulin 0.1 unit/kg via deep IM injection.
- Treat the hypertonic dehydration of DKA according to the established principles of the treatment of any chronic hypertonic dehydration (i.e. slowly, with deficit replacement given gradually over 48 hours).
- Evaluate the state of dehydration separately from the degree of the ketoacidosis (by physical examination, blood urea nitrogen, glucose level, and the predicted serum sodium concentrations).
- Ignore the amount of urine output unless it becomes scant.
- Assume the serum potassium concentration will fall as the ketoacidosis improves, and plan accordingly.
- Replace magnesium, phosphorus, and potassium deficiencies.
- Add glucose to the rehydration solution once the serum glucose is <300 mg/dL.
- Calculate the predicted sodium for each measured sodium-glucose level:
  (1) The predicted sodium value should remain approximately the same with each paired serum sodium and glucose determination.
  (2) Calculation at the bedside: For every 100-mg/dL decrease in the concentration of glucose during treatment, the serum sodium should increase by approximately 1.6 mEq/L.
- Ensure a gradual but progressive decrease in the blood urea nitrogen during treatment.
- Have hypertonic mannitol readily available (within minutes).
- Have a high index of suspicion for the development of raised ICP if the neurological status deteriorates during therapy.
- Try to identify possible triggers of DKA.
- Contact an appropriate accepting physician such as a pediatric intensivist or diabetologist who will facilitate admission to an appropriate unit.

BOX 14-7. DON'TS OF DIABETIC KETOACIDOSIS

- Don't assume each episode is exactly like every other episode and therefore warrants identical treatment.
- Don't treat nonshock as if shock were present.
- Don't assume dry oral mucous membranes signify clinically significant dehydration.
- Don't treat children as adults by giving 1 to 2 liters of isotonic saline solution in the first 1 to 2 hours.
- Don't try to volume resuscitate to normal skin perfusion, particularly when the blood pH is very low; good pulses in the feet with appropriate blood pressure are sufficient.
- Don't wait beyond the first treatment hour to give continuous intravenous short-acting insulin. An IV push of insulin is insufficient to treat DKA, as is insulin by the subcutaneous route.
- Don't continue insulin pump therapy if the patient presents in DKA (switch to continuous IV insulin).
- Don't mask the neurologic status of the patients who are vomiting by giving neurotropic antiemetics (e.g., promethazine, ondansetron).
- Don't mask potential underlying concomitant gastrointestinal diseases (e.g., appendicitis, pancreatitis) by giving antiemetics, analgesics, or anxiolytics.
- Don't treat the hypertonic dehydration of DKA as an isotonic/hypotonic dehydration (i.e., over 24 hours).
- Don't assume a low blood pH means severe dehydration.
- Don't replace urine output milliliter for milliliter.
- Don't ignore the serum magnesium and phosphorus concentrations.
- Don't miss the diagnosis of new-onset diabetes by failing to obtain an adequate history, by assuming polyuria/polydipsia can be known from the history, or by failing to recognize nonspecific signs and symptoms such as weight loss, vaginal candidiasis, and generalized malaise.
- Don't use actual weight to calculate fluid and electrolyte needs in the obese patient.
- Don't give oral fluids during DKA.
- Don't withhold or decrease insulin during DKA because the serum glucose is <250 mg/dL. Add glucose to the IV fluid instead.
- Don't forget the signs and symptoms of raised ICP while managing DKA.
- Don't rely on a head CT scan to make the diagnosis of raised ICP.
- Don't worry about worsening the dehydration if you think mannitol is needed (if you think the patient has raised ICP, give mannitol).

DIAGNOSIS

THYROID STORM

SYNONYMS

Thyrotoxic crisis
Accelerated hyperthyroidism

Definition and Etiology

1. The terms hyperthyroidism, thyrotoxicosis, thyrotoxic crisis, and thyroid storm describe the continuum of disease that results from hyperfunction of the thyroid gland.
2. Thyroid storm is a severe thyrotoxicosis and occurs due to sudden release of thyroid hormone into the circulation.
3. The mechanisms responsible for the progression of thyrotoxicosis to thyroid storm are unclear.
4. Thyrotoxicosis is defined as elevated concentrations of free thyroxine (T_4) and/or free triiodothyronine (T_3).
5. Thyrotoxicosis may be due to either
   a. Increase in thyroid hormone synthesis and release (hyperthyroidism) *or*
   b. Increased T_4 and/or T_3 concentrations *without hyperthyroidism* (i.e., without an increase in thyroid hormone synthesis)

Associated Clinical Features

1. Thyroid storm is seen less commonly in children than in adults.
2. The diagnosis of thyroid storm is based on clinical findings.
3. Standard thyroid function tests cannot differentiate thyrotoxicosis from thyroid storm because thyroid hormone levels are not diagnostic in these conditions. Thyroid function tests are also usually not available as emergency

laboratory tests. However, when they are performed, the results include:

a. Generally elevated values of both T_4 and T_3 (some patients with thyrotoxicosis may only have elevated values of T_3)
b. An increase in serum values of free T_4 or an elevated free thyroxine index
c. A decrease in thyroid-stimulating hormone (TSH)

Consultation

Endocrinology (usually consulted after the patient is admitted)

Emergency Department Treatment and Disposition

1. The patient requires ICU monitoring during initial phases of therapy.
2. Supportive measures:
   a. Control of hyperpyrexia with a cooling blanket, ice packs, and acetaminophen
   b. Do not us aspirin, as it displaces T_4 from thyroid-binding protein.
   c. Treatment of the precipitating event (e.g., infection)
   d. Replace fluid deficits.
3. When the diagnosis is strongly suspected, specific therapy is started immediately without waiting for laboratory confirmation.
   a. Beta-blocker therapy (e.g., propranolol) to block adrenergic effects
   b. Inhibit biosynthesis of new thyroid hormone
      1) Propylthiouracil (PTU) or methimazole (when the patient is allergic to PTU)
      2) PTU should be administered before iodine (to inhibit synthesis).
   c. To decrease release of preformed thyroid hormone
      1) Iodine (blocks thyroid hormone release)
      2) Glucocorticoids (e.g., hydrocortisone or dexamethasone (blocks conversion of T_4 to T_3)

Clinical Pearls: Thyroid Storm

1. Thyroid storm is a rare but a potentially life-threatening manifestation of thyrotoxicosis (an abrupt, severe exacerbation of thyrotoxicosis). If not recognized early and treated aggressively, it can lead to death.
2. Graves' disease is the most common etiology of thyroid storm.
3. Thyroid storm occurs most frequently in patients with severe thyrotoxicosis who develop an intercurrent infection or undergo surgery.
4. The classic presentations of thyrotoxicosis (thyroid storm) include hyperpyrexia, tachyarrhythmias, anxiety, extreme restlessness, and heat intolerance.
5. There are no definitive laboratory tests to differentiate thyroid storm from uncomplicated thyrotoxicosis; thyroid storm is a clinical diagnosis. Patients with thyroid storm may rapidly deteriorate with shock and coma; thus emergency treatment should not await laboratory confirmation.

BOX 14-8. THYROID STORM

- *Thyroid disorders that lead to thyroid storm:*
  - (1) Graves' disease (Fig. 14-3)
  - (2) Toxic multinodular goiter
  - (3) Toxic thyroid adenoma
  - (4) Factitious thyrotoxicosis (exogenous thyroid hormone ingestion)
  - (5) Thyroiditis
- *Precipitating factors for thyroid storm:*
  - (1) Infection
  - (2) Trauma
  - (3) Surgery
  - (4) Diabetic ketoacidosis
  - (5) Withdrawal of antihyperthyroid medications
  - (6) Iodine administration
  - (7) Thyroid hormone ingestion
  - (8) Other drugs (e.g., lithium)
  - (9) Idiopathic
  - (10) Cerebrovascular accident
  - (11) Pulmonary embolism
  - (12) Myocardial infarction

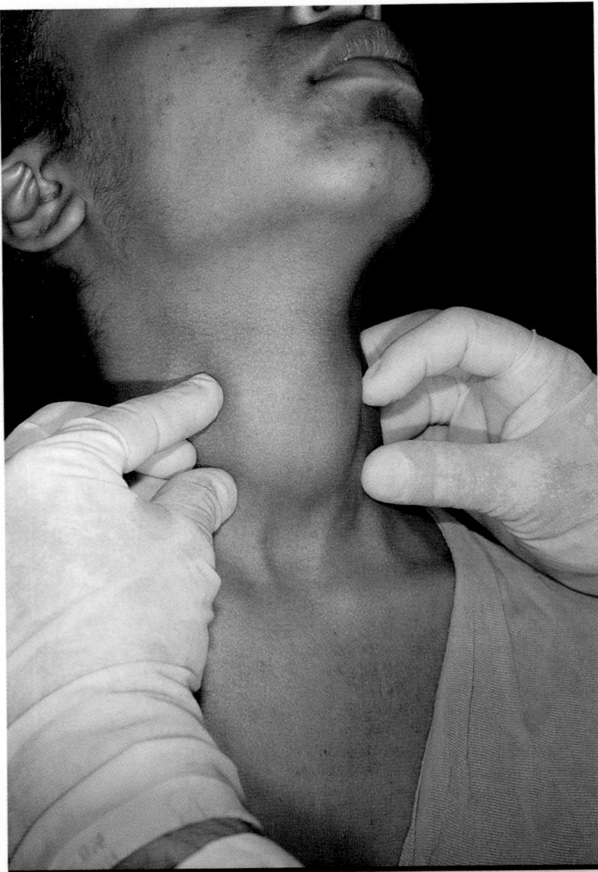

Figure 14-3. Goiter in Graves' Disease

Most cases of thyroid storm are secondary to Graves' disease. Goiter (a feature of Graves' disease) will be seen in most patients with thyroid storm. Sudden onset of hyperpyrexia (105.9°F), tachycardia/palpitation (HR 160 bpm), profuse sweating, and extreme restlessness were the presenting signs of this 16-year-old girl who was known to have Graves' disease. Her serum T4 value was 53.7 μg/dL (normal, 4.7 to 11.4), total T3 value was 391 ng/dL (normal, 45 to 137), free T4 value was 5.25 ng/dL (normal, 0.7 to 1.85), and TSH value was 0.027 mIU/mL (normal, 0.4 to 4.6).

BOX 14-9. CLINICAL FEATURES OF THYROID STORM

- *Cardinal presenting features:*
  (1) Fever (almost invariably present; often severe and in excess of temperature elevation expected from the intercurrent illness)
  (2) Tachycardia (out of proportion to the degree of fever)
  (3) Acute metabolic encephalopathy (extreme restlessness, agitation, psychosis, delirium, confusion, stupor, or coma)
- *Other presenting features:*
  (1) Arrhythmias, palpitations
  (2) Profuse sweating (warm moist skin)
  (3) Heat intolerance
  (4) High-output congestive heart failure
  (5) Cardiogenic shock
  (6) Goiter
  (7) Proptosis, lid retraction
  (8) Diarrhea
  (9) Abdominal pain
  (10) Jaundice
  (11) Tremulousness
  (12) Nausea and vomiting
  (13) Stroke

DIAGNOSIS

HYPOCALCEMIA

Definition

A total serum calcium (Ca) value <7 mg/dL or an ionized Ca value <3.5 mg/dL

Laboratory Evaluation

1. Total serum Ca, ionized Ca, phosphorus, magnesium, electrolytes, blood urea nitrogen, creatinine, total protein, and albumin
2. Exclude hypocalcemia associated with hypoalbuminemia.
   a. For every 1 g/dL decrease in serum albumin, there is a drop in the protein-bound Ca fraction of 0.8 mg/dL.
   b. Example: a patient with a serum albumin level of 1.5 g/dL could have a total serum Ca value of 2 mg/dL $[(4-1.5) \times 0.8]$ below the normal concentration *without* an actual reduction of serum ionized Ca concentration.
3. Additional tests (as indicated) include serum amylase, alkaline phosphatase, parathyroid hormone, and vitamin D levels (25-hydroxyvitamin D and 1,25-$(OH)_2$ vitamin D).
4. Electrocardiogram (prolonged QTc interval; see page ??)

Consultation

Endocrinology (usually obtained after hospitalization; e.g., for parathyroid-related hypocalcemia, vitamin D–related hypocalcemia)

Emergency Department Treatment and Disposition

1. With continuous cardiac monitoring, calcium gluconate 10% is given intravenously slowly at a dose of 1 to 2 mL/kg to patients presenting with hypocalcemic seizures or tetany. Cessation of symptoms and shortening of the QTc interval (if prolonged) are endpoints in the ED. Subsequently the patient will need hospitalization in the ICU for either continuous IV infusion or repeated boluses of Ca therapy.
2. Specific therapy of hypocalcemia depends on the underlying etiology (e.g., vitamin D therapy for vitamin D–deficiency rickets; Fig. 14-4).
3. Patients presenting with hyperventilation-induced carpopedal spasm should breathe slowly into and out of a paper bag. Rebreathing of CO_2 leads to a decrease in serum pH with a subsequent increase in ionized Ca. These patients can be discharged home once the precipitating cause for the anxiety attack has been appropriately addressed and follow-up has been arranged.

Clinical Pearls: Hypocalcemia

1. Recurrent croup in an afebrile child without signs or symptoms of upper respiratory tract infection may be secondary to tetany.
2. Hyperventilation-induced alkalosis leading to hypocalcemia is one of the common etiologies of tetany seen in the ED.
3. Repeated doses of phosphate-containing enemas may lead to significant elevations of serum phosphorus that can reciprocally reduce serum Ca values, and the patient may develop hypocalcemic seizures or tetany.

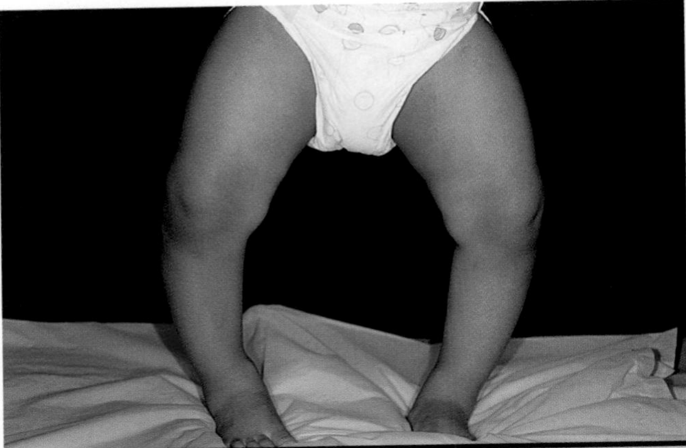

Figure 14-4. Bow Legs in Vitamin D–Deficiency Rickets Presenting with a Seizure due to Hypocalcemia

A 14-month-old toddler presented with one episode of febrile seizure. The nutritional history consisted of a strict vegan diet and the patient was still being breast-fed with no vitamin D supplementation. His physical examination showed bow legs, rachitic rosary, and prominent wrists. Hypocalcemia (Ca, 6.5 mg/dL), hypophosphatemia (PO_4, 2.1 mg/dL), and elevated serum alkaline phosphatase (1850 units/L) confirmed the clinical diagnosis of rickets due to vitamin D deficiency. He received vitamin D therapy (high-dose or "stoss" therapy) that was followed by normalization of all his abnormal laboratory values. *Important:* Take a detailed history and do a complete physical examination in all patients presenting with febrile seizures. Fever can reduce the seizure threshold in patients with preexisting metabolic conditions, and such patients can be mistakenly given a diagnosis of febrile seizures, thus overlooking a treatable cause of the seizures.

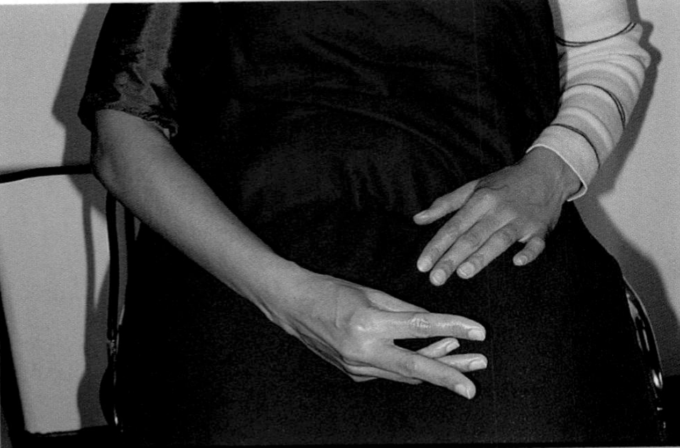

Figure 14-5. Positive Trousseau's Sign (Latent Tetany); Carpopedal Spasm (flexion at wrist and metacarpophalangeal joints, extension at interphalangeal joints with adduction of thumb into palm).

An 18-year-adolescent female patient presented with difficulty breathing and chest pain. She was noted to be hyperventilating. She developed carpopedal spasm when an attempt was made to obtain her blood pressure. She confessed having an "anxiety/panic attack". She was instructed to breath slowly in and out of a paper bag given to her and symptoms improved shortly afterwards.

BOX 14-10. SIGNS AND SYMPTOMS OF HYPOCALCEMIA

- Hypocalcemic tetany (hyperexcitability of the central and peripheral nervous systems)
  - (1) Manifest tetany = carpopedal spasm
    - a. Upper extremity: flexion at wrist and at metacarpophalangeal joints, extension at interphalangeal joints, adduction of thumb into palm
    - b. Lower extremity: feet held adducted and extended (talipes equinovarus)
  - (2) Latent tetany
    - a. Positive Chvostek's sign: contraction of orbicularis oris with twitching of the upper lip or entire mouth when the facial nerve is tapped just anterior to external auditory meatus
    - b. Positive peroneal sign: tapping the peroneal nerve where it passes over the head of the fibula leads to dorsiflexion and abduction of the foot secondary to contraction of the peroneal muscles
    - c. Positive Trousseau's sign: carpopedal spasm provoked by ischemia when blood pressure cuff is maintained at just above systolic pressure for 2 to 3 minutes
- Seizures
  - (1) *Usually generalized, brief but recurrent, without loss of consciousness in between seizures*
  - (2) May be focal seizures
  - (3) Postictal state may be seen after a prolonged series of seizures
- Laryngospasm (high-pitched inspiratory stridor); may lead to apnea, cyanosis
- ECG changes (prolonged QTc interval)
- Muscle cramps
- Sensory manifestations (tingling and numbness of hands, feet, perioral region)
- Behavioral changes (irritability, lethargy, psychosis, depression)
- Poor feeding, lethargy, cyanosis, vomiting (neonates)
- Increased intracranial pressure and papilledema (long-standing hypocalcemia)

CHAPTER 15

GASTROINTESTINAL DISORDERS

Binita R. Shah / David Tran
Edited by Binita R. Shah

DIAGNOSIS ESOPHAGEAL FOREIGN BODY

Definition

An esophageal foreign body (FB) is a foreign object lodged in the esophagus.

Etiology

1. Most children with impacted FBs have a structurally and functionally normal esophagus (unlike adults who may have intrinsic strictures or neuromuscular conditions).
2. Entrapment of FBs occurs at sites of *normal* anatomic narrowing of the esophagus.
3. If a FB is lodged at any other site, underlying esophageal disease should be suspected. Children with prior surgery (e.g., repair of a tracheoesophageal fistula) or strictures (e.g., secondary to caustic ingestion or esophagitis due to recurrent gastroesophageal reflux) are at increased risk for recurrent FB lodgments.
4. Patients presenting with food bolus impaction often have underlying esophageal pathology that is directly responsible for the impaction.

Associated Clinical Features

1. The esophagus is a common site for entrapment of FBs (Fig. 15-1).
2. Most lodged esophageal FBs in children are blunt or smooth objects; the most common esophageal FBs are coins (50 to 75%).
3. Most ingested coins pass into the esophagus rather than into the airway.
4. Pennies are the most frequently swallowed coins, followed by quarters, dimes, and nickels. This probably is due to the frequency with which pennies are accessible to children.
5. Other swallowed FBs include toys, crayons, marbles, beads, batteries, wood, glass, chicken or fish bones, and a large bolus of food. Less commonly, sharp objects (e.g., screws, pins) are involved.
6. Older children who ingest FBs often have psychiatric or neurologic disorders and ingest items other than coins.
7. Conventional imaging studies include:
   a. A single frontal radiograph that includes the neck, chest, and entire abdomen can be made to locate the FB (radiopaque FBs are readily seen).
   b. If the FB is below the diaphragm, usually no additional views are required (in the absence of any prior GI pathology or surgery).
   c. If the FB is above the diaphragm, both anteroposterior and lateral views of the chest are required to precisely locate the FB (tracheal versus esophageal impaction; Figs. 15-4 and 15-5) and to confirm that the FB is not in fact two or more adherent objects (e.g., multiple coins stacked on top of each other may simulate a single coin on an AP radiograph).
8. For clinically suspected radiolucent FBs (e.g., plastic objects, food boluses):
   a. A barium swallow may be needed to outline radiolucent FBs in asymptomatic patients in whom perforation is not a concern (barium coats the FB and esophagus, reducing the effectiveness of subsequent endoscopy and increasing the risk of aspiration).
   b. If an esophageal leak is suspected, water-soluble contrast solution should be used.
9. CT scan
   a. CT scanning with coronal and sagittal reconstructions may be considered for special cases in identifying FBs (e.g., impacted bony FBs).
   b. Gives information about the FB size, type, location, and orientation with respect to other anatomic structures
   c. Helps in patients with positive plain films and negative esophagoscopy to look for a FB that has migrated from the intraluminal to extraluminal space

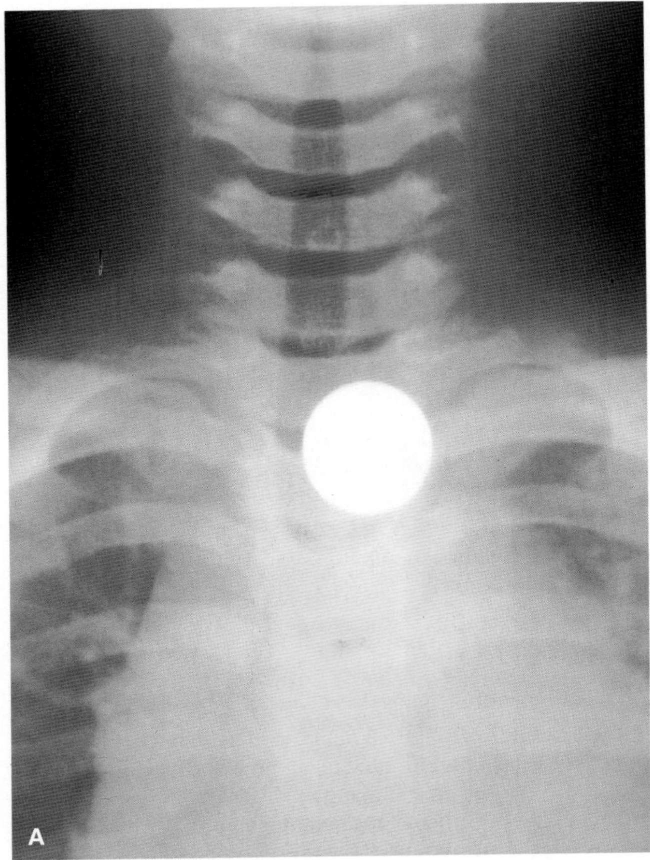

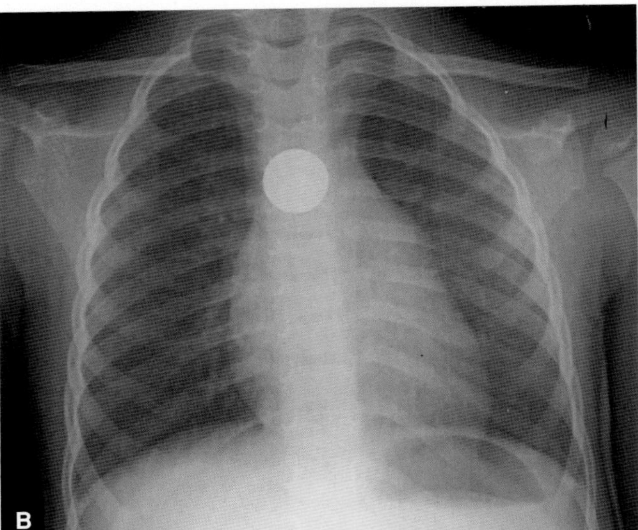

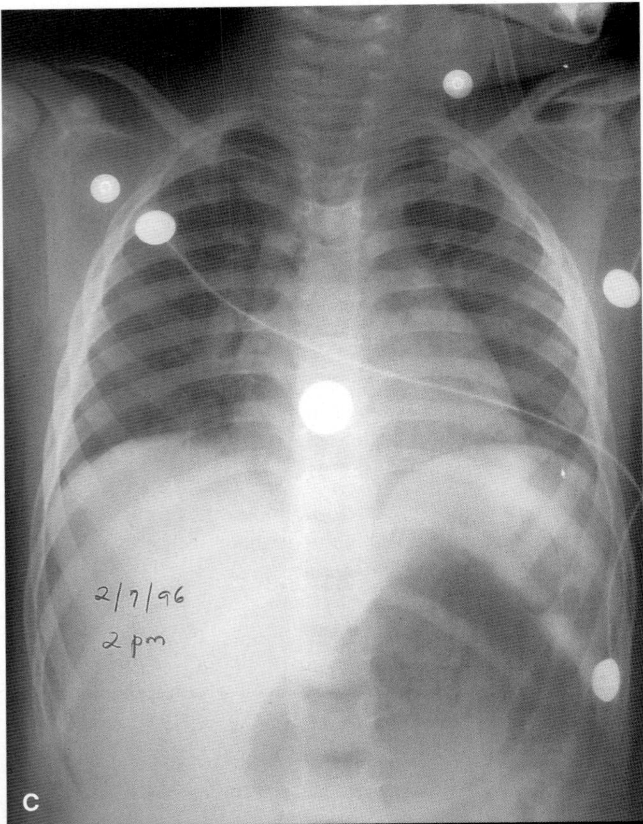

Figure 15-1. The Three Most Common Locations Where an Esophageal FB Becomes Lodged (Sites of Normal Anatomic Narrowing of the Esophagus)

A. *Proximal esophagus* at the cricopharyngeus muscle or upper esophageal sphincter at the thoracic inlet (defined as the area between the clavicles on a chest x-ray) is the *most common location of entrapment*. B. *Mid-esophagus* at the level of the aortic arch (the aortic arch and carina overlap the esophagus). C. *Distal esophagus* just proximal to the gastroesophageal junction.

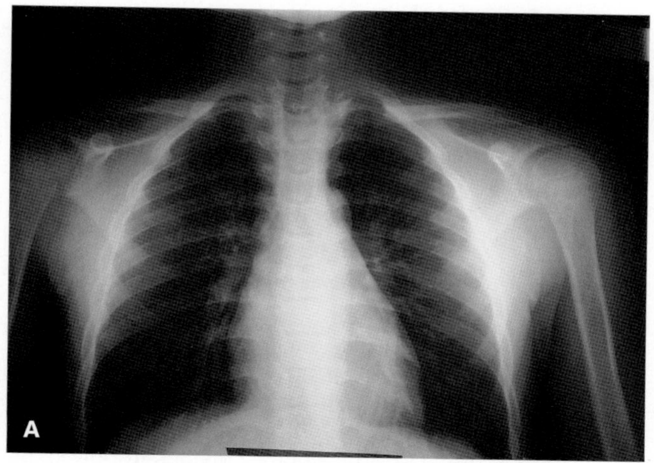

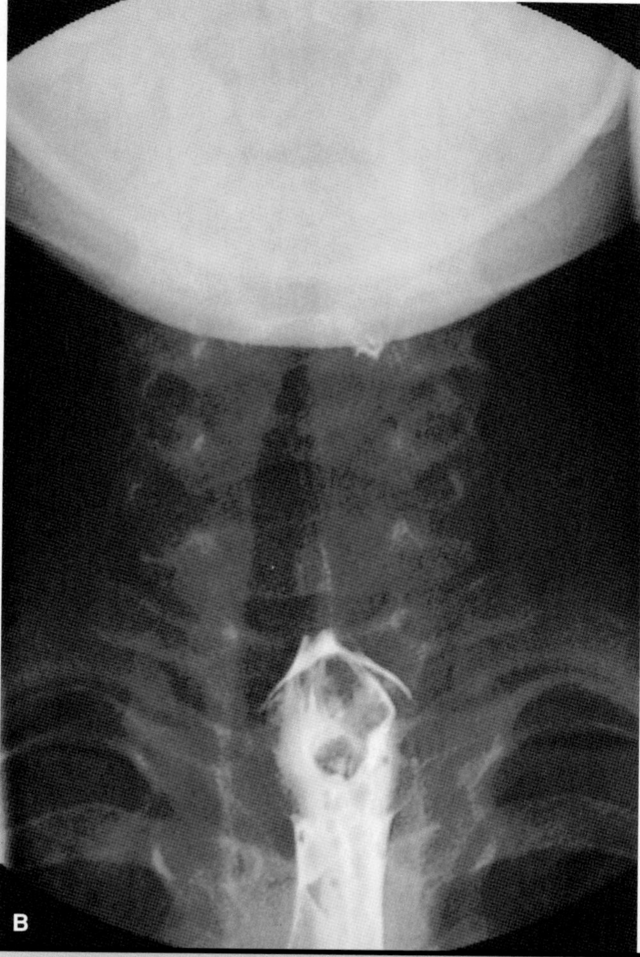

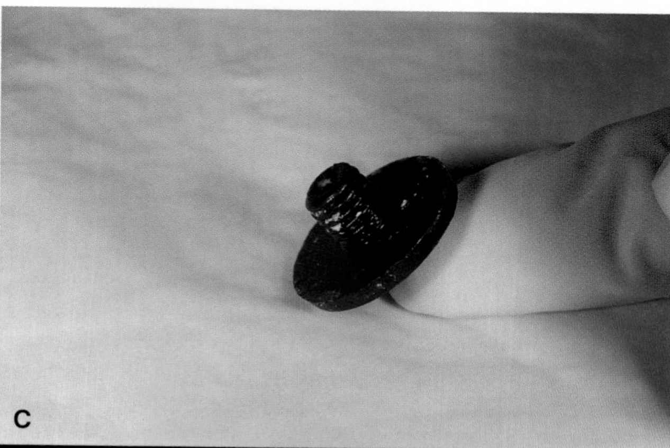

Figure 15-2. Radiolucent Esophageal Foreign Body

A. This 8-year-old boy presented with a history of drooling and swallowing a piece of a toy 12 hours prior to presenting to our ED. He was seen at another institution and was sent home because his chest and neck X-rays were negative. He was brought to our ED because of persistent drooling and vomiting. His chest radiograph (as seen here) was negative. *B*. A limited double contrast barium swallow showing a disc like structure with a central protrusion at the level of T1-T2 esophagus (upper thoracic esophagus). There is no evidence of perforation or obstruction. *C*. Foreign body that was removed by direct endoscopy under general anesthesia is shown.

d. Helps in identifying complications (e.g., esophagoaortic fistulous tract)

10. A hand-held metal detector (HHMD) for the initial screening may be used.
    a. An alternative approach to initial screening radiographs in asymptomatic patients
    b. Helps in detecting and localizing metal FBs
    c. Detects aluminum FBs (low radiodensity objects, such as the tab top from a soda can) or thin razor blades or pins that are missed by radiography
    d. The patient should be free of metallic hardware, implants, glasses, and jewelry.
    e. Undress the patient and pass the detector slowly over entire abdomen and torso.
    f. This method has no side effects and no radiation.
    g. If HHMD is positive, radiographs are ordered to confirm the presence of a FB.
    h. If HHMD negative, no radiographs are necessary.

Consultations

Radiology, surgery, or gastroenterology (depending on the therapeutic intervention required), and anesthesiology.

Emergency Department Treatment and Disposition

1. Emergent removal of a FB by operative endoscopy is recommended if:
    a. A sharp object is involved (e.g., open safety pins, straight pins; risk of perforation)
    b. A disc battery is involved (risk of corrosive injury; see Figs. 15-11 and 15-12)
2. In symptomatic patients, the FB should be removed immediately.
3. Repeat the radiograph just prior to any therapeutic intervention to make sure that the object has not passed spontaneously into the stomach.
4. The method of choice to retrieve the coin or other FB will depend on the location, duration of impaction, clinical condition of the patient, prior history of esophageal disease, and availability of a consultant (a skilled radiologist, surgeon, or gastroenterologist). Options include rigid endoscopy with forceps extraction under general anesthesia (GA), or flexible fiberoptic nonoperative endoscopy, extraction by Foley catheter, or advancement using a bougie dilator (with or without fluoroscopy).
5. Rigid endoscopy with forceps extraction under GA (*standard method of choice*):
    a. Allows controlled removal of FBs including removal of objects that are sharp or embedded in the mucosa
    b. Allows visualization of the esophagus (to check for mucosal injury or underlying pathology)
    c. Indications include patients with airway compromise, those with prolonged impaction of the FB, or those with a prior history of esophageal disease or surgery.
7. Flexible fiberoptic nonoperative endoscopy:
    a. No risk of GA; patient may need sedation
    b. Indications include patients without respiratory distress (airway control is not guaranteed with this procedure) and for FBs in place <24 hours.
8. Extraction by Foley catheter (by a radiologist under fluoroscopic guidance):
    a. Only for FBs that are smooth or blunt objects (e.g., coin) in place <24 hours.
    b. No risk of GA and usually no hospitalization is required.
    c. A Foley catheter is passed beyond the coin and a balloon is inflated with contrast media, followed by removal of both the coin and the catheter at the same time.
    d. May be considered for patients *without* airway compromise (clinically or radiographically) or underlying esophageal pathology.
9. Advancement using bougie dilator (with or without fluoroscopy):
    a. Only for FBs that are smooth or blunt (e.g., coin)
    b. Only for a single FB ingestion in place <24 hours
    c. The FB is pushed into the stomach in a patient in an upright or prone position, followed by its confirmation in the stomach by a radiography.
    d. May be considered for patients *without* respiratory distress or esophageal pathology or a prior history of FB ingestion
5. Await spontaneous passage (expectant management; e.g., coin impaction at the lower esophageal sphincter [LES])
    a. A blunt FB at the LES often passes spontaneously within several hours of ingestion.
    b. Done only in an *asymptomatic, healthy child* (normal esophageal anatomy [no prior history of esophageal surgery or injury])
    c. *History of coin lodged in esophagus <24 hours*
    d. Allows patient to eat or drink
    e. Repeat radiograph in several hours to confirm the spontaneous passage through the LES
    f. If the patient fails the tests of eating and time (no progression of the FB from the LES to the stomach), the patient is a candidate for endoscopic removal of the FB.
6. Indications for thoracotomy for removal of a FB include poor endoscopic visualization of the FB because of inflammatory tissue or herald bleeding during endoscopy.

Clinical Pearls: Esophageal Foreign Bodies

1. Coins are the most common esophageal FBs in children.
2. A history of swallowing a FB may be present; however, absence of such history *does not exclude* the possibility of

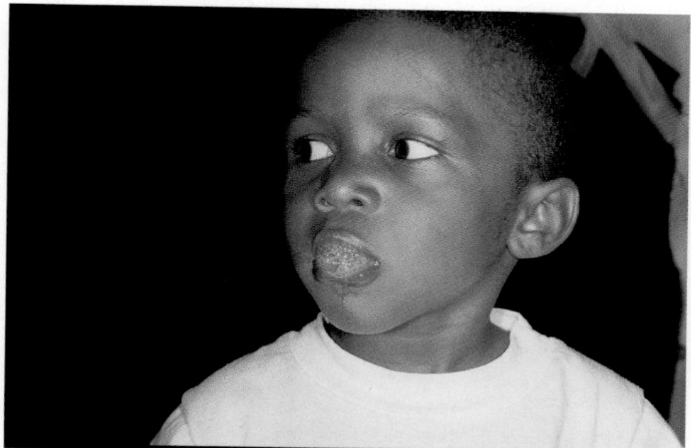

Figure 15-3. Drooling as a Presenting Sign of an Esophageal Foreign Body

A 30-month-old afebrile child presented with a sudden onset of drooling and an inability to eat solid foods of 12 hours' duration. There was no history of any witnessed episode of choking, gagging, or FB ingestion. Based on his history, an esophageal FB was suspected and radiographs were obtained (see Fig. 15-4). Drooling is a very common and consistent sign seen with a high-grade obstruction.

a FB (*in the majority of patients such episodes are usually not witnessed by a caretaker*).

3. The most common symptoms of an esophageal FB are drooling or dysphagia (Fig. 15-3). The presence of symptoms at the time of evaluation often predicts the presence of an esophageal FB; however, absence of symptoms does not rule it out.
4. The initial radiograph provides extremely valuable information including size, shape, orientation, location, and type of FB (e.g., coin, battery; Fig. 15-4).
5. Suspect an underlying esophageal disease if a child presents with an FB lodged in an unusual location, other than the normal anatomical narrowing sites.
6. Since impacted esophageal FBs can lead to serious complications (and even death), *a FB lodged in the esophagus must be removed*. Under no circumstances should a FB or food bolus impaction be allowed to remain in the esophagus beyond 24 hours from presentation (impacted disc batteries or sharp objects must be removed emergently).
7. When the duration of an esophageal FB is unknown, it should be retrieved by rigid endoscopy under general anesthesia.
8. The majority of FBs ingested by children are radiopaque, in contrast to FB inhalation, in which case the majority of FBs are radiolucent.
9. Persistent symptoms related to the esophagus in cases of suspected FB ingestion must be pursued with endoscopy, even after an apparently unrevealing radiographic evaluation.

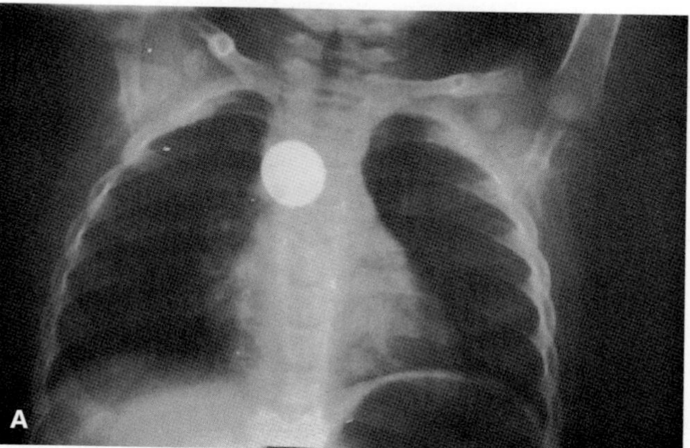

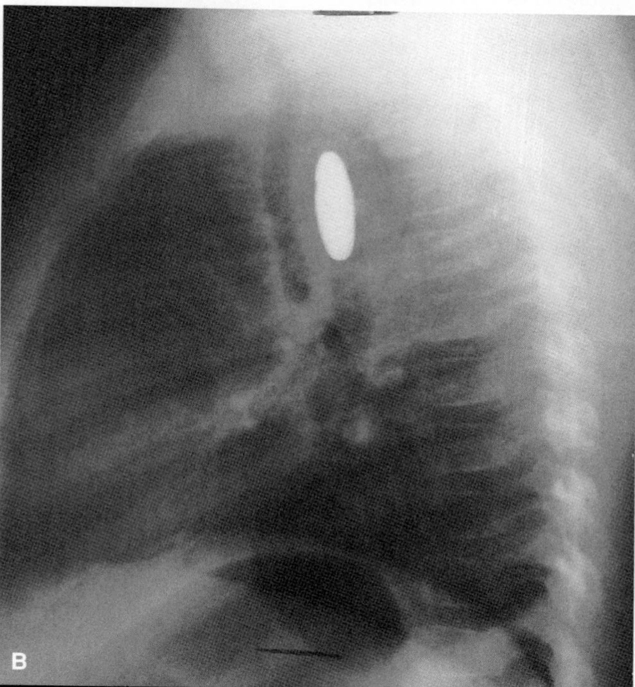

Figure 15-4. Classic Orientation of an Esophageal Foreign Body on Radiographs

A. Frontal view of chest showing an esophageal coin lodged at the level of the aortic arch. The coin in the esophagus will lie in the coronal plane (i.e., the coin is seen as a disk on a frontal view) since the opening into the esophagus is much wider in this orientation. *B*. Note the sagittal orientation of the coin on a lateral film (i.e., the coin is seen from the side and posterior to the tracheal air column).

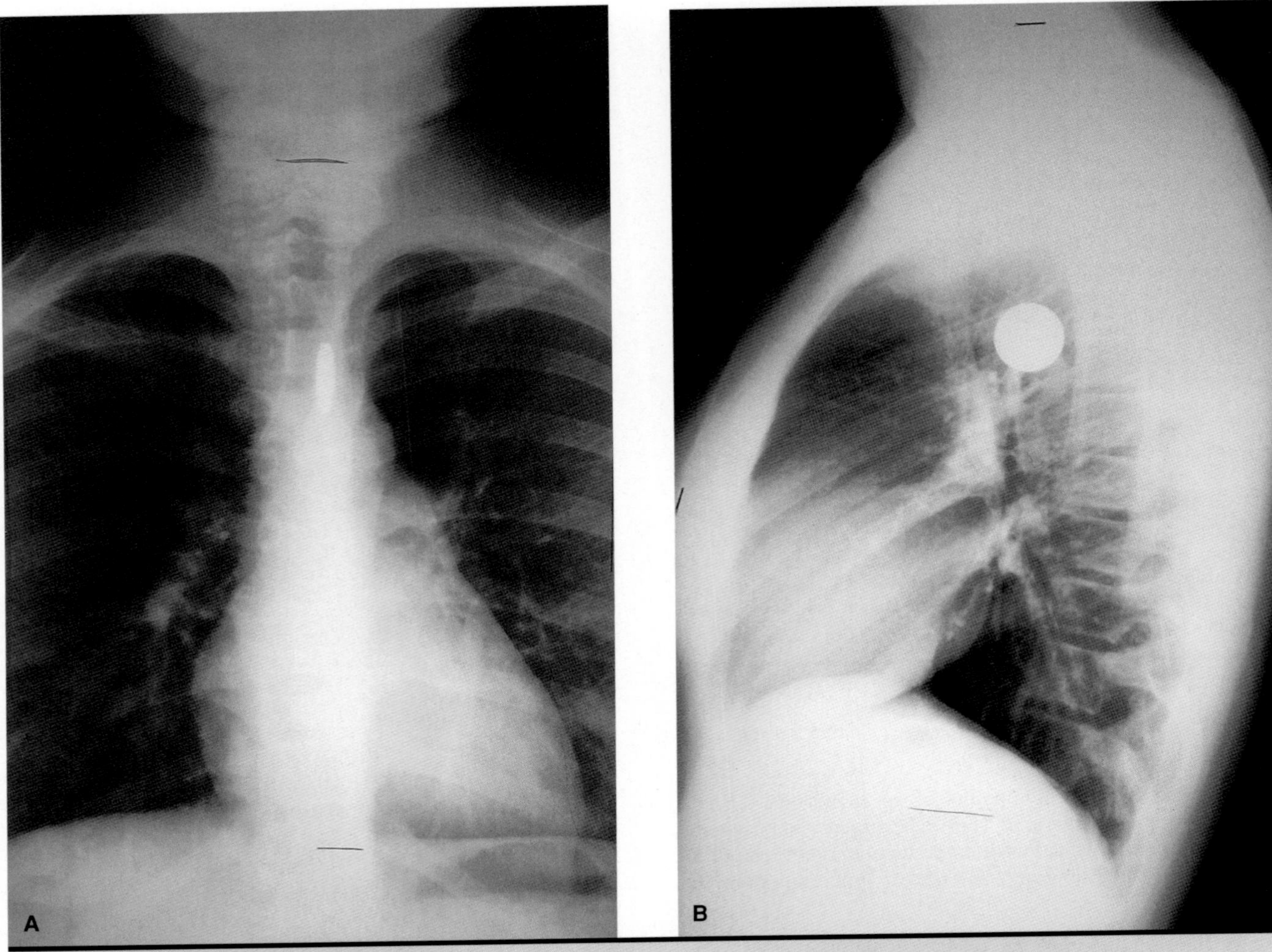

Figure 15-5. Esophageal Foreign Body Mimicking a Tracheal Foreign Body

Frontal and lateral views of the chest showing a coin at the thoracic inlet. When a coin gets lodged in the trachea, the orientation of the coin is *opposite* that seen with an esophageal coin (see Fig. 15-4). With the configuration of the tracheal rings and with incomplete cartilage posteriorly, a coin in the trachea appears in the sagittal orientation (i.e., the coin is seen from the side) in a frontal view, and in the coronal orientation (i.e., the coin is seen as a disk) on a lateral view (*B*). However, as seen here, this rule is not always correct. These radiographs actually show an impacted esophageal coin that mimics the orientation that is classically seen with a coin lodged in the trachea. The normal diameter of a dime is 17 mm, the penny is 18 mm, the nickel is 20 mm, and the quarter is 24 mm. The normal tracheal airway caliber as measured on chest radiograph ranges from 13 to 25 mm (sagittal diameter) in men and from 10 to 23 mm in women; thus, any one these coins can be potentially aspirated into an adult trachea.

BOX 15-1. CLINICAL FEATURES OF ESOPHAGEAL FOREIGN BODIES

Location of esophageal FBs:

- Entrapment of FBs occurs at the sites of normal anatomic narrowing of the esophagus.
- The three most common locations where a FB becomes lodged:
  (1) Proximal esophagus at the cricopharyngeus muscle (C6) or upper esophageal sphincter at the thoracic inlet (T1): about 70%
  (2) Mid-esophagus at the level of the aortic arch (T4; the aortic arch and carina overlap the esophagus): about 15%
  (3) Distal esophagus (at level 2 to 4 vertebral bodies cephalad to the gastric bubble; gastroesophageal junction): about 15%

Epidemiology, signs and symptoms:

- 80% of all FB ingestions occur in children <5 years of age
- Peak incidence of FB ingestion: 6 months to 3 years of age
- Sudden history of choking, gagging, or coughing (provoked by swallowing a FB)
- History of swallowing a FB (in some cases, there is no such history)
- Asymptomatic (7 to 35% of patients with proven esophageal FBs are asymptomatic)

Most common presentations:

(1) Drooling or excessive salivation

(2) Retching

(3) Dysphagia (young infants will refuse solid food but may take liquids)

(4) Chest or neck pain (older patients)

(5) Discomfort on swallowing (odynophagia)

(6) Vomiting

(7) Hematemesis

(8) Localization or a FB body sensation (older patients)

(9) Respiratory signs and symptoms: cough, stridor, wheezing, respiratory distress (from external compression of the trachea or larynx), or aspiration (saliva, food)

Uncommon presentations:

(1) Symptom-free period followed by edema or inflammation (signs and symptoms of esophageal obstruction)

(2) Fever (secondary to complications)

(3) Pain (worsening chest pain, pain radiating to neck)

(4) Crepitus (in the neck and upper chest due to perforation)

(5) Shock secondary to perforation

BOX 15-2. COMPLICATIONS OF ESOPHAGEAL FOREIGN BODIES

- Impaction of a FB for a prolonged period (weeks, months, or years)
- Mucosal scratching or abrasions, ulceration, and granulation at the point of impaction
- Esophageal necrosis (button batteries)
- Airway obstruction (wheezing, stridor from external tracheal obstruction)
- Lobar atelectasis
- Regurgitation and lodging of a FB in the trachea
- Extraluminal migration of a FB
- Formation of esophageal strictures
- Esophageal diverticulum
- Esophageal perforation leading to:
  (1) Paraesophageal abscess
  (2) Mediastinitis
  (3) Pericarditis
  (4) Pericardial tamponade
  (5) Pneumothorax
  (6) Pneumomediastinum
  (7) Tracheoesophageal fistula
  (8) Esophageal-aortic fistula
  (9) Death (related to any of the above)

(Modified and reproduced with permission from: Munter DW: Disorders of the esophagus. In: Howell JM, Altieri M (eds). *Emergency Medicine*. WB Saunders, Philadelphia, 1998, p. 319.)

DIAGNOSIS FOREIGN BODIES IN THE STOMACH AND LOWER GASTROINTESTINAL TRACT

Definition

An ingestion of a foreign object into the gastrointestinal tract (GI) that occurs either accidentally or intentionally.

Associated Clinical Features

1. Foreign bodies (FBs) in GI tract can be seen in all age groups. However, FB ingestion is more commonly seen in pediatric, psychiatric, or incarcerated patients or patients with risk-taking behaviors. Risk of ingestion increases after consumption of alcohol or cold liquids (due to a decrease in oral sensory acuity).
2. Ingestion of multiple FBs and repeated episodes are not uncommon.
3. The most common foreign objects ingested are:
   a. Young children: coins, toys, jewels, marbles, buttons, batteries (see Fig. 15-10).
   b. Older children, teenagers, and adults: fish or chicken bones, a large bolus of food, toothpicks, sharp objects (e.g., needles, pins, nails; Figs. 15-6, 15-7, and 15-8)
4. Body packing (e.g., cocaine or heroin wrapped in plastic or well-concealed in condoms) or body stuffing (hurried ingestion of poorly prepared packages of illicit drugs in the face of imminent arrest) may be seen in drug trafficking (see Figs. 17-8 through 17-10).
5. Where a FB is retained in the GI tract depends on:
   a. Shape and size of the FB
   b. Diameter of GI tract including normal anatomic sites of narrowing or angulation at the following locations: esophagus, pylorus, duodenum, ligament of Treitz, ileocecal valve, appendix, hepatic and splenic flexures of the colon and rectum (the level of the cricopharyngeus muscle and ileocecal valve are the most clinically significant)
   c. Any other location of congenital (e.g., webs, diaphragms, diverticula) or acquired narrowing
   d. Patients with a prior surgical history (e.g., pyloromyotomy) are prone to impaction.
   e. GI motility
6. After ingestion, usually FBs are found:
   a. About 55 to 62% of cases: below the diaphragm
   b. About 20 to 30% of the cases: esophagus
   c. About 10 to 20% of reported ingestions: FBs cannot be found
7. Imaging studies:
   a. About 90% of ingested FBs are radiopaque and are readily seen on radiographs.
   b. To locate the FB, a single frontal radiograph that includes the neck, chest, and entire abdomen can be ordered. Additional lateral views help in confirming type, location/orientation, and number of ingested objects. Free mediastinal or peritoneal air is also identified on radiographs.
   c. If the FB is below the diaphragm, usually no additional views are required if the FB is not sharp (in the absence of any prior GI pathology or GI surgery).
   d. An esophagogram with contrast may be indicated in asymptomatic patients for clinically suspected radiolucent FBs with nonvisualization of FBs on radiograph (e.g., aluminum tab, plastic toy, food bolus, most glass, and wood).

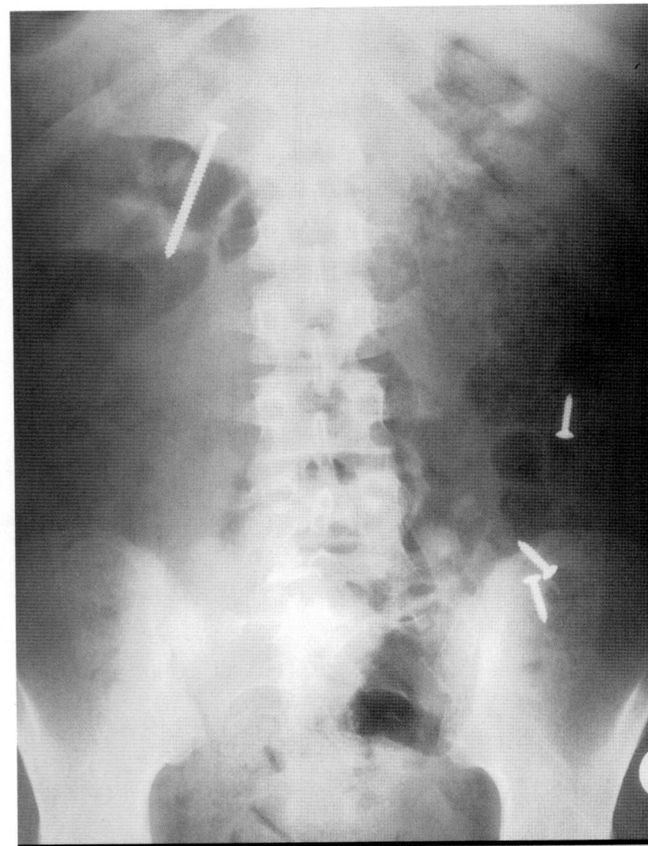

Figure 15-6. Nail Ingestion

A flat plate of the abdomen showing several nails scattered throughout the intestines. These nails were intentionally ingested by an adolescent psychiatric patient. She remained asymptomatic and passed these nails over a period of 72 hours.

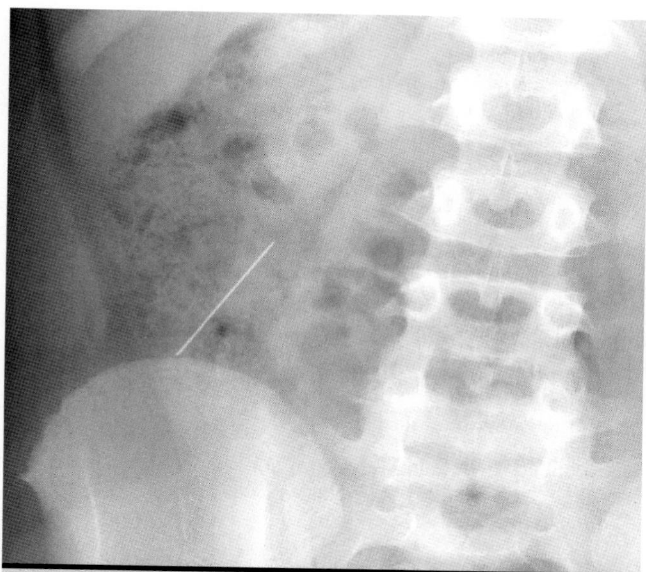

Figure 15-7. Pin Ingestion

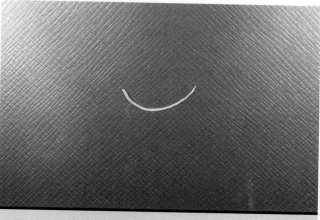

A linear metallic density (straight pin) is seen in the right lower quadrant, possibly in the ascending colon. This 11-year-old child presented with a history of accidentally swallowing a pin followed by abdominal pain. His first radiograph showed the pin in the stomach. He was admitted and underwent serial abdominal examinations and daily radiographs. He passed this pin after 6 days without developing any complications. A sharp pointed object lodged in the esophagus is a medical emergency and needs removal endoscopically. Even though the majority of sharp objects that enter the stomach pass through the remaining GI tract without any problem, the risk of complications in such patients is high (about 35%). Thus, sharp objects that are either in the stomach or proximal duodenum should be removed endoscopically (if this can be done safely). Otherwise these patients need very close monitoring.

e. CT scanning with coronal and sagittal reconstructions may be considered in special cases for identifying FBs, especially impacted bony FBs, visualizing low-density objects, and identifying complications (e.g., adjacent soft tissue inflammation or abscess formation).

Consultations

Radiology, surgery, or gastroenterology (depending on the therapeutic interventions)

Emergency Department Treatment and Disposition

1. Conservative outpatient management is recommended for most FBs that have already passed the esophagus and entered the stomach (exception: sharp FBs).
   a. Most FBs will pass through the intestine in 4 to 6 days; however, some may take as long as 3 to 4 weeks.

Figure 15-8. Fish Bone

An adolescent girl presented to the ED with a complaint of something stuck in back of her throat after eating fish for dinner. Radiographs of the neck and chest were negative for the presence of any radiopaque FB. This impacted fish bone was removed by direct laryngoscopy from the hypopharynx. Chicken or fish bones are often poorly visualized because of their varying degree of calcification. Only 29 to 50% of endoscopically-proven bones are seen on plain radiographs.

   b. Instruct parents to observe the stools for the appearance of the ingested FB. Even though this is an unpleasant task, most parents are willing to accept it (tell the parent to think of the FB as if it were a diamond ring that was swallowed by the child, and the parent is trying to retrieve it).
   c. Educate parents about the warning signals (vomiting, abdominal pain, melena, or hematemesis) and advise them to report to a physician immediately if such symptoms develop.
   d. In the absence of symptoms, weekly radiographs may be considered to follow the progression of small blunt objects not observed to pass spontaneously.
   e. Stool softeners, cathartics, and special diets have no proven benefit in the management of ingested FBs.
2. Objects that may require removal by endoscopy:
   a. Sewing needles or open safety pins (increased risk of perforation)
   b. A FB longer than 6 cm or wider than 2 cm in infants (such FBs usually will not pass through the pylorus)
   c. Oval shaped FBs >5 cm in diameter or >2 cm in thickness tend to lodge in the stomach in older children and adults.
   d. Foreign objects like toothbrushes or spoons that are >6 to 10 cm in length may have difficulty passing through the duodenum.
   e. Objects that remain in the same location for >1 week after passing from the stomach
3. Once a FB has passed the ligament of Treitz, it cannot be removed endoscopically.

4. Perform serial abdominal examinations and radiographs for a patient with a sharp or long object that already has passed out of the stomach.
5. Immediate surgical consultation is required for patients presenting with symptoms related to FB ingestion (e.g., signs of perforation, bleeding, fever, vomiting, abdominal pain).
6. Body packets usually pass through the GI tract spontaneously. They are usually not removed endoscopically because of the risk of rupture. Surgery is indicated for patients presenting with signs of rupture, obstruction, or if there is a failure to progress. Patients are admitted for close monitoring (both for passage of packets as well as toxicity). Whole-body irrigation with polyethylene glycol or laxatives can be used to facilitate passage.

Clinical Pearls: Foreign Bodies in the Stomach and Lower GI Tract

1. Coins are the FBs most frequently swallowed by children.
2. The majority of FBs that reach the GI tract will pass spontaneously. The lower esophageal sphincter is the narrowest passage in the GI tract through which a FB must pass. Once a swallowed FB reaches the stomach of a child with a normal GI tract, it is unlikely to lead to any complications, and about 95% of the FBs will pass through the remainder of the GI tract in an average time of 5 days.
3. A prophylactic laparotomy is not indicated for the retrieval of the FB; surgery is indicated for patients who develop complications due to ingestion.
4. Ingestion of unusual FBs may suggest an underlying abnormality (e.g., ingestion of multiple screws by a patient suffering from a psychiatric illness, or toothbrush ingestions and bulimia in adolescents).
5. Retained fish bones are commonly identified by direct vision of the mouth and pharynx with the use of a tongue blade and good light source.
6. Suspect child neglect with a repeated history of FB ingestions in children.

BOX 15-3. CLINICAL FEATURES OF FOREIGN BODIES IN THE STOMACH AND LOWER GASTROINTESTINAL TRACT

- 80% of all FB ingestions occur in children <6 years of age.
- Peak incidence of FB ingestion: 6 months to 6 years of age

Signs and symptoms:

(1) Completely asymptomatic (symptoms uncommon when a swallowed FB has already passed through the gastroesophageal sphincter)

(2) Sudden history of choking, coughing, or gagging provoked by ingestion of a FB

(3) History of a swallowed FB

(4) Occasionally, history of passing a FB in the stool (and the patient presents to the ED for evaluation)

(5) Complaints of pain at the site of impaction of the FB by older children/adolescents

(6) Abdominal pain

(7) Vomiting

(8) Abdominal distention

(9) Abdominal mass, if FB is a bezoar (a mass of undigested vegetable matter [phytobezoar], milk curds [lactobezoar], or hair [trichobezoar])

(10) Hematochezia

(11) Usually unremarkable physical examination (unless the patient is presenting with complications related to FB ingestion)

(12) Swelling, tenderness, crepitus, or erythema in the neck (oropharyngeal or proximal esophageal perforation)

(13) Signs or symptoms of toxicity from illicit drugs such as narcotics, due to rupture of packets or obstruction caused by packets

Complications related to FB ingestion:

A. Bowel perforation
   (1) Frequency estimated to be <1%.
   (2) Frequency is increased (about 15 to 35%) with sharp or pointed metallic objects like animal or fish bones, bread bag clips, toothpicks, straightened paper clips, or needles.
   (3) Sites of perforation: areas of previous surgery, areas of acute angulation or sites of anatomic narrowing (e.g., pylorus, duodenum, ileocecal valve, appendix)
   (4) Complications related to perforation: peritonitis, hemorrhage, abscess formation, inflammatory tumors, and death

B. Bowel obstruction

BOX 15-4. RETAINED FISH BONES

- Impaction of swallowed fish bones is common in countries where fish are a major dietary resource.
- Common presenting complaint: a bone or something stuck in the throat
- Symptoms often due to minor mucosal injury (e.g., abrasion or laceration)
- Common sites where a bone may get lodged: tonsils, base of tongue, or posterior pharyngeal wall
- *Diagnosis made by any of the following:*
  (1) Direct inspection of the mouth, oropharynx, and hypopharynx
  (2) Indirect laryngoscopy
  (3) Fiberoptic pharyngoscopy
- A bone is identified in only 20 to 30% of such patients (fish or chicken bones are poorly visualized on radiographs because of their varying degrees of calcification)
- A lateral plain radiograph with soft tissue technique may show the presence of a bone.
  (1) Plain radiographs are *not* useful in the diagnosis of fish bone lodgment.
  (2) Radiolucent fish skeleton: commonly eaten fish like salmon, mackerel, or trout
  (3) Radiopaque fish skeleton: fish like cod, haddock, and halibut (however, the radiograph may still be negative)
- A retained fish bone rarely passes spontaneously once it becomes lodged in the mucosa, and usually requires removal.
- Local anesthetic spray may aid in the evaluation and removal of a retained bone.

BOX 15-5. CLINICAL FEATURES OF ANORECTAL FOREIGN BODIES

- *Anorectal FBs result from:*
  (1) Retrograde introduction of a FB due to sexual practices (most common; Fig. 15-9)
  (2) Lodgment of a FB in the rectum after passing through the proximal GI tract (e.g., fish bone)
- *Presenting signs and symptoms include:*
  (1) Patients are usually reluctant to admit to a history of a self-introduced FB.

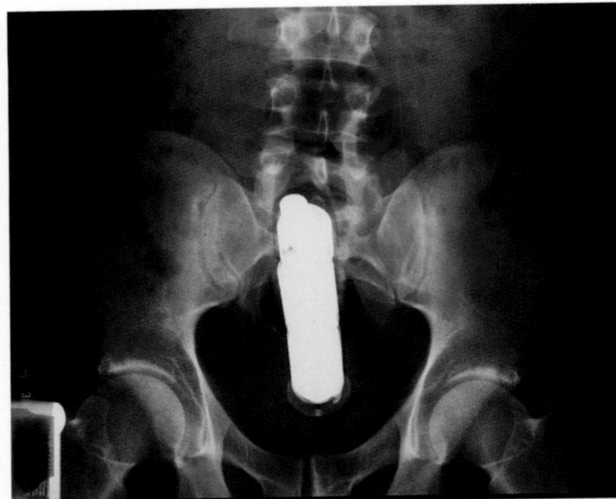

Figure 15-9. Rectal Foreign Body

This vibrator was inserted into his rectum by a 21-year-old homosexual patient. He presented to the ED because he could not retrieve the vibrator. Attempts to remove it in the ED with sedation/analgesia failed, and he required laparotomy.

  (2) Anal pain
  (3) Constipation
  (4) Rectal bleeding
  (5) Inability to void (due to large objects impinging on the urethra)
  (6) Signs of peritonitis (anorectal perforation)
  (7) Poor sphincter tone
  (8) FB may be palpated on digital rectal examination
  (9) Bloody discharge on digital rectal examination
- Plain abdominal radiograph
  (1) Detects radiopaque anorectal FB
  (2) Free intraperitoneal air suggests anorectal perforation.
- A contrast study (preferably using water-soluble contrast medium for patients with possible perforation) for patients with a negative radiograph
- *Caution:* Use of enemas or cathartics to facilitate passage of an anorectal FB may increase the risk of perforation (especially with sharp FBs).
- Various management options (as indicated with either sedation/analgesia or general anesthesia)
  (1) Digital extraction (lubricate digit with lidocaine jelly)
  (2) Use an anoscope or vaginal speculum for visualization of the FB, followed by forceps-aided removal of the FB.
  (3) Sigmoidoscopy with forceps-aided removal of FB
  (4) Laparotomy

DIAGNOSIS BATTERY INGESTIONS

Definition

Accidental or intentional ingestion of cylindrical or button battery (or batteries)

Associated Clinical Features

1. Both cylindrical and button batteries are commonly found in most households. Some examples include cylindrical batteries for toys and cameras and button batteries for hearing aids, games, watches, calculators, cameras, remote control devices, phones, musical greeting cards, and talking story books (Fig. 15-10).
2. Disk or button battery ingestion is common. Batteries are often placed accidentally in the ear or nose by children.
3. Both the size and the chemical composition are important in determining the possible consequences and management of ingested batteries.
   a. Button cells range in diameter from 6.8 to 23 mm.

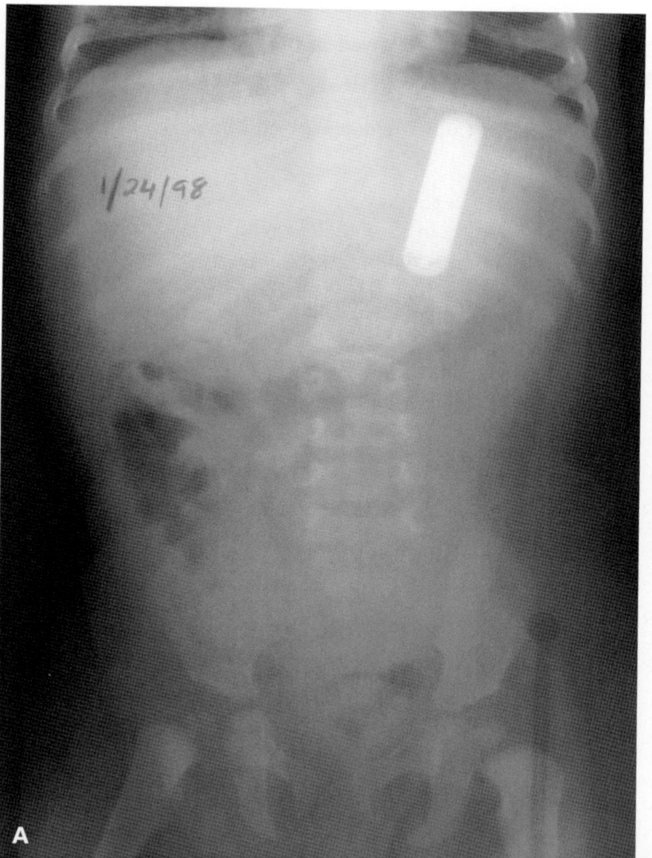

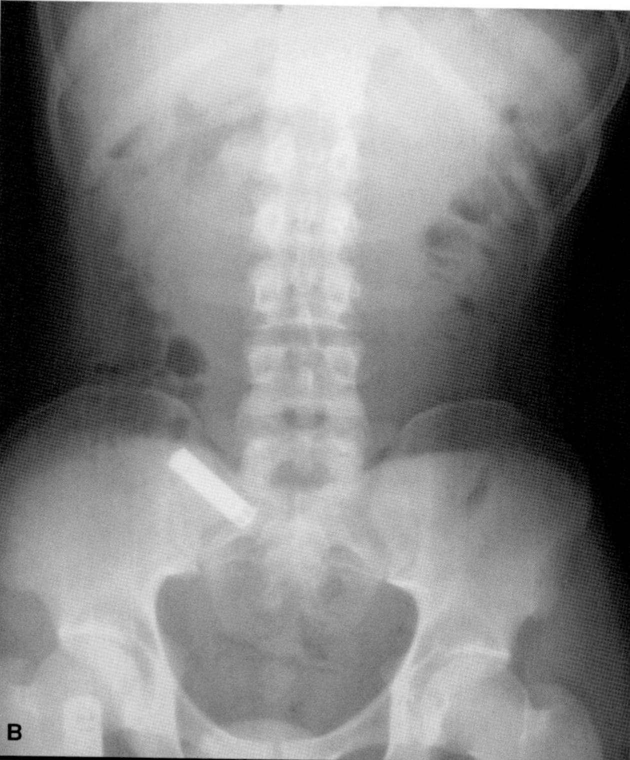

Figure 15-10. Cylindrical Battery Ingestion

A. Frontal view of the abdomen showing a cylindrical battery lodged in the stomach. This was accidentally found in this 5-month-old infant when a chest radiograph was obtained for suspected pneumonia. Serial radiographs over 72 hours showed failure of progression of the battery beyond the stomach (arrested transit). Because of the failure to progress and unknown exact time of ingestion, this battery (which turned out to be a severely corroded AAA battery) was removed endoscopically. *B*. An adolescent psychiatric patient was brought to the ED because he confessed to intentionally swallowing a battery 24 hours before this radiograph was obtained. He was completely asymptomatic. He passed the battery 48 hours after this radiograph was obtained.

   b. The most popular button batteries are 7.9 or 11.6 mm in diameter.
   c. Most batteries that become lodged in the esophagus and cause tissue injury are large batteries (20 to 23 mm, about the size of a quarter).

4. Chemical composition of commonly used batteries:
   a. Metallic salts (e.g., mercury, lithium, nickel, zinc, cadmium, silver, manganese) and concentrated alkali media (e.g., sodium or potassium hydroxide)
   b. Lithium cells (both larger diameter and higher voltage) are more often associated with adverse effects.
   c. Mercuric oxide cells (more likely to rupture in the GI tract; legislation enacted in 1996 bans the marketing of mercury oxide button cells in the United States)

5. Mucosal injury from battery impaction results from liquefaction necrosis (due to release of concentrated alkali), direct pressure necrosis, and local electrical current discharge.

6. A radiograph must be obtained promptly to determine the location of the battery. Posteroanterior (PA) and lateral views of the neck and chest, and if required a PA view of the abdomen are obtained.

7. Heavy metal poisoning (including mercury) is unlikely. Blood or urine mercury levels are not indicated unless a mercury oxide battery ruptures in the GI tract or radiopaque droplets are seen in the gut.

Consultation

Emergent consultation with surgeon or gastroenterologist for batteries lodged in the esophagus or patients with signs of GI tract injury

Emergency Department Treatment and Disposition

1. Hospitalize all patients with batteries lodged in the esophagus and all symptomatic patients with signs of injury to the GI tract (see below).
2. Determine the battery's diameter and chemical composition from the code printed on an identical battery. For assistance and to report all battery ingestions, call the National Button Battery Ingestion Hotline (National Capital Poison Center, Washington, DC) at (202) 625-3333 (call collect). After passage or retrieval, ingested batteries are mailed to the poison center to determine the extent of corrosion, crimp area dissolution, and pitting (reporting allows collection of case data and refinement of clinical management recommendations).
3. Do not induce vomiting with syrup of ipecac
   a. Risk of perforation of esophagus or stomach in the presence of mucosal burns
   b. Risk of aspiration in the tracheobronchial tree during retrograde movement of the battery during ipecac-induced emesis
4. Batteries lodged in the esophagus must be removed *emergently.*
   a. By endoscopy under direct visualization (allows visualization of the esophageal mucosa)
   b. Observation and reevaluation over several days after removal of the battery for possible complications that may not be evident soon after removal
   c. Removal using the Foley catheter technique should be avoided.
      1) Does not allow direct visualization of esophageal mucosa
      2) Risk of esophageal perforation may be increased
   d. Indications for thoracotomy for removal:
      1) Poor endoscopic visualization of a battery because of inflammatory tissue
      2) Herald bleeding during endoscopy
5. For a battery that has passed beyond the esophagus, battery retrieval is indicated for
   a. Symptomatic patients with significant signs of injury to the GI tract (e.g., hematochezia, abdominal pain, tenderness, or radiographic signs of battery rupture). Minor GI symptoms (e.g., transient vomiting, stool discoloration [in the absence of GI bleeding]) usually do not mandate retrieval.
   b. Failure of a large battery (e.g., 20 mm or larger) to pass through the pylorus (if a battery does not pass from the stomach within 48 hours, it is unlikely to pass)
6. If a battery has passed beyond the esophagus and the patient is asymptomatic
   a. The patient can be followed closely as an outpatient and should be encouraged to resume a regular diet and normal activity in order to promote GI transit. The patient should be followed closely by inspection of the stools and by radiographs (if indicated for 7 to 14 days postingestion to confirm the passage of the battery if it has not been observed in the stool).
   b. Consider more frequent radiographs (once or twice weekly) if a 15.6-mm diameter mercury oxide cell was ingested (high incidence of rupture of the battery in the GI tract).
7. Pharmacologic therapy (e.g., metoclopramide [enhances gastric passage] in combination with a histamine antagonist [to limit corrosive damage and local injury]) is usually not recommended due to a lack of significant efficacy. Routine use of antibiotics and steroids is also not recommended.
8. Most batteries pass without any complications through the GI tract (Box 15-7 and Box 15-9).

Clinical Pearls: Ingestion of Cylindrical and Button Batteries

1. Hearing aid batteries are the batteries most frequently ingested by children.
2. Location of the ingested battery *must be determined promptly* by a radiograph.
3. Batteries lodged in the esophagus *should be removed emergently* by endoscopy under direct visualization or by surgery.

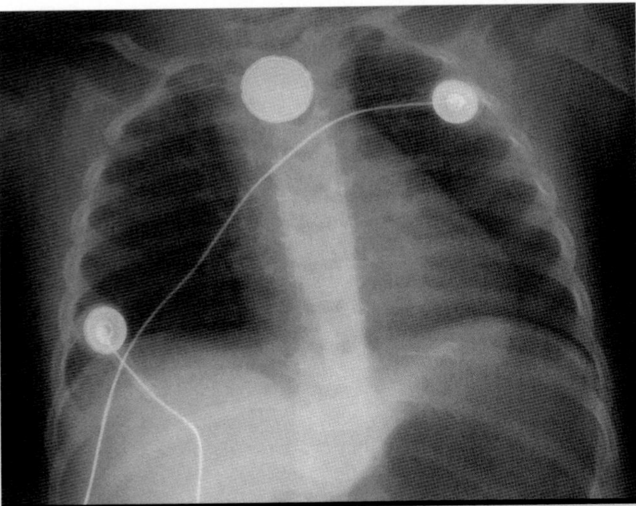

Figure 15-11. Button Battery Mimicking a Coin on Radiography

An impacted battery was seen in the esophagus at the thoracic inlet in this 18-month-old infant who presented with persistent cough, noisy breathing of 72 hours' duration, and high fever of 48 hours' duration. His radiograph showed an impacted battery which was initially misidentified as a coin by both the physician and radiologist. During an attempt to endoscopically remove this battery in the operating room, he had a massive hemorrhage followed by cardiopulmonary arrest. Intense esophageal inflammation was seen at the site of impaction and he had also developed a tracheoesophageal fistula. (Reproduced with permission from: Shah BR, Laude TL: Ingestion of cylindrical and button (disc) batteries. In: *Atlas of Pediatric Clinical Diagnosis*. WB Saunders, Philadelphia, 2000, p. 394.)

4. Batteries are radiopaque and button batteries appear the same as does an impacted coin (both are round densities), but a three-dimensional appearance suggests a battery (Figs. 15-11 and 15-12).

5. It is unsafe and contraindicated to induce vomiting with syrup of ipecac with battery ingestion.

6. Most cases of battery ingestion follow a benign course if the battery has not lodged in the esophagus.

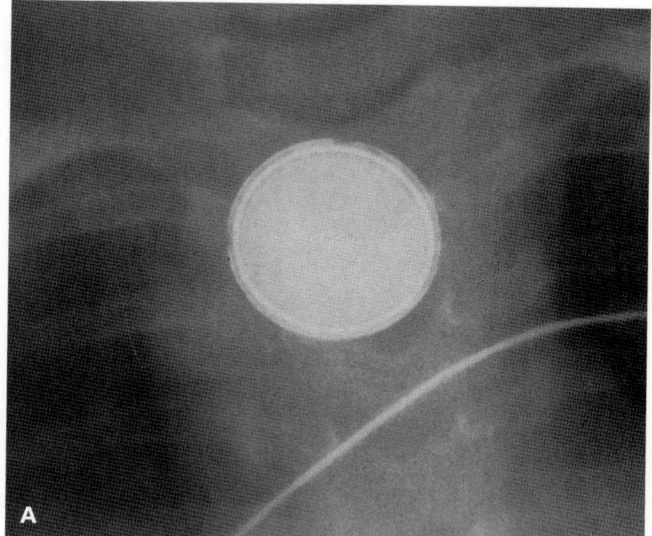

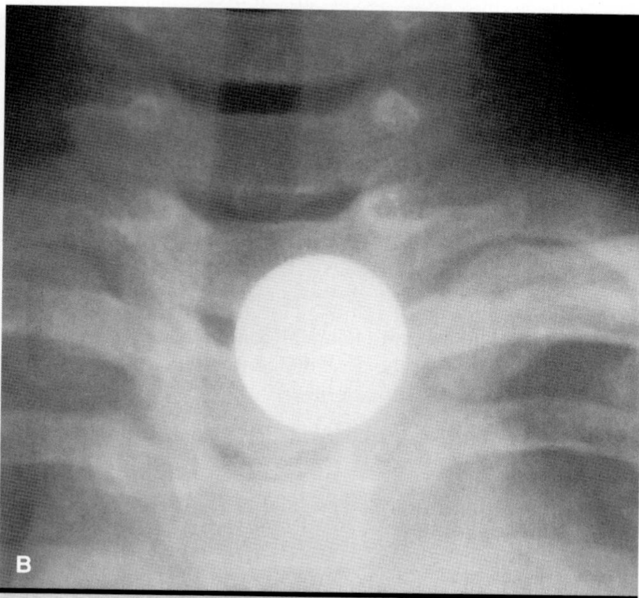

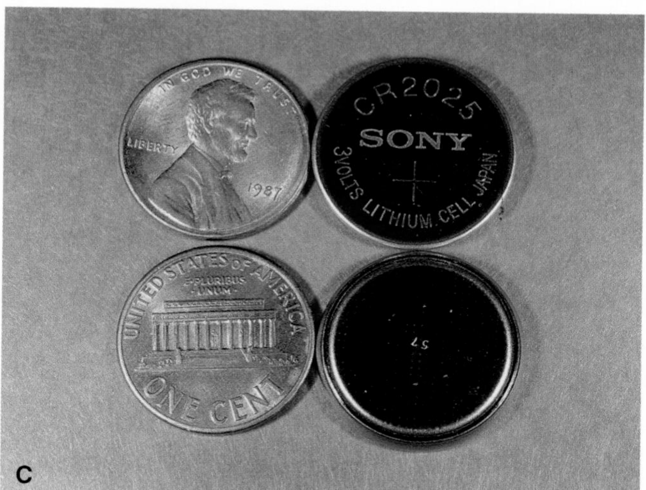

Figure 15-12. Interpreting Radiography in Battery and Coin Ingestion

A. Compare the magnified views of the battery seen here (from the same patient seen in Fig. 15-11) with a coin (*B*) from a different patient. These images clearly demonstrate the radiologic differences between a battery, with a lucent center and serrated three-dimensional appearance, and a coin, which has homogenous density and smooth edges. *C*. Here, compare the size and appearance of a button battery with that of a penny. (Reproduced with permission from: Shah BR, Laude TL: Ingestion of cylindrical and button (disc) batteries. In: *Atlas of Pediatric Clinical Diagnosis*. WB Saunders, Philadelphia, 2000, p. 394.)

BOX 15-6. CLINICAL FEATURES OF BATTERY INGESTION

- Most ingestions are accidental (rarely is there suicidal intent).
- Most ingestions occur in children <5 years of age (peak between 1 and 2 years of age).
- The most frequently ingested batteries are hearing aid batteries (batteries are often removed by children from their own hearing aids, and subsequently are ingested).
- Ingestion may involve multiple button batteries.
- About 80% of patients with battery ingestions remain completely asymptomatic (thus, there can be difficulty in making the diagnosis based on clinical signs and symptoms).
- Both the size and chemical composition are important in determining the possible consequences and management of ingested batteries.
- A sudden history of choking, coughing, or gagging may be present.
- Burns in the oral mucosa and pharynx (if a battery was chewed)
- Signs and symptoms suggestive of esophageal impaction of battery
  (1) Drooling
  (2) Fever and irritability
  (3) Vomiting
  (4) Refusing food/dysphagia (young infants will take liquids but refuse solid food)
  (5) Respiratory signs (tracheal compression): stridor, tachypnea, wheezing, respiratory distress
  (6) Retrosternal pain or discomfort
  (7) Odynophagia
- Signs and symptoms suggestive of GI tract injury due to battery ingestion
  (1) Abdominal pain, tenderness, cramps
  (2) Hematochezia
  (3) Vomiting, diarrhea
  (4) Bloody, dark, or discolored stools
- Nickel hypersensitivity producing skin rashes (if ingested button batteries are nickel-plated)

BOX 15-7. COMPLICATIONS RELATED TO BATTERY LODGMENT IN THE GASTROINTESTINAL TRACT

- *Esophageal impaction:*
  (1) Pressure necrosis
  (2) Leakage of contents producing caustic injury (liquefaction necrosis)
  (3) Esophageal burns (seen as early as 4 hours after ingestion)
  (4) Electrical injury by conduction to surrounding tissues (from a battery that is not exhausted)
  (5) Esophageal perforation (seen as early as 6 hours postingestion)
  (6) Esophageal stenosis
  (7) Tracheoesophageal fistula
  (8) Tension pneumothorax
  (9) Hemothorax
  (10) Mediastinitis
  (11) Esophageal-aortic fistula
  (12) Perforation through the aortic arch or its branches
  (13) Massive exsanguination
  (14) Death (from complications related to esophageal perforation)
  (15) Aspiration of the battery into tracheobronchial tree
- *Impaction in the GI tract beyond the esophagus:*
  (1) Leakage or rupture of the cell
  (2) Tissue injury *without* leakage as a result of direct current flow from an intact button cell
  (3) Ulceration leading to perforation
  (4) Impaction leading to obstruction, that can lead to perforation in certain locations (e.g., Meckel's diverticulum)
  (5) Heavy metal absorption (e.g., from a split mercuric oxide cell [usually a cell 15.6 mm in diameter])

BOX 15-8. DIFFERENTIAL DIAGNOSIS OF BATTERY INGESTION

- Respiratory signs and symptoms due to other etiologies (e.g., bronchiolitis, asthma, airway obstruction due to FB aspiration)
- GI signs and symptoms from other etiologies (e.g., gastroenteritis, bacterial enteritis, food poisoning, surgical abdomen [intussusception, volvulus])
- Other ingestions (e.g., caustic ingestion, esophageal FB, food impaction)
- Other esophageal diseases (e.g., esophagitis, gastroesophageal reflux)

BOX 15-9. GASTROINTESTINAL TRANSIT TIME OF 1366 INGESTED BATTERIES

- Passage within 24 hours: 22.6% of cases
- Passage within 48 hours: 61.3% of cases
- Passage within 72 hours: 78% of cases
- Passage within 94 hours: 86.4% of cases
- Passage >1 week: 4.5% of cases
- Passage >2 weeks: 1.1% of cases
- Of a total of 2382 cases of battery ingestion, GI transit time was known for 1366 cases.

(Reproduced with permission from: American Association of Poison Control Centers National Data System, Washington, DC, 1992.)

DIAGNOSIS CONSTIPATION

Definitions

1. Constipation is defined as difficulty in defecation, usually from incomplete defecation resulting in abnormalities of frequency, size, consistency, or ease of passage of stool.
   a. Normal pattern of defecating varies considerably between infants and children. Usually between 2 and 20 weeks of age, bowel movements for breast-fed babies are 3/day, and bottle-fed babies are 2/day. Older children (like adults) have a broad range of bowel frequency, varying between 3 times/week to 3 times/day.
   b. Passing hard, large-diameter stools or pelletlike stools or passing fewer than 3 stools/week associated with pain or excessive straining are features of constipation (Fig. 15-13).
2. Encopresis is fecal soiling associated with a solidified fecal impaction in the rectum. Passage of stool occurs in the underwear (children >4 years) as a result of chronic constipation.

Associated Clinical Features

1. Any of the following features may be present, depending on the underlying etiology of the constipation:
   a. Failure to thrive (e.g., Hirschsprung's disease; Fig. 15-14)
   b. Developmental delay (e.g., cerebral palsy)
   c. Dimple or tuft of hair on lower back (e.g., spina bifida occulta, meningomyelocele)
   d. Symptoms and signs of hypothyroidism
2. Hirschsprung's disease (HD) results from an absence of ganglionic cells in the bowel wall extending proximally from the anus for a variable distance. The aganglionic segment is limited to the rectosigmoid (75%), entire colon (10%), or entire intestine (rare).

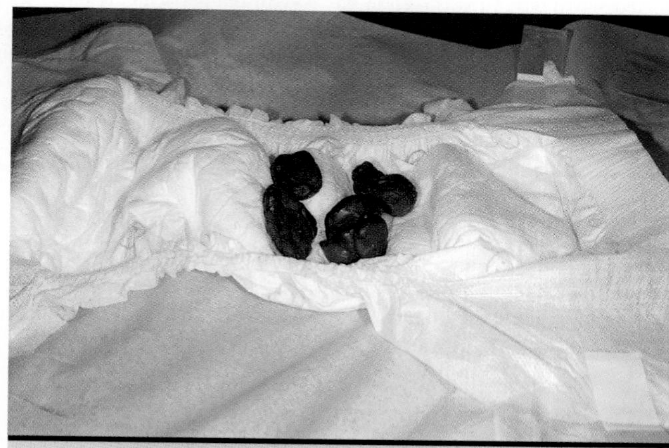

Figure 15-13. Constipation

Passing lumpy or hard, large-diameter stools, pelletlike stools, or passing fewer than 3 stools/week associated with pain or excessive straining are features of constipation. Excessive crying and passing hard stools were the complaints in a 18-month-old infant who presented with fecal impaction. During his rectal examination, very hard stool was felt in the ampulla and after manual disimpaction he passed this stool.

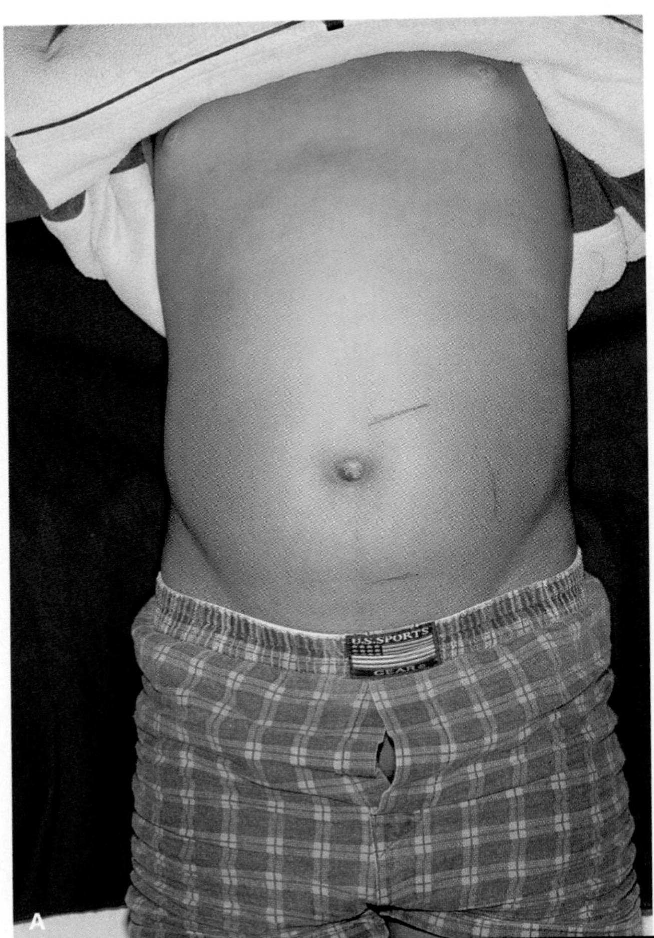

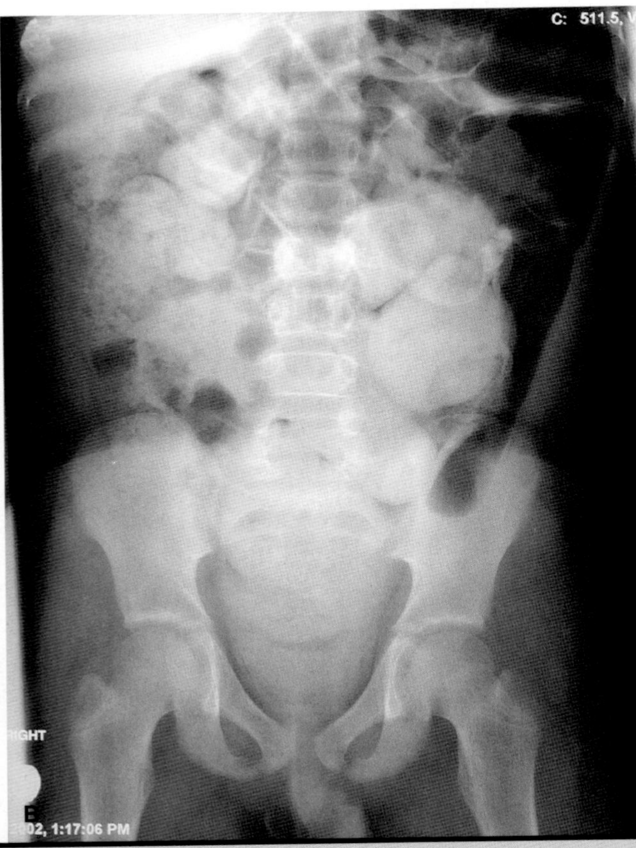

Figure 15-14. Hirschsprung's Disease

A. Abdominal distension is seen in this 10-year-old boy who presented with abdominal pain, vomiting, and a chronic history of constipation since 3 weeks of age. He had a very protuberant abdomen with a palpable abdominal mass (shown by the marks) in the left lower quadrant. He had received numerous enemas and suppositories in various EDs, including two prior hospitalizations (ages 6 and 9) for fecal impaction. He was supposed to undergo a rectal biopsy but missed several appointments at the GI clinic. *B*. This frontal radiograph of the abdomen in the same patient shows gross dilation of the rectum and sigmoid colon secondary to distal rectal obstruction. Also seen is mild dilation of more proximal colonic loops. A rectal biopsy confirmed the diagnosis of an aganglionic segment in the rectosigmoid region.

3. A plain abdominal radiograph is not performed routinely. When performed:
   a. Confirms diagnosis of constipation in an obese patient in whom an abdominal exam may be difficult to perform.
   b. Can be used as a teaching aid for children and parents
4. To exclude organic causes, various studies that are helpful include thyroid function tests, serum calcium levels, barium enema, rectal suction mucosal biopsy, anorectal manometry, and spinal MRI. These tests are not routinely preformed. They are only indicated based on history and physical examination suggesting an organic etiology.

Consultations

Gastroenterology, radiology, and surgery, if clinical suspicion of HD

Emergency Department Treatment and Disposition

1. The majority of the patients with constipation can be managed as outpatients and do not require hospitalization.
2. In patients with fecal impaction, medications are either given orally or per rectum. Rarely a patient may require manual disimpaction.

a. Oral agents for disimpaction include stimulants (e.g., bisacodyl or senna), osmotic agents (e.g., magnesium citrate, lactulose, magnesium hydroxide), lubricants (e.g., mineral oil), or lavage (e.g., polyethylene glycol).
b. Medications that can be given rectally for disimpaction include stimulants (e.g., bisacodyl, glycerin suppositories) or osmotic agents (e.g., phosphate enemas).

3. Use of Fleet enema (either saline or phosphate):
   a. Use adult-sized enemas in children >2 years old and pediatric-sized enemas in children <2 years of age.
   b. Do not use more than 1 enema per day (especially phosphate enemas).
   c. Patient may require 1 enema/day for 3 to 5 days
   d. *Hyperphosphatemia is an important side effect related to phosphate enema use and can lead to hypocalcemia* (avoid repeated dosing or using adult-sized enemas for young children).

4. Maintenance therapy includes:
   a. Stool softeners and lubricants (e.g., mineral oil, corn syrup, milk of magnesia)
   b. Osmotic laxative (e.g., polyethylene glycol 3350)
   c. Carbohydrate agents (e.g., Malt soup extract or lactulose) for infants
   d. Mineral oil is used for children >1 year old.
      1) Cheap and effective
      2) *Do not use in neurologically impaired children or in infants* (risk of aspiration and lipoid pneumonia)
      3) Dose: 1 to 2 tablespoons bid for children 1 to 3 years and 2 to 3 tablespoons for children >3 years of age
      4) Chilling it and mixing it with food (e.g., yogurt) may improve its taste.

5. Encourage consumption of a high-fiber diet including fruits, vegetables, cereals, and grains, as well as drinking plenty of fluids.

6. Treat any underlying aggravating condition (e.g., anal fissures).

7. Consider hospitalization for patients presenting with severe abdominal pain and abdominal mass (related to constipation) that does not respond to colonic enema and if the patient remains symptomatic. During hospitalization, the patient usually is treated with administration of polyethylene glycol or repeated high colonic enemas.

8. Behavioral modification includes:
   a. Teach the child not to wait to have a bowel movement. Instead, encourage the child to sit on the toilet for 10 minutes after breakfast and dinner (at the same time each day) in order to establish a routine for defecation.
   b. Encourage the child to read a story or listen to music while sitting on the toilet.

9. Infants with constipation can also be treated with prune juice or barley malt extract.

10. A follow-up with the primary care provider is important for ongoing maintenance therapy.

Clinical Pearls: Constipation

1. Functional or nonorganic (idiopathic) causes constitute 90 to 95% of cases of childhood constipation.

2. Later age of onset, normal growth, normal anal placement and anal wink, presence of stool in the anal canal and fecal soiling are features of functional constipation.

3. Absence of stool in the rectal vault and expulsion of foul-smelling liquid stool on withdrawal of a finger are features of HD.

4. A history of passing hard stools with blood streaks or fresh blood on the toilet paper after wiping suggests an anal fissure.

5. A rectal examination is essential in the evaluation of a patient with constipation.

6. *Important note:* Repeated doses of adult-sized enemas in a child can lead to significant hyperphosphatemia and hypocalcemia (we treated a 4-year-old child who received three doses of adult enemas in 2 days who presented with an afebrile seizure, serum calcium of 5 mg/dL, and serum phosphorus of 20 mg/dL).

BOX 15-10. ETIOLOGY AND DIFFERENTIAL DIAGNOSIS OF CONSTIPATION

- *Common causes:*
  (1) Diet (lack of fiber)
  (2) Anal fissure
  (3) Functional constipation
  (4) Hypothyroidism
  (5) Hirschsprung's disease
- *Uncommon causes:*
  (1) Anal atresia
  (2) Anal stenosis
  (3) Anteriorly displaced anus
  (4) Cerebral palsy
  (5) Hypercalcemia
  (6) Disorders of the spinal cord (e.g., spinal dysraphism, meningomyelocele, spina bifida occulta, spinal tumor)
  (7) Ovarian pathology (e.g., teratoma)
  (8) Ectopic or malpositioned anus
  (9) Hypotonia
  (10) Infant botulism
  (11) Lead poisoning
- *Medications associated with constipation:*
  (1) Antacids (containing aluminum)
  (2) Cough medications (containing codeine)
  (3) Elevated Mg^{2+} in neonate (mother given Mg^{2+} during labor)
  (4) Opiates
  (5) Anticholinergics
  (6) Antidepressants

(Modified and reproduced with permission from: Shah BR, Laude TL: Hirschsprung disease. In: *Atlas of Pediatric Clinical Diagnosis*. WB Saunders, Philadelphia, 2000, p. 342.)

BOX 15-11. CLINICAL FEATURES SEEN WITH CONSTIPATION

Symptoms and signs:

- History of delayed passage of meconium in neonates (e.g., HD; see Box 15-12)
- History of enterocolitis (e.g., HD; see Box 15-12)
- History of constipation since birth (e.g., HD; see Box 15-12)
- Abdominal pain
- Straining
- Withholding stools
- Painful defecation
- Lumpy or hard stools
- Decreased frequency of defecating
- Sensation of incomplete evacuation
- Tenesmus
- Blood-streaked stools
- Fecal soiling
- Anorexia
- Weight loss (e.g., HD)
- Irritability
- Abdominal distension (from either a colon filled with stool or bowel obstruction due to impaction)
- Palpable fecal masses on abdominal examination
- Voluntarily increased anal tone due to contraction of the external sphincter (e.g., fear of pain due to anal fissure)
- Malpositioned anus (e.g., anteriorly displaced anus)
- Marked decrease in anal tone (e.g., spina bifida)
- Presence of anal fissure
- Fistula or abscess (e.g., perianal streptococcal cellulitis)
- Rectal examination (may reveal any of the following)
  (1) Stenosis
  (2) A normal-length canal with rectal ampulla filled with stool (suggests functional or acquired megacolon)
  (3) A long, tight canal with the rectal ampulla empty (suggests HD)

BOX 15-12. CLINICAL FEATURES OF HIRSCHSPRUNG'S DISEASE (HD)

- Delayed passage of meconium in newborns
  (1) About 94% of patients with HD fail to pass meconium within the first 24 hours after birth.
  (2) About 90% of normal full-term neonates pass meconium within 24 hours after birth, and about 99% pass it within 48 hours after birth.
- Enterocolitis
  (1) Most commonly seen between the second and fourth weeks of life
  (2) Abdominal distention
  (3) Vomiting
  (4) Explosive diarrhea (following digital rectal exam) that rapidly becomes bloody
  (5) High fever
  (6) Lethargy
  (7) Colonic perforation
  (8) Peritonitis and shock
- Complete intestinal obstruction (bilious vomiting, abdominal distention, obstipation)
- Chronic constipation frequently requiring enemas, suppositories, or rectal stimulation
- Rectal exam
  (1) Tight anal canal (as opposed to functional constipation, which has a wide rectal vault)
  (2) Empty rectal vault (no stool palpable)
  (3) Small-caliber (not dilated) distal rectal vault
  (4) Explosive release of foul-smelling liquid feces may result from withdrawal of the examiner's finger.

DIAGNOSIS GASTROINTESTINAL BLEEDING

Definitions

1. Hematemesis is the vomiting of bright red blood; in contrast, hemoptysis is expectoration of blood of pulmonary origin.
2. Coffee-grounds vomitus results from alteration of blood by gastric acid.
3. See Box 15-13 for types of rectal bleeding.

Etiology and Associated Clinical Features

1. In general, a lesion proximal to the ligament of Treitz causes upper GI bleeding.
2. Hemorrhage proximal to the ileocecal valve usually produces melena (tarry stools).
3. The source of hematochezia (bloody stools) is located in the lower intestine or due to rapid transit of upper GI bleeding.
4. Causes of GI bleeding vary significantly. The most common causes in pediatric age groups tend to be age-specific.
   a. Neonatal period:
      1) The most common cause of upper GI bleeding in neonates is idiopathic.
      2) Benign anal or rectal lesions are the most common causes of lower GI bleeding in neonates.
      3) Necrotizing enterocolitis should be suspected in a premature or full-term infant that presents with abdominal distension, bilious vomiting, and lower GI bleeding.
      4) Midgut volvulus is a true surgical emergency in a neonate that presents with bilious vomiting, abdominal pain, and melena.
   b. Infant (30 days to 1 year of age):
      1) Upper GI bleeding in an infant is commonly caused by esophagitis or peptic ulcer disease.
      2) *Campylobacter, Salmonella, Shigella*, or *Yersinia* can all cause hematochezia.
      3) Intussusception is most frequently diagnosed in this age group. Patients usually present with intermittent abdominal pain, vomiting, and guaiac-positive or currant-jelly stool (Fig. 15-15).
   c. Children (1 to 12 years of age):
      1) Esophageal varices may cause massive hematemesis (Fig. 15-16). Most varices are secondary to extrahepatic portal hypertension and most variceal bleeding will stop spontaneously.
      2) Juvenile polyps are the most frequent cause of lower GI bleeding.
      3) Infectious diarrhea is a common cause of lower GI bleeding.
      4) Meckel's diverticulum can cause massive hematochezia. It follows the "rule of 2s" (it is seen in

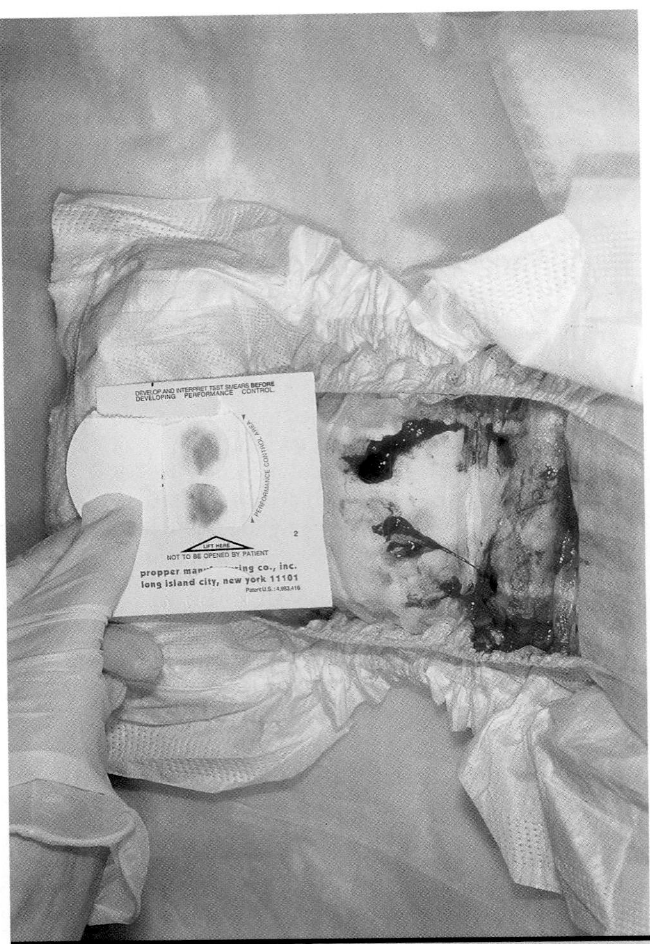

Figure 15-15. Bleeding per Rectum: Intussusception

This currant-jelly stool was passed by a 8-month-old infant who was brought to the ED with complaints of vomiting, lethargy, and intermittent episodes of crying of 12 hours' duration (he was seen at another ED and was sent home with a diagnosis of acute gastroenteritis). He had ileocolic intussusception that was not reduced by barium enema and he required surgical reduction.

about 2% of population, 45% of symptomatic patients are less than 2 years old, and the anatomical location is about 2 feet proximal to the ileocecal valve).

5) Henoch-Schönlein purpura (HSP) and hemolytic-uremic syndrome (HUS) can cause lower GI bleeding in this age group. Bleeding results from generalized vasculitis of the GI tract in HSP and thrombosis of small mucosal vessels in HUS.

d. Adolescence (13 to 19 years of age):

1) Peptic ulcer disease and esophagitis are the most common causes of upper GI tract bleeding (Fig. 15-17).
2) Anal fissures and juvenile polyps are the most common causes of lower GI tract bleeding.
3) Inflammatory bowel disease and infectious diarrhea should be considered in this age group with lower GI tract bleeding.

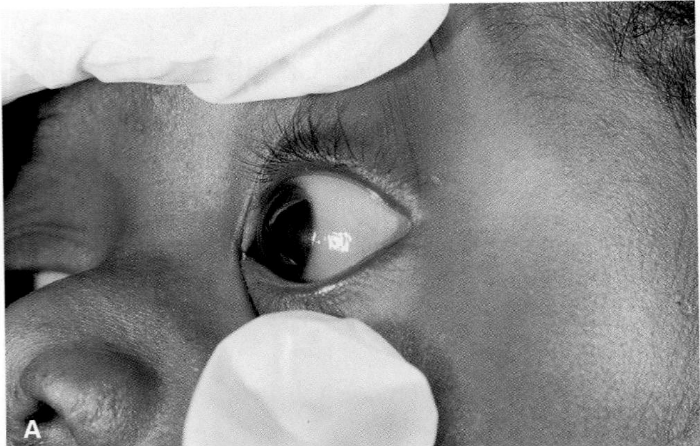

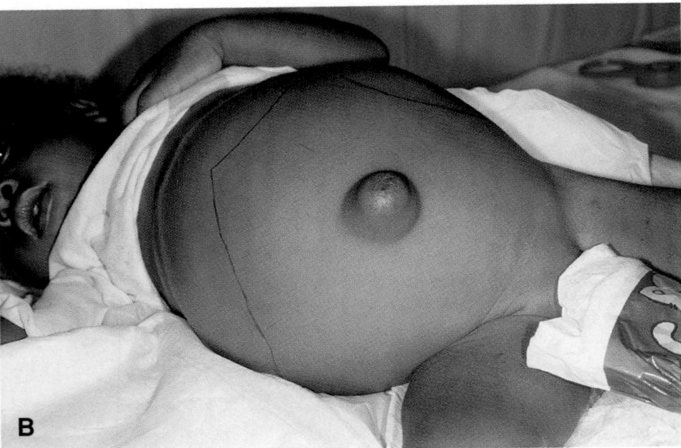

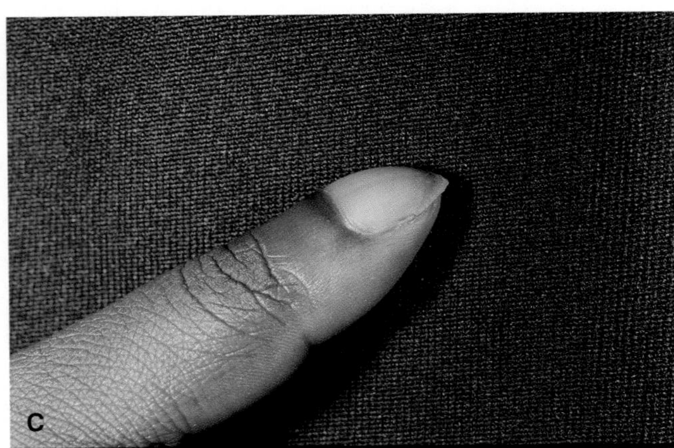

Figure 15-16. Biliary Atresia

Marked jaundice (*A*) and hepatosplenomegaly with ascites (*B*) and clubbing (*C*) are seen in a patient with untreated biliary atresia with portal hypertension and esophageal varices. In such children, sudden massive hemorrhage may result from rupture of varices.

5. The diagnostic work-up should focus on the potential hemodynamic instability of the patient secondary to GI bleeding. Laboratory tests should minimally include CBC, PT/PTT, and type and cross-match of blood (for massive hemorrhage). Other tests (as clinically indicated) include

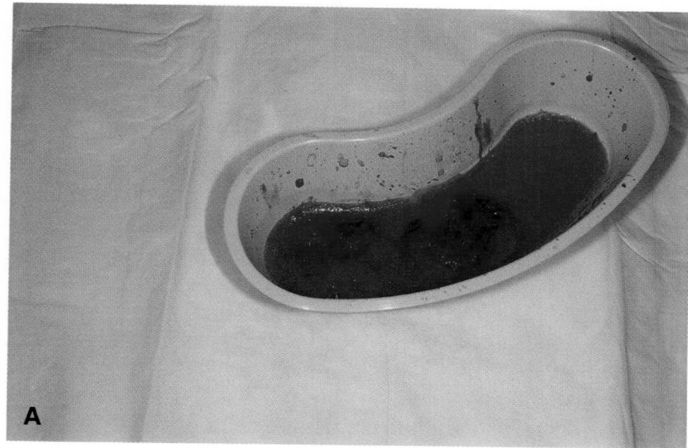

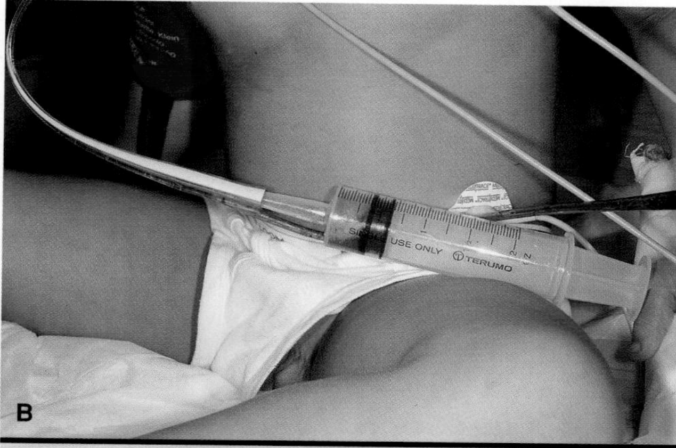

Figure 15-17. Upper GI Bleeding: Peptic Ulcer Disease

An 8-year-old child was brought to the ED with a sudden history of vomiting blood. Nasogastric lavage showed fresh blood (*A*). He was lavaged with room-temperature normal saline until the aspirate was clear. Coffee-ground-appearing material is seen during lavage in part *B*. Endoscopic examination showed the presence of gastritis (due to *H. pylori*) and superficial ulcers. His father also had peptic ulcer disease.

serum electrolytes, liver enzymes, bilirubin, total protein and albumin, and stool culture (to exclude common bacterial pathogens in patients with rectal bleeding). Apt-Downey test can differentiate swallowed maternal blood from infant blood.

6. Plain radiographs of the abdomen can help to diagnose pneumoperitoneum (perforation in acute ulcers), toxic megacolon, or pneumatosis intestinalis.
7. Additional tests (as indicated) include Meckel's scan (technetium^{99m} pertechnetate; localizes functional gastric mucosa in Meckel's diverticulum) and a contrast study of the small intestine (Crohn's disease or other pathology).

Consultations

Gastroenterologist and surgeon (as soon as possible for unstable or complicated cases)

Emergency Department Treatment and Disposition

1. Hemodynamically unstable patients require stabilization of vital signs including two large-bore intravenous lines to infuse a bolus of normal saline or lactated Ringer's (or if indicated, central or intraosseus infusion may be used), continuous cardiac and pulse oximetry monitoring, and oxygen therapy. Hemodynamically unstable patients should be admitted to the PICU.
2. Nasogastric (NG) intubation should be performed in patients with suspected upper GI bleeding.
   a. NG lavage can identify blood in the stomach and helps in determining if bleeding has ceased or is ongoing.
   b. An absence of blood in the lavage fluid does not exclude upper GI bleeding; likewise the presence of blood does not identify the origin of bleeding (which may be anywhere from the mouth to the duodenum proximal to the ligament of Treitz).
   c. Administer a room-temperature normal saline lavage until the aspirate is clear (chilled water may produce hypothermia).
   d. Lavage does not stop the bleeding.
   e. Lavage reduces the volume of blood and thus facilitates upper endoscopy.
3. Modality of treatment depends on the etiology of the GI bleed.
4. Pharmacotherapy for upper GI bleeds in children is similar to that of adults.
5. Empiric therapy with acid-reducing and cytoprotective medications is justified in children with upper GI bleeding because these bleeds are predominantly secondary to peptic ulcer disease.
6. Antibiotic therapy should be administered to patients with hemorrhagic gastritis or gastroduodenal ulceration that is associated with *Helicobacter pylori* to prevent relapsing infection.
7. Octreotide or vasopressin may be useful in suspected cases of variceal bleeding.
8. Endoscopy (esophagogastroduodenoscopy) is the preferred procedure for evaluation and treatment of upper GI bleeding. Perform flexible sigmoidoscopy and colonoscopy (or full colonoscopy) for patients with rectal bleeding, as indicated.
9. Angiography is used diagnostically and therapeutically in selected cases that involve massive hemorrhage (e.g., patients with massively bleeding ulcers whose stomachs cannot be lavaged enough to allow endoscopy). Angiography can demonstrate the site of bleeding and can permit injection of vasoconstrictors or thrombotic agents to control the bleeding.
10. Allergic colitis (milk protein-induced colitis) in infancy responds to diet restriction and hydrolyzed protein formula.

11. Most pediatric GI bleeding is minor and patients can be discharged from the ED for outpatient work-up and follow-up.

Clinical Pearls: Gastrointestinal Bleeding

1. Most GI bleeding in pediatric patients is self-limited. Massive uncontrollable bleeding is rare and usually spontaneously decreases early in its course.
2. Meckel's diverticulum is the most important source of small bowel hemorrhage in children, and can present with painless massive hematochezia; while intestinal duplication is the second most important source of small bowel hemorrhage.
3. Many cases of painless upper GI bleeding are due to esophageal varices.
4. Epigastric abdominal pain that awakens the child from sleep is associated with peptic ulcer disease, gastritis, or esophagitis.
5. Hematemesis following a paroxysm of vomiting suggests a Mallory-Weiss tear or prolapsed gastropathy.
6. A well-appearing (absence of hemodynamic instability) neonate or infant presenting with regurgitation of milk mixed with blood usually suggests maternal blood swallowed at the time of delivery or during breast-feeding.
7. A well-appearing (absence of hemodynamic instability) formula-fed or breast-fed infant presenting with blood-streaked mucus in the stool (and negative stool culture) usually suggests milk protein–induced colitis.

BOX 15-13. TYPES OF RECTAL BLEEDING

- *Melena*
  (1) Black, tarry stool
  (2) Usually with a distinct odor
  (3) Blood present in the GI tract for a prolonged period; degradation of hemoglobin by colonic flora
  (4) Blood usually from lesions proximal to the ileocecal valve and often above the ligament of Treitz
- *Hematochezia*
  (1) Bright red blood per rectum *or* maroon-colored stool
  (2) Usually from colonic source
  (3) Rarely upper GI hemorrhage with very rapid GI transit time
- *Occult blood*
  (1) Presence of blood in the stool that is not grossly detectable
  (2) False-positive results: meat, ferrous sulfate, fresh red berries, tomatoes, turnips, horseradish
  (3) False-negative results: vitamin C, outdated reagent or card

BOX 15-14. CONDITIONS MISTAKEN FOR GASTROINTESTINAL BLEEDING

- *Hematemesis*
  (1) Commercial dyes #2 and #3 ("Frankenberry stool")
  (2) Swallowed maternal blood at delivery or during breast-feeding
  (3) Bleeding from nose, mouth, or pharynx
  (4) Swallowed nonhuman blood
- *Melena*
  (1) Iron preparations
  (2) Licorice
  (3) Blueberries
  (4) Spinach
  (5) Beets
  (6) Bismuth (e.g., Pepto-Bismol)
  (7) Lead
  (8) Charcoal
  (9) Dirt
  (10) Swallowed nonhuman blood
- *Hematochezia*
  (1) Menstruation
  (2) Commercial dyes #2 and #3
  (3) Ampicillin
  (4) Hematuria

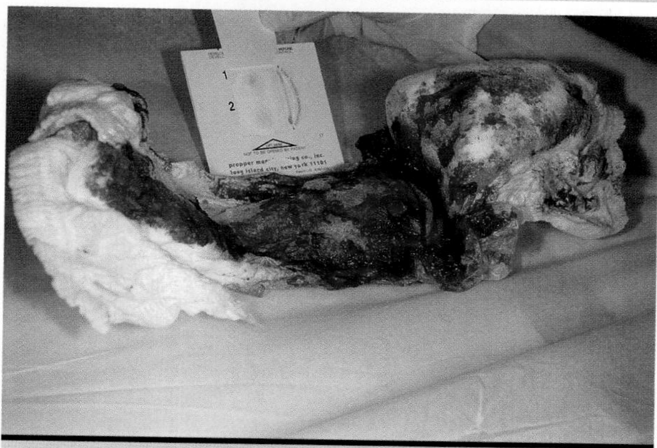

Figure 15-18. Ingestion of Beets That Can be Mistaken for Bleeding per Rectum

Grossly bloody-appearing stool was passed by this toddler, who was rushed to the ED by a very frightened mother. The patient was completely asymptomatic. As shown, a stool guaiac test was negative. The mother gave a history of feeding him beets for the past 2 days. This is a good example of how a lot of unnecessary and some potentially dangerous tests can be avoided with a thorough history and negative guaiac test in a well-appearing infant.

(Reproduced with Permission from: Squires, RH Jr: Gastrointestinal bleeding. *Pediatr Rev* 1999;20:95.)

BOX 15-15. CLINICAL FEATURES OF GASTROINTESTINAL BLEEDING

- Pallor
- Tachycardia
- Signs of circulatory impairment (depending on the amount of blood loss)
  (1) Peripheral pulses: rapid, thready, weak, or absent
  (2) Discrepancy in volume between peripheral and central pulses
  (3) Skin perfusion: color pale, blue, or mottled; cool extremities
  (4) Prolonged capillary refill (>2 seconds)
  (5) Irritable, lethargic, confused, or decreased level of consciousness
  (6) Diminished response to pain
  (7) Postural hypotension
  (8) Decreased pulse pressure of >20 mmHg
  (9) Decreased or no urinary output
- Abnormal physical findings may suggest underlying etiology
  (1) Splenomegaly, prominent abdominal vessels (e.g., chronic liver disease)
  (2) Clubbing (e.g., chronic liver disease, inflammatory bowel disease)
  (3) Purpura with abdominal pain, arthralgia/arthritis, hematuria (e.g., HSP)
  (4) Intermittent abdominal pain, vomiting (bilious or nonbilious), and guaiac positive or currant-jelly stool (e.g., intussusception)
  (5) Bloody or guaiac positive stools with abdominal pain, growth failure, and anorexia (e.g., inflammatory bowel disease)
  (6) Intense erythema/cellulitis around the anus (e.g., perianal streptococcal disease)
- Abnormal laboratory tests may suggest underlying etiology
  (1) Low Hgb/Hct and mean corpuscular volume (e.g., chronic blood loss)
  (2) Low platelet count (e.g., sepsis, hypersplenism, HUS)
  (3) Elevated liver enzymes (e.g., liver disease leading to esophageal varices or hypersplenism)
  (4) Prolonged PT/PTT (e.g., acute hemorrhage, liver disease, disseminated intravascular coagulation)

BOX 15-16. ETIOLOGY AND DIFFERENTIAL DIAGNOSIS OF GASTROINTESTINAL BLEEDING

Age	*Upper GI*	*Lower GI*
Birth to 1 month	Idiopathic Gastritis Stress ulcers Esophagitis Swallowed maternal blood Congenital blood dyscrasia Vascular malformation	Anal fissure Upper GI bleeding Midgut volvulus Necrotizing enterocolitis Swallowed maternal blood Infectious colitis Milk allergy Blood dyscrasia Intestinal duplication
1 month to 1 year	Gastritis Esophagitis Stress ulcer Mallory-Weiss tear Vascular malformation Duplication Munchausen's syndrome by proxy	Anal fissure Intussusception Meckel's diverticulum Infectious diarrhea Milk allergy Duplication Pseudomembranous colitis
1 to 12 years	Esophageal varices Peptic ulcer disease Stress ulcer NSAIDs Gastritis Mallory-Weiss tear Foreign body Esophagitis	Polyps Anal fissure Infectious diarrhea Meckel's diverticulum HSP HUS Intussusception Pseudomembranous colitis Perianal streptococcal dermatitis
Adolescent	Peptic ulcer disease Gastritis Esophageal varices Mallory-Weiss tear Esophagitis Stress ulcer	Polyps Anal fissure Hemorrhoids Inflammatory bowel disease Infectious disease Foreign body

Modified and Reproduced with Permission Ochsenschlager DW: Gastrointestinal bleeding. In: Barkin RM (ed). *Pediatric Emergency Medicine.* Mosby, St. Louis, 1997, p. 812.

BOX 15-17. PRINCIPLES OF PHARMACOTHERAPY IN PATIENTS WITH GI BLEEDING

- *Acid reduction*
  (1) Magnesium hydroxide and aluminum hydroxide suspension
  (2) Ranitidine (H_2-receptor antagonist)
  (3) Omeprazole (proton pump inhibitor)
- *Cytoprotection*
  (1) Sucralfate
  (2) Misoprostol
- *Vasoconstriction*
  (1) Octreotide (somatostatin analog)
  (2) Vasopressin
- *Antibiotic*
  (1) Amoxicillin
  (2) Clarithromycin
  (3) Metronidazole

Suggested Readings

Alcaraz A, Lopez-Herce J, Serina C: Gastrointestinal bleeding following ketorolac administration in a pediatric patient. *J Pediatr Gastroenterol Nutr* 1996;23:479.

Berezin S, Newman LJ: Lower gastrointestinal bleeding in infants owing to lymphonodular hyperplasia of the colon. *Pediatr Emerg Care* 1987;3:164.

Broderick A, Kleinman RE: Constipation. In: Burg FD (ed). *Gellis and Kagan's Current Pediatric Therapy,* 17th ed. Elsevier, Philadelphia, 2002, 622.

Chaibou M, Tucci M, Dugas MA et al: Clinically significant upper gastrointestinal bleeding acquired in a pediatric intensive care unit: A prospective study. *Pediatrics* 1998;102:933.

Cox K, Ament ME: Upper gastrointestinal bleeding in children and adolescents. *Pediatrics* 1979;63:408.

Eisen GM, Baron TH, Dominitz JA et al: Guideline for the management of ingested foreign bodies. *Gastrointest Endosc* 2002;55:802.

Goyal A, Treem WR, Hyams JS: Severe upper gastrointestinal bleeding in healthy full-term neonates. *Am J Gastroenterol* 1994;89:613.

Hicsonmez A, Karaguzel G, Tanyel FC: Duodenal varices causing intractable gastrointestinal bleeding in a 12-year-old child. *Eur J Pediatr Surg* 1994;4:176.

Litovitz T: Button batteries. In: Ford ?? (ed). *Clinical Toxicology,* 1st ed. WB Saunders, Philadelphia, 2001, p. 1027.

Henneman PL. Gastrointestinal Bleeding In Marx JA: *Rosen's Emergency Medicine: Concepts and Clinical Practice*, 5th ed. Mosby, St. Louis, 2002, p. 194.

Meyerovitz MF, Fellows KE: Angiography in gastrointestinal bleeding in children. *Am J Roentgenol* 1984;143:837.

Ochsenschlager DW: Gastrointestinal bleeding. In: Barkin RM (ed). *Pediatric Emergency Medicine.* Mosby, St. Louis, 1997, p. 812.

Victor FL: Gastrointestinal bleeding in infancy and childhood. *Gastroenterol Clin* 2000;29:37.

Schafermeyer RW: Pediatric abdominal emergencies. In: Tininalli JE et al (eds). *Emergency Medicine.* McGraw-Hill, New York, 2000, p. 846.

Siafakas C, Fox VL, Nurko S: Use of octreotide for the treatment of severe gastrointestinal bleeding in children. *J Pediatr Gastroenterol Nutr* 1998;26:356.

Squires RH: Gastrointestinal bleeding. *Pediatr Rev* 1999;20:95.

Victor FL: Gastrointestinal bleeding in infancy and childhood. *Gastroenterol Clin* 2000;29:37.

CHAPTER 16

NEPHROLOGY

Anup Singh / Binita R. Shah
Edited by Binita R. Shah

DIAGNOSIS PROTEINURIA

Definition

1. Protein is normally found in the urine of healthy children and adults.

2. The upper limit of normal protein excretion in healthy children is up to 150 mg/day and in healthy adults is up to 200 mg/day. Since albumin has a relatively small molecular size, it tends to become the dominant constituent in proteinuria. Tamm-Horsfall mucoprotein, a mucoprotein produced in the distal tubule, makes up the remainder of normal urinary protein.

Associated Clinical Features

1. Use of a urine dipstick to detect proteinuria
   a. Dipstick readings are graded as negative, trace, 1+ (closest to 30 mg/dL), 2+ (closest to 100 mg/dL), 3+ (closest to 300 mg/dL), and 4+ (>2000 mg/dL).
   b. Dipstick proteinuria reflects primarily albuminuria. It is less sensitive for other forms of proteinuria (e.g., low-molecular-weight proteins, Bence Jones protein).
   c. Dipsticks also detect amounts of protein that fall in the normal range due to high sensitivity.
   d. False-positive dipstick tests are seen with gross hematuria, concentrated urine, alkaline urine (pH >8), or contamination with chlorhexidine or certain medications (e.g., phenazopyridine therapy).

2. Persistent proteinuria needs to be quantitated by a more precise method (sulfosalicylic acid) in a timed urine collection (12- or 24-hour collection) since dipstick analysis cannot accurately measure protein excretion. The sulfosalicylic acid method will detect as little as 10 mg/100 mL of protein, whereas the dipstick is not reliable for less than 20 to 30 mg/100 mL.

3. Urinary protein excretion can be estimated by measuring the ratio of urinary protein (Pr) to creatinine (Cr) concentrations in a random specimen (a semiquantitative measurement).
   a. Urinary Cr excretion is constant in patients with relatively normal renal function.
   b. Urinary Pr excretion is also constant in patients with most disease states.
   c. Determination of the ratio is helpful in quantitating proteinuria when a timed urine collection is not practical (see Box 16-1 for normal values).

4. Characteristics of Orthostatic (postural) proteinuria
   a. Children excrete normal or slightly increased amounts of protein in the supine position.
   b. Protein excretion increases 10-fold or more in the upright position.
   c. Absence of hematuria
   d. Normal values of creatinine clearance and C3 complement

5. As indicated (e.g., patients with 3+ or 4+ proteinuria) laboratory tests should include serum electrolytes, blood urea nitrogen (BUN), serum creatinine, total protein, albumin, lipid profile, and complement (C3). Urine culture and renal ultrasound may be considered for patients with suspected urinary tract infection or congenital renal anomalies.

Consultation

Nephrology consultation in patients with heavy proteinuria

Emergency Department Treatment and Disposition

1. Hospitalize patients with severe nephrosis. With a first episode of nephrosis, the family needs to be educated about the chronic relapsing nature of the disease, home monitoring of urine by dipstick, and diet and complications related to both the disease and the therapy.

2. All other patients with proteinuria (with normal blood pressure and urine output) can be sent home with a follow-up appointment with their primary care provider.
3. In general, urinalysis is not reliable during acute illness, unless there are other symptoms and signs that point to diseases related to the kidneys. Thus, patients with only one abnormality on UA (in the absence of symptoms and signs that point to the kidneys) can be discharged to be followed up by their primary care provider.

Clinical Pearls: Proteinuria

1. Not all proteinuria is pathological.
2. Exclude hematuria when evaluating patients with proteinuria in the ED.
3. Proteinuria on a screening urinalysis is not an uncommon finding in children. It may indicate a completely benign condition (e.g., febrile illness, exercise, or exposure to cold) or it may be the first clue to a significant renal parenchymal disease (e.g., nephrotic syndrome or glomerulonephritis; Fig. 16-1).
4. Heavy proteinuria (3+ or 4+ on dipstick) is typically seen in patients with nephrotic syndrome, while patients with fever or dehydration usually have mild proteinuria (trace to 1+).
5. Orthostatic proteinuria is proteinuria seen only in the upright position. It is probably the most common cause of functional proteinuria and accounts for 15 to 20% of healthy young men who have proteinuria on routine urinalysis.
6. Heavy proteinuria is an essential element of nephrotic syndrome. Other laboratory abnormalities seen in nephrotic syndrome include hypoproteinemia, hypoalbuminemia, and hyperlipidemia (increased cholesterol, triglycerides, and low-density and very-low-density lipoproteins).

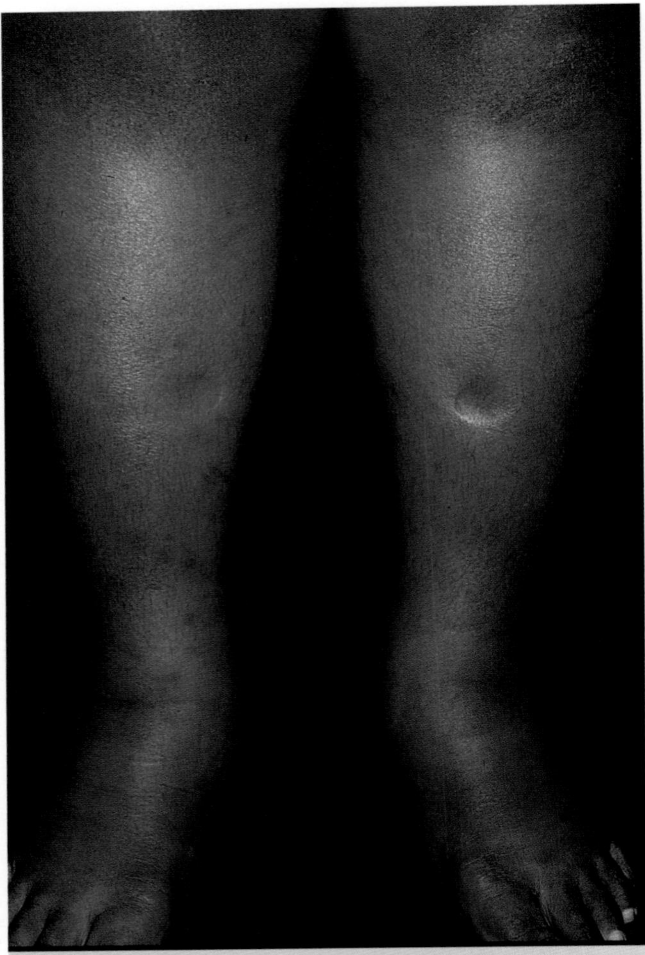

Figure 16-1. Bilateral Pitting Edema in Nephrotic Syndrome

Facial puffiness and difficulty putting on shoes (swelling around the ankles due to edema) were the presenting complaint of this patient. Urinalysis in this patient showed 3+ protein (closest to 300 mg/dL) and microscopic hematuria. Heavy proteinuria (3 + or 4 + on dipstick) is typically seen in patients with nephrotic syndrome. Depth of color of the dipstick reaction increases in a semiquantitative manner with increasing urinary protein concentrations. A diagnosis of focal segmental glomerulosclerosis was confirmed in this patient by renal biopsy.

BOX 16-1. PROTEIN EXCRETION IN URINE

- Upper limit of normal protein excretion in healthy children = $<$4 mg/m^2 per hour in 24 hours
- Upper limit of normal protein excretion in healthy children = up to 150 mg/24 hours
- Upper limit of normal protein excretion in healthy adults = up to 200 mg/24 hours
- Normal urine protein:creatinine ratio (mg/mg) = $<$0.5 in children $<$2 years
- Normal urine protein:creatinine ratio (mg/mg) = $<$0.2 in older children
- Nephrotic-range proteinuria (any of the following):
  (1) Proteinuria $>$40 mg/m^2 per hour in 24 hours (normal $<$4 mg/m^2 per hour in 24 hours) or $>$50 mg/kg per 24 hours
  (2) Urine protein:creatinine ratio (mg/mg) $>$2 (normal ratio: infant $<$0.5, child $<$0.2)

BOX 16-2. VARIOUS ETIOLOGIES OF PROTEINURIA

Nonpathologic (functional) proteinuria

- Febrile
- Severe dehydration, shock
- Severe acidosis
- Severe muscular exertion
- Pregnancy
- Seizures
- Orthostatic (postural) proteinuria
- Congestive heart failure

Pathologic proteinuria

- Proteinuria due to glomerular diseases
  (1) Glomerulonephritis
  (2) Nephrotic syndrome (e.g., minimal change NS, focal segmental glomerulosclerosis)
  (3) Membranous nephropathy (e.g., systemic lupus erythematosus)
  (4) IgA nephropathy
- Proteinuria with acute tubulointerstitial nephritis (ATIN)
  (1) Immune-mediated ATIN (e.g., sarcoidosis, Sjögren's syndrome)
  (2) Drug-related ATIN (e.g., antibiotics such as penicillin, ampicillin, methicillin, cephalosporins, sulfonamides, and rifampin, and the nonsteroidal anti-inflammatory drugs naproxen and ibuprofen)
  (3) Infection-related ATIN (e.g., streptococcal disease, toxoplasmosis, syphilis, *Rickettsia*)
- Obstructive uropathy
- Destructive parenchymal lesions (tumor, infection, infarct)
- Cystic diseases
- Heavy metal poisoning (e.g., mercury, gold, lead)

Postrenal proteinuria

(protein added to the urine at some point beyond the renal parenchyma)

- Infection of renal pelvis or ureter
- Cystitis
- Urethritis or prostatitis
- Contamination with vaginal secretions (suggested by the presence of moderate to large numbers of squamous epithelial cells in urine sediment)

DIAGNOSIS HEMATURIA

Definitions

1. Hematuria is either gross (visible to the naked eye) or microscopic (detected only by dipstick followed by confirmation of red blood cells [RBCs] by microscopic examination of the urine sediment).
2. Zero to five RBCs per high-power field (hpf) detected on urinalysis is considered within normal limits. Microscopic hematuria is defined as >5 RBCs/hpf in the sediment from 10 mL of centrifuged freshly voided urine.

Associated Clinical Features

1. A thorough history, physical examination, and some baseline laboratory tests as clinically indicated will help in diagnosing most common causes of hematuria. Not all children with hematuria will require the same tests.
   a. In a patient presenting with urinary frequency, urgency, dysuria, abdominal pain (suprapubic or costovertebral angle tenderness, fever), and hematuria, exclude UTI by performing urine culture.
   b. In a patient with trauma presenting with hematuria or blood at the urethral meatus, exclude abdominal/renal/urethral trauma
2. Family history of renal failure and hearing loss suggests hereditary nephritis or Alport's syndrome.
3. Urolithiasis presenting as hematuria
   a. Rare in children
   b. Severe colicky, episodic flank or abdominal pain with hematuria (either gross or microscopic) suggests nephrolithiasis.
   c. Patients may have a medical condition that predisposes to stone formation (e.g., hypercalciuria, hyperoxaluria, or cystinuria).
   d. Family history is often positive for nephrolithiasis.
4. Gross hematuria that originates from the upper urinary tract (e.g., poststreptococcal glomerulonephritis)
   a. Urine is either brown or cola-colored (brown color of urine is produced because hemoglobin is converted to hematin by the acidic urine).
   b. Urine may contain RBC casts.

5. Gross hematuria that originates from the lower urinary tract (bladder and urethra [e.g., hemorrhagic cystitis])
   a. Urine is red-pink
   b. Usually terminal hematuria
   c. Passage of blood clots
6. Gross glomerular hematuria with proteinuria (greater than 2+) suggests glomerulonephritis.
7. Examination of RBCs under the microscope also helps in determining the etiology.
   a. Dysmorphic cells are seen with upper tract bleeding.
   b. Presence of casts suggests parenchymal disease.
8. Urine dipstick changes color either on the basis of a peroxidase reaction or orthotoluidine blue reaction (Hemastix).
   a. It detects hemoglobin and thus urinary RBCs.
   b. It also gives a positive reaction in the presence of myoglobin.
   c. Dipstick testing cannot differentiate between RBCs, free hemoglobin, and myoglobin.
   d. Potential false-negative reactions may be seen with highly concentrated urine and urine containing high levels of ascorbic acid.
   e. Certain drugs and foods cause a red, brown, or orange coloration of the urine. However, dipstick is negative in such cases.
9. Usual laboratory tests that are done in patients with hematuria include CBC, urine culture, serum creatinine and C3 values, and 24-hour urine collection (or a random urine specimen) for creatinine, protein, and calcium (determine urine calcium:creatinine ratio).
10. Additional laboratory tests (as indicated) include throat culture for group A beta-hemolytic streptococci and antistreptolysin O or streptozyme tests (serologic evidence for streptococcal infection), screening for sickle cell disease and work-up for collagen diseases (e.g., antinuclear antibody test).
11. As indicated, radiographic evaluation includes:
    a. Kidney-ureter-bladder (KUB) film if urolithiasis is suspected (KUB will show larger stones that contain calcium)
    b. Renal and bladder sonography if KUB is negative and there is a strong suspicion of stones
    c. Spiral CT scan (thin cuts) without contrast may be indicated if both KUB and sonography are negative and there is a strong suspicion of stones.
    d. Ultrasonography for clinically suspected nephrocalcinosis or malignancy

Consultation

As indicated, nephrology (e.g., patients with a clinical diagnosis of acute poststreptococcal glomerulonephritis [APSGN] presenting with edema, hypertension, or oliguria) or urology (e.g., patients presenting with renal injury from trauma)

Emergency Department Treatment and Disposition

1. Most children with hematuria do not require hospitalization. Some examples of patients who will require hospitalization include:
   a. Patients presenting with hematuria with hypertension, oliguria, or pulmonary edema due to APSGN
   b. Patients presenting with hematuria due to renal injury from trauma
   c. Patients with hematuria due to papillary necrosis due to sickle hemoglobinopathy (Fig. 16-2)
   d. Patients with urolithiasis requiring aggressive hydration and pain management
2. If history or physical examination is not suggestive of any obvious cause of hematuria, the patient can be referred to a primary care physician (or nephrologist) for evaluation for diagnoses such as hypercalciuria, nephrocalcinosis, benign familial hematuria, or hereditary nephritis.
3. For patients presenting with hematuria from urolithiasis
   a. Pain management as indicated
   b. Smaller stones (3 mm or less) in distal ureter usually pass spontaneously following aggressive hydration

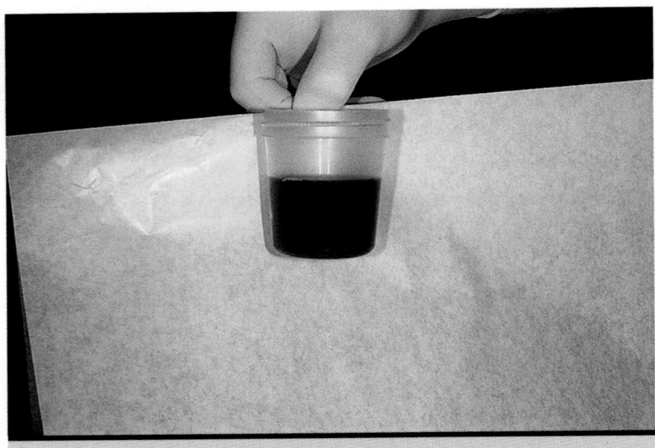

Figure 16-2. Gross Hematuria in Sickle Cell Disease

Gross hematuria is not an uncommon feature of sickle cell anemia, sickle cell trait, and Hb-SC disease. Sudden onset of painless hematuria was a presenting complaint in this 17-year-old patient with sickle cell anemia. His urinalysis showed 1 + protein and microscopic examination of the urine showed many RBCs and was negative for WBCs and bacteria. Patients with either sickle cell disease or sickle cell trait may develop ischemia in the renal papillae resulting in necrosis. Predisposing factors for necrosis include sickle cell crisis, dehydration, hypoxemia, and use of nonsteroidal anti-inflammatory drugs. Patients may present with flank pain and painless hematuria. Blunting or cavitation of the papillary tip is best diagnosed by intravenous pyelography. The hematuria is usually painless and self-limited. Treatment is supportive, including adequate hydration and pain management. Papillary necrosis may predispose patients to repeated urinary tract infections or may progress to chronic renal insufficiency.

c. Larger stones (usually >5 mm in adolescents and >3 mm in children) usually do not pass spontaneously and may require urology consultation for lithotripsy.
d. Send the stone for analysis if collected.

Clinical Pearls: Hematuria

1. *A dipstick cannot differentiate between RBCs, free hemoglobin, and myoglobin.*
2. A microscopic examination of the urine is required to confirm the presence of RBCs. Absence of any RBCs in urine with a positive dipstick reaction suggests either hemoglobinuria or myoglobinuria.
3. An occasional RBC on microscopic examination of the urine may be seen in most children. Further testing is required if examination reveals >5 RBCs/hpf.
4. Tea or cola-colored urine, RBC casts, and dysmorphic RBCs are pathognomonic for glomerular bleeding (e.g., APSGN).
5. Common nonglomerular causes of hematuria include UTI, urolithiasis, hypercalciuria, and anatomic abnormality.
6. Common glomerular causes of hematuria include APSGN, IgA nephropathy, Alport's syndrome, and membranoproliferative glomerulonephritis (MPGN).
7. Most causes of hematuria in children represent medical conditions that often will require referral to a pediatric nephrologist.

BOX 16-3. DIFFERENTIAL DIAGNOSIS OF COLA-COLORED OR DARK RED URINE

- Blood (red blood cells or hemoglobin [hemoglobinuria])
- Myoglobinuria
- Porphyrinuria
- Urates
- Ingestion of medication
  (1) Aminopyrine
  (2) Chloroquine
  (3) Deferoxamine
  (4) Ibuprofen
  (5) Methyldopa
  (6) Nitrofurantoin
  (7) Pyridium
  (8) Phenazopyridine
  (9) Phenolphthalein
  (10) Rifampin
  (11) Rhodamine B
  (12) Sulfasalazine
  (13) Furazolidone
  (14) Diphenylhydantoin
- Ingestion of food
  (1) Azo dyes
  (2) Beets
  (3) Blackberries
  (4) Red food coloring agents
- Dark brown or black urine
  (1) Alkaptonuria
  (2) Melanin
  (3) Methemoglobinuria
  (4) Tyrosinosis
  (5) Homogentisic acid

BOX 16-4. VARIOUS ETIOLOGIES OF HEMATURIA (GROSS OR MICROSCOPIC HEMATURIA)

- Infectious (bacterial, viral, tuberculosis)
  (1) Pyelonephritis
  (2) Cystitis (e.g., hemorrhagic cystitis from adenovirus)
  (3) Urethritis
- Acute postinfectious glomerulonephritis (e.g., acute poststreptococcal glomerulonephritis)
- IgA nephropathy (recurrent gross hematuria)
- Henoch-Schönlein purpura
- Benign familial hematuria (recurrent gross hematuria)
- Membranous glomerulopathy (e.g., systemic lupus erythematosus [SLE])
- Membranoproliferative glomerulonephritis (e.g., SLE)
- Rapidly progressive glomerulonephritis
- Hemolytic uremic syndrome
- Alport's syndrome (recurrent gross hematuria)
- Exercise-induced
- Hematologic (thrombocytopenia, coagulopathies, sickle cell disease and trait)
- Renal vein thrombosis
- Hypercalciuria (recurrent gross hematuria)
- Nephrocalcinosis (e.g., vitamin D intoxication)
- Nephrolithiasis
- Trauma
- Congenital (polycystic kidney, multicystic dysplasia)
- Interstitial nephritis from drugs (e.g., nonsteroidal anti-inflammatory drugs)
- Malignancy (e.g., Wilms' tumor)

DIAGNOSIS MINIMAL CHANGE NEPHROTIC SYNDROME

SYNONYMS

Historically known as lipoid nephrosis, nil disease, foot process disease, and idiopathic nephrotic syndrome

Definition

The term nephrosis or nephrotic syndrome (NS) applies to heavy proteinuria, hypoproteinemia (hypoalbuminemia), edema, and hyperlipidemia.

Etiology

1. Primary or idiopathic (90% of cases)
   a. Minimal change nephrotic syndrome ([MCNS]): most common type (80%)
   b. Focal segmental glomerulosclerosis: 10% (Fig. 16-3)
   c. Diffuse mesangial hypercellularity (DMH): 4%
   d. Membranoproliferative glomerulonephritis (MPGN): 6%
2. Secondary (10% of cases)
   a. Associated with systemic diseases (e.g., systemic lupus erythematosus, Henoch-Schönlein purpura, IgA nephropathy)
   b. Associated with infections (e.g., syphilis, hepatitis, malaria)

Pathogenesis and Associated Clinical Features

1. An increase in glomerular capillary wall permeability results in protein loss, which is primarily albumin. Hypoalbuminemia leads to a decrease in plasma oncotic pressure, permitting transudation of intravascular fluid into the interstitial space.
2. Depleted intravascular volume activates the renin-angiotensin-aldosterone system (reabsorption of sodium in distal tubules) and release of antidiuretic hormone (reabsorption of water in collecting ducts). Reabsorbed sodium and water are lost into the interstitial space secondary to reduced oncotic pressure and thus edema is worsened.
3. Hypoalbuminemia and low oncotic pressure stimulate protein synthesis in the liver, including synthesis of lipoproteins.
4. Laboratory tests include:
   a. High hemoglobin and hematocrit (hemoconcentration) and thrombocytosis
   b. Serum values of electrolytes usually normal (hyponatremia may be seen due to hyperlipidemia [pseudohyponatremia])
   c. Serum values of creatinine may be elevated in 25%.

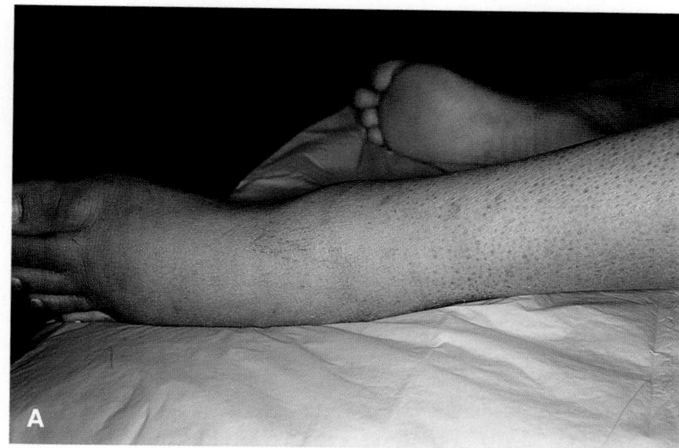

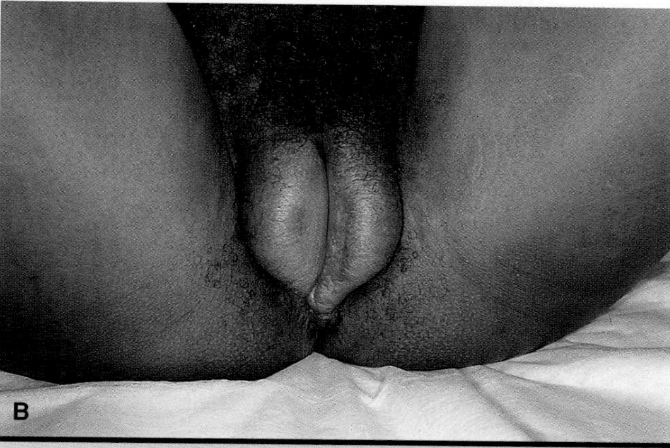

Figure 16-3. Focal Segmental Glomerulosclerosis

Severe edema of the lower extremity and edema of the vulva is seen in a 10-year-old girl who presented with hypoalbuminemia, heavy proteinuria, microscopic hematuria, and hypertension.

d. Serum complement values usually normal.
e. Hypocalcemia (secondary to hypoalbuminemia; ionized fraction normal)

6. Renal biopsy is usually *not* indicated to confirm the diagnosis of MCNS. It is usually indicated for children whose initial presentation suggests a diagnosis *other than* MCNS. Some examples include:
   a. Infants <12 months or children >10 years old
   b. Presence of azotemia (not secondary to hypovolemia)
   c. Decreased serum complement
   d. Gross hematuria (in absence of infection)
   e. Persistent hypertension
7. Complications include infections (e.g., spontaneous bacterial peritonitis, sepsis, cellulitis secondary to skin breakdown from edema), respiratory compromise due to ascites and/or pleural effusion, hypercoagulability leading to venous thrombosis (e.g., deep veins in the legs/pelvis, pulmonary, renal), and rarely arterial thrombosis (e.g., pulmonary). Hemoconcentration and use of diuretics increase the risk of thrombosis.

Consultation

Pediatric nephrology

Emergency Department Treatment and Disposition

1. Hospitalize all cases of severe nephrosis.
2. Hospitalize all patients with a first episode of nephrosis for diagnosis and provide family education (e.g., education about the chronic relapsing nature of the disease, home monitoring of urine by dipstick, diet, and complications related to both the disease and therapy).
3. Specific therapy includes
   a. Prednisone therapy for a period of 8 to 12 weeks (dose: 2 mg/kg per day or 60 mg/m^2 per day [maximum 60 mg/day]) given orally every morning in one dose or in two divided doses, preferably after meals for the first 4 weeks followed by 40 mg/m^2 per day [maximum 40 mg/day] given every other day for weeks five through twelve).
   b. The majority of children (80 to 85%) will respond with remission of proteinuria and resolution of edema by 4 weeks (average time: about 2 weeks).
4. Salt and fluid restriction is used for symptomatic edema. If indicated, diuretics (e.g., spironolactone, furosemide) are also used during periods of edema.
5. A child with relapse (presence of proteinuria >1+ on urinary dipstick on three consecutive days)
   a. Treat with 60 mg/m^2 per day until the urine is protein-free for 3 consecutive days
   b. Followed by prednisone 40 mg/m^2 every other day for 4 to 8 weeks
6. Patients with MCNS usually have repeated relapses until the disease resolves spontaneously toward the end of the second decade of life.
7. Most children with MCNS do not develop progressive renal disease. It is essentially a benign disorder.

Clinical Pearls: Minimal Change Nephrotic Syndrome

1. The term nephrotic syndrome applies to heavy proteinuria, hypoproteinemia (hypoalbuminemia), and edema.
2. Minimal change NS is the most common variety of primary NS.
3. Heavy proteinuria is an essential element of NS. Proteinuria from other causes (e.g., transient proteinuria associated with fever, dehydration, or exercise) or orthostatic proteinuria rarely exceeds 1 g/24 hours and is not associated with edema.

4. Children with periorbital edema due to NS are misdiagnosed as having angioedema (allergic reaction) in approximately 30% of cases on initial presentation. Absence of itching and a positive urine dipstick for proteinuria should alert to the possibility of NS in such children.
5. Edema is gravity-dependent; thus, early morning periorbital/facial edema may not be apparent by the time the child is seen later in the day.
6. Despite the edematous appearance with fluid and salt retention, some children are actually intravascularly depleted and injudicious use of diuretics can lead to shock or acute renal failure.
7. Overwhelming infection is one of the major causes of death. Presence of fever, leukocytosis, abdominal pain, and rebound tenderness in an edematous patient with ascites suggest spontaneous peritonitis.

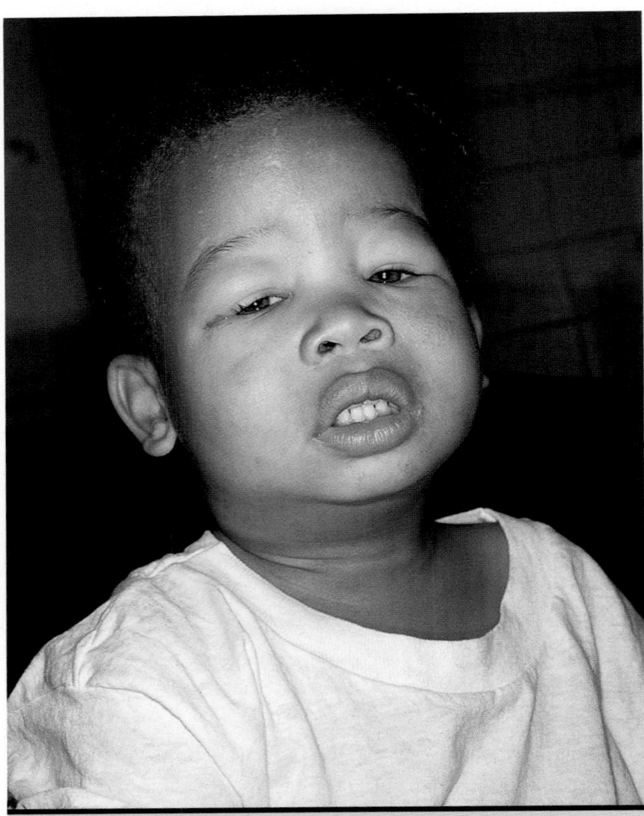

Figure 16-4. Minimal Change Nephrotic Syndrome

A 15-month-old infant presented with periorbital and facial edema associated with hypoalbuminemia and heavy proteinuria. This photo was taken soon after he woke up in the morning. Facial and periorbital edema are usually seen on arising in the morning. Edema is gravity-dependent; thus, early morning periorbital/facial edema may not be apparent by the time the child is seen later in the day. Edema also involves dependent areas such as the feet and legs, scrotum, and sacrum.

BOX 16-5. CLINICAL FEATURES OF MINIMAL CHANGE NEPHROTIC SYNDROME

- Age at presentation
  (1) Pre–school-aged children between 2 and 6 years old
  (2) About 80% of children <6 years old
  (3) Median age at diagnosis: 2.5 years
- Presenting signs and symptoms
  (1) Most common sign heralding diagnosis: edema (often periorbital edema; Fig. 16-4)
  (2) Edema is gravity-dependent
  (3) Pedal edema (difficulty putting on shoes)
  (4) Leg (pretibial) edema
  (5) Ascites (or increased abdominal girth)
  (6) Edema of scrotum, penis or vulva, sacrum
  (7) Weight gain due to edema, ascites
  (8) Hypertension (10% of cases)
  (9) Oliguria
  (10) Pleural effusion
  (11) Abdominal pain, diarrhea, vomiting (bowel wall edema)
- Laboratory
  (1) Hypoalbuminemia (serum albumin <2.5 g/dL)
  (2) Nephrotic-range proteinuria:
    a. Proteinuria >40 mg/m^2 per hour (normal: <4 mg/m^2 per hour)
    b. Urine protein:creatinine ratio (mg:mg) >2 (normal: infants <0.5, children <0.2)
  (3) Hyperlipidemia (elevated cholesterol, triglycerides, and low-density and very-low-density lipoproteins)
  (4) Elevated blood urea nitrogen (15 to 30%)
  (5) Urinalysis
    a. High specific gravity (intravascular volume depletion)
    b. Proteinuria 3 + or 4 +
    c. Microscopic hematuria (20 to 25%); gross hematuria (rare)
    d. Lipid droplets and broad waxy casts

BOX 16-6. DIFFERENTIAL DIAGNOSIS OF MINIMAL CHANGE NEPHROTIC SYNDROME

- Differential diagnosis of edema
  (1) Periorbital edema due to infections (e.g., sinusitis)
  (2) Periorbital edema due to allergies (e.g., angioedema following insect bite)
  (3) Proteinuria from other causes
  (4) Protein-losing enteropathy
  (5) Kwashiorkor (protein calorie malnutrition)

DIAGNOSIS ACUTE POSTSTREPTOCOCCAL GLOMERULONEPHRITIS

SYNONYMS

Acute proliferative glomerulonephritis
Acute postinfectious glomerulonephritis

Definition

Acute poststreptococcal glomerulonephritis (APSGN) or acute postinfectious glomerulonephritis (APGN) is characterized by an abrupt onset of one or more features of acute nephritic syndrome that includes hematuria, proteinuria, volume overload, hypertension, and azotemia.

Etiology

1. The specific pathogenesis is not fully understood.
2. The elements necessary for the production of the disease include certain unknown host factors and infection with nephritogenic strains of group A beta-hemolytic streptococci (GABHS). It is hypothesized that there is deposition of antigen in the glomeruli that activates the immune response and release of cytokines. Other organisms have been implicated and thus the term acute postinfectious glomerulonephritis is used (Box 16-7).

Associated Clinical Features

1. Pyoderma and pharyngitis are the most common antecedent infections of APGN.
2. Streptococcal pharyngitis occurs more commonly in children between 5 and 15 years of age, most commonly in the winter and spring months. Impetigo occurs most commonly in the summer and the fall.
3. A latent period exists from the onset of the primary infection to the development of the nephritis. Approximately 20% of school-age children are carriers of streptococci; thus some children may present with the disease without any identifiable prodrome.
   a. In children with acute pharyngitis, the latent period is approximately 7 to 14 days.
   b. In contrast, children with impetigo could have a latent period of up to 6 weeks.
4. The prognosis of APSGN is excellent, with about 95% of patients recovering spontaneously and 5% developing chronic glomerulonephritis.
5. Gross hematuria usually disappears in a few days. Microscopic hematuria may persist for 1 to 2 years. The C3 usually returns to normal values in 6 to 8 weeks.
6. Recurrences of APSGN are extremely rare.

Emergency Department Treatment and Disposition

1. Children with obvious edema, hypertension, and azotemia warrant hospitalization because of possible noncompliance with salt and water restriction and progression of fluid overload.
2. The treatment approach to a child with ASPGN is mostly supportive.
   a. Confirm the diagnosis.
   b. Bed rest is unnecessary and impractical.
   c. *Fluid restriction is a must.* Fluid intake should be limited to insensible water loss equivalent.

d. Salt intake should be decreased to one-third to one-half of the usual intake.
e. Surveillance for and control of hypertension, hyperkalemia, acidemia, and hyperphosphatemia

3. Hypertension should be treated quickly and appropriately. Furosemide is effective in inducing diuresis and thus decreasing volume expansion. Angiotensin-converting enzyme inhibitors have been shown to be effective in some cases even though peripheral plasma renin levels are normal in the majority of cases.

4. Severe hyperkalemia is usually rare except in children with severe azotemia. Mild to moderate hyperkalemia could be treated with potassium restriction and exchange resin. Severe hyperkalemia may need temporization with bicarbonate administration, insulin and glucose infusion, and finally with appropriate hemodialysis.

5. Patients sent home should have close outpatient monitoring that includes monitoring of volume overload, development of hypertension, deterioration of renal function, and development of hyperkalemia.

6. Penicillin or other antistreptococcal antibiotic therapy
   a. Antibiotic therapy is given to all patients who either did not receive therapy for preceding GABHS infection, or who have evidence of ongoing GABHS infection.
   b. Antibiotic therapy does *not* affect the natural course of APSGN. Antibiotic therapy is recommended to prevent the spread of nephritogenic strains of GABHS.
   c. Family members of patients with APSGN should be cultured for GABHS and treated if culture is positive.

Clinical Pearls: Acute Poststreptococcal Glomerulonephritis

1. APSGN is a delayed nonsuppurative sequela of pharyngeal or skin infection with certain nephritogenic GABHS strains.

2. APSGN is the most common type of acute nephritis.

3. APSGN is one of the most common glomerular causes of gross hematuria in children.

4. Most children with APSGN will manifest with edema and gross hematuria at presentation.

5. Acute nephritic syndrome associated with hypocomplementemia and antecedent streptococcal infection strongly suggests the diagnosis of APSGN.

6. The hallmark of APSGN is hematuria and urinary RBC casts, with only minimal to moderate proteinuria. Multiple microscopic examinations may be needed to identify the presence of RBC casts.

BOX 16-7. ORGANISMS IMPLICATED AS POSSIBLE ETIOLOGIC FACTORS FOR ACUTE POSTINFECTIOUS GLOMERULONEPHRITIS

Bacteria:
- Group A beta-hemolytic streptococci
- *Streptococcus viridans*
- *Streptococcus pneumoniae*
- *Staphylococcus aureus*
- *Staphylococcus epidermidis*
- *Corynebacterium*
- Atypical mycobacteria
- *Mycoplasma*
- *Brucella*
- Meningococcus
- *Leptospira*

Viruses:
- Varicella
- Rubeola
- Epstein-Barr virus
- Cytomegalovirus
- Influenza

Others:
- Toxoplasmosis
- *Rickettsia*
- *Trichinella*

Reproduced with permission: Barbara Cole and Luis Salinas-Madrigal, Acute proliferative Glomerulonephritis and Cresentic Glomerulonephritis, page 670, table 41.2. Pediatric Nephrology 4th edition, T. Martin Baratt, Ellis Avner and William Harmon editors. Lippincott, Williams and Wilkins publisher. 1999.

BOX 16-8. CLINICAL FEATURES ASSOCIATED WITH ACUTE POSTSTREPTOCOCCAL GLOMERULONEPHRITIS

- Most common in children aged 5 to 12 years
- Uncommon <3 years of age
- Most children will manifest with edema (seen in 85% of cases) and gross hematuria at presentation.
- Hematuria (Fig. 16-5)
  (1) Most common presentation
  (2) Either gross hematuria (seen in 30 to 50% of cases) or microscopic hematuria
  (3) Either tea-colored or cola-colored urine
  (4) Painless hematuria (*unlike hemorrhagic cystitis from adenoviral infection*)
- Renal involvement (severity varies from asymptomatic microscopic hematuria with normal renal function to acute renal failure)
- Hypertension (seen in 50 to 90% of cases)
- Oliguria (common)
- Hypertensive encephalopathy (headache, somnolence or coma, seizures; seen in about 10% of cases)
- Congestive heart failure and respiratory distress due to volume overload (dyspnea, orthopnea, rales, pulmonary edema)
- Predominantly nephrotic picture (anasarca and severe ascites; seen in about 10 to 20% of cases)
- Laboratory findings
  (1) Elevated BUN and serum creatinine (decreased GFR)
  (2) Acidosis and life-threatening hyperkalemia (with severe azotemia)
  (3) C3 and CH50 generally low at onset of disease and rise back to normal in 6 to 8 weeks
  (4) C4 usually normal or slightly decreased
  (5) Hyperphosphatemia and hypocalcemia (with renal failure)
  (6) Evidence of GABHS infection
    a. A positive throat culture for GABHS (represents either acute infection or carrier state)
    b. A rising antibody titer to streptococcal antigen(s) confirms a recent streptococcal infection (antistreptolysin O [ASLO] titers usually elevated with pharyngitis, but may be normal with impetigo).
    c. Streptozyme test (a slide agglutination test that detects antibodies to ASLO, deoxyribonuclease [DNase B], hyaluronidase, streptokinase, and nicotinamide adenine dinucleotide)
- Urinary findings
  (1) Increased RBCs and WBCs
  (2) RBC casts, granular casts, and hyaline casts
  (3) Proteinuria may be present (but large amounts uncommon).
  (4) Increased osmolarity

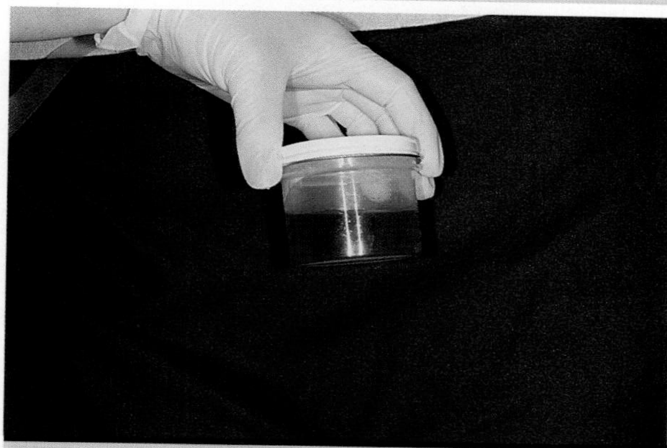

Figure 16-5. Hematuria in Acute Poststreptococcal Glomerulonephritis

Tea- or cola-colored urine, RBC casts, and dysmorphic RBCs are pathognomonic for glomerular bleeding. Two weeks following a sore throat, this 10-year-old boy presented with a sudden onset of painless hematuria. His urinalysis showed 1 + proteinuria and had many RBCs on microscopic examination with some RBC casts. His serum complement was decreased.

BOX 16-9. DIFFERENTIAL DIAGNOSIS OF ACUTE POSTSTREPTOCOCCAL GLOMERULONEPHRITIS

- Hematuria from other etiology (see Box 16-4)
- IgA nephropathy
- Membranoproliferative glomerulonephritis
- Hereditary nephritis
- Systemic lupus erythematosus
- Henoch-Schönlein purpura
- Other conditions associated with hypocomplementemia (e.g., SLE, membranoproliferative glomerulonephritis, shunt nephritis, subacute bacterial endocarditis)

DIAGNOSIS URINARY TRACT INFECTION

SYNONYMS

Acute pyelonephritis
Acute cystitis

Definitions

1. Urinary tract infection (UTI) is an acute inflammation of the urinary system or parts thereof.
2. Acute pyelonephritis denotes infection involving the upper urinary tract (e.g., kidneys). Acute cystitis indicates infection limited to the lower urinary tract (e.g., urinary bladder).

Etiology

1. Bacterial species implicated as causative agents for UTI:
   a. *Escherichia coli* (85 to 90%)
   b. *Klebsiella* spp. (2 to 4%)
   c. *Proteus* spp. (3%)
   d. *Enterococcus* spp. (2%)
   e. *Staphylococcus* spp. (2%)
   f. *Pseudomonas* spp. (<1%)
2. The body's main protection against the development of UTI is the ability of the urinary bladder to wash out contaminating organisms. In children with UTI, there is a disruption of these mechanisms either due to some anatomical defect, physiologic dysfunction, or due to the ability of the offending organism to overcome normal host factors (uroepithelial adherence).
3. Almost all UTIs are ascending infections except in the neonatal period.
4. Risk factors for UTI include
   a. Anatomical abnormalities
      1) Vesicoureteral reflux
      2) Obstruction
      3) Duplex collecting system
      4) Ureterocele
      5) Foreign body
      6) Constipation
   b. Physiologic dysfunction
      1) Daytime urinary frequency syndrome or irritable bladder
      2) Lazy bladder syndrome or bladder hyporeflexia
      3) Detrusor dysergia
      4) Hinman's syndrome (pseudoneurogenic bladder)
   c. Bacterial and other host factors
      1) Bacterial fimbriae
      2) Increased uroepithelial cell receptivity

Associated Clinical Features

1. UTI is responsible for 5% of fevers in infants with no evident source from history and physical examination.

2. The prevalence of UTIs in infants and children presenting in the ED varies by sex, race, degree of fever, and circumcision status.
   a. The highest prevalence of UTIs is in girls and uncircumcised males.
   b. Screen for UTI in girls <12 months old presenting with fever >39°C or fever of >2 days' duration without an apparent source of infection.
3. Diagnosis of UTI should be made by urine culture.
4. A bag specimen for urine culture is 100% sensitive, but false-positive results are seen in as many as 85%. A negative urine culture obtained by a bag specimen rules out UTI, provided the child did not receive antibiotics prior, and a cleansing agent (e.g., povidone-iodine solution) did not contaminate the sample.
5. Obtain urine by suprapubic aspiration or transurethral catheterization and send for urinalysis and culture (have a sterile container ready during the procedure in the event the infant voids during manipulation) (Fig. 16-6).
   a. Suprapubic aspiration (SPA) has gone out of favor.
      1) Gold standard
      2) Any number of colonies growing is considered significant.
      3) Requires technical expertise
      4) May be the only option for a boy with a tight phimosis
   b. Transurethral catheterization
      1) 95% sensitive and 99% specific
      2) >10,000 colonies of single organism indicates infection is likely

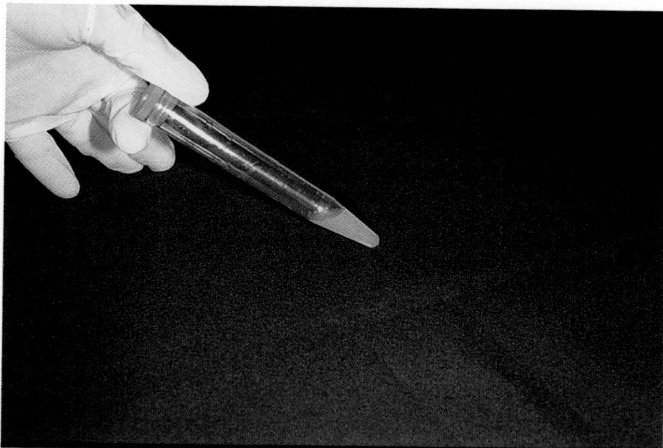

Figure 16-6. Cloudy Urine in Urinary Tract Infection

Irritability and fever were the presenting complaints of this 3-month-old uncircumcised male infant. He had hyperbilirubinemia with total bilirubin/direct bilirubin of 18/8 mg/dL. Urine was obtained by catheterization and had a cloudy appearance, was nitrite- and leukocyte esterase–positive, and had many bacteria and pyuria on microscopic examination. Subsequent urine culture was positive for *E. coli*.

6. Urinalysis
   a. Urinalysis should not substitute for a urine culture.
   b. It is most meaningful if done on fresh urine.
   c. The following are suggestive of infection and assist in selecting individuals warranting antibiotic treatment while waiting for the results of the urine culture.
      1) Positive leukocyte esterase or nitrite test
      2) More than 5 WBCs/hpf on a properly spun specimen
      3) Bacteria present on an unspun gram-stained specimen
   d. Presence of leukocyte esterase or WBCs in the urine is suggestive of an inflammatory response; however, there are many false-positive results (e.g., fever from other sources or vulvovaginitis can give false-positive results).
   e. A positive nitrite test indicates the presence of nitrate-reducing bacteria in the urine (e.g., *E. coli*). False-negative results may be seen in infants because of insufficient reduction time or in children with frequent voiding. Contaminating bacteria may cause a false-positive result in an improperly stored or handled specimen.
7. Evaluation
   a. Identification of the risk factor for the development of UTI is important to prevent future infection.
   b. The probability of developing renal scars increases with the number of infections.
   c. The younger the child at the time of infection, the higher the probability of an anatomical lesion, with vesicoureteral reflux being the most common.
   d. The following tests are commonly ordered:
      1) Renal ultrasound: a good screening test for significant structural anomalies (e.g. hydronephrosis, renal asymmetry).
      2) DMSA scan: commonly used to identify active infection or scars (to identify scars, the test has to be done 6 months after the active infection)
      3) Voiding cystogram: preferably done after the infection is treated; it is used to identify urinary reflux, bladder wall structural abnormalities, and urethral narrowing or valves.

Emergency Department Treatment and Disposition

1. Hospitalize patients with any of the following:
   a. Febrile UTI in infants <2 months old
   b. Any child with clinically suspected pyelonephritis
   c. Any adolescent with clinically suspected pyelonephritis if:
      1) Ill or toxic appearance
      2) Vomiting
      3) Increased creatinine
      4) Patients with underlying conditions
2. In a child with fever who is not so ill that antibiotic therapy is immediately needed:
   a. Obtain urine as above (obtain by the most convenient way possible and do a urinalysis).

b. If urinalysis is suggestive of infection, obtain urine by transurethral catheterization or SPA.
c. If urinalysis is negative, it is reasonable to observe a child without antibiotics. However, a negative urinalysis does not rule out UTI.

2. Children with fever assessed to be sufficiently ill to warrant immediate antibiotic therapy:
   a. Obtain urine by SPA or transurethral catheter.
   b. Start IV antibiotics once the specimen is obtained.
   c. Common *intravenous antibiotics* used for treatment of UTI:
      1) Ceftriaxone (dose: 75 mg/kg once a day) *or* cefotaxime (dose: 150 mg/kg per day divided every 6 hours) *or* cefazolin (dose: 50 mg/kg per day divided every 6 hours) *or* gentamicin (dose: 7.5 mg/kg per day divided every 8 hours) *or* tobramycin (dose: 5 mg/kg per day divided every 8 hours)
      2) Ampicillin should not be used as a first-line medication (resistance of *E. coli* to ampicillin is as high as 30 to 40% in some centers).

3. Common oral medications for treatment of UTI (treat for 7 to 10 days)
   a. amoxicillin-clavulanate (dose: 20 to 40 mg/kg per day in two divided doses)
   b. trimethoprim-sulfamethoxazole (TMP-SMX) (dose: 8 to 10 mg/kg per day of TMP in two divided doses)
   c. Cefixime (dose: 8 mg/kg per day once a day)
   d. Cefpodoxime proxetil (dose: 10 mg/kg per day in two divided doses)

4. Empirical therapy for cystitis in adolescents
   a. TMP-SMX (first-line therapy) *or* cephalosporin *or* nitrofurantoin
   b. Duration: 7 days

5. Short-term treatment of UTI in young children is not recommended because of the high risk of scarring from undiagnosed or inadequately treated UTI in infants and children, and differentiation of cystitis and acute pyelonephritis is at times difficult.

6. Common medications used for prophylaxis of UTI include:
   a. Amoxicillin (dose: 10 mg/kg orally at night) *or*
   b. TMP-SMX (dose: 1 to 2 mg/kg of TMP at night) *or*
   c. Nitrofurantoin (dose: 1 to 2 mg/kg orally at night)

Clinical Pearls: Urinary Tract Infection

1. In the ED, UTI is prevalent in febrile infants without a definitive source for fever.
2. The highest prevalence of UTI is in girls and uncircumcised males.
3. Infants <1 year old with fever without an apparent source should be considered at risk for UTI.
4. Female infants between 1 and 2 years old with fever without an apparent source should be considered at risk for UTI.
5. Urethral catheterization or suprapubic aspiration are the best methods for diagnosing UTI.

BOX 16-10. CLINICAL FEATURES OF URINARY TRACT INFECTION

- Clinical features of cystitis (inflammation of bladder)
  (1) Dysuria
  (2) Frequency
  (3) Urgency
  (4) Lower abdominal pain
  (5) If signs and symptoms not recognized early, it will progress to pyelonephritis
- Clinical features of pyelonephritis (inflammation of kidney)
  (1) High fever
  (2) Abdominal/flank pain
  (3) Costovertebral angle tenderness (older children)
  (4) Irritability, vomiting, decreased feeding (younger children)
  (5) Usually elevated ESR
  (6) Usually elevated C-reactive protein
- Special circumstances: neonates and infants
  (1) Usually present with unexplained fever and irritability
  (2) Infants not able to express initial discomfort associated with cystitis/urethritis other than being described as cranky
  (3) Majority of cases have pyelonephritis at presentation (febrile UTI will show pyelonephritis on nuclear scan)
  (4) Some infants may have foul-smelling urine.
  (5) Hyperbilirubinemia (neonates; especially direct hyperbilirubinemia)
  (6) Poor feeding
  (7) Vomiting and diarrhea (neonates)

BOX 16-11. DIFFERENTIAL DIAGNOSIS OF URINARY TRACT INFECTION

- Hypercalciuria
- Urethritis
- Gastroenteritis
- Appendicitis
- Urolithiasis

DIAGNOSIS HYPERTENSIVE EMERGENCIES

Definitions

1. Hypertensive emergencies occur when there is elevation of systemic blood pressure 30% above normal for age and sex, accompanied by end-organ involvement (e.g., *hypertensive encephalopathy, congestive heart failure, and renal failure*).
2. Hypertensive urgency is a term used to denote severe elevations of BP in children without any signs or symptoms of end-organ involvement.

Associated Clinical Features

1. Hypertensive emergencies may present with either signs and symptoms of hypertensive encephalopathy or congestive heart failure (Box 16-12).
2. Laboratory evaluation includes urinalysis with microscopy and basic metabolic panel.
3. Additional tests include serum renin and aldosterone levels, renal sonogram (once blood pressure is reasonably controlled), and thyroid function testing (if applicable).

Emergency Department Treatment and Disposition

1. Severe hypertension with no evidence of end-organ involvement (hypertensive urgency):
   a. Gradual control of blood pressure to baseline usually in 24 hours; 20% reduction in the first 2 hours
   b. Ideally, children should be admitted for close monitoring and titration of response to medication. Some children may be sent home, only if BP has shown an appropriate response, and compliance with medication and follow-up with a pediatric nephrologist is assured.
   c. Familiarize yourself with contraindications and side effects before initiating therapy. Therapeutic options include:
      1) IV labetalol: start with lower dose; 0.2 to 1 mg/kg/dose via slow IV push every 10 minutes and titrate to response (maximum bolus 20 mg); onset of action 1 to 5 minutes and duration is variable, approximately 6 hours
      2) IV enalaprilat: 0.005 to 0.01 mg/kg/dose every 8 to 24 hours
      3) IV hydralazine (weaker vasodilator): 0.1 to 0.2 mg/kg/dose every 4 to 6 hours (maximum 20 mg/dose)
      4) Oral nifedipine (effective but may cause severe hypotension, palpitations, and headaches; thus, use with caution): 0.25 to 0.5 mg/kg/dose (10-mg capsule has 0.34 mL of solution); take with a small amount of juice or water; onset of action 30 minutes; may give second dose if no response
2. Hypertensive encephalopathy: All children should be admitted and monitored in the PICU with continuous blood pressure monitoring. The target should be a 30% drop in blood pressure in the first 8 hours and normalization of BP in 24 to 48 hours.
   a. Sodium nitroprusside (ideal, but may take time to prepare)
      1) Rapid onset and short duration of action
      2) Requires ICU setting with arterial line
      3) Follow thiocyanate levels and development of metabolic acidosis if used long term.
      4) Usual dose is 0.3 to 8 μg/kg per minute

b. IV labetalol: start as above, and then start continuous infusion of 0.4 to 1 mg/kg per hour
c. Diazoxide
   1) Must be given as rapid IV push
   2) Onset of action 1 to 5 minutes and duration is variable (2 to 12 hours)
   3) Usual dose is 1 to 3 mg/kg up to max dose of 150 mg/dose
   4) Repeat every 5 to 15 minutes
   5) Caution: may cause dramatic drop of blood pressure and hyperglycemia
d. Nicardipine infusion (limited experience with children): rapid onset and 3-hour duration; dose is 0.5 to 5 μg/kg per minute via continuous IV infusion.

Clinical Pearls: Hypertensive Emergencies

1. Infants with severe hypertension will present with poor feeding and respiratory distress.
2. Older children with hypertension complaining of headache, nausea, or dizziness may be in the early stage of encephalopathy and could progress to frank seizures (Fig. 16-7).
3. Essential hypertension is rare in prepubertal children and rarely causes hypertensive emergencies. Look for a renal or renovascular cause.
4. Always take blood pressure readings in all four extremities during the initial evaluation to check for vascular diseases (e.g., coarctation of the aorta, Takayasu's arteritis, and mid-aortic syndromes).

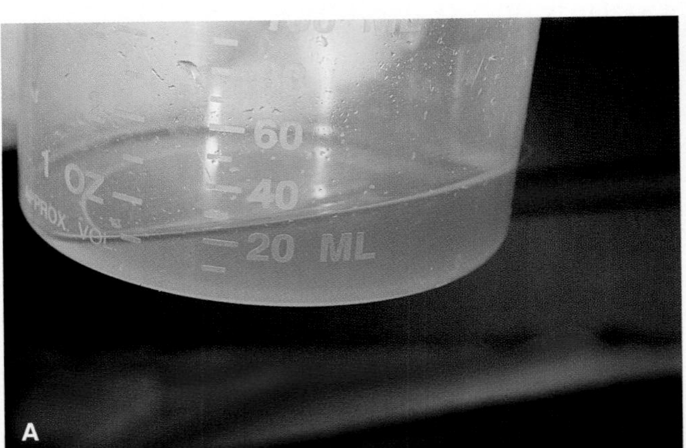

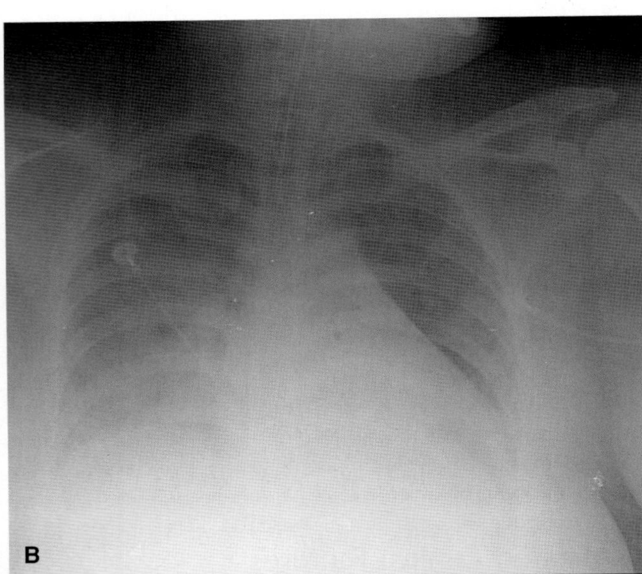

Figure 16-7. Acute Poststreptococcal Glomerulonephritis Presenting with Hematuria, Congestive Heart Failure and Hypertensive Encephalopathy.

A. Gross hematuria. A previously healthy 16-year-old girl presented with severe hypertension with a generalized tonic-clonic seizure. Other findings included gross hematuria, oliguria, hypocomplementemia, and renal insufficiency following a "strep throat" 2 weeks prior to the current illness. *B*. Cardiomegaly with pulmonary edema. Her chest x-ray shows cardiomegaly, obscured costophrenic angles, and bilateral hazy opacification of the lung with greater involvement of the right side.

BOX 16-12. CLINICAL FEATURES OF HYPERTENSIVE EMERGENCIES

- Signs and symptoms of hypertensive encephalopathy
  (1) Headache, dizziness, nausea
  (2) Altered mental status
  (3) Blurred vision, cortical blindness
  (4) Focal neurologic deficits
  (5) Seizures
  (6) Stroke (rare in children but has been reported)
- Signs and symptoms of congestive heart failure
  (1) Young infants: poor feeding and respiratory distress (often mistaken for sepsis), hepatomegaly (almost always present)
  (2) Older children: usually present with variable degree of respiratory distress, lethargy, hepatomegaly, and edema of lower extremities

BOX 16-13. CONDITIONS THAT COMMONLY PRESENT WITH HYPERTENSIVE EMERGENCIES

- Acute glomerulonephritis
- Systemic vasculitis
- Renal artery stenosis
- Neural crest tumors
  (1) Pheochromocytoma
  (2) Neuroblastoma
  (3) Paraganglioma

BOX 16-14. DIFFERENTIAL DIAGNOSIS OF HYPERTENSIVE EMERGENCIES

- Altered level of consciousness (various etiologies; see Box 13-4)
- Status epilepticus (various etiologies; see Box 13-22)
- Seizure disorder (various etiologies; see Box 13-18)
- Raised intracranial pressure (various etiologies)
- Central nervous system trauma with intracranial hemorrhage or edema

Suggested Readings

Cole B, Madrigal L: Acute proliferative Glomerulonephritis and Cresentic Glomerulonephritis. In: Barrett TM, Avner E, Harmon W (eds). *Pediatric Nephrology,* 4th ed. Lippincott Williams & Wilkins, Baltimore, 1999;670.

Gorelick MH, Shaw KN: Screening tests for urinary tract infection in children: A meta-analysis. *Pediatrics* 1999;104(5). URL: http://www.pediatrics.org/cgi/content/full/104/5/e54; *urinary tract infection, diagnostic tests, urinalysis, pyuria, bacteriuria, meta-analysis.*

Patel HP, Bissler JJ: Hematuria in children. *Pediatr Clin North Am* 2001;48:1591.

Roth KS, Amaker BH, Chan JCM: Nephrotic syndrome: Pathogenesis and management. *Pediatr Rev* 2002;23:237.

Shaw K, McGowan KL, Gorelick MH, Schwartz JS: Screening for urinary tract infection in infants in the emergency department; Which test is best? *Pediatrics* 1998;101(6). URL: http//www.pediatrics.org/cgi/content/full/101/6/e1; *urinalysis, Gram stain, dipstick, UTI, rapid screening, febrile infants.*

CHAPTER 17

TOXICOLOGY

Ronak R. Shah / Mark Su / Robert Hoffman / Kumarie Etwaru

Edited by Mark Su

DIAGNOSIS THE POISONED PATIENT: GENERAL APPROACH AND GASTROINTESTINAL DECONTAMINATION

Background

1. Incidence of pediatric poisoning follows a biphasic curve.
   a. About 85 to 90% of cases in children occur between the ages of 1 and 6 years. Most cases are single-agent exposures (frequently nontoxic household products) that are unintentionally ingested in small amounts (Fig. 17-1).
   b. About 10 to 15% of cases occur in adolescents. These cases usually involve multiple pharmaceutical agents that are intentionally ingested, often in the context of a suicide attempt.
2. Most reported exposures among pharmaceutical agents in children <6 years of age include analgesics, cough and cold preparations, cardiovascular agents, topical preparations, sedative hypnotic agents, and antidepressants (Figs. 17-2 and 17-3). Exposures to household cleaners, cosmetics, and plants are among the leading nonpharmaceutical agents.
3. Caustics, iron products, prescription medications, and toxic alcohols are among reported toxins that potentially cause significant toxicity (small doses induce great toxicity).

Emergency Department Evaluation

1. The most important factor in successfully treating a patient with a toxicologic exposure is to recognize that there is a toxicologic etiology of the patient's condition.
2. Often, when a patient presents with an ingestion, the nature of the poison or even the existence of a poisoning may be uncertain. Poisoning must be considered in the differential diagnosis of multiple conditions, especially when a patient presents with any of the following: cyanosis, shock, vomiting, diarrhea, hypothermia or hyperthermia, abnormal behavior, or altered mental status.
3. Historical key points include:
   a. Identification of the toxin; the patient or the patient's caretakers may be able to directly identify the involved toxin due to a known exposure (e.g., medications taken, intentional overdose attempt, substance abuse, exposure to occupational chemicals). Further historical information that is often helpful includes:
      1) Prehospital health care workers may search the patient's home for medication containers or report the presence of other possible toxins at the time of arrival in the ED.
      2) A sample of the substance ingested (e.g., similar mushrooms, plants) may be available.
      3) Interview the patient's family members for additional clues.
      4) In cases of potential carbon monoxide poisoning (CO), the local fire department may also be dispatched to determine the presence and concentration of CO in a building.
      5) Look for all medications and potentially toxic household products present in the home. All products that cannot readily be accounted for may have been ingested.
      6) A poison control center or product manufacturer should be contacted if the ingredients of a product are unknown. Review of drug and chemical databases (i.e., Poisindex) is also useful.
      7) Maintain a high level of suspicion and always search for occult coingestions (e.g., acetaminophen) in adolescents.
      8) Route of exposure; toxicity from various substances can occur via multiple routes of exposure (e.g., dermal, rectal, ocular, parenteral, or transplacental). The route of exposure will likely affect the severity of toxicity.
      9) Amount of exposure; patients may report the exact amount. Other times it may be necessary to search through medication containers and count the number of remaining pills or measure approximate quantities of liquid. Comparison with the expected amount may reveal a discrepancy.

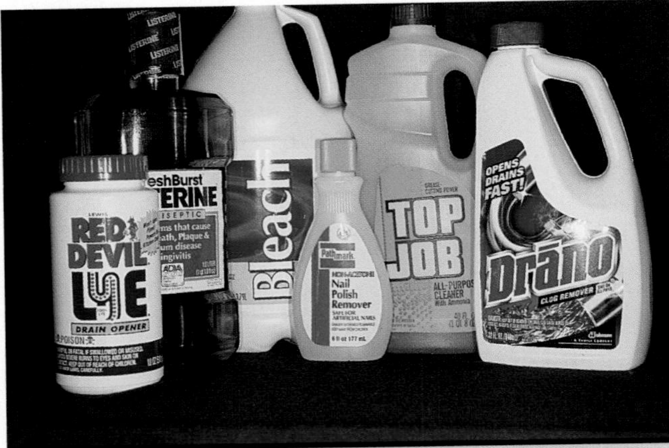

Figure 17-1. Household Products Frequently Ingested by Children

Household cleaners, cosmetics, and plants are among the leading nonpharmaceutical agents ingested by children. Some of these products contain sodium hydroxide (e.g., Drano, lye), 21.6% alcohol, methyl salicylate (e.g., Listerine), and sodium hypochlorite (e.g., bleach).

b. Determination of symptoms since ingestion will aid in recognition of toxidromes (see below) as well as determination of degree of toxicity.
c. Any treatment and attempts at decontamination prior to hospital arrival
d. Past medical history and comorbidities; focus on the patient's medications including herbal supplements, over-the-counter medications, and alternative medical therapies.
e. Intent of exposure; unintentional or intentional? This may aid in assessing the reliability of the history given by the patient.
f. Consider child abuse in children younger than 1 year of age, repeated episodes of ingestion, or if the child's developmental level and skills preclude performance of the described events (e.g., a child too young to open childproof containers).

4. A thorough physical examination beginning with vital signs should be performed.
   a. This will aid in identifying other nontoxicologic causes of a patient's illness.
   b. Attempt to identify toxidromes (toxicologic syndromes) which are a characteristic constellation of signs and symptoms seen with certain poisons. Toxidromes help in the diagnosis and management of acutely ill patients, especially when a history of poisoning is lacking. Examples of compounds categorized by their associated toxidromes include:
      1) Anticholinergics: atropine, tricyclic antidepressants (TCAs), antipsychotics, antihistamines, phenothiazines, and antispasmodics
      2) Sympathomimetics: amphetamines (phenylpropanolamine, ephedrine, methamphetamine), cocaine, methyl xanthines (e.g., caffeine, theophylline)
      3) Opioids: heroin, methadone, morphine, codeine, meperidine
      4) Sedative-hypnotics: barbiturates, benzodiazepines, ethanol
      5) Cholinergics: organophosphates and carbamate insecticides
      6) Hypermetabolics: salicylates

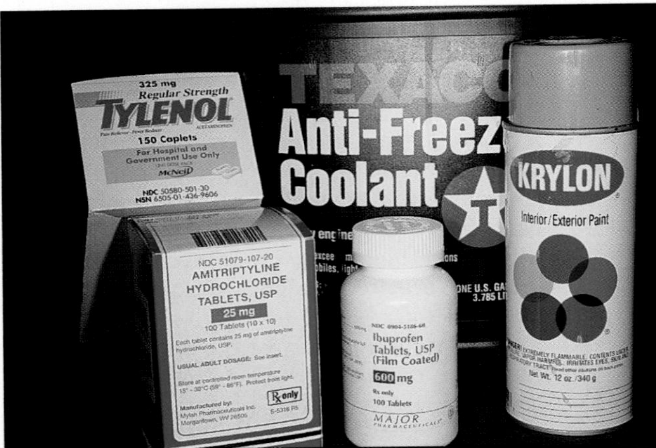

Figure 17-2. Medications and Poisons Frequently Ingested by Adolescents

Among the top pharmaceutical agents that are intentionally ingested in the context of a suicide attempt by adolescents include analgesics, sedative-hypnotics, tricyclic antidepressants, antihistamines, and ethylene glycol.

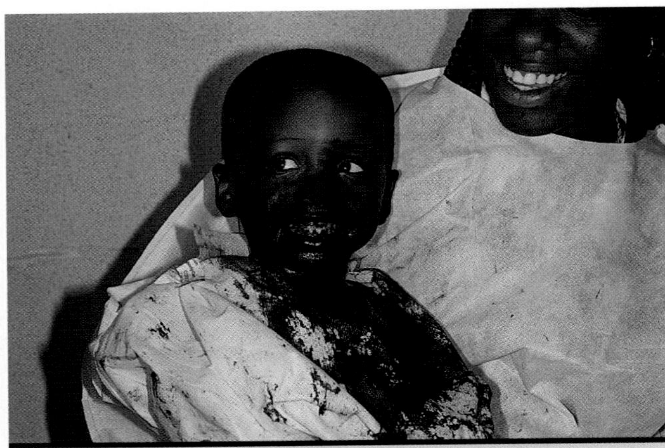

Figure 17-3. Activated Charcoal Administration

A 3-year-old child presented after accidentally drinking 4 ounces of Dimetapp liquid (grape flavor) 1 hour prior to arrival in the ED. He was completely asymptomatic. As seen here, AC is poorly accepted by young children and often there is a battle between the hospital staff and the child over its administration. AC should *not* be routinely administered in the management of a poisoned patient.

   7) Withdrawal: opioids, benzodiazepines, ethanol cocaine

5. Laboratory studies should be performed, *if clinically indicated,* for diagnosis or to guide therapy (see specific chapters for agents and laboratory studies that may prove useful in management).
   a. Serum electrolytes including glucose, BUN, and creatinine (determine renal function as well as calculation of anion gap)
   b. Serum osmolality; substances that cause an increased osmolal gap include ethanol, methanol, isopropyl alcohol, and ethylene glycol (osmolal gap = measured serum osmolality − calculated osmolality)
   c. Toxicology screens (either urine or serum) may occasionally help in determining occult coingestions; however, they are almost never helpful in the acute management because most detected agents are supportively managed. Often, however, they are requested by consultants (e.g., psychiatry) or the admitting physicians and may be performed to facilitate disposition and long-term management.
   d. All patients with an intentional overdose should have serum acetaminophen and salicylate levels determined.
   e. All females of childbearing age should have a pregnancy test performed.
   f. For gastric aspirate/vomitus, note appearance, pills, odor (e.g., camphor); and test for occult blood in the stool.

6. Radiographic studies may be useful for management. Chest radiographs may show pulmonary edema or aspiration pneumonitis consistent with hydrocarbon exposure. Abdominal radiographs may show radiopaque substances. Radiographs may confirm the diagnosis with a high index of suspicion (e.g., iron), and help to evaluate the efficacy of gastrointestinal decontamination. The absence of visible tablets does not exclude ingestion.

Emergency Department Treatment and Disposition

1. All patients should be properly decontaminated externally prior to entry into the ED to protect health care personnel and to prevent contamination of the ED. Although rarely indicated, this involves removal of all clothing and washing the skin to remove agents.

2. Treatment of all patients must begin with stabilization of airway, breathing, and circulation (ABCs) based on abnormal vital signs *before* any diagnostic tests are performed.

3. Attempt to identify a specific toxidrome when possible. It must be emphasized that one should focus on *treating the patient, not the poison*. Patients may have more than one type of exposure or ingestion, complicating the identification of distinct toxidromes.

4. Motor seizures are generally well-controlled by benzodiazepines. If the toxic agent is known, seizures may be controlled with specific therapy (e.g., pyridoxine for acute isoniazid toxicity). Anticonvulsants are rarely used in the treatment of toxin-induced seizures.

5. Patients with altered mental status should be evaluated for all causes of altered sensorium including nontoxicologic causes (e.g., infection, electrolyte imbalance, trauma; see mnemonic COMATOSE PATIENT, Box 13-4).

6. Unresponsive patients may empirically be given IV thiamine 100 mg (in adolescents), followed by IV dextrose (1 g/kg) and IV naloxone (1 to 2 mg, may be repeated several times) and observed for a response.

7. Gastrointestinal decontamination in the management of the poisoned patient includes:
   a. Syrup of ipecac-induced emesis
      1) There is no evidence from clinical studies that ipecac improves outcome of poisoned patients.
      2) Ipecac should *not be routinely administered* in the ED.
      3) Insufficient data exist to support ipecac administration soon after poison ingestion. Ipecac results in emesis roughly 20 minutes after its administration; thus its administration may impair delivery of other oral therapies (e.g., activated charcoal or antidotes such as *N*-acetylcysteine).
      4) Other complications include persistent emesis, lethargy, or diarrhea.
      5) Contraindications: ingestion of caustics or hydrocarbons with a high risk for aspiration, and patients with an unprotected airway (e.g., obtunded, seizing); children under 6 months of age
   b. Orogastric lavage
      1) *It should not be routinely performed* in the management of poisoned patients. Under no circumstances should it be used to punish patients.
      2) Insufficient evidence exists that it improves clinical outcome.
      3) Possible indications include potentially life-threatening ingestion of a poison in which a definitive antidote is lacking. The greatest benefit is likely to be seen in the patient who presents within 60 minutes of ingestion. Patients presenting after 60 minutes may also benefit because of delayed gastric emptying.
      4) Contraindications include ingestion of caustics, hydrocarbons, and foreign bodies; bleeding diathesis, and an unprotected airway.
      5) Complications include aspiration pneumonia, gastrointestinal perforation, laryngospasm, and emesis.
   c. Activated charcoal (AC; see Fig. 17-3)
      1) AC should *not* be routinely administered in the management of all poisoned patients.
      2) Administration may be considered if a patient has ingested a potentially toxic amount of a poison that is known to be adsorbed by AC.
      3) It is likely to be most effective if administered within 60 minutes of ingestion, but may also be given after 60 minutes if there is delayed gastric emptying, possible bezoar formation, and enteroheptic or enteroenteric circulation of the toxin.

4) AC adsorbs many toxins. It does not adsorb acids, alkalis, lithium, iron (most metals), alcohols, or hydrocarbons.
5) It is given orally as a slurry in water or fruit juice (also by nasogastric or orogastric tube).
6) Usual single dose (children/adults): 1 to 2 g/kg up to 50 g or 10:1 ratio of AC:drug is ideal.
7) Multiple-dose AC (0.5 to 1 g/kg every 4 to 6 hours) should be considered if a patient has ingested a large quantity of agents that decreases gastric motility (e.g., anticholinergics, enteric-coated preparations), theophylline, phenobarbital, carbamazepine, quinine, or dapsone. Patients should have good GI motility as evidenced by normal bowel sounds and passage of stool (i.e., no evidence of GI obstruction).
8) Contraindications: intestinal obstruction or perforation, altered sensorium (absent gag reflex/unprotected airway), caustics (may obscure endoscopic visualization of gastroesophageal injury)
9) Complications: pulmonary aspiration, intestinal obstruction, constipation, charcoal bezoars

d. Cathartics (sorbitol, magnesium sulfate, or magnesium citrate)
1) Administration of a cathartic alone has *no* role as a method of gut decontamination.
2) Routine use of a cathartic with AC is *not* recommended.
3) If desorption of ingestant from AC is a possibility, a single dose of cathartic may be given to an adolescent who has ingested a large amount of drugs.
4) Complications: nausea, vomiting, diarrhea, abdominal pain; dehydration with electrolyte disturbances (with multiple doses)
5) Contraindications: absent bowel sounds, ingestion of caustics or gastrointestinal irritants

e. Whole bowel irrigation (WBI)
1) *WBI should not be routinely used in the management of the poisoned patient.*
2) May be considered in patients who have ingested foreign bodies, packets containing toxins, iron, sustained-release or enteric-coated tablets
3) It is commonly performed by the continuous administration of a bowel cleansing solution containing polyethylene glycol electrolyte solution (PEG ELS) via an oral or nasogastric tube. It is given at a rate of 0.5 L/hour until the rectal effluent is clear. In larger children and adolescents, it should be given at a rate of 1 to 2 L/hour.
4) No significant adverse effects of prolonged WBI with PEG ELS have been demonstrated.

8. Specific antidotes
a. Prophylactic use of antidotes is not recommended. There are indications for the use of specific antidotes, depending on the toxin, because of potentially serious side effects with inappropriate administration.
b. Life-threatening poisonings such as opioids cholinergics, TCAs, methemoglobinemia, CO, and cyanide require simultaneous use of an antidote with the initial stabilization of vital signs.
c. Other antidotes are not usually required immediately, and if indicated, can be administered once the diagnosis is confirmed.

9. Consider hospital admission if:
a. The patient manifests significant toxicity.
b. The patient has suicidal intent (psychiatric/social services intervention).
c. Patients in whom identification of poison is unclear or acutely ill patients requiring emergency stabilization
d. Patients requiring further management such as urinary alkalinization (e.g., salicylates, phenobarbital), hemodialysis (e.g., methanol, ethylene glycol, salicylates, lithium), or whole-bowel irrigation (e.g., iron)
e. Observation and possible treatment for substances that have delayed toxicity

10. Consider discharge to home all patients with unintentional ingestion if :
a. The patient has received appropriate counseling and social service intervention.
b. The product or drug has been identified and is determined to be benign.
c. The amount ingested is less than the smallest amount known to produce toxicity (*be careful with this; the history is often unreliable*).
d. The patient has no signs of toxicity since the time of ingestion.
e. The time elapsed since the ingestion is greater than the longest interval known between ingestion and peak toxicity.
f. Child abuse/neglect is not considered likely.

Clinical Pearls: Poisoning

1. Unintentional poisonings are commonly encountered medical emergency in young children.

2. There are insufficient data on poisoned patients demonstrating improved patient outcome from any type of GI decontamination. The removal of a toxin before it is absorbed may prevent or mitigate toxicity. Two important questions that need to be answered in ED are: "Has the child ingested a toxic dose?" and "What is the time since ingestion?"

3. Gastric lavage should *not* be considered unless the patient has ingested a potentially life-threatening amount of a poison.

4. AC should *not* be routinely administered in the management of a poisoned patient. Administration may be considered if a patient has ingested a potentially toxic amount of a poison that is known to be adsorbed by AC. In most cases, a nasogastric tube should not be placed for the sole purpose of AC administration.

5. WBI should NOT be routinely used in the management of the poisoned patient. It may be considered in patients presenting with potentially toxic ingestion of iron, lead, packets of illicit drugs, sustained-release or enteric-coated tablets.

BOX 17-1. THE POISONED PATIENT: TOXICOLOGIC CLUES AND TESTS TO PERFORM AT THE BEDSIDE

- Therapeutic response to oxygen = CO poisoning
- Cyanosis unresponsive to O_2 = methemoglobinemia
- Chocolate brown blood = methemoglobinemia
- Therapeutic response to glucose = hypoglycemic agents, alcohols, salicylates
- Therapeutic response to naloxone = opiates
- Coma: alcohol, sedative hypnotics, opiates, TCAs, anticholinergics, CO, salicylates, isoniazid, organophosphates, anticonvulsants, antihistamines, clonidine, PCP, phenothiazines (see mnemonic COMATOSE PATIENT, page ???)
- Respiration
  (1) Bradypnea: opiates, alcohol, benzodiazepines, clonidine, barbiturates
  (2) Tachypnea: salicylates, sympathomimetics, methanol, ethylene glycol, theophylline, caffeine, cocaine
  (3) Wheezing: organophosphates
  (4) Kussmaul: salicylates, methanol, ethylene glycol
- Pulse
  (1) Bradycardia: beta-blockers, calcium channel blockers, clonidine, digoxin, sedative hypnotics, opiates, organophosphates, phenylpropanolamine
  (2) Tachycardia: anticholinergics, sympathomimetics (cocaine, amphetamines, over-the-counter [OTC] cold remedies), theophylline, caffeine, iron, salicylate, TCAs, levothyroxine
  (3) Arrhythmias: anticholinergics, TCAs, phenothiazines, beta-blockers, organophosphates, CO, cyanide (CN)
- Blood pressure
  (1) Hypotension: beta-blockers, calcium channel blockers, clonidine, opiates, iron, TCAs, phenothiazines, CO, CN
  (2) Hypertension: phenylpropanolamine (OTC cold remedies), sympathomimetics, phencyclidine (PCP), cocaine, amphetamines, anticholinergics, antihistamines
- Temperature
  (1) Hypothermia: alcohol, opiates, benzodiazepines, clonidine, barbiturates, phenothiazines, TCAs, CO, antidepressants, hypoglycemic agents
  (2) Hyperthermia: sympathomimetics, anticholinergics, salicylates, TCAs, cocaine, amphetamines, theophylline, phenothiazines
- Bedside glucose analysis
  (1) Hyperglycemia: salicylates, iron, isoniazid
  (2) Hypoglycemia: hypoglycemic agents, alcohols, salicylates
- Analysis of arterial blood gases
  (1) CO: normal Po_2, normal hemoglobin saturation and normal pulse oxymetry
  (2) Methemoglobinemia: normal or increased Po_2, decreased hemoglobin saturation and decreased pulse oxymetry
  (3) Carboxyhemoglobin and methemoglobin levels
- ECG: terminal 40-msec frontal plane QRS vector, prolonged QRS = TCAs
- Urine ferric chloride assay (1 ml of urine + few drops of 10% ferric chloride): purple = salicylates, phenothiazines
- Urine:
  (1) Calcium oxalate crystals = ethylene glycol
  (2) Ketones = acetone, isopropyl alcohol, salicylates
- Urine fluoresces under Wood's lamp: ethylene glycol from antifreeze (fluorescein)
- Gastric contents deferoxamine test: (deferoxamine + hydrogen peroxide added to gastric contents yields a rose color) = iron
- Skin
  (1) Cherry red = CO, anticholinergics, CN
  (2) Blue/cyanosis = methemoglobinemia
  (3) Flushing = anticholinergics, sympathomimetics, alcohol, antihistamines
  (4) Hot, dry skin = anticholinergics, antihistamines
  (5) Diaphoresis = sympathomimetics, salicylates, cocaine, PCP, organophosphates, barbiturates
  (6) Jaundice = acetaminophen, mothballs (naphthalene), heavy metals
- Odor
  (1) Acetone = isopropanol, methanol, chloroform, salicylate
  (2) Wintergreen = methyl salicylate
  (3) Alcohol = ethanol, isopropyl alcohol, methanol
  (4) Garlic = organophosphates, arsenic, thallium, phosphorus
  (5) Coal gas = CO
  (6) Bitter almond = CN
  (7) Rotten eggs = hydrogen sulfide
  (8) Fruity = isopropanol, ethanol, amyl nitrite, diabetic ketoacidosis

BOX 17-1. THE POISONED PATIENT: TOXICOLOGIC CLUES AND TESTS TO PERFORM AT THE BEDSIDE (CONTINUED)

(9) Mothballs = Camphor, naphthalene
(10) Petroleum = Petroleum distillate
(11) Pears = chloral hydrate

- Extrapyramidal signs (rigidity, dysphonia, torticollis, oculogyric crisis) = phenothiazines
- Myoclonus/rigidity = phenothiazines, anticholinergics, haloperidol
- Nystagmus = phenytoin, PCP, alcohol, barbiturates, sedative-hypnotics, carbamazepine, CO
- Psychosis/delirium = PCP, anticholinergics, phenothiazines, cocaine, heroin, sympathomimetics, LSD, marijuana, ethanol, antihistamines
- Ataxia = alcohol, phenytoin, barbiturates, benzodiazepines, CO
- Fasciculations = organophosphates
- Paralysis = organophosphates, botulinum toxin, carbamates, heavy metals
- Blindness = methanol

BOX 17-2. MNEMONICS FOR POISONINGS

A. *Increased anion gap metabolic acidosis:*

MUD PILES	*ACIDOSIS*
*M*ethanol	*A*lcohols (methanol, ethylene glycol)
*U*remia	*C*arbon monoxide or *C*yanide
*D*iabetic ketoacidosis	*I*ron
*P*henformin, *P*araldehyde	*D*iabetic ketoacidosis
*I*ron, *I*soniazid	*O*ther (uremia, paraldehyde)
*L*actic acidosis (caused by CO, CN, seizure, shock)	*S*eizures or shock (lactic acidosis)
*E*thylene glycol	*I*soniazid
*S*alicylates	*S*alicylates

B. *Anticholinergics:*
- *Hot* as a hare (febrile)
- *Red* as a beet (flushed skin)
- *Blind* as a bat (mydriasis)
- *Mad* as a hatter (delirium)
- *Dry* as a bone (decreased secretions)

C. *Cholinergics: DUMBELS*
- *D*iarrhea
- *U*rination
- *M*iosis
- *B*ronchorrhea/*B*ronchospasm
- *E*mesis
- *L*acrimation
- *S*alivation

D. *Miosis: COPS*
- *C*lonidine, *C*holinergics
- *O*piates (except meperidine and diphenoxylate/atropine sulfate), *O*rganophosphates
- *P*henothiazines, *P*hencyclidine
- *S*edative-hypnotic coma (barbiturates, benzodiazepines, ethanol)

E. *Mydriasis: WASH*
- *W*ithdrawal (sedative-hypnotic, opioid, ethanol)
- *A*nticholinergics (atropine)
- *S*ympathomimetics
- *H*allucinogens

F. *Radiopaque substances: COCAINE*
- *C*ocaine packets
- *O*piate packets
- *C*hloral hydrate
- *A*rsenic (heavy metals, lead, mercury)
- *I*ron
- *N*euroleptics (phenothiazines, tricyclic antidepressants)
- *E*nteric-coated preparations (e.g., aspirin)

G. *Drugs or chemicals producing seizures: CAMPHOR BALLS*
- *C*amphor, *C*ocaine, *C*arbon monoxide, *C*yanide, *C*affeine, *C*lonidine, *C*arbamazepine
- *A*mphetamines, *A*nticholinergics (tricyclic antidepressants, antihistamines)
- *M*ethylxanthines (theophylline)
- *P*henothiazines or *P*hencyclidine
- *H*ypoglycemic agents (oral insulin), *H*eavy metals (e.g., lead)
- *O*pioids (propoxyphene, meperidine), *O*rganophosphates
- *R*odenticides (strychnine, thallium, arsenic)
- *B*arbiturates, *B*enzodiazepines (withdrawal seizures)
- *A*lcohols (methanol, ethylene glycol), ethanol (withdrawal seizure)
- *L*idocaine
- *L*ithium
- *S*alicylates

(Reproduced with permission from: Shah BR: Child poisoned by unknown substance. In: Finberg L, Kleinman RE (eds). *Saunders Manual of Pediatric Practice*. WB Saunders, Philadelphia, 2002, p. 1158.)

BOX 17-3. MEDICATIONS AND TOXINS FOR WHICH QUANTITATIVE SERUM CONCENTRATIONS AID IN THE MANAGEMENT OF A POISONED PATIENT

- Medications
  - (1) Acetaminophen
  - (2) Salicylates
  - (3) Iron
  - (4) Carbamazepine
  - (5) Phenobarbital
  - (6) Phenytoin
  - (7) Valproic acid
  - (8) Theophylline
  - (9) Ethanol
  - (10) Methanol
  - (11) Ethylene glycol
  - (12) Digoxin
  - (13) Lithium
- Toxins
  - (1) Carboxyhemoglobin
  - (2) Methemoglobin

BOX 17-4. EXAMPLES OF POISONS AND THEIR ANTIDOTES

Poison	*Antidote*
Acetaminophen	*N*-Acetylcysteine
Anticholinergics	Physostigmine
Benzodiazepines	Flumazenil
Beta-blockers	Glucagon
Carbon monoxide	Oxygen/hyperbaric oxygen
Carbamate insecticide	Atropine
Cyanide	Cyanide antidote kit (amyl nitrate, sodium nitrate, sodium thiosulfate)
Digoxin	Digibind
Ethylene glycol	Ethanol, fomepizole
Iron	Deferoxamine
Isoniazid	Pyridoxine
Lead, Copper, Arsenic	DMSA, calcium disodium edetate (EDTA), dimercaprol, penicillamine
Methanol	Ethanol, Fomepizole
Methemoglobinemia	Methylene blue
Opioids	Naloxone
Organophosphate insecticides	Atropine, pralidoxime
Phenothiazines	Diphenhydramine
Salicylate	Sodium bicarbonate (alkalinize urine)
Tricyclic antidepressants	Sodium bicarbonate (alkalinize serum)

(Reproduced with permission from: Shah BR: Child poisoned by unknown substance. In: Finberg L, Kleinman RE [eds]. *Saunders Manual of Pediatric Practice*. WB Saunders, Philadelphia, 2002, p. 1158.)

DIAGNOSIS ACETAMINOPHEN TOXICITY

Background and Pharmacokinetics

1. Acetaminophen is also known as *N*-acetyl-*p*-aminophenol (APAP) or paracetamol and is available in many OTC preparations. Although it is very safe with therapeutic use, overdose can lead to hepatic necrosis, fulminant hepatic failure and death.
2. APAP is available in two major formulations (by itself) and in a multitude of combination preparations.
   a. Immediate-release (serum concentrations usually peak within 1 hour)
   b. Extended-release (serum concentrations usually peak between 1 and 2 hours)
3. Therapeutic doses
   a. Children: 10 to 15 mg/kg per dose with maximum dosage 80 mg/kg per day
   b. Adults: 325 to 1000 mg/dose every 4 to 6 hours with maximum dosage of 4 g/day
   c. Therapeutic serum concentrations range from 10 to 20 μg/mL
4. At therapeutic doses of APAP
   a. Rapidly and completely absorbed from the GI tract
   b. The elimination half-life ranges from 2 to 4 hours in normal healthy patients, but may be prolonged in patients with underlying hepatotoxicity or in massive ingestions.
   c. 90% metabolized in the liver to glucuronide and sulfate conjugates which are excreted in urine
   d. 5% excreted unchanged in urine
   e. 5% metabolized via hepatic cytochrome P450 oxidase system to a highly reactive, toxic intermediate, *N*-acetyl-*p*-benzoquinoneimine (NAPQI)
      1) NAPQI binds to hepatocyte macromolecules resulting in oxidative injury and hepatic necrosis.
      2) Normally with nontoxic doses, NAPQI is quickly conjugated with hepatic glutathione to form cysteine and mercaptate compounds (nontoxic and excreted in urine).
5. With toxic doses of APAP
   a. Glucuronidation and sulfation pathways become saturated; this leads to increased metabolism via the cytochrome P450 system and subsequent increased production of NAPQI.
   b. Glutathione stores are depleted and hepatic injury occurs.
6. Liver damage from NAPQI occurs with excessive intake of acetaminophen.
   a. Approximate minimal toxic dose (single-dose ingestion): 150 mg/kg for a child or 7.5 g to 10 g for an adult.
   b. Virtually all patients who ingest doses >350 mg/kg develop severe liver toxicity unless treated.
7. The following conditions may increase the likelihood of liver damage from APAP:
   a. Decreased capacity for glucuronidation or sulfation (e.g., Gilbert's syndrome)
   b. Depleted glutathione stores (e.g., malnourishment, chronic alcoholism)
   c. Increased cytochrome P450 activity
      1) Many drugs (e.g., carbamazepine, phenobarbital, phenytoin, rifampin, isoniazid) induce cytochrome P450 activity, predisposing to greater toxicity.
      2) Chronic ethanol use also induces cytochrome P450 activity.

Emergency Department Evaluation

1. Important considerations in the history include dose, time of ingestion, intent, coingestants, comorbid conditions that may predispose to development of hepatotoxicity (as mentioned above), pattern of ingestion (i.e., single or repeat dosing), and formulations that decrease GI motility (e.g., combination preparations containing anticholinergic agents such as diphenhydramine or opioids such as codeine).
2. Laboratory tests should include serum acetaminophen concentration, CBC, glucose, electrolytes, BUN, creatinine, prothrombin time, International Normalized Ratio (INR), liver enzymes (ALT, AST), serum bilirubin and serum lactate and phosphate values. A urine pregnancy test should be obtained in female patients of reproductive age.
3. Once a serum acetaminophen level has been obtained 4 hours post ingestion, the Rumack-Matthew nomogram (Fig. 17-4) should be used to characterize the risk of toxicity.

Differential Diagnosis of Hepatotoxicity

1. Viral hepatitis (usually a positive serology and aminotransferase levels <3000 IU/L)
2. Other drug- or toxin-induced hepatitis (e.g., isoniazid, carbamazepine, *Amanita phalloides* mushroom, phenytoin)
3. Alcoholic hepatitis
4. Hepatobiliary disease
5. Reye's syndrome
6. Ischemic hepatitis (usually following a prolonged period of hypotension; e.g., during CPR)

Consultations

1. Poison control center for patients who have developed signs and symptoms of hepatotoxicity (i.e., metabolic acidosis, hepatic encephalopathy, coagulopathy, or renal insufficiency),

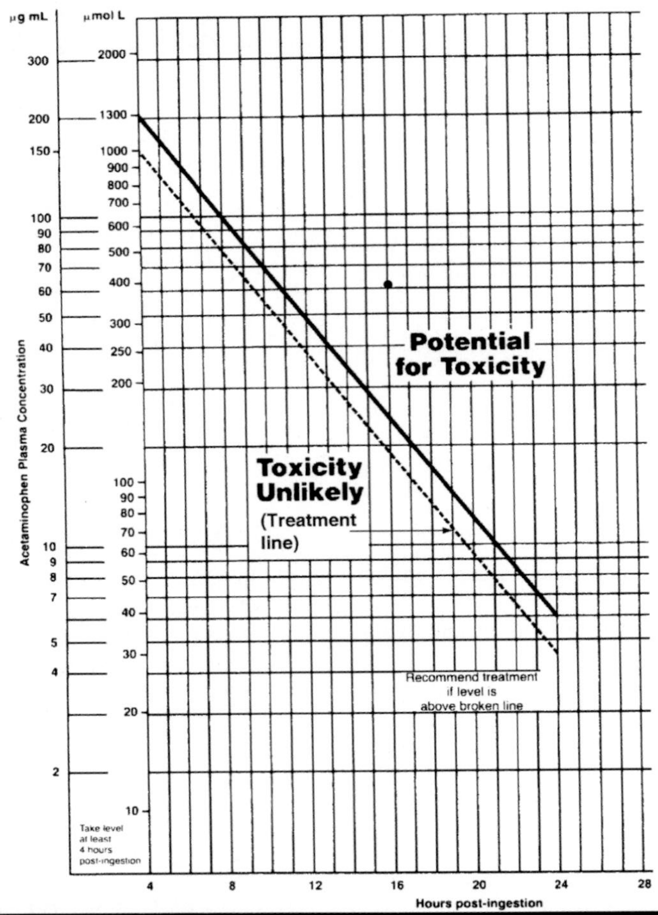

Figure 17-4. Acetaminophen Toxicity Nomogram (Rumack-Matthew Nomogram)

The nomogram shows the plasma acetaminophen concentration versus time after acetaminophen ingestion. (Reprinted, with permission, from Management of Acetaminophen Overdose. McNeil Products, 1986.)

1. The risk of toxicity is best evaluated by comparing the serum acetaminophen concentration to the time of ingestion. Example: A 15-year-old female presented to ED 16 hours postingestion of 32.5 g of APAP (100 tablets of 325 mg each). Her serum acetaminophen value was 62 μg/mL and aminotransferase levels were mildly elevated (AST 368 IU/L and ALT 295 IU/L). The patient's serum APAP concentration was plotted on the nomogram (see above) and found to be in the "Potential for Toxicity" area. Therapy with oral NAC was initiated. Over the next 3 days, her aminotransferases continued to rise to a peak AST of 7600 IU/L, and she developed a coagulopathy (INR of 2.5). Her aminotransferases began to trend downward after day 5 of admission and she had a full recovery.
2. After a single, acute overdose of an immediate-release preparation, serum acetaminophen concentrations should be measured between 4 and 24 hours after ingestion, and results should be plotted on the nomogram to determine the need for antidotal therapy.
3. Serum levels drawn before 4 hours may not represent peak concentrations and still should be checked at 4 hours postingestion. The optimal level is drawn at 4 hours after ingestion or as soon after 4 hours as possible. (The 4-hour level is not necessarily the peak. In fact, many people who overdose probably have much higher APAP concentrations prior to 4 hours.)
4. Values that fall above the "upper line or original line" in the "*Potential for Toxicity*" area on the nomogram, represent a 60% incidence of severe hepatotoxicity and 5% mortality, if left untreated.
5. "Lower line" or "broken line" that runs parallel to the upper line has been arbitrarily lowered by 25% (in order to add greater sensitivity), and represents acetaminophen concentration considered to be toxic in the United States. (The "upper line" is still used in the United Kingdom and other locations.) Values that fall below the "lower line" are associated with "*Toxicity Unlikely*" and an absence of mortality.
6. There is currently insufficient evidence to support using the nomogram to assess probability of toxicity from sustained-release preparations of acetaminophen. However, if a 4-hour level is in the "Potential for Toxicity" area, treatment should be implemented. Also, this is a rare setting in which a second APAP level may be drawn 4 to 6 hours later, if the initial level is in the "Toxicity Unlikely" area. If the second level is in the "Potential for Toxicity" area, treatment should be implemented.
7. The nomogram is also not useful if the time of ingestion is uncertain, if ingestion occurred more than 24 hours before presentation, or if repeated ingestion has occurred.

for patients presenting with ingestion of extended-release preparations, those presenting more than 24 hours postingestion, or when oral *N*-acetylcysteine (NAC) therapy cannot be successfully administered

2. Liver transplantation center for patients progressing to fulminant hepatic failure for possible liver transplant
3. Psychiatry consultation for all cases of intentional ingestion

Emergency Department Treatment and Disposition

1. All patients who have a toxic APAP level require a full course of NAC therapy and should be admitted. Patients with signs and/or symptoms of significant hepatotoxicity should be admitted to the ICU.
2. Patients presenting after 24 hours following an overdose and with evidence of hepatotoxicity should be started on NAC because it is still effective. Patients should be admitted for supportive care.
3. Indications for transfer to a liver transplantation center in patients who develop fulminant hepatic failure include:
   a. Arterial pH <7.3 after fluid resuscitation OR
   b. Grade III or IV encephalopathy
   c. Creatinine >3.3 mg/dL
   d. INR >2 to 3

Clinical Pearls: Acetaminophen Toxicity

1. Acetaminophen is the most widely used analgesic-antipyretic in the United States and accounts for more overdoses and overdose fatalities per year than any other pharmaceutical agent.
2. Since APAP preparations are commonly used, all patients presenting with an intended overdose of medication should have a serum APAP concentration checked.
3. Severe acetaminophen toxicity may produce fulminant hepatic failure 3 to 5 days postingestion.
4. A 10-kg infant can be poisoned by a 15-mL bottle of 80 mg/0.8 mL preparation (15 mL contains 1500 mg of APAP, or 150 mg/kg).

BOX 17-5. CLINICAL FEATURES OF ACETAMINOPHEN TOXICITY

Stage/time	*Signs and symptoms*
I (0.5 to 24 hours)	Nausea, vomiting, diaphoresis, pallor, lethargy, malaise; laboratory studies usually normal
II (24 to 72 hours)	Stage I symptoms resolve; subclinical elevations in AST, ALT; may develop right upper quadrant tenderness with hepatomegaly
III (72 to 96 hours)	Stage I symptoms will appear with jaundice, confusion (encephalopathy); marked *elevation* of hepatic enzymes, serum ammonia, bilirubin, and coagulation time; acute renal failure (acute tubular necrosis); death from multiorgan failure most common in this stage
IV (4 days to 2 weeks)	Generalized recovery may take several weeks for full resolution of signs and symptoms and laboratory abnormalities; histologic recovery lags behind clinical recovery and may take up to 3 months

BOX 17-6. MANAGEMENT OF ACETAMINOPHEN TOXICITY

- Gastrointestinal decontamination: administer activated charcoal (AC) if patient tolerates it
  (1) Preferred method of decontamination for all patients who present within 4 hours of ingestion
  (2) AC avidly adsorbs APAP and significantly reduces its absorption if given early.
  (3) AC does bind to NAC; however, the dose of NAC given over the full 72-hour course usually exceeds the amount needed; consequently, *binding of NAC by AC is not clinically significant.*
  (4) Dose: 1 to 2 g/kg for a child and 50 g for adolescent/adult
  (5) Multiple doses not required (may be used for coingestions)
- Measure serum acetaminophen concentration at 4 hours, and perform other tests as mentioned in the text.
- Administer NAC if the serum concentration is above the treatment line on the Rumack-Matthew nomogram (Fig. 17-4).
- If the plasma concentration is below the treatment line on the nomogram, NAC is unnecessary and the patient may be managed supportively.
- N-Acetylcysteine (NAC)
  (1) Specific antidote for treatment of APAP poisoning
  (2) NAC is a glutathione precursor and prevents toxicity by detoxifying NAPQI.
  (3) *Start NAC if >150 mg/kg APAP has been ingested, the patient is symptomatic, or other tests are abnormal* (however, there is no need to do this if you can get the APAP level reduced within 8 hours of ingestion).
  (4) If given within 8 hours of ingestion, NAC is extremely efficacious and serious hepatotoxicity and death do not occur (regardless of the initial dose and serum concentration).
  (5) *NAC is also beneficial for late presentations;* patients presenting after 24 hours following overdose and with evidence of hepatotoxicity should be started on NAC because a beneficial effect still exists.
  (6) Both routes of NAC administration (PO or IV [not FDA-approved]) are similar in efficacy.
  (7) Current recommended dosing regimen of NAC is administration over 72 hours
  (8) Give a 140-mg/kg loading dose, followed by a maintenance dose of 70 mg/kg every 4 hours for a total of 17 additional doses.
  (9) If the patient is asymptomatic and test results are normal, there is little risk of complications from oral NAC; NAC treatment may be stopped.
  (10) NAC [20% solution] has a noxious rotten-egg-like taste and odor that can lead to nausea and vomiting; these adverse effects may be minimized by mixing NAC in soda or fruit juice (make a 1:4 ratio to produce a 5% solution to improve the taste; a chilled preparation is more palatable).
  (11) Antiemetic drugs may be given to help patients with oral intolerance.

DIAGNOSIS SALICYLATE TOXICITY

Background and Pharmacokinetics

1. The most commonly used salicylate is acetylsalicylic acid (ASA; aspirin). Many over-the-counter preparations contain salicylates, including Ben-Gay and Pepto-Bismol, as well as the highly concentrated salicylate product, oil of wintergreen (Figs. 17-5 and 17-6).
   a. 1 mL of pure oil of wintergreen (methyl salicylate) contains 1400 mg of salicylate.
   b. 15 mL of original strength Pepto-Bismol contains 262 mg of salicylate.
2. Therapeutic serum concentrations range from 15 to 30 mg/dL.
3. In a large ingestion, the protein binding capacity is exceeded (normally it is 99% bound), hepatic metabolism pathways become saturated, the half-life increases to 6 to 12 hours (normal, 2 to 3 hours), and urinary excretion becomes the primary mode of elimination.
4. Clinical findings include nausea and vomiting due to direct irritation of the GI mucosa, hyperpnea and tachyphea leading to respiratory alkalosis due to direct stimulation of the medullary respiratory center, and intracellular effects (e.g., uncoupling of mitochondrial oxidative phosphorylation, inhibition of Krebs cycle enzymes, and stimulation of gluconeogenesis, glycolysis, and lipid metabolism). There is increased production of ketoacids (acetoacetic and beta-hydroxybutyric acids), lactic acid, and pyruvic acid.

Emergency Department Evaluation

1. Important considerations in the history include amount, time of ingestion, intent, possibility of coingestants, and

type of preparation (i.e., immediate-release versus enteric-coated).

2. ASA tablets may occasionally form concretions (bezoars) resulting in delayed and prolonged absorption. Enteric-coated preparations also result in delayed absorption.
3. Laboratory tests should include CBC, serum electrolytes, glucose, BUN, creatinine, arterial blood gases, liver transaminases, coagulation studies, serum calcium and ketone concentrations. The patient must be evaluated for coingestions (e.g., acetaminophen).
4. The serum salicylate concentration 6 hours after an overdose may reflect the peak concentration; however, since the time of ingestion often is unknown, obtain a salicylate level upon presentation, followed by additional levels every 2 hours for the first 4 to 8 hours to determine the trend. In patients who already have a toxic concentration, follow serial concentrations every hour until a consistent decrease is noted.
5. Urinalysis should be done to determine urinary pH. Obtain a urine pregnancy test in females of reproductive age.
6. Radiographs of the abdomen may demonstrate enteric-coated tablets (other salicylates containing magnesium or bismuth salts may also appear on x-ray). A chest radiograph may show acute lung injury (ALI).

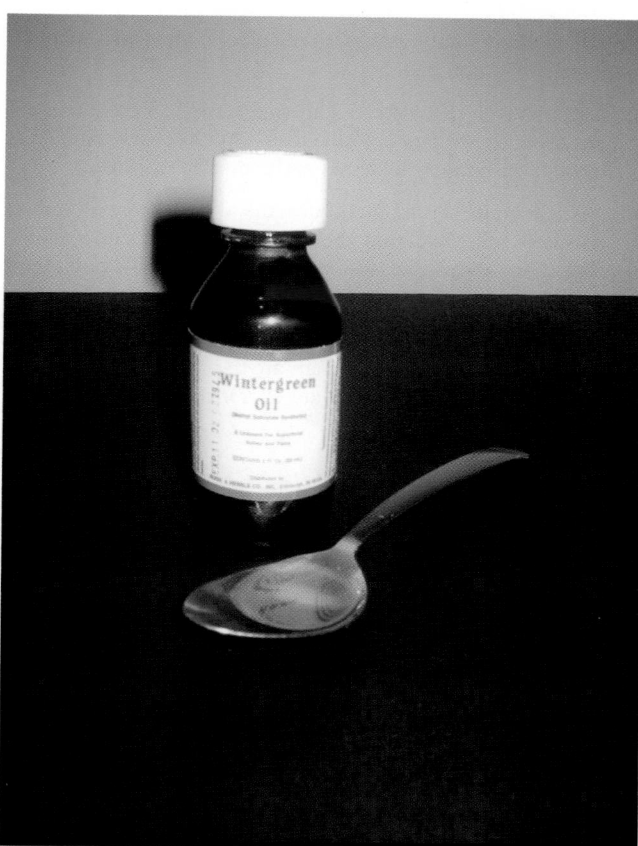

Figure 17-5. Oil of Wintergreen

This sweet-smelling product contains 100% methyl salicylate. One teaspoon of oil of wintergreen contains 7000 mg of methyl salicylate (equivalent to 21.5 tablets of aspirin, each containing 325 mg). In a 10-kg child, the minimum toxic salicylate dose of about 150 mg/kg body weight can almost be achieved with ingestion of 1 mL (1 mL = 1400 mg of methyl salicylate = 140 mg/kg for a 10-kg child). As little as 1.5 mL (2100 mg) can kill a small child; thus, ingestion of this preparation is potentially very dangerous.

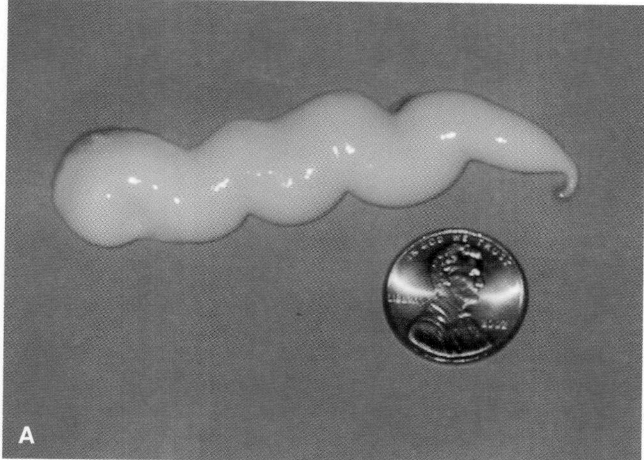

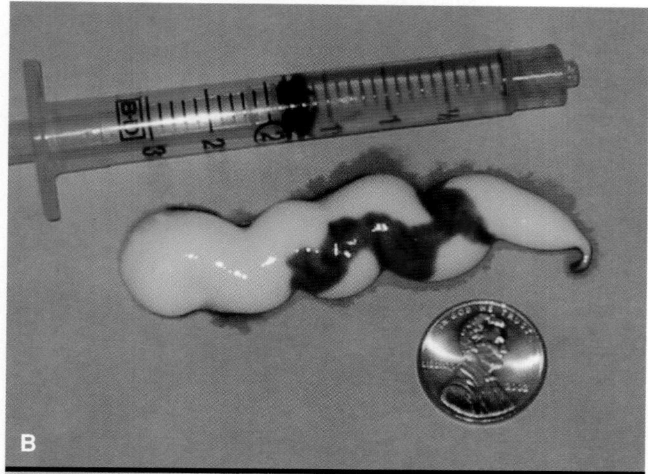

Figure 17-6. Positive Ferric Chloride Reaction with Salicylate-Containing Topical Cream

A. A 14-month-old Chinese boy was found unconscious with vomitus on the floor of his grandmother's bedroom. An open tube of a topical rubefacient was also in the room, and the parents reported that the vomitus smelled like the rubefacient (a very strong, pleasant smell of wintergreen or mint). A sample of the rubefacient balm was available (most of the package label was worn off, and the remaining label, printed in Chinese, did not identify the ingredients). *B*. Positive ferric chloride reaction. Application of ferric chloride to the product yielded a purple color (positive ferric chloride test). In its natural state, ferric chloride is translucent brown, and upon reaction with salicylate it produces a purple hue.

Differential Diagnosis

1. Other toxins that may cause an increased anion gap metabolic acidosis (see MUDPILES or ACIDOSIS mnemonics, Box 17-2).
2. Hypoglycemia from other etiologies (e.g., oral hypoglycemic agents, alcohol ingestion)
3. Diabetic ketoacidosis (similar signs and symptoms: hyperglycemia, ketoacidosis, polyuria)
4. Gastroenteritis (similar signs and symptoms: vomiting, dehydration, electrolyte abnormalities)

Consultations

Poison center, nephrology (hemodialysis), psychiatry (suicidal intent), and rarely gastroenterology (possible endoscopic removal of aspirin bezoars) as indicated

Emergency Department Treatment and Disposition

1. Nearly all patients with salicylate poisoning are volume depleted (secondary to vomiting, urinary diuresis, and hyperpyrexia) and should be resuscitated with IV crystalloid solution. Electrolyte abnormalities should be corrected (e.g., add potassium supplementation to IV fluids after urine output is established).
2. If the patient has significant gastrointestinal bleeding, administer blood products such as packed red blood cells as indicated.
3. Gastric endoscopy may rarely be required for bezoar removal if serum salicylate levels continue to rise despite alkalinization.
4. Admit all symptomatic patients for repeat doses of AC, urinary alkalinization, observation, and supportive care.
5. All patients presenting with suicidal intent should have a psychiatric evaluation.
6. The patient may be medically cleared if he or she is asymptomatic, has been observed for 4 to 6 hours, serum salicylate levels have significantly declined to the nontoxic range, no significant acid-base abnormalities are present, and the patient has not ingested an enteric-coated preparation.

Clinical Pearls: Salicylate Toxicity

1. Severity of poisoning and aggressiveness of therapy is determined by clinical and metabolic abnormalities and not based on absolute serum salicylate concentration (unless very high [>100 mg/dL]).
2. Salicylate toxicity produces metabolic acidosis with an increased anion gap.
3. Children with salicylate toxicity may initially present without an apparent respiratory alkalosis. Adolescents and adults develop respiratory alkalosis early after an overdose.
4. An acidemic serum facilitates the distribution of undissociated salicylate into the brain, while systemic alkalization increases the ionized fraction of salicylate, and decreases salicylate entry into brain and other tissues.
5. Alkalinization of the urine leads to intratubular ionization of salicylate. The resulting ions are trapped in renal tubules, leading to increased salicylate excretion in the urine.

BOX 17-7. CLINICAL FEATURES OF SALICYLATE TOXICITY

Clinical features:

• Vital signs	Tachypnea, tachycardia, hypotension, hyperpyrexia
• HEENT	Tinnitus
• Cardiovascular	Hypotension, shock, dysrhythmias (severe poisoning)
• Pulmonary	Tachypnea, hyperventilation, ALI, respiratory depression (severe poisoning)
• Gastrointestinal	Nausea, vomiting, hepatotoxicity
• Renal/electrolytes	Dehydration, acute renal failure (severe poisoning)
• Neurologic	Lethargy, agitation, confusion, seizures, coma, cerebral edema, encephalopathy
• Hematologic	Coagulopathies, disseminated intravascular coagulation, platelet aggregation irreversibly inhibited

Laboratory features:

- Respiratory alkalosis (may or may not be present in children)
- Mixed respiratory alkalosis and metabolic acidosis
- Metabolic acidosis
- Hypoglycemia or hyperglycemia
- Hyponatremia or hypernatremia
- Hypokalemia
- Hypocalcemia
- Prolonged prothrombin time
- Proteinuria
- Positive urine ketones
- Urine ferric chloride test positive (purple color) (see Fig. 17-6)

Prediction of acute toxicity: (use of the Done nomogram is *not* recommended)

- 150 mg/kg or less = usually no toxicity
- 150 to 300 mg/kg = mild to moderate toxicity
- 300 to 500 mg/kg = severe toxicity
- >500 mg/kg = potentially lethal
- Chronic ingestion of >100 mg/kg per day may cause toxicity.

BOX 17-8. MANAGEMENT OF SALICYLATE TOXICITY

- Stabilize ABCs, including appropriate treatments for altered mental status, seizures, cerebral edema, or ALI as indicated.
- Treat hypoglycemia and administer IV crystalloid if patient is volume depleted
- Decrease temperature with external cooling.
- Consider GI decontamination.
  (1) Gastric lavage if patient demonstrates significant signs and symptoms of toxicity or a potentially toxic amount of ingestion is reported
  (2) Administer activated charcoal (dose: 1 to 2 g/kg; up to 50 g maximum).
  (3) Multiple-dose AC (dose: 0.5 to 1 g/kg) every 4 to 6 hours for an additional one to two doses (AC binds neutral agents better than ionized agents, and salicylic acid may not be adsorbed by AC in the alkaline milieu of the small intestine)
  (4) Consider whole-bowel irrigation if an enteric-coated preparation was ingested or if a pharmacologic bezoar is suspected.
- Urinary alkalinization
  (1) Begin urinary alkalinization if the patient is significantly symptomatic and/or serum salicylate is >70 mg/dL.
  (2) Enhances urinary excretion of salicylate (as urine pH increases from 5 to 8, renal clearance increases by a factor of more than 50 times)
  (3) Indications: patients with large ingestions and signs and symptoms of severe toxicity, or development of a metabolic acidosis
  (4) Contraindications: patients with encephalopathy, cerebral edema, blood pH >7.55, renal failure, or serum sodium >150 mEq/L
  (5) First give IV bolus of sodium bicarbonate 1 to 2 mEq/kg followed by 3 ampules of $NaHCO_3$ (132 mEq) mixed in 1 L of D_5W and infused at a rate equivalent to 1.5 to 2 times the maintenance fluid rate
  (6) Urine pH should be checked hourly and $NaHCO_3$ infusion should be titrated to maintain a urine pH between 7.5 and 8.
  (7) Continue alkalinization until the patient demonstrates clinical improvement and the serum salicylate acid levels decline to the nontoxic range.
- Consider hemodialysis for all severely poisoned patients, including those with progressive clinical deterioration, respiratory acidosis, rising salicylate levels despite GI decontamination and urinary alkalinization, end-organ damage characterized by hypotension, ALI, cerebral edema, altered mental status, seizures, or oliguric renal failure.

DIAGNOSIS

IRON TOXICITY

Background

1. Iron is a commonly used dietary supplement. It is found in several different forms for use. Each form varies in the amount of elemental iron. Ferrous fumarate, ferrous gluconate, and ferrous sulfate contain 33%, 12%, and 20% elemental iron, respectively.
2. Most children's multivitamin tablets contain 10 to 18 mg elemental iron per tablet, while adult multivitamins may contain up to 65 mg elemental iron per tablet.

Pharmacokinetics/Toxicity

1. When attempting to determine if a toxic dose has been ingested, it is important to determine the amount of elemental iron ingested. For example, a patient ingesting 10 tablets of ferrous sulfate (each tablet is 325 mg, 20% elemental iron [65 mg elemental iron/tablet]) has ingested a total amount of 650 mg of elemental iron.
2. Signs of toxicity usually begin to develop with ingestions >20 mg/kg.
3. Free iron is highly toxic. Normally, iron is tightly bound to proteins including ferritin (as stored in tissues) and transferrin (serum). Ferritin and transferrin allow for storage and transport of iron, respectively.
4. In overdose, the iron-binding capacity of these proteins is overwhelmed and free iron accumulates. As a consequence, iron exerts toxicity on multiple organs including the heart and liver. Mechanisms of iron toxicity include:
   a. Irritation to the gastrointestinal (GI) mucosa because of its corrosive effects
   b. Impaired oxidative phosphorylation in mitochondria

c. Production of oxygen free radicals which leads to cell death
d. Venodilation
e. Increased capillary permeability
f. Disruption of coagulation factor formation leading to coagulopathy
g. Direct myocardial depression
h. Metabolic acidosis (mostly lactic) occurs as a result of poor tissue perfusion, anaerobic metabolism, and liberation of an unbuffered proton when ferrous iron is converted to ferric iron during absorption from the GI tract.

Emergency Department Evaluation

1. History should focus on determining the specific preparation involved, dosage, timing of exposure, and symptoms following ingestion.
2. Physical examination should focus on vital signs, cardiopulmonary assessment, abdominal signs, and neurological status.
3. Obtain serum electrolytes, BUN, Cr, salicylate, and acetaminophen levels.
4. Although iron toxicity is generally a clinical diagnosis, serum iron concentrations 4 to 6 hours following ingestion can be determined in an asymptomatic patient or immediately in a symptomatic patient.
   a. Normally, serum iron concentrations will peak within a few hours of ingestion and then will decline as iron distributes to tissues. Patients with declining serum iron concentrations are not necessarily improving.
   b. Patients with tablets confirmed on abdominal radiography may have serial serum iron concentrations measured (Fig. 17-7).

Differential Diagnosis

1. Other etiologies of acute GI injury (e.g., poisoning by acetaminophen, salicylates, mushrooms, heavy metals, theophylline, and NSAIDs)
2. Acute gastroenteritis (e.g., *Salmonella*, *Shigella*, viral)
3. Increased anion gap metabolic acidosis from other etiologies (see MUDPILES and ACIDOSIS mnemonics, Box 17-2).
4. Acute hepatitis (various etiologies)
5. Acute surgical abdomen

Consultations

Poison control center and psychiatry (suicidal intent)

Emergency Department Treatment and Disposition

1. Admit all patients presenting with persistent symptoms of GI toxicity, altered mental status, cardiovascular instability, or those in whom GI decontamination is unsuccessful. Moderately and severely ill patients admitted to an intensive care unit.
2. Patients may be discharged from the ED 6 hours postingestion provided they are asymptomatic or demonstrate minimal toxicity, there are no tablets seen on abdominal radiography, their serum iron level is <500 μg/mL, and they have been evaluated by psychiatry (if indicated).

Clinical Pearls

1. Emesis should *not* be induced in patients because of iron toxicity-induced GI irritation.
2. Declining serum iron concentrations may reflect iron uptake into cells and should not be used as a sign of clinical improvement or response to therapy.
3. A serum iron concentration becomes unreliable in patients receiving deferoxamine.
4. Patients presenting with moderate to severe hypovolemia due to vomiting and diarrhea should receive aggressive fluid resuscitation.
5. Iron toxicity is generally a clinical diagnosis and treatment should *not* be delayed while awaiting serum iron concentrations.
6. The typical course of iron toxicity involves clinical resolution of symptoms up to 24 hours following ingestion ("deceptive quiescence") followed by rapid clinical deterioration. Iron toxicity is generally categorized in stages. The quiescent phase usually refers to stage II iron poisoning, in which the GI symptoms resolve but the patient is still clinically ill (e.g., metabolic acidosis is progressing).

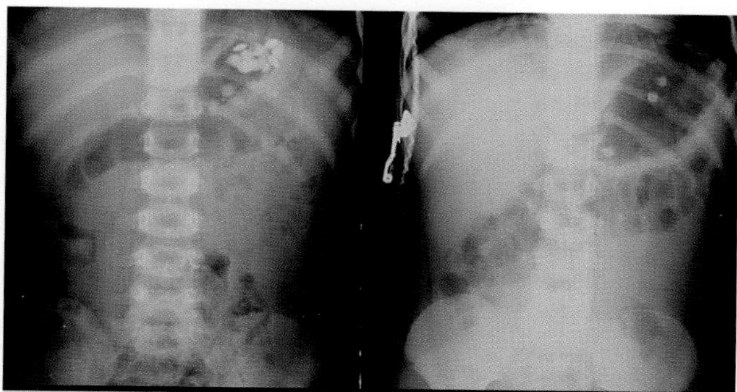

Figure 17-7. Radiopaque Tablets in Iron Poisoning

A flat plate of the abdomen showing the presence of radiopaque tablets (*left panel*) in a 2-year-child who presented about 1 hour after the ingestion of a number of ferrous sulfate tablets. Gastric lavage was performed (whole-bowel irrigation was not used for GI decontamination of such cases in the past). The right panel shows a radiograph taken shortly after the lavage, showing removal of almost all of the tablets. At the present time, whole-bowel irrigation would be the method of choice for GI decontamination in such patients. Identification of radiopaque tablets confirms the diagnosis in a patient with a suspected iron overdose, and helps guide gastric decontamination in such cases.

BOX 17-9. CLINICAL FEATURES OF IRON TOXICITY

Stage/time	*Signs and symptoms*
I (0 to 6 hours)	Abdominal pain, vomiting, diarrhea, melena, hematemesis and hematochezia (direct corrosive effects of iron on GI mucosa), hypovolemic shock (may be a presenting sign)
II (6 to 24 hours)	Resolution of clinical signs (deceptive quiescence), progression of metabolic acidosis
III (up to 72 hours)	Shock from hypovolemia, hypotension, and cardiac failure, metabolic acidosis worsens, hyperglycemia, lethargy, seizures, coma, fulminant hepatic failure, coagulopathy, hyperammonemia, hypoglycemia
IV (3 days to weeks)	Gastric outlet obstruction (e.g., pyloric or duodenal stenosis due to strictures/scarring)

Potential toxicity

- <20 mg/kg of elemental iron ingestion = insignificant or mild
- 20 to 60 mg/kg of elemental iron ingestion = moderate
- >100 mg/kg of elemental iron ingestion = potentially lethal

Serum iron values

- Serum iron concentrations will be elevated 4 to 6 hours postingestion
  (1) <300 μg/dL = rarely symptomatic
  (2) 300 to 500 μg/dL = usually signs of GI toxicity and mild systemic toxicity
  (3) >500 μg/dL = *increased risk of severe systemic toxicity and increased mortality*
  (4) >1000 μg/dL = potentially fatal
- Obtain serial iron concentrations on patients with tablets visible on abdominal radiograph.

Laboratory values

- White blood cell count >15,000 cells/μL (specific, but not sensitive)
- Serum glucose >150 mg/dL (specific, but not sensitive)
- Increased anion gap metabolic acidosis (see ACIDOSIS and MUDPILES mnemonics, Box 17-2)
- Obtain abdominal radiograph to evaluate for presence of iron-containing tablets
  (1) Absence of tablets does not rule out ingestion of a toxic dose of iron.
  (2) Multivitamin tablets and liquid preparations containing iron may not be visible on radiography.
- Serum total iron-binding capacity (TIBC) may be falsely increased (*this test is no longer recommended*).
- Deferoxamine challenge test will result in rose-colored urine (*this test is no longer recommended*)
  (1) Deferoxamine binds free iron in tissues and plasma to form ferrioxamine, which is then excreted in urine.
  (2) A color change is considered a positive test, which may be due to free iron (not necessarily from ingestion).

BOX 17-10. MANAGEMENT OF IRON TOXICITY

- Stabilize ABCs including appropriate treatment of hypovolemic shock, hypotension, respiratory distress, hypoglycemia, and altered mental status.
- GI decontamination
  (1) Consider gastric lavage in patients who present following a large ingestion or patients with moderate to severe symptoms (e.g., hematemesis, shock) Lavage may not be necessary or even indicated because significant iron toxicity has prominent vomiting. Furthermore, iron tablets may not fit through the lavage tube.
  (2) Activated charcoal does not effectively bind iron, but may be given if coingestions are suspected.
  (3) Consider whole-bowel irrigation in patients with rising serum iron levels or pills on radiography.
- Specific antidote: deferoxamine mesylate
  (1) Iron chelating agent that binds free iron in tissues and plasma to form ferrioxamine which is then excreted in urine
  (2) Indicated in patients with serum iron >500 μg/dL 4 to 6 hours postingestion or patients with signs of significant toxicity such as repeated vomiting, increased anion gap metabolic acidosis, altered mental status, hypotension, or GI bleeding
  (3) Relatively contraindicated in patients with renal insufficiency or renal failure (ferrioxamine may be removed by hemodialysis)
  (4) Dosage: up to 15 mg/kg per hour via continuous IV infusion which then may be titrated upward or downward based on the patient's course (should start slowly then increase to this rate)
  (5) If infused rapidly, may cause hypotension or exacerbate underlying hypotension; other complications include ARDS and infection (e.g., *Yersinia enterocolitica*).
  (6) Deferoxamine is safe in pregnancy.

DIAGNOSIS — OPIOID TOXICITY

Background

1. Opioids are found legally in a variety of forms including morphine, meperidine, codeine, oxycodone, methadone, hydromorphone, propoxyphene, and fentanyl.
2. Opioids are used medically primarily as analgesics. Some are also selectively used as antitussive agents. They are available in oral as well as intravenous preparations.
3. Heroin and its derivatives are available and illicitly purchased on the street. Heroin use has had a recent resurgence, partially due to the increased availability of higher-purity heroin.
4. "Body packing" refers to the practice of intentional transport of opioids (or other contraband) inside a body cavity (Figs. 17-8 and 17-9). "Body stuffing" implies haphazard ingestion of contraband, usually in an attempt to evade arrest. Body packing is accomplished via ingestion of packets (wrapped in condoms, latex, or tape) containing the illicit drug. Packets ingested during body packing are generally well-designed with multiple layers to prevent leakage of contents. This is not the case in body stuffing.

Pharmacokinetics and Toxicity

1. Many opioids are rapidly absorbed by all routes except for some which are not significantly absorbed through the GI tract. Most are metabolized in the liver with 90% excreted in the urine as inactive compounds. They act at several central nervous system (CNS) receptors and some peripheral receptors, all of which are responsible for their different physiological effects.
2. Therapeutic and toxic doses vary with the agent being used, as well as the tolerance of the individual. Tolerance is defined as an individual's requirement for more frequent use in increasing doses to achieve the same physiological effect.
3. Opioid toxicity is characterized by the classic triad of CNS depression, pupillary miosis, and respiratory depression.
   a. Mu (μ) receptor stimulation results in supraspinal analgesia, respiratory depression, decreased GI motility, and euphoria.
   b. Kappa (κ) receptor stimulation results in sedation and miosis.

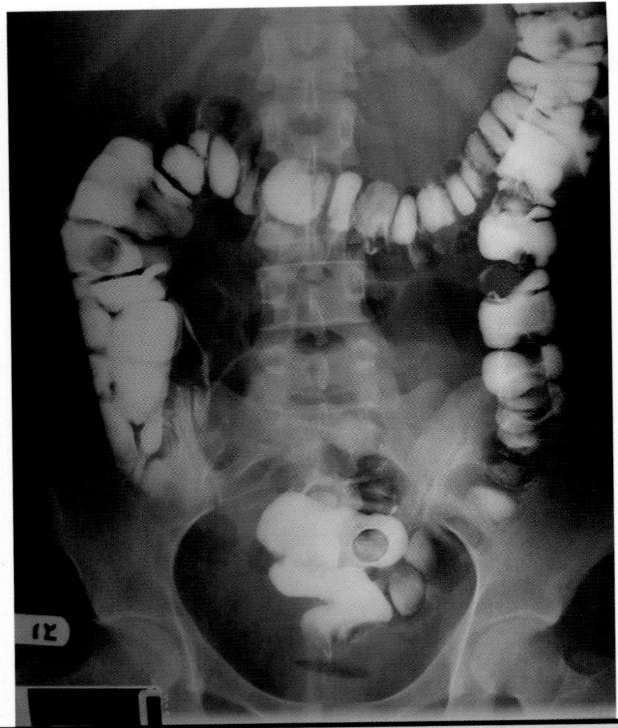

Figure 17-8. Heroin Packets

Delayed images of an upper GI series showing multiple filling defects within contrast-filled loops of large bowel (seen in the rectum and just below the hepatic flexure). Subsequently these packets were found to contain heroin.

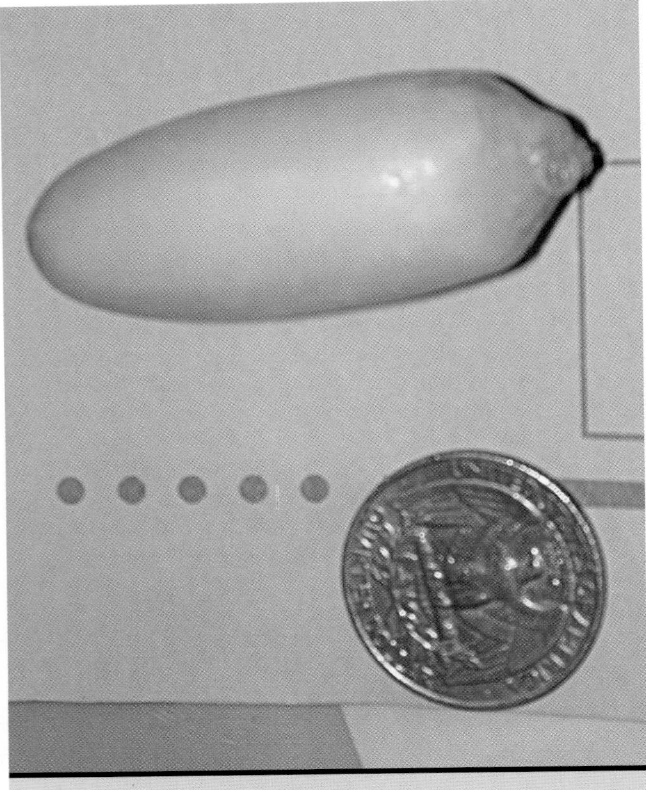

Figure 17-9. Heroin Packet

Heroin packet recovered from a "mule" or "body packer."

c. Delta (δ) receptor stimulation results in modulation of the μ receptors and dopaminergic neurons.

4. Toxicity from other impurities (e.g., quinine, strychnine) may occasionally result from illicit heroin use.

5. Body packing may result in prolongation or delay of symptoms of toxicity due to slow leakage of opioids from tightly wrapped packages.

Emergency Department Evaluation

1. History should focus on the particular agent involved, dosage, timing, symptoms since exposure, and determination if the patient is a chronic opioid user or opioid dependent.

2. Physical examination should immediately address airway patency, adequacy of ventilation, and respiratory effort.

Differential Diagnosis

1. Altered mental status from other toxic etiologies (e.g., hypoglycemia, antidepressants, benzodiazepines, ethanol, anticonvulsants, antihistamines, muscle relaxants, antipsychotics; see COMATOSE PATIENT mnemonic, page 523)

2. Miosis from other etiologies (e.g., pontine hemorrhage, cholinergics [organophosphate insecticides], clonidine and imidazolines, and phenothiazines; see COPS mnemonic, page 625).

3. Bezoars (or other cylindrically shaped foreign bodies) may appear on radiographs of body packers. Body packers may present with signs of obstruction and an acute surgical abdomen.

Consultations

Poison control center, psychiatry (intentional ingestion), and gastroenterologist and/or surgery for body packers

Emergency Department Management and Disposition

1. All patients presenting with prolonged duration of symptoms or severe symptoms need to be hospitalized. Older patients who use short-acting opioids do not need admission, especially if they present with respiratory depression that has resolved. Consider admission to an ICU for continuous monitoring and additional doses of naloxone as indicated for patients with persistent altered mental status,

recurrent respiratory depression, hypoxia, hypotension, or dysrhythmias.

2. All young children presenting with opioid toxicity should be hospitalized. Older patients may be discharged from the ED if they are asymptomatic following a 6-hour observation period, and have been evaluated by psychiatry (if indicated).

Clinical Pearls: Opioid Toxicity

1. Opioid toxicity is characterized by the *classic triad* of CNS depression, pupillary miosis, and respiratory depression.
2. Pediatric patients may have unusual sensitivity to opioids and may display signs of toxicity at therapeutic doses.
3. Many preparations of opioids contain ASA or APAP and patients should be evaluated for toxicity from these combination products.
4. When administering naloxone to a chronic user of opioids, it may be prudent to initially start with small doses of naloxone for diagnostic and therapeutic purposes. This approach will decrease the likelihood of precipitating acute withdrawal in the patient. Clinicians should be prepared to deal with consequences of withdrawal symptoms if they do occur.
5. Body packers may also place packets containing contraband in their ears, vagina, or rectum. A careful inspection of all body cavities is warranted in this situation.

BOX 17-11. CLINICAL FEATURES OF OPIOID TOXICITY

Signs and symptoms:

Vitals	Hypothermia or hyperthermia, hypotension
Neurological	Miosis (meperidine less consistently), mydriasis (diphenoxylate with atropine), lethargy, coma, tremors, seizures (especially propoxyphene)
Cardiovascular	Hypotension, bradycardia, dysrhythmias, heart block
Pulmonary	Respiratory depression, direct pulmonary toxicity causing acute lung injury (ALI; previously referred to as noncardiogenic pulmonary edema), respiratory arrest, bronchospasm, pneumonitis
Gastrointestinal	Decreased motility, constipation, ileus
Renal	Urinary retention (diphenoxylate with atropine), myoglobinuria, acute tubular necrosis (ATN)

Laboratory values:

- Obtain serum electrolytes, glucose, BUN, Cr (evaluate for other etiologies of altered mental status)
- ABG may show hypoxia, hypercapnia, and metabolic acidosis (lactic).
- Urine drug screen may be positive for opiates (some opioids may require specific screens for detection); synthetic opioids (e.g., fentanyl) may not be detected by urine drug screens.
- Aspirin (ASA) or acetaminophen (APAP) levels may be elevated with preparations containing either ASA or APAP (e.g., Percodan, which is oxycodone plus aspirin, or Percocet, which is oxycodone plus acetaminophen).
- Elevated serum creatinine (ATN or renal failure from rhabdomyolysis)
- Elevated serum creatine kinase (seizures or rhabdomyolysis)
- Abdominal radiograph may show packets in body packers.
- Chest x-ray may show ALI or pneumonitis.

BOX 17-12. COMPARISON OF OPIOID AND SEDATIVE-HYPNOTIC TOXICITY

	Opioids	*Sedative-hypnotics*
Vital signs	Bradypnea, bradycardia, hypotension, hypothermia	Bradypnea, bradycardia, hypotension, hypothermia
Pupils	Miosis (except meperidine)	Mydriasis, miosis (early)
CNS	Lethargy to coma	Coma, nystagmus, ataxia
Other	Acute lung injury, track marks	Bullae
Antidote	Naloxone	Flumazenil (for benzodiazepine only)

(Reproduced with permission from: Shah BR: Child poisoned by unknown substance. In: Finberg L, Kleinman RE (eds). *Saunders Manual of Pediatric Practice*. WB Saunders, Philadelphia, 2002, p. 1158.)

BOX 17-13. MANAGEMENT OF OPIOID TOXICITY

- Stabilize ABCs, including appropriate treatment of altered mental status, hypoglycemia, seizures, pulmonary edema, and hypotension.
- Consider antidote if possibility of opioid toxicity (see Box 17-14)
- GI decontamination
  (1) Consider gastric lavage if presenting within 1 hour of ingestion (e.g., in the setting of a massive Percodan or propoxyphene overdose)
  (2) Administer activated charcoal (dose: 1 to 2 g/kg up to max 50 g)
- Patients in whom body packing is suspected and patients are asymptomatic
  (1) Whole-bowel irrigation (WBI) with 2 L/hour of polyethylene glycol solution
  (2) WBI can be discontinued if the GI tract is empty as verified by radiographic contrast study, such as upper GI series with small bowel follow-through

BOX 17-14. ANTIDOTES TO OPIOID TOXICITY

Naloxone

- Opioid antagonist that immediately reverses effects of opioids
- *No* significant side effects in treatment of acute overdose except opioid withdrawal symptoms in dependent patients
- Give IV, IM, and SC sublingually or endotracheally (however, it is not necessary to give naloxone if the patient is already intubated).
- Time of onset of effects: 1 to 2 minutes
- Duration of action: 60 to 90 minutes
- Must continue observation for re-sedation (or other complications) once naloxone wears off
- For patients with apnea or hypoventilation
  (1) Initial dose: 1 to 2 mg (patients of all ages except neonates)
  (2) Additional dose: 2 mg every 2 minutes until a therapeutic response is seen or to a total of 10 mg
- Patients with CNS depression without respiratory depression
  (1) Initial dose: 0.1 to 0.4 mg.
  (2) Additional dose (up to 2 mg) as required to a total of 10 mg
- Failure to respond to 10 mg of naloxone excludes opiates as a sole cause of respiratory depression.
- Opioid-dependent patients
  (1) Titrate to avoid opioid withdrawal
  (2) Smaller initial dose of 0.05 mg, then increase gradually to 0.4 mg, then repeat every minute to a total of 2 mg
- Opioid withdrawal symptoms
  (1) Note: Opioid withdrawal is *not* acutely life-threatening and is distinctly characterized by a normal mental status (an exception is neonates whose mothers abused opioids during pregnancy; they may develop withdrawal seizures 1 to 2 weeks after birth).
  (2) Signs and symptoms: GI, tachycardia, anxiety/restlessness, hyperpnea, diaphoresis, hypertension, sialorrhea, mydriasis

Nalmefene

- Similar doses as naloxone
- Effect lasts longer (4 to 6 hours)

DIAGNOSIS COCAINE TOXICITY

Background

1. Cocaine (benzoylmethylecgonine) is derived from the coca plant by a complex process that results in the purified hydrochloride salt form. This form is bioavailable via multiple routes but is most often used via nasal insufflation and intravenously.
2. When extracted using a basic solvent such as ammonia, cocaine hydrochloride can be converted into the freebase or crack form resulting in higher purity (85 to 90%). These forms are water insoluble but heat stable, and therefore are smoked for inhalation through the lungs.
3. Cocaine is also used as a topical anesthetic and vasoconstrictor. It is available in solutions containing 4 to 10% cocaine for use in medical procedures. It is also often combined with tetracaine and epinephrine ("adrenaline") to create the topical anesthetic TAC.

Pharmacokinetics and Toxicity

1. Inhalational and IV routes result in a peak effect within 5 minutes, while insufflation produces a peak effect in 20 minutes. The half-life of cocaine is 0.5 to 1.5 hours, as it is hydrolyzed to metabolites that have half-lives as long as 8 hours.
2. Cocaine causes an increase in the concentration of norepinephrine at neuronal synapses by increasing its release from the presynaptic membrane in both the peripheral as well as central nervous systems. It also inhibits reuptake of norepinephrine at the presynaptic membrane of neurons in the sympathetic nervous system.
3. The effects of cocaine result from the hyperadrenergic state induced by increased norepinephrine levels. Although short-lived, euphoria is the usual impetus for recreational cocaine use. Patients may develop severe agitation, muscular rigidity, and hyperthermia.

4. Cocaine also has moderate effects on CNS release and reuptake of both serotonin and dopamine.
5. Patients vary greatly in dosages required to produce toxicity. In children, as little as 1 mL of a 4% solution applied nasally has resulted in death.
6. Body packers and stuffers may be exposed to extremely high doses of cocaine if a container containing cocaine ruptures (for more on body packers and body stuffers, see opioid toxicity).
7. Maternal cocaine use during pregnancy is associated with an increased risk of spontaneous abortion, placental abruption, fetal prematurity, low birth weight, congenital intestinal atresia, and necrotizing enterocolitis.
8. The *cocaine washout syndrome* refers to the state of persistent lethargy and altered mental status that may follow prolonged and intense cocaine use. This is due to depletion of CNS catecholamines and may manifest as coma. The patient's condition usually improves over several hours with supportive care.

Emergency Department Evaluation

1. The history should focus on the amount, route, timing, form, and frequency of cocaine use. It is important to determine the symptoms expressed. Witnesses should be questioned concerning seizure activity or alteration in mental status.
2. Physical examination should focus on vital signs in addition to a complete assessment of the cardiac, pulmonary, and neurologic status of the patient.
3. The history should also focus on specific organ system complaints.
   a. Patients complaining of chest pain should have an evaluation for myocardial ischemia or pulmonary pathology (e.g. pnemothorax)
   b. Patients complaining of headache or presenting with seizures should have an evaluation for intracranial hemorrhage.
   c. Patients with fever should be evaluated for possible occult infection.
4. Patients should be evaluated for other occult ingestions (if suicidal ideation is suspected).

Differential Diagnosis

1. Other toxicologic agents that may produce physiologic stimulation include amphetamines, caffeine, oral decongestants, thyroid hormone (not acutely), beta-adrenergic agonists, ergot alkaloids, and monoamine oxidase (MAO) inhibitors.
2. Neuroleptic malignant syndrome, malignant hyperthermia, and serotonin syndrome may similarly present with muscular rigidity, hyperthermia, and altered mental status.
3. Other nontoxicologic etiologies that may present with similar signs and symptoms include hypoglycemia, pheochromocytoma, hyperthyroidism, alcohol or sedative-hypnotic withdrawal, or acute psychosis.

Consultations

Poison control center and psychiatry (for suicidal ideation)

Emergency Department Management and Disposition

1. Body stuffers who swallow small amounts of poorly packed contraband in an effort to evade arrest, may often be treated with activated charcoal and supportive care.
2. Body packers usually swallow large quantities of well-packaged contraband for illegal transportation (Fig. 17-10). If asymptomatic, these patients should be treated with whole-bowel irrigation. If symptomatic, these patients will require emergent surgical intervention to remove the offending packets.

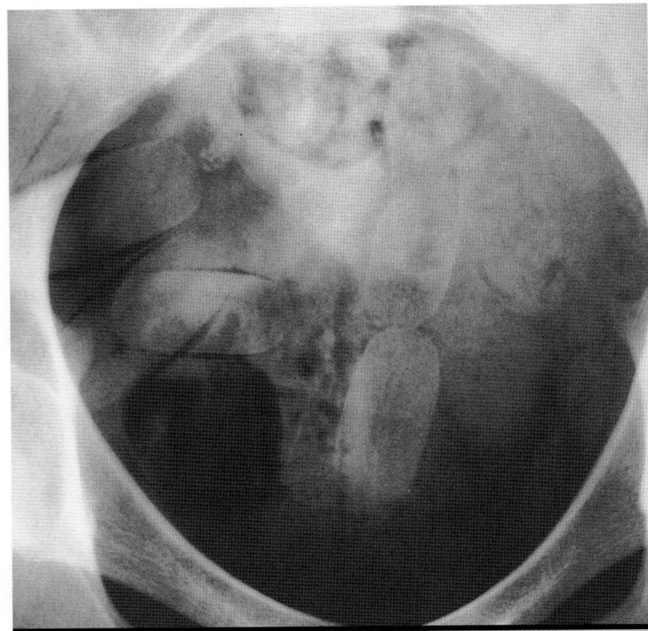

Figure 17-10. Radiopaque Packets Seen with Body Packing

Magnified frontal projection of the pelvis reveals multiple well-defined radiopaque densities within the pelvic bowel loops. Note the air around some of the individual packets. This implies that the packets were not tightly sealed, and there is a risk of spontaneous perforation of such packets. This adolescent patient was arrested and brought to the ED directly from the airport as a suspected drug dealer. This patient was completely asymptomatic. Whole-bowel irrigation was performed with polyethylene glycol solution. Subsequently these packets were analyzed and were found to contain cocaine. "Body packing" refers to the practice of intentional transport of opioids (or other contraband) inside a body cavity. "Body stuffing" implies haphazard ingestion of contraband, usually in an attempt to evade arrest. These forms of transport are accomplished via ingestion of packets (wrapped in condoms, latex, or tape) containing the illicit drug. Packets ingested during body packing are generally well designed, with multiple layers to prevent leakage of contents. This is not the case in body stuffing.

3. Patients presenting with symptoms that do not resolve quickly or patients presenting with severe toxicity or serious sequelae of cocaine intoxication should be admitted. All patients presenting with myocardial ischemia, hyperthermia, intracranial hemorrhage, or cocaine washout syndrome should be admitted to an ICU for monitoring and management.
4. Patients presenting with mild toxicity may be discharged upon clinical improvement. They should be referred for drug counseling.
5. All young children presenting with cocaine intoxication should be admitted.

Clinical Pearls

1. Beta-blockers should *never* be used to control heart rate or hypertension due to cocaine intoxication. These agents will likely exacerbate cocaine-induced coronary vasospasm.
2. Haloperidol should not be used to control agitation in patients suspected of cocaine intoxication because it may lower the seizure threshold and impair the body's ability to dissipate heat.
3. Benzodiazepines are highly effective, and are the treatment of choice for almost all forms of acute cocaine intoxication, including initial management of psychomotor agitation, hyperthermia, seizures, tachycardia, hypertension, dysrhythmias, and ischemic chest pain.

BOX 17-15. CLINICAL FEATURES OF COCAINE TOXICITY

Signs, symptoms, and complications:

- Vital signs: tachycardia, hypertension, hyperthermia, hypotension, severe hyperthermia, shock
- HEENT: mydriasis, epistaxis; cocaine residue on nasal septum; nasal septal perforation with chronic use
- Cardiovascular: myocardial ischemia (due to coronary vasospasm, thrombus formation, platelet activation, inhibition of fibrinolysis, premature atherosclerosis, and increased myocardial oxygen consumption during episodes of tachycardia and hypertension); aortic dissection; fatal dysrhythmia; sudden cardiac arrest; with chronic cocaine use, congestive heart failure, myocarditis, dilated cardiomyopathy
- Pulmonary: exacerbation of asthma (inhalation of particulate matter); pneumothorax; pneumomediastinum or pulmonary edema (acute lung injury) with deep Valsalva maneuvers
- Gastrointestinal: bowel ischemia and infarction (splanchnic vasospasm); necrotizing enterocolitis in neonates
- Renal: acute renal failure (due to renal infarction or rhabdomyolysis)
- Musculoskeletal: rhabdomyolysis (due to agitation, seizures, or hyperthermia)
- Neurologic: psychomotor agitation and seizures; intracranial hemorrhage or cerebral infarction
- Psychiatric: euphoria, psychosis, and mania (common); neonatal withdrawal manifesting as jitteriness, irritability

Laboratory values (as indicated):

- CBC may show elevated WBC (in patients with hyperthermia, suggests occult infection or demargination)
- Serum electrolytes, BUN, Cr, and glucose (to exclude other etiologies of altered mental status and seizures and for assessment of dehydration and/or acute renal insult)
- Serum and urine drug screen will be positive for cocaine metabolites.
- ECG may show tachycardia, dysrhythmias, or signs of acute myocardial ischemia or infarction.
- Chest radiograph may show pulmonary edema, pneumothorax, or pneumomediastinum.
- Abdominal radiographs may show packets containing cocaine, ileus; thumbprinting or bowel gas in intestinal wall suggests bowel infarction
- Head CT may demonstrate intracranial hemorrhage or cerebral infarction.
- Lumbar puncture may demonstrate subarachnoid hemorrhage.
- Creatine kinase may be elevated (suggests rhabdomyolysis).
- Elevated CK-MB or troponin (suggests myocardial injury)
- Elevated LFTs and coagulopathy (may occur following hyperthermia)
- Serum ASA, APAP levels, and urine drug screen for possible coingestions

BOX 17-16. MANAGEMENT OF COCAINE TOXICITY

- Stabilize ABCs, including appropriate treatment for seizures, pneumothorax, cardiac dysrhythmias, cerebral infarction, intracranial hemorrhage, pulmonary edema, and rhabdomyolysis.
- Management is primarily supportive and includes control of hypertension, psychomotor agitation, and hyperthermia.
- GI decontamination usually not recommended because cocaine is rarely ingested (unless body packer or body stuffer; for management of body packers, see opioid toxicity Box 17-13).
- Benzodiazepines for agitation
- Haloperidol *contraindicated* (may lower seizure threshold and impair the body's ability to dissipate heat)
- Lowering of core temperature and muscle relaxation with benzodiazepines for hyperthermia
- Aggressive IV hydration to ensure adequate urinary output
- Evaluate for myocardial ischemia or infarction
  (1) Standard therapy (O_2, nitrates, aspirin, and morphine) for patients with ischemia or infarction
  (2) Beta-blockers contraindicated (may exacerbate cocaine-induced coronary vasospasm)
  (3) Consider phentolamine or nitrate therapy for hypertension.
  (4) Reperfusion therapy via percutaneous cardiac catheterization (rather than thrombolysis) for patients with ischemia or infarction
- Sodium bicarbonate and lidocaine for cardiac dysrhythmias

DIAGNOSIS METHEMOGLOBINEMIA

Background, Pathophysiology, and Toxicity

1. Methemoglobin (MetHb) is hemoglobin in which the normally reduced ferrous ion (Fe^{2+}) is oxidized to the ferric form (Fe^{3+}). This process prevents the binding of oxygen (O_2) to this abnormal hemoglobin (Hgb).
2. MetHb causes tissue hypoxia, as it cannot bind O_2 and results in a leftward shift of the O_2 dissociation curve, impairing normal Hgb from unloading O_2 to the peripheral tissues. Thus, symptoms of methemoglobinemia are related to decreased O_2 delivery to the tissues.
3. Under normal circumstances, serum MetHb concentration is maintained at 1 to 2% by normal physiologic protective mechanisms. The enzyme NADH methemoglobin reductase, located in the erythrocyte, is most responsible for counteracting the oxidation process that produces MetHb. NADPH methemoglobin reductase is an additional enzyme that also reduces MetHb, although it is much less active under normal physiologic conditions.
4. A serum MetHb concentration above 2% is termed methemoglobinemia, and occurs due to multiple etiologies.
   a. Oxidative stress due to sepsis, toxins, or drugs (e.g., nitrates, topical anesthetics, aniline dyes, quinine, sulfonamides, hydrocarbons), and food additives containing nitrites or nitrates
   b. Congenital hemoglobinopathy, such as hemoglobin M (makes hemoglobin more susceptible to oxidative stress)
   c. Congenital deficiency of NADH methemoglobin reductase
5. MetHb concentration typically correlates well with the severity of symptoms. The degree of toxicity is also related to the presence of underlying anemia. At any given MetHb concentration, patients with a baseline anemia will present with more severe symptoms because they have less normal hemoglobin. Some of the oxidants that cause methemoglobinemia also cause hemolysis. Although the occurrence of methemoglobinemia does not necessarily lead to hemolysis, in the setting of methemoglobinemia, there is an increased risk of hemolysis and vice versa.

Emergency Department Evaluation

1. History should focus on possible exposure and on past medical history to determine if the patient has underlying conditions that may predispose to methemoglobinemia.
2. Physical examination should focus on vital signs, degree of cyanosis, and assessment of neurological and cardiopulmonary status.
3. Serum glucose-6-phosphate dehydrogenase (G6PD) determination should be done to exclude deficiency (usually

performed at a later time after the acute condition resolves).

4. Serum acetaminophen and salicylate concentrations should also be obtained if the exposure is intentional.

Differential Diagnosis

1. Cyanosis from other etiology (e.g., cardiac, pulmonary); cyanosis from methemoglobinemia may be differentiated from other causes of hypoxia by its unresponsiveness to supplemental O_2, and a normal Po_2 on arterial blood gas (Fig. 17-11).
2. Carbon monoxide poisoning (patients usually not cyanotic)
3. Sulfhemoglobinemia (differentiated from methemoglobinemia by ABG with co-oximetry)

Consultations

Poison control center, psychiatry (intentional drug ingestions), and hematology (evaluation for underlying conditions that predispose to developing methemoglobinemia)

Emergency Department Treatment and Disposition

1. Decontamination of the patient is vital to prevent further exposure to the offending agent.
2. GI decontamination remains controversial in the management of MetHb toxicity. However, gastric lavage may be considered for massive ingestions in which ongoing toxicity is expected.
3. Consider administering one dose of activated charcoal (dose: 1 to 2 g/kg).
4. Use of methylene blue (a weak oxidant) in patients with G6PD deficiency or known NADPH methemoglobin reductase deficiency may not be effective or may precipitate massive hemolysis; however, it has been effectively used in some patients. Methylene blue should therefore be used judiciously in this setting and the clinician should be aware of possible adverse effects or the potential inefficacy (Fig. 17-12).
5. All patients (especially infants and young children) presenting with significant methemoglobinemia requiring therapy with methylene blue admitted to an ICU for continuous monitoring and supportive care.

Clinical Pearls: Methemoglobinemia

1. Patients with methemoglobinemia may present with profound cyanosis with minimal symptoms.
2. Methemoglobinemia must be considered in all patients *presenting with cyanosis in spite of a normal Po_2 determination from ABG or cyanosis unresponsive to supplemental O_2 therapy.*
3. Methemoglobinemia is characterized by *normal O_2 saturation and normal Po_2 on ABG with metabolic acidosis (lactic acidosis).* Pulse oximetry in such patients is usually around 80 to 90% or may be lower (pulse oximetry only measures the ratio of OxyHb to DeoxyHb, and does not account for other forms of hemoglobin).
4. Neonates are prone to developing methemoglobinemia because of lower levels of NADH methemoglobin reductase and the presence of fetal Hgb, which is more readily oxidized than the adult form of Hgb.
5. Nitrate ingestion is one of the most common causes of methemoglobinemia. Nitrates get converted to nitrites

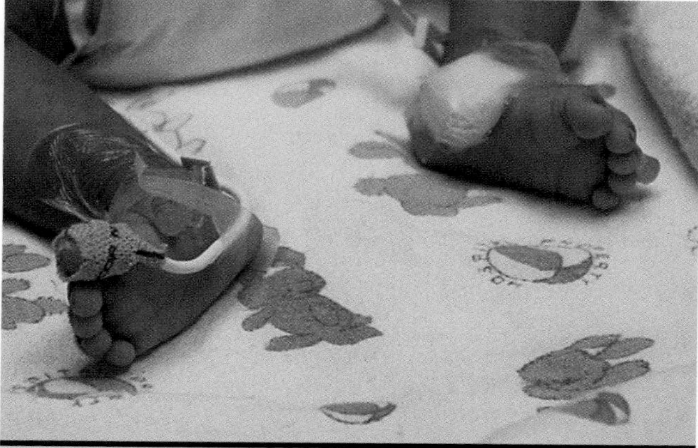

Figure 17-11. Methemoglobinemia

An infant presenting with dusky discoloration of the entire body. He presented with hypovolemic shock due to acute gastroenteritis and methemoglobinemia. Infants with diarrhea may develop methemoglobinemia without any exogenous toxic exposures. His ABG while receiving 100% oxygen by nasal cannula showed: pH 7.176, Pao_2 271.4 mmHg, Pco_2 19.7 mmHg, O_2 saturation (100%), HCO_3 7 mmol/L, BE −20 mmol/L, and the MetHb value was 27.6%.

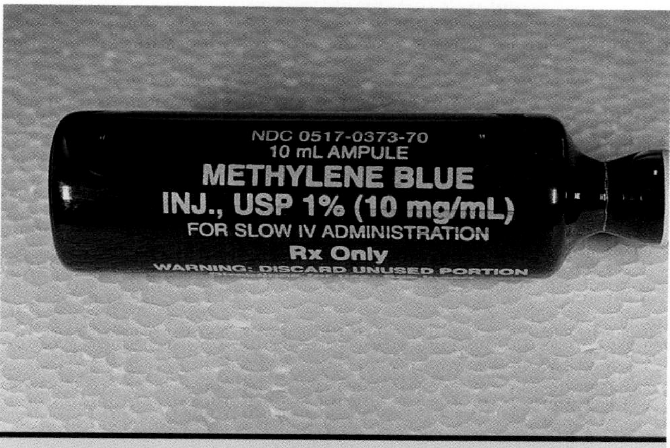

Figure 17-12. Methylene Blue

An antidote for methemoglobinemia is available as 1% methylene blue (10 mg/mL) for IV administration.

(powerful oxidizing agents) by GI bacteria, especially in neonates. Patients taking nitrate medications, or drinking well water contaminated by fertilizer are prone to developing methemoglobinemia.

6. Administration of methylene blue may cause hemolysis, methemoglobinemia, or a significant decrease in O_2 saturation on pulse oximetry (due to the presence of the methylene blue) in the blood.

7. Sulfhemoglobin is incorrectly detected by co-oximetry as MetHb, and will produce falsely elevated MetHb levels. Sulfhemoglobinemia should be suspected in cyanotic patients not responding to O_2 therapy and in those failing to improve after treatment with methylene blue.

BOX 17-17. CLINICAL FEATURES OF METHEMOGLOBINEMIA

- Vital signs: tachycardia, tachypnea, hypotension (when severe)
- Cardiovascular: dysrhythmias and arrest (severe cases)
- Pulmonary: dyspnea
- Gastrointestinal: nausea, vomiting
- Neurologic: lethargy, confusion, coma, seizures (when severe)
- Hematologic: chocolate-brown blood, hemolysis (Fig. 17-13)
- Dermatologic: persistent cyanosis

Laboratory values

- Bedside screening tests
  (1) Place 1 drop of the patient's blood on white filter paper or a bed sheet along with a drop of normal blood and allow it to dry. If the patient has methemoglobinemia, it will dry to a chocolate-brown color, while normal blood will dry to a red color.
  (2) Mix the patient's blood vigorously with O_2 in a syringe. Venous blood containing MetHb will remain brownish in color, while normal venous blood will turn bright red upon mixing with O_2.
- Pulse oximetry
  (1) Only detects OxyHb and DeoxyHb, and cannot detect other forms of hemoglobin
  (2) Pulse oximetry readings are usually decreased, with O_2 saturations of 80 to 90% (may be lower in many patients)
- Arterial blood gas (ABG) measurements

  Standard ABG:

  (1) Measures PO_2 which represents the dissolved O_2 content of blood
  (2) O_2 saturation by ABG is calculated from PO_2 based on pH and temperature. It assumes that only normal Hgb is present and *does not account for MetHb, COHb or sulfhemoglobin.*
  (3) In methemoglobinemia *a normal PO_2 and falsely normal (or elevated) O_2 saturation is seen with metabolic acidosis (lactic acidosis).*

  ABG analysis with co-oximetry:

  (1) It is required to determine the actual O_2 saturation.
  (2) It identifies different forms of hemoglobin (OxyHb, DeoxyHb, MetHb) based on their varying wavelengths.
- Saturation gap = difference between O_2 saturation measured by standard ABG and that obtained from co-oximetry, or the difference between O_2 saturation by standard ABG and pulse oximetry
- Elevated MetHb concentration
- CBC (to assess underlying anemia if hemolysis is suspected)
- Serum electrolytes, glucose, BUN, and Cr to evaluate acid-base status (elevated anion gap acidosis due to lactic acidosis)

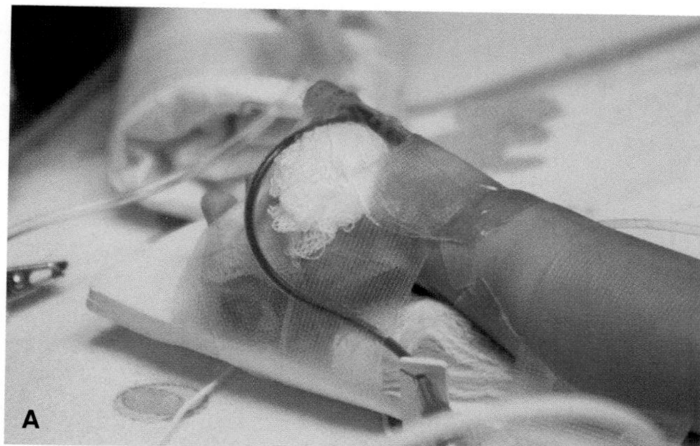

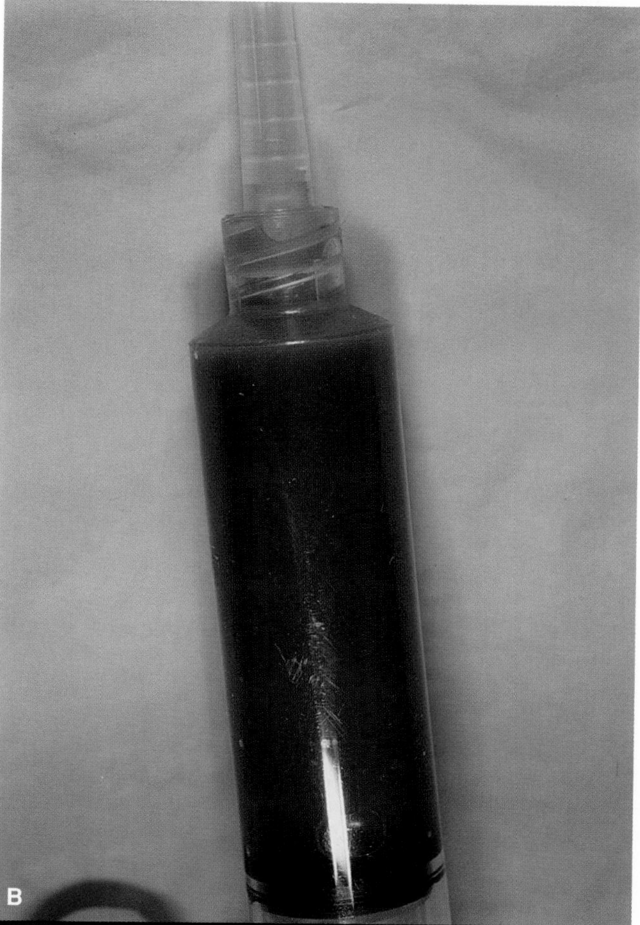

Figure 17-13. Chocolate-Colored Blood in Methemoglobinemia

A. Blood containing MetHb has a distinct chocolate-brown color and provides an important clue to the diagnosis. Arterial blood from the patient in Fig. 17-11 is shown. *B*. A 23-day-old neonate presenting with hypovolemic shock with methemoglobinemia also had chocolate-brown blood. His MetHb value was 40.2% and ABG showed pH of 7.02 with severe metabolic acidosis (HCO_3 of 2.8 mmol/L and BE −26.7 mmol/L). He was resuscitated with IV fluids followed by IV methylene blue. This was followed by an immediate marked improvement in cyanosis, metabolic acidosis, and peripheral perfusion.

BOX 17-18. MANAGEMENT OF METHEMOGLOBINEMIA

Predictors of toxicity (based on serum MetHb concentrations):

- <2% = normal
- 2 to 20% = mild, asymptomatic cyanosis (in a nonanemic patient)
- 20 to 50% = moderate, symptomatic (headache, dyspnea on exertion, tachycardia, dizziness, weakness, mild hypertension and tachypnea)
- 50 to 70% = severe (CNS depression, metabolic acidosis, cardiac dysrhythmias)
- >70% = fatal (severe hypoxia and death)

Management principles:

- Stabilize ABCs, including appropriate treatment of respiratory distress and cardiovascular instability.
- Decontaminate the patient via removal of clothing and vigorous washing of exposed surfaces if cutaneous exposure
- Evaluate for causes of methemoglobinemia.
- ECG, chest radiograph, and cardiac monitoring
- Do not rely on standard pulse oximetry to monitor the patient's status.
- May consider performing filter-paper test at bedside
- Specific antidote: methylene blue
  (1) Acts as a substrate of NADPH methemoglobin reductase, thus converting MetHb back to normal hemoglobin
  (2) Indications: asymptomatic patients with MetHb concentration of >20% and rising *or symptomatic patients* regardless of MetHb concentration *or* If MetHb level unavailable or pending in a patient with persistent cyanosis despite therapy with supplemental oxygen
  (3) Initial dose: 1 to 2 mg/kg (0.1 to 0.2 mL/kg 1% solution) IV over 5 minutes
  (4) Clinical improvement should be seen within 1 hour.
  (5) Urine will turn blue or green after its administration.
  (6) If the patient has not improved following the first dose, repeat measurement of serum MetHb concentration, and then repeat dose of methylene blue to a maximum dose of 7 mg/kg within 3 hours.
- Consider hyperbaric oxygen or exchange transfusion.
  (1) In patients in whom methylene blue may be harmful (e.g., G6PD deficiency) *or*
  (2) Patients not responding to methylene blue *or*
  (3) Patients with MetHb concentration >70%

DIAGNOSIS ORGANOPHOSPHATE AND CARBAMATE INSECTICIDE TOXICITY

Background

1. Organophosphates and carbamates are commonly found in pesticides. Exposures usually occur inadvertently in an agricultural setting or via accidental or intentional ingestion of household products.

2. In recent years, the threat of chemical warfare has brought attention to the highly toxic nerve agents sarin, soman, and tabun. Nerve agents are a class of organophosphates.

3. Pharmaceutical uses:
   a. Organophosphates: malathion is used to treat head lice
   b. Carbamates: pyridostigmine and neostigmine (treatment for myasthenia gravis), physostigmine (treatment for anticholinergic toxicity), and donepezil (treatment of Alzheimer's disease)

Pharmacokinetics and Toxicity

1. Organophosphates bind to the active site of acetylcholinesterase and inactivate it by phosphorylation.
   a. This leads to excessive acetylcholine at synapses in both central and peripheral nervous systems, leading to postsynaptic excitation.
   b. This initial binding is reversible, but then the bond may undergo the process of "aging" and may become irreversible.
   c. All organophosphates differ in the speed of this aging process.
   d. In general, nerve agents may quickly age, making them treatment difficult.

2. Carbamates also bind to acetylcholinesterase and inactivate it; however, this effect is reversible. Carbamates also poorly penetrate the central nervous system (CNS). Thus, their toxicity is similar to that of organophosphates, but generally of shorter duration and usually lacking signs and symptoms of CNS involvement (physostigmine is an exception).

3. The severity and extent of toxicity is dependent on the specific agent, dose, and route of exposure. Inhaled agents lead to rapid symptomatology, while skin absorption may be prolonged or delayed.
   a. Symptoms can occur in 5 minutes with inhaled agents.
   b. Agents with higher lipid solubility may produce delayed, prolonged, or cyclical toxicity.

4. Excessive acetylcholine at muscarinic receptors leads to hyperactivity of the parasympathetic nervous system. This results in the classic DUMBELS symptoms, resulting from smooth muscle contraction and exocrine gland stimulation (For expansion of mnemonic DUMBELS, see page 654).

5. Nicotinic receptor activation
   a. Sympathetic ganglion hyperactivity results in autonomic instability via stimulation of the adrenal gland, resulting in increased secretion of catecholamines.
   b. Neuromuscular junction hyperactivity manifests with striated muscle abnormalities of ineffectual muscle contraction, twitching, weakness, and ultimately paralysis.

6. CNS neurons are directly affected, resulting in impaired nerve impulse transmission.

7. The *intermediate syndrome* refers to a constellation of symptoms that develop 1 to 4 days following acute organophosphate poisoning despite therapy with atropine and pralidoxime.
   a. Signs and symptoms: cranial nerve palsies, nuchal weakness, acute respiratory paralysis, proximal limb weakness, and depressed reflexes. This condition may last up to 15 days (most patients recover).
   b. Occurs more commonly with organophosphates that are highly fat-soluble (possibly due to the release of organophosphates from tissue reservoirs after treatment with atropine and oximes)

8. A delayed peripheral neuropathy may develop 1 to 3 weeks following acute organophosphate exposure. This neuropathy may result from organophosphate inhibition of a neuronal esterase, causing axonal and myelin degeneration. It results in a distal flaccid paralysis which has a variable recovery (often months to years) and occasionally may be permanent.

Emergency Department Evaluation

1. History should focus on the agent, amount, time, and route of exposure.

2. Physical examination should focus on vital signs, with careful attention to cardiovascular and neuromuscular status. The patient's respiratory effort and motor strength should be carefully monitored. The amount of respiratory secretions should be noted.

3. If the exposure is intentional, serum acetaminophen and salicylate levels should also be obtained.

Differential Diagnosis

1. Other direct-acting cholinergic agents (e.g., pilocarpine, bethanechol, and urecholine) producing identical symptomatology

2. Nicotine poisoning from tobacco ingestion (symptoms of nicotinic receptor hyperactivity)

3. Opioid toxicity (miosis, respiratory depression, lethargy, bradycardia)

4. Bradycardia from other drugs (e.g., digitalis, calcium channel blockers, beta-blockers)
5. Nontoxic causes (e.g., Eaton-Lambert syndrome, myasthenia gravis)
6. Muscarine-containing mushrooms (e.g., *Clitocybe*, *Inocybe*)

Consultations

Poison control center, psychiatry (for suicidal attempts or homicidal intentions)

Emergency Department Treatment and Disposition

1. Decontamination of the patient is of the utmost importance to prevent further toxicity to the patient and to prevent toxic exposure of health care providers. The patient's clothes must be removed and all exposed surfaces washed thoroughly. Health care providers must be careful not to become exposed, as transdermal absorption of organophosphates may occur.
2. Admit all patients who present with significant symptoms requiring treatment, or those with evolving toxicity (Fig. 17-14). It may be preferable to admit to the ICU for close observation and monitoring of CNS and cardiopulmonary status.
3. Most asymptomatic patients with unintentional exposures may be discharged to home after a 6-hour observation period. However, some organophosphates may present with delayed toxicity, especially if the route of exposure was dermal.
4. For organophosphate toxicity, both atropine and pralidoxime are given as antidotes. Atropine and pralidoxime given together have synergistic effects against signs and symptoms of cholinesterase inhibition, thus decreasing atropine requirements.
5. For carbamate toxicity, atropine alone is usually adequate therapy; however, pralidoxime may also be given for significant carbamate toxicity. Pralidoxime should be given if there is any uncertainty concerning the identification of the toxic agent involved, because organophosphate and carbamate toxicity may be indistinguishable.

Clinical Pearls: Organophosphate and Carbamate Pesticide Toxicity

1. If a patient requires intubation, paralytic agents (e.g., succinylcholine) may have their duration of action increased by organophosphate toxicity.
2. Death usually occurs from respiratory failure. Physicians should have a low threshold to perform endotracheal intubation and mechanically ventilate patients early in the course of treatment.
3. Atropine dosing should be given until the drying of secretions is noted and should *not* be titrated to tachycardia or mydriasis.
4. Organophosphate agents vary greatly in the symptoms they produce. Nerve agents will mostly present with nicotinic and CNS effects rather than muscarinic effects.

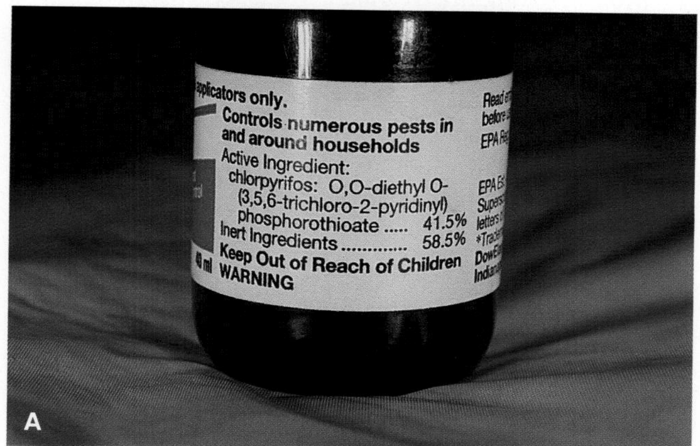

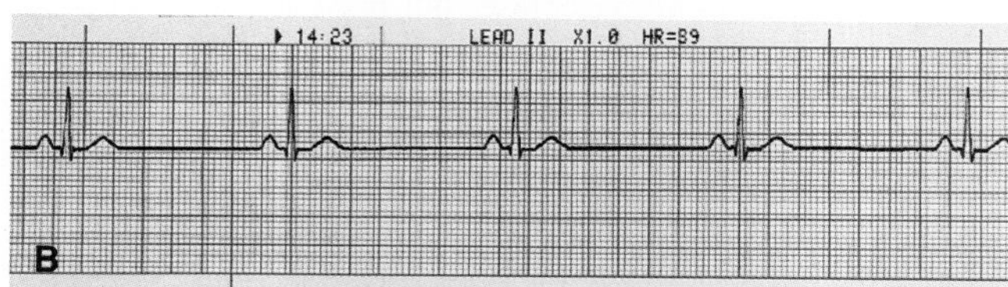

Figure 17-14. Organophosphate Insecticide Toxicity

A. A 10-year-old child was brought to the ED with a history of lethargy and numerous episodes of vomiting which started shortly after receiving a liquid preparation thought to be cough syrup (given to him by his grandmother). Actually what he received was a commercial pesticide containing chlorpyrifos and "inert" ingredients (pesticides contain hydrocarbon solvent carriers such as petroleum distillates and aromatic hydrocarbons as "inert" ingredients. The hydrocarbon diluent may contribute to the overall picture of toxicity). *B*. The patient had bradycardia, increased salivation, and bilateral diffuse rales with wheezing and miosis. Gastric lavage was performed and a petroleumlike odor was noted from the gastric contents. He received one dose of activated charcoal. He received a total of 16 doses of atropine within the first 6 hours after admission to the ICU to remain free of respiratory secretions. Two hours after arrival in the ED, he also became disoriented and developed tongue fasciculations. He was started on pralidoxime. Both atropine and pralidoxime were continued for the next 36 hours until he was fully oriented with an absence of any respiratory secretions.

BOX 17-19. ORGANOPHOSPHATE AND CARBAMATE INSECTICIDES TOXICITY

Clinical features

Muscarinic (DUMBELS)	*Nicotinic (sympathetic)*	*Nicotinic (neuromuscular)*	*CNS (CARDS)*
*D*iarrhea, *D*iaphoresis	Diaphoresis	Fasciculations	*C*onfusion, *C*oma
*U*rination	Tachycardia	Weakness	*A*taxia, anxiety
*M*iosis	Mydriasis	Cramps	*R*espiratory depression
*B*ronchospasm, *B*radycardia	Hypertension	Paralysis	*D*epression
*E*mesis	Pallor		*S*eizures
*L*acrimation			
*S*weating, *S*alivation			

- Other signs and symptoms: garlic odor, fever, tenesmus, blurred vision, heart block, dysrhythmias

Laboratory tests

- RBC cholinesterase activity (in general these tests are not very useful clinically because the results do not come back in a timely fashion)
  (1) Decreased activity
  (2) RBC cholinesterase activity is more specific than plasma cholinesterase, but may not correlate well with the level of toxicity.
  (3) Many limitations to its use (i.e., serum AChE activity may not reflect tissue AChE activity)
  (4) Organophosphates vary in their ability to affect RBC cholinesterase and plasma cholinesterase.
  (5) There is a wide range of variability in AChE activity in the normal population.
- Plasma pseudocholinesterase activity
  (1) Decreased activity
  (2) Less expensive and much more widely available test
  (3) Can be used in lieu of RBC cholinesterase activity
- CBC may show leukocytosis (normal differential) and elevated hematocrit (large fluid losses).
- Serum electrolytes may show an anion gap acidosis from poor tissue perfusion.
- Hyperglycemia
- Hypokalemia
- Hypomagnesemia
- Increased BUN:Cr ratio, suggesting prerenal azotemia
- ABG may show acidosis (lactic).

Predictors of toxicity: RBC or plasma cholinesterase activity

- 50 to 90% of normal = no toxicity
- 20 to 50% of normal = mild toxicity (nausea/vomiting, fatigue, salivation, sweating, abdominal cramps, headache)
- 10 to 20% of normal = moderate toxicity (generalized weakness, difficulty speaking, fasciculations, miosis)
- <10% of normal = severe toxicity (coma, miosis, flaccid paralysis, cyanosis, pulmonary edema)

BOX 17-20. MANAGEMENT OF ORGANOPHOSPHATE AND CARBAMATE INSECTICIDE TOXICITY

- Decontaminate the patient as quickly as possible.
- Stabilize ABCs, including appropriate treatment of pulmonary edema, respiratory distress, altered mental status, and hypotension as indicated.
- Obtain ECG, pulse oximetry, and chest radiograph, and perform continuous cardiac monitoring.
- Obtain serum electrolytes, glucose, calcium, magnesium, and phosphorus.
- Consider gastric lavage if the patient has presented within 1 hour of ingestion and is not already vomiting.
- Administer 1 dose of activated charcoal (dose: 1 to 2 g/kg; max 50 g)
- Specific antidotes: atropine (effective at treating muscarinic toxicity) and pralidoxime (effective at treating both nicotinic and muscarinic effects)
- Administer atropine
  (1) Give to all patients with bronchorrhea or bradycardia
  (2) Competitively blocks acetylcholine at muscarinic receptors, preventing excessive parasympathetic stimulation
  (3) No effect on neuromuscular junction (nicotinic receptors)
  (4) Dose: 0.05 mg/kg IV (adult dose: 2 to 5 mg; minimum dose 0.1 mg in children)
  (5) Repeat dose (or double dose) in 5 to 15 minutes as needed until pulmonary secretions are controlled.
  (6) *Titrate atropine dose to clearing of oral and bronchial secretions.*
  (7) *Do not* titrate atropine dose to mydriasis or tachycardia.
  (8) Large amounts of atropine may be required.
- Administer pralidoxime
  (1) Patients with significant toxicity who receive atropine should also be given pralidoxime.
  (2) *Only given after atropinization* (atropine acts quickly, is more readily available, and is given first to decrease respiratory secretions and distress; pralidoxime has a greater delay to onset of effect)
  (3) Pralidoxime works by dephosphorylating acetylcholinesterase (thus reactivating it).
  (4) Given as IV boluses (effects seen within 10 minutes)
  (5) Dose: 25 mg/kg (up to 1 g) IV over 30 minutes
  (6) Repeat dose (25 to 50 mg/kg) in 1-hour if fasciculations persist.
  (7) Repeat the dose at 6- to 12-hour intervals for the following 48 hours as needed.
  (8) May be given as a continuous infusion (10–20 mL/kg/hr)

DIAGNOSIS CAMPHOR TOXICITY

Background

1. Camphor is a volatile organic compound used as an ingredient in many over-the-counter liniments, antipruritics, cold remedies, antiseptics, topical anesthetics, and aphrodisiacs. A few examples include liniments (e.g., Ben-Gay, Children's Vaporizing Rub, Vicks VapoRub, Deep Down Rub) and liquid preparations (e.g., Campho-Phenique; one of the most widely available preparations, contains 10.8% camphor). Camphor is also found in moth repellents, lacquers, varnishes, explosives, embalming fluid, and cosmetics. Many of these products do not have child safety protective mechanisms. Although federal regulations have limited the camphor content of products manufactured in the United States, this does not hold true for foreign products.
2. There is no definitive therapeutic role for camphor in medicine.

Pharmacokinetics and Toxicity

1. The precise mechanism of camphor toxicity is unknown. It acts as a central nervous system stimulant and as an irritant to tissues.
2. Camphor toxicity can occur through inhalation, ingestion, or dermal absorption.
3. Although significant toxicity is rare, death has been reported.

Emergency Department Evaluation

1. The history should focus on dosage, time, route, intent of exposure, and symptoms since exposure.
2. Physical examination should focus on assessment of neurological status, odor of camphor on breath (described as pungent or fragrant), and signs of dermal irritation.
3. Serum camphor levels are not readily available.

Emergency Department Treatment and Disposition

1. Patients who are asymptomatic 6 hours postexposure may be discharged after appropriate decontamination and psychiatric evaluation (if indicated).
2. Admit any patient who presents with significant signs of toxicity (e.g., seizures or altered mental status) from camphor exposure for continued monitoring and supportive care.

Consultations

Poison control center and psychiatry (intentional ingestion)

Clinical Pearls: Camphor Toxicity

1. In its liquid form, camphor has been reported to have potential morbidity with ingestion of as little as 50 mg/kg, and a potentially fatal dose of 100 mg/kg (in a single case report, 5 mL of a 1 g/5 mL preparation of camphor caused the death of a toddler weighing 10 kg).
2. Consider camphor toxicity in any patient in the differential diagnosis of toxin-induced seizures (especially in patients who have access to over-the-counter preparations containing camphor).
3. Patients with camphor toxicity may abruptly seize without antecedent signs or symptoms of camphor toxicity. Seizures rarely occur after dermal contact or inhalation exposure.
4. Camphor-induced seizures occasionally may be recurrent or invariably prolonged (status epilepticus). Status epilepticus with respiratory depression is often the cause of morbidity and mortality.

BOX 17-21. CLINICAL FEATURES OF CAMPHOR TOXICITY

Signs and symptoms

- Vital signs: tachycardia
- HEENT: burning sensation in oropharynx, visual disturbances (veiling, darkening, or flickering), camphor odor on breath
- Cardiovascular: cardiovascular collapse (severe overdose)
- GI: nausea, vomiting, burning sensation in mouth, epigastric burning, hepatitis (mild transaminitis)
- Neurologic: headache, fasciculations, confusion, delirium, coma, tremors; seizures usually seen within 5 minutes or within 1 to 2 hours postingestion (may be significantly delayed for solid camphor products, which must dissolve prior to GI absorption); rarely seizures are prolonged or recurrent (status epilepticus) (Fig. 17-15)

Management principles

- Treatment is mainly supportive and symptomatic (*no specific antidote*).
- Stabilize ABCs, including appropriate treatment for seizures and altered mental status.
- Decontaminate the patient to prevent continuing exposure.
- Do not induce emesis (liquid products are often rapidly absorbed; mental status may be depressed, with increased risk of aspiration)
- Consider gastric lavage if a large quantity of a liquid product was ingested and the patient presents to the hospital soon after the exposure.
- Administer 1 dose of activated charcoal (dose: 1 to 2 g/kg) if the patient has good mental status (use caution, as the patient's mental status may quickly deteriorate).
- Evaluate serum electrolytes, BUN, Cr, glucose, and liver function tests.
- Consider other causes of altered mental status in patients in whom the history is unclear (see mnemonic COMATOSE PATIENT, Box 13-4).

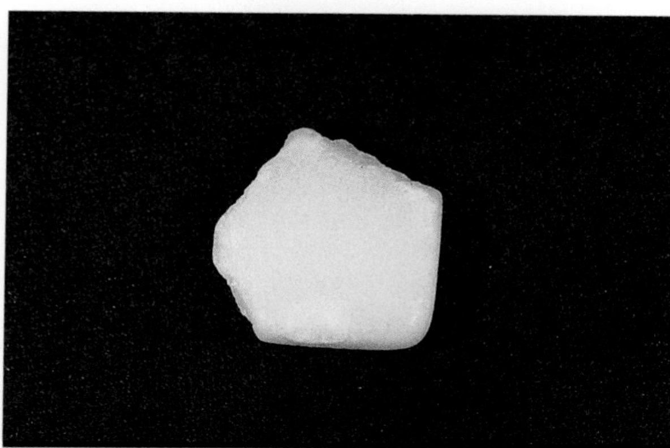

Figure 17-15. Camphor Cube

An 13-month-old previously healthy toddler presented with afebrile status epilepticus (a generalized tonic-clonic seizure lasting about 30 minutes). During stabilization, he vomited gastrointestinal contents that had an odor of camphor. His seizures were controlled by IV diazepam followed by a loading dose of IV phenobarbital (if the patient continues to seize, phenobarbital may be the preferred anticonvulsant, as it enhances hepatic enzymes that metabolize camphor). His mother found the infant chewing on this camphor cube (shown here with a portion eaten away). The mother was using camphor cubes at home as moth repellent.

BOX 17-22. DIFFERENTIAL DIAGNOSIS OF DRUGS OR CHEMICALS PRODUCING SEIZURES

Mnemonic *CAMPHOR BALLS*

- *C*amphor, *C*ocaine, *C*arbon monoxide, *C*yanide, *C*affeine, *C*lonidine, *C*arbamazepine
- *A*mphetamines, *A*nticholinergics (tricyclic antidepressants, antihistamines), *A*spirin
- *M*ethylxanthines (theophylline)
- *P*henothiazines or *P*hencyclidine
- *H*ypoglycemic agents (oral insulin), *H*eavy metals (e.g., lead)
- *O*pioids (propoxyphene, meperidine), *O*rganophosphates
- *R*odenticides (strychnine, thallium, arsenic)
- *B*arbiturates, *B*enzodiazepines (withdrawal seizures)
- *A*lcohols (methanol, ethylene glycol), *E*thanol (withdrawal seizure)
- *L*idocaine
- *L*ithium
- *S*alicylates

(Reproduced with permission from: Shah BR: Child poisoned by unknown substance. In: Finberg L, Kleinman RE (eds). *Saunders Manual of Pediatric Practice*. WB Saunders, Philadelphia, 2002, p. 1158.)

DIAGNOSIS CASTOR BEAN AND ROSARY PEA INGESTION

Background

1. *Ricinus communis* is a large, leafy plant that may be green or red, that produces soft-spined fruits that contain castor beans. The beans are hard, shiny, and colored with grey and brown streaks (Fig. 17-16).
2. *Abrus precatorius* is a high-climbing, woody, green vine found in India, Florida, and the Caribbean (Fig. 17-17). It produces a fruit known as the jequirty pea (also known as the rosary pea, Indian bean, crab's eye, Buddhist's rosary bead, and prayer bead), which is hard and may be bright red with a black center, black with a white center, or white with a black center.
3. Both seeds are used commercially as decorative pieces in jewelry. The rosary pea, because of its distinctive coloring, may also be used on toy dolls as eyes.
4. *Ricinus communis* is also the source of castor oil, which is used as a purgative and as a lubricant for engines.

Pharmacokinetics and Toxicity

1. All parts of the plants are toxic, but the seeds contain the highest concentration of cellular toxins (*ricin* in the castor bean, *abrin* in the rosary pea), which inhibit protein synthesis and lead to cellular demise.
2. Ingestion of either kind of seed rarely results in toxicity. Toxicity requires the hard outer casing to be broken via chewing or digestion followed by GI absorption.
3. Anecdotally, castor beans have been regarded as highly lethal with only one bean sufficient to cause death in a child. Fortunately, toxicity is generally limited by poor GI absorption.
4. Abrin from the rosary pea is also poorly absorbed from the GI tract.

Emergency Department Evaluation

1. The history should focus on identification of the seed ingested (if observed by a caretaker), the number of seeds ingested, and the timing of ingestion. Asking patients if they actively chewed the seed may be helpful as well. The history should also focus on analyzing symptoms that develop postexposure.
2. Physical examination should focus on vital signs, mental status, and proper evaluation of the abdomen.

Differential Diagnosis

1. Toxicologic causes of diarrhea include ingestion of organophosphates and other cholinergic agents.
2. Infectious causes of gastroenteritis should also be considered.
3. Other toxicologic causes of seizures (e.g., camphor, caffeine, cocaine, tricyclic antidepressants, amphetamines, anticholinergics, opioids; see mnemonic CAMPHOR BALLS, Box 17-2).

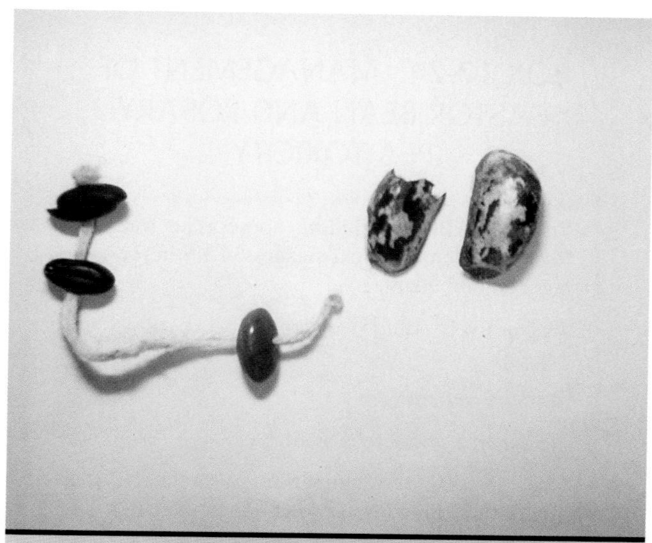

Figure 17-16. Bracelet Made with Castor Bean Seeds

One of the seeds from this bracelet was chewed and eaten by a 1-year-old infant, who was rushed to the ED with swelling of the lips and new onset of wheezing shortly after chewing the seed. He was readmitted with anaphylaxis (hypotension, angioedema, and wheezing) about 2 weeks after the first admission, again after chewing the seeds from a similar necklace (a necklace made of castor beans that was purchased with this bracelet as a matching set). Allergic reactions, as seen in this patient, are well recognized and reproducible with patch testing. The castor plant flourishes in warm climates, including the southwestern United States and Mexico. It produces clusters of pods containing seeds. Castor bean seeds are almond-sized and glossy with a mottled black, dark brown, gray and white coating.

4. Other etiologies of CNS depression (e.g., ethanol, benzodiazepines, barbiturates or other sedative-hypnotics)

Consultations

Poison control center and psychiatry consult (intentional ingestion)

Emergency Department Evaluation and Disposition

1. This is potentially a very toxic ingestion; however, because of its rare occurrence insufficient data are available with regard to optimal management.

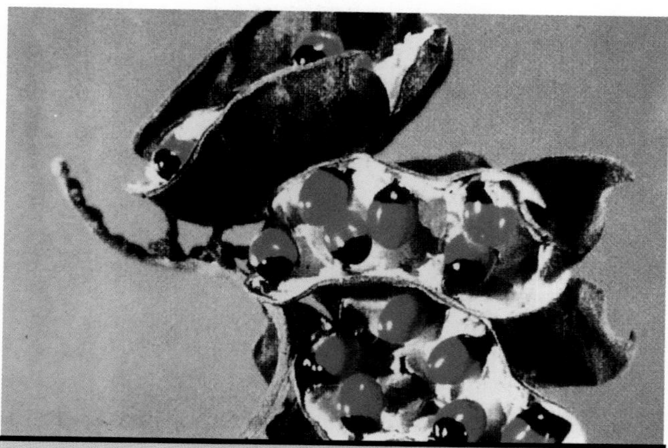

Figure 17-17. Rosary Pea (*Abrus precatorius*)

The fruit is a pea-shaped pod approximately 4 cm in length. When opened and dried, 3 to 5 scarlet pea-sized seeds with a small black spot at the point of attachment are found. As seen here, these seeds are glossy and colored bright red and black. The rosary pea contains the toxalbumin abrin. *Abrus precatorius* has many common names including jequirty pea, rosary pea, Indian bean, Buddhist's rosary bead, prayer bead, and crab's eye. It thrives in the tropical climates of South and Central America, the Caribbean, and Florida. (Reproduced with permission from: Plants by Shih RD and Goldfrank LR. In: *Goldfrank's Toxicologic Emergencies,* 6th edition. New York, McGraw-Hill, 1998, p. 1104.)

2. All patients presenting following ingestion of castor beans or rosary peas should be admitted for observation and supportive care.

Clinical Pearls: Castor Bean and Rosary Pea Ingestion

1. Seeds of both these plants are very attractive and are used for ornamental purposes to make necklaces and rosaries. They contain large amounts of the toxalbumins ricin (*R. communis*) and abrin (*A. precatorius*).
2. Ingestion of intact seeds rarely results in toxicity. However, severe toxicity results if toxins are released by chewing the seeds followed by absorption in the GI tract.
3. Any child with a history of ingesting a rosary pea or castor bean should undergo GI decontamination.

BOX 17-23. CASTOR BEAN AND ROSARY PEA TOXICITY

- Symptoms typically are seen within 2 to 10 hours after toxalbumin ingestion.
- Symptoms may be delayed up to 48 hours following rosary pea ingestion.

Signs and symptoms

- Vital signs: tachycardia, hypotension, shock (severe fluid loss or hemorrhage)
- Cardiac: cardiac dysrhythmias
- Gastrointestinal: severe vomiting and diarrhea (may become bloody), colicky abdominal pain, GI hemorrhage
- CNS: CNS depression, seizures, cerebral edema
- Hematology: hemolysis
- Systemic: multiorgan injury (may be seen within 24 hours), hepatic failure, renal insufficiency, lethargy, stupor, seizures, death; allergic reactions including anaphylaxis

Laboratory values

- CBC and type and cross-match in patients with GI bleeding (CBC may show elevated WBC count and anemia secondary to GI hemorrhage)
- Serum electrolytes may show elevated BUN and Cr, suggesting dehydration.
- Coagulation studies (PT, PTT, INR) may demonstrate coagulopathy.

BOX 17-24. MANAGEMENT OF CASTOR BEAN AND ROSARY PEA TOXICITY

- Stabilize ABCs, including appropriate treatment for hypovolemic shock, seizures, CNS depression, and cerebral edema.
- Aggressively fluid resuscitate all hypovolemic patients.
- Supportive treatment
- No specific antidote is available.
- Consider GI decontamination (as indicated, with any of the following; for details see page 621)
  (1) Activated charcoal (dose: 1 to 2 g/kg up to max 50 g)
  (2) Gastric lavage in patients presenting soon after ingestion and demonstrating any sign of toxicity
  (3) Whole-bowel irrigation is ideal to decrease GI transit time for the seeds.

DIAGNOSIS ANTICHOLINERGIC DRUG AND PLANT TOXICITY

Background

1. Many pharmacologic agents (e.g., antiparkinsonism drugs, antihistamines, belladonna alkaloids, neuroleptics, and tricyclic antidepressants) and naturally occurring plants (jimson weed [Fig. 17-18], nutmeg, potatoes, and deadly nightshade) may produce anticholinergic toxicity.
2. Plant substances are readily available and may be abused, especially by adolescents interested in experimentation.

Pharmacokinetics/Toxicity

1. The toxic dosage varies according to the agent involved.
2. Exposure primarily occurs through ingestion, intra-ophthalmic use, or inhalation.
3. Patients may present with initial symptoms suggestive of blockade of peripheral muscarinic acetylcholine receptors. At higher dosages, CNS effects may be seen that suggest blockade of subcortical muscarinic receptors.
4. Even at high doses, the neuromuscular junction remains relatively spared and unaffected.

Emergency Department Evaluation

1. The history should focus on the agent involved, dosage, and timing of exposure. Careful attention must be paid not only to prescribed medications, but to over-the-counter medications as well. The history should also include a determination of possible plant ingestion.

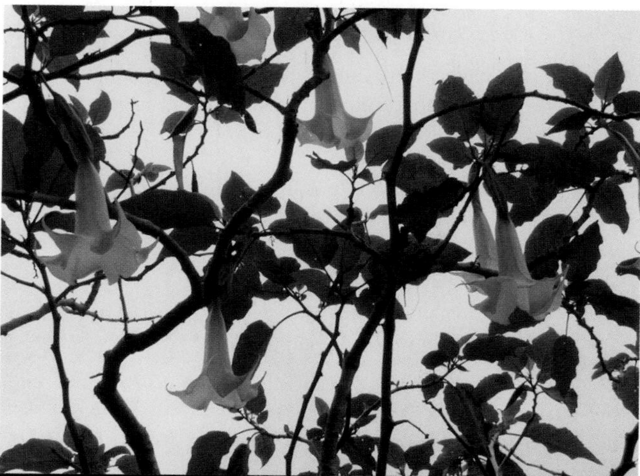

Figure 17-18. Jimson Weed Plant with White Trumpet-Shaped Flowers

Both the leaves and the seeds have anticholinergic properties. Many plants contain belladonna alkaloids (atropine and scopolamine). These plants are often used as hallucinogens or as asthma remedies. Jimson weed contains atropine, hyoscyamine, and stramonium. Other plants with anticholinergic properties include henbane and mandrake.

2. Physical examination should focus on vital signs, pupillary reactivity, skin characteristics, bowel and bladder function, and determination of neurologic status.

Differential Diagnosis

1. Ingestion of sympathomimetic agents may mimic anticholinergic agent toxicity (Box 17-26).
2. Often, anticholinergic toxicity may be subtle. For example, a patient admitting to heroin use may not be aware that scopolamine was added as a contaminant. Being unaware of this may lead a clinician to falsely conclude that a patient's mental status is due strictly to heroin.
3. Patients may be incorrectly diagnosed with ethanol intoxication.

Consultations

Poison control center and psychiatric evaluation (if suicidal ideation)

Emergency Department Management and Disposition

1. Admit all patients who display signs of toxicity, including tachycardia, altered mental status, seizures, sedation, or hyperthermia. Patients should be admitted to a setting with cardiac monitoring available. After physostigmine administration, all patients should be admitted to an ICU.
2. Patients may be discharged from the ED if they are asymptomatic following a 6- to 12-hour observation period (or 4 to 6 hours after their last dose of benzodiazepine), and if they have received appropriate GI decontamination and psychiatric evaluation (if indicated).

Clinical Pearls: Anticholinergic Drug and Plant Toxicity

1. Many medications, including over-the-counter preparations, contain agents with anticholinergic properties. A careful history should be obtained in all patients displaying signs of anticholinergic toxicity.
2. Anticholinergic toxicity can be recognized using the mnemonic: *red as a beet, hot as a hare, blind as a bat, dry as a bone, and mad as a hatter* (e.g., flushed skin, hyperthermia, mydriasis, dry mouth, urinary retention, agitation along with tachycardia and diminished bowel sounds).
3. Because of the widespread availability of plants with anticholinergic activity, patients should be referred to substance abuse counseling to help prevent future repetition of events.
4. Patients with suspected tricyclic antidepressant ingestion should not be given physostigmine.

BOX 17-25. CLINICAL FEATURES OF ANTICHOLINERGIC TOXICITY

Signs and symptoms

- Red as a beet, hot as a hare, blind as a bat, dry as a bone, and mad as a hatter

  Red as beet = flushed skin
  Hot as hare = hyperthermia
  Blind as bat = mydriasis with blurred vision
  Dry as bone = skin and mucous membranes dry
  Mad as hatter = agitation

- Vital signs: sinus tachycardia (*in the absence of tachycardia, question this diagnosis*), hyperthermia (occasionally significant)
- Skin: warm, dry, and flushed; mucous membranes dry
- Cardiovascular: tachycardia (dysrhythmias rare)
- Gastrointestinal: decreased bowel sounds, constipation, and ileus
- Genitourinary: urinary retention
- Musculoskeletal: psychomotor agitation, rhabdomyolysis
- Neurologic: mydriasis (blurred vision), agitation, altered mental status, CNS depression, coma, seizures, hallucinations

Laboratory values

- Obtain serum electrolytes, glucose, aspirin, and acetaminophen levels for coingestions
- Elevated BUN and Cr (dehydration or renal injury from rhabdomyolysis)
- Elevated creatine kinase (rhabdomyolysis)
- Elevated urine specific gravity
- ECG
  (1) Sinus tachycardia
  (2) May show dysrhythmias
  (3) Widening of QRS interval or an R wave in aVR suggests tricyclic antidepressant toxicity (see Figs. 17-28 through 17-30) or other Na^+ channel blocker toxicity

BOX 17-26. COMPARISON OF SYMPATHOMIMETICS AND ANTICHOLINERGICS

	Sympathomimetics	*Anticholinergics*
Vital signs	Tachyarrhythmias, hypertension/tachycardia, hyperthermia	Tachyarrhythmias, hypertension/hypotension, hyperthermia,
Pupils	Mydriasis	Mydriasis
CNS	Hyperalert/agitation, hallucinations, delirium/psychosis	Coma/agitation/delirium, hallucinations, extrapyramidal movements
Skin	Severe sweating	Dry, hot, flushed
Urine	Normal	Retention
Gastrointestinal	Increased bowel sounds	Decreased bowel sounds (ileus)

(Reproduced with permission from: Shah BR: Child poisoned by unknown substance. In: Finberg L, Kleinman RE (eds). *Saunders Manual of Pediatric Practice*. WB Saunders, Philadelphia, 2002, p. 1157.)

BOX 17-27. MANAGEMENT OF ANTICHOLINERGIC TOXICITY

- Stabilize ABCs, including appropriate treatment for altered mental status, agitation, CNS depression, cardiac dysrhythmias, and seizures.
- Decontaminate eyes with vigorous irrigation with normal saline (if indicated).
- GI decontamination
  (1) Gastric lavage if presenting within 1 hour of ingestion
  (2) Administer one dose of activated charcoal (dose: 1 to 2 g/kg) for patients presenting after 1 hour postingestion (AC is preferred method of decontamination).
  (3) *Decreased GI motility may permit both gastric lavage and administration of AC to have increased efficacy despite a delay in implementation.*
- Take measures to control patient presenting with agitation to prevent self-harm or harm to others.
- Specific antidote: physostigmine
  (1) May be used as a diagnostic agent to determine if altered mental status is due to anticholinergic toxicity or from other causes
  (2) It is a reversible inhibitor of acetylcholinesterase.
  (3) It can penetrate the CNS and thus reverse central anticholinergic toxicity.
  (4) Indications for its use include severe agitation, extrapyramidal movement disorders, recurrent or refractory seizures, severe hallucinations, or refractory dysrhythmias.
  (5) It can produce profound cholinergic effects.
  (6) Contraindicated in patients with severe cardiac or peripheral vascular disease, asthma, bowel obstruction, or urinary tract obstruction
  (7) Contraindicated in patients with known tricyclic antidepressant ingestion or findings suggestive of this (ECG changes, see Figs. 17-28 through 17-30)
  (8) During its administration, the patient must have cardiac monitoring; atropine must be available at the bedside with preparation for endotracheal intubation.
  (9) Given as a slow IV push (over 2 to 5 minutes) of 0.02 mg/kg (up to 2 mg) repeated every 5 to 10 minutes as necessary until life-threatening anticholinergic symptoms resolve
  (10) If the patient develops adverse reactions to physostigmine, atropine should be administered in a dose equal to half the amount of physostigmine given.

DIAGNOSIS PHENOTHIAZINE TOXICITY

Background

Phenothiazines (e.g., prochlorperazine, chlorpromazine, thioridazine), often referred to as neuroleptics, are medications commonly used as antiemetics, antipsychotics, and anxiolytics.

Pharmacokinetics and Toxicity

1. Phenothiazines act as competitive inhibitors at many receptor types including dopaminergic, serotonergic, cholinergic, histaminic, and α_1 and α_2 adrenergic receptors.
   a. Antipsychotic effects are believed to be related to inhibition of dopaminergic receptors and are likely to be mediated by serotonergic receptors.
   b. Occurrence of extrapyramidal movement disorders may be related to decreased dopaminergic activity in the basal ganglia.
2. Therapeutic and toxic doses vary according to the agents being used.
3. Extrapyramidal adverse effects
   a. Dystonic reaction
   b. Akathisia: typically seen between 5 and 60 days after starting neuroleptic therapy; patients are restless and may complain that their "body wants to jump out of its skin." Treatment includes decreasing the dose of neuroleptic and administering anticholinergic agents and benzodiazepines.
   c. Parkinsonism: typically seen within 2 to 3 months of starting neuroleptic therapy. Patients may present with resting tremor, bradykinesia, a shuffling gait, or mask-like facies. Treatment involves decreasing the neuroleptic dose and administering anticholinergic agents.
   d. Tardive dyskinesia: may develop months to years following initiation of neuroleptic therapy; patients typically have involuntary buccolinguomasticatory movements and choreoathetoid movements. This condition is usually irreversible but may respond to discontinuing, decreasing, or increasing the dose of neuroleptic agent

or occasionally administration of cholinergic agents (e.g., physostigmine).

e. Neuroleptic malignant syndrome: may be seen within days to weeks of starting neuroleptic therapy. Patients may present with hyperthermia, muscular rigidity, autonomic instability, and altered mental status ranging from extreme confusion to catatonia. Rhabdomyolysis may occur. Specific treatment (aside from stabilization of ABCs and supportive care) includes rapid cooling, and pharmacologic agents such as benzodiazepines, dantrolene, and dopamine agonists such as bromocriptine and amantadine.

4. CNS depression is commonly seen. In large overdoses (especially thioridazine and mesoridazine), seizures and cardiac dysrhythmias may occur.

Emergency Department Evaluation

1. History should focus on determining the agent involved, as well as the dose, time of ingestion, chronicity of ingestion, and intent. The patient's mental status may impede obtaining a thorough history.
2. Physical examination should focus on vital signs, including measurement of orthostatic blood pressure and assessing cardiovascular and neurologic status.

Differential Diagnosis

1. Other agents causing CNS depression; especially important are those that impair cardiac conduction (e.g., tricyclic antidepressants, type Ia antidysrhythmics)
2. Other etiologies of CNS depression (e.g., meningitis, intracranial hemorrhage, cerebral ischemia)
3. Electrolyte imbalances leading to cardiac conduction abnormalities

Consultations

Poison control center and psychiatry (for patients with intentional overdose as well as for those patients displaying toxicity from phenothiazines administered for the treatment of psychiatric disorders)

Emergency Department Management and Disposition

1. Admit all patients presenting with acute overdose. Patients presenting with cardiovascular instability or CNS depression should be admitted to an ICU for monitoring and treatment.
2. Even though patients with acute dystonic reactions may have responded to the therapy (e.g., diphenhydramine), exposure to extended-release products may require admission for extended observation.
3. Patients may be discharged from the ED after appropriate GI decontamination if they do not develop seizures, hypotension, or ECG changes after a 6-hour observation period. Evaluation by a psychiatrist should be performed (if indicated).

Clinical Pearls: Phenothiazine Toxicity

1. Phenothiazine toxicity presents with extrapyramidal signs (most common) and anticholinergic signs.
2. Response to parenteral diphenhydramine or benztropine mesylate potentially serves both as a diagnostic as well as a therapeutic test in patients presenting with extrapyramidal signs (Fig. 17-19).
3. Patients may develop signs of toxicity while receiving therapeutic doses or overdose of phenothiazines. Signs and symptoms may develop acutely or after chronic therapy.
4. A previous history of extrapyramidal signs is strongly associated with recurrence upon repeat challenge of the drug.
5. Phenothiazines may cross-react with urine drug screens as tricyclic antidepressants, resulting in a false-positive test.

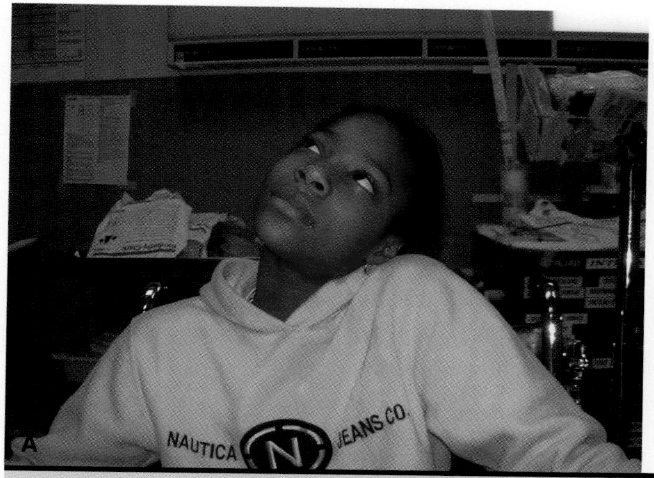

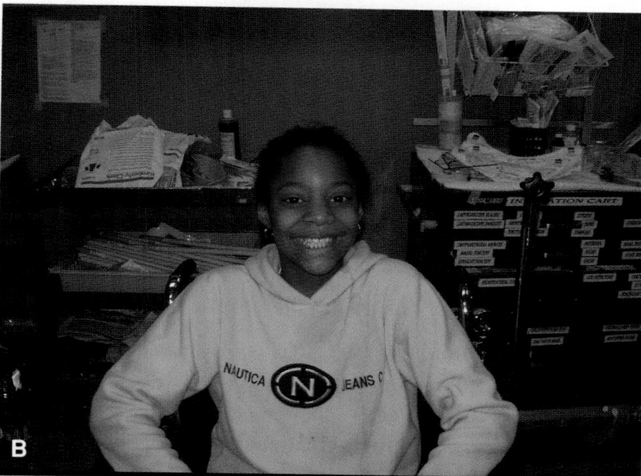

Figure 17-19. Dystonic Reaction

A. Extrapyramidal signs seen here such as torticollis, inability to speak, and trismus were the presenting complaints in this girl who was brought to the ED from school. There was no history available when she arrived at the ED. Based on her clinical findings, phenothiazine toxicity was suspected. *B*. Dramatic improvement after IV diphenhydramine. Extrapyramidal signs are very frightening to caregivers (especially in a previously healthy child without any history of ingestion), and following the dramatic improvement, treating physicians are often lauded as heroes. Subsequently we learned that this patient's uncle was receiving mesoridazine for nervousness, and the patient confessed to taking her uncle's medication.

BOX 17-28. CLINICAL FEATURES OF PHENOTHIAZINE TOXICITY

- Toxicity may be classified as:
  (1) CNS effects (primarily mediated by dopaminergic and serotonergic actions)
  (2) Non-CNS effects (mediated by cholinergic and adrenergic actions)
- Toxicity may occur with therapeutic doses.
- Extrapyramidal signs
  (1) Most common presentation of toxicity
  (2) Associated with either an acute ingestion or as side effects of chronic treatment
  (3) May be intermittent and delayed up to 24 hours from ingestion
  (2) Typically seen within 1 to 5 days of starting neuroleptic therapy
  (3) Signs and symptoms: *patient awake and alert,* oculogyric crisis, torticollis, opisthotonos, trismus, difficulty speaking, facial grimacing, chorealike movements
  (4) Responds to therapy with anticholinergics (diphenhydramine or benztropine)
- Anticholinergic signs and symptoms

  *R*ed as a beet, *H*ot as a hare, *B*lind as a bat, *D*ry as a bone, *M*ad as a hatter (see Box 17-25)
- Vital signs: tachycardia, hypertension or hypotension, hyperthermia, or hypothermia (rare)
- Cardiovascular: ECG changes include prolonged QT interval, QRS widening, AV block, fatal dysrhythmias (severe toxicity)
- Gastrointestinal: constipation, ileus, cholestatic or hepatocellular jaundice
- Renal: urinary retention
- Hematologic: agranulocytosis, anemia
- Musculoskeletal: rhabdomyolysis
- Other neurologic: CNS depression, seizures, coma, miosis, delirium/psychosis

Laboratory values:

- Serum electrolytes, glucose, BUN, and creatinine
- Elevated transaminase and bilirubin may be seen
- Elevated creatine kinase (rhabdomyolysis)
- Increased serum creatinine (rhabdomyolysis-induced renal failure)
- Urine may be red, pink, purple, orange, or rust-colored.
- Urine phenothiazine colorimetric testing may be used and may suggest presence of phenothiazine (limited availability).
- Abdominal x-ray may show radiopaque phenothiazine tablets.
- If indicated, acetaminophen and salicylate levels to evaluate for occult ingestion

BOX 17-29. MANAGEMENT OF PHENOTHIAZINE TOXICITY

- Stabilize ABCs, including appropriate treatment of cardiac dysrhythmias, altered mental status, and hypotension with IV fluid therapy.
- Continuous ECG and cardiac monitoring
- Benzodiazepines (e.g., diazepam or lorazepam) for control of seizures
- Consider GI decontamination
  (1) Gastric lavage for large ingestions and recent ingestions *or*
  (2) Administration of activated charcoal (dose: 1 to 2 g/kg up to max 50 g)
- For cardiac dysrhythmias such as widened QRS complex of >100-msec duration (see tricyclic antidepressant toxicity, Figs. 17-28 through 17-30)
  (1) Sodium bicarbonate ($NaHCO_3$) 1 to 2 mEq/kg as an IV bolus for QRS widening, and repeat as necessary to narrow QRS interval
  (2) Care must be taken because QT prolongation may also occur with phenothiazine toxicity, and $NaHCO_3$ administration may actually exacerbate this condition by causing hypokalemia.
  (3) ABG analysis to monitor acid-base status (especially patients with ECG or mental status changes); arterial pH should not exceed 7.55 when administering sodium bicarbonate
- Central anticholinergic syndrome may require physostigmine.
- For patients presenting with acute dystonic reactions
  (1) Diphenhydramine (dose: IV or IM 1 mg/kg; IV given over 1 to 2 minutes [rapid push may cause seizures]) *or*
  (2) Benztropine mesylate (dose: IV or IM 0.5 to 1 mg for toddlers and 1 to 2 mg for adolescents)
- To prevent recurrence of extrapyramidal symptoms
  (1) Diphenhydramine (dose: 5 mg/kg per day divided qid; maximum 300 mg/d) *or*
  (2) Benztropine mesylate (dose: 0.5 mg bid for toddler and 1 mg bid for adolescents) is given orally.

DIAGNOSIS ACUTE ISONIAZID TOXICITY

Background

1. Isoniazid (INH) is an antimicrobial agent used to treat active tuberculosis or for prophylaxis in the event of a positive tuberculin skin test (purified protein derivative; PPD).
2. INH is also found in Rifamate (capsules which contain 150 mg of INH with 300 mg of rifampin).

Pharmacokinetics and Toxicity

1. A toxic dose of INH is believed to be between 30 and 40 mg/kg. Ingestion of 80 to 150 mg/kg produces severe CNS symptoms. Seizures are frequent manifestations of acute INH neurotoxicity. The dose of INH that can cause convulsions is variable, and may occur with ingestion of 40 mg/kg or less. Acute ingestion of 2 to 3 g causes acute toxicity in most individuals, and ingestion of 10 to 15 g frequently causes death if untreated or inappropriately treated.
2. INH and its metabolites produce toxicity by creating pyridoxine deficiency and a subsequent reduction in the synthesis of γ-aminobutyric acid (GABA; Fig. 17-20).

Emergency Department Treatment and Evaluation

1. The history should focus on determining the preparation involved, the dosage, timing of exposure, and symptoms following ingestion.
2. Physical examination should focus on vital signs, cardiopulmonary assessment, abdominal pain, and neurological status.
3. Laboratory studies may be obtained to assess for renal function, acid-base status, rhabdomyolysis, and other causes of seizure activity. INH serum levels may be obtained to

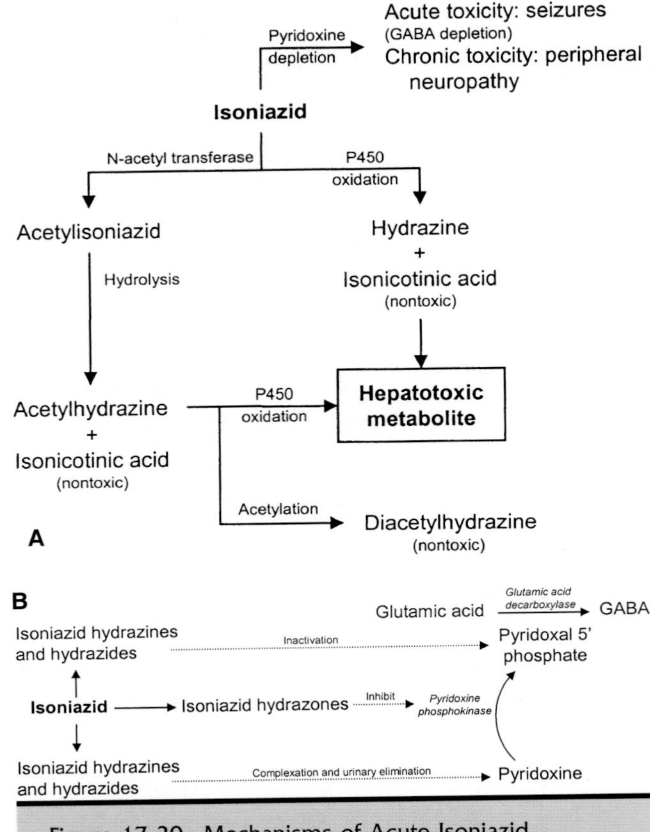

Figure 17-20. Mechanisms of Acute Isoniazid Neurotoxicity

A. The effect of isoniazid on pyridoxine, leading to reduced activation and a diminished supply of pyridoxine. *B*. The mechanism of the inactivation of pyridoxal 5′-phosphate resulting in the reduction of the synthesis of GABA. GABA is the main inhibitory neurotransmitter of the CNS and a decrease in the availability of GABA (with resultant loss of its vital inhibitory influence) is the presumed etiology of isoniazid-induced seizures. Isoniazid also enhances inactivation of GABA via transamination. (Reproduced with permission from: Osborn HH: Antituberculous agents. In: *Goldfrank's Toxicologic Emergencies*, 6th ed. New York, McGraw-Hill, 1998, p. 729.)

confirm the diagnosis, but results are not available in a clinically useful time frame.

4. If indicated, consider chest radiographs, head CT, and lumbar puncture to evaluate for other causes of altered mental status and seizures.

Differential Diagnosis

1. Other causes of increased anion gap metabolic acidosis (see mnemonics ACIDOSIS and MUDPILES, Box 17-2).
2. Other toxicologic causes of seizure activity with anion gap acidosis (due to lactic acidosis) include lidocaine, tricyclic antidepressants, neuroleptic agents, hypoglycemic agents, sympathomimetic agents, and local anesthetics (see mnemonic CAMPHOR BALLS, page 658).
3. Nontoxicologic causes of seizure activity with anion gap acidosis include hypoglycemia, hypoxia, sepsis, meningitis, and intracranial hemorrhage.

Consultations

Poison control center and psychiatry (if suicidal intent)

Emergency Department Treatment and Disposition

1. Treatment should focus on immediate treatment of seizures and airway management.
2. Admit all patients who present with altered mental status, seizures, or other signs of serious toxicity to an ICU for continuous monitoring and supportive care.

Clinical Pearls: Acute Isoniazid Toxicity

1. Acute INH toxicity is characterized by the classic triad of refractory seizures, coma, and increased anion gap metabolic acidosis.
2. *Consider acute INH toxicity in any patient presenting with seizures (with or without fever) that are refractory to conventional anticonvulsant therapy.*
3. In a patient with known access to INH, seizures should be considered to be caused by INH toxicity unless proven otherwise.
4. INH-induced seizures are usually generalized tonic-clonic seizures and often progress to status epilepticus.
5. Acute INH toxicity usually occurs as a result of an intentional ingestion.
6. Acute INH toxicity causes an increased anion gap metabolic acidosis, a lactic acidosis due to seizure activity.
7. Acute INH toxicity can cause hyperglycemia, ketonemia, glycosuria, ketonuria, elevated beta-hydroxybutyrate and can mimic diabetic ketoacidosis.

BOX 17-30. CLINICAL FEATURES OF ACUTE ISONIAZID TOXICITY

Clinical signs and symptoms:

- Classic triad of acute INH toxicity: refractory seizures, coma, and increased anion gap metabolic acidosis
- Vital signs: hyperthermia, tachycardia, hypotension (severe toxicity)
- HEENT: optic neuritis (chronic therapy), nystagmus, mydriasis, photophobia, blurred vision
- Cardiovascular: tachycardia, cyanosis, hypotension and shock in severe intoxication
- Pulmonary: Kussmaul's respirations (as a response to metabolic acidosis), respiratory depression (from seizure activity)
- Gastrointestinal: nausea, vomiting
- Neurologic: dizziness, seizures (frequently occur within the first 2 hours postingestion, refractory in nature), coma or altered mental status, slurred speech, hyper- or areflexia, psychosis, hallucinations, peripheral neuropathy (chronic overdose)
- Fluids and electrolytes: increased anion gap metabolic acidosis, hyperglycemia, ketonemia, lactic acidosis
- Renal: anuria or oliguria

Laboratory values:

- ABG with serum electrolytes will reveal increased anion gap metabolic acidosis.
- Hyperglycemia, ketonemia, glycosuria, and ketonuria may be present (*mimics diabetic ketoacidosis*)
- Elevated liver enzymes (in up to 40% of patients taking therapeutic doses of INH)
- Elevated serum creatinine (with prolonged seizure activity resulting in rhabdomyolysis)
- Elevated urine myoglobin (with rhabdomyolysis)
- Elevated serum creatine kinase (with rhabdomyolysis)
- Increased serum INH levels (helps in confirming diagnosis, but results are not available in a clinically useful time frame)

BOX 17-31. MANAGEMENT OF ACUTE ISONIAZID TOXICITY

- Stabilize ABCs, including treatment of hypotension, altered mental status, and seizures.
- Consider GI decontamination
  (1) Gastric lavage in patients presenting with large ingestion or signs of toxicity within 1 hour of ingestion
  (2) Activated charcoal (dose: 1 to 2 g/kg up to maximum of 50 g)
- Obtain serum electrolytes, ABG, creatine kinase, LFTs, and urinalysis to evaluate acid-base status and to evaluate for rhabdomyolysis.
- *Specific antidote: pyridoxine* (Fig. 17-21)
  (1) Pyridoxine is also referred to as vitamin B6.
  (2) Repletes pyridoxine deficiency created by INH
  (3) Indicated for the treatment of seizures induced by known INH overdose or for empiric use in patients presenting with seizures of unknown origin refractory to benzodiazepines and other conventional anticonvulsants
  (4) If the amount of INH ingested is known, pyridoxine should be given on a gram-for-gram basis (*1 gram of pyridoxine for every gram of INH*).
  (5) If the amount of INH ingested is unknown, an empiric dose of pyridoxine of 70 mg/kg to a maximum of 5 g (adult dose) should be given over 15 to 30 minutes.
    a. If seizures persist: the 70-mg/kg dose (maximum of 5 g) should be repeated.
    b. If seizures continue to persist despite administration of a total of 70 mg/kg (or 10 grams) of pyridoxine, reconsider the diagnosis (multiple large doses of pyridoxine should be avoided).
  (6) If no IV pyridoxine is available, crushed vitamin B_6 tablets can be given orally as a slurry (1 gram for each gram of INH ingested).
  (7) Adverse effects of pyridoxine therapy (usually in the setting of chronic administration) include delayed peripheral neuropathy and ataxia, seizures, or paralysis, which reverse following discontinuation of pyridoxine. Death has also been reported after very high doses.

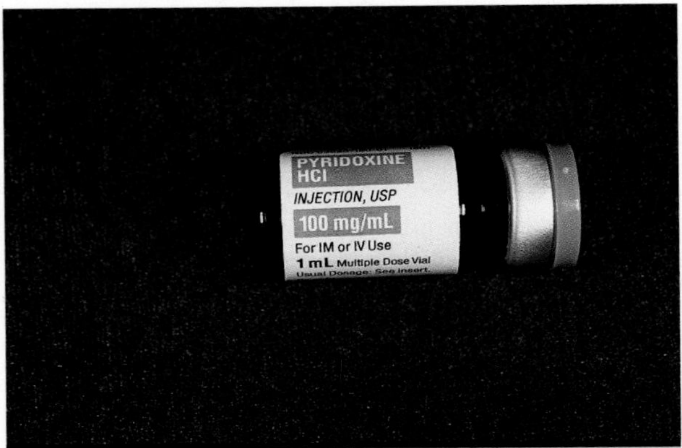

Figure 17-21. Pyridoxine, an Antidote for Isoniazid-Induced Seizures

Dose for pyridoxine is 1 gram per gram of isoniazid ingested, or 70 mg/kg if the quantity is unknown. Shown above is 100 mg/mL vial of pyridoxine; however in many hospitals, the only available concentration is 50 mg of pyridoxine per 1-mL vial. Thus in a patient presenting with an unknown amount of isoniazid ingestion, 100 vials need to be used to provide 5 grams of pyridoxine. This may quickly deplete hospital stores. *Do not lose your patience while opening 100 vials for a patient presenting with status epilepticus thought to be due to acute isoniazid toxicity.* For example: A 14-year-old girl was brought to the ED in status epilepticus from school. She continued to seize after IV diazepam and a loading dose of phenytoin. During a quick differential diagnosis of her refractory seizures, her ABG showed severe metabolic acidosis (pH 6.987 and BE −18.3 mmol/L) and increased anion gap metabolic acidosis (Na^+ 140 mmol/L, K^+ 3.1 mmol/L, Cl^- 105 mmol/L, HCO_3^- 10 mmol/L, anion gap 25), which led to a possible diagnosis of an acute isoniazid-induced seizure. She received 5 g of pyridoxine and her seizures were controlled. When her mother arrived at ED, we learned that this patient was recently diagnosed with a positive PPD test, and she was receiving 300 mg of isoniazid daily. She had an argument with her stepfather and subsequently she took a total of 20 tablets of isoniazid (a total dose of 6000 mg = 110 mg/kg for her weight) with the intent of killing herself.

DIAGNOSIS

DRUGS OF ABUSE

Background

1. Commonly abused drugs discussed here can be broadly classified as stimulants, sedatives, or hallucinogens.
   a. Stimulants include "ecstasy" (3,4-methlenedioxymethamphetamine, or MDMA) (Fig. 17-22), methamphetamine (Fig. 17-23), ephedra, and other products.
   b. Depressants discussed here include PCP and ketamine (Fig. 17-24), which are similar in chemical structure and clinical effect; γ-hydroxybutyrate (GHB) and analogues including GBL and butanediol; nitrous oxide; marijuana; and heroin and other opiates.
   c. Hallucinogens discussed here include LSD, mescaline, and psilocybin (hallucinogenic mushrooms).

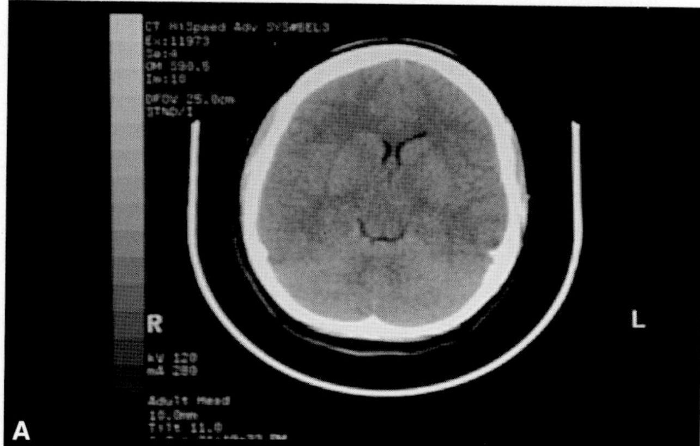

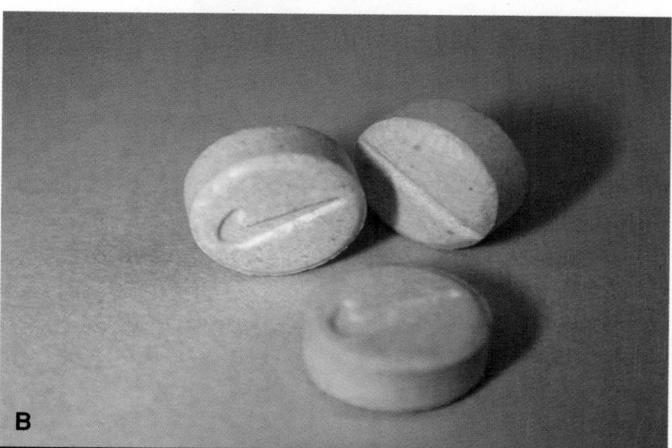

Figure 17-22. Ecstasy-Induced SIADH.

A. Head CT of a young woman who experienced ecstasy-induced SIADH shows effacement of the brain with disappearance of gyri and sulci as well as slit ventricles. Her serum sodium was 119 mmol/L. She had taken the drug at a party the previous evening, and was brought to the ED by college roommates who noticed her to be delirious the following morning. *B*. Ecstasy tablets seized in New York City.

2. The clinical effect of a substance is the result of both its pharmacologic action and the individual's response to it. Thus although PCP is a sedative, a user may become very agitated.
3. Certain drugs including PCP, ketamine, dextromethorphan, and MDMA may cause distortion of sensory perception or hallucinations, in addition to stimulation or sedation.
4. Although the percentage of high school students surveyed who admit to abusing drugs has been declining over the past 5 years, the youngest age at which drug use is occurring has been decreasing. Children as young as 7 and 8 years of age are capable of volitionally abusing drugs.
5. Drugs of abuse come from a variety of sources:
   a. Legitimate and illegitimate sources of pharmaceuticals such as oxycodone or methylphenidate

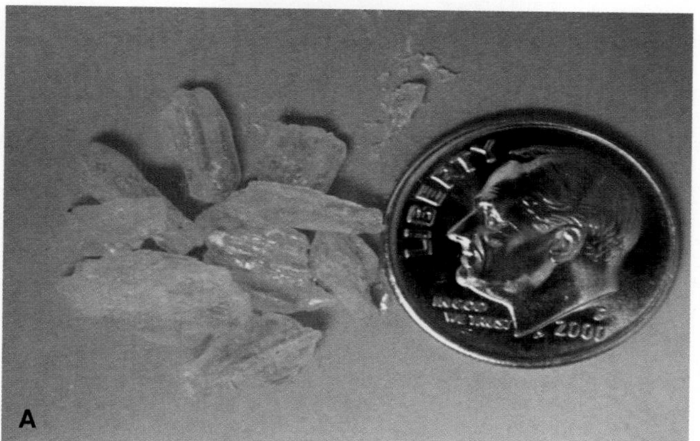

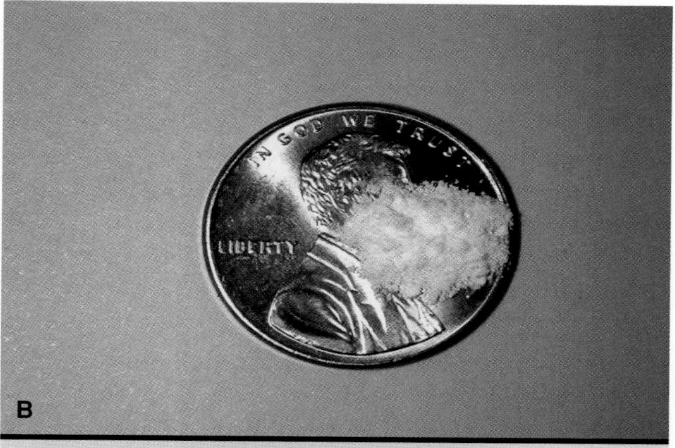

Figure 17-23. Methamphetamine

A. Methamphetamine in crystalline form. *B*. Methamphetamine on a penny. This small amount approximates that typically used to maintain euphoria or a "high" over a 24-hour period.

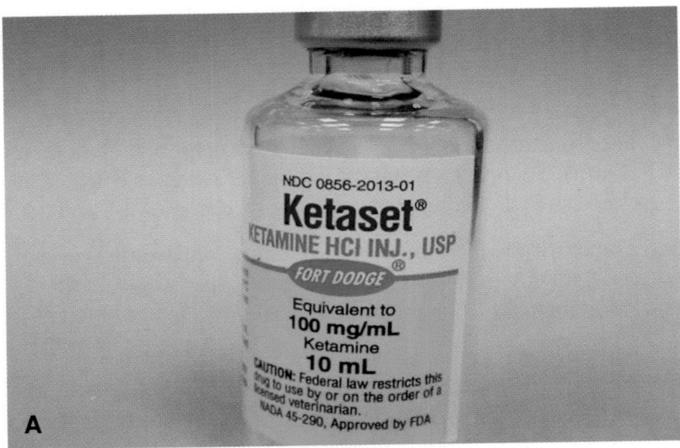

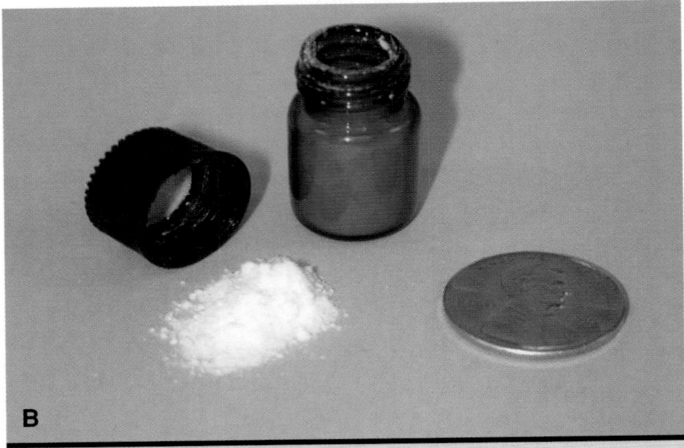

Figure 17-24. Ketamine

A. Ketamine hydrochloride. Veterinary ketamine in commercially available form is commonly diverted for illegitimate use. *B*. "Cooked" ketamine. Ketamine that was heated to precipitate the active ingredient from the liquid solution.

b. Dextromethorphan, ephedra, and nitrous oxide are legal over-the-counter agents. Hallucinogenic mushrooms (*Psilocybe* spp.) may be foraged in the wild. Children without access to "harder drugs," particularly adolescents in rural areas, may prefer these types of easy-to-obtain agents.
c. Marijuana, MDMA, methamphetamine, PCP, ketamine, GHB, heroin, and LSD are typically purchased through drug dealers.

Pharmacokinetics

1. Amphetamines, PCP, ketamine, dextromethorphan, and heroin:
   a. Rapid absorption after use by any route
   b. Peak concentrations occur within minutes to 2 hours, with variable half-lives.
   c. Undergo hepatic metabolism and renal elimination with variable half-lives.
2. GHB and nitrous oxide:
   a. Ultrarapid absorption, minimal metabolism, and rapid excretion
   b. Nitrous oxide clearance is typically complete within minutes, and a patient presenting to the hospital is rare due to its rapid elimination by the body (unless toxicity occurred from in-hospital use of nitrous oxide).
3. LSD, mescaline and psilocybin: delayed absorption of a typically miniscule quantity of drug with inconsequential metabolism
4. Marijuana (Fig. 17-25):
   a. Rapid absorption after smoking and delayed (approximately 1 to 2 hours) absorption after ingestion
   b. Undergoes extensive hepatic metabolism, and the half-life varies according to previous exposure

Emergency Department Evaluation

1. The history should focus on determining the agent involved, the dose, time of ingestion, and intent. Use of drugs of abuse with intent of suicide or self-harm is significantly different than recreational use, and warrants psychiatric consultation. The patient's mental status may impede obtaining a thorough history.
2. Physical examination should focus on vital signs, including evaluation for CNS toxicity and observation of mental status.

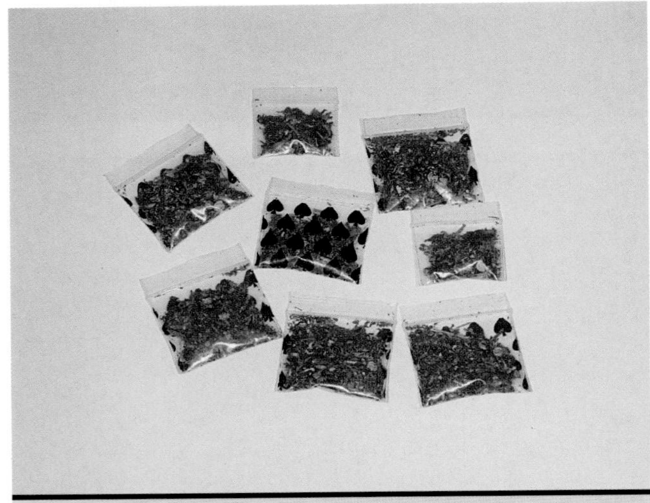

Figure 17-25. Marijuana

Marijuana leaves in small plastic bags (a total of 8 bags) were found on an adolescent male who was brought to the ED with a stab wound to the chest. Marijuana refers to material obtained from the leaves and flowers of the Indian hemp plant, *Cannabis sativa*. A few examples of other names by which it is known include pot, weed, smoke tea, joint, hashish, Colombian ganga, ace, bush, rope, Jamaican, and Panama red. Marijuana is the most commonly used illegal substance in the Unites States. After nicotine, alcohol, and caffeine, marijuana is probably the most commonly abused substance in the world.

Differential Diagnosis

1. Other agents causing CNS depression; ethanol is a readily accessible drug and is often used in conjunction with these drugs of abuse.
2. Other etiologies of CNS depression (e.g., meningitis, intracranial hemorrhage, cerebral ischemia; see mnemonic COMATOSE PATIENT, Box 13-4).

Consultations

Poison control center and psychiatry (suicidal intent)

Emergency Department Management and Disposition

1. In rare cases, GI decontamination (see page 621) may be of potential benefit. It is uncommon to have a patient who has ingested such a drug within the previous hour, which is the window of time typically considered appropriate to perform GI decontamination.
2. Amphetamines:
   a. Cases involving significant hypertension or any end-organ manifestation of hypertensive injury (e.g., cerebrovascular accident, myocardial ischemia, infarction) may be treated with calcium channel antagonists, nitrates, or a combined regimen of an alpha-blocker and beta-blocker.
   b. Use of a beta-blocker alone without another agent to cause vasodilation is dangerous and contraindicated because it may cause a dramatic rise in blood pressure.
3. Patients with CNS or respiratory depression, cardiovascular toxicity requiring treatment, cardiac dysrhythmias, or systemic toxicity resulting from toxicity should be admitted to an ICU for monitoring.

Clinical Pearls: Drugs of Abuse

1. Even with a history of using drugs, all patients with altered mental status should have assessment of serum glucose, and further neurologic investigation such as head CT should be considered as necessary.
2. Agitation, hallucinations, or psychosis may be very distressing for patients, parents, and staff, but these symptoms typically resolve within hours and are not life-threatening.
3. *Agitation or psychosis should be treated with benzodiazepines, not antipsychotics.*
4. Cardiovascular toxicity and respiratory depression are the typical mechanisms by which drugs of abuse may cause severe morbidity or mortality.
5. In hypertensive patients, administration of a beta-blocker without simultaneous use of another agent to lower blood pressure, such as an alpha-blocker, may cause a dramatic rise in blood pressure and end-organ damage such as a cerebrovascular accident.
6. Drugs of abuse or toxicology screening are incapable of aiding the clinical management of patients and should never be used for this purpose. Except for forensic purposes, these tests lack utility and should not be routinely used.
7. Except for cocaine, toxicity from drugs of abuse does not result in seizures. Patients experiencing seizures should be evaluated for other toxicities (e.g., tricyclic antidepressant ingestion; see mnemonic CAMPHOR BALLS, Box 17-22) or medical problems (e.g., intracranial hemorrhage).

BOX 17-32. GENERAL CHARACTERISTICS OF TOXICITY DUE TO DRUGS OF ABUSE

Clinical manifestations:

(1) Stimulants: cardiovascular and CNS stimulation, psychomotor agitation, hallucinations

a. Vital signs: tachycardia, hypertension
b. Cardiovascular: typically sinus tachycardia, may have fatal dysrhythmias (severe toxicity)
c. Gastrointestinal: vomiting
d. Neurologic: hyperaltertness, restlessness, agitation, psychosis, hallucinations

(2) Depressants: respiratory and CNS depression

a. Vital signs: bradycardia, hypotension
b. Cardiovascular: typically sinus bradycardia
c. Gastrointestinal: bowel motility diminished with opioids, vomiting with other drugs
d. Neurologic: somnolence, lethargy, coma, nystagmus (PCP, ketamine)

Laboratory values

- Serum glucose (always indicated, especially in patients with altered mental status)
- Serum electrolytes, glucose, BUN, Cr, anion gap, and urine myoglobin (evaluation for metabolic derangement and rhabdomyolysis)
- 12-lead ECG
- Obtain serum acetaminophen and salicylate levels for coingestions (suicidal intent)
- A diagnosis of toxicity from drugs of abuse is always clinical:

(1) Drugs-of-abuse screening or toxicology testing may be incapable of confirming or disproving intoxication with abusable drugs.
(2) Toxicology lab testing should not be routinely used in cases of suspected drug of abuse toxicity and should never be used to guide clinical management.
(3) Toxicology lab testing should only be routinely used for forensic purposes (e.g., in children too young to volitionally use abusable drugs, in whom the presence of such drugs would corroborate child abuse).
(4) Qualitative determination of the presence of a limited number of drugs of abuse may be performed (useful for forensic purposes only).

BOX 17-33. TOXICITY OF SELECTED DRUGS OF ABUSE

- *Amphetamines:* (increased sympathomimetic activity and general increase of catecholamine release including norepinephrine, epinephrine, dopamine, and to a lesser extent serotonin)
  (1) CNS stimulation: insomnia, hyperalertness, agitation or psychosis, seizures (rare)
  (2) "Tweaking," severe agitation and psychosis that occurs with methamphetamine binging, poses a danger to both the unrestrained patient and others.
  (3) Cardiovascular stimulation: hypertensive emergency, cerebrovascular accident, intracranial hemorrhage, myocardial infarction
  (4) Metabolic stimulation: hyperthermia, rhabdomyolysis, disseminated intravascular coagulation (DIC)
- *MDMA (ecstasy):*
  (1) General toxic effects of other amphetamines
  (2) Unique toxicity includes syndrome of inappropriate secretion of antidiuretic hormone (SIADH; particularly in females) and life-threatening serotonin syndrome (Fig. 17-22)
- *GHB:*
  (1) Dose-dependent CNS depression (activity at GABA receptors)
  (2) Patients typically comatose with normal vital signs
  (3) Often causes myoclonus that may be misinterpreted as seizures
  (4) May cause respiratory depression that rarely requires endotracheal intubation (respiratory depression is unique in that it typically lasts minutes to several hours, after which patients abruptly awake to baseline health status)
- *Heroin:*
  (1) Active at opioid receptors
  (2) Classic opioid toxidrome (miosis, respiratory depression, and CNS depression)
- *LSD, mescaline, and psilocybin:*
  (1) Hallucinogen toxicity typically comes to the attention of physicians when a patient has a psychiatric disturbance (e.g., a "bad trip"). This may involve overwhelming fear, anxiety, and agitation.
  (2) Minor toxicity of hallucinogens includes nausea.
- *PCP, ketamine, and dextromethorphan:*
  (1) Sedation (antagonism at NMDA receptor) and dysphoria or hallucinosis (binding at opioid receptor)
  (2) Use of these agents may result in a clinical state anywhere on a spectrum between coma and agitated delirium.
  (3) PCP is associated with greater agitation and delirium, whereas dextromethorphan is associated with sedation and coma.
  (4) Nystagmus is typical with ketamine or PCP toxicity (*clinical clue in diagnosis*).
- *Dextromethorphan:*
  (1) Occasionally results in respiratory depression for which naloxone therapy may be attempted
  (2) May cause choreoathetosis, myoclonus, or other movement disorder (particularly in children)
- *Marijuana:*
  (1) Marijuana lacks severe acute toxicity, in contrast to other drugs of abuse.
  (2) Adverse clinical effects might include somnolence or sedation.
  (3) Other signs and symptoms from marijuana use are likely to be the result of marijuana laced with other drugs.
  (4) The most common adulterant in marijuana is PCP (PCP-laced marijuana may be referred to by a number of street names, including "*dip*", "*wet*", "*hydro*", or "*illy*", as well as numerous others).

BOX 17-34. MANAGEMENT OF TOXICITY DUE TO DRUGS OF ABUSE

- Stabilize the ABCs, including assessment of serum glucose.
- Continuous cardiac and ECG monitoring
- Supportive care is the mainstay of subsequent therapy (most patients require only assessment and observation).
- Respiratory depression resulting from opioids should be treated with a brief period of assisted ventilation followed by parenteral naloxone with repeat dosing as needed.
- As indicated, endotracheal intubation and ventilatory support for patients who have ingested GHB (typically only necessary for 1 to 4 hours)
- Agitation
  (1) Regardless of its etiology, agitation or psychosis is treated similarly.
  (2) Even the most agitated delirium is likely to improve within hours.
  (3) *Must* ensure that agitation is not the result of other causes (e.g., hypoglycemia, hypoxia)
  (4) Control agitation, psychosis, or unpleasant hallucinations with benzodiazepines (e.g., diazepam or lorazepam). Both agitation or anxiety should be treated with escalating doses of parenteral benzodiazepines for sedation.
  (5) Avoid the use of antipsychotic drugs such as haloperidol (risk of hyperthermia in an agitated patient).
  (6) The duration of agitation in most patients with toxicity from drugs of abuse is typically brief and does not warrant antipsychotic use.
- Amphetamines
  (1) The main goal of treatment is supportive care and maintenance of vital signs within acceptable limits.
  (2) Use of IV benzodiazepines is the first-line therapy (may improve both agitation and cardiovascular stimulation).
  (3) Treat cardiovascular stimulation with an agent that will counteract both the inotropic and vasoconstrictive effects of amphetamines (e.g., calcium channel blockers, nitrates, or a combination of alpha-blockers and beta-blockers).

DIAGNOSIS

CAUSTICS

Background

1. Caustics are agents that cause both functional and histologic damage on contact with body tissues.
2. Most cases occur in the pediatric population, especially in children less than 5 years old.
3. Caustic substances are commonly associated with extremes of pH such as strong acids (low pH) and strong alkalis (bases; high pH). However, they are a diverse group of agents and other factors besides pH determine the potential for tissue injury. Examples of various caustic agents are listed in Box 17-35.

Pathophysiology and Toxicity

1. Factors affecting the extent of injury from caustic agents include specific type of agent ingested (i.e., acid or alkali, solid or liquid, and its concentration), the amount, the duration of tissue contact, and the presence of food in the stomach.
2. Intrinsic properties of the particular caustic agent such as pH or titratable reserve are also important. *Titratable reserve* is the amount of neutralizing substance that is required to bring the agent to a physiologic pH. The larger the titratable reserve, the greater the caustic potential.
3. Acids cause coagulation necrosis and tend to form an eschar that theoretically may limit tissue penetration. This potential mitigating factor to tissue damage is insignificant, however, because perforation does in fact occur.
4. Alkalis cause liquefactive necrosis and result in a deeper burn. In general, solid alkalis may readily adhere to the oropharynx and upper esophagus, while liquid alkalis are more likely to cause injury to the distal esophagus and stomach (Fig. 17-26).
5. Acids may be systemically absorbed and cause hemolysis of red blood cells (RBCs) and/or acidemia.
6. Anatomic areas of narrowing such as the upper part of the esophagus near the cricopharyngeus muscle, the mid-esophagus near the aortic arch, and the distal esophagus

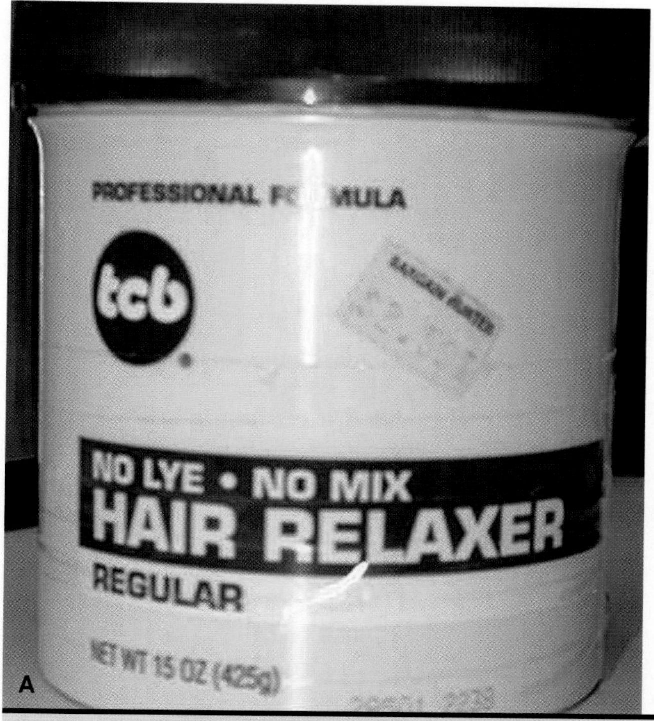

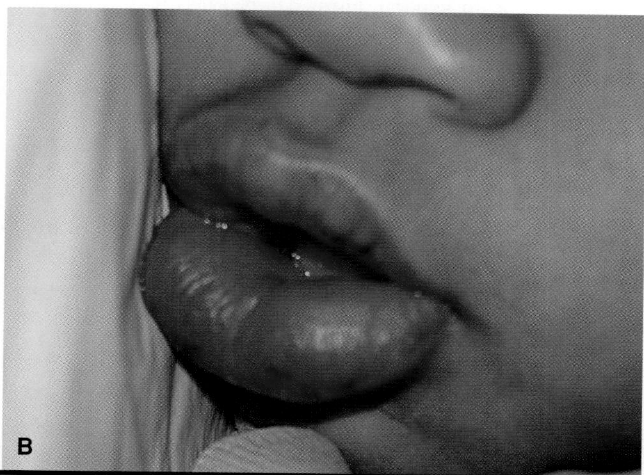

Figure 17-26. Caustic Injury

A. A 16-month-old boy was found with the container on the left, and with the substance from the container on his mouth and hands. Lithium hydroxide, a strong base, was noted to be one of the major ingredients. He was brought to the ED about 4 hours after the exposure. He was noted to be drooling and had two episodes of emesis. *B*. Physical examination revealed oropharyngeal burns with erythema and swelling of the lips as shown. Fiberoptic laryngoscopy was performed and there was no evidence of edema of the patient's vocal cords or hypopharynx. Endoscopy revealed no evidence of injury and he was admitted to the ICU. One day later he was able to eat and drink without difficulty and was discharged home.

proximal to the lower esophageal sphincter, are all sites that are predisposed to injury from caustic agents.

Emergency Department Evaluation

1. The history should focus on determining the agent involved, the amount and time of ingestion, and intent. The patient's mental status may impede obtaining a thorough history.
2. Contact with any external or internal tissue surface by a caustic agent can result in injury.
3. Initial stabilization of the ABCs is crucial because injury occurs so rapidly. Two large-bore IVs may be necessary to administer fluids.
4. Acute complications include:
    a. Airway injury
    b. Aspiration
    c. Gastrointestinal perforation and/or hemorrhage
    d. Acidosis (from systemic absorption of acids) resulting in hemolysis, myocardial depression, and shock; tissue necrosis
    e. Death
5. Long-term or delayed complications include:
    a. GI strictures that may result in repeated hospitalizations, nutritional deficiencies, and multiple esophageal dilatations
    b. Pyloric obstruction and impaired gastric function
    c. Other laryngotracheal and pharyngeal injuries such as stenosis or reflux can contribute to further morbidity and patient discomfort.
    d. Squamous cell carcinoma of the esophagus; alkaline injury of the esophagus is reported to increase the risk of the development of this complication 1000-fold, with a latency of 25 to 40 years.

Consultations

Poison control center, gastroenterology, surgery, and psychiatry (if intentional)

Emergency Department Management and Disposition

1. If a solid has been ingested, a small quantity of water may be given to dissolve and subsequently wash away the agent.

This will also be effective therapy if the caustic material becomes lodged in an area of anatomic narrowing.

2. Critically ill patients may benefit from surgical intervention to remove necrotic tissue. However, unless there is obvious perforation, presence of peritoneal signs, or persistent hypotension, there are no other reliable indications for surgery.
3. Various endoscopic grading systems of gastrointestinal burns exist. In general, burns can be classified as follows:

Clinical Pearls: Caustics

1. Most tissue injury from caustic agents occurs immediately upon contact with tissue.
2. Dilution or neutralization is *not* recommended for liquid agents.
3. *Absence of obvious burns on physical examination does not exclude significant distal injury.*

Grade	Findings/prognosis	Implications
Grade 0	No injury	No stricture formation
Grade 1	Hypertension or edema of mucosa	No stricture formation
Grade IIA	Submucosal lesions, ulcerations and exudates	Usually no stricture formation
Grade IIB	Circumferential	Often develop strictures
Grade III	Deep ulcers; necrosis	Almost always develop strictures; other complications

4. Treatment with both steroids and antibiotics of grade IIB esophageal burns within 24 hours of injury may prevent stricture formation.
   a. Prednisone 1 to 2 mg/kg per day to a maximum of 60 mg/day, tapered over a 3-week course, has been recommended.
   b. Choice of antibiotic should be one that is effective against oral flora.
5. All patients presenting with symptoms with or without clinically evident oropharyngeal burns need to be admitted. All patients with intentional ingestions also need to be admitted for endoscopy.

4. Child abuse should be suspected in exposures in very small children and infants.
5. Endoscopic evaluation should be performed within 24 hours if possible.
6. Patients with significant caustic injuries to the GI tract require long-term follow-up for many years to monitor development of complications.

BOX 17-35. HOUSEHOLD CAUSTIC SUBSTANCES

Chemical agent	*Commercial applications*
Acetic acid	Permanent wave neutralizers, photographic stop bath
Acids (tungstic, picric, tannic)	Industrial use
Ammonia (ammonium hydroxide)	Toilet bowl cleaners, metal cleaners and polishes, hair dyes and tints, anti-rust products, jewelry cleaners, floor strippers, glass cleaners, wax removers
Benzalkonium chloride	Detergents
Boric acid	Roach powders, water softeners, germicide
Cantharides (Spanish fly)	Aphrodisiac (in animals), hair tonic, illicit abortifacient
Formaldehyde, formic acid	Deodorizing tablets, plastic menders, fumigant, embalming agent
Hydrochloric acid (muriatic acid)	Metal and toilet bowl cleaners
Hydrofluoric acid	Anti-rust products, glass etching, microchip etching
Iodine	Antiseptics
Mercuric chloride	Preservative
Methylethyl ketone peroxide	Industrial synthetic agent
Oxalic acid	Disinfectants, household bleach, metal cleaning liquids, anti-rust products, furniture polish
Phenol (creosol, creosote)	Antiseptics, preservatives
Phosphoric acid	Toilet bowl cleaners
Phosphorus	Matches, rodenticides, fireworks, insecticides
Potassium permanganate	Illicit abortifacient, antiseptic solution
Selenious acid	Gun bluing
Sodium hydroxide (lye)	Detergents, Clinitest tablets, paint removers, drain cleaners and openers, oven cleaners
Sodium borates, carbonates, phosphates, and silicates	Detergents, electric dishwasher preparations, water softeners
Sodium hypochlorite	Bleaches, cleaners
Sulfuric acid	Automobile batteries, drain cleaners
Zinc chloride	Soldering flux

BOX 17-36. CLINICAL FEATURES OF CAUSTIC EXPOSURE

Signs and symptoms

- Pain is usually the first symptom.
- Most caustic agents are ingested and may result in pain localized to the oropharynx, chest, and abdomen.
- Upper airway injury may result in development of stridor.
- Rapid deterioration of respiratory status may occur.
- GI effects include nausea, vomiting, drooling, and inability to swallow.
- *Although signs of physical injury around the mouth and oropharynx may be visualized, significant esophageal injury may still be present in the absence of physical examination findings.*
- *Burns may be seen on the face and upper chest (i.e., "dribble burns").*
- Ocular injury may occur, and examination of the eyes for pH, abrasions, and ulcers is very important.
- Chest examination may reveal subcutaneous emphysema, abnormal breath sounds, and pericardial friction rub (Hamman's crunch).
- Abdominal examination may show pain or tenderness, and peritoneal signs may be present (peritoneal signs may not be detectable if acute perforation occurs early in the course).

Laboratory values

- Obtain serum electrolytes, glucose, BUN, Cr, urinalysis
- Serial CBCs may show decreasing hemoglobin/hematocrit indicative of hemorrhage, or decreasing platelets due to development of disseminated intravascular coagulation.
- Serial PT, INR, and PTTs may show coagulopathy.
- Arterial blood gas may show metabolic acidosis or respiratory alkalosis.
  (1) Metabolic acidosis may be lactic or nonlactic (from systemic absorption of acids).
  (2) Respiratory alkalosis may result from hyperventilation.
- Electrolytes may reveal anion gap acidosis.
  (1) From a lactic acidosis *or*
  (2) From systemic absorption of an acid (with an anion not taken into account by the anion gap; e.g., sulfuric acid) or non–anion gap acidosis (e.g., systemic absorption of chloride from hydrochloric acid)
- ECG may show tachycardia, dysrrhythmias, or acute myocardial ischemia or infarction.
- Chest and abdominal radiographs may show pneumomediastinum, pneumothorax, subcutaneous emphysema, pleural effusions, or pneumoperitoneum.
- Coingestants (e.g., acetaminophen) and subsequent toxidromes should be sought for patients who present with intentional ingestion.
- Type and screen for blood products if indicated.
- Imaging studies such as contrast studies with Gastrografin or barium and computed tomography are not useful in the acute setting.

BOX 17-37. MANAGEMENT OF CAUSTIC EXPOSURES

- Stabilize ABCs, including appropriate treatment of airway injury and hypotension.
- Intubation may be necessary for patients with respiratory distress (although injury usually occurs immediately, airway obstruction may progress over several hours).
- External decontamination is usually accomplished by copious irrigation with water.
- Gastrointestinal decontamination
  (1) Emesis should not be induced because tissue injury may be exacerbated by re-exposing potentially damaged areas.
  (2) In almost all cases, GI decontamination via gastric lavage or activated charcoal should *not* be performed.
    a. Activated charcoal should *not* be given because of its inability to adsorb most caustics, and if emergent endoscopy is performed, it will obscure the visualization of damaged tissue.
    b. Patients with very large ingestions (determined by history and presentation to the hospital within 30 to 60 minutes) might benefit from orogastric lavage (this is controversial and there is a definite increased risk of gastrointestinal perforation).
- Request immediate consultation services.
- Endoscopy is a useful diagnostic procedure in caustic ingestions.
  (1) Emergent endoscopy should be performed in children with unintentional ingestions if they have two of the following: vomiting (inability to drink), drooling, or stridor.
  (2) All patients with intentional suicidal ingestions should have endoscopy performed.
  (3) Optimal time to perform endoscopy is controversial, but it should be performed within 24 hours of injury.

DIAGNOSIS ETHANOL TOXICITY

Background

1. Ethanol, commonly referred to as alcohol, is one of the most frequently used and socially accepted drugs in the world. Ethanol abuse is a significant social disease afflicting many adults.
2. Ethanol is responsible for the most yearly toxicologic deaths in the 15- to 45-year-old age group.
3. In young children, ethanol exposures are usually unintentional and significant toxicity occasionally occurs. Common household products containing ethanol include mouthwashes, antitussive medications, perfumes and colognes.
4. In adolescents, intentional abuse of ethanol-containing beverages is extremely common and much more likely to be dangerous.
5. Ethanol concentration is expressed in various units, usually proof or percent. In the United States, *percent* refers to 1/2 of the *proof* value (i.e., 80 proof = 40% ethanol). In general discourse, *proof* is commonly used, but in science, percentage (or milligrams per deciliter) is used as the unit of concentration.

Pharmacokinetics and Toxicity

1. Pure ethanol is a colorless liquid hydrocarbon.
2. The mechanism of action in the CNS is not completely clear but is likely to be a combination of multiple receptor effects (i.e., GABA agonism, NMDA antagonism, etc).
3. Ethanol is rapidly absorbed from the gastrointestinal tract with a peak concentration usually occurring within 60 minutes of ingestion. Absorption may be delayed depending on the presence of food, coingestion of other drugs, and individual physiology.
4. Ethanol is primarily metabolized in the liver by alcohol dehydrogenase to acetaldehyde (using NAD^+ as a cofactor), which is converted to acetic acid by aldehyde dehydrogenase (also using NAD^+ as a cofactor). Other enzyme systems play a role in ethanol metabolism with chronic use, but are of little clinical significance in non–ethanol-dependent individuals unless the serum ethanol concentrations are very high.

Emergency Department Evaluation

1. The history should focus on determining the agent involved, the amount, time of ingestion, intent, possibility

of coingestants, and awareness of possible factors delaying absorption. The patient's mental status may impede obtaining a thorough history.

2. Depending on the age of the patient, quantity ingested, and the individual, clinical manifestations can be markedly different. In general, increasing concentrations of ethanol will result in CNS depression and occasionally respiratory depression. Occasionally, paradoxical CNS stimulation may occur from CNS disinhibition.
3. In cases of massive ingestions, respiratory depression, loss of protective reflexes, coma, and death may occur.
4. Laboratory tests should include serum chemistry (including calcium, magnesium, and phosphate), ketones, CBC, and ethanol concentration.
5. Coingestants (e.g., acetaminophen) and subsequent toxidromes should be sought in patients who present with intentional ingestion.

Differential Diagnosis

1. Altered mental status/coma from other etiology (see mnemonic COMATOSE PATIENT, page ???)
2. Overdose of other sedative-hypnotic agents (e.g., GHB, benzodiazepines, barbiturates)
3. Hypoglycemia from other etiology (e.g., oral hypoglycemia agents, salicylates)
4. Infection (e.g., meningitis, sepsis)
5. Head trauma
6. Ingestion of other alcohols (e.g., methanol, ethylene glycol)

Consultations

Poison control center and psychiatry (if intentional or suspected abuse)

Emergency Department Evaluation and Treatment

1. In patients with persistent altered mental status, other etiologies besides ethanol intoxication should be considered (see mnemonic COMATOSE PATIENT, Box 13-4).
2. Although individual variation exists, ethanol intoxication in non–alcohol dependent individuals is usually apparent at a blood ethanol concentration of 50 mg/dL.
3. Supportive care (i.e., intravenous fluids, warm blankets) is the mainstay of therapy.
4. Patients with simple intoxication may be discharged home after a period of observation.
5. Patients with hemodynamic instability, persistent altered mental status, and hypoglycemia should be admitted to the ICU for continuous monitoring and management. Patients with coingestants (especially with suicidal intent) should also be hospitalized.

Clinical Pearls: Ethanol Toxicity

1. Ethanol intoxication should be considered early in the differential diagnosis of altered mental status and/or hypoglycemia.
2. Ethanol metabolism interferes with gluconeogenesis and significant hypoglycemia may occur, especially in young children with low glycogen stores. Acute neuroglycopenia is known to cause generalized tonic-clonic seizures. Hypoglycemia in adolescents and healthy adults is less frequent.
3. Significant head or neck trauma may be overlooked in trauma patients who are intoxicated. Have a low threshold to perform a head CT to look for intracranial hemorrhage.
4. No measures of enhanced elimination of ethanol other than hemodialysis are effective at removing ethanol from the body.
5. Parents should be educated on proper storage of ethanol-containing beverages (Fig. 17-27). Older children may need to be referred for substance abuse counseling.
6. Toxic alcohols (i.e., methanol and ethylene glycol) may present in a similar manner to ethanol intoxication, but these patients can develop a persistent non-lactate, non-ketotic, anion gap metabolic acidosis. Suspicion of these agents must be high to prevent misdiagnosis.

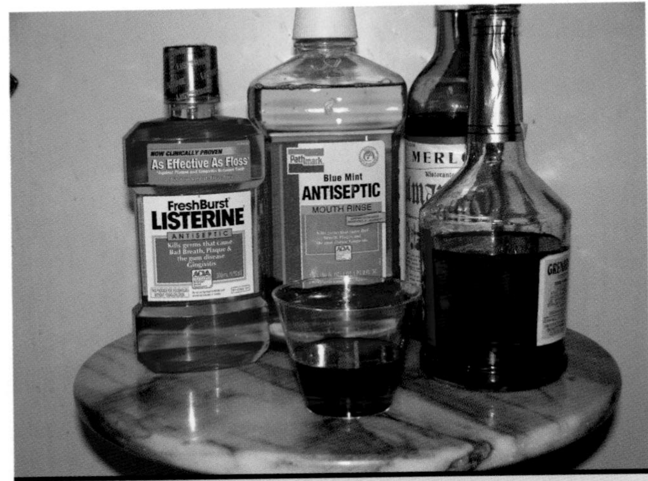

Figure 17-27. Common Sources of Ethanol for Young Infants and Children

Common household products containing ethanol that are accidentally ingested by infants and young children include mouthwashes, antitussive medications, perfumes and colognes. Alcohol content of these preparations varies significantly (e.g., the alcohol content in mouthwash varies from 5% to almost 30%). Accidental ingestion of wine from left over wine glasses after parties (especially New Year's or Christmas Eve) is a common cause of a toddler presenting with hypoglycemic seizures.

BOX 17-38. CLINICAL FEATURES OF ETHANOL TOXICITY

Clinical features:

- Vital signs: bradypnea, tachycardia, hypotension, hypothermia
- HEENT: head and neck trauma, nystagmus
- Cardiovascular: hypotension, reflex tachycardia, dysrhythmias (e.g., atrial fibrillation), myocardial depression, vasodilatation
- Pulmonary: hypoventilation, pulmonary edema, respiratory depression (severe poisoning)
- Gastrointestinal: nausea, vomiting, gastritis, pancreatitis
- Renal/electrolytes: dehydration
- Neurologic: lethargy, excitation, agitation, confusion, ataxia, delirium, seizures, coma
- Skin: flushing, urticaria, hypothermia

Laboratory features:

- Hypoglycemia
- Hyponatremia or hypernatremia
- Hypokalemia
- Hypocalcemia
- Hypomagnesemia
- Hyperamylasemia
- Hyperlipidemia
- Osmolar gap
- Elevated liver transaminases

BOX 17-39. MANAGEMENT OF ETHANOL TOXICITY

- Stabilize ABCs, including appropriate treatments for altered mental status (hypotension and reflex tachycardia may be prominent).
- A bedside fingerstick glucose
  (1) Must be performed on all patients with altered mental status
  (2) Give empiric treatment with IV dextrose if fingerstick glucose unavailable.
  (3) Treat hypoglycemia in adolescents with IV D_{50} (dose: 1 g/kg or 1 to 2 mL/kg)
  (4) Treat hypoglycemia in infants/children with IV D_{25} (dose: 2 to 4 mL/kg; D_{25} is made by diluting D_{50} with sterile water 1:1)
- Administer IV crystalloid if patient is volume depleted
- Obtain an ECG to detect any cardiac dysrhythmias and electrolyte disturbances.
- Cover patients with warm blankets.
- Gastrointestinal decontamination
  (1) Unnecessary and ineffective in most cases
  (2) Gastric lavage may be beneficial if a massive dose is suspected and respiratory depression has occurred.
  (3) Consider in patients presenting with a recent ingestion or serious coingestion.
- Consider hemodialysis for most severe cases (e.g., massive overdose with respiratory depression).

DIAGNOSIS TRICYCLIC ANTIDEPRESSANT TOXICITY

Background

1. Tricyclic antidepressants (TCAs; e.g., imipramine, amitriptyline, desipramine, nortriptyline) are commonly used medications for the treatment of various disorders including depression, nocturnal enuresis, anxiety disorders, attention-deficit/hyperactivity disorder (ADHD), and migraine headaches.
2. TCAs inhibit CNS reuptake of norepinephrine, serotonin, and dopamine. Although not clearly demonstrated, their mechanism of action for the treatment of depression may be due to an increase in CNS catecholamines.
3. Not all TCAs have three rings; hence the more accurate term *cyclic antidepressants* is often used.

Pharmacokinetics/Toxicity

1. There is rapid absorption from the gastrointestinal tract. Peak concentrations occur 2 to 8 hours after administration of a therapeutic dose. Most TCAs undergo extensive first-pass metabolism. However, after overdose, bioavailability may be increased as these metabolic pathways become saturated.
2. TCAs are highly lipophilic and in general have large volumes of distribution (15 to 40 L/kg). They are also largely protein bound. TCAs are metabolized by the cytochrome P450 enzyme system in the liver. Very little is excreted in the feces and urine.
3. Toxicity from TCAs may be mostly attributed to cardiovascular and CNS effects. Toxicity may occur with therapeutic doses as well, but usually is less clinically significant.

Emergency Department Evaluation

1. History should focus on determining the agent involved, dose, time of ingestion, and intent. The patient's mental status may impede obtaining a thorough history.
2. Physical examination should focus on vital signs, including evaluation for anticholinergic effects and observation of mental status.

Differential Diagnosis

1. Other agents causing CNS depression; especially important are those that impair cardiac conduction (e.g., type Ia antidysrhythmics, phenothiazines)
2. Other etiologies of CNS depression (e.g., meningitis, intracranial hemorrhage, cerebral ischemia)
3. Electrolyte imbalance leading to cardiac conduction abnormalities

Consultations

Poison control center and psychiatry (if indicated)

Emergency Department Management and Disposition

1. If patients have seizures, cardiac dysrhythmias, or CNS depression, they should be admitted to an ICU for monitoring and treatment.
2. Patients may be discharged from the ED after appropriate GI decontamination if they do not develop seizures, hypotension, or ECG changes after a 6-hour observation period. Evaluation by a psychiatrist should be performed for patients with intentional ingestion.

Clinical Pearls: Tricyclic Antidepressant Toxicity

1. TCAs are among the most common causes of reported deaths from pharmaceutical products in the United States.
2. TCAs have a low toxicity threshold and ingestion of small amounts may be toxic in young children.
3. TCA toxicity presents with cardiovascular and CNS effects.
4. A 12-lead ECG is the best diagnostic test to determine if a patient has significant toxicity from TCAs (Figs. 17-28, 17-29, and 17-30). A QRS duration of >100 msec is suggestive of TCA toxicity.
5. Physostigmine should not be given to reverse anticholinergic toxicity from TCAs because of potential deleterious cardiovascular consequences.

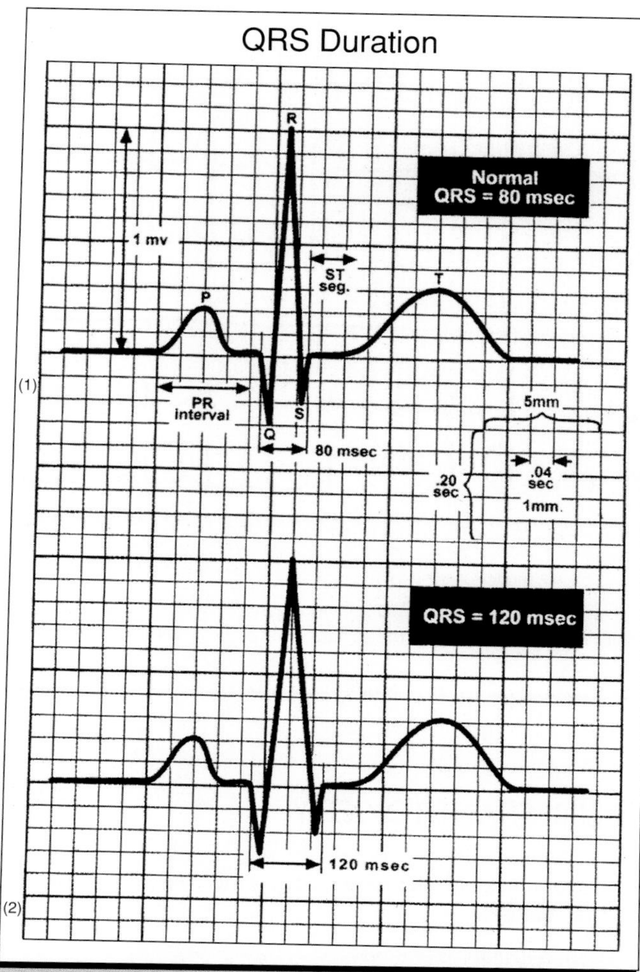

Figure 17-28. QRS Duration in Tricyclic Antidepressant Toxicity

Example of QRS widening on electrocardiography. (Reproduced with permission from: McGuigan ME: Poisoning potpourri. *Pediatr Rev* 2001;22:295.)

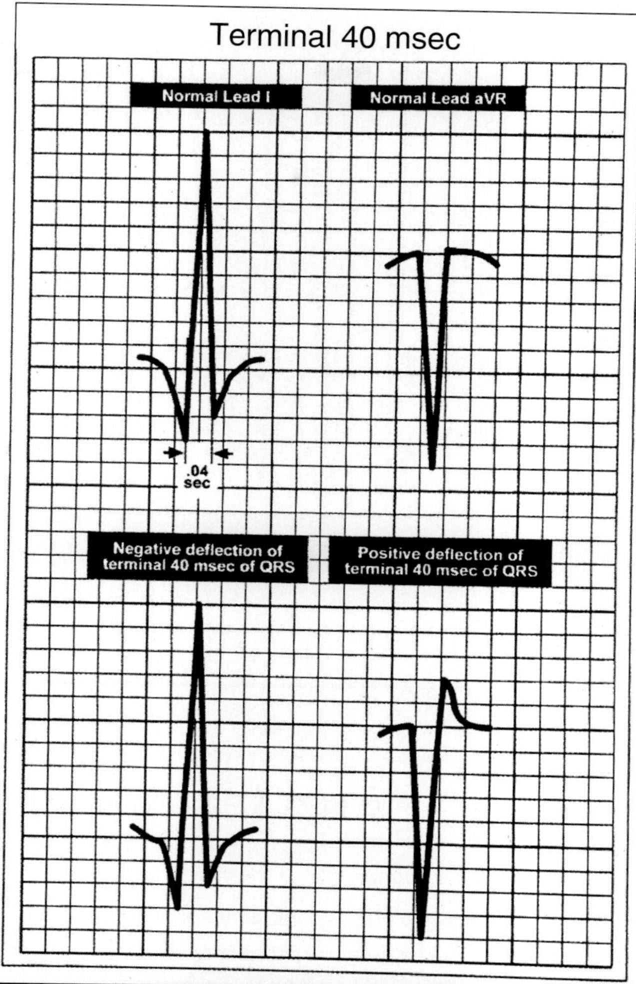

Figure 17-29. Terminal 40 msec

Right axis deviation of the terminal 40 ms of the QRS complex. (Reproduced with permission from: McGuigan ME: Poisoning potpourri. *Pediatr Rev* 2001;22:295.)

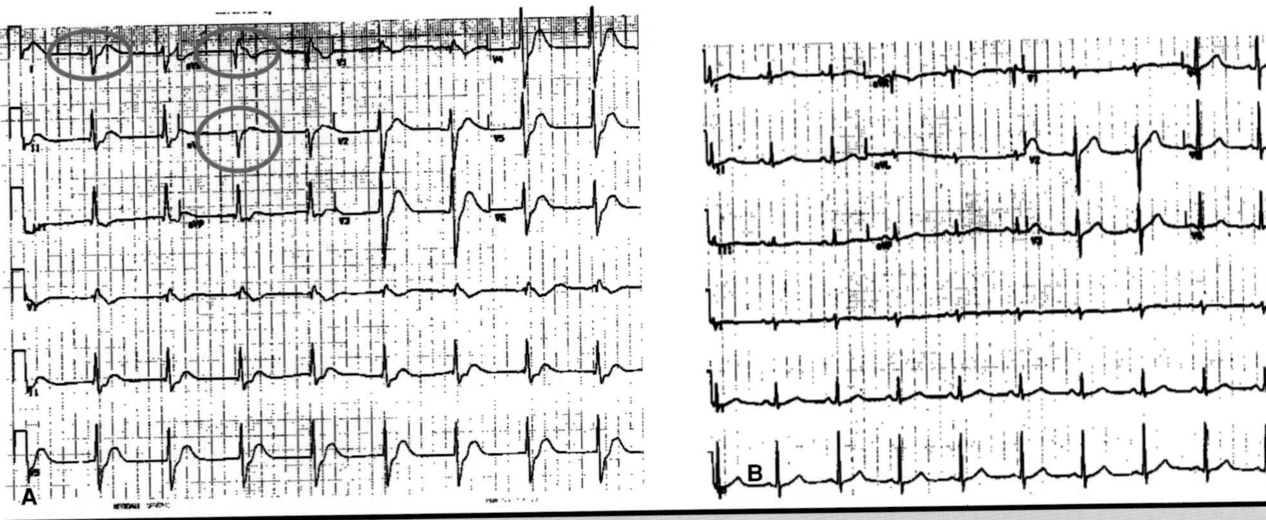

Figure 17-30. Tricyclic Antidepressant Toxicity.

A. Electrocardiogram of patient after overdose of amitriptyline. QRS duration of 160 ms, and terminal 40 ms axis changes in leads I, aVL, and aVR (circled in red) are seen. *B*. Electrocardiogram of the same patient after treatment with sodium bicarbonate, demonstrating narrowing of QRS complex (QRS duration 80 ms).

BOX 17-40. TRICYCLIC ANTIDEPRESSANT TOXICITY

Clinical manifestations:

- Anticholinergic effects: central and peripheral effects

  Mnemonic: *H*ot as a hare, *B*lind as a bat, *D*ry as a bone, *R*ed as a beet, *M*ad as a hatter

  (1) Central effects: lethargy, delirium, hallucinations, seizures, coma
  (2) Peripheral effects: dry skin, tachycardia, mydriasis, decreased bowel sounds, urinary retention

- Neurologic effects

  (1) Depressed or altered mental status
  (2) Seizures (secondary to anticholinergic toxicity and GABA antagonism)

- Cardiovascular effects

  (1) Sodium channel blockade: Type Ia antidysrhythmic (quinidine-like); conduction delays and myocardial depression, prolonged PR and QRS intervals, QTc prolongation, rightward shift in axis of terminal 40 ms of QRS complex, wide complex ventricular dysrhythmias (ventricular tachycardia, torsades de pointes, ventricular fibrillation)
  (2) Alpha-adrenergic blockade: hypotension due to vasodilatation
  (3) Tachycardia (due to anticholinergic effect and reflex response secondary to vasodilatation)

- Vital signs: tachycardia, hypotension
- Gastrointestinal: decreased GI motility (i.e., constipation and ileus)
- Renal: urinary retention
- Neurologic: myoclonus, CNS depression, seizures, coma

Laboratory values:

- A 12-lead electrocardiogram should be obtained as soon as possible.

  (1) QRS interval highly predictive of toxicity
  (2) In a landmark study, about 30% of patients with a QRS duration >100 ms had seizures, and the incidence of ventricular dysrhythmias was about 50% in patients with a QRS duration of >160 ms.
  (3) In the setting of an acute TCA overdose, terminal 40 ms right axis changes (S wave in leads I and aVL and R in aVR) had positive predictive value of 66%, and a negative predictive value of 99%.

- Quantitative measurement of TCA plasma concentration may be performed (usually of limited utility in the acute setting because plasma concentrations may not correlate with clinical toxicity)
- Obtain serum electrolytes, glucose, BUN, Cr
- Urinalysis
- Obtain serum acetaminophen and salicylate levels to evaluate for occult coingestion.

BOX 17-41. MANAGEMENT OF TRICYCLIC ANTIDEPRESSANT TOXICITY

- Stabilize ABCs, including appropriate treatment of hypotension, cardiac dysrhythmias, and altered mental status, with continuous cardiac and ECG monitoring.
- Intubation may be necessary for patients who are severely ill.
- Hypotension is managed initially with intravenous fluids and/or $NaHCO_3$ and then vasopressors if hypotension persists.
- Benzodiazepines (e.g., diazepam or lorazepam) for initial control of seizures (phenytoin contraindicated because no benefit is observed and it may be potentially harmful based on animal models)
- Consider GI decontamination.
  (1) Perform gastric lavage if patients have life-threatening toxicity or a history of a large ingestion.
  (2) Activated charcoal (dose: 1 to 2 g/kg) should be given with caution because patients may have a rapid deterioration in mental status.
- Sodium bicarbonate ($NaHCO_3$)
  (1) Given to patients with signs of significant toxicity and a prolonged QRS duration (>100 ms) on 12-lead ECG
  (2) Dose: 1 to 2 mEq/kg as an IV bolus for QRS interval widening
  (3) Perform a 12-lead ECG immediately after sodium bicarbonate administration to determine if a therapeutic effect has occurred.
  (4) If patients have a therapeutic response to $NaHCO_3$ as demonstrated on ECG by a decrease in QRS duration, serum alkalinization should be performed (create "normal bicarb" and infuse at a rate of 1.5 to 2 times maintenance; the IV solution is created by mixing 2 to 3 ampules [44 to 50 mEq/ampule] in 1 liter of D_5W).
  (5) ABG analysis to monitor acid-base status (especially in patients with ECG or mental status changes); arterial pH should not exceed 7.55 when administering bicarbonate
  (6) Hyperventilation and/or hypertonic saline may also be useful if alkalinization cannot be tolerated.

DIAGNOSIS HYDROCARBON AND NAPHTHALENE TOXICITY

Background, Pharmacokinetics, and Toxicity

1. Hydrocarbons (HCs) are a group of diverse organic compounds made up of hydrogen and carbon atoms, and typically have from 1 to 60 carbon atoms. Physical properties of HCs vary by the number of carbon atoms and molecular structure. Two different classes (with multiple subclasses) of HCs exist:
   a. Aliphatic (straight or branched chains) and cyclic (closed rings)
   b. Two subclasses, halogenated HCs and the aromatic HCs, are particularly important because of their unique toxicity.
   c. In general, aliphatic HCs have very little intrinsic toxicity; however, halogenated HCs are potentially cardiotoxic.
   d. Aromatic HCs such as benzene (one ring), naphthalene (two rings), and derivatives (toluene, phenol, styrene) are also a particularly toxic subclass of the cyclic HCs, with adverse effects on multiple organ systems.
2. Occupational exposures to HCs are extremely common in adults. Almost half of all unintentional exposures in children under 6 years of age are due to HCs (Fig. 17-31).
3. Exposure to HCs commonly occurs through inhalation, ingestion, or dermal routes.
   a. Inhalation of HCs for the purposes of intentional abuse occurs in an attempt to achieve a euphoric state (Fig. 17-32).
   b. Several terms are used to describe intentional inhalation including sniffing, bagging, and huffing, each differing in its exact method of inhalation.
   c. These various techniques of HC abuse result in exposure to vapor concentrations over a hundred times higher than those set as industrial safety standards.
4. Many common household products contain HCs including solvents, polishes, felt-tipped markers, glues, paints, car waxes, stain removers, and paint thinners.
5. The most common serious side effect of most liquid HCs is pulmonary aspiration. Viscosity of the HC is one factor in determining the risk of aspiration, with a higher risk

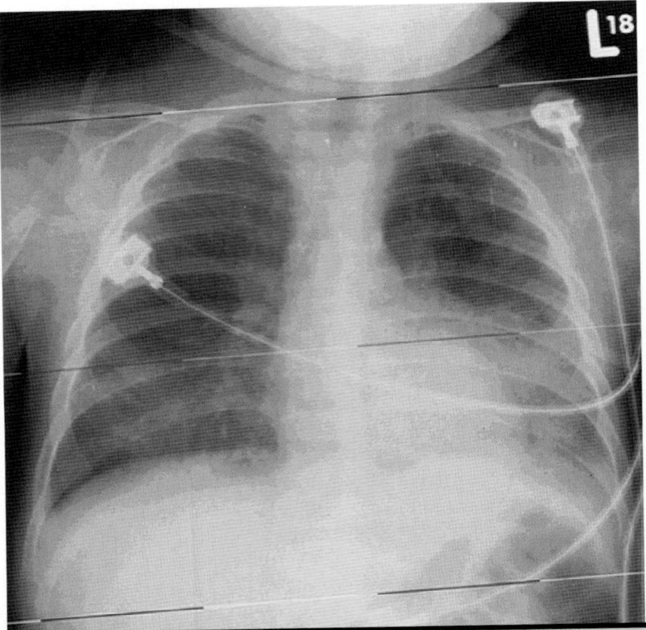

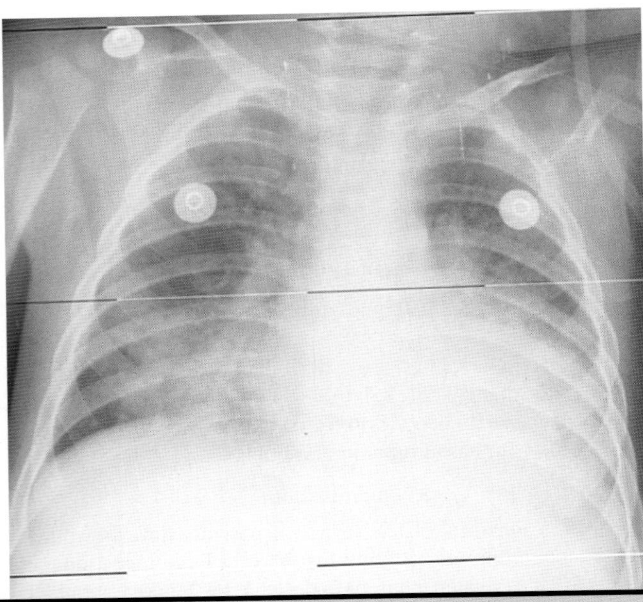

Figure 17-31. Hydrocarbon Pneumonitis

An 18-month-old male was found by his parents coughing with an open bottle of paraffin lamp oil next to him. He also had paraffin oil spilled on his clothing. He presented with persistent coughing and several episodes of vomiting. He was tachypneic with O_2 saturation of 90% on room air. He was admitted to the PICU. He experienced progressive respiratory distress and hypoxia due to hydrocarbon pneumonitis. These serial chest x-rays demonstrate pneumonitis that progressed over a 4-day period (pulmonary damage reaches its peak about 3 days after aspiration).

associated with less viscous materials. Other properties, such as surface tension and volatility, are also important considerations.

a. Some examples of low-viscosity aliphatic HCs include gasoline, kerosene, lighter fluid, and mineral spirits.

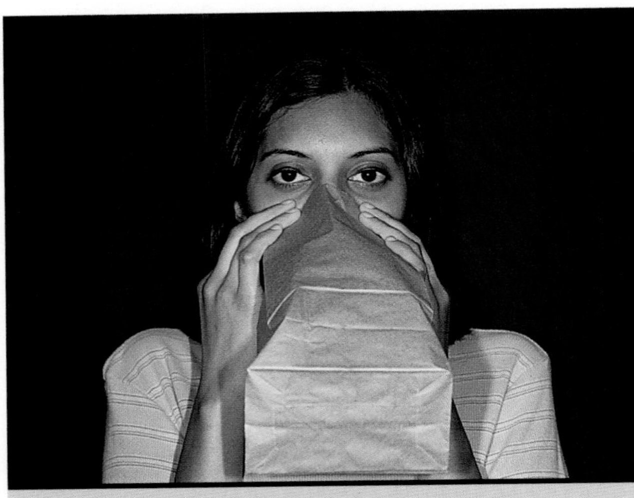

Figure 17-32. Bagging Hydrocarbon Abuse

This is common among adolescents because of the ease of acquisition of products such as paints, model glue, and various solvents. Two methods of HC abuse include huffing and bagging, as demonstrated in the photo.

b. Some examples of low-viscosity aromatic HCs include benzene, toluene, and xylene.

c. Some examples of high-viscosity aliphatic HCs include motor oil, grease, paraffin, and petroleum jelly.

6. The molecular weight of HCs is important in predicting systemic absorption after ingestion. Lower-molecular-weight compounds are more readily absorbed compared to higher-molecular-weight compounds.

7. Rapid distribution to the brain by certain HCs occurs, and clinical effects are seen within minutes of exposure. Chronic use of toluene and other solvents can lead to irreversible CNS damage.

8. Myocardial irritation and depression from the halogenated HCs predisposes to the development of cardiac dysrhythmias. Sudden death from ventricular fibrillation can occur.

9. Significant hepatic toxicity may result from exposure to chlorinated HCs (e.g., carbon tetrachloride, chloroform).

10. Naphthalene or paradichlorobenzene (PDB) are commonly found in moth repellent products such as mothballs, flakes, and crystals in 100% concentrations. In the United States, mothballs usually consist of naphthalene or PDB. In many other countries, camphor mothballs are legal products and they can be easily obtained in the United States despite laws against their use. Although adverse effects are reported, the majority of PDB mothball ingestions are inconsequential (for camphor toxicity, see page 652).

11. Naphthalene may precipitate methemoglobinemia in patients, especially those with decreased ability to handle oxidative stress (e.g., G6PD deficiency).

Emergency Department Evaluation

1. A thorough history should be obtained, with attempts made to identify the agent involved, the route of exposure, timing, intent, amount of exposure, and symptoms since the exposure occurred.
2. Physical examination should focus on vital signs and assessment of neurologic and cardiopulmonary status.

Differential Diagnosis

1. Consider other toxicologic causes of CNS depression (examples include exposure to ethanol, opiates, benzodiazepines, and hypoglycemic agents).
2. Consider other causes of altered mental status (examples include infection, trauma, and cerebral ischemia).
3. Consider other causes of methemoglobinemia (examples indude nitrites, benzocaine, dapsone, topical anesthetics, and exposure to well water in neonates).
4. Consider other causes of increased anion gap metabolic acidosis (see mnemonic MUDPILES, Box 17-2).

Consultations

Poison control center and psychiatry (intentional ingestion)

Emergency Department Management

1. Patients who have ingested a small amount of HC and are asymptomatic require only observation and do not require any intervention. Patients who remain asymptomatic following a 6-hour observation period may be discharged (following psychiatric evaluation if self-harm was intended).
2. All symptomatic patients should undergo laboratory tests for the evaluation and monitoring of their respiratory status. Patients who have signs of altered mental status, cardiac dysrhythmias, or respiratory insufficiency should be admitted to an ICU for continuous monitoring and supportive care.
3. Patients exposed to naphthalene mothballs
    a. Admit if any signs of acute hemolytic anemia or methemoglobinemia are present.
        1) Remove the toxin.
        2) Oxygen therapy and close monitoring of vital signs including cardiac and pulse oximetry
        3) Packed red blood cell transfusion is usually indicated for hemodynamically unstable or symptomatic patients with a hemoglobin value of ≤6 g/dL or patients with hemoglobin between 6 and 9 g/dL with ongoing hemolysis (e.g., ongoing hemoglobinuria).
        4) Patients should receive parenteral hydration to maintain adequate urine output and urinary alkalinization, if indicated (to prevent renal damage from precipitation of hemoglobin in renal tubules).
    b. Follow asymptomatic patients with G6PD deficiency at presentation (i.e., no evidence of hemolytic anemia/hemolysis) (Fig. 17-33).
        1) Hemolysis usually occurs at least a day or two after exposure.
        2) Perform initial screen for hemolysis by doing CBC and peripheral smear.
        3) Follow these patients very closely with serial CBCs and peripheral smears.

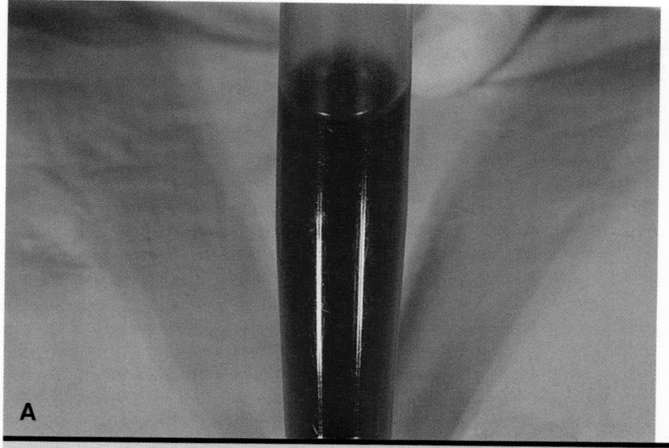

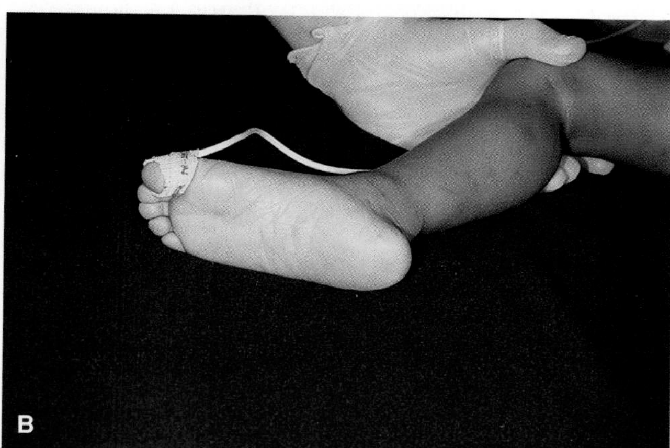

Figure 17-33. Acute Hemolytic Anemia in a Child with G6PD Deficiency Following Exposure to Naphthalene Mothballs

A. Reddish urine (hemoglobinuria) and extreme pallor (*B*) in a 2-year-old African-American male child who presented with lethargy, poor feeding, and a hemoglobin value of 5 g/dL. Two days prior to his presentation to the ED, he was found playing with naphthalene mothballs that his mother was using as moth repellent. His peripheral smear showed signs of hemolysis. Ingestion of less than one naphthalene mothball by a patient with G6PD deficiency can result in significant toxicity.

4) Educate patients to immediately bring the child to the ED if there is onset of dark urine, pallor, jaundice, or any symptoms of anemia (e.g., weakness, lethargy).

c. In asymptomatic patients who are not G6PD deficient, small quantities of naphthalene are well tolerated and patients can be sent home with close outpatient follow-up.

Clinical Pearls: Hydrocarbon and Naphthalene Toxicity

1. Ingestion of less than one naphthalene mothball by a patient with G6PD deficiency can cause significant toxicity.
2. Neonates without G6PD deficiency may develop hemolytic anemia or methemoglobinemia upon exposure to naphthalene mothballs (neonates have increased fetal hemoglobin, which is more susceptible to the formation of methemoglobin). They also have decreased levels of NADH methemoglobin reductase and are therefore unable to convert methemoglobin back to hemoglobin.
3. Parents should be advised to remove all naphthalene or camphor mothballs from the home (Fig. 17-34). Cedar or paradichlorobenzene mothballs are safe alternatives.
4. Gasoline, kerosene, lighter fluid/naphtha, mineral oil, and Varsol 1 are among the most common HC exposures reported in the United States (gasoline being the most common).
5. GI decontamination may result in increased risk of aspiration pneumonitis and should be performed with caution in patients with HCs ingestions.
6. Adolescents presenting with apparent ethanol intoxication may be abusing volatile hydrocarbons.

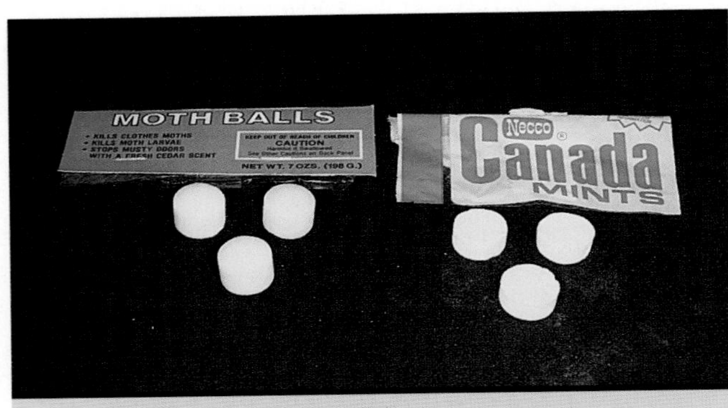

Figures 17-34. Candy Look-Alikes

As seen here, a naphthalene mothball could easily be mistaken for candy and be accidentally ingested. (Reproduced with permission from: Shah BR, Laude TL: Acute hemolytic anemia and glucose-6-phosphate dehydrogenase deficiency. In: *Atlas of Pediatric Clinical Diagnosis*. Philadelphia, WB Saunders, 2000, p. 249.)

BOX 17-42. HYDROCARBON TOXICITY

Clinical signs and symptoms:

- Vital signs: tachycardia, bradycardia, tachypnea, bradypnea, hypoxia, fever (within a few hours after exposure, due to tissue damage)
- HEENT: eye pain, irritation, lacrimation, blurred vision; residual paint or inhalational agents may be seen around the nose and mouth
- Cardiovascular: dysrhythmias including ventricular fibrillation
- Pulmonary: dyspnea, cough, chest tightness, and hypoxia may be seen immediately; bronchitis, interstitial pneumonitis, pulmonary edema, aspiration pneumonia
- GI: nausea, vomiting, abdominal pain, hepatotoxicity (chloroform, carbon tetrachloride)
- Hematologic: development of disseminated intravascular coagulation
- Neurologic: CNS depression or excitation
- Metabolic: renal tubular acidosis (toluene)

Laboratory values:

- Chest radiograph may show pulmonary edema, aspiration pneumonia, or pneumonitis
- *Important: findings on chest radiography lag behind findings on physical examination, and may not reveal abnormalities until 4 to 6 hours after aspiration.*
- Arterial blood gas analysis, pulse oximetry, and peak flow measurements will confirm hypoxia, hypercarbia, and respiratory acidosis.
- CBC in chronic exposure may demonstrate aplastic anemia or leukemia (benzene).
- Serum electrolytes, BUN, and creatinine may demonstrate acute renal failure.
- Liver function tests may demonstrate elevated transaminases, suggesting hepatic injury.
- Serum acetaminophen level to evaluate for occult coingestion in cases of intentional exposures

BOX 17-43. MANAGEMENT OF HYDROCARBON TOXICITY

- Management of HC exposures is largely supportive.
- It is extremely important to perform external decontamination prior to the patient's arrival in the ED (patients may still have HCs on their clothing and skin which present a potential risk to emergency personnel).
- All health care personnel should have adequate skin and respiratory protection.
- Stabilize ABCs, including appropriate treatment of respiratory distress, seizures, coma, and cardiac dysrhythmias as indicated.
- Gastric lavage (gastrointestinal tract decontamination)
  - (1) Gastric emptying via gastric lavage remains controversial.
  - (2) Performing gastric lavage may result in an increased risk of aspiration or development of pneumonitis.
  - (3) If lavage is to be performed, it should be done with a small nasogastric tube (18F, not the conventional large-bore tubes).
  - (4) Consider gastric lavage if significant systemic toxicity is likely based on history and if the patient presents to the hospital soon after ingestion.
  - (5) It is recommended that lavage be performed only in specific circumstances:
    - a. If the ingested HC has an inherent toxicity (e.g., carbon tetrachloride)
    - b. The HC has been ingested with another potentially fatal toxin.
    - c. A large amount of HC has been ingested (>30 mL).
- Activated charcoal
  - (1) Does not effectively adsorb HCs; most HCs are also not absorbed through the GI tract; thus AC has limited utility
  - (2) Administration of AC may also cause gastric distention, which may result in emesis with risk of aspiration and development of pneumonitis.
  - (3) Consider administration of AC (dose: 1 to 2 g/kg) orally if the patient has a known coingestion.
  - (4) If the patient ingested a caustic agent, do not administer AC.
- Use of prophylactic antibiotics and steroids is not recommended.

BOX 17-44. NAPHTHALENE TOXICITY

Clinical signs and symptoms of acute toxicity (toxicity due to oral, inhalational, and dermal exposure):

- Hematology: hemolytic anemia (especially in patients with G6PD deficiency; pallor, weakness, poor feeding, jaundice, dark urine), methemoglobinemia, hemolysis (fragmented RBCs, Heinz bodies, reticulocytosis, anisocytosis, poikilocytosis)
- Renal: hemoglobinuria
- GI: nausea, vomiting, diarrhea, abdominal pain
- CNS: lethargy, seizures

Laboratory values:

- CBC with peripheral smear and reticulocyte count
- Bilirubin
- G6PD level
- Serum electrolytes including BUN, creatinine (evaluate renal function)
- Methemoglobin level
- Type and screen (for patients with acute hemolysis)
- Ascertain exposure:
  (1) Naphthalene: white, dry, faintly radiopaque balls that float in saturated salt solution, but sink in water
  (2) Paradichlorobenzene: white, wet, densely radiopaque balls that sink in saturated salt solution and water
  (3) Camphor: wet, oily, crystalline, radiolucent, and readily floats in saturated salt solution and water; odor of camphor is an important clue in identification of unknown ingestion

Management principles:

- Gastrointestinal decontamination for naphthalene ingestion
  (1) Emesis (syrup of ipecac can be given for ingestion of a small number of mothballs if the patient presents within first 1 to 2 hours following ingestion)
  (2) Do not induce emesis if there is possible camphor mothball ingestion (risk of seizures from camphor).
  (3) Activated charcoal to prevent further absorption (dose: 1 to 2 g/kg)
  (4) Mothballs are often larger than orogastric tubes and gastric lavage usually has no benefit.
  (6) Whole-bowel irrigation may be considered to prevent further absorption if ingestion is significant.
  (7) Avoid fatty meals (increase absorption).
- Cutaneous exposure
  (1) Remove and discard contaminated clothes (clothes may serve as a reservoir for reexposure).
  (2) For removal of naphthalene from skin or fabrics, soap and water is required (water alone does not adequately remove it).

Suggested Readings

Belson MG, Simon HK: Utility of comprehensive toxicologic screens in children. *Am J Emerg Med* 1999;17:221.

Boehnert MT, Lovejoy FH: Value of the QRS duration versus the serum drug level in predicting seizures and ventricular arrhythmias after an overdose of tricyclic antidepressants. *N Engl J Med* 1985;313:474.

Chiang W: Amphetamines. In: *Goldfrank's Toxicologic Emergencies,* 7th ed. Stamford, CT, Appleton & Lange, 2002, p. 1020.

Ernst AA, Jones K, Nick TG, et al: Ethanol ingestion and related hypoglycemia in a pediatric and adolescent emergency department population. *Acad Emerg Med* 1996;3:46.

Lewis RK, Palaucek FP: Assessment and treatment of acetaminophen overdose. *Clin Pharmacol* 1991;10:765.

Liebelt EL, Francis PD: Cyclic antidepressants. In: *Goldfrank's Toxicologic Emergencies,* 7th ed. Stamford, CT, Appleton & Lange, 2002, p. 847.

Litovitz TL, Klein-Scwartz W, et al: 1997 Annual Report of the American Association of Poison Control Centers Toxic Exposure Surveillance System. *Am J Emerg Med* 1998;16:443.

Molupus JL, Nadkarni M: Massive embolic myocardial infarction in a teenager. *Pediatr Emerg Care* 2002;18:101.

Niemann JT, Bessen HA, Rothstein RJ, Laks MM: Electrocardiographic criteria for tricyclic antidepressant cardiotoxicity. *Am J Cardiol* 1986;57:1154.

Olmedo R: Phencyclidine and ketamine. In: *Goldfrank's Toxicologic Emergencies,* 7th ed. Stamford, CT, Appleton & Lange, 2002, p. 1034.

Pentel P, Peterson CD: Asystole complicating physostigmine treatment of tricyclic antidepressant overdose. *Ann Emerg Med* 1980;9:588.

Porter RS: Alcohol and injury in adolescents. *Pediatr Emerg Care* 2000;16:316.

Rao RB, Hoffman RS: Caustics and batteries. In: *Goldfrank's Toxicologic Emergencies,* 7th ed. Stamford, CT, Appleton & Lange, 2002, p. 1323.

Riordan M, Rylance G, Berry K: Poisoning in children 4: Household products, plants, and mushrooms. *Arch Dis Child* 2002;87:43.

Rumack BH, Matthew H: Acetaminophen poisoning and toxicity. *Pediatrics* 1975;55:871.

Schaffer SB, Hebert AF: Caustic ingestion. *J La State Med Soc* 2000;152:590.

Shannon M, Liebelt EL: Toxicology reviews: Targeted management strategies for cardiovascular toxicity from tricyclic antidepressant overdose: The pivotal role for alkalinization and sodium loading. *Pediatr Emerg Care* 1998;14:293.

Tucker JR, Ferm RP. Lysergic acid diethylamide and other hallucinogens. In: *Goldfrank's Toxicologic Emergencies*, 7th ed. Stamford, CT, Appleton & Lange, 2002, p. 1046.

Trong T, Boyer EW: Club drugs, smart drugs, raves, and circuit parties: An overview of the club scene. *Pediatr Emerg Care* 2002;18:216.

Yip L: In: *Goldfrank's Toxicologic Emergencies*, 7th ed. Stamford, CT, Appleton & Lange, 2002, p. 1323.

CHAPTER 18

ENVIRONMENTAL EMERGENCIES

Michael Lucchesi / Ronak R. Shah / Karen Santucci / Binita R. Shah / M. Douglas Baker / Lewis Kohl
Edited by Michael Lucchesi

DIAGNOSIS

BURNS

Mechanism of Injury

1. There are four types of burns: chemical, radiation, electrical, and thermal. This section will concentrate on the most common mechanism, thermal injury.
2. The extent of injury depends on the amount of heat, the medium by which it is delivered (gas, liquid, or vapor), and the duration of contact with the tissue.
   a. Temperatures below 45°C rarely cause cell damage.
   b. Temperatures greater than 50°C denature proteins.

Associated Clinical Features

1. First-degree: partial thickness; involves the outer layer of the epidermis
2. Second-degree: partial thickness; extends into the dermis (Fig. 18-1)
3. Third-degree: full thickness; hair follicles, sweat glands, and other adnexal structures are involved (Fig. 18-2)
4. Fourth-degree: involves subcutaneous tissue, muscle, fascia, and bone.
5. Erythema and tenderness are present with first- and second-degree burns.
6. Blistering is caused by at least a second-degree burn.
7. Paresthesias (lack of tactile sensation) is diagnostic of third-degree burns.

Laboratory

1. Most burns are minor and do not require x-rays or blood work.
2. Significant burns (>10% of the body surface area; BSA) should prompt screening labs: CBC, electrolytes, glucose, BUN, creatinine, CPK and urinalysis.
3. Any history or signs (carbonaceous sputum, hoarse voice, or evidence of hypoxia) of significant smoke inhalation should prompt a chest x-ray, venous carboxyhemoglobin level, and pulse oximetry.

Complications

1. For major thermal injuries (>20% BSA) and significant burns (>10% BSA) in patients with other medical conditions, the possibility of multiorgan failure needs to be anticipated.
2. All burn patients should be evaluated for carbon monoxide poisoning.
3. Significant electrical burns to the mouth may be followed (usually in 7 to 10 days) by delayed bleeding from the labial artery (Fig. 18-3).

Consultation

1. Burn victims are trauma patients and should be considered for trauma evaluation.
2. Second-degree burns over >10% BSA should always be presented to a burn center for a potential referral.
3. Burns on the face, hands, or genitalia should always be presented to a burn center for a potential referral (Fig. 18-4).
4. Circumferential burns of an extremity need to be followed extremely closely with urgent referral to orthopedics to monitor for compartment syndrome (Fig. 18-5).

Emergency Department Treatment and Disposition

1. All burn patients should receive analgesics as soon as possible, upon arrival in the ED.
2. Minor burn patients (<10% BSA, with no airway involvement and no involvement of hands, face, or genitalia) can be managed with local wound care.
3. All burns should be irrigated with copious amounts of room temperature normal saline.
4. In patients who are being discharged home with second-degree burns, the involved skin below the clavicles should be covered with silver sulfadiazine (if not allergic to sulfa) and a sterile dressing.

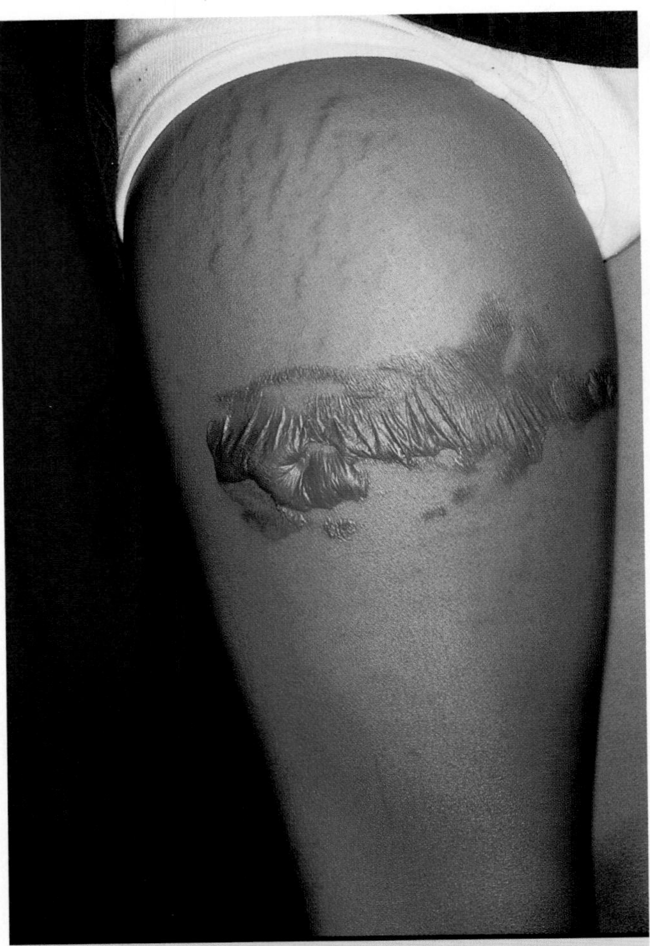

Figure 18-1. Second-Degree Burn with Blistering

An image of a 10-year-old boy who sustained a second-degree burn to the anterior surface of the upper thigh from a hot iron.

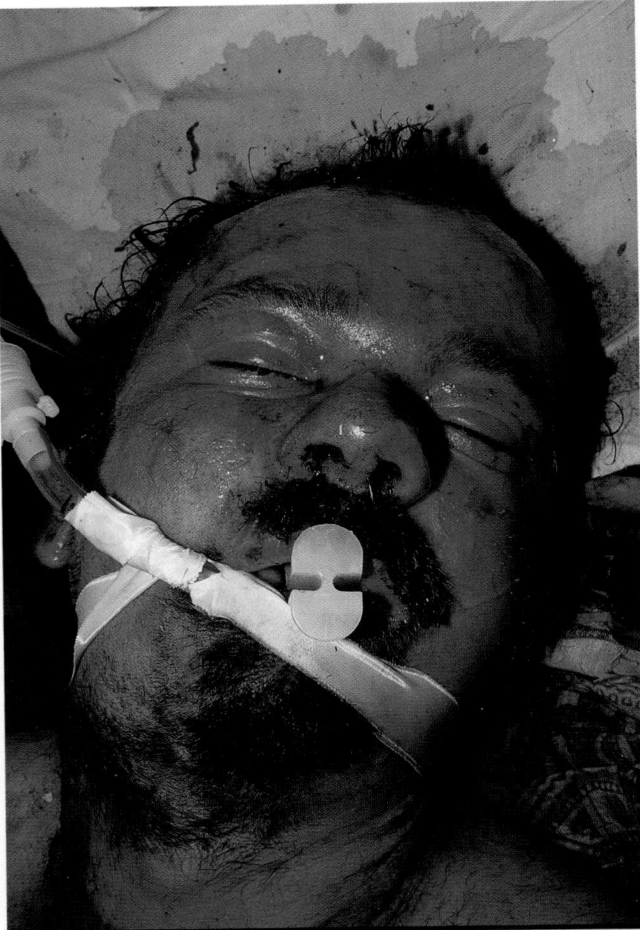

Figure 18-2. Second- and Third-Degree Burns to the Face

Picture of a young man with second- and third-degree burns to the face. His oropharyngeal burns and carbonaceous sputum necessitated intubation upon arrival in the ED. This patient was also found to have a carboxyhemoglobin level of 32%. After initial resuscitation and stabilization, he was transported to a hyperbaric chamber.

5. Blisters over joints should be débrided.
6. Bacitracin ointment should be applied to second-degree burns above the clavicles.
7. Major burn patients should be resuscitated in the ED and transferred to a burn center. These criteria define a major burn patient:
   a. Greater than 10% BSA
   b. Greater than 5% third-degree
   c. Involvement of the hands, face, or genitalia
8. This is the formula for calculating the amount of Ringer's lactate needed for initial resuscitation for burn shock: 2 to 4 mL/kg × body weight in kilograms × percentage of BSA burned = total lactated Ringer's required. Half should be given in the first 8 hours after the burn occurred, and half in the following 16 hours. Increased fluid resuscitation should be dictated by urine output. A urine output of 1 mL/kg per hour should be maintained.

Clinical Pearls: Burns

1. When burn patients die, it is usually secondary to inhalational injury.
2. Children with a large percentage of BSA burned often become hypothermic and need to be kept warm.
3. All burn patients need strict scrutiny of their tetanus immunization status, and if in doubt vaccine should be given.
4. All burn patients should initially receive supplemental oxygen until it is determined they don't need it.

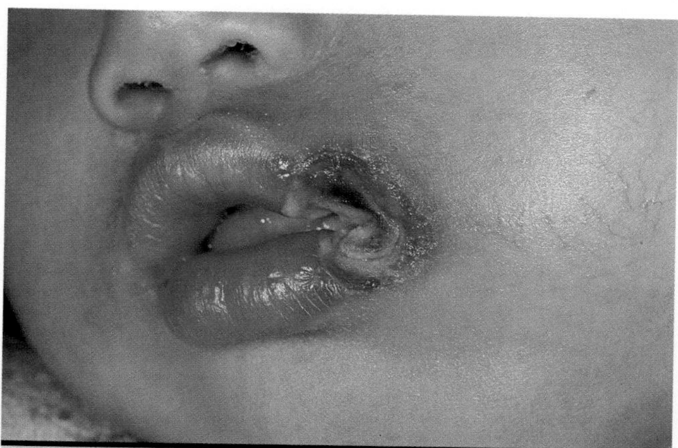

Figure 18-3. Electrical Burn

An image of a 2-year-old male who sustained a third-degree burn to the commissure of the mouth after biting down on an electrical cord. This picture was taken on a follow-up visit 3 days after he was initially treated. He had several additional follow-up visits in which his oral cavity was scrutinized for an eschar and possible delayed bleeding from the labial artery.

5. An indoor fire in an enclosed space have a high suspicion of inhalational injury.
6. Hypoglycemia is common in pediatric burn patients.
7. Children <5 years of age with significant burns need maintenance fluids plus that recommendation for burn shock.
8. Ten percent of burns in children are secondary to abuse (see Figs. 1-22 and 1-24).

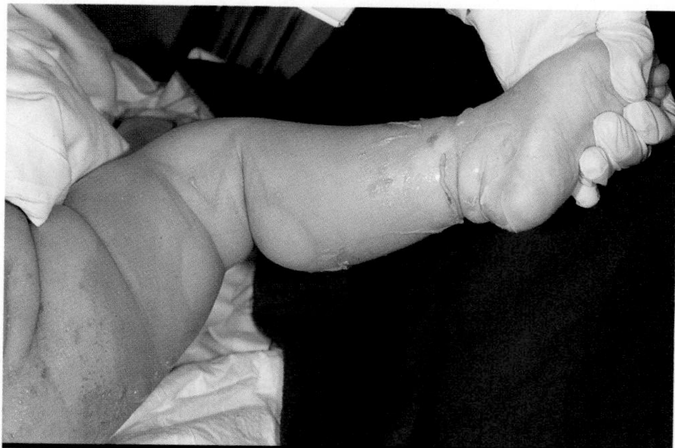

Figure 18-5. Circumferential Burns of the Leg

An image of a 9-month-old child who sustained circumferential burns to the ankle, calf, and thigh after being burned with a hot liquid. The baby had not yet started walking, which led to the ED staff to consider child abuse. The pattern of the burn is consistent with a splash injury and not a submersion injury.

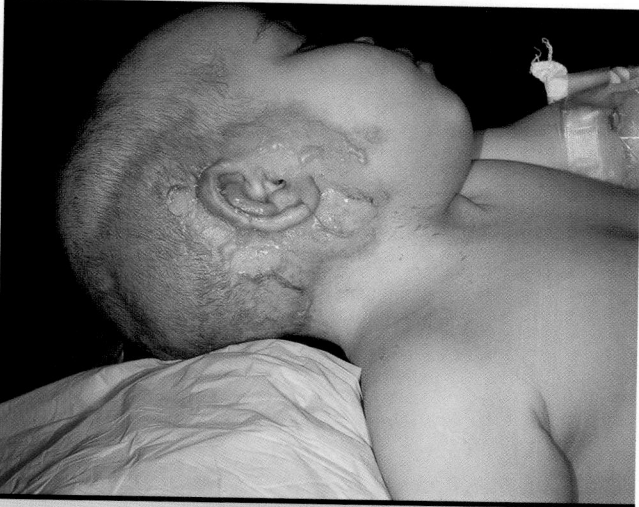

Figure 18-4. Second-Degree Burns

An image of a 2-year-old boy who sustained second-degree burns to the side of his face, ear, and head after pulling down a cup of hot coffee from a table.

BOX 18-1. CARBON MONOXIDE POISONING

- Outside fires (those not in the confines of a building or vehicle) rarely raise carbon monoxide (CO) levels.
- Carbon monoxide has an affinity for hemoglobin 200 times that of oxygen.
- Venous CO levels are as accurate as arterial levels.
- A good pulse oximetry level (>96%) *and* a normal venous CO level (<5%) significantly lowers the possibility of inhalation injury.
- Half-life of carboxyhemoglobin:
  Room air = 330 minutes
  F_{IO_2} 100% = 90 minutes
  Hyperbaric chamber = 20 minutes

BOX 18-2. DIFFERENTIAL DIAGNOSIS OF BURNS

- Upper airway obstruction
- Myofascial trauma
- Hemorrhagic shock
- Pulmonary injury
- Staphylococcal scalded skin syndrome (see Figs. 3-24 to 3-27)
- Toxic epidermal necrolysis (see Figs. 7-8 and 7-9)

DIAGNOSIS PERIPHERAL COLD INJURIES

Definitions

1. Frostbite is local tissue destruction resulting from exposure to extreme cold.
2. Hypothermic injury can be either central (core) or peripheral. It can be a systemic problem or a local one. Hypothermia can be accidental or due to an intentional drop in ambient temperature, causing injury.
3. Depending on the temperature and the duration of the insult, peripheral cold injuries can range from chilblain (a superficial form of peripheral cold injury), to frostnip (an initial response to cold injury) with reversible skin changes including blanching and numbness, to true frostbite that involves deep structures such as muscle, bone, and tendon.

Pathophysiology

1. Peripheral cold injuries almost always effect the distal areas: fingers, toes, nose, and ears (Figs. 18-6, 18-7, 18-8, and 18-9).
2. Tissue damage occurs through several mechanisms:
   a. Direct cell damage from intracellular ice crystal formation
   b. Indirect cell damage occurs via intracellular dehydration due to extracellular ice crystal formation.
   c. Microvascular vasoconstriction and thrombosis occurs due to erythrocyte sludging.
   d. Direct cell death due to extreme cold
   e. Reperfusion inflammation due to edema and thrombosis

Associated Clinical Features and ED Evaluation

1. The history should focus on determining exposure temperature, duration, wind velocity, apparel worn, and underlying cardiovascular and neurologic diseases.
2. Physical examination should focus on vital signs, the ABC's of resuscitation, and assessment of the degree of associated hypothermia.
3. Laboratory studies are usually not needed. Systemically hypothermic patients can show an acidosis, but for the most part peripherally-injured patients will not have any abnormal laboratory values. Consider obtaining a CBC, electrolytes, and

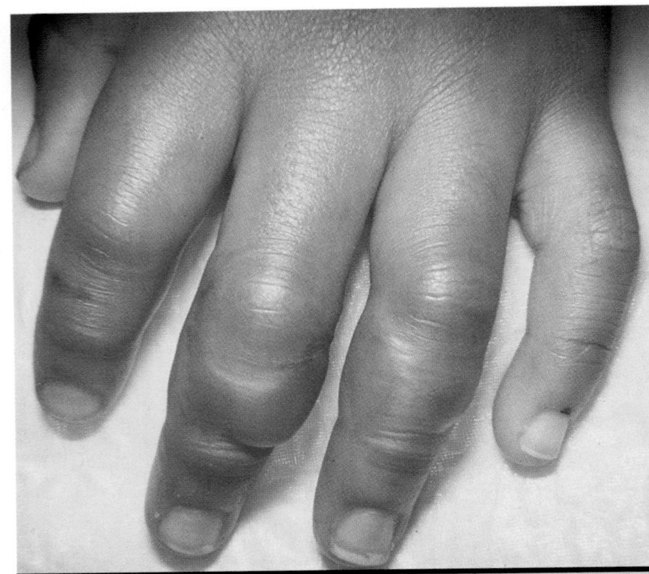

Figure 18-6. Superficial Frostbite

Here we see the hand of a 5-year-old who was playing in the snow for several hours and sustained superficial frostbite to the second, third, and fourth digits. The picture was taken several hours after the injury occurred.

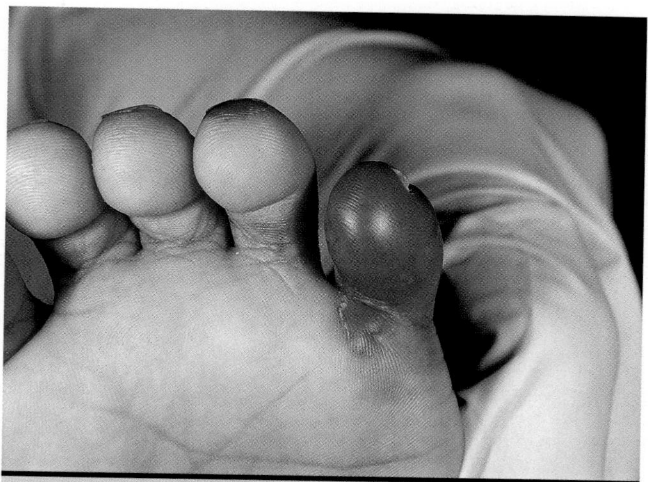

Figure 18-7. Deep Frostbite

An image of the fifth toe of an 8-year-old who was ice skating at night for several hours with tight skates. The picture was taken hours after the injury and it turned out to be deep frostbite with eventual mummification and autoamputation.

serum myoglobin values for severe cases. Gram's stain and culture may be required in cases of severe frostbite of exposed areas when infection is suspected.

Complications

1. Sepsis
2. Local infection

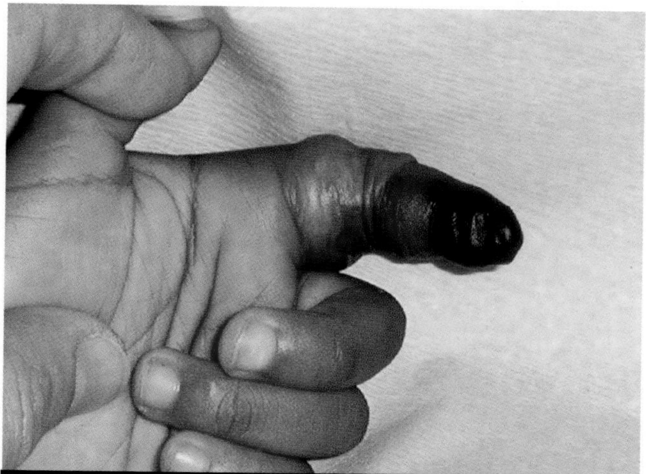

Figure 18-8. Deep Frostbite

An image of the index finger of a 6-year-old with deep frostbite several weeks after the injury. The child had gone sleigh riding with his family at night. He was wearing a torn glove on that hand and had gone unsupervised for several hours.

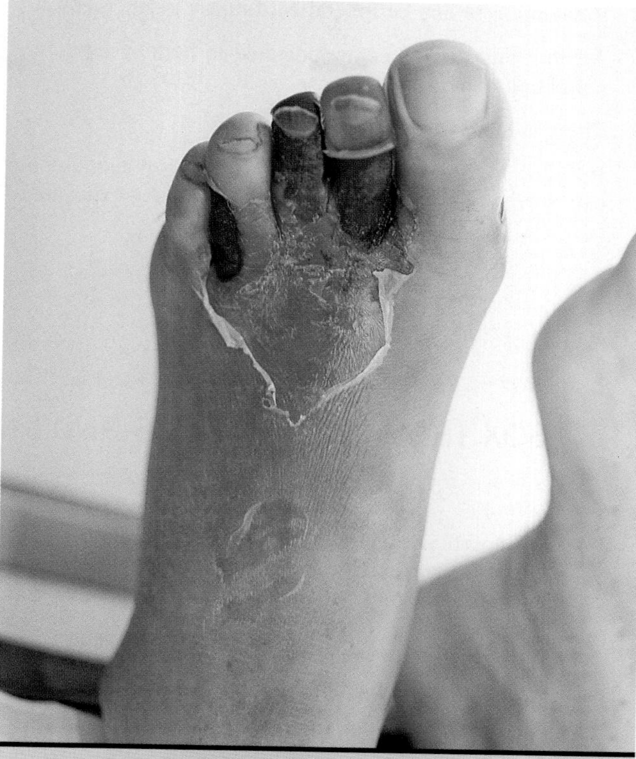

Figure 18-9. Deep Frostbite

An image of the foot of 17-year-old male several weeks after he sustained deep frostbite to his second, third, fourth, and fifth toes. Note the irregular pattern of demarcation which required eventual surgical débridement.

3. Loss of function
4. Autoamputation

Consultation

Consider surgical consultation for severe cases which may require wound débridement or amputation.

Emergency Department Treatment and Disposition

1. Treat any degree of underlying hypothermia.
2. Treatment efforts should be focused on rapid rewarming of affected areas and supportive care.
3. All patients should be admitted for observation and supportive care unless frostbite is very superficial and painless.

Clinical Pearls: Peripheral Cold Injuries

1. Dry rewarming (e.g., near an open fire) is uneven, dangerous, and should be avoided.
2. Frostnip is the only peripheral cold injury that should be treated at the scene.

3. Rewarming of any peripheral cold injury is emergent.
4. Alcohol ingestion is contraindicated in both systemic and peripheral cold injuries.
5. There is more susceptibility to reinjury.
6. Be sure to remove the patient from all potential cold exposure prior to rewarming efforts. Continued exposure to cold after rewarming may lead to refreezing and much more extensive tissue damage.
7. Be sure to treat any degree of underlying hypothermia.
8. Frostbitten areas may take up to 6 months to become apparent.
9. Time for reperfusion should be maximized before amputation is considered.

BOX 18-3. CLINICAL SIGNS AND SYMPTOMS OF PERIPHERAL COLD INJURIES

- *Frostnip*
  (1) Superficial, reversible ice crystal formation
  (2) No tissue destruction
  (3) Transient numbness and paresthesias resolve with rewarming.
  (4) No long-term sequelae
- *Chilblain (perniosis)*
  (1) Mild dry-cold injury that occurs after repetitive cold exposure
  (2) "Cold sores" may progress to plaques, nodules, or ulcerations.
  (3) Accompanied by pruritus, edema, and erythema
- *Superficial frostbite*
  (1) The skin is white or waxy in appearance.
  (2) Loss of sensation to pain, temperature, or light touch
  (3) Burning or stinging sensation
  (4) Rewarming results in return of neurologic function and hyperemia.
  (5) No tissue destruction, no long-term sequelae
- *Deep frostbite*
  (1) Involvement of subcutaneous tissue, muscle, or bone
  (2) Patient complains of clumsiness and numbness in the affected area.
  (3) No sensation to deep pain or temperature
  (4) Severe pain and burning sensation in affected areas after rewarming
  (5) Decreased mobility even after rewarming
  (6) Post-rewarming edema may begin within 3 hours and last up to 7 days.
  (7) Within 24 hours large, clear, fluid-filled blisters appear.
  (8) After 24 hours, small hemorrhagic blisters develop if deeper injury has occurred.
  (9) Eschar formation within 2 weeks
  (10) Mummification within 6 weeks (a blackened, hard, dry gangrene, and clear demarcation of the area appears within weeks)

BOX 18-4. DIFFERENTIAL DIAGNOSIS OF PERIPHERAL COLD INJURIES

- Paronychia
- Local ischemia
- Trauma-related injury
- Vasculitis

BOX 18-5. MANAGEMENT PRINCIPLES FOR FROSTBITE

- Stabilize the ABC's including management of hypothermia, cardiac dysrhythmias, intoxication, head injury, and hypoglycemia.
- After systemic hypothermia has been ruled out, peripheral injuries should be treated.
- Remove all restrictive and wet garments, which may cause continued cold exposure.
- Initiate rapid rewarming of affected areas with immersion in water at 40 to 42°C for 10 to 30 minutes.
- Rapid rewarming should be stopped when the area is warm, erythematous, and pliable.
- Analgesia should be provided for reperfusion pain.
- Nonsteroidal anti-inflammatory drugs (NSAIDs) are controversial but may be used to inhibit effects of released prostaglandins on skin necrosis.
- Clear blisters may be débrided or aspirated to remove inflammatory mediators that can worsen tissue destruction.
- Hemorrhagic blisters must be left intact.
- Aloe vera cream may be applied to intact blisters to inhibit inflammatory mediators.
- Tetanus prophylaxis should be administered.
- The affected extremity should be elevated, splinted, and dressed with a dry sterile dressing (change dressing two to four times daily).
- Antibiotic prophylaxis against staphylococci, streptococci, and pseudomonal species should be considered for severe frostbite cases (e.g., penicillinase-resistant penicillin, cephalosporins, or quinolones)
- Although salicylates, NSAIDs, and aloe vera are controversial in terms of benefit, they are not known to be detrimental.

DIAGNOSIS

SPIDER BITES

Definitions and Etiologies

1. Spiders are in the phylum Arthropoda, class Arachnida. There are approximately 200 species of spiders that have been identified and associated with significant envenomations. Significant clinical syndromes produced by their bites are discussed here.
2. In North America alone there are eighteen genera of spiders that produce envenomations that require intervention.
3. Brown recluse spider (*Loxosceles reclusa*; violin or fiddleback spider)
   a. There are thirteen species of *Loxosceles* in the United States, but *L. reclusa* is the most common.
   b. Like the black widow spider, the female is clearly more dangerous than the male.
   c. The classic identifying mark for this spider is the brown violin-shaped mark on the dorsum of its cephalothorax.
   d. This is a small spider measuring about 6 to 12 mm in length and its pigmentation ranges from gray to orange or reddish brown.
   e. This spider is found in the southern United States and generally inhabits darkened areas like woodpiles, basements, and closets.
4. Black widow spider (*Latrodectus mactans*; hourglass spider)
   a. Widow spiders live in temperate and tropical latitudes.
   b. They live in small crevices, under decks, in woodpiles, and under and around houses and outbuildings.
   c. The female is larger than the male (about 2.5 to 3.5 cm) and has a distinct red hourglass-shaped mark on its ventral surface. The female is also more venomous than the male and is most toxic in the summer.
   d. There are five species of known widow spiders in the United States:
      1) *Latrodectus mactans* (black widow)
      2) *Latrodectus hesperus* (western black widow)
      3) *Latrodectus variolus* (northern black widow)
      4) *Latrodectus bishopi* (red widow [southern U.S.])
      5) *Latrodectus geometricus* (brown widow)

Associated Clinical Features

1. The true incidence of venomous spider bites is unknown.
2. There are no specific tests to diagnose brown recluse spider envenomation. However, patients with systemic signs require monitoring of CBC including platelet count, coagulation profile, serum electrolytes, creatinine, BUN, and urinalysis.
3. There are no specific tests to diagnose black widow spider envenomation.

Consultation

Poison center for patients with systemic toxicity (e.g., patients with black widow spider bites requiring antivenin therapy)

Emergency Department Treatment and Disposition

1. For brown recluse spider bites
   a. While local treatment of the lesion is controversial, the best management of the necrotic site most likely includes local cleansing, splinting (for immobilization), attention to tetanus prophylaxis, and pain management.
   b. There is no indication for prophylactic antibiotics.
   c. Some advocate early use of dapsone (leukocyte inhibitor).
   d. Routine use of steroids has not been proven effective.
   e. Patients with systemic manifestations from the bite or evidence of an expanding necrotic lesion should be admitted for observation.
   f. With hemolysis, maintaining good urine output, alkalinization of urine with intravenous administration of sodium bicarbonate to keep the urine pH >7, and close monitoring of renal function and hematocrit are required.
2. For widow spider bites
   a. The mainstay of treatment involves establishing an airway and supporting respiration and circulation if the patient's status is compromised.
   b. Attention must be paid to wound management and updating tetanus immunization if needed.
   c. It may benefit the patient to apply ice to the bite area.
   d. Pain control with salicylates, NSAIDs, or even opioids if necessary
   e. Calcium gluconate 10% solution
      1) It has been given IV over 10 minutes for treatment of muscle cramps in the past
      2) Its use has fallen out of favor, as most controlled studies have not shown a benefit.
   f. Antivenin (available as a crude hyperimmune horse serum)
      1) Indicated for severe envenomations that are unresponsive to other treatments
      2) Some indications include life-threatening hypertension, tachycardia, respiratory difficulty, or members of high-risk groups, such as pediatric, elderly, and pregnant patients.
      3) Rapid complete resolution of symptoms occurs after antivenin administration.
      4) May precipitate anaphylaxis and serum sickness
   g. Hospitalization is recommended for all pediatric patients, patients requiring IV analgesics to control the pain, and patients with hypertension or other autonomic symptoms.

Clinical Pearls: Spider Bites

1. All patients with brown recluse spider bites should be monitored for evidence of hemolysis, renal failure, or coagulopathy (Fig. 18-10). Children are more likely to develop these systemic effects.
2. The hallmark of black widow spider envenomation is muscle cramping, usually affecting the abdomen, back, and chest.
3. The venom produced by the black widow spider is one of the most potent known venom.
4. Classically, the shorter the time to the onset of symptoms following black widow spider bite, the more severe the envenomation is. The populations at greatest risk are infants, elderly, chronically ill, and pregnant women.

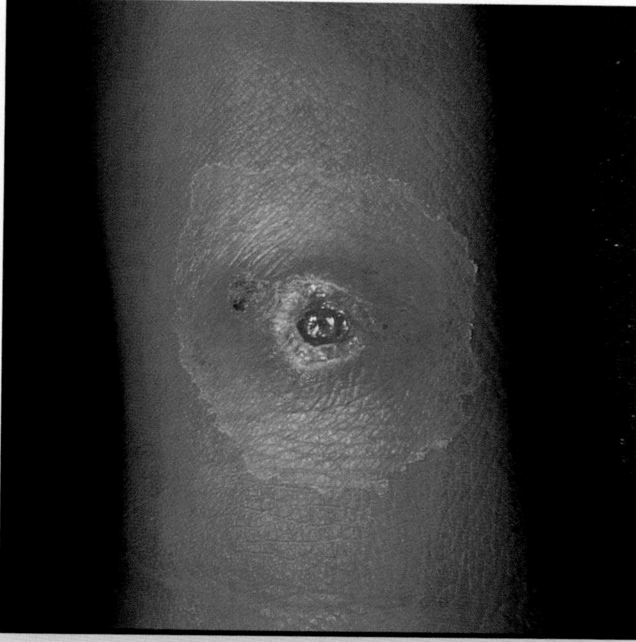

Figure 18-10. Brown Recluse Spider Bite

Extremities are the most commonly affected sites. This patient presented with local cutaneous necrosis following the bite. This was followed by ulceration (as seen here).

BOX 18-6. CLINICAL FEATURES OF BROWN RECLUSE SPIDER BITES

- Extremities are the sites most commonly affected.
- May present as local cutaneous necrosis
- Bite initially painless but eventually blisters, bleeds, and ultimately ulcerates 2 to 8 hours later
- If the wound goes untreated, the lesion may enlarge for up to a week.
- Granulation and healing may take up to 2 months.
- More severe systemic symptoms and signs associated with the bite include:
  (1) Fever and chills
  (2) Nausea
  (3) Morbilliform rash
  (4) Arthralgias
  (5) Myalgias
  (6) Seizures
  (7) Coma
  (8) Hemolysis
  (9) Thrombocytopenia
  (10) Disseminated intravascular coagulopathy
  (11) Renal failure
- A constellation of symptoms known as *loxoscelism* includes gangrenous slough at the site of the bite, nausea, malaise, fever, hemolysis, and thrombocytopenia.

BOX 18-7. CLINICAL FEATURES OF BLACK WIDOW SPIDER BITE

- Majority of bites seen on the extremities
- The bite of a widow spider may be associated with a sharp pain (pinprick sensation) or may be painless.
- The local reaction is limited and two red dots will appear at the bite site.
- A bite by a female spider produces latrodectism.
- Effects due to neurotoxin
  (1) Primary site of action is at the neuromuscular junction
  (2) It causes release and inhibits reuptake of acetylcholine and norepinephrine, resulting in overstimulation of motor endplates.
  (3) Symptoms develop 15 minutes to several hours after the bite.
- Muscle cramps and rigidity
  (1) Hallmark of widow spider envenomation
  (2) Seen 30 to 90 minutes after the bite and peaks in 3 to 12 hours
  (3) Occurs at the site of inoculation initially, but may involve other muscle groups (e.g., chest, abdomen, face)
  (4) Involvement of abdominal muscles: abdominal pain and rigidity without peritoneal signs
  (5) Involvement of chest muscles: grunting and respiratory distress
  (6) Waxing and waning course
- Classic "facies latrodectismica" is characterized by
  (1) Sweating
  (2) Contortion
  (3) Grimacing
- Autonomic symptoms include
  (1) Hypertension
  (2) Tachycardia
  (3) Nausea or vomiting
  (4) Diaphoresis
- Other symptoms that have been reported include
  (1) Weakness
  (2) Headache
  (3) Periorbital edema
  (4) Hyperesthesias
  (5) Ptosis
  (6) Hyperreflexia
  (7) Seizure or tremors
  (8) Arthralgias

BOX 18-8. HOBO SPIDER BITES (*TEGENARIA AGRESTIS*)

- Background
  (1) This spider is also known as the aggressive house spider.
  (2) Small brown spiders with gray markings
  (3) Most commonly encountered in midsummer through fall
  (4) The male is the aggressor (unlike the black widow and brown recluse).
- Clinical features
  (1) Initial bite painless
  (2) An expanding area of erythema and blistering ensues
  (3) A necrotic ulcer forms
  (4) Healing may be prolonged (some cases reportedly took 45 days to 3 years to heal completely).
  (5) Associated systemic symptoms may include nausea, vomiting, fatigue, amnesia, and visual disturbances.
- Emergency Department Treatment and Disposition
  (1) Local wound care should be emphasized.
  (2) Systemic steroids may be of some value.

BOX 18-9. FUNNEL WEB SPIDER BITES (*ATRAX* AND *TRECHONA* SPECIES)

- Background
  (1) They have a potent neurotoxin.
  (2) They are found in Queensland, New South Wales, Victoria, and Tasmania.
  (3) These spiders are large (5 cm).
  (4) Male's venom more potent than female's venom.
- Clinical features
  (1) Children are particularly susceptible to the spider's neurotoxin.
  (2) Death can occur as soon as 4 hours post-envenomation.
  (3) The toxin, atraxotoxin (a neurotoxin), causes release of the neurotransmitters acetylcholine, norepinephrine, and epinephrine.
  (4) Widespread muscle fasciculations are seen early on accompanied by piloerection.
  (5) Tachycardia, dysrhythmias, hypertensive crisis, coma, cholinergic crisis, apnea, and other untoward events develop moments later.
  (6) Within several hours, progression to hypotension, pulmonary edema, and respiratory depression may ensue.
- Emergency Department Treatment and Disposition
  (1) The bite of this spider requires immediate prehospital measures.
  (2) Immobilize the affected limb and apply a tourniquet proximal to the bite.
  (3) Antivenin (of rabbit origin) is available in Australia. It is given IV (two ampules every 15 minutes, repeated to effect).
  (4) Atropine, muscle relaxants, sedatives, and antihypertensive agents are all recommended treatments.

DIAGNOSIS ANAPHYLAXIS

Definitions

1. Anaphylaxis is a clinical syndrome with a systemic reaction following antigen exposure in a sensitized person.
2. It is a type 1 IgE-mediated hypersensitivity reaction involving multiple organ systems (e.g., cutaneous, respiratory, cardiovascular, gastrointestinal, or central nervous system).
3. Two or more systems must be involved to make a diagnosis of anaphylaxis.
4. The term *anaphylactoid reaction* indicates a non-IgE-mediated reaction. It requires no immunologic memory (thus, degranulation of mast cells may occur on first exposure to an allergen).
5. An anaphylactoid reaction is clinically indistinguishable from true anaphylaxis and treatment for both disorders are same.

Epidemiology and Pathogenesis

1. The estimated rate of fatal anaphylaxis from any cause is 0.4 per million persons (about 500 incidents per year in the United States).
2. The estimated rate of fatal anaphylaxis from penicillin is 1 per 7.5 million injections.
3. *Hymenoptera* venom causes an estimated 50 deaths per year in the United States.
4. Exposure to a sensitizing agent leads to the formation of specific IgE antibodies that become affixed to receptors on tissue mast cells and peripheral basophils. Upon re-exposure, the sensitizing antigen cross-links specific IgE antibodies. Bridging of adjacent receptors initiates a cascade of biochemical events that leads to a discharge of the inflammatory mediators histamine, leukotrienes, and prostaglandins. Potent proinflammatory cytokines and chemokines are also released from the mast cells after their activation. Inflammatory mediators exert physiologic effects on the cardiovascular system, respiratory tract, gastrointestinal tract, mucus glands, and skin.

Associated Clinical Features

1. Signs and symptoms vary in both severity (mild urticaria to shock and death) and the spectrum of organ system involvement. Major manifestations include cutaneous, respiratory, cardiovascular, and gastrointestinal symptoms (Figs. 18-11 and 18-12).
2. Usual clinical course
   a. About 80% of patients present with a predictable uniphasic course, in which signs and symptoms occur early, but there is a good response to therapy, and the patients remain symptom-free thereafter.
   b. A biphasic course is seen in about 20% of patients. A second episode of anaphylaxis, that can occur up

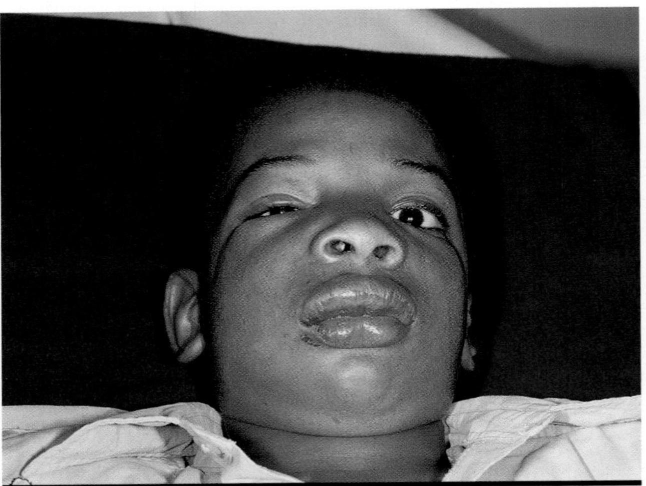

Figure 18-11. Anaphylaxis

Right-sided periorbital and facial swelling and lip swelling (angioedema), wheezing, hoarseness of the voice, and urticaria were the presenting complaints in this child after eating peanuts. Angioedema usually involves the loose connective tissues of the ear or the periorbital or perioral areas, but may involve the oropharynx or extremities.

to 8 hours following apparent recovery from the initial event, is seen in these patients.

c. Anaphylaxis rarely can take a protracted course and symptoms may persistent for about 3 weeks.

3. Clinical diagnosis of anaphylaxis is straightforward in a patient who manifests the full-blown syndrome after exposure to an identifiable provocative agent.

4. The diagnosis may be less obvious in patients presenting with symptoms and signs limited to one or two organ systems. A detailed medical history with particular attention given to the types of symptoms experienced and potential triggers encountered is of paramount importance in establishing the diagnosis of anaphylaxis and identifying its cause.

5. When the diagnosis is unclear, laboratory tests may be helpful in making a diagnosis.
   a. Acute systemic mast cell degranulation leads to a rise in plasma histamine that can be detected by measuring urinary histamine metabolites following the episode.
   b. Measurement of serum beta-tryptase (representing mast cell degranulation) may also help in arriving at the diagnosis.
   c. Demonstration of elevated serum tryptase levels at the time of the acute reaction with a subsequent fall to the normal range strongly support the diagnosis of anaphylaxis.

Emergency Department Treatment and Disposition

1. It is critical to think of anaphylaxis as one end of a spectrum of clinical disorders that includes asthma, urticaria, and angioedema. Since there is no way to predict how rapidly a reaction will progress, all patients with suspected anaphylactic reaction should receive an immediate assessment of the stability of their airway, breathing, and circulation (ABCs).

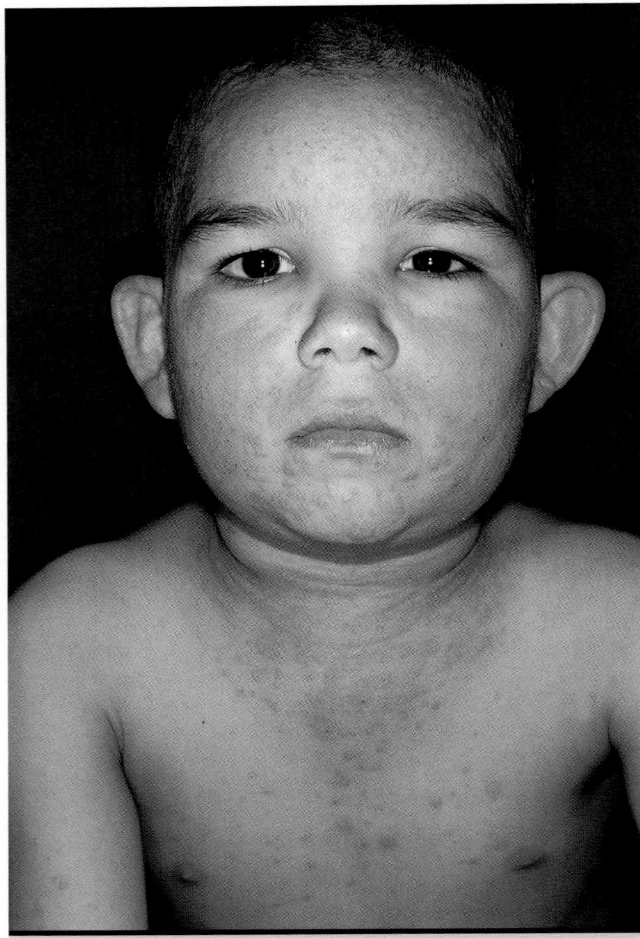

Figure 18-12. Acute Allergic Reaction

Acute onset of pruritic, erythematous rash, bilateral periorbital edema, and swelling of the ear were the presenting complaints of this child. At the time these pictures were made, the etiology of this acute allergic reaction was unclear.

2. Anaphylaxis with life-threatening presentations requires *simultaneous evaluation and management of the ABCs* based on a rapid examination and often a minimal history.
   a. Establish a secure airway (if required) followed by 100% oxygen, continuous pulse oximetry, and cardiac and blood pressure monitoring.
   b. Some examples of indications for endotracheal intubation include the presence of stridor, drooling, labored breathing, altered mental status, and signs of potential airway compromise (e.g., voice change, perioral/lingual edema, or shortness of breath).
   c. Two large-bore IVs should be placed.
   d. Monitor arterial blood gases.

3. Epinephrine is the critical first-line therapy for anaphylaxis, *regardless of cause*.
   a. For mild reactions with good perfusion (e.g., urticaria, bronchospasm):
      1) Give subcutaneously (dose: 0.01 mL/kg or 0.01 mg/kg [max 0.5 mL] of 1:1000 concentration)
      2) Duration of action of epinephrine is short.
      3) The dose can be repeated every 15 to 20 minutes as needed in the face of persistent or reappearing symptoms.
   b. For moderate to severe reactions (e.g., angioedema, hypotension, laryngeal edema):
      1) Give via intramuscular, intravenous, or intraosseous route (dose: 0.1 mL/kg [max 10 mL] of 1:10,000 concentration) *or*
      2) Given via endotracheal route (dose: 0.1 mL/kg [max 5 mL] of 1:1000 concentration)
   c. For circulatory collapse and hypotension:
      1) The patient should receive an IV fluid bolus (20 mL/kg) of crystalloid (lactated Ringer's or normal saline).
      2) Repeat boluses may be necessary to compensate for the marked peripheral vasodilation and third-spacing that may accompany anaphylaxis.
      3) An intravenous epinephrine or dopamine infusion may be required for patients with hypotension that is refractory to fluids.
      4) The patient should be placed in the Trendelenburg position (head 30° below the feet).

4. Racemic epinephrine (2.25% diluted in 2.5 mL of normal saline) may be used in patients with signs and symptoms of airway compromise.

5. For bronchospasm:
   a. Inhaled β_2-agonist such as nebulized albuterol (dose: 2.5 mg <30 kg; 5 mg for >30 kg; repeat dose every 20 minutes for 1 to 2 hours *or* 0.5 mg/kg per hour by continuous nebulization [15 mg/hour maximum dose]) *or*
   b. IV aminophylline (dose: 4 to 6 mg/kg in saline drip every 6 hours or 0.9 to 1.1 mg/kg per hour as continuous infusion) may be used.

6. As clinically indicated, the following measures should be carried out:
   a. The offending antigen must be removed whenever possible (e.g., stop antibiotic infusion).
   b. Removal of the insect's stinger may be best accomplished by flicking it out with a credit card (use of the tweezers or forceps may actually release more venom).
   c. To delay systemic absorption of the allergen, apply a tourniquet proximal to the injection or sting site.
   d. Split the dose of epinephrine, with 0.1 mL directly infiltrated SC into the allergen injection or sting site, and the remainder administered into the contralateral arm.

7. Patients undergoing treatment with β-adrenergic blocking agents may not respond to epinephrine and may require glucagon (dose: 1 to 5 mg given IV as an initial bolus followed by a continuous infusion titrated against blood pressure, if required)

8. Antihistamines as adjunctive therapy:
   a. Antihistamines do not reverse end-organ effects or hypotension in patients with anaphylaxis.
   b. They block further release of histamine and provide symptomatic relief in anaphylactic reactions accompanied by urticaria and angioedema.
   c. A combination of H_1- and H_2-receptor blocking agents can be synergistic in effect and should be used.
      1) Examples of H_1-blocking agents: diphenhydramine and hydroxyzine
      2) Examples of H_2-blocking agents: cimetidine and ranitidine
      3) Diphenhydramine (most commonly used) can be given IV, IM, or orally (dose: 1 to 2 mg/kg every 4 to 6 hours [50-mg maximum single dose]).
      4) Cimetidine is given IV slowly over 15 minutes (dose: 5 mg/kg every 6 to 8 hours [300-mg maximum single dose]) or ranitidine is given IV slowly over 15 minutes (dose: 1 mg/kg every 6 to 8 hours [50-mg maximum single dose]).

9. Corticosteroids as adjunctive therapy
   a. Corticosteroids do not play a role in the immediate reversal of anaphylaxis since their onset of action is delayed for 4 to 6 hours. However, they inhibit or lessen biphasic and protracted anaphylactic reactions including bronchospasm with their anti-inflammatory properties.
   b. Given IV as hydrocortisone (dose: 5-mg/kg bolus) or methylprednisolone (dose: 2-mg/kg bolus followed by 2 mg/kg per day divided every 6 hours) or orally (e.g., prednisone 2-mg/kg bolus [60-mg maximum single dose] followed by once-daily dose)

10. All patients with moderate to severe reactions requiring resuscitation must be hospitalized and observed for 24 to 48 hours, even in the absence of persistent symptoms.

11. All patients with milder reactions:
   a. Must be observed for at least 6 to 8 hours, even if they have had a prompt response to the initial therapy.
   b. Some patients may experience biphasic reactions with recurrence of signs and symptoms (after initial resolution) within this period of time
   c. Antihistamines and steroids are prescribed orally for the next 72 hours if the patient's condition improves and remains stable (e.g., patients with angioedema, urticaria, and minimal bronchospasm).

12. Patients may be referred to an allergist for desensitization immunotherapy (e.g., anaphylaxis from insect stings).

13. Patient/parent education and prevention:
   a. Educate them regarding possible future recurrences; *be prepared*.
   b. Previous episodes of mild anaphylaxis do not guarantee that future episodes will not be life-threatening.
   c. Counsel about avoidance of precipitating allergens if they have been identified (e.g., nuts, fish).
   d. A patient with severe reactions should wear a MedicAlert bracelet that indicates precipitating agents if known, in the event of recurrent anaphylaxis.

e. Insect exposure should be avoided and patients should be instructed to avoid wearing things that attract insects (e.g., perfumes, bright-colored clothes).
f. Latex-free gloves and catheters should be used for patients allergic to latex.
g. Parents and older children should be given a prescription and educated in detail about self-administering epinephrine (e.g., EpiPen JR, Ana-Kit).
h. Printed patient information is available from the Asthma and Allergy Foundation of America and MedicAlert tags from the MedicAlert Foundation.

Clinical Pearls: Anaphylaxis

1. Anaphylaxis is a potentially life-threatening manifestation of an IgE-mediated hypersensitivity reaction involving two or more organ systems.
2. Life-threatening features of anaphylaxis include upper airway obstruction (laryngeal, pharyngeal, and lingual edema) and hypotensive shock (profound vasodilation and increased vascular permeability).
3. Epinephrine is the mainstay of therapy for anaphylaxis regardless of the cause.

BOX 18-10. COMMON ETIOLOGIES OF ANAPHYLAXIS AND ANAPHYLACTOID REACTIONS

- *IgE-mediated (anaphylaxis)*
  (1) Insect venom (*Hymenoptera* venom: honeybees, bumblebees, hornets, wasps, fire ants, yellow jackets)
  (2) Drugs (penicillin [leading cause], sulfonamides, cephalosporins, topical anesthetics)
  (3) Foods (nuts [walnuts, pecans], peanuts, legumes, seafood (fish, shellfish), eggs, milk, monosodium glutamate, soybeans, mollusks)
  (4) Latex (gloves, catheters, balloons, condoms)
  (5) Blood products (especially in IgA-deficient patients)
  (6) Vaccines (avian-based: measles, mumps, influenza, yellow fever)
  (7) Allergenic extracts for immunotherapy or skin testing (pollens, dust mite, venom)
  (8) Exercise (jogging)
- *Non–IgE-mediated (anaphylactoid reactions)*
  (1) Aspirin
  (2) NSAIDs
  (3) Radiocontrast media
  (4) Dextran
  (5) Succinylcholine

Key points

- The most common offending agents that induce anaphylaxis are drugs.
- Among the many drugs that have been implicated, beta-lactam antibiotics top the list.
- Latex allergy is more common in high-risk groups such as patients with spinal bifida or those who have undergone repeated genitourinary surgical procedures.

BOX 18-11. CLINICAL FEATURES OF ANAPHYLAXIS

- *Cutaneous*
  (1) Pruritus
  (2) Warmth, flushing, erythema
  (3) Urticaria
  (4) Angioedema
- *HEENT*
  (1) Conjunctival itching, lacrimation, injection, or chemosis
  (2) Sneezing, rhinorrhea
  (3) Stridor, hoarseness
  (4) Edema of the lips, tongue, pharynx, larynx, or nasal turbinates that impairs ventilation and swallowing
  (5) Tingling in the lips, itching of the mouth and throat
- *Respiratory*
  (1) Chest pain, tightness, dyspnea, cough
  (2) Wheezing, intercostal and subcostal retractions, bronchorrhea
- *Circulatory*
  (1) Faintness
  (2) Palpitations, tachycardia, arrhythmias
  (3) Hypotension
  (4) Cardiopulmonary arrest
- *GI*
  (1) Nausea, vomiting
  (2) Abdominal cramps
  (3) Bloating, diarrhea, tenesmus
- *CNS*
  (1) Dizziness, syncope
  (2) Seizures
  (3) Altered level of consciousness
  (4) "Sense of impending doom"
- *GU*
  (1) Genital edema
  (2) Uterine cramps
  (3) Urinary urgency

Key points

- Any route of exposure (oral, parenteral, or inhalational) can cause anaphylaxis.
- Time between exposure to the inciting antigen and onset of symptoms:
  (1) Usually minutes to hours (*a majority of symptoms occur within 30 minutes*)
  (2) The interval depends on the route, quantity, and rate of administration of the antigen, and the sensitivity of the host.
  (3) In general, the more rapid the onset the more severe the overall course.
  (4) Risk factors include a previous history of anaphylaxis, atopy or asthma.

BOX 18-12. DIFFERENTIAL DIAGNOSIS OF ANAPHYLAXIS

- Vasovagal syncope
  (1) Pallor, bradycardia
  (2) *Absence of cutaneous or respiratory findings*
- Shock from other etiologies (e.g., septic, cardiogenic, toxic shock syndrome)
- Other causes of airway obstruction
  (1) Foreign body aspiration
  (2) Infections (e.g., retropharyngeal abscess, croup, epiglottitis or bacterial tracheitis)
- Hereditary angioedema
  (1) C1 esterase deficiency
  (2) Painless, pruritus-free angioedema *without* urticaria, flushing or respiratory findings
- Serum sickness (usually several days after exposure to the inciting agent)
- Scombroid poisoning
  (1) Due to ingestion of dark-meat fish such as tuna or mackerel
  (2) Release of a histamin-like mediator
- Systemic mastocytosis
- Pheochromocytoma
  (1) Hypotensive attacks with tachycardia
  (2) *Absence* of urticaria, flushing or wheezing
- Panic attacks
- Metastatic carcinoid (flushing syndromes)
- Vocal cord dysfunction

DIAGNOSIS ANIMAL BITES

Introduction

1. Children are common victims of bites by mammals. Their inexperience as animal handlers, aggressiveness of play, and relative physical weakness of youth contribute to their vulnerability.
2. Although rarely a cause of death, mammalian bites are a source of substantial morbidity. Cosmetic and infectious complications can be minimized by understanding the pathophysiology of these injuries, and proper principles of medical management.

Epidemiology

1. Animal bites constitute a worldwide problem of epidemic proportions. In the United States, incidence rates have been reported to be on the order of 2 to 3.5 million per year. Animal bites account for between 0.5 and 1.2% of all ED visits.
2. While the vast majority of bites are probably trivial and go unreported, serious injuries frequently occur. Though infrequent, fatalities from animal bites do occur. Reviews of published epidemiologic data, nationwide newspaper articles, electronic news files, and vital records consistently demonstrate disproportionately higher death rates in infants and young children.
3. In a review of data from the Humane Society of the United States regarding dog bite–related fatalities, Sacks and colleagues (1989) noted a disproportionate association with specific breeds of dogs. While more than 25 breeds of dogs were involved in 238 human dog bite–related fatalities from 1979 through 1998, more than half involved pit bulls or Rottweilers (Figs. 18-13 and 18-14). However, the authors noted that other breeds also bite and might cause fatalities at equal or higher rates, based on their proportion of the total population of dogs.
4. Children and young adults are most often the victims of nonfatal bites. The highest incidence has consistently been in schoolchildren 5 to 14 years old, who tend to overexcite, mistreat, or unintentionally threaten house pets. Though making up only 20% of the population, this age group accounts for one-third to one-half of all domestic animal bite injuries.
5. Males sustain dog bite injuries twice as frequently as do females, perhaps due to their greater tendency toward active and aggressive play. On the other hand, girls are twice as likely as boys to be bitten by cats.
6. Most animal bites are caused by dogs, which account for 90% of injuries, while slightly under 10% are caused by cats. Miscellaneous species, primarily rodents and rabbits, are responsible for the remaining small number. German shepherds are implicated in up to half of all incidents, which far exceeds their population proportion in the community (this disproportion may be due in part to the tendency for observers to identify any large dog as a "shepherd"). The pit bull is also often implicated or identified as the biting animal.

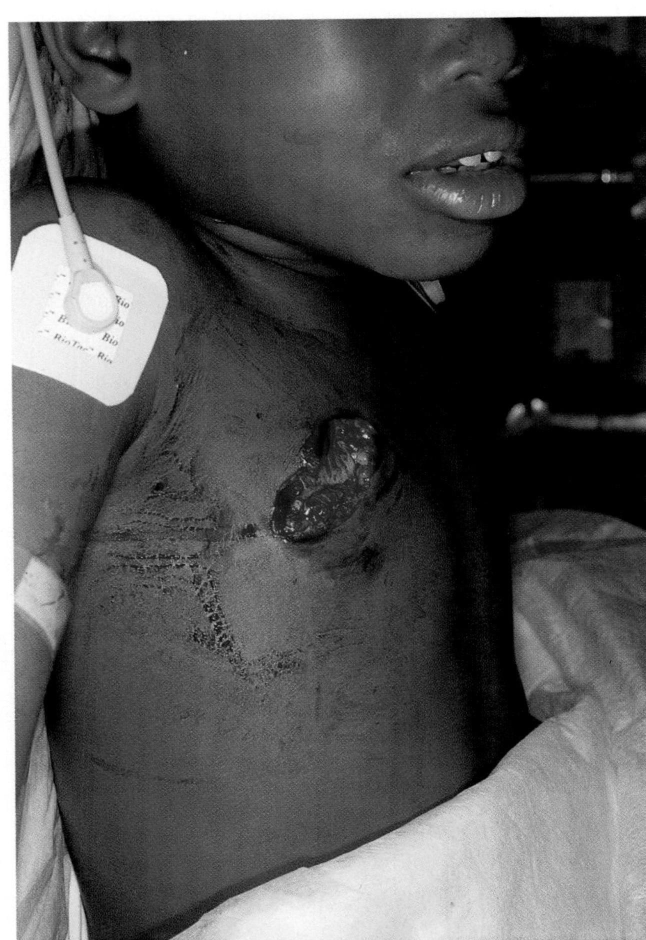

Figure 18-13. Dog Bites by a Pit Bull

Dog bite wounds cause a spectrum of tissue injuries that vary from scratches and abrasions to contusions and lacerations. Dog bites occur in the head and neck area in 60 to 70% of victims 5 years and younger, and in 50% of those who are 10 years and younger.

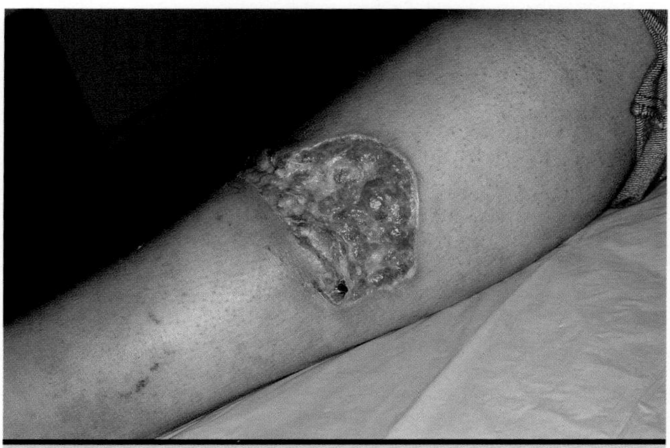

Figure 18-14. Dog Bites by a Pit Bull

This picture was taken 2 weeks after the dog bite.

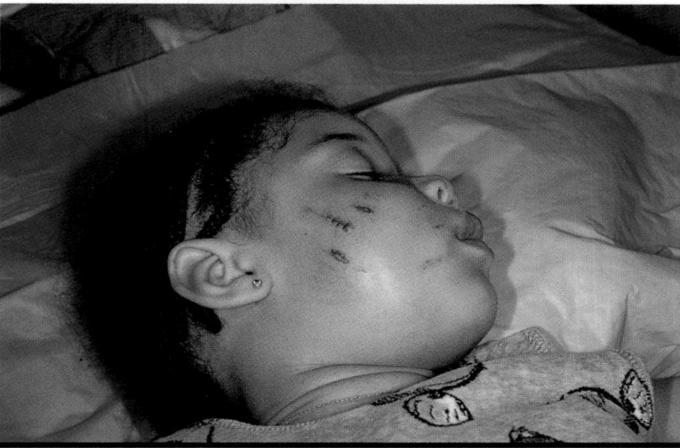

Figure 18-15. Cellulitis in a Dog Bite

Intense local tenderness, severe pain (greater than clinical signs indicated), and rapidly spreading erythema were seen in this febrile patient who came back to the ED 12 hours after being discharged from the ED following a bite by a German shepherd that was owned by the family.

7. The dogs that most often bite people are not strays or wild dogs, but rather pets well known to the victim, owned by the family (15%) or neighbors (75%).

8. In areas with distinct temperature variations, most dog bites occur during spring and summer months, when opportunities are greatest for contact between children and animals in streets, parks, and playgrounds. This seasonality is absent or diminished in climates with little temperature variation such as California and Florida.

Microbiology of Infection

1. Approximately 5% of dog bites and 15 to 50% of cat bites become significantly infected (Fig. 18-15).

2. Microorganisms isolated from infected wounds are normally present on body surfaces as well as the mouths of biting animals. However, it is believed that animal saliva, rather than the victim's skin flora, is the major source of bacteria isolated from bite-wound cultures.

3. A wide variety of bacteria are present in dog bite injuries.
   a. The importance of indigenous oral flora of the biting animal is well illustrated by the high incidence of infections due to *Pasteurella* species following dog and cat bites.
   b. *P. canis* and other pasteurella species have been identified in up to 50% of infected dog bites.
   c. *P. multocida* and other pasteurella species have been identified in up to 80% of infected cat bites.
   d. These gram-negative facultatively anaerobic rods have been found in the oral cavities of one-half to two-thirds of dogs and cats. Multiple biotypes have been identified, but serve no practical clinical significance; all are susceptible to penicillin.
   e. Other common isolates from infected bite wounds include streptococci, *Staphylococcus epidermidis*, and some enteric bacteria.
   f. *Staphylococcus aureus* has also been identified as an important cause of infection following bite injuries (especially human), having been isolated from 10 to 40% of these wounds. Anaerobes have also been regularly isolated when carefully sought.
   g. Bite wound infections are usually polymicrobial in nature. A study of the infected wounds of 50 patients with dog bites and 57 patients with cat bites yielded a median of five bacterial isolates per culture (range, 0 to 16).

Emergency Department Treatment and Disposition

1. The same basic principles of care apply to all animal bites:
   a. Cleansing and surgical débridement
   b. Proper wound exploration and repair
   c. Immobilization and elevation of larger injured areas
   d. Administration of tetanus prophylaxis when required
   e. Evaluation for rabies prophylaxis
   f. Administration of antibiotics in selected cases
   g. Close follow-up care

2. Since almost all animal bites are contaminated, meticulous wound toilet is essential.
   a. Copious irrigation of wounds from dog bites was associated in one study with a drop in the infection rate from 69 to 12%.

b. Lacerations and avulsions are best cleansed with moderate pressure irrigation utilizing copious amounts of water, normal saline or Ringer's lactate solution delivered via a large syringe through a 19-gauge nozzle.
c. Effective irrigation of puncture wounds is technically difficult; incision and drainage may actually increase tissue destruction.

3. The suturing of bite wounds is controversial.
   a. In recent years, the consensus has changed from a policy of never suturing such wounds to one of closing them with good surgical wound toilet.
   b. Both retrospective and prospective studies have shown lower (not statistically significant) rates of infection in sutured as opposed to nonsutured wounds. A recent study of 145 consecutive patients with bite wounds receiving primary closure (mean age of patient, 21 years) demonstrated a 6% rate of infection.
   c. Tissue adhesives should not be used to close bite wounds, since such closure traps in any remaining bacterial pathogens.

4. The utilization of antibiotics in the management of bite wounds varies by case.
   a. In the presence of an obvious infection, administration of penicillin plus a penicillinase-resistant penicillin would seem to be the best treatment.
   b. A combination of amoxicillin and clavulanic acid or clindamycin are also effective as an alternate regimen.
   c. Effectiveness of antibiotic prophylaxis in dog bites
      1) The effectiveness of antibiotic prophylaxis in fresh wounds that appear to be free of infection is less well established. Awareness of the high incidence of wound contamination has led many to advocate the use of prophylactic antibiotics for wounds seen within the first 24 hours. However, efficacy has not been established by adequate studies.
      2) Two investigations utilizing narrow-spectrum antibiotics in dog bites (one protocol excluded facial injuries) demonstrated equal rates of infection in both antibiotic-treated and control groups. All infected bites in both studies occurred in wounds of the hands.
      3) Another study of dog bite wounds in children thought to be at low risk for subsequent infection showed no statistically significant difference in infection rates when treatment with prophylactic antibiotics was compared to treatment with local care only. In the same study, however, a trend toward higher infection rates in full-thickness wounds was seen.
      4) In a meta-analysis of eight randomized trials, investigators found that the relative risk of infection after prophylactic antibiotic treatment was 0.56 (95% confidence interval, 0.38 to 0.82).
   d. Effectiveness of antibiotic prophylaxis in cat bites (Fig. 18-16)
      1) Research regarding the efficacy of prophylactic antibiotics following cat bites is scant.
      2) A significant reduction in the frequency of infection with prophylactic antibiotic use was shown in one small prospective study of cat bite wounds.

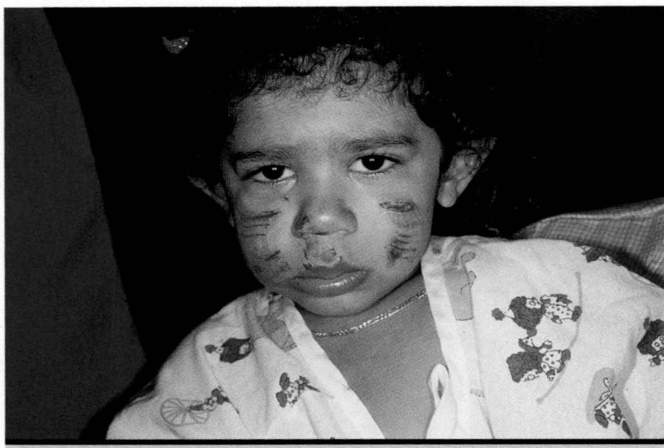

Figure 18-16. Cat Scratches

This 3-year-old girl presented with bilateral scratches and puncture wounds (around the lips) inflicted by the cat owned by her family. Cat scratches are most commonly seen on the upper extremities or periorbital region. Cat bites are located on upper extremities in two-thirds of the cases and usually consist of puncture wounds rather than lacerations or contusions.

      3) In a descriptive report of 186 consecutive patients presenting with cat bite (or scratch) wounds that were managed according to a standardized protocol, 148 patients had initially uninfected wounds. Of those, 101 were administered antibiotics, and 47 were not. The patient infection rate was 2% for those receiving oral antibiotics, versus 6% for those not receiving oral antibiotics.
   e. At present, the use of prophylactic antibiotics would seem best limited to specific instances in which the risk of infection or residual deformity is high. These include:
      1) Puncture wounds, particularly cat bites, which cannot be adequately irrigated or débrided
      2) Deep wounds of the hand
      3) Complicated facial wounds, where excess scarring due to infection would be unacceptable
      4) Bites in immunocompromised hosts
      5) Bites intended for delayed primary closure
   f. There is no advantage in treating patients who present more than 24 hours after injury with an wound that does not appear to be infected.

5. Hand wounds following mammalian bites
   a. Hand wounds present a special problem, as 30% or more become infected.
   b. Because of the presence of avascular tendon sheath spaces, the propensity for spread of infection, and potential for significant morbidity, the safety of suturing is much less certain. While some authors recommend that hand wounds not be sutured, it is common practice to repair them at the time of the injury.
   c. It is especially important that these wounds be meticulously cleansed prior to repair.
   d. After repair, prophylactic antibiotics are commonly prescribed for these patients.

6. Tetanus prophylaxis following mammalian bites
   a. Tetanus prophylaxis should be given when indicated. Most children are completely immunized and have antitoxin levels high enough to obviate the need for boosters more often than every 5 years. Those not fully immunized may require adsorbed tetanus (and diphtheria) toxoid at the time of injury.
   b. Tetanus immune globulin, of human origin, is the product of choice for passive immunization. It is required only for dirty wounds in children with inadequate or uncertain immunization status.
7. The need for rabies prophylaxis depends entirely on the species of biting animal and experience with rabies in the community. Local health authorities should be consulted when there is doubt. For complete discussion of the epidemiology, pathophysiology, and prevention in humans, see page 708.

Clinical Pearls: Animal Bites

1. Animal bites present a significant potential for morbidity in childhood. Most injuries are trivial; however, infections and fatalities do occur.
2. Many injuries could be avoided by proper parental education of children regarding their behavior in the presence of animals (Fig. 18-17). Most instances of animal bite, when impartially investigated, turn out to be the fault of the child, not the animal.
3. Bite wound infections are usually polymicrobial in nature.
4. Hand wounds tend to become infected more often than those located elsewhere. Considering the complexity of the hand's structure and the ease with which infection spreads along contaminated tissue planes, function can be easily compromised or destroyed. Thus every bite of the hand should be considered potentially serious.

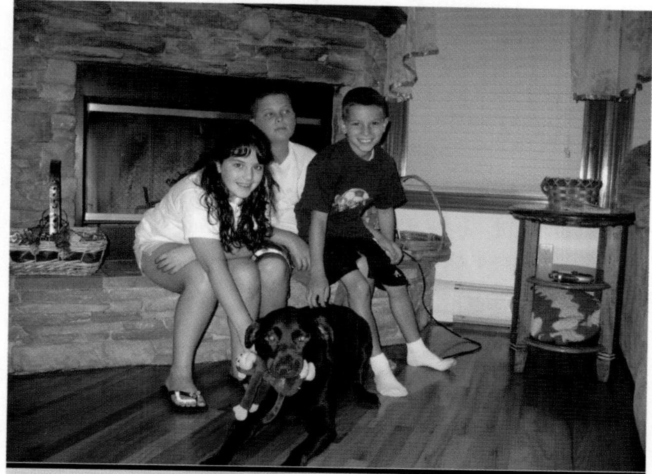

Figure 18-17. The "Bear"; sometimes a teddy and sometimes a grisly, but always a "Bear". The Lucchesi family children with their dog who is biting a stuffed monkey but not the children!!.

The dogs that most often bite people are not strays or wild dogs, but rather pets well known to the victim and owned by the family (15%) or neighbors (75%). Many injuries could be avoided by proper parental education of children regarding their behavior in the presence of animals. When impartially investigated most instances of animal bites turn out to be the fault of the child, not the animal.

BOX 18-13. CHARACTERISTICS OF INFECTIONS IN DOG AND CAT BITES

- Risk factors for infection include
  (1) Nature of the wounds inflicted (dog bites versus cat bites; see below)
  (2) Location of the wound (e.g., hand wounds tend to become infected more often than those located elsewhere)
  (3) Type of wound (deep punctures and crushes have higher infection rates)
  (4) Age of the wound (delay of >24 hours in seeking medical care)
- Dog bites
  (1) Dogs may exert from 150 to 450 pounds per square inch of pressure during a bite.
  (2) Dog bites, while generally presenting as lacerations or avulsions, are also crush injuries with areas of devitalization more extensive than can be appreciated by simple inspection of the wound.
  (3) Larger wounds can be easily cleansed and débrided and are paradoxically less likely to become infected than are minor lacerations or puncture wounds, which quickly close over the bacterial inoculum.
- Cat bites
  (1) Cats are capable of far less biting force than dogs.
  (2) A cat's sharp teeth penetrate more deeply, often inoculating organisms several centimeters into tissues; as a consequence, deep tissue infections may follow seemingly trivial cat bites

BOX 18-14. CLINICAL FEATURES OF INFECTIONS FOLLOWING ANIMAL BITES

- General signs of infection following animal bites:
  (1) They almost always become apparent between 12 and 72 hours postbite (earlier if pasteurella is involved; see below)
  (2) Redness, swelling, and tenderness around the site of injury
  (3) Often accompanied by purulent or serosanguineous drainage
  (4) Restricting the infection to the hand may be difficult, since most lymphatic drainage is through the dorsal subcutaneous space, and puffiness of this area may develop even when the infection is located elsewhere.
- Infections due to pasteurella
  (1) These infections display a more rapid and virulent course than those due to staphylococci or streptococci.
  (2) Redness and extensive swelling usually begin within 12 to 18 hours of the injury (6 to 12 hours earlier) when pasteurella is an infecting agent.
  (3) Intense local tenderness and severe pain (greater than clinical signs indicate) accompany these findings.
  (4) Regional lymphadenopathy (one-third of patients)
  (5) Low-grade fever (one-fourth of patients)
  (6) Penicillin treatment is effective, but deep tissue infections such as tenosynovitis, osteomyelitis, and septicemia can occur.

MANAGEMENT RABIES EXPOSURE AND VACCINE PROPHYLAXIS

Epidemiology

1. Infection with rabies virus produces an acute illness with rapidly progressive central nervous system manifestations (including anxiety, dysphagia, and seizures) that is almost invariably lethal.
2. In spite of the recent attention focused on rabies in some geographic areas, in the United States the number of cases detected in humans has steadily declined since 1950. This decline reflects the widespread vaccination of domestic pets, and the availability of effective immunoprophylaxis after exposure to a rabid animal.
3. Most of the United States, including all of the East Coast, is an endemic area for rabies.
   a. Raccoons, skunks, foxes, coyotes, and bats are common vectors. However, any warm-blooded wild or domestic carnivore can transmit the virus.
   b. Exempt are rabbits and most small rodents, including squirrels and mice. When infected experimentally with rabies, most rodents do not shed the virus in their saliva.
   c. Although unusual, transmission has been documented from house pets, including dogs, cats, and ferrets.
4. Despite the intense focus on rabies in raccoons in the eastern United States, no human deaths have been attributed to the raccoon rabies virus variant. However, case reports involving domestic cats and dogs have reemerged coincident with the surge in the raccoon population during the past 20 years. Of the 42 cases of rabies in humans diagnosed in the United States from 1980 to 1997, 13 were related to rabid animals outside of the United States, and 26 involved bats.

Pathophysiology

1. Rabies virus is an RNA virus classified in the Rhabdovirus family. It is concentrated in animal saliva.
2. Modes of transmission include
   a. Most cases occur following introduction of the virus into an open wound.
   b. Another, but much less common method of infection is direct mucosal exposure.
   c. It is also conjectured that exposure to high concentrations of airborne virus (as might occur in a cave that is densely inhabited by bats) can result in infection; however, there have been no confirmed cases of transmission to humans by that route.
   d. Transmission has also rarely occurred in the laboratory (airborne), and by transplantation of corneas from patients dying of undiagnosed rabies.
   e. Person-to-person transmission by bites has not been documented, although the virus has been isolated from the saliva of patients.

Prevention

1. Many states or commonwealths require rabies vaccinations for at-risk pets (i.e., pets that could possibly become exposed to rabies). The vaccine is generally required every 2 years for dogs and cats. In some animals, the vaccine could be effective for more than 2 years. The longevity of effectiveness of the vaccine in humans is variable.
2. The American Academy of Pediatrics Red Book (2000) lists current recommendations for administration of rabies vaccines. When a child presents with a complaint of an animal bite from a mammal, the managing physician should attempt to determine the nature of the animal and its rabies status.
   a. If the biting animal is known to have up-to-date vaccination status, then the bitten child need not receive prophylactic vaccines.
   b. If the biting animal is a wild animal unavailable for examination, it should be regarded as rabid and immunization of the bitten child should proceed (see below).
   c. If the biting animal is healthy and available (captive), but its vaccine status cannot be verified or is not up-to-date, the following steps should be taken:
      1) *Biting mammal that is healthy and captive:*
         i. The animal can be sacrificed and the brain inspected for rabies, *or*
         ii. The animal can be quarantined for 10 days and observed for suspicious behavior.
      2) *Bitten child:*
         i. The child can be administered rabies prophylaxis (see below), *or*
         ii. The child can await administration of rabies prophylaxis pending results of the rabies tests listed above.
3. Rabies prophylaxis requires administration of two agents.
   a. Rabies immune globulin (RIG) provides temporary passive immunization.
   b. Agents like human diploid cell vaccine (HDCV), and Rab Avert produce longer-acting (active) protection from the virus. The development of newer vaccines has markedly reduced the incidence of reactions previously associated with postexposure prophylaxis with duck embryo vaccine.
4. Passive immunization
   a. It is accomplished by administering RIG only once, on the day of initial presentation, at a dose of 20 IU/kg.
   b. The one exception is a person who has been immunized previously with rabies vaccine and has a documented adequate rabies antibody titer.
   c. The Centers for Disease Control and Prevention currently recommends that the entire dose of RIG should be infiltrated into the soft tissues surrounding the bite site.
   d. If that is impractical, the amount unable to be infiltrated traditionally has been injected into a large muscle distant from the injection site for the active vaccine (e.g., gluteus or quadriceps on the opposite side of the body).
5. Active immunization
   a. It is accomplished by administering HDCV (or any other brand) in five separate doses.
   b. Regardless of the child's weight or age, the dose is 1 ml, injected into the deltoid muscle.
   c. Single doses should be administered on days 0, 3, 7, 14, and 28, with day 0 being the day of initial presentation.
   d. With HDCV administration, there is a 6% incidence of serum sickness–like (type III) hypersensitivity reactions to booster doses given months or years after the primary series.
   e. Purified chick embryo cell culture (PCEC; RabAvert) vaccine has been developed for use in patients who develop sensitivity to one of the other vaccines. The brands are equally effective; they differ only in the cell lines used for vaccine production.
   f. If a child develops an allergic reaction to HDCV, one of the other brands should be substituted.
   g. All brands are expensive (the charge to the patient for the active vaccine alone [5 doses] is approximately $725). To be effective, all five doses must be given.
   h. If there is any patient-related deviation from the schedule, the manufacturer should be contacted for advice about the proper method of completion. The toll-free number is printed on the vaccine container.
6. *Bat exposures* deserve a special footnote.
   a. Between 1980 and 2000, 26 of 42 human rabies cases diagnosed in the United States were bat variants.
   b. Because bat teeth are quite small, their bites can be imperceptible, both in terms of noticeable pain and visible evidence on the skin.
   c. If anyone believes that they could have been bitten by a bat (including physical contact without a perceived bite), regardless of the findings on physical examination, rabies prophylaxis should be provided.
   d. Rabies prophylaxis should also be administered to anyone who has an open wound or mucous membrane that could have become contaminated with saliva or other potentially infectious material, or who has occupied the same closed space with a bat during a time of altered perception (e.g., asleep, intoxicated, developmentally immature, mentally impaired), regardless of the findings on physical examination.
7. All animal bites are supposed to be reported to the local animal control agency. Animal shelters are often capable of quarantining the biting animal. The police generally need not be contacted unless no one is available at the local animal shelter, and the animal needs to be located for quarantine or sacrifice.

Clinical Pearls: Rabies Exposure and Vaccine Prophylaxis

Local health authorities should be consulted when there is doubt about the local rabies status of a particular species of biting animal.

DIAGNOSIS HUMAN BITES

Introduction and Epidemiology

1. While not as common as dog bites, bites by humans are common occurrences in childhood. Human bites are reported to account for 1 per 600 pediatric ED visits, which is approximately one-third the rate of bites by other mammals.
2. Of those who present to the ED with human bite injuries, 5% require suturing and 5% to 30% (average, 15%) develop infection.
3. Overall, there is an even distribution of bites among males and females. However, in children younger than 10 years, males are more commonly bitten, while in older children (>10 years) bites of females are more commonly reported. Of all human bites involving children younger than 16 years, more than half (58%) occur in children older than 10 years. It is postulated that this likely reflects an increased frequency of fighting within this segment of the pediatric population.
4. As are animal bites, human bites are reported to occur more often during the summer months and during evening hours. However, in the preschool segment of the pediatric population, both summer and autumn were high-incidence seasons.

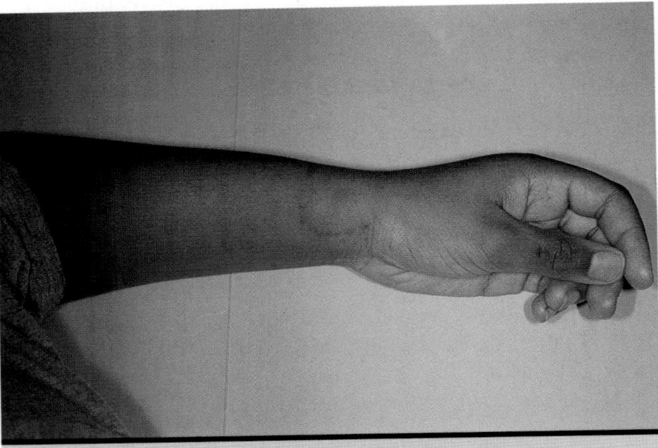

Figure 18-18. Human Bite

An 11-year-old girl presented with a human bite sustained during a fight at school. Most human bite injuries in children are minor. Abrasions (as seen here) account for two-thirds to three-quarters of bite injuries in children. Bites are most commonly seen on the upper extremities.

Associated Clinical Features

1. Children sustain their injuries most often during fights (61%) or play (26%).
2. Most human bite injuries in children are minor (Fig. 18-18).
   a. Abrasions account for two-thirds to three-quarters of bite injuries in children.
   b. The remainder are evenly distributed between punctures and lacerations.
3. Most injuries are located above the waist (see Box 18-15).

Microbiology of Infection

1. As is the case for other mammalian bites, the bacteria most commonly isolated from infected human bites are those found in the saliva of the biter.
2. Infected human bites are typically polymicrobial, and often involve staphylococci, streptococci, enteric organisms, gram-negative organisms, and/or anaerobes.
3. *Eikenella* species are also common pathogens in infected human bites.
4. Factors that seem to increase the likelihood of development of subsequent infection include:
   a. Delay in initial care >20 hours
   b. Occurrence of bites during fights and sports events (i.e., crush injuries)
   c. Presence of punctures or deep lacerations
   d. Suture closure of deep wounds
   e. Larger intraoral bites

Emergency Department Treatment and Disposition

1. The general principles of care of other mammalian bites also apply to human bites. These include:
   a. Thorough cleansing and appropriate débridement
   b. Proper wound exploration and repair
   c. Immobilization and elevation of larger injured areas
   d. Tetanus prophylaxis and antibiotic administration in selected cases
   e. Close follow-up care
2. All human bites must be managed as contaminated wounds.
   a. To avoid infection, meticulous wound toilet is essential.
   b. Wounds should be cleansed with copious amounts of water or saline delivered through a large-bore needle (or equivalent). When it comes to irrigation of this type of wound, more is better.
3. The suturing of human bite wounds is somewhat controversial. Although these are contaminated wounds, it is possible to surgically repair most of those that require closure. While most studies fail to show statistically significantly higher infection rates in surgically closed human bite wounds, many indicate trends in that direction.

BOX 18-15. HUMAN BITE WOUNDS IN CHILDREN (N = 322)

Location of wound		*Body part*	
Upper extremities	42%	Finger	17%
Head and neck	32%	Forearm	12%
Trunk	20%	Cheek	12%
Lower extremities	4%	Breast	9%
Genitalia	4%	Forehead	6%
		Chest	5%

(Reproduced with permission from: Baker MD, Moore SE: Human bites in children: A six-year experience. *Am J Dis Child* 1987;141:1285.).

4. Use of antibiotics
   a. It seems prudent to carefully cleanse all human bite wounds, and to administer antibiotics to patients whose wounds are at particularly high risk for development of infection. Sutured wounds are generally considered to be among the latter group.
   b. For nonsutured human bite wounds, the utilization of prophylactic antibiotics for wounds that appear to be uninfected is controversial. The use of antibiotics in this manner would seem best limited to specific instances in which the risk of infection or residual deformity is high. These include:
      1) Deep puncture wounds
      2) Sutured full-thickness wounds
      3) Full-thickness wounds of the hand
      4) Wounds caused by high impact (i.e., sports-related or fight-related) that likely contain crushed tissue.
      5) Intraoral bite wounds (a study in children showed a trend [though statistically insignificant] toward higher infection rates in longer, deeper lacerations)
   c. There seems to be no advantage in administering antibiotics to patients who present more than 24 hours after injury with wounds that appear to be uninfected.
   d. Contusions and abrasions resulting from human bites generally do not become infected.
   e. If antibiotics are indicated, agent(s) should be selected that provide broad-spectrum coverage.
      1) The combination of amoxicillin and clavulanic acid is generally effective against the organisms that contaminate human bite wounds.
      2) Clindamycin is an effective alternative.
5. Tetanus prophylaxis should be considered in all bite wounds and should be given when indicated.
6. Proper attention should always be paid to protection, immobilization, and elevation of any significant injury. A properly structured three-layer dressing should be applied to any full-thickness wound to enhance wound healing.
7. Appropriate follow-up care (within 36 hours) should also be arranged for these patients.

Clinical Pearls: Human Bites

1. All human bites must be managed as contaminated wounds.
2. Infection is the most common type of morbidity associated with human bites. If not aggressively treated, human bite infections can lead to serious permanent dysfunction of the injured area.

DIAGNOSIS VENOMOUS MARINE ANIMALS

Stinging Marine Animals: Corals, Sea Anemones, Hydroids, and Fire Coral

Background

1. This group includes cnidarians (phylum Cnidaria) and sponges.
2. Cnidarians are members of the massive phylum Coelenterata.
   a. Of this group, cnidarians are distinguished by possessing microscopic offensive and defensive weaponry in their tentacles: nematocysts.
   b. Nematocysts are toxin-filled sacs, and each contains a coiled poison dart (cnidocil). When stimulated by contact or by osmotic force (when a saltwater nematocyst is exposed to fresh water), the nematocyst discharges the cnidocil, firing it at high velocity (over 20 meters per second). The cnidocil can penetrate skin, and the venomous contents of the sac are injected into the victim (Figs. 18-19 and 18-20).
   c. The cnidarians include corals, sea anemones, hydroids, fire coral, jellyfish, and the Portuguese man-of-war.
3. Class Anthozoa
   a. Hard corals (order Scleractinia) and soft corals (order Alcyonacea)
      1) Corals are the building blocks of marine reefs.
      2) Hard corals are stonelike and can be quite sharp and unpleasant for the unwary swimmer or diver. Some hard corals are also the dwellings of stinging hydroids, as well as a variety of other creatures that bite.
      3) Soft corals are plantlike, and in places like the South Pacific can even form treelike structures. Although corals possess nematocysts, these are usually unable to penetrate human skin. Occasionally, though, contact with soft corals can cause envenomation (Fig. 18-21).

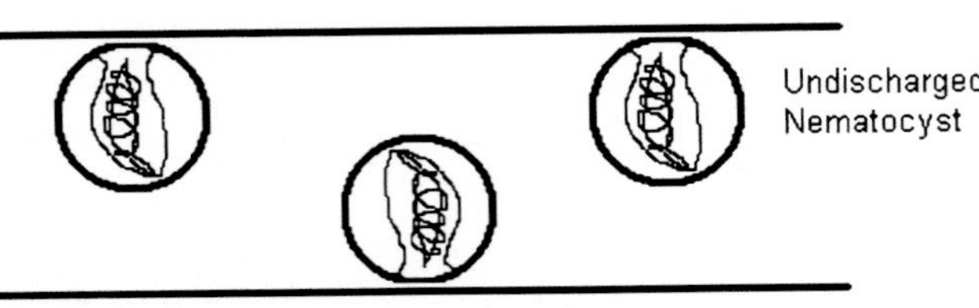

Figure 18-19. Nematocysts

Representation of coiled, undischarged nematocysts in a section of tentacle.

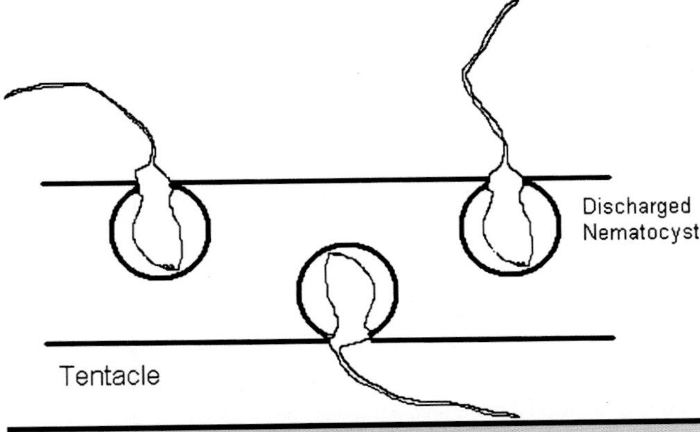

Figure 18-20. Discharged Nematocysts

Representation of discharged nematocysts in a section of tentacle.

   b. Sea anemones (class Actinaria)
      1) These are flowerlike creatures that capture food with nematocyst-covered tentacles (Fig. 18-22).
      2) Although most anemone nematocysts cannot penetrate human skin, there are more poisonous varieties that can cause painful stings, rashes, and itching on contact. In particular, there are Indo-Pacific varieties that can cause severe skin and even systemic reactions.
4. Class Hydrozoa
   a. Fire coral (order Milleporina): Fire coral or false coral is a hydrozoan that grows in plantlike colonies in shallow tropical waters, and is the bane of divers and snorkelers (Fig. 18-23).
   b. Hydroids: Hydroids are radially symmetrical organisms that live singly (Fig. 18-24) or form fernlike colonies (Fig. 18-25), and their sting can be painful (Fig. 18-26).

Mechanism of Injury

1. Thousands of nematocysts can burst and fire toxin-laden cnidocils at high velocity into the skin.
2. In the case of hard corals, lacerations and abrasions can occur.

Laboratory Tests

1. Nonspecific
2. In rare, severe envenomations, evidence of organ failure may be seen.
3. Complications include long-term skin changes, such as hyper- and hypopigmentation and eschar formation.

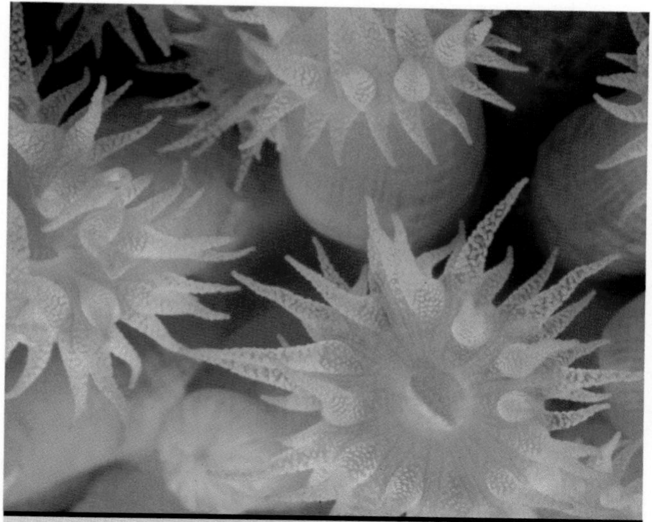

Figure 18-21. Orange Cup Coral

An example of a soft coral with tentacles. Photo taken in Bonaire, the Netherlands Antilles.

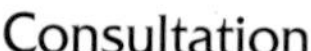

Consultation

Experts in marine envenomation may be sought through local poison control centers or through the Divers Alert Network (1-919-684-8111; 1-919-684-4326 collect).

Emergency Department Treatment and Disposition

1. Treatment should begin in the field. All tentacles must be removed.
2. Rinsing the wound immediately with vinegar may prevent further discharge of nematocysts, but its effectiveness with this group is less clear than with the cubomedusa jellyfish.
3. Baking soda has been advocated by some to reduce wound pain when applied shortly after the sting.
4. In the ED, the wound should be cleansed with normal saline.
5. Tetanus status should be assessed, and toxoid administered if no there was no vaccination in the previous 5 years.
6. Mild local reactions may be treated with antihistamines and topical corticosteroids.

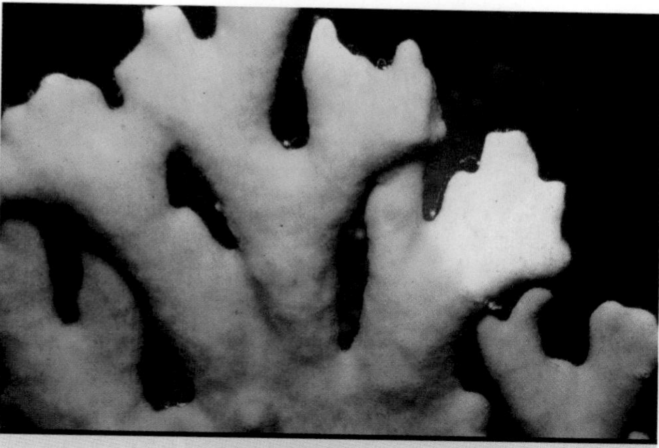

Figure 18-23. Fire Coral

Photo taken in Bonaire, Netherlands Antilles.

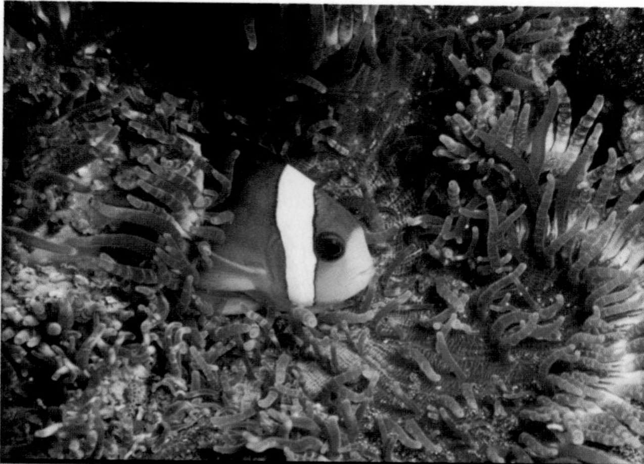

Figure 18-22. Sea Anemone

Clownfish living symbiotically in a venomous sea anemone. Photo taken in Papua New Guinea.

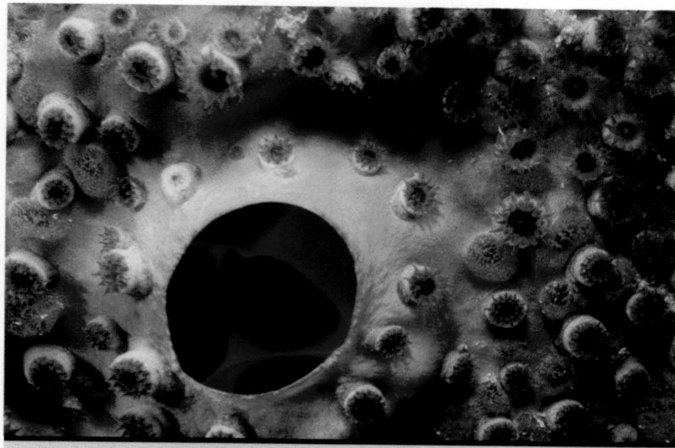

Figure 18-24. Hydroids

Hydroids living on a sponge. Photo taken in Fiji.

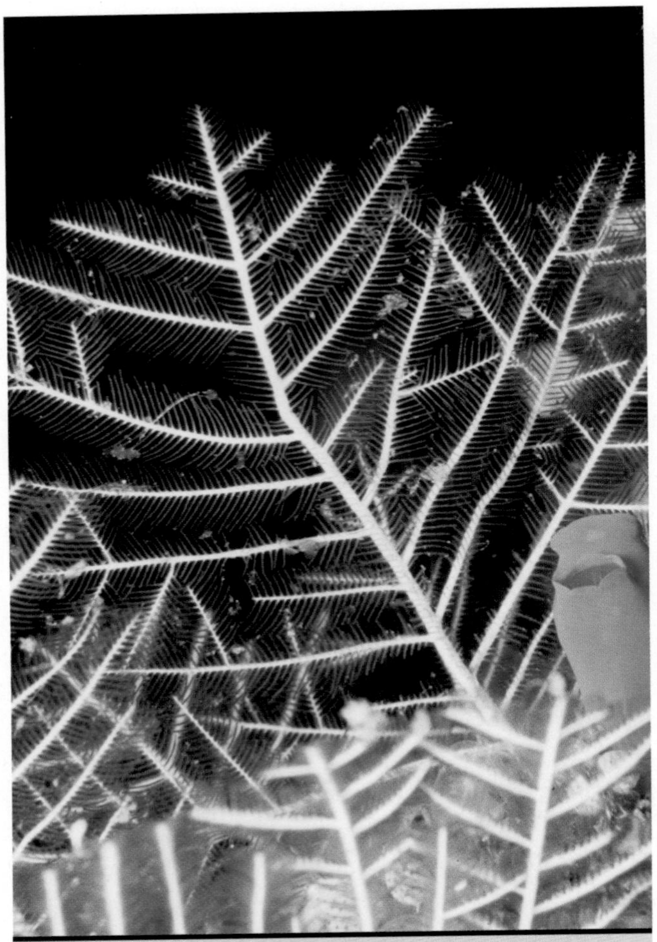

Figure 18-25. Stinging Hydroids

Photo taken in Komodo, Indonesia.

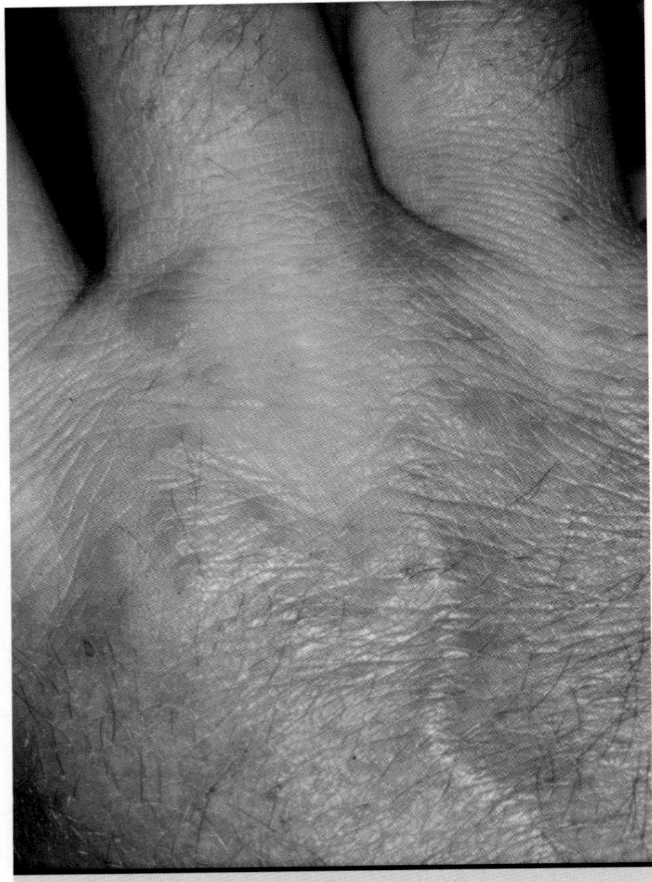

Figure 18-26. Hydroid Injury

A hand 24 hours after touching the hydroids shown in Fig. 18-25.

7. More severe skin reactions may require systemic corticosteroids. A 5- to 10-day course of prednisolone is normally adequate.
8. Patients without evidence of a systemic reaction 4 to 6 hours postenvenomation may be discharged.
9. Patients with evidence of systemic illness will most likely require admission.
10. Lacerations and abrasions due to contact with hard corals must be cleansed well.
    a. Lacerations should be rinsed with saline under pressure, if possible.
    b. Lacerations should be x-rayed for foreign body. All foreign bodies and devitalized tissue must be removed.
    c. Lacerations should not undergo tight primary closure, due to the propensity for infection; approximation with adhesive strips or delayed closure is preferred.
    d. Antibiotics are not normally indicated for immunocompetent patients.
11. Dermatologist follow-up is indicated for more severe skin reactions.

Clinical Pearl: Stinging Marine Animals (Corals, Sea Anemones, Hydroids, and Fire Coral)

Vinegar may be of benefit.

BOX 18-16. CLINICAL FEATURES OF INJURIES FROM STINGING MARINE ANIMALS (CORALS, SEA ANEMONES, HYDROIDS AND FIRE CORAL)

- Immediate burning sensation of the skin
- Local erythema and urticaria; sometimes lesions are pale at the center
- Less commonly edema, local skin hemorrhage, vesiculation, and desquamation can occur.
- Secondary bacterial infections can occur rarely.
- Systemic illness occurs rarely
  (1) Anaphylaxis
  (2) Nausea, vomiting, paresthesias
  (3) Altered mental status, cardiovascular collapse
  (4) Renal and hepatic failure

BOX 18-17. DIFFERENTIAL DIAGNOSIS OF INJURIES FROM STINGING MARINE ANIMALS (CORALS, SEA ANEMONES, HYDROIDS AND FIRE CORAL)

- Stings by other cnidarians (box jellyfish, Portuguese man-of-war)
- Anaphylactic/anaphylactoid reactions (from other etiology)
- Delayed hypersensitivity reaction
- Cold urticaria
- Sunburn
- Insect bite

Stinging Marine Animals: Box Jellyfish, True Jellyfish, and Portuguese Man-of-War

Background

1. This section describes stinging marine animals, including true jellyfish (scyphozoans), the box jellyfish (cubozoan jellyfish) and the Portuguese man-of-war.
   a. Portuguese man-of-war or bluebottle (*Physalia* species)
      1) The Portuguese man-of-war is found around the world.
      2) Although it appears to be a jellyfish, it is actually a collection of specialized hydroids that live in a colony.
      3) It consists of a float at the top, and long, stinging tentacles that can be 10 meters long that are used to catch fish (Fig. 18-27).
      4) Swimmers and divers can be envenomated when these animals are blown near shores and reefs.
      5) Beachgoers can be envenomated by tentacles that have washed ashore, even days later.
   b. Box jellyfish (cubozoan jellyfish)
      1) The box jellyfish family includes the world's most dangerous jellyfish, and these creatures are amongst the most dangerous venomous animals in the world.
      2) *Chironex fleckeri*, the Australian box jellyfish, is the most feared of all (Fig. 18-28).
      3) Serious stings from these jellyfish can be lethal in a matter of minutes.
      4) These animals have literally changed the way Australians see and use their beaches and coastal areas.
      5) Children are at particular risk.
   c. True jellyfish (scyphozoans)
      1) They are distributed throughout the world, including the arctic and antarctica.
      2) They vary from millimeters to 2 meters across.
      3) Most true jellyfish have stinging tenacles, and stings vary from mildly irritating to life threatening.

Mechanism of Injury

1. When jellyfish tentacles containing thousands or even millions of nematocysts comes into contact with skin, the nematocysts burst and fire toxin-laden cnidocils at high velocity into the flesh.
2. The venom is neurotoxic, cardiotoxic, and dermonecrotic.

Complications

1. Long-term skin changes, such as hyper- and hypopigmentation, lichenification, and keloid and eschar formation have been reported
2. Full-thickness dermal necrosis can occur with box jellyfish envenomation.
3. Multiorgan failure may occur post–severe envenomation.

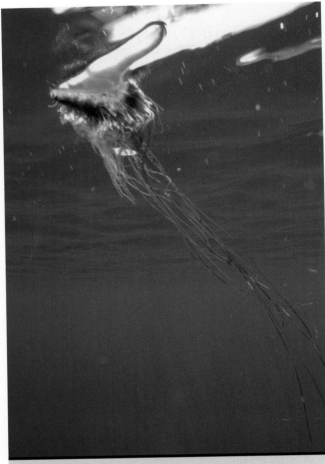

Figure 18-27. Portuguese Man-of-War or Bluebottle

(Photo by Paul Sutherland/Sutherlandimages.com)

Consultation

1. Experts in marine envenomation may be sought through local poison control centers or through the Divers Alert Network (1-919-684-8111; 1-919-684-4326 collect).
2. Burn specialists may be required for management of severe dermal necrosis.

Emergency Department Treatment and Disposition

1. Treatment should begin in the field. All tentacles must be removed.
   a. Immediately rinse the wounds with seawater (if the water is known to be free of tentacles).
   b. Rinsing the wound immediately with vinegar may prevent further discharge of nematocysts, and may inactivate the venom.
   c. Other agents, such as alcohol, papain, urine, and ammonia have not been found to be terribly effective, and in the case of alcohol may worsen envenomation.

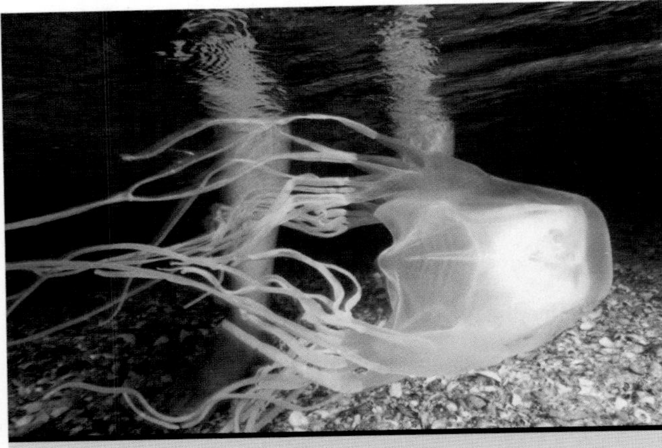

Figure 18-28. Australian Box Jellyfish

Chironex fleckeri at the foot of a bather. (Photo by Paul Sutherland/Sutherlandimages.com)

   d. Tentacles may be scraped off with a credit card or paper plate if necessary; some recommend covering the area with clean beach sand first.
   e. In cases of box jellyfish or severe *Physalia* or jellyfish sting:
      1) Soak the area for at least 30 seconds with vinegar (5% acetic acid).
      2) Remove tentacles while wearing gloves (not thin latex gloves), or use another tool.
      3) Do not crush the tentacles.
      4) Soak the area in vinegar, or place a vinegar-soaked cloth on the wound.
      5) *Note:* In cases of stinging by the Portuguese man-of-war (*Physalia physalis*) in or near Australia, *vinegar may increase nematocyst discharge and should not be used.*
      6) If severe envenomation by the box jellyfish occurs, an antivenin may be available at the beach for IV or IM use (sheep-derived immunoglobulin).
      7) If antivenin is not available, pressure and immobilization may be utilized until definitive care is available. *Remember: All tentacles must be removed first.*
2. In the ED, critical care must be available.
   a. In severe envenomation, antivenin should be administered in the ED if it was not given in the field.
   b. Dermonecrotic injuries (essentially chemical burns) can be treated with silver sulfadiazine.
   c. In the ED, the wound should be cleansed with normal saline.
   d. Tetanus status should be assessed, and toxoid administered if 5 years have passed since the last update.
   e. Mild local reactions may be treated with antihistamines and topical corticosteroids.
   f. More severe skin reactions may require systemic corticosteroids. A 5- to 10-day course of prednisolone is normally adequate.

g. Patients without evidence of systemic reaction 4 to 6 hours postenvenomation may be discharged.
h. Patients with evidence of systemic illness who show improvement must be observed for 6 to 8 hours, since rebound illness has been reported.
i. Patients with systemic signs will most likely require admission.
j. Antibiotics are not normally indicated for immunocompetent patients.

3. Dermatologist follow-up is indicated for more severe skin reactions

Clinical Points: Stinging Marine Animals (Box Jellyfish, True Jellyfish and Portuguese Man-of-War)

1. Antivenom is available for *Chironex fleckeri* envenomation.
2. Vinegar may be of benefit.

BOX 18-18. CLINICAL FEATURES OF BOX JELLYFISH, TRUE JELLY FISH AND PORTUGUESE MAN-OF-WAR ENVENOMATION

- Immediate burning sensation of the skin
- The pain can be intense.
- Overwhelming pain in case of Australian box jellyfish envenomation.
- Local erythema and urticaria
- The tentacles leave markedly erythematous marks on the skin where they made contact (Fig. 18-29).
- These marks can have a beaded appearance.
- Edema, local skin hemorrhage, vesiculation, and desquamation can occur.
- Systemic illness can occur.
  (1) Anaphylaxis
  (2) Nausea, vomiting, paresthesias
  (3) Altered mental status
  (4) Respiratory distress
  (5) Cardiovascular collapse
  (6) Death from severe box jellyfish envenomation can occur in minutes

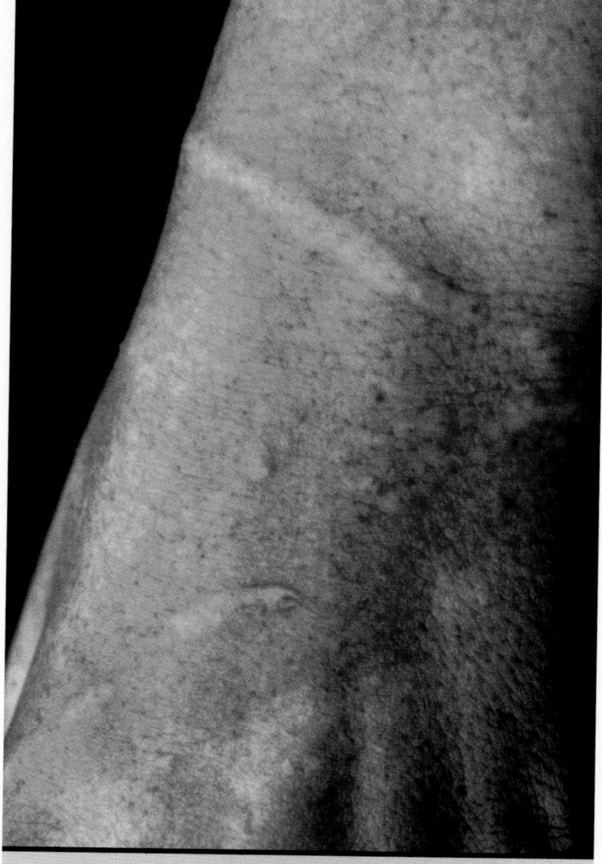

Figure 18-29. Jellyfish Injury

Tentacle prints on the hand of a researcher. (Photo by Paul Sutherland/Sutherlandimages.com)

Stinging Marine Animals: Sponges (Phylum Poriphera)

Background

1. Sponges are simple, multicellular animals that are elastic in nature with a matrixlike skeleton composed of silicon dioxide and calcium carbonate.
2. They are frequently home to a host of other animals that are also capable of biting and stinging (see Fig. 18-24).

Mechanism of Injury

1. There are three ways sea sponges can hurt the unwary:
   a. They can penetrate the skin with silicate or calcite spicules, which can be coated with toxin. This causes a spicule or irritant dermatitis.
   b. They can cause a contact dermatitis very much like that from poison ivy.
   c. They can be home to stinging cnidarians, particularly hydroids, which sting.

Laboratory Tests

Nonspecific

Complications

1. Resolution may take a week or more, and desquamation may occur.
2. Erythema multiforme has been reported.

Consultation

Experts in marine envenomation may be sought through local poison control centers or through the Divers Alert Network (1-919-684-8111; 1-919-684-4326 collect).

Emergency Department Treatment Disposition

1. In general it is not possible to distinguish which of the three mechanisms of injury are responsible for the patient's reaction, so we treat for all three.
2. Treatment is preferably begun in the field.
   a. The affected area should be rinsed with vinegar, if it is available.
   b. The area should then be gently patted dry and adhesive tape applied over the affected skin.
   c. Removing the tape may remove much of the spicular material.
   d. The area should then be soaked in vinegar for 20 to 30 minutes.
3. In the ED, wounds must be well cleansed with normal saline.
   a. For mild reactions, topical steroids may prevent or reduce secondary inflammation.
   b. Tetanus status must be evaluated and updated if necessary.
   c. Severe skin reactions may require treatment with a tapering course of oral steroids.
   d. Antibiotics would rarely be indicated, except where deep tissue penetration or injury has occurred.
   e. Urticaria and itching may respond to antihistamine therapy.
4. Dermatologist follow-up is indicated for more severe skin reactions

Clinical Pearls: Stinging Marine Animals (Sponges)

1. Remove sharp spicules with adhesive tape.
2. Vinegar may be of benefit.

BOX 18-19. CLINICAL FEATURES OF SPONGE INJURIES

- After contact with a sponge, burning is the most common symptom.
- With very stiff sponges abrasions may occur and spicules may be felt (they feel like splinters in the skin).
- Itching may develop within 20 minutes.
- Urticaria, edema, and vesiculation may occur.
- Systemic symptoms are rare (e.g., nausea, vomiting, fever, chills, malaise).
- Anaphylactoid reactions have been reported.

BOX 18-20. DIFFERENTIAL DIAGNOSIS OF SPONGE INJURIES

- Stings from a hydroid, fire coral, or jellyfish
- Cold urticaria

Stabbing Marine Animals: Starfish, Sea Urchins, and Crown-of-Thorns Starfish

Background

1. Stabbing marine animals include:
   a. Echinoderms (starfish and sea urchins)
   b. The crown-of-thorns starfish (*Acanthaster planci*)
      1) Crown-of-thorns starfish are large (up to 60 cm across), dangerous looking, multi-armed animals (Fig. 18-30).
      2) The arms are covered with thick, sharp spines. The spines are coated with toxins, which are surrounded by a thin skinlike integument.
   c. Sea urchins (family Diadematidae)
      1) Sea urchins are round animals with bodies that bristle with spines (Fig. 18-31).
      2) Depending on the species, the spines can be razor sharp and may contain toxins.
      3) They are found worldwide, but as with all toxic marine animals, the most dangerous are found in the Indo-Pacific.

Mechanism of Injury

1. Sharp spines become embedded in skin or joints.
2. In the case of the crown-of-thorns starfish and certain urchins, envenomation may also occur. Urchins may also have venemous pedcellariae, small tulip-like structures at the base of the spine that can bite and envenomate.
3. The venom coating the spines of the sea star is forced into the tissue, as is the integumentary sheath, seawater, particulate matter, and microorganisms.

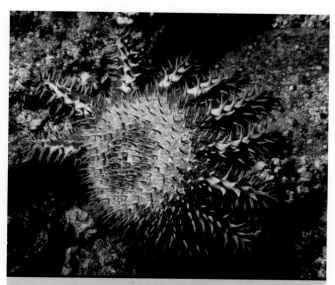

Figure 18-30. Crown-of-Thorns Starfish

The crown-of-thorns starfish (*Ancanthaster planci*) is found in Red Sea and Indo-Pacific coral reefs. These starfish are especially abundant in Australia's Great Barrier Reef. Photo taken at Cocos Island, Costa Rica.

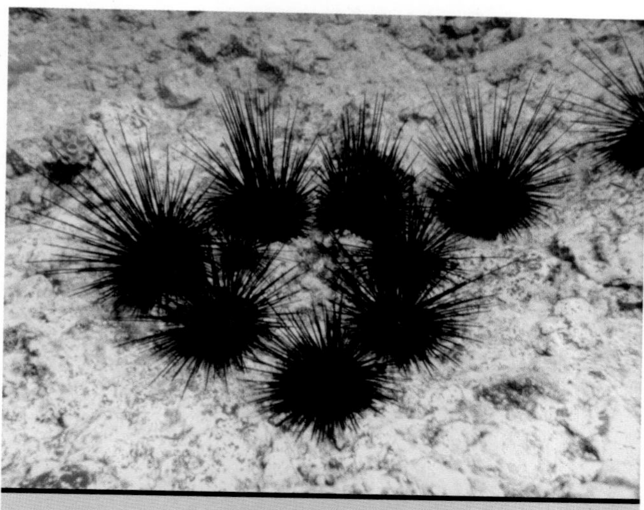

Figure 18-31. Sea Urchins

Sea urchins, like the ones seen here, are radially symmetrical creatures covered with sharp spines. Photo taken in Cocos Island, Costa Rica

Laboratory Tests

Nonspecific

Complications

1. Acute and chronic wound and joint infections
2. Death can occur rarely with severe envenomations.

Consultation

Experts in marine envenomation may be sought through local poison control centers or through the Divers Alert Network (1-919-684-8111; 1-919-684-4326 collect).

Emergency Department Treatment and Disposition

1. Treatment should begin in the field. Visible spines should be carefully removed (they fracture easily).
2. Immersion in hot water (114°F/45.6°C) for 30 to 90 minutes may relieve the pain. Always test the water before placing the injured body part in it.
3. Tetanus toxoid update should be given for those not vaccinated within the past 5 years.
4. Foreign bodies must be sought with radiographs and/or sonography.
5. Wounds must be cleansed and débrided aggressively. The spines crumble easily and the clinician should avoid crushing them.
6. All foreign material must be removed. Penetrated joints should be addressed in an operating room setting.

7. Antibiotics such as quinolones, that have activity against marine organisms are indicated for deep penetrations.
8. Care for envenomations is supportive. No antivenin is available.

Clinical Pearls: Stabbing Marine Animals (Starfish, Sea Urchins, and Crown-of-Thorns Starfish)

1. Painful injuries are treated with heat.
2. Perform radiography to look for foreign bodies.

BOX 18-21. CLINICAL FEATURES OF INJURIES FROM STABBING MARINE ANIMALS (STARFISH, SEA URCHINS, AND CROWN-OF-THORNS STARFISH)

- Immediate pain and burning at the site of the stab
- Erythema and swelling may follow, particularly with starfish envenomation.
- Nausea and vomiting may occur, particularly with starfish envenomation.
- Systemic effects such as hypotension, neuromuscular weakness, respiratory failure, and death occur rarely.

BOX 18-22. DIFFERENTIAL DIAGNOSIS OF INJURIES FROM STABBING MARINE ANIMALS (STARFISH, SEA URCHINS, AND CROWN-OF-THORNS STARFISH)

- Stab injuries by venomous fish
- Stab injuries by stingray

Stabbing Marine Animals: Stingray

Background

1. Stingrays are cartilaginous fish, and are found worldwide (Fig. 18-32).
2. They have sharp barbs on their tails, which are coated with venom and covered by an integumentary sheath (Fig. 18-33).
3. Although they are not aggressive creatures, they spend much of their time hidden in the sand. When stepped on or frightened, they whip their tails forward, stabbing the barb into whatever disturbed it.
4. In addition to envenomating their victims, deaths have occurred from chest, neck, and abdominal penetrating injuries.

Mechanism of Injury

1. The sharp, venom-coated barb is forcefully driven into the tissues.
2. Venom that coats the spine is forced into the tissue, as are the integumentary sheath, seawater, particulate matter, and microorganisms.

Laboratory Tests

Nonspecific

Complications

1. Pneumo- and hemothorax and visceral injury have been reported.
2. Acute and chronic wound and joint infections
3. Death can occur rarely with severe envenomations.

Consultation

Experts in marine envenomation may be sought through local poison control centers or through the Divers Alert Network (1-919-684-8111; 1-919-684-4326 collect).

Emergency Department Treatment and Disposition

1. Treatment should begin in the field.
2. Immersion in hot water (114°F/45.6°C) for 30 to 90 minutes may relieve the pain.

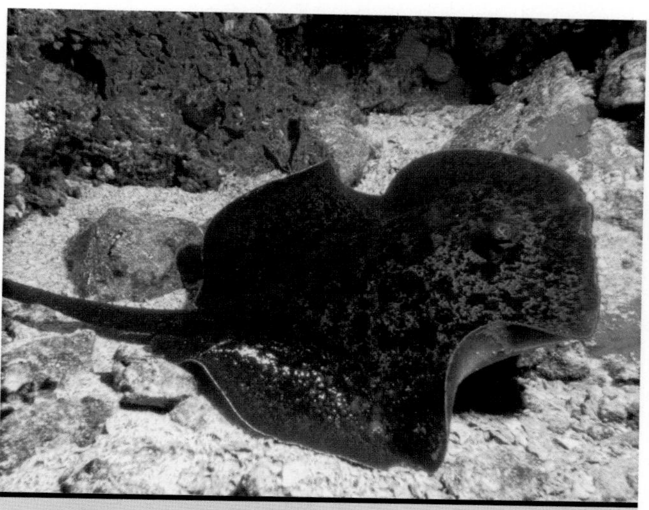

Figure 18-32. Stingray

Photo taken in Cocos Island, Costa Rica.

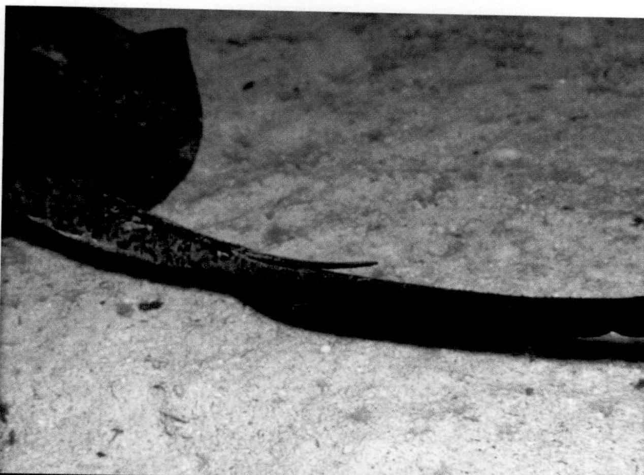

Figure 18-33. Barb on a Stingray's Tail

3. Stingray barb injury must be treated as if it were a stab wound. Evidence of visceral injury must be sought.
4. Tetanus toxoid should be updated for patients who have not been vaccinated within the previous 5 years.
5. Foreign bodies must be sought with radiography, sonography, or MRI.
6. Wounds must be cleansed and débrided aggressively.
7. All foreign bodies must be removed. Penetrated joints should be addressed in an operating room setting.
8. Antibiotics such as quinolones, that have activity against marine organisms are indicated for deep penetrations.
9. Patients should be observed for 6 hours postinjury, after which neurologic involvement is unlikely to occur.
10. Care for envenomations is supportive. No antivenin is available.

Clinical Pearls: Stabbing Marine Animals (Stingray)

1. Painful stab injuries are treated with heat to reduce pain.
2. Perform radiography to check for foreign bodies.

BOX 18-23. CLINICAL FEATURES OF STINGRAY INJURY

- Immediate pain and burning at the site of the stab, and pain may spread up the involved limb.
- Swelling and whitish, bluish, or red discoloration may follow.
- Nausea, vomiting, diaphoresis, and diarrhea may occur.
- Systemic effects, such as hypotension, neuromuscular weakness, respiratory failure, and death occur rarely.

BOX 18-24. DIFFERENTIAL DIAGNOSIS OF STINGRAY INJURY

- Stab injuries by other venomous fish
- Stab injury by sea urchin or crown-of-thorns starfish
- Cone shell envenomation

Stabbing Marine Animals: Stonefish and Scorpionfish (Family Scorpaenidae)

Background

1. Members of the scorpionfish family are found in all tropical oceans.
2. Family members vary from the beautiful lionfish (Fig. 18-34), to the unusual frogfish (Fig. 18-35), the camouflaged scorpionfish (Fig. 18-36), and the bizarre devilfish (Fig. 18-37).
3. They all have defensive spines along the back and belly; these are coated with poison and covered with an integumentary sheath.
4. When alarmed, the fish makes the spines erect, in an effort to frighten or injure their enemies.
5. The stonefish (*Synanceja* spp.) is by far the most venomous and dangerous of these creatures (Fig. 18-38).
6. Lionfish are frequently kept pets in marine aquaria, and a child could easily be envenomated if he or she places a hand in the tank.

Mechanism of Injury

1. Sharp spines become embedded in skin or joints.
2. Venom that coats the spines is forced into the tissue, as are the integumentary sheath, seawater, particulate matter, and microorganisms.

Complications

1. Acute and chronic wound and joint infections
2. Death can occur rarely with severe envenomations.

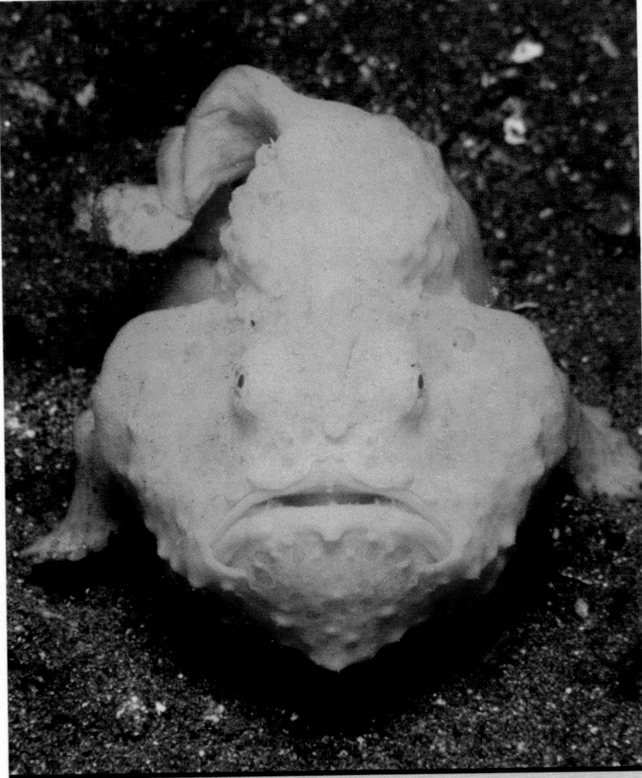

Figure 18-35. Frogfish

Photo taken in Fiji.

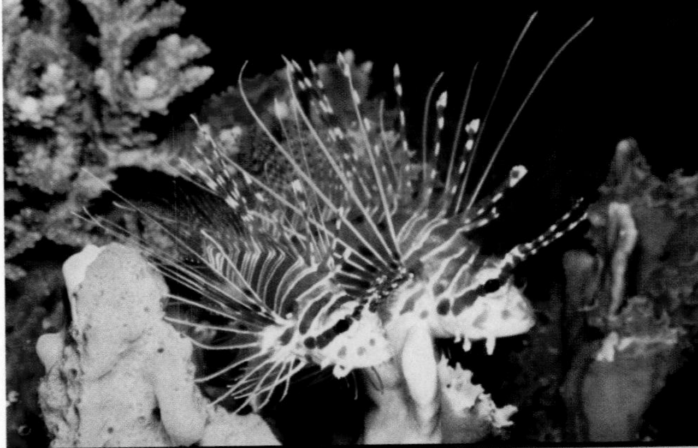

Figure 18-34. Pair of Lionfish

Photo taken in Fiji.

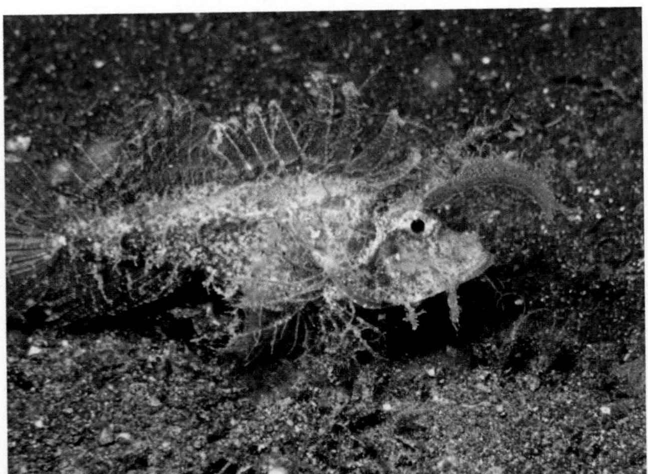

Figure 18-36. Ambon Scorpionfish (*Pteroidichthys amboinensis*)

Photo taken in Northern Sulawesi, Indonesia.

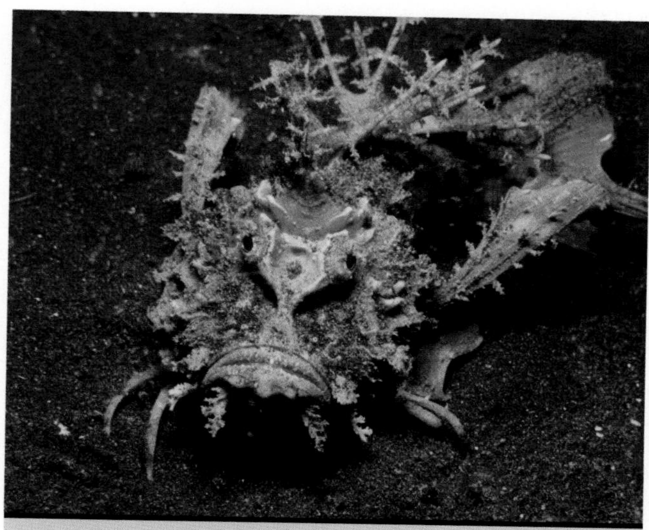

Figure 18-37. Devilfish (Genus *Inimicus*)

This creature is locally known as the devilfish, due to its painful sting. Photo taken in Northern Sulawesi, Indonesia.

Consultation

Experts in marine envenomation may be sought through local poison control centers or through the Divers Alert Network (1-919-684-8111; 1-919-684-4326 collect)

Emergency Department Treatment and Disposition

1. Treatment should begin in the field.
2. Immersion in hot water (114°F/45.6°C) for 30 to 90 minutes may relieve the pain, but narcotic analgesics in liberal doses will likely be required for stonefish injury.
3. Tetanus toxoid should be updated for those not vaccinated within the past 5 years.
4. Foreign bodies must be sought with radiography, sonography, or MRI.
5. Wounds must be cleansed and débrided aggressively.
6. All foreign bodies must be removed. Penetrated joints should be addressed in an operating room setting.
7. Antibiotics such as quinolones, that have activity against marine organisms are indicated for deep penetrations and wounds that occurred more than 6 to 12 hours earlier.
8. Care is supportive, except in the case of severe stonefish envenomation.
9. Stonefish antivenom is produced by CSL, Ltd. of Australia, from the venom of *Synanceja trachynis*), and may be available for use in the Indo-Pacific region to treat systemic intoxication.

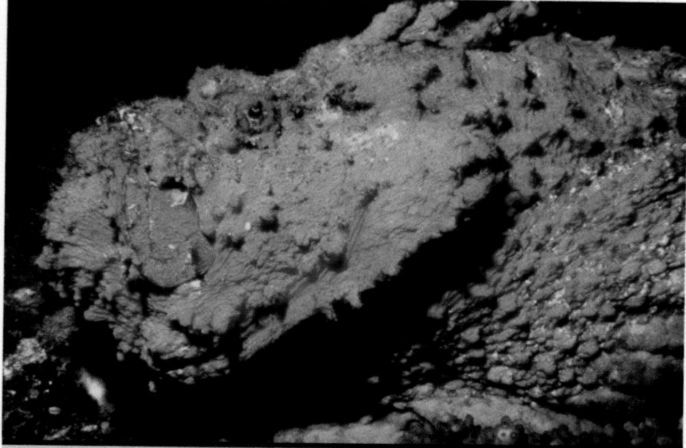

Figure 18-38. Stonefish (Genus *Synanceja*)

The stonefish is among the most dangerous fish in the sea. (Copyright Carl Roessler.)

Clinical Pearls: Stabbing Marine Animals (Stonefish and Scorpionfish)

1. Painful stab injuries are treated with heat.
2. Perform radiography to check for foreign bodies.
3. Antivenom is available for stonefish envenomation.

BOX 18-25. CLINICAL FEATURES OF STONEFISH AND SCORPIONFISH ENVENOMATION

- Immediate pain and burning at the site of the wound
- Pain can be intense and unrelenting in the case of stonefish envenomation.
- Erythema and swelling may follow.
- Nausea and vomiting may also occur.
- Stonefish venom (more so than scorpionfish venom) can depress the neurologic and cardiovascular systems and can cause hemolysis and increased vascular permeability.
- Systemic effects such as hypotension, neuromuscular weakness, respiratory failure, and death occur rarely.

BOX 18-26. DIFFERENTIAL DIAGNOSIS OF STONEFISH AND SCORPIONFISH ENVENOMATION

- Stab injuries by urchins and starfish
- Stab injuries by stingray

Stabbing Marine Animals: Cone Shells (Family Conidae)

Background

1. Cone shells are snail-like mollusks that inhabit tropical waters.
2. Species of the Indo-Pacific region are the most dangerous. They often have beautiful shells, making them attractive to children (Fig. 18-39). Unfortunately, they are carnivorous animals that hunt and have a highly venomous bite.
3. The venom apparatus (the tooth) is contained in its proboscis (Fig. 18-40); thus the wound it inflicts is known as a bite. The proboscis can reach any part of the shell, making no part of the animal safe to touch.
4. Cone shell venom is an extremely lethal set of neurotoxins that can paralyze its prey.

Mechanism of Injury

A venomous tooth held inside the proboscis injects venom into prey, or an unfortunate human body part.

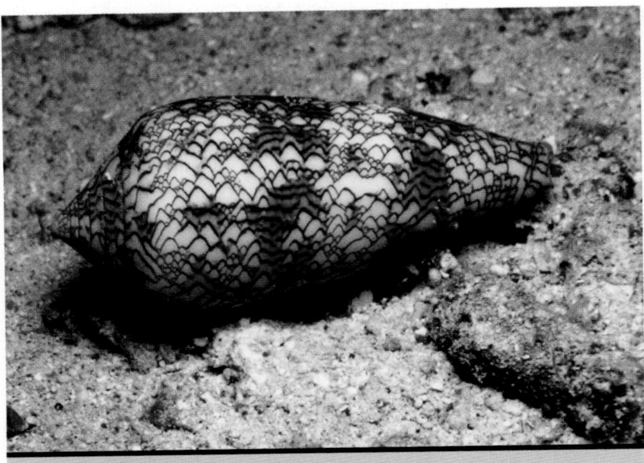

Figure 18-39. Cone Shell at Rest

Photo taken in Papua New Guinea.

Complications

1. Neurologic impairment may persist for days or weeks.
2. Prolonged mechanical ventilation may be required.
3. All marine injuries carry the risk of infection.

Consultation

Experts in marine envenomation may be sought through local poison control centers or through the Divers Alert Network (1-919-684-8111; 1-919-684-4326 collect).

Emergency Department Treatment and Disposition

1. Injuries will likely be sustained in remote areas, making field management essential.
2. The pressure/immobilization technique has been recommended.
   a. Place a gauze pad (sterile if available) over the bite or sting site.
   b. Starting at the site, wrap the entire extremity with an elastic bandage (Ace wrap). The wrap should be snug, as when wrapping a sprained ankle, but circulation should not be impeded, and should be checked frequently. You are trying to impede lymphatic circulation.
   c. Splint the extremity, and if an arm is involved, place in a sling.
   d. If possible, keep the bite/stab/sting site at the level of the heart.
   e. Keep the patient as still as possible to delay circulation of the venom.
   f. Do not remove the dressing until resuscitative equipment and medication are available, but do check the wound/extremity regularly if there is extended transport time to definitive care.

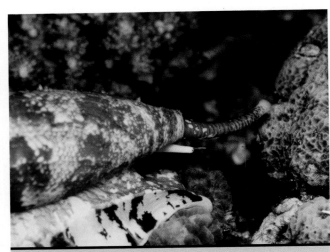

Figure 18-40. Cone Shell Hunting with Its Proboscis Extended

Photo taken in Papua New Guinea.

3. Application of heat for 30 to 90 minutes has been suggested (114°F/45.6°C), but the pressure bandage should be left in place.
4. Respiratory support must be maintained.
5. Peak activity of venom is within the first 12 hours, but neurologic deficits may persist for days.
6. Treatment in the ED is supportive.
7. Patients without respiratory weakness should be observed for 8 to 10 hours, and are unlikely to deteriorate after this period.
8. Tetanus toxoid should be administered where appropriate.
9. The wound must be carefully cleansed and checked for foreign bodies. Radiography should be considered.
10. Antibiotics may be considered for deep injuries, for wounds over joints, and in patients with immune impairment or with significant comorbidities such as diabetes mellitus.

Clinical Pearls: Stabbing Marine Animals (Cone Shells)

1. Neurotoxic venom
2. The pressure/immobilization technique may be of value.
3. Applying heat may help control pain.

BOX 18-27. CLINICAL FEATURES OF CONE SHELL BITES

- Initially the wound may be asymptomatic, but sharp pain or stinging is more common.
- Numbness, pallor, and/or cyanosis surrounding the wound may follow.
- Nausea and vomiting may occur.
- In severe envenomation numbness or paresthesias may proceed up the extremity.
- Perioral numbness may be an early sign of systemic intoxication.
- Cranial nerve dysfunction
- Voluntary and involuntary muscle paralysis develop, leading to respiratory failure.
- The patient may remain alert while paralyzed, if respirations are maintained.
- Hypotension, cardiac failure, cerebral edema, coma, and death occur rarely.

BOX 18-28. DIFFERENTIAL DIAGNOSIS OF CONE SHELL BITES

- Blue-ringed octopus bite
- Jellyfish envenomation
- Stab by a venomous fish
- Stingray envenomation
- Guillain-Barré syndrome
- Decompression sickness with neurologic involvement

Biting Marine Animals: Blue-Ringed Octopus

Background

1. Blue-ringed octopuses are small (<25 cm), shy animals found throughout the Indo-Pacific region. They are found in tide pools and among coral rubble and rocks. They are beige to brown animals that are covered by blue rings that glow when the animal is excited, fascinating children and the unwary (Fig. 18-41).
2. The octopus' parotid glands produce a highly potent venom that is transmitted by a bite. The chief component of the venom is a tetrodotoxin-like agent that blocks cellular sodium channels and produces neuromuscular paralysis.
3. The octopuses must be handled or stepped on to induce them to bite.

Mechanism of Injury

Bite with chitinous beak

Laboratory Tests

1. Laboratory findings are nonspecific.
2. Coagulation studies should be performed, as the venom may have anticoagulant properties.

Complications

All marine injuries carry the risk of infection.

Consultation

Experts in marine envenomation may be sought through local poison control centers or through the Divers Alert Network (1-919-684-8111; 1-919-684-4326 collect).

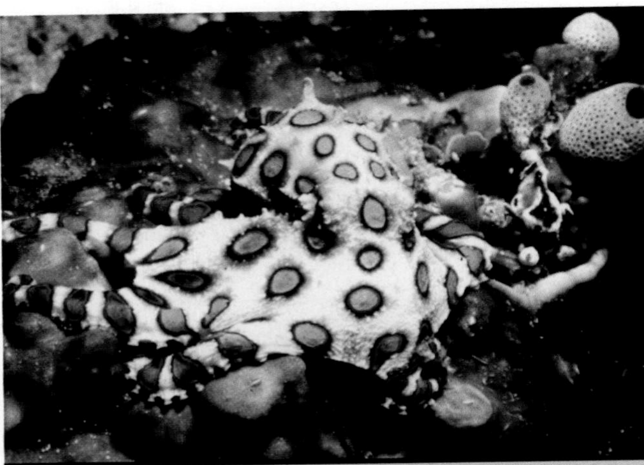

Figure 18-41. Blue-Ringed Octopus

(Copyright Carl Roessler.)

Emergency Department Treatment and Disposition

1. Bites are usually sustained in remote areas, making field management essential.
2. The pressure/immobilization technique has been recommended (see treatment section under cone shell envenomation).
3. Treatment in the ED is supportive.
4. Respiratory support must be maintained.
5. Peak activity of venom is within the first 12 hours, but neurologic deficits may persist for 3 to 4 days.
6. Patients without respiratory weakness should be observed for 8 to 10 hours, and are unlikely to deteriorate after this period.
7. Tetanus toxoid should be administered where appropriate.
8. The wound must be carefully cleansed.
9. Antibiotics may be considered for deep injuries, for bites over joints, and in patients with immune impairment or with significant comorbidities such as diabetes mellitus.

Clinical Pearls: Biting Marine Animals (Blue-Ringed Octopus)

1. A paralyzed victim may be fully alert.
2. The pressure/immobilization technique may be of value.

BOX 18-29. CLINICAL FEATURES OF BLUE-RINGED OCTOPUS BITES

- Initially the bite may be asymptomatic.
- Numbness or pain at the bite site may occur.
- In less than 30 minutes, pruritus, erythema, and urticaria may develop in the involved limb.
- Nausea and vomiting may be seen in severe envenomations.
- By 30 minutes, facial numbness and weakness ensue.
- Cranial nerve dysfunction
- Voluntary and involuntary muscle paralysis develop, leading to respiratory failure.
- The patient may remain alert while paralyzed, if respirations are maintained.
- Hypotension may occur, but is not a consistent feature.

BOX 18-30. DIFFERENTIAL DIAGNOSIS OF BLUE-RINGED OCTOPUS BITES

- Cone shell envenomation
- Guillain-Barré syndrome
- Decompression sickness with neurologic involvement

Suggested Readings

Aghababian RV, Conte JE Jr.: Mammalian bite wounds. *Ann Emerg Med* 1980;9:79.

Altieri M, Brasch L: Antibiotic prophylaxis in intraoral wounds. *Am J Emerg Med* 1986;4:507.

American Academy of Pediatrics. Rabies. In: (Peter G, ed). *2000 Red Book: Report of the Committee on Infectious Diseases*, 25th ed. Elk Grove Village, IL, American Academy of Pediatrics, 2000, p. 475.

American Academy of Pediatrics: Tetanus. In: (Peter G, ed). *2000 Red Book: Report of the Committee on Infectious Diseases*, 25th ed. Elk Grove Village, IL, American Academy of Pediatrics, 2000, p. 563.

Avner JR, Baker MD: Dog bites in urban children. *Pediatrics* 1991;88:55.

Baker MD, Moore SE: Human bites in children: A six year experience. *Am J Dis Child* 1987;141:1285.

Battle WE, Stowe EC, Schmitt AM: Aerobic bacterial flora of oral and nasal fluids of canines with reference to bacteria associated with bites. *J Clin Microbiol* 1978;7:223.

Beck AM, Loring H, Cockwood R: The ecology of dog bite injury in St. Louis, Missouri. *Public Health Rep* 1975;90:262.

Berzon DR, Farber RE, Gordon J et al: Animal bites in a large city: A report on Baltimore, Maryland. *Am J Public Health* 1972;62:422.

Berzon DR: The animal bite epidemic in Baltimore, Maryland: Review and update. *Am J Pub Health* 1978;68:593.

Boenning DA, Fleisher GR, Campos JM: Dog bites in children: Epidemiology, microbiology and penicillin prophylactic therapy. *Am J Emerg Med* 1983;1:17.

Brogan TV, Bratton SL, Dowd MD et al: Severe dog bites in children. *Pediatrics* 1995;96:947.

Brook I: Microbiology of human and animal bite wounds in children. *Pediatr Infect Dis J* 1987;6:29.

Callaham M: Dog bite wounds. *JAMA* 1980;244:2327.

Callaham ML: Prophylactic antibiotics in common dog bite wounds: A controlled study. *Ann Emerg Med* 1980;9:410.

Callaham ML: Treatment of common dog bites. Infection Risk Factors. *JACEP* 1978;7:83.

Centers for Disease Control and Prevention: Rabies prevention–United States, 1999. Recommendations of the Advisory Committee on Immunization Practices (ACIP). *MMWR Morb Mortal Wkly Rep* 1999;48(RR-1):1.

Centers for Disease Control and Prevention: Rabies vaccine, adsorbed: A new rabies vaccine for use in humans. *MMWR Morb Mortal Wkly Rep* 1988;37:217.

Chen E, Hornig S, Shepherd SM, Hollander JE: Primary closure of mammalian bites. *Acad Emerg Med* 2000;7:157.

Chun Y-T, Berkelhamer JE, Herold TE: Dog bites in children less than 4 years old. *Pediatrics* 1982;69:119.

Cummings P: Antibiotics to prevent infection in patients with dog bite wounds: a meta-analysis of randomized trials. *Ann Emerg Med* 1994;23:535.

Dire DJ: Cat bite wounds: Risk factors for infection. *Ann Emerg Med* 1991;20:973.

Dire DJ, Hogan DE, Walker JS: Prophylactic oral antibiotics for low-risk dog bite wounds. *Pediatr Emerg Care* 1992;8:194.

Douglas LG: Bite wounds. *Am Fam Physician* 1975;11:93.

Earley MJ, Bardsley AF: Human bites: A review. *Br J Plastic Surg* 1984;37:458.

Elenbaas RM, McNabney WK, Robinson WA et al: Evaluation of prophylactic oxacillin in cat bite wounds. *Ann Emerg Med* 1984; 13:155.

Elenbaas RM, McNabney WK, Robinson WA, et al: Prophylactic oxacillin in dog bite wounds. *Ann Emerg Med* 1982;11:248.

Faulkner LC: Dimensions of the pet population problem. *Am J Vet Med Assoc* 1975;166:477.

Feder HM, Stanley JD, Barbera JA: Review of 59 patients hospitalized with animal bites. *Pediatr Infect Dis J* 1987;6:24.

Fishbein DB, Yenne KM, Dreesen DW et al: Risk factors for systemic hypersensitivity reactions after booster vaccinations with human diploid cell rabies vaccine: a nationwide prospective study. *Vaccine* 1993;11:1390.

Fleisher GR: The management of bite wounds. *N Engl J Med* 1999;340:138.

Francis DP, Holmes MA, Brandon G: *Pasteurella multocida* infections after domestic animal bites and scratches. *JAMA* 1975;233:42.

Garrard J, Leland N, Smith D: Epidemiology of human bites to children in a day care center. *Am J Dis Child* 1988;142:643.

Goldstein EJC, Citron DM, Wield B et al: Bacteriology of human and animal bite wounds. *J Clin Microbiol* 1978;8:667.

Goldstein EJC, Citron DM, Finegold SM: Dog bite wounds and infection: A prospective clinical study. *Ann Emerg Med* 1980;9:508.

Goldstein EJC, Reinhardt JF, Murray PM, Finegold SM: Outpatient therapy of bite wounds: demographic data, bacteriology, and a prospective, randomized trial of Amoxicillin/clavulinic acid versus penicillin ± dicloxacillin. *International Journal of Dermatology* 1987;26:123–127.

Graber MA: Anaphylaxis. In: (Dambro MR, ed). *Griffith's 5-Minute Clinical Consult*. Baltimore, Lippincott Williams & Wilkins, 2001, p. 40.

Hawkins LG: Local *Pasteurella multocida* infections. *J Bone Joint Surg Am* 1969;51:362.

Hubbert WT, Rosen MN: *Pasteurella multocida* infection due to animal bites. *Am J Public Health* 1970;60:1103.

Jaffe AC: Animal bites. *Pediatr Clin North Am* 1983;30:405.

Jarvis WR, Banko S, Snyder E et al: *Pasteurella multocida* osteomyelitis following dog bites. *Am J Dis Child* 1981;135:625.

Joint Task Force on Practice Parameters: The diagnosis and management of anaphylaxis. Joint Task Force on Practice Parameters, American Academy of Allergy, Asthma and Immunology, American College of Allergy, Asthma and Immunology, and the Joint Council of Allergy. Asthma and Immunology. *J Allergy Clin Immunol* 1998;101:S465.

Kauffman FH, Goldman BJ: Rabies (review). *Am J Emerg Med* 1986;4:525.

Kizer KW: Epidemiologic and clinical aspects of animal bite injuries. *JACEP* 1979;8:134.

Lauer EA, White WC, Lauer BA: Dog bites: A neglected problem in accident prevention. *Am J Dis Child* 1982;136:202.

Lee JLH, Buhr AJ: Dog bites and local infection with *Pasteurella septica*. *Br Med J* 1960;2:169.

Levinson AI: Anaphylaxis and serum sickness. In: (Rakel RE, ed). *Conn's Current Therapy*, 53rd ed. Philadelphia, WB Saunders, 2001, p. 773.

Lindsey D, Christopher M, Hollenbach J, et al: Natural course of the human bite wound: Incidence of infection and complications in 434 bites and 803 lacerations in the same group of patients. *J Trauma* 1987;27:45.

Mann RJ, Hoffeld TA, Farmer CB: Human bites of the hand: Twenty years of experience. *J Hand Surg* 1977;2:97.

March SM: Infections due to dog and cat bites. *Pediatr Infect Dis* 1982;1:351.

Marr JS, Beck AM, Lugo JA: An epidemiologic study of the human bite. *Public Health Rep* 1979;94:514.

Messenger SL, Smith JS, Rupprecht CE. Emerging epidemiology of bat-associated cryptic cases of rabies in humans in the United States. *Clin Infect Dis* 2002; 35:738–747.

Moore RM, Zehmer RB, Moulthrop JI, et al: Surveillance of animal bite cases in the United States, 1971–1972. *Arch Environ Health* 1977;32:267.

Ordog GJ: The bacteriology of dog bite wounds on initial presentation. *Ann Emerg Med* 1986;15:1324.

Parks BJ, Hawkins LG, Horner RL: Bites of the hand. *Rocky Mt Med J* 1974;71:85.

Peeples E, Boswick JA Jr., Scott FA: Wounds of the hand contaminated by human or animal saliva. *J Trauma* 1980;20:383.

Pinckney LE, Kennedy LA: Traumatic deaths from dog attacks in the United States. *Pediatrics* 1982;69:193.

Sacks JJ, Lockwood R, Hornreich J, Sattin RW: Fatal dog attacks, 1989–1994. *Pediatrics* 1996;97:891.

Sacks JJ, Sattin RW, Bonzo SE: Dog bite-related fatalities from 1979 through 1988. *JAMA* 1989;262:1489.

Sacks JJ, Sinclair L, Gilchrist J et al: Breeds of dogs involved in fatal human attacks in the United States between 1979 and 1998. *J Am Vet Med Assoc* 2000;217:836.

Schmidt DR, Heckman MD: *Eikenella corrodens* in human bite infections of the hand. *J Trauma* 1983;23:478.

Schultz RC, McMaster WC: The treatment of dog bite injuries, especially those of the face. *Plast Reconstr Surg* 1972;49:494.

Schweich P, Fleisher G: Human bites in children. *Pediatr Emerg Care* 1985;1:51.

Strassburg MA, Greenland S, Marron JA et al: Animal bites: Patterns of treatment. *Ann Emerg Med* 1985;10:193.

Talan DA, Citron DM, Abrahamian FM et al: Bacteriologic analysis of infected dog and cat bites. *N Engl J Med* 1999;340:85.

Thompson HG, Svitek V: Small animal bites: The role of primary closure. *J Trauma* 1973;13:20.

Tindall JP, Harrison CM: *Pasteurella multocida* infections following animal injuries, especially cat bites. *Arch Dermatol* 1972;105:412.

Trott A: Care of mammalian bites. *Pediatr Infect Dis J* 1987;6:8.

Winkler W: Rodent rabies in the United States. *J Infect Dis* 1972;126:565.

CHAPTER 19

ORTHOPEDICS

Michael Lucchesi

DIAGNOSIS — FRACTURES: OVERVIEW

Mechanism of Injury

1. Fractures are caused by a high-energy force directed against bone. Fractures can be caused by either blunt trauma or penetrating trauma.
2. Although there are many similar types of fracture patterns, their shapes and sizes are determined by the amount of energy absorbed by the bone, the focus of the energy, and the mass and resistance of the bone.

Associated Clinical Features

1. Obvious deformities may or may not be present, depending on the degree of angulation of the fracture. Deformity may also be present if there is an associated joint dislocation.
2. Swelling and tenderness are almost always present. Fractures are painful and as long as the patient has an intact mental status and there is no associated nerve damage, the patient will complain of pain and have tenderness upon palpation.
3. Ecchymosis may not appear for many minutes to hours. This is dependent upon the amount of associated tissue damage, the thickness and integrity of the overlying skin, and the degree of vascular injury.
4. Contamination of the wound in open fractures may occur with material from the environment such as dirt, sand, or glass. These wounds are always contaminated with the normal bacterial skin flora. Additional bacterial contamination is present when the wounds and subsequent fractures are caused by bites such as the classic boxer's fracture or dog bite.
5. Retained foreign bodies are a possibility in any open wound or open fracture. Not all foreign bodies are radiopaque. The ability to see glass, a common wound contaminant, on an x-ray is dependent on its size and lead content.
6. Ligamentous injuries are often associated with all types of fractures, particularly when the fracture occurs at the ends of bones, in proximity to joints, or in areas with known ligamentous insertions.

Radiology

If there is suspicion of a fracture, plain films are indicated. X-rays should be selected so that the entire injured area can be evaluated. The bones and joints being evaluated should also be studied at various different angles, as often fractures may be present on one view but not on a different view of the same bone.

Complications

1. Neurovascular compromise
   a. Neurovascular compromise to the immediate area or the area distal to the fracture site may occur.
   b. Manifested by a decrease in sensation, motor strength and /or pulses
   c. The degree of neurovascular compromise depends on the direct damage to the vessels or nerves at the fracture site or pressure applied subsequently due to swelling (thus neurovascular deficits may progress over time after the injury, as swelling increases).
      1) Vascular compromise may occur at the time of injury due to injury to the intima of the vessel with subsequent thrombus formation, or subsequently due to pressure applied from outside the vessel.
      2) Neurologic deficits may occur if there is direct injury to the nerve, or subsequently due to extrinsic pressure from swelling. Physical damage done to the nerve will produce immediate loss of motor function or sensation distal to the injury. A deficit resulting from this type of injury is usually permanent without surgical intervention. The possibility of successful surgical repair depends on the size of the damaged nerve and the amount and type of injury sustained.
2. Compartment syndrome
   a. A feared complication of fractures or any type of injury to an extremity in which neurovascular bundles travel in closed compartments
   b. Crush injuries to the extremities should be closely watched for the development of compartment syndrome.

c. The mechanism is such that edema and swelling cause an increase in pressure of closed fascial compartments. Once the pressure in the closed compartments begins to rise to the point where there is further vascular congestion or compromise, compartment syndrome becomes a possibility. Oxygen (O_2) delivery to the injured area is already compromised due to edema. Further impairment of O_2 delivery causes further cell death and necrosis. A vicious cycle is set in motion as decreased O_2 delivery causes further necrosis, edema, and swelling. The increase in swelling causes further vascular compromise and still worsening O_2 delivery.
d. Compartment syndrome can occur in multiple parts of the body.
   1) Seen with highest frequency in anterior and posterior compartments of the thighs and calf, peroneal compartments of the legs, and volar and dorsal compartments of the forearm
   2) Seen less frequently in interossei of the hands and the compartment of the gluteus medius
e. The "five P's" used to clinically diagnose compartment syndrome:
   1) *Pain* and *paresthesias* occur first, followed by
   2) *Pallor*, *pulselessness*, or *paralysis* (irreversible damage has already been done once these signs are seen)

3. Nonunion of the fracture site can often occur if the fractured bony parts are not placed in close proximity. It also occurs to a much greater extent in bones that have a tenuous blood supply, such as the femoral neck and the scaphoid bone of the wrist.

4. Osteomyelitis
   a. A dreaded complication of open fractures
   b. Although it may occur by hematogenous spread or be associated with peripheral vascular disease, it occurs with greatest frequency secondary to a contiguous focus of infection.
   c. Inoculation occurs when there is a contiguous pathway from the outside environment to the bone in an open fracture. Often fractured bones protrude through the skin momentarily and then retract.

5. Fat embolism
   a. Fat embolism occurs with significant frequency in patients who sustain major trauma. Luckily, only one-third of the time are the emboli large enough to have clinical significance.
   b. Patients who sustain fat embolism syndrome usually present with signs of pulmonary embolism.

6. Post-traumatic reflex dystrophy
   a. A painful complication of trauma or infection involving the extremities
   b. Emergency medicine physicians may see patients in the period weeks to months after injury, with complaints of weakness and/or pain in an extremity.
   c. Although no emergent treatment is necessary, recognition of this condition is necessary and early rehabilitation prior to muscle atrophy can minimize long-term morbidity.

7. Volkmann's ischemic contracture
   a. An end result of ischemic injury to muscle or nerves in an extremity
   b. Ischemic insult is usually secondary to trauma
   c. Volkmann's ischemic contracture is synonymous with irreversible damage.
   d. It is rare for this complication to occur without preceding compartment syndrome.

Consultation

Orthopedic consultation should be obtained for all fractures. Patients with open fractures need emergent orthopedic consultation and often will have their wounds irrigated by the consultant in the operating room.

Emergency Department Treatment and Disposition

1. All patients with fractures should be given analgesics, should have their fracture elevated, and cold compresses should be applied after other more serious injuries have been ruled out.

2. For the prevention of osteomyelitis in patients with open fractures, intravenous antibiotics should be given as soon as possible upon arrival to the ED.

3. Involvement with the consultant should occur in a timely fashion. After adequate immobilization and consultation, most isolated closed extremity fracture patients can be sent home with expeditious follow-up.

4. All patients with open fractures should be admitted to the hospital for closer observation and continued parenteral antibiotics.

Clinical Pearls: Fractures

1. A violation of the skin overlying a fracture should be considered and treated as an open fracture until proven otherwise.

2. If there is suspicion of a foreign body, use of a radiologic marker in the area of the laceration or puncture may be helpful.

3. Wounds should be explored and irrigated only by someone with expertise in open wound care.

4. Mechanisms of injury that do not fit the injury pattern, particularly spiral long bone fractures, should alert the practitioner to the possibility of child abuse.

5. Occult fractures should be immobilized and when occurring in the area of the physis should be treated like Salter-Harris type I fractures.

BOX 19-1. TYPES OF FRACTURES

Open fractures

- Fractures with either perforation or avulsion of the skin and soft tissue overlying a fracture site
- Perforation or laceration often caused by sharp bony fragments forcing their way through the skin
- Open fractures have a high propensity towards infection.

Closed fractures

- Skin and soft tissue overlying the fracture are intact.

Complete fractures

- A fracture that causes a complete separation or discontinuity of the bone

Incomplete fractures

- A fracture that does not extend completely through the bone leaving a portion of the cortex intact

Occult fractures

- A fracture that is not immediately radiologically apparent but clinically has a high index of suspicion due to physical findings
- These fractures can often be detected on follow-up radiologic studies.

Transverse fractures

- A fracture that occurs perpendicular to the long axis of the bone

Oblique fractures

- A fracture that occurs at an angle not perpendicular to the long axis of the bone

Comminuted fractures

- A fracture composed of more than two fragments with a typical shattered appearance; often the pieces are large and form a typical Y or T shape.

Avulsion fractures

- A fracture in which a fragment of bone is pulled away from the cortex at the site of tendon insertion
- Often the bone fragment is extremely small and may be seen as a chip or flake in proximity to a bony tuberosity.

Impacted fractures

- Fractures in which the fragmented segments are driven into each other
- The fracture may be complete or incomplete.
- The fracture line may not appear as a lucency but as a more dense area.

Torus fractures

- A type of incomplete fracture in which one side of the cortex of a long bone buckles outward
- Fractures typically occur at the base of long bones.
- A fracture named after a term from Greek architecture in which a *torus* is typically the bump at the base of a column
- These fractures are often subtle on x-ray.

BOX 19-2. FRACTURES WITH SPECIAL CONSIDERATIONS

Epiphyseal fractures (see Box 19-3)

Spiral fractures

- A fracture that occurs down the shaft of a long bone in a circumferential manner
- The mechanism of injury for this type of fracture is usually a twisting around the long axis of the bone.
- Often seen in child abuse cases

Greenstick fractures

- Fractures limited to infancy and early childhood
- The fracture occurs along the shaft of a long bone through one side of the cortex in a transverse manner, then abruptly runs along the longitudinal axis of the bone without disrupting the opposite cortex.
- A fracture similar to the pattern of breaking a green stick

Stress fractures

- Seen in healthy people, usually athletes, in response to a repeated stress
- Originally termed "march fractures" (due to their predominance in military recruits)
- Often these fractures are not radiologically apparent until weeks after symptoms appear.
- Eventually these fractures manifest as a thin line of radiolucency or a periosteal callus without an underlying fracture.

Pathologic fractures

- Fractures occurring in diseased bone with characteristically minor injury
- Fractures are often transverse and surrounded by areas of demineralized bone.
- Often seen in metastatic bony disease, areas with bone cysts, or in patients with osteogenesis imperfecta

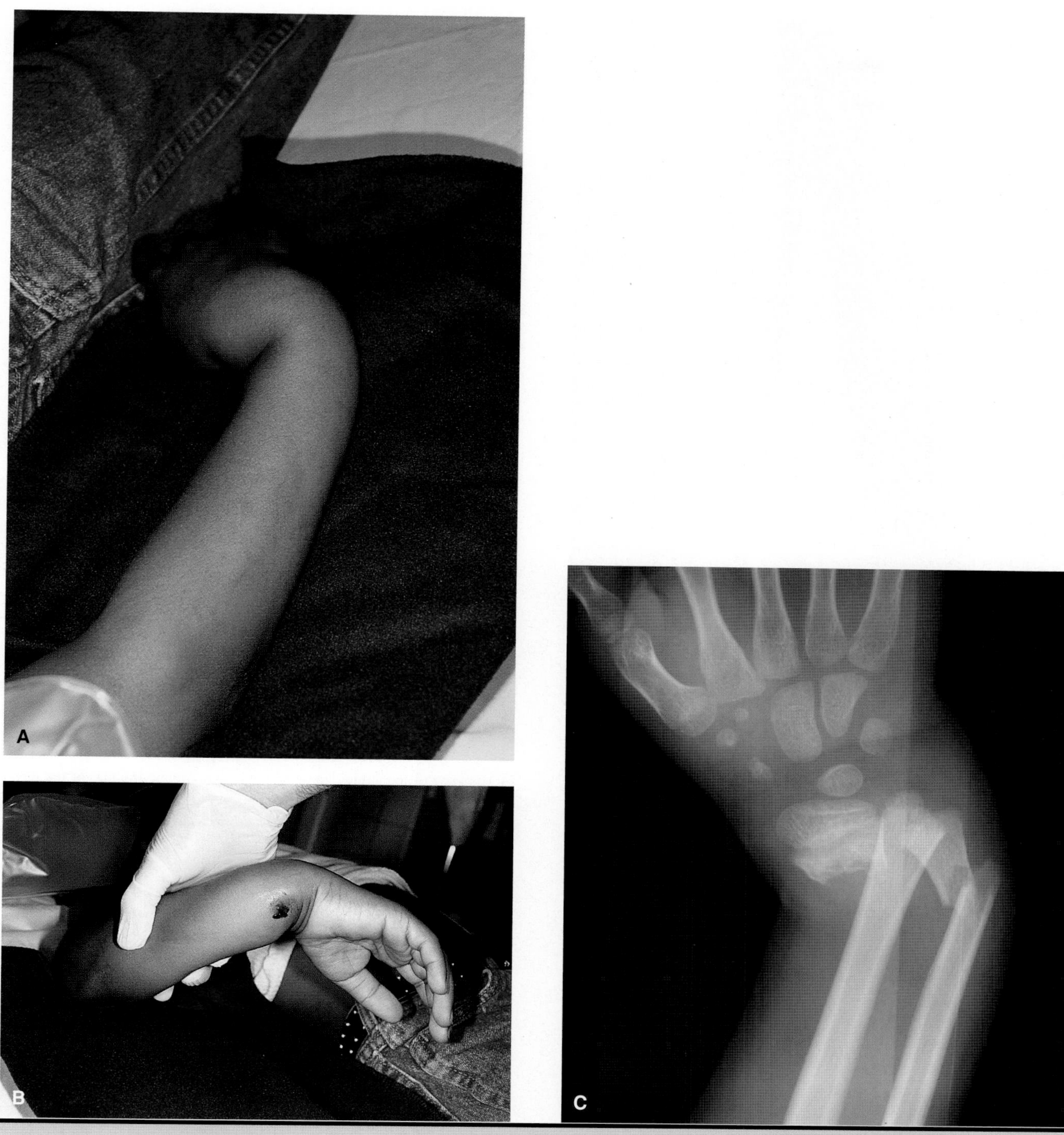

Figure 19-1. Open Fractures

A. A picture of a wrist showing obvious severe deformity. *B*. A puncture wound at the site of the deformity is diagnostic for an open fracture. *C*. X-ray demonstrating a markedly displaced fracture of the distal radius and ulna. There is also a dislocation of the distal radioulnar joint.

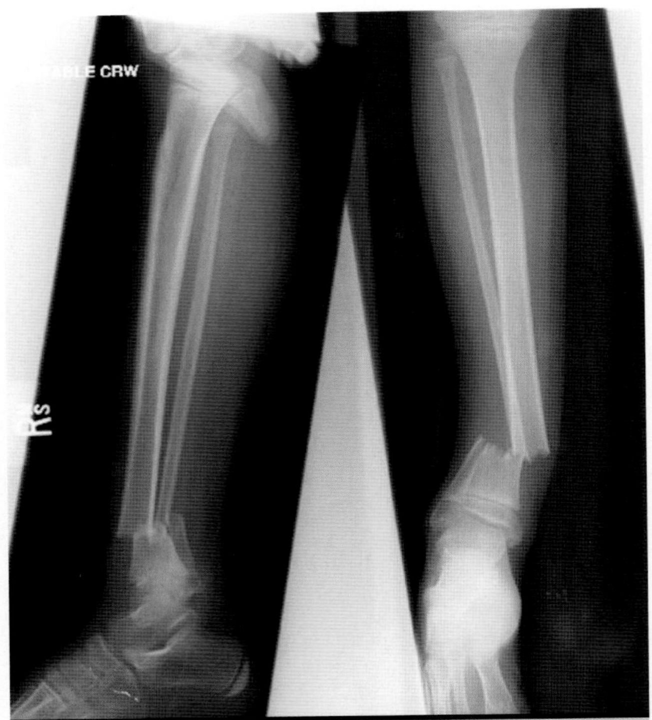

Figure 19-2. Complete Fracture

Two views (AP and lateral) of a complete transverse fracture of the distal tibial and fibular shafts. The two views demonstrate the posterior and lateral displacement of the distal segments.

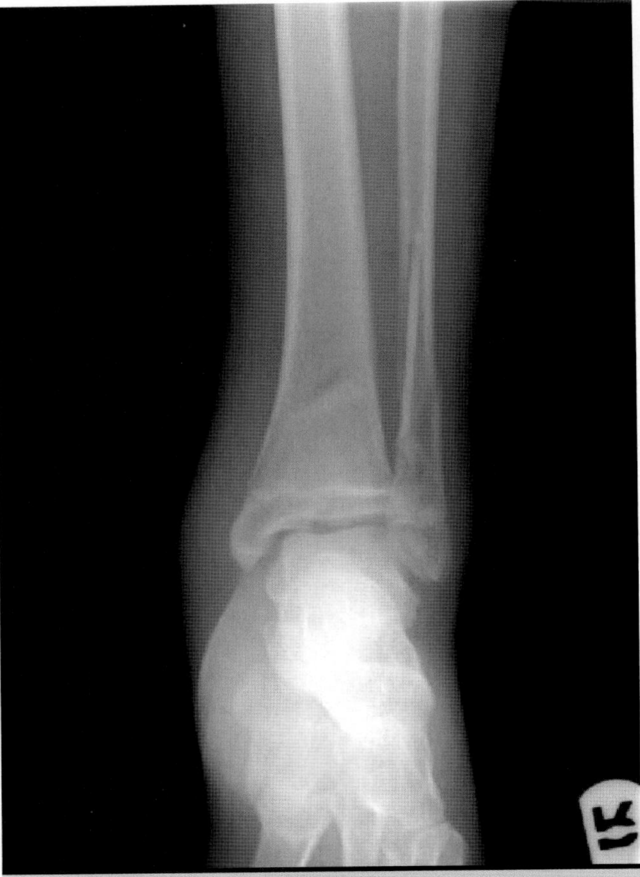

Figure 19-3. Incomplete Fracture

Mortis view of the ankle demonstrates an incomplete fracture of the distal tibia.

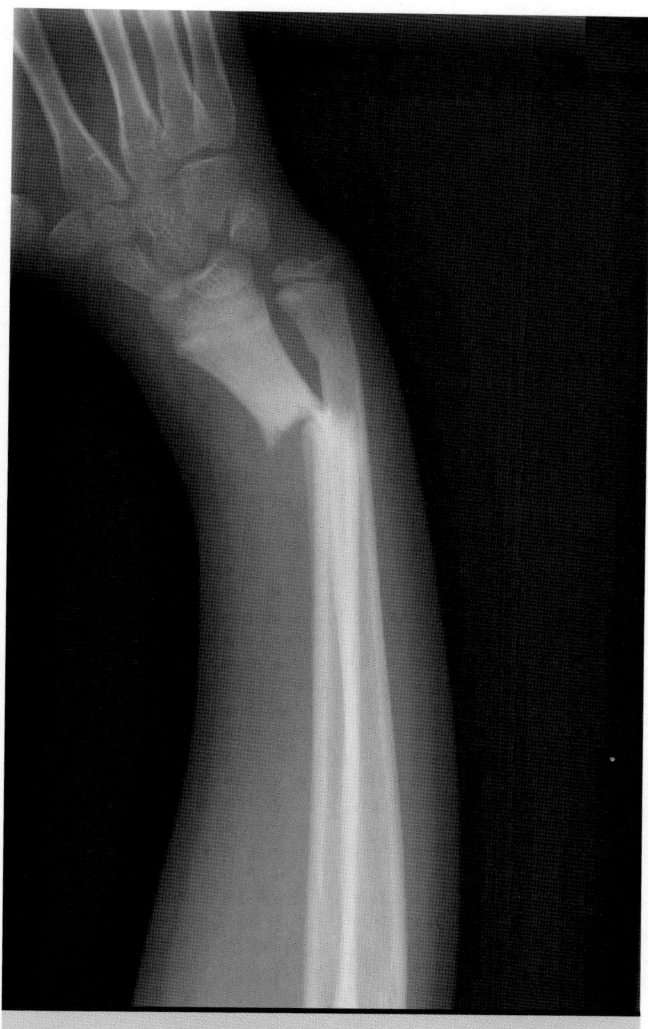

Figure 19-4. Transverse Fracture

A transverse, medially displaced angulated fracture of the distal radial diaphysis is seen, associated with adjacent soft tissue swelling. There is also an incomplete fracture of the distal ulna and a subluxation of the radiocarpal joint.

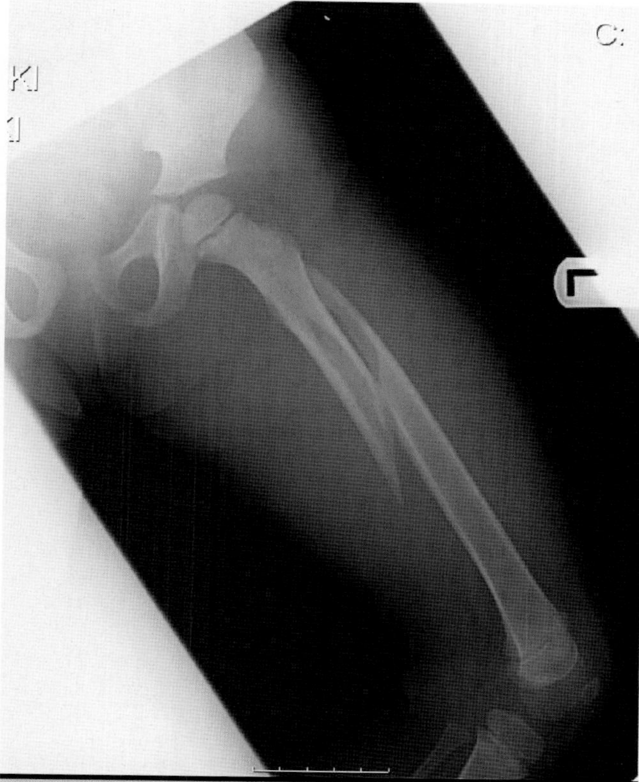

Figure 19-5. Oblique Fracture

There is an oblique fracture through the midportion of the left femoral shaft. This patient is a 3-year-old female. In the absence of a significant dependable mechanism, child abuse should be strongly considered.

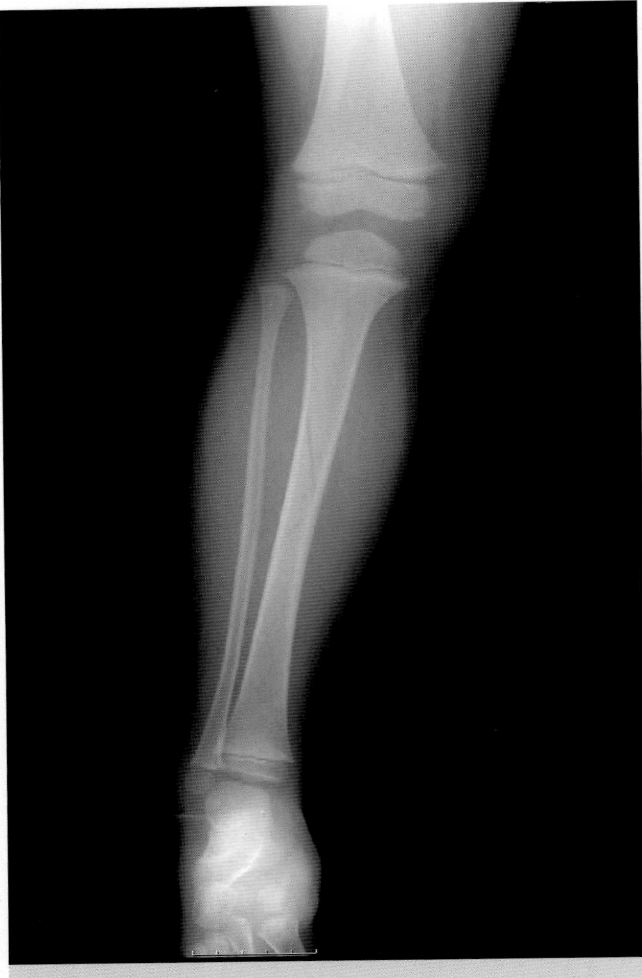

Figure 19-6. Spiral Fracture

A nondisplaced spiral fracture of the mid-shaft of the tibia.

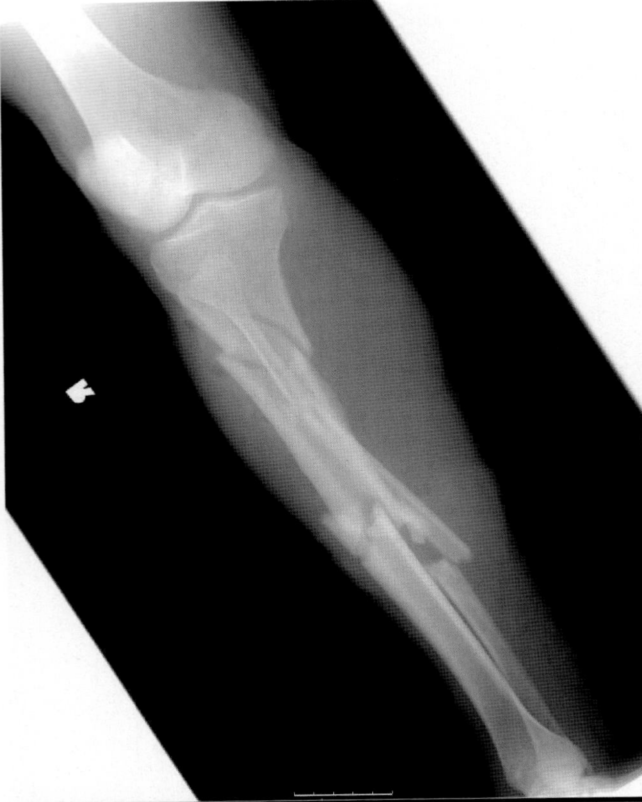

Figure 19-7. Comminuted Fracture

An x-ray of a pedestrian struck by a car. There are comminuted fractures of the proximal tibia and fibular mid-shaft with lateral angulation of the bone fragments. There are also fractures of the proximal and distal fibular mid-shaft.

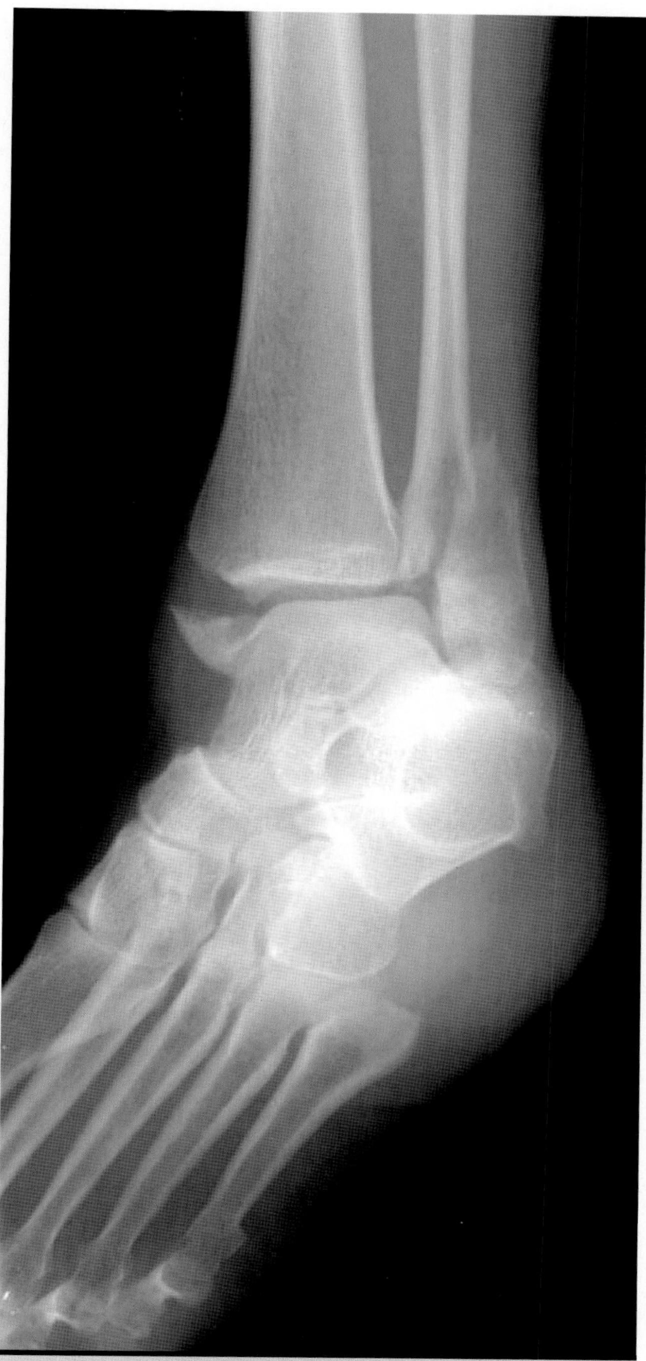

Figure 19-8. Avulsion Fracture

X-ray demonstrates an avulsion fracture of the medial malleolus and an oblique fracture of the lateral malleolus (bimalleolar fracture).

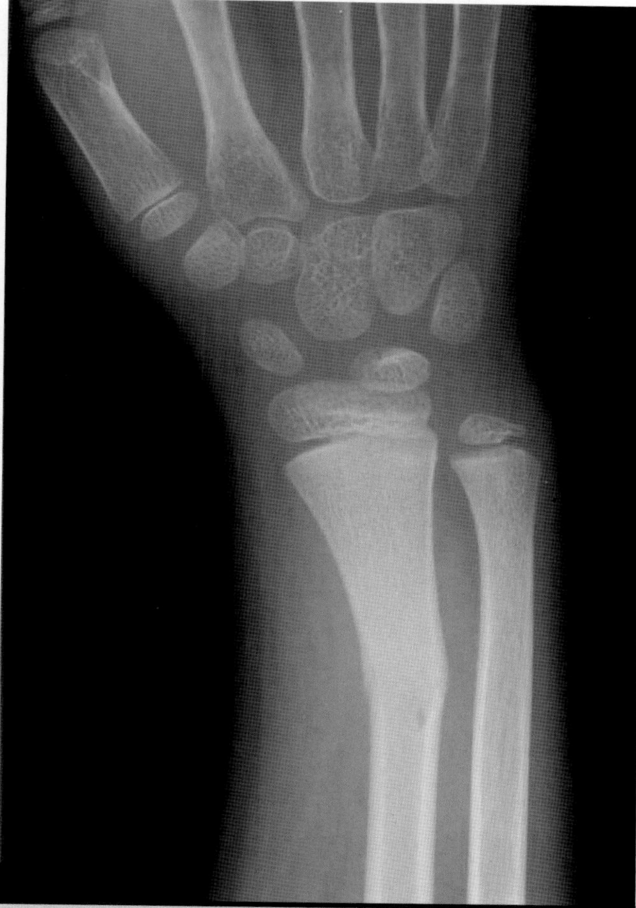

Figure 19-9. Greenstick Fracture

An x-ray demonstrating a greenstick fracture of the distal radius. Note the slight fragmentation on the lateral side.

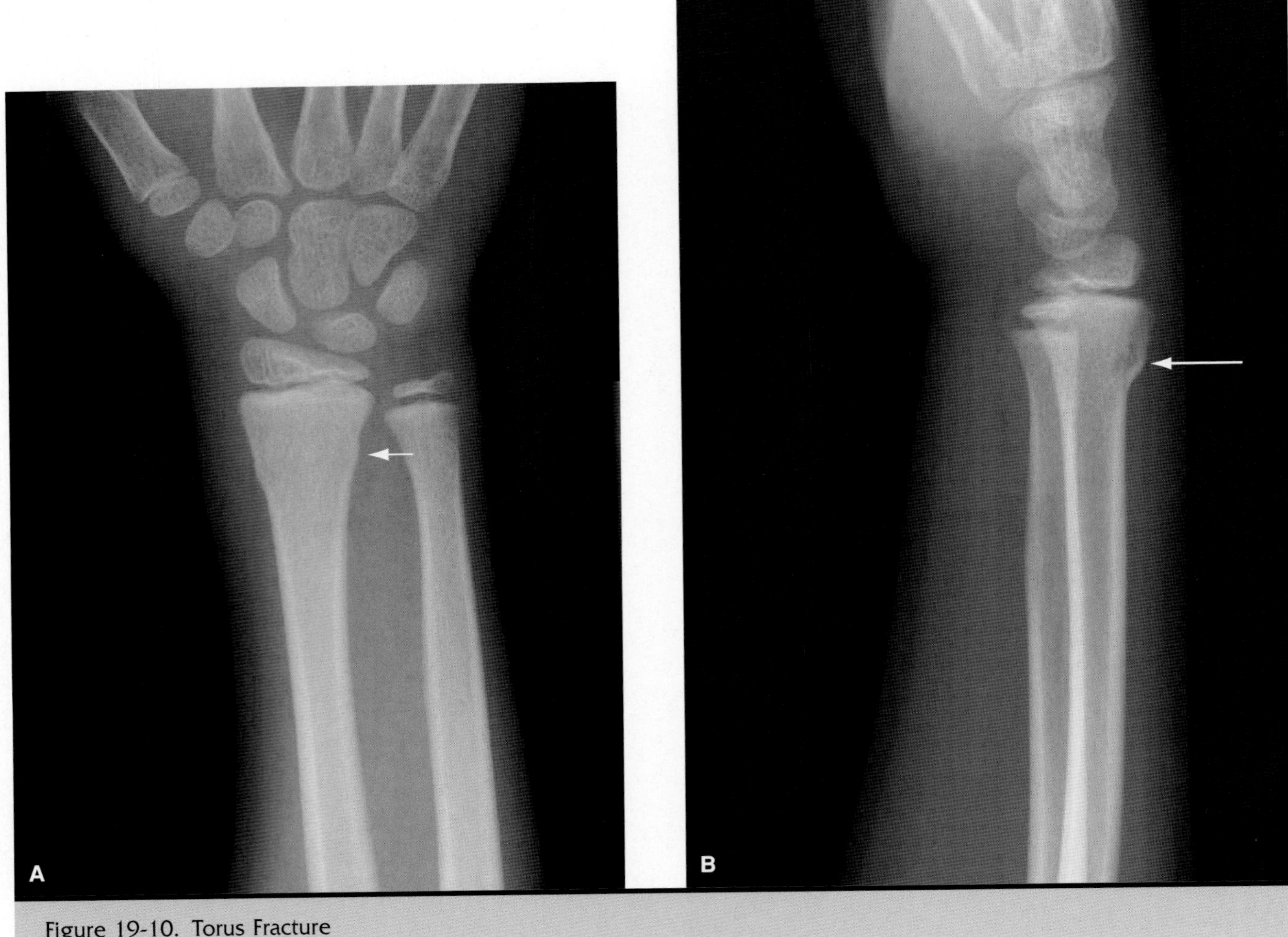

Figure 19-10. Torus Fracture

A. Anteroposterior x-ray of the wrist with a subtle torus fracture. *B*. Lateral x-ray of the same wrist with an obvious buckle or torus fracture.

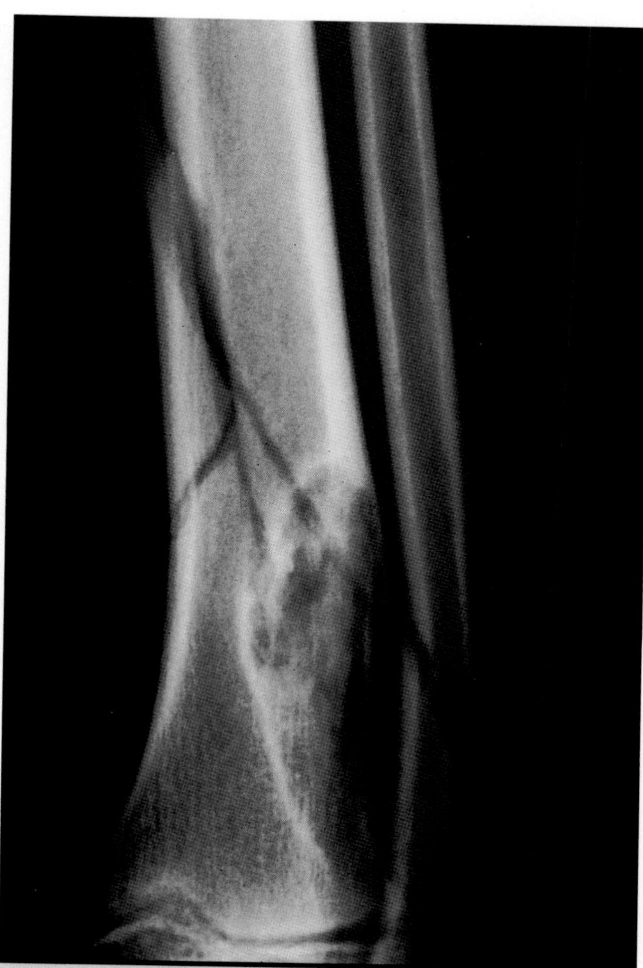

Figure 19-11. Pathologic Fracture

Anteroposterior radiograph of the leg shows a comminuted fracture through an abnormal expansile benign-appearing lytic lesion (bone cyst), in the lateral aspect of the distal tibia. An oblique fracture of the fibula is also seen.

BOX 19-3. EPIPHYSEAL FRACTURES

Salter-Harris classification (Fig. 19-12)

- Most widely used classification for epiphyseal fractures
- This classification gives a general prognosis for the risk of premature closure of physes, as well as generalized treatment guidelines.
- There are five types which are differentiated by location and involvement of the physeal growth plate.

Type I:

- The fracture line goes through the physis, not involving the epiphysis or the metaphysis.
- Usually managed by closed reduction, as the joint space is not involved and perfect alignment is not required

Type II:

- The fracture line goes through a portion of the physis and extends through the metaphysis on either side of the bone.
- Fractures not involving the joint space are generally managed by closed reduction.
- *Exception: A type II fracture of the distal femur requires anatomical alignment by either open or closed technique.*

Type III:

- The fracture line goes through a portion of the physis and extends through the epiphysis into the joint space on either side of the bone.
- Fractures usually require open alignment of the physis and the articular surface.

Type IV:

- The fracture line goes through a portion of the metaphysis, extends through the physis, and also involves a portion of the epiphysis and thus enters the joint space.
- Fractures require open alignment of the physis and the articular surface.

Type V:

- This fracture is a crush injury, compressing the physis.
- The fracture is not always initially recognized.
- Often diagnosed in retrospect with premature physeal closure

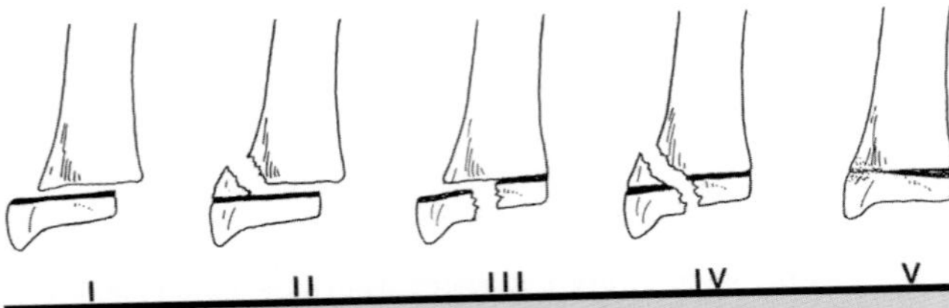

Figure 19-12. Schematic Drawings of Epiphyseal Fractures Based on the Salter-Harris Classification

(Reproduced with permission from: Tintinalli JE, Ruiz E, Krome RL: *Emergency Medicine: A Comprehensive Study Guide*, 4th ed. New York, McGraw-Hill, 1996, p. 1211).

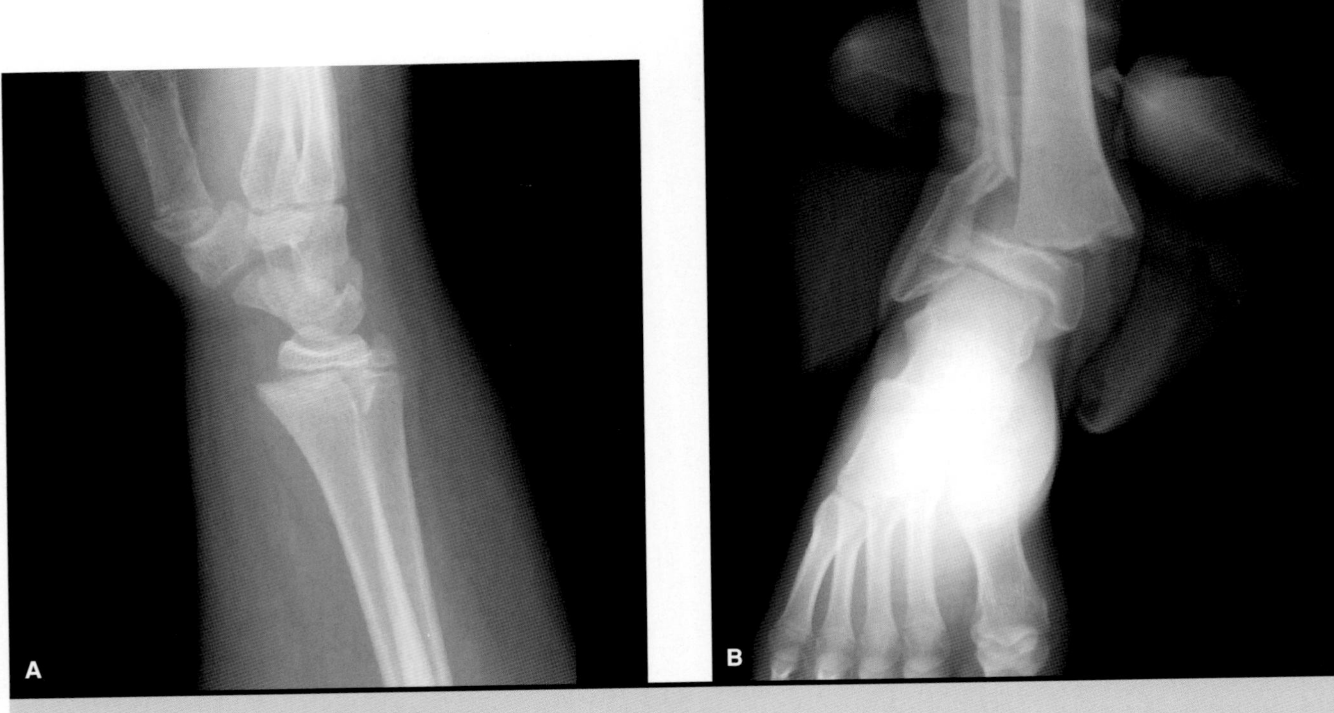

Figure 19-13. Salter-Harris Type II Fracture

A. Salter-Harris type II fracture of the distal radius. *B*. Salter-Harris type II fracture of the distal tibia with complete disruption of the physis and displacement of the metaphysis relative to the epiphysis. There is also a comminuted angulated fracture of the distal fibular metaphysis that does not involve the physis. The x-ray is of a 13-year-old boy who had his ankle run over by a car.

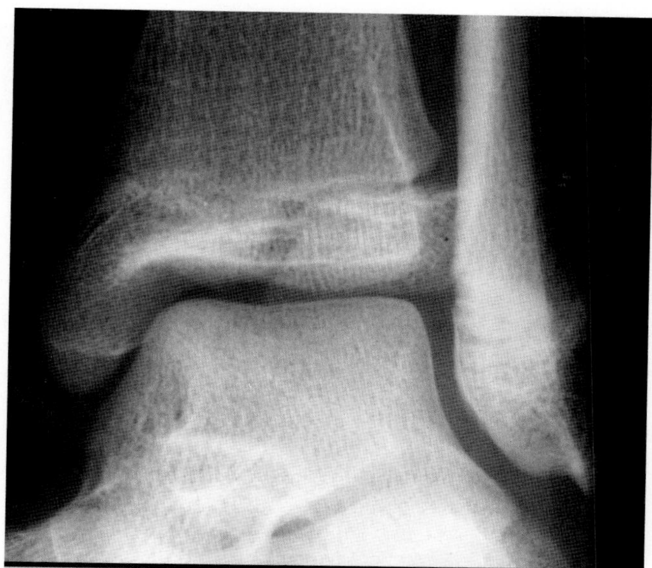

Figure 19-14. Salter-Harris Type III Fracture

An x-ray of a Salter-Harris type III fracture of the lateral portion of the distal tibia. Note the intra-articular component extending through the growth plate and the medial epiphysis of the tibia.

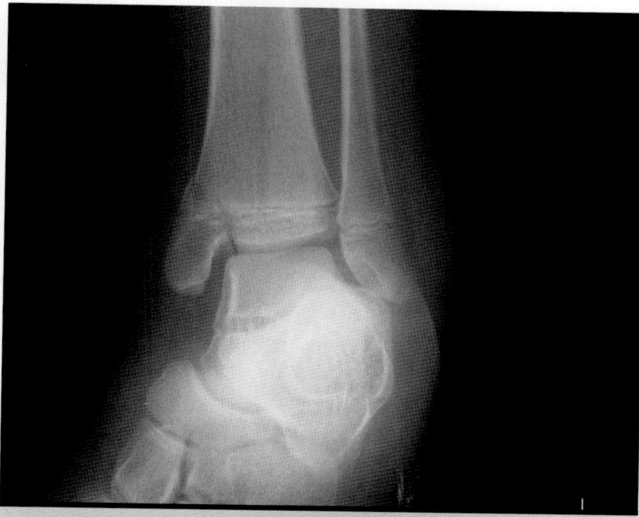

Figure 19-15. Salter-Harris Type IV Fracture

X-ray of a Salter-Harris type IV fracture of the medial malleolus.

DIAGNOSIS HAND INJURIES AND INFECTIONS

Introduction

1. The pediatric emergency medicine physician will see multiple cases of injuries and infections of the hand. Appropriate evaluation requires a thorough history and physical examination.
2. Significant morbidity can be associated with certain fractures if they are not recognized, treated properly, and referred early. Several key points must be kept in mind.
   a. The hand is a highly sophisticated instrument in which multiple bones move in coordination around a fixed center.
   b. The second and third metacarpal bones are relatively immobile and act as the stabilizing center around which all other bones move.
   c. Significant injuries may appear relatively minor.
   d. Evaluation of the hand must include examination and documentation of neural, motor, and vascular integrity.
   e. When considering the metacarpals and phalanges, different degrees of angulation may be acceptable, but rotational malalignment should never be.

Phalanx Fractures

Mechanism of Injury

Phalangeal fractures (Fig. 19-16) often occur from a fall on an outstretched hand, although they can also occur from a crush injury. Distal phalangeal fractures in particular are most often secondary to crush injuries.

Radiology

1. Any injury that results in swelling to the hand should be evaluated radiographically.
2. Often chip or avulsion fractures will not produce a great degree of swelling and may go undetected if radiographs are not taken.

Complications

1. Osteomyelitis is often associated with open fractures, which includes nail plate lacerations and fractures associated with drained subungual hematomas (Fig. 19-17).

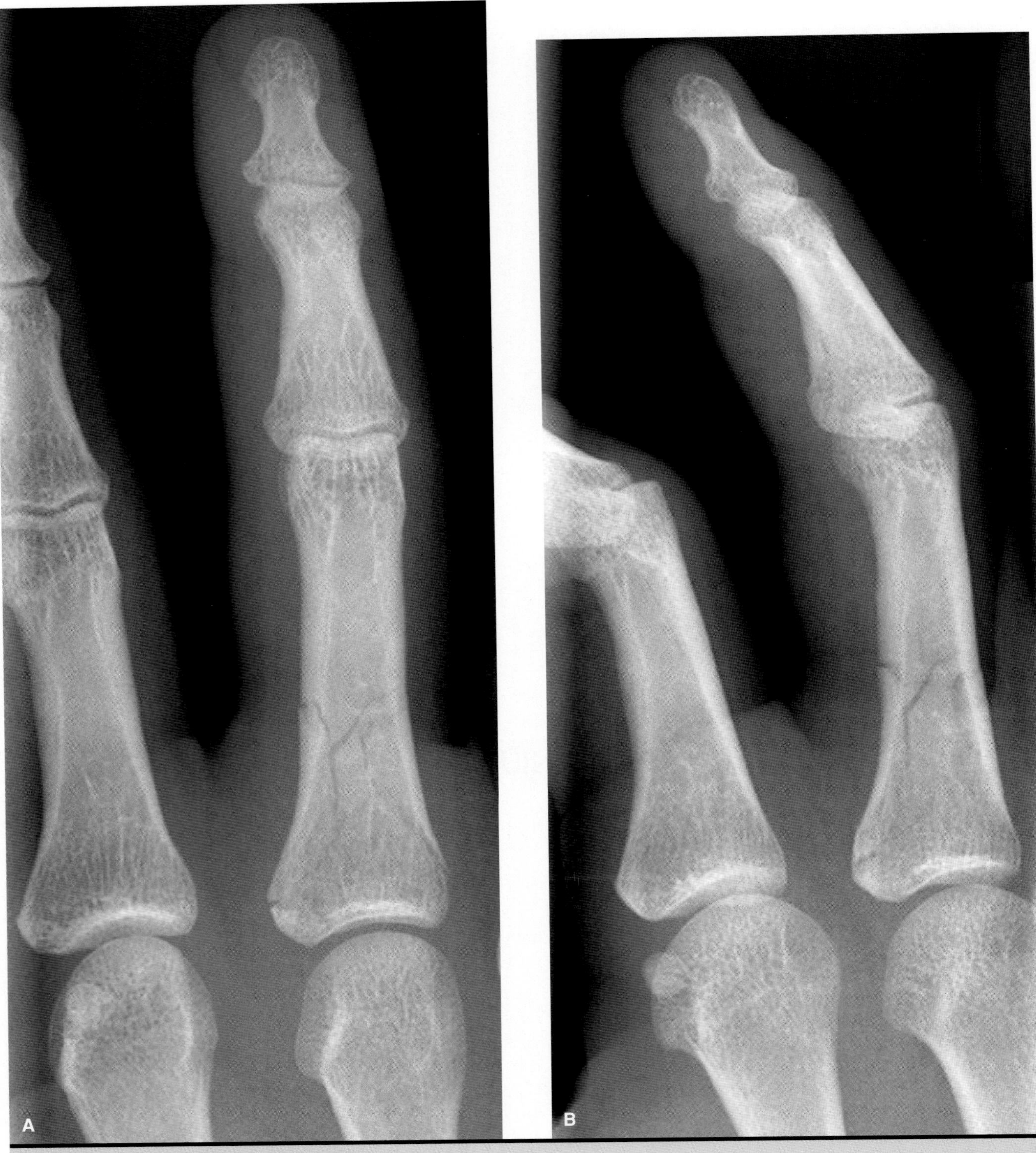

Figure 19-16. Proximal Phalanx Fracture

A. An AP view of a comminuted nondisplaced intra-articular fracture of the proximal phalanx of the middle finger that was sustained from a crush injury to the MCP joint. *B*. An oblique view of the same fracture with poor demonstration of the intra-articular component.

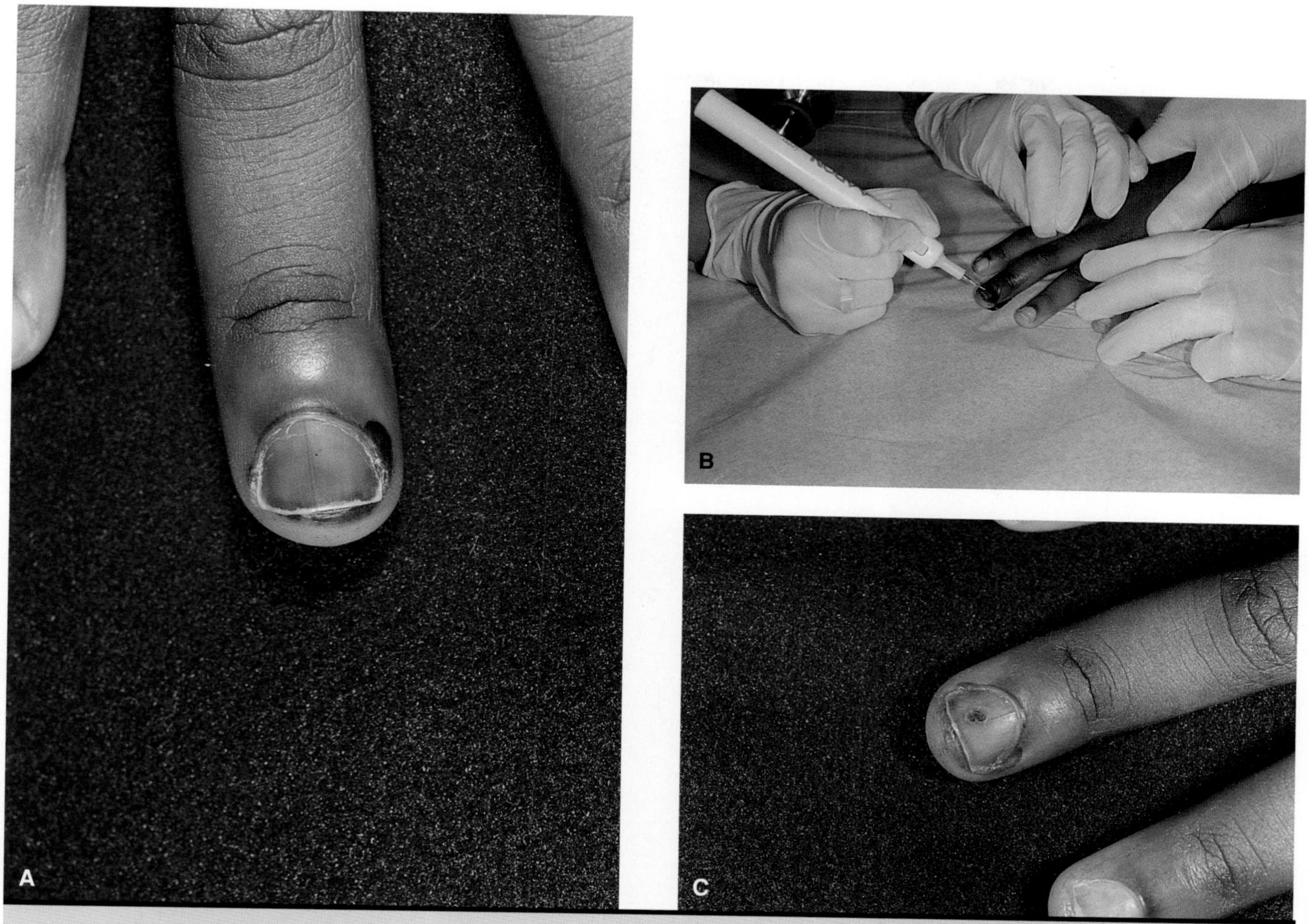

Figure 19-17. Subungual Hematoma

A. A picture of a 100% subungual hematoma, which was sustained from a crush injury to the distal phalanx. There was no underlying tuft fracture. *B*. Drainage of the subungual hematoma using cautery. *C*. Postdrainage of the subungual hematoma, ready for gauze dressing.

2. Swan-neck deformity results from an intra-articular avulsion fracture or tendon tear of the dorsal surface of the distal phalanx (Fig. 19-18). If the injury is not initially treated properly, a hyperextension deformity of the proximal interphalangeal joint with simultaneous flexion of the distal interphalangeal joint may occur. The resultant swan-neck appearance of the finger is the reason for its name.
3. Subungual hematoma is the most common complication of trauma to the distal phalanx. Most subungual hematomas do not have to be drained. Drainage is most often done for pain control. Hematomas of greater than 50% of the nail should be drained for pain control. Those of less than 50% can be managed conservatively, unless the patient is having a considerable amount of pain. Subungual hematomas can be drained by cautery through the nail or careful drilling through the nail with an 18-gauge needle.

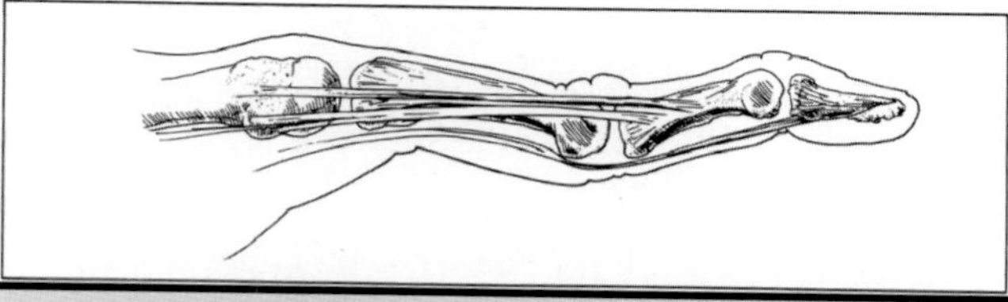

Figure 19-18. Swan-Neck Deformity

An illustration of a swan-neck deformity that results from the improper treatment of a dorsal avulsion fracture of the distal phalanx. A hyperextension deformity will occur at the proximal interphalangeal joint, with a slight flexion of the distal interphalangeal joint. This is secondary to an imbalance between the ruptured and the unopposed distal flexor tendon. (Reproduced with permission from: Simon RR, Koenigsknecht SJ: *Emergency Orthopedics: The Extremities*, 4th ed. New York, McGraw-Hill, 2001, p. 107.)

4. A nailbed laceration occasionally occurs with distal phalanx injuries. Most nailbed lacerations should be repaired. Identification and repair of a nailbed laceration implies evaluation with removal of the entire nail after digital block.

Consultation

1. This should be performed on all open fractures, fractures involving the joint space, and fractures that involve any degree of digit rotation or any significant degree of angulation.
2. In general, because of the increased mobility from the second to the third to the fourth to the fifth metacarpal bones, a higher degree of angulation is tolerated with greater mobility.
3. Angulation of 30 to 40 degrees can be tolerated for the fifth metacarpal, 30 degrees for the fourth metacarpal, 20 degrees for the third metacarpal, and 10 degrees for the second metacarpal.
4. When in doubt, the emergency department physician should consult a hand specialist.

Emergency Department Treatment and Disposition

1. Most closed phalanx fractures can be managed by an emergency medicine physician.
2. Intra-articular fractures, comminuted fractures, or open fractures should have urgent/emergent orthopedic consultation.

BOX 19-4. CLINICAL FEATURES OF PHALANX FRACTURES

- Tenderness in particular on axial loading (Fig. 19-19)
- Angulation off the longitudinal axis of the bone
- Rotational deformity
- Tuft fractures of the distal phalanges may be longitudinal, transverse, comminuted, or transverse with displacement.

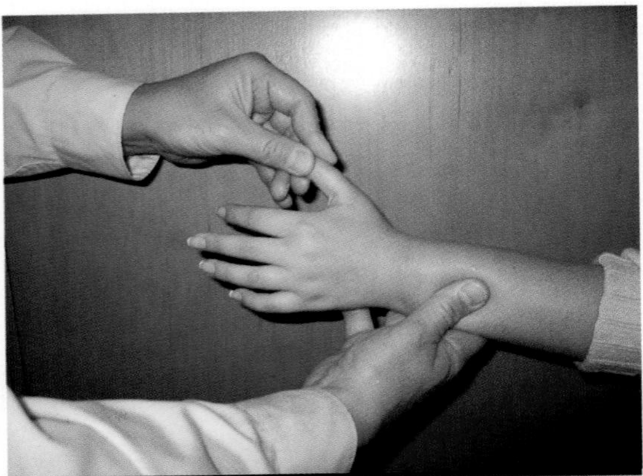

Figure 19-19. Axial Loading of a Digit

An image demonstrating the proper technique of axial loading of the thumb.

BOX 19-5. CLINICAL PEARLS: PHALANX FRACTURES

- Lacerations over any joints on the dorsum of the hand must be thoroughly scrutinized to be sure that the dorsal hood is not violated, which would mean it is an open joint, necessitating emergent consultation.
- Any pain on axial loading should necessitate radiographic evaluation.
- There is a high association of hand and wrist injuries with phalanx fractures.

Tuft Fractures

Definition

The tuft or the distal portion of the distal phalange is located directly beneath the nailbed. Most fractures of the distal phalange do not involve the distal interphalangeal (DIP) joint space.

Mechanism of Injury

These usually occur from a crush injury to the distal finger (Fig. 19-20).

Clinical Features

1. Swelling, pain, erythema
2. Usually associated with a subungual hematoma

Laboratory and Radiography

Standard x-rays of the digit

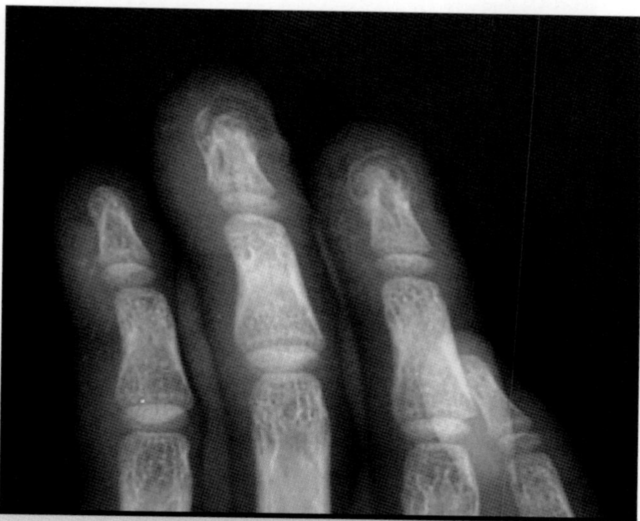

Figure 19-20. Tuft Fracture

This x-ray is of a 5-year-old boy whose hand was caught in a closing door. It demonstrates tuft fractures of the third and fourth digits. The tuft fracture of the long finger is more displaced than the more subtle fracture of the ring finger.

Complications

1. Extension into the joint space
2. Extensor or flexor tendon rupture

Consultation

1. All fractures should be referred for orthopedic follow-up.
2. Fractures involving the joint space should have orthopedic follow-up in 48 to 72 hours.
3. Open fractures require orthopedic consultation in the ED.

Emergency Department Treatment and Disposition

1. Cautery drainage of a subungual hematoma as necessary
2. Hairpin aluminum splinting for comfort

BOX 19-6. DIFFERENTIAL DIAGNOSIS OF TUFT FRACTURES

- Felon
- Paronychia
- Cellulitis
- Foreign Body
- Onychomycosis

BOX 19-7. CLINICAL PEARLS: TUFT FRACTURES

- Axial loading of the finger will always elicit pain.
- Always evaluate the other digits.
- Always evaluate the wrist, in particular looking for scaphoid tenderness.

Paronychia

Definition

An infection involving the fold of the nail (Fig. 19-21)

Clinical Features

Swelling, tenderness, and fluctuance at the base of the nail

Etiology

1. Associated with nail biting
2. Can also be caused by any penetrating injury at the base of the nail

Radiology

Radiographic evaluation is not necessary unless there is a recent history of significant trauma.

Complications

1. Spread of infection proximally
2. Felon (infection of the volar surface of the distal phalanx pulp space)

Emergency Department Treatment and Disposition

After adequate anesthesia with a digital block, incision and drainage with a no. 11 blade scalpel sliding up the nail proximally

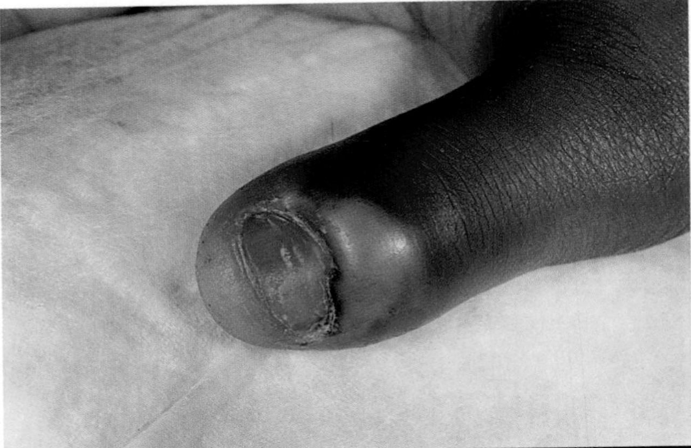

Figure 19-21. Paronychia

This image shows paronychia of the thumb with localized cellulitis, which was drained after digital block.

BOX 19-8. DIFFERENTIAL DIAGNOSIS OF PARONYCHIA

- Contusion
- Retained foreign body
- Tuft fracture
- Hair-tourniquet syndrome (Fig. 19-22)

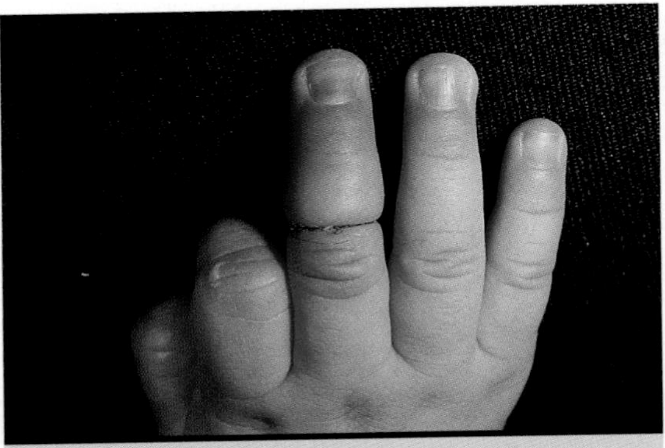

Figure 19-22. Hair-Tourniquet Syndrome

A 4-month-old child who presented with inconsolable crying was found to have a hair wrapped around the middle finger. The finger is edematous, erythematous, and could be mistaken as infected. One or more hairs may be wrapped around one or more times. A thorough inspection is required after removal of the hair to see if any strands remain.

BOX 19-9. CLINICAL PEARL: PARONYCHIA

- For best drainage, a digital block should be used.

Interphalangeal Joint Dislocation

Mechanism of Injury

Usually the result of a pull and twist of an isolated finger or a fall on a hand with the fingers locked in extension

Clinical Features

1. Hyperextension of the proximal or distal interphalangeal joint
2. Angulation of the proximal or distal interphalangeal joint
3. Inability to flex the affected joint

Radiology

X-rays of the digit in at least two views

Complications

1. Articular surface fracture
2. Ligamentous tear
3. If associated with a laceration, an open joint

Consultation

Hand/orthopedic specialist on any suspicion of an open joint or in dislocations associated with fractures

Emergency Department Treatment and Disposition

1. Open joints need irrigation in the operating room and admission to the orthopedic service.
2. Open joints also need intravenous antibiotics as soon as possible upon presentation to the ED, and certainly within 2 to 3 hours of injury.
3. Isolated dislocations without an associated fracture or open joint should be reduced by the emergency physician.
   a. One attempt at axial traction of the distal phalanx can be made without digital block in very young children who have a simple dislocation without phalangeal overlap.
   b. All other dislocations should be reduced with the same axial traction after appropriate anesthesia (digital block) (Fig. 19-23).

BOX 19-10. CLINICAL PEARLS: INTERPHALANGEAL JOINT DISLOCATION

- Most can be reduced in the ED
- After successful reduction the finger should be splinted using a commercial aluminum splint with the interphalangeal joints at 15 to 20 degrees of flexion.
- Postreduction x-rays should always be obtained to assure proper alignment with splinting.

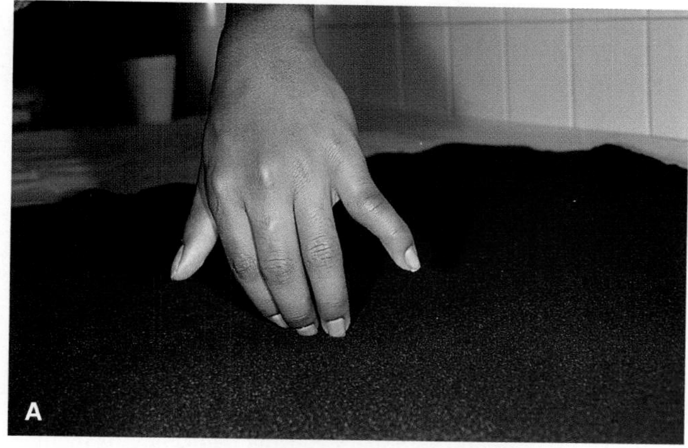

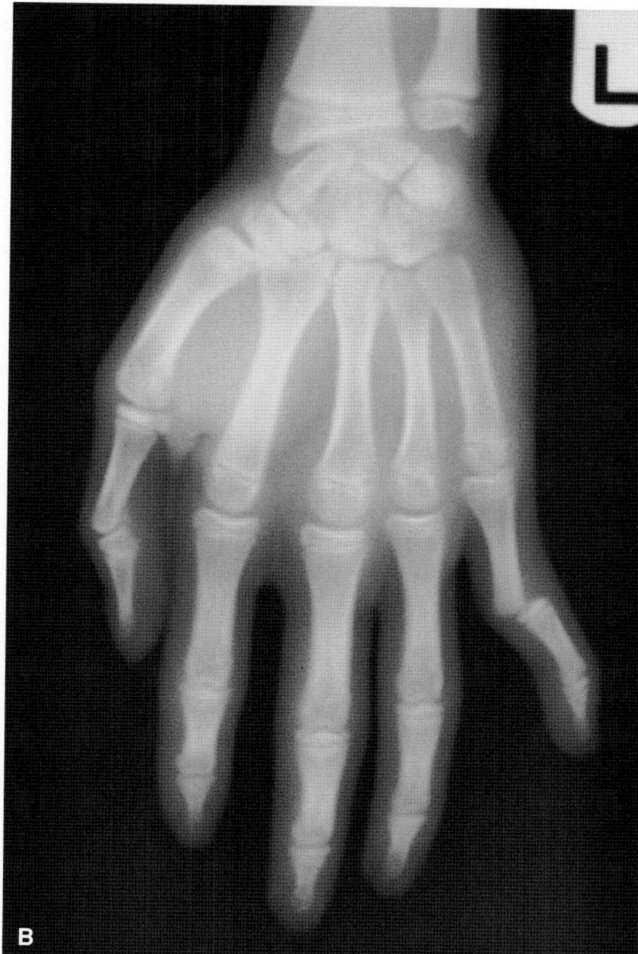

Figure 19-23. Interphalangeal Joint Dislocation

A. Picture of obvious PIP deformity of the fifth digit. *B*. X-ray of the finger demonstrates PIP dislocation, which was easily reduced with axial traction after digital block.

Flexor Tenosynovitis

Mechanism of Injury

Usually a result of a puncture wound along the volar aspect of the digit

Clinical Features and Etiology

1. Kanavel's signs seen in flexor tenosynovitis include:
   a. Symmetrical swelling of the finger (Fig. 19-24)
   b. Tenderness over the flexor tendon sheath
   c. Pain with passive extension
   d. The finger is held in a flexed position.
2. The most common pathogens causing tenosynovitis include *Staphylococcus aureus*, and *Streptococcus* spp., followed by *Pseudomonas* spp.

Radiology

Standard x-rays of the digit should be done to rule out occult fracture or foreign body.

Complications

1. Osteomyelitis
2. Septic arthritis
3. Ascending cellulitis
4. Joint fibrosis and limited mobility

Consultation

Flexor tenosynovitis requires emergent consultation in the ED.

Emergency Department Treatment and Disposition

1. Admission to the hospital
2. Elevation
3. Intravenous oxacillin therapy (or clindamycin therapy for patients who are allergic to penicillin)
4. Possible incision and drainage in the operating room

BOX 19-11. DIFFERENTIAL DIAGNOSIS OF FLEXOR TENOSYNOVITIS

- Occult fracture
- Osteomyelitis
- Retained foreign body

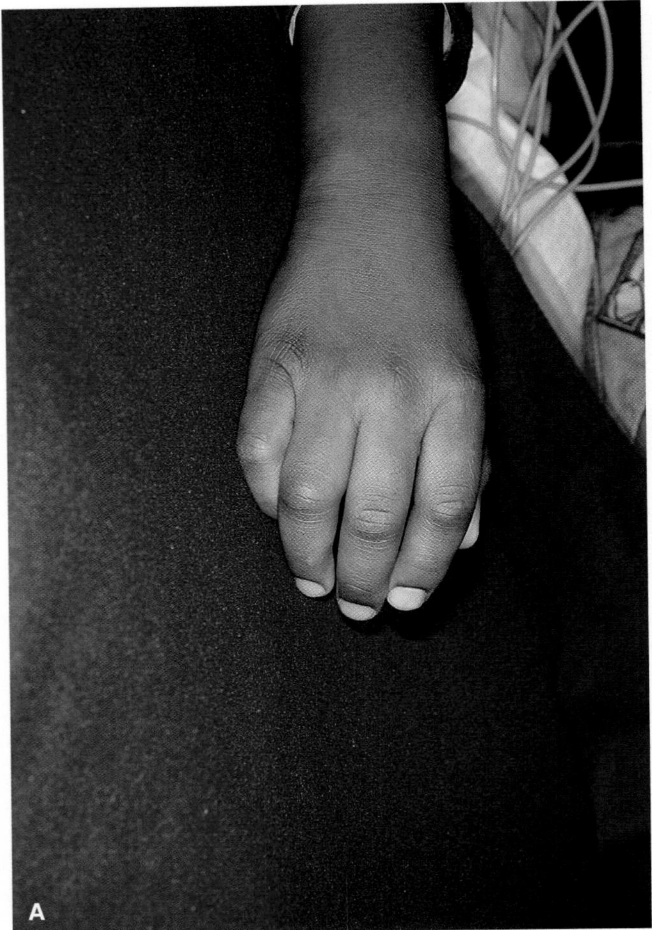

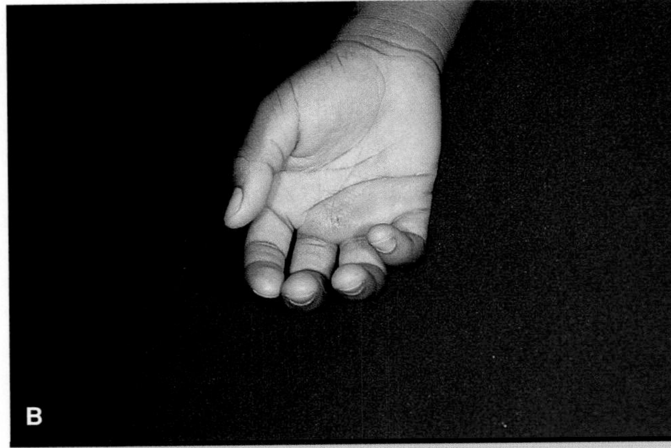

Figure 19-24. Flexor Tenosynovitis

A. Dorsal view of a hand with fusiform swelling of the third and fourth digits in a patient with tenosynovitis. *B*. Palmar view of the same child demonstrates the swelling of the third and fourth digits, caused by a puncture wound to the palm over the MCP joint.

BOX 19-12. CLINICAL PEARLS: FLEXOR TENOSYNOVITIS

- With no barriers to the spread of infection, the entire tendon sheath usually becomes involved.
- At the flexor creases, the tendons are near the surface of the skin and are more susceptible to penetrating injury.
- *Staphylococcus aureus* and *Streptococcus* spp. are the most common causative agents, followed by *Pseudomonas* spp.

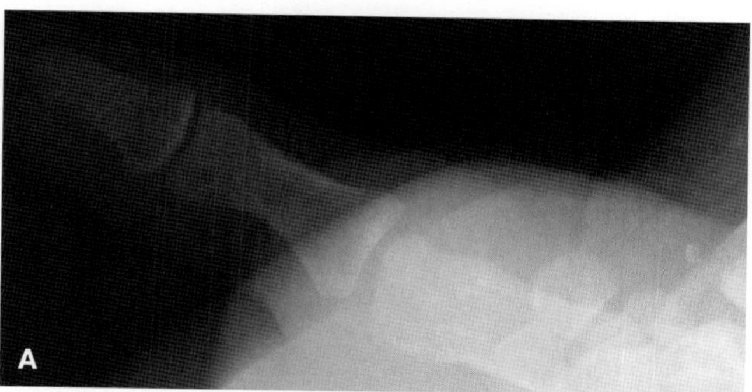

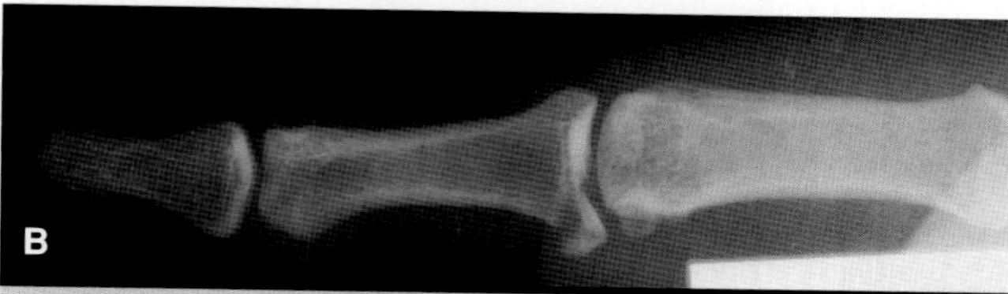

Figure 19-25. Gamekeeper's Thumb

A. An x-ray demonstrating a gamekeeper's thumb with lateral angulation of the first proximal phalanx shaft with respect to the first metacarpal, resulting in widening of the medial aspect of the MCP joint. *B*. An x-ray of an avulsion fracture of the ulnar collateral ligament of the thumb off the proximal phalanx.

Gamekeeper's Thumb

Definition

A tear of the ulnar collateral ligament of the metacarpophalangeal joint (MCP) of the thumb

Mechanism of Injury

1. The name originally was given to this occupational ligamentous injury of the thumb because gamekeepers would kill fowl by snapping the birds' necks with their hands. By holding the bird's neck with two hands and ulnarly deviating both wrists, strain is placed on the ulnar collateral ligament of the MCP joint of the thumb.
2. As this is no longer a common occupation, this injury is more often associated with falling on an outstretched hand and is now referred to as skiers thumb.

Radiology

1. This injury may not be apparent on x-ray.
2. Appears as an avulsion fracture of the base of the proximal phalanx on the medial side (Fig. 19-25)

Complications

1. Decreased range of motion of the thumb and functionality of the hand
2. Decreased strength of the pincer grip

Emergency Department Treatment and Disposition

1. All injuries should be immobilized with splinting.
2. After immobilization, closed injuries can be sent home with orthopedic or hand specialist follow-up in 48 to 72 hours.

BOX 19-13. CLINICAL FEATURES OF GAMEKEEPERS THUMB

- Lateral deviation of the thumb at the MCP joint
- Tenderness over the MCP joint
- Inability to oppose the index finger and the thumb

BOX 19-14. CLINICAL PEARLS: GAMEKEEPER'S THUMB

- The diagnosis can be made by looking for laxity of greater than 20 degrees of the ulnar collateral ligament with the thumb in full extension. Due to the pain this will cause, the examination should only take place after local anesthesia with 2% lidocaine *without epinephrine*.

Mallet Finger

Definition

Mallet fractures are a result of a dorsal avulsion fracture in which the extensor mechanism of the distal interphalangeal joint (DIP) is destroyed, leaving the DIP joint in partial flexion.

Mechanism of Injury

1. Mallet fractures may occur if there is forced flexion of the distal phalanx when the finger is in taut extension.
2. This particular type of fracture is often seen as a result of playing basketball or baseball when the ball hits and creates axial loading of an outstretched finger (Fig. 19-26).

Radiology

1. Standard x-rays of the digit should be performed.
2. Avulsion fracture may not be apparent on x-ray.

Complications

1. Inability to fully extend the DIP joint
2. Swan-neck deformity (see Fig. 19-18)

Emergency Department Treatment and Disposition

1. Splinting of the digit with the DIP in hyperextension and the PIP in 45 degrees of flexion
2. Patients can be discharged with orthopedic or hand specialist follow-up in 72 to 96 hours.

BOX 19-15. CLINICAL FEATURES OF MALLET FINGER

- At rest, the DIP joint is held in excessive flexion.
- Inability of the patient to fully extend the DIP joint
- Tenderness over the DIP joint

BOX 19-16. CLINICAL PEARLS: MALLET FINGER

- A fairly common injury
- Appropriate splinting and follow-up leads to a good outcome.

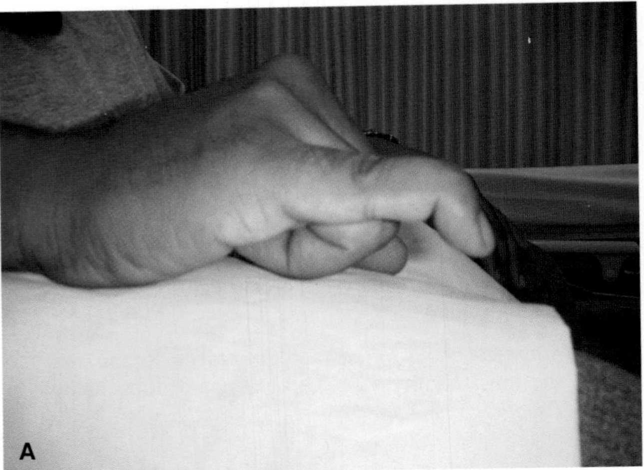

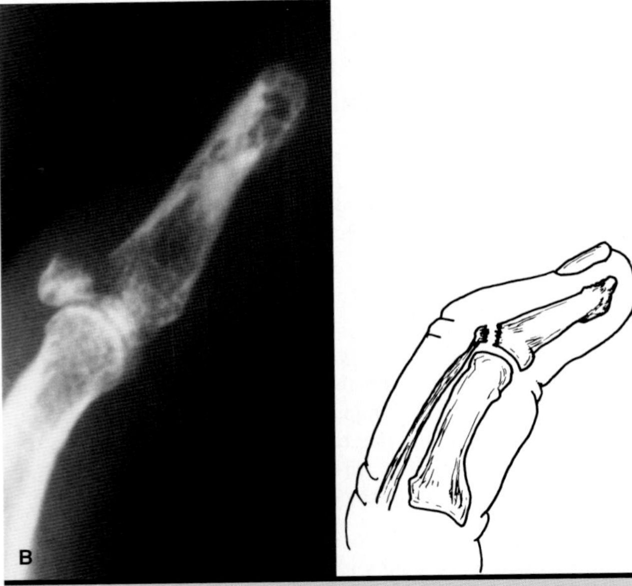

Figure 19-26. Mallet Finger

A. An image of the fifth digit of an adolescent who sustained a direct blow to the tip of his finger while playing basketball. The youth was unable to extend the DIP joint. *B*. An x-ray and drawing demonstrates how forced flexion of the DIP joint causes avulsion of the extensor tendon from the base of the distal phalanx. The associated avulsion fracture is occasionally seen and is demonstrated nicely on this lateral x-ray. (Part *B* reproduced with permission from: Wilks M, Meldon S: The hand. In: Schwartz DT, Reisdorff EJ (eds). *Emergency Radiology*. New York, McGraw-Hill, 2000, p. 40.)

Bennett's Fracture and Rolando's Fracture

Definitions

1. Bennett's fracture: transverse fracture of the base of the first metacarpal, which extends into the joint and is associated with a metacarpal dislocation
2. Rolando's fracture: similar to a Bennett's fracture except that the metacarpal fracture is comminuted

Mechanism of Injury

Usually seen with a fall on an outstretched hand; often associated with high-impact sports such as skiing

Radiology

1. Standard x-rays of the hand, thumb, and wrist (Fig. 19-27)
2. Scaphoid x-rays to evaluate for fracture

Complications

1. Nonunion
2. Arthritis
3. Limited range of motion
4. Decreased grip strength

Consultation

Orthopedics or hand surgery should always be consulted immediately, while the patient is in the ED, as these fractures require open reduction internal fixation.

Emergency Department Treatment and Disposition

1. Ice, elevation, and analgesics in the ED
2. Definitive treatment requires surgical repair.

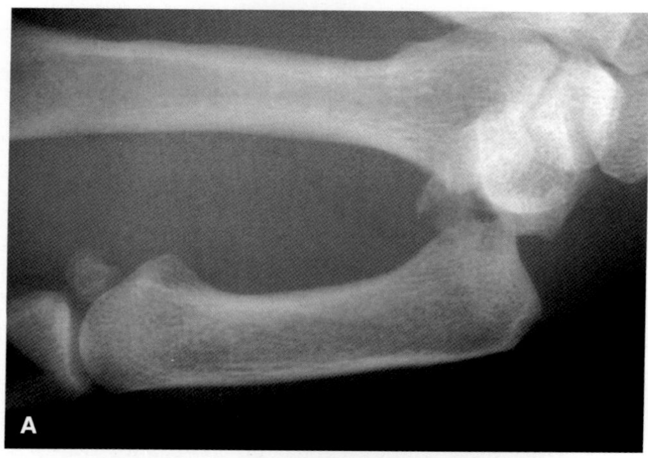

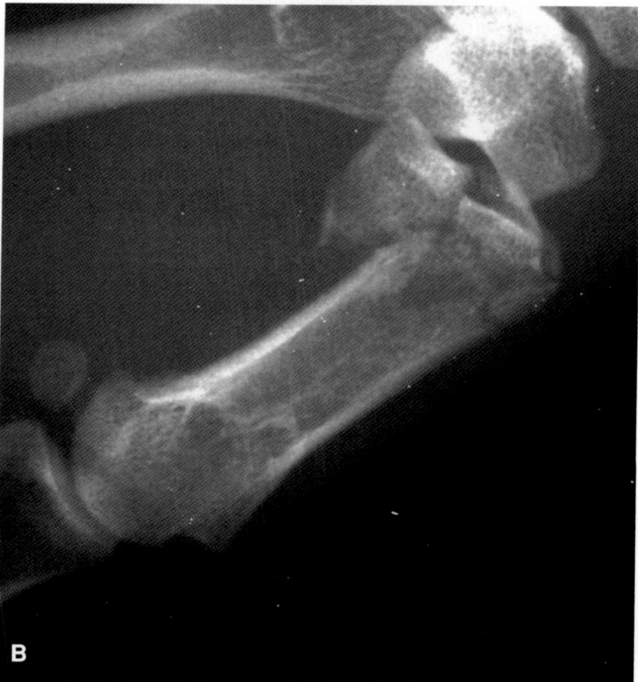

Figure 19-27. Bennett's and Rolando's Fractures

A. An x-ray of an intra-articular fracture at the base of the thumb metacarpal; the pull of the abductor pollicis tendon displaces the thumb carpometacarpal joint. *B*. An x-ray of the thumb demonstrating a Rolando's fracture with an intra-articular comminuted fracture of the base of the first metacarpal.

BOX 19-17. CLINICAL FEATURES OF METACARPAL FRACTURES (BENNETT'S AND ROLANDO'S FRACTURES)

- Tenderness and swelling over the base of the thenar eminence
- Inability to adduct or abduct the thumb
- Pain on movement of the wrist

BOX 19-18. CLINICAL PEARLS: METACARPAL FRACTURES (BENNETT'S AND ROLANDO'S FRACTURES)

- These are serious hand injuries with a high incidence of morbidity.
- Orthopedic evaluation is absolutely necessary.
- The carpal bones, in particular the scaphoid, need to be evaluated for injury.
- Often these injuries will require CT scan for evaluation of the carpal bones and to facilitate repair by the orthopedic surgeon.

Boxer's Fracture

Definition

Fracture of the neck of the fourth or the fifth metacarpal bone; these are the most common metacarpal fractures. The distal portion of the bone almost always has a volar angulation.

Mechanism of Injury

It's commonly called the "boxer's fracture," though some argue that it's virtually never seen in patients who wear boxer's gloves, and often the object struck is a wall rather than another boxer (Fig. 19-28).

Clinical Features

1. The patient will always have swelling and tenderness over the distal portion of the fifth metacarpal.
2. Metacarpal neck fractures typically involve comminution of the anterior cortex resulting in volar angulation of the metacarpal head.
3. Often the neutral position of the pinky will be normal unless there is extreme volar angulation or any rotational component.

Radiology

Standard x-rays of the hand that include an anteroposterior (AP) and a lateral. The lateral is essential to determine the amount of volar angulation.

Complications

1. Fractures isolated to the metacarpal neck have few complications.
2. Due to the mobility of the fifth metacarpal-carpal joint, angulation up to 40 degrees is well tolerated. If not reduced, angulation of greater than 40 degrees or any rotational deformity will result in an inability to maintain the normal tucked-in position of a clenched hand. This will lead to further vulnerability to injury of the fifth digit.

Consultation

All open fractures, intra-articular fractures, or fractures with a rotational component should have orthopedic/hand specialist consultation in the ED. Human bites (clenched fist injuries) should also have ED consultation.

Emergency Department Treatment and Disposition

1. A patient with a classic boxer's fracture can be treated in the ED with an ulna gutter splint, be discharged, and have orthopedic/hand specialist follow-up within the next week.
2. Angulation of greater than 40 degrees for the fifth or 30 degrees for the fourth digit, or any rotational deformity requires orthopedic/hand specialist consultation in the ED.

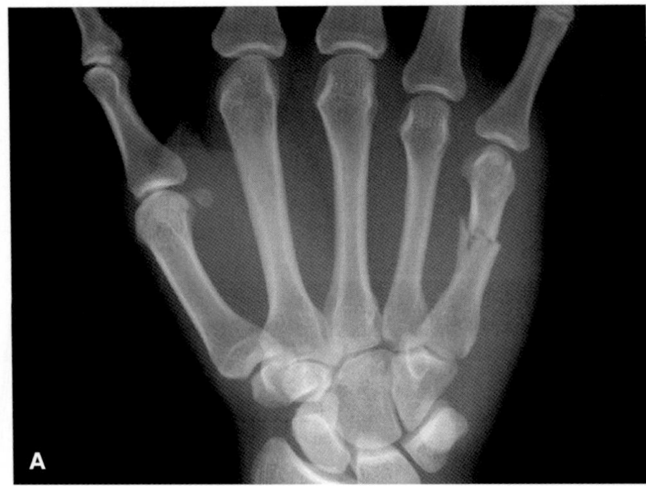

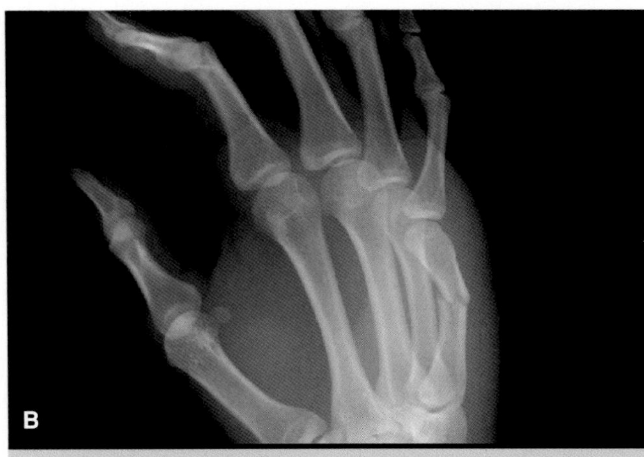

Figure 19-28. Boxer's Fracture

A. AP view of comminuted fifth metacarpal, boxer's fracture. *B*. Oblique view of the same fracture demonstrates the anterior angulation.

BOX 19-19. CLINICAL PEARLS: BOXER'S FRACTURE

- Most common metacarpal fracture
- Almost always involve the fifth metacarpal
- If the fracture of the fifth metacarpal is not angulated >40 degrees, does not involve the articular surface, and does not have any rotational component, it can be managed with a volar splint and orthopedic/hand specialist referral within 1 week.
- Clinched fist-to-mouth injuries resulting in a puncture/laceration over the fourth or fifth MCP joints need, at minimum, antibiotics in the ED, scrutiny for involvement of the MCP joint, and admission when associated with a fracture.

DIAGNOSIS OTHER UPPER EXTREMITY INJURIES

Fractures of Carpal Bones (Scaphoid or Navicular Fracture)

Mechanism of Injury

The most common fractures of the carpal bones are of the scaphoid or navicular. This may occur by either falling on an outstretched hand or after seemingly minor trauma.

Clinical Features

1. On physical exam there are three maneuvers that must be performed to clinically rule out a scaphoid fracture. If any one of these three maneuvers causes pain in the area of the anatomic snuffbox, a scaphoid fracture should be highly suspected.
   a. Snuffbox tenderness is best assessed with the thumb fully flexed into the palm and the second through fifth digits flexed over it. At this point the wrist is actively flexed medially into ulnar deviation. With this manipulation, the scaphoid is easily palpated in the snuffbox.
   b. The second maneuver is axial loading of the thumb (see Fig. 19-19). For this the thumb is kept in the extended position, and the examiner holds it by the distal phalanx and gently pushes it into its origin. The proximal phalanx sits on the scaphoid and with injury this will elicit pain.
   c. The third maneuver is forced supination (Fig. 19-29). The patient is asked to shake hands with the examiner and to resist the examiner's attempts to force the hand into supination.

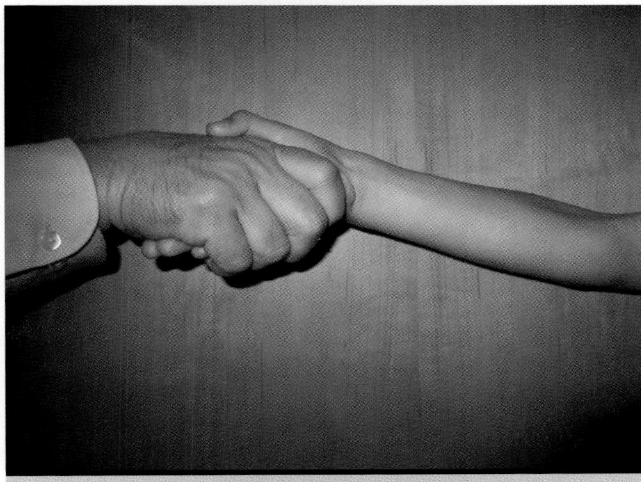

Figure 19-29. Forced Supination of the Wrist.

This picture shows a handshake demonstrating forced supination of the wrist.

Radiology

1. Standard x-rays of the wrist should be performed (Fig. 19-30).
2. If there is any suspicion, a scaphoid or navicular view should also be performed.

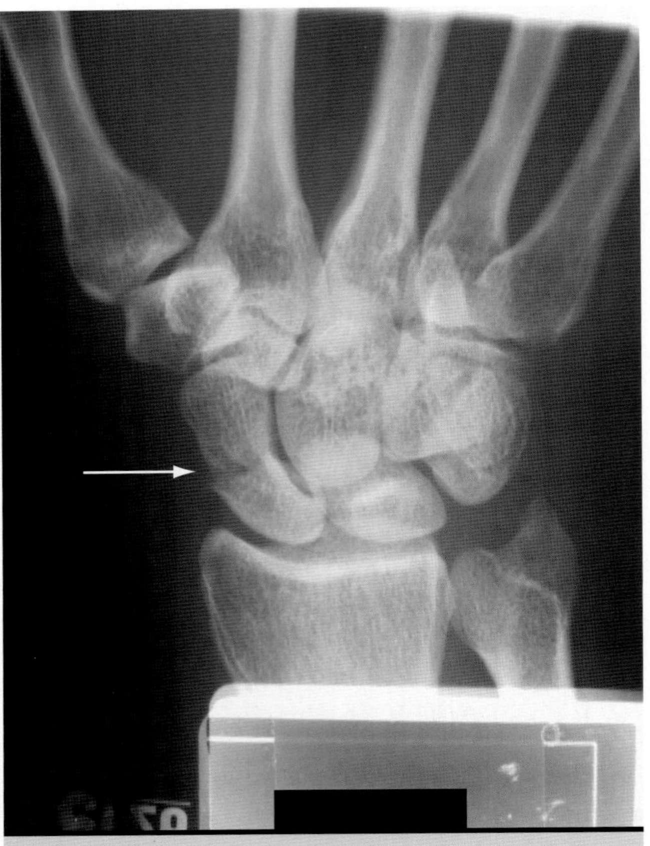

Figure 19-30. Scaphoid Fracture

AP radiograph of the wrist demonstrates a transverse fracture through the body of the scaphoid.

Complications

1. The most common complication of a scaphoid/navicular fracture is nonunion.
2. Nonunion of the scaphoid requires open pinning with subsequent decreased mobility.

Consultation

All radiologically apparent injuries of the carpal bone's fractures or dislocations should have emergent orthopedic consultation in the ED.

Emergency Department Treatment and Disposition

1. Radiologically-apparent carpal fractures or dislocations require orthopedic consultation in the ED for a long arm thumb spica splint or cylindrical cast.
2. Non–radiologically-apparent injuries to the wrist with point tenderness should be immobilized with urgent orthopedic referral.
3. Any patient with pain with direct palpation of the area of the snuffbox, axial loading of the thumb, or forced supination should be immobilized in a thumb spica splint.

BOX 19-20. CLINICAL PEARLS: SCAPHOID OR NAVICULAR FRACTURES

- The blood supply of the scaphoid bone is paradoxical, coming from the palmar arch and the dominant ulnar artery. Therefore distal scaphoid fractures heal better than proximal scaphoid fractures.
- X-rays may not detect a scaphoid fracture for weeks.

Lunate and Perilunate Dislocations

Mechanism of Injury

Extreme hyperextension of the wrist is the usual cause.

Clinical Features

1. A protruding deformity on the dorsum of the wrist with a dorsal lunate or a dorsal perilunate dislocation
2. A concavity over the dorsum of the wrist with volar lunate or volar perilunate dislocations
3. With a perilunate dislocation, the lunate remains in anatomic position. The remainder of the hand is displaced either volar or dorsally.

Radiology

1. Standard x-rays should be taken, but the lateral of the hand is particularly important (Figs. 19-31 and 19-32). On the lateral, look for alignment of (proximally to distally) the distal radius, the proximal border of the lunate, and the proximal border of the capitate.
2. With lunate dislocation, x-rays show that the capitate is aligned and the lunate is displaced, resembling a spilled teacup.

Complications

1. Undiagnosed wrist dislocations could result in neurologic or vascular compromise as well as severe mobility limitations.
2. Median nerve injury
3. Scaphoid fractures

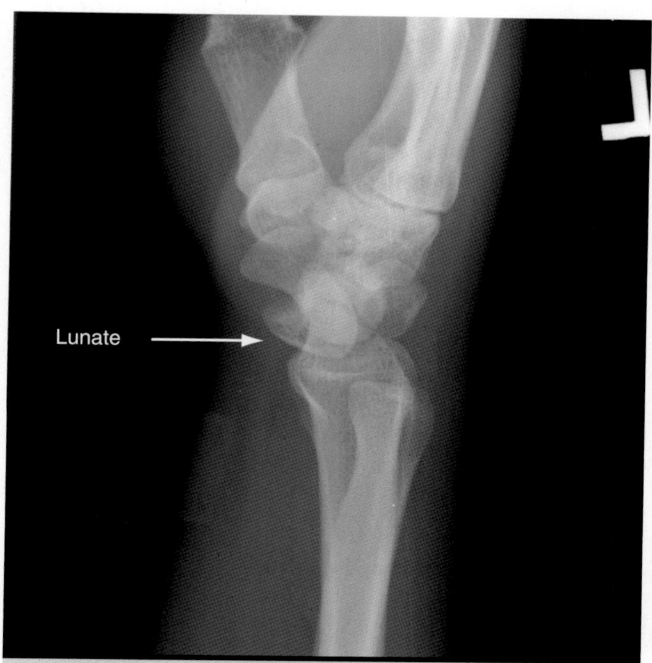

Figure 19-31. Lunate Dislocation

Lateral x-ray of the wrist demonstrates a lunate dislocation with the classic spilled teacup orientation. The lunate is displaced in the volar direction. The capitate, which can be dimly seen through the silhouette of the lunate is still in line with the distal radius.

Consultation

All wrist dislocations require emergent consultation in the ED.

Emergency Department Treatment and Disposition

Wrist dislocations should be elevated, iced, and immobilized while waiting for emergent consultation.

BOX 19-21. CLINICAL PEARLS: LUNATE AND PERILUNATE DISLOCATIONS

- Perilunate dislocation is the most common wrist dislocation.
- The lunate usually dislocates volarly.

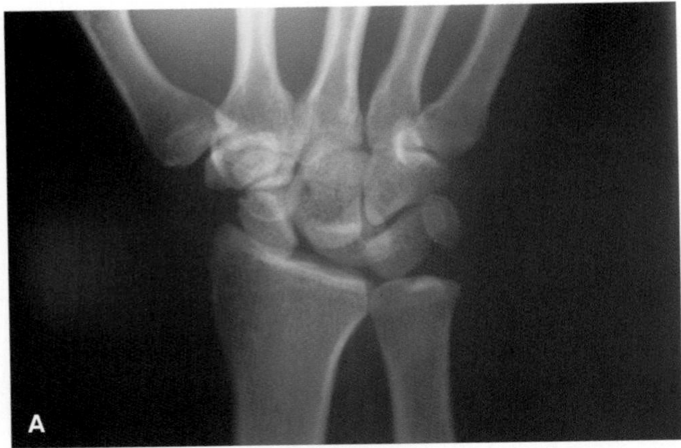

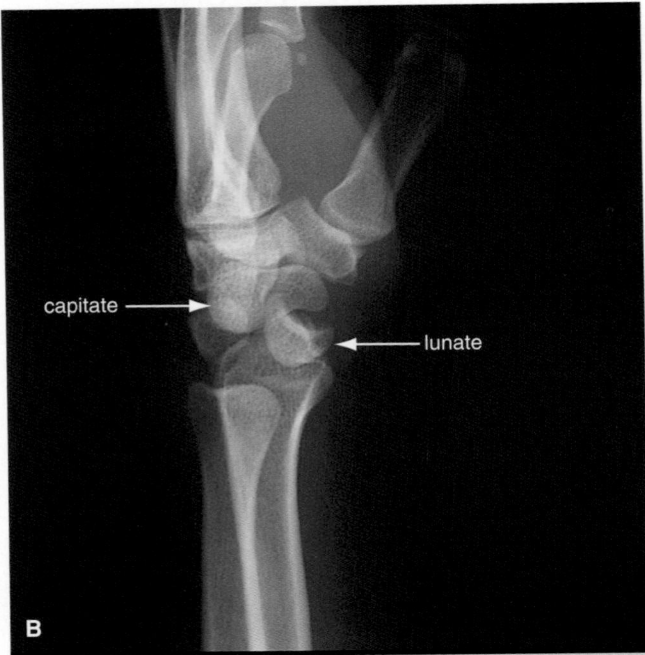

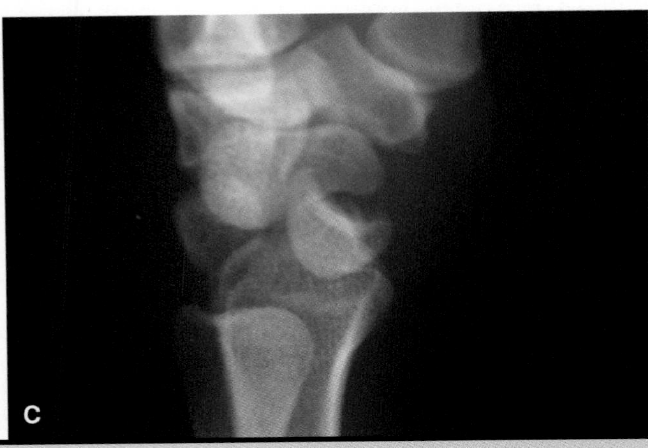

Figure 19-32. Perilunate Dislocation

A. AP radiograph of the wrist, showing the subtle finding of the lunate out of line with the capitate. *B*. Lateral view of the wrist demonstrating the lunate in line with the distal radius and the capitate posterior to its normal alignment with the lunate. *C*. A closer lateral view of the wrist demonstrates the perilunate dislocation more clearly.

Distal Radius Fractures

Mechanism of Injury

Wrist fractures often occur from a fall on an outstretched hand, as are phalanx fractures (Fig. 19-33). To a much lesser extent they can also occur from a crush injury.

Clinical Features

1. The most common upper extremity injury
2. When angulation occurs posteriorly it is referred to as a Colles fracture.
3. When angulation occurs anteriorly it is referred to as a Smith's fracture.
4. There is often a simultaneous ulnar styloid fracture.

Complications

1. Seen infrequently, but includes tendon damage
2. Subsequent arthritis is also a complication and occurs much more frequently when the articular surface of the distal radius is involved.
3. Injuries of the epiphysis may result in growth arrest with subsequent instability of the radioulnar joint.

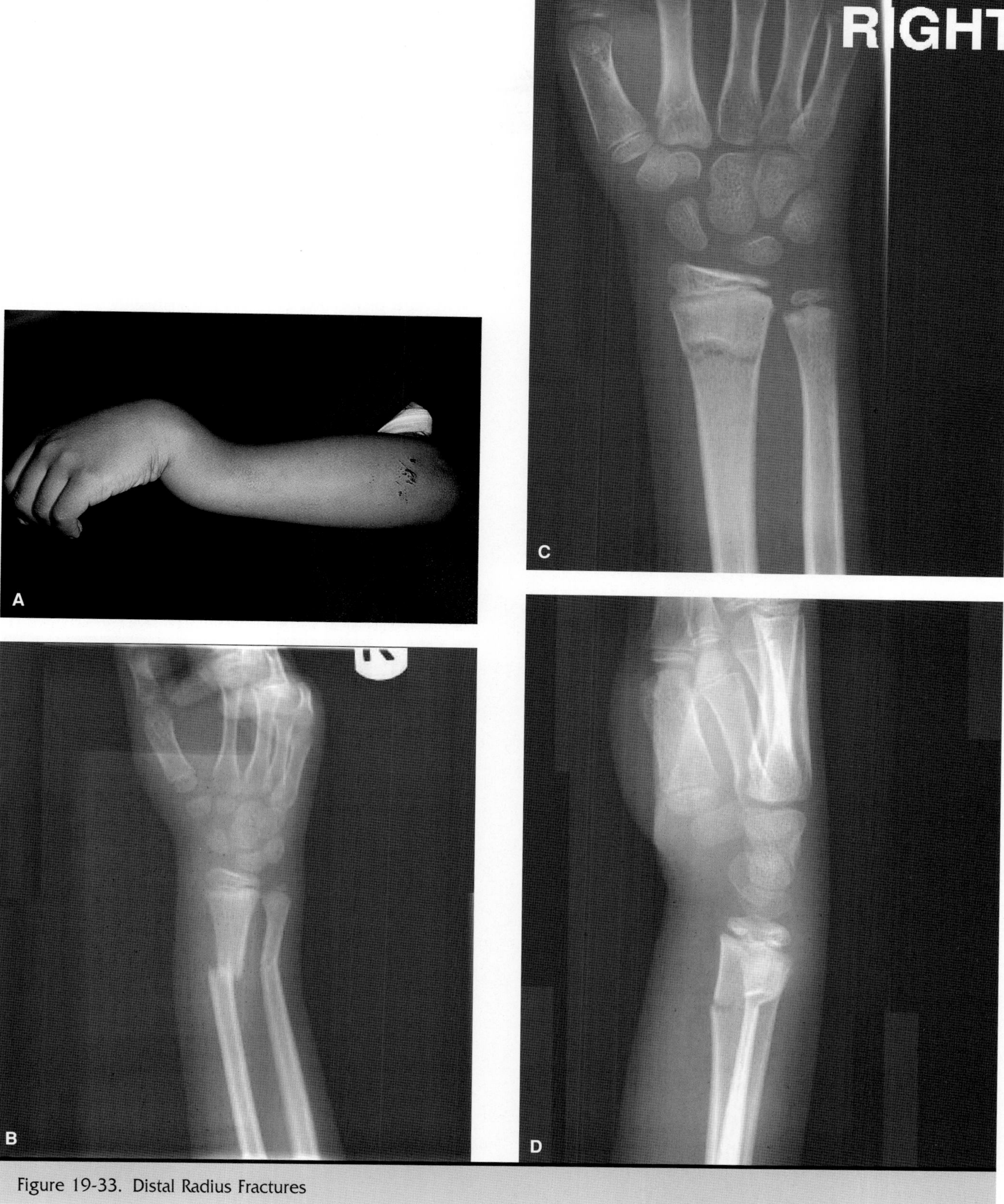

Figure 19-33. Distal Radius Fractures

A. A photograph of the wrist of a child who fell from a fence, showing an obvious "dinner fork" deformity. *B*. X-ray demonstrates a transverse fracture of the distal shaft of the radius and ulna. Dorsal and lateral angulation and distraction are noted, causing the deformity seen clinically. *C* and *D*. AP and lateral views of the wrist with an isolated distal radius (Colles fracture) in a different patient.

Consultation

Orthopedic consultation for displaced or angulated fractures involving the articular surface

Emergency Department Treatment and Disposition

1. Torus fractures and nondisplaced, nonangulated fractures not involving the articular surface can be splinted with expeditious orthopedic referral.
2. All other distal radius fractures should have emergent orthopedic consultation in the ED.
3. Definitively done by closed reduction

> **BOX 19-22. CLINICAL PEARLS: DISTAL RADIUS FRACTURES**
>
> - Often referred to as a "dinner fork" deformity
> - Due to a fall on an outstretched hand
> - Must test for median nerve injury

Galeazzi's Fracture Dislocation and Monteggia's Fracture Dislocation

Definitions

1. Galeazzi's fracture dislocation: fracture of the distal radial shaft associated with a distal radioulnar dislocation (Fig. 19-34)
2. Monteggia's fracture dislocation: fracture of the proximal third of the ulna with a radial head dislocation (Fig. 19-35)

Mechanism of Injury

Fall on the arm

Clinical Features

1. Tenderness on palpation
2. Swelling and deformity may be minimal.

Radiology

Complete x-rays of the radius and ulna as well as the wrist should be obtained.

Complications

1. Neurovascular complications with Galeazzi's fracture dislocations are uncommon.
2. Monteggia's fracture dislocations are associated with radial nerve injury.

Consultation

Orthopedic specialists should be consulted in the ED.

Emergency Department Treatment and Disposition

1. Immobilization, elevation, and ice are indicated in the ED.
2. Both Galeazzi's fracture dislocation and Monteggia's fracture dislocation require open reduction and internal fixation in the operating room.

> **BOX 19-23. CLINICAL PEARL: FOREARM FRACTURES**
>
> - Usually both the radius and ulna are injured.

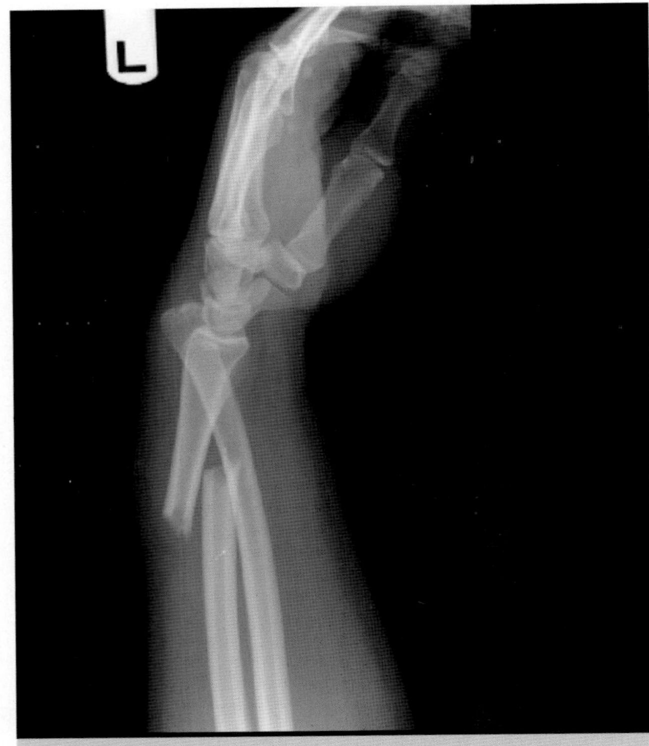

Figure 19-34. Galeazzi's Fracture

A lateral x-ray of the wrist and distal forearm demonstrating a distal radial fracture and radioulnar dislocation.

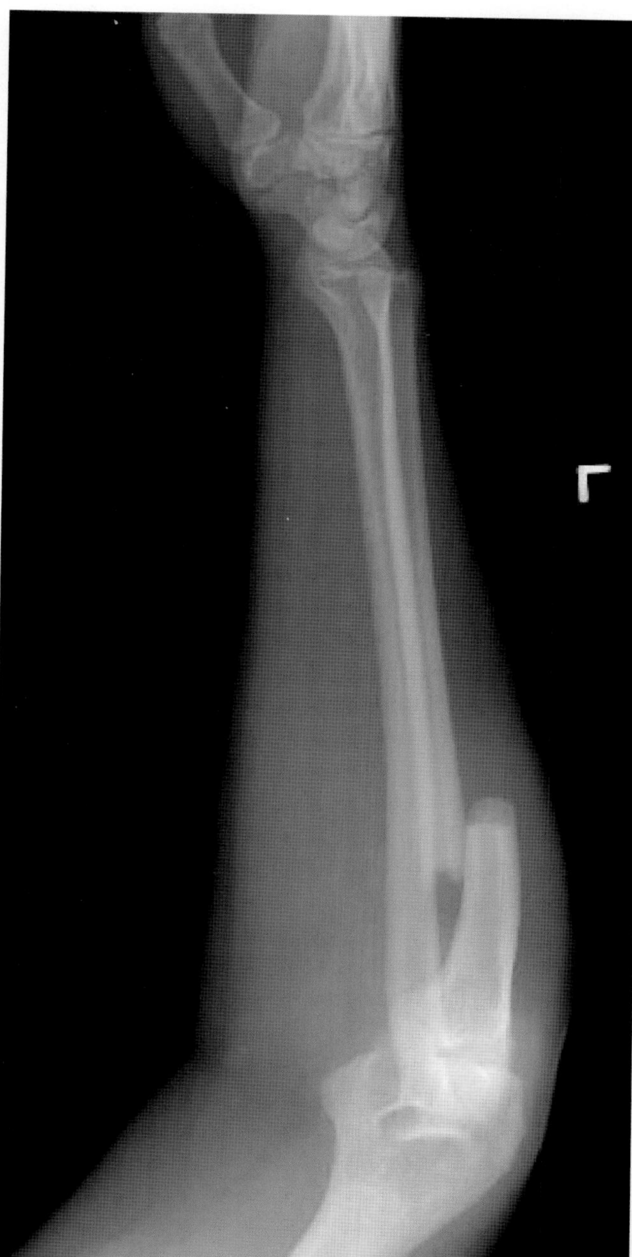

Figure 19-35. Monteggia's Fracture

A lateral x-ray of the forearm demonstrates a fracture of the proximal ulna with a radial head dislocation.

Olecranon Fracture

Mechanism of Injury

Usually due to a direct blow to the elbow

Clinical Features

1. Tenderness and swelling over the posterior elbow
2. Pain on flexion and extension of the elbow

Radiology

X-rays of the elbow including AP and lateral views (Fig. 19-36)

Complications

Associated with ulnar nerve injury

Consultation

Fractures with greater than 2 mm of displacement need orthopedic consultation in the ED and referral for open reduction and internal fixation.

Emergency Department Treatment and Disposition

1. Ice, elevation, and immobilization while waiting for definitive diagnosis
2. Nondisplaced fractures can be splinted with the elbow in 90 degrees of flexion with a referral to orthopedics in the next several days.

BOX 19-24. CLINICAL PEARLS: OLECRANON FRACTURE

- Caused by a direct blow; consider child abuse
- Must test for ulnar nerve injury
- Even minimal displacement requires emergent orthopedic consultation and surgical repair.

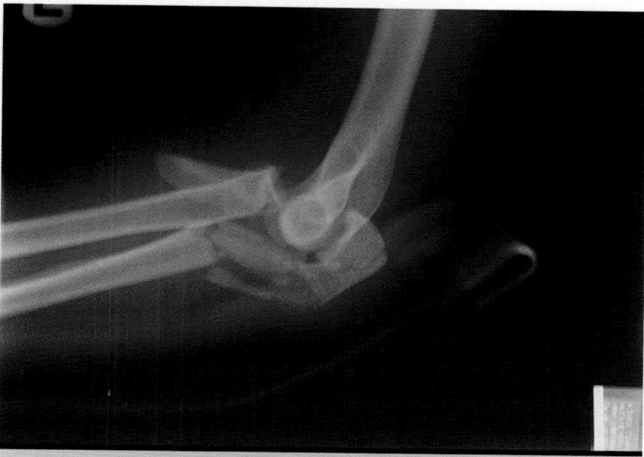

Figure 19-36. Olecranon Fracture

A lateral x-ray of a comminuted fracture of the olecranon process. There is also a radial head dislocation. The radial head itself does not appear to be fractured.

Radial Head Fracture

Mechanism of Injury

Usually due to a fall on an outstretched hand

Definitions of Types of Radial Head Fractures

1. Type I: involves less than one-third of the articular surface with displacement of less than 1 mm (nondisplaced or marginal fractures)
2. Type II: displacement of over 1 mm or depression of over 3 mm with over one-third of the articular surface involved

Clinical Features

1. Tenderness on palpitation of the radial head
2. Pain is worse with supination of the arm.

Radiology

1. Standard x-rays of the elbow should be performed (Fig. 19-37).
2. A fracture may not be apparent.
3. Fat pad signs are often the only evidence of a fracture (Fig. 19-38).
   a. A small anterior fat pad may be normal.
   b. A "sail sign" or a large anterior fat pad is abnormal.
   c. A posterior fat pad suggests a fracture.

Complications

1. Neurovascular complications are rare in minimally displaced radial head fractures.
2. Myositis ossificans in this area can occur when radial head or neck fractures are accompanied by elbow dislocation.

Consultation

Most fractures can be immobilized and referred within several days to orthopedics.

Emergency Department Treatment and Disposition

1. Nondisplaced fractures can be splinted, placed in a sling, and referred to orthopedics within several days.
2. Comminuted or displaced fractures require ice, elevation, and immobilization in the ED with emergent evaluation by orthopedics.

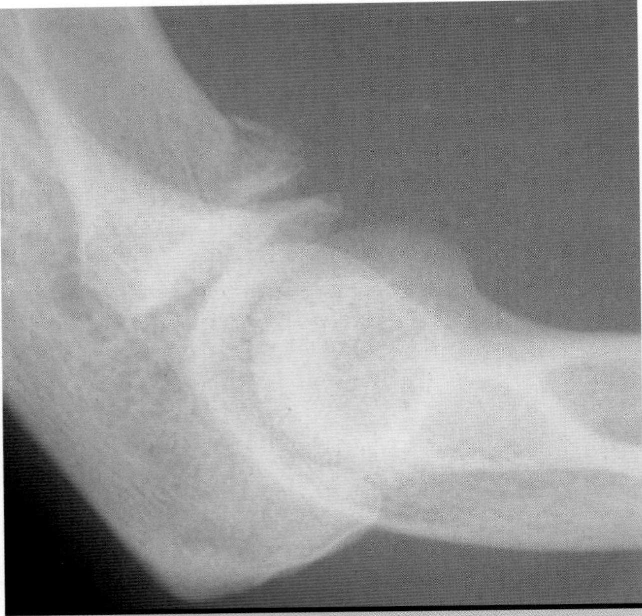

Figure 19-37. Radial Head Fracture

An x-ray of an obvious radial head fracture with mild displacement, (type II). In actuality most radial head fractures are not obvious and are of the type I variety.

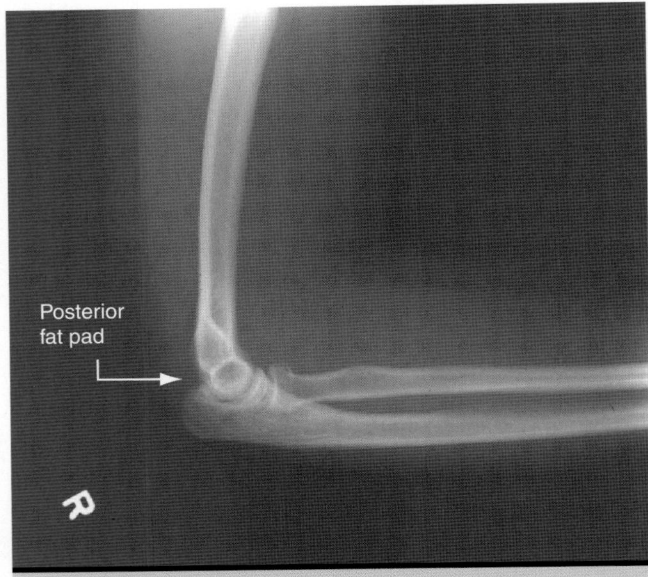

Figure 19-38. Lateral Elbow Sign and Posterior Fat Pad

The lateral x-ray of the elbow shows that the normal flat shape of the anterior fat pad is now flared out. The abnormal posterior fat pad is also present.

BOX 19-25. CLINICAL PEARLS: RADIAL HEAD FRACTURE

- Evaluate for point tenderness of the lateral distal elbow over the radial head.
- On the lateral x-ray of the elbow, small, thin fat pads are normal.
- Wide anterior fat pads suggest a fracture.
- Any posterior fat pad suggests a fracture.
- Radial neck fractures, which are also common in children, are usually buckle fractures that can easily be overlooked on x-rays.

Supracondylar Fracture

Mechanism of Injury

Fall on an outstretched hand, typically in children from 3 to 15 years of age

Clinical Features

The elbow is usually swollen, with tenderness over both the lateral and medial epicondyles.

Radiology

1. With suspicion of a supracondylar fracture, four views of the elbow should be obtained including an AP of the forearm, AP of the humerus, lateral of the forearm, and lateral of the humerus.
2. X-rays may show the fracture line, an anterior fat pad sign (displaced anterior fat pad), a posterior fat pad, or an abnormal anterior humeral line (Figs. 19-39).
3. The anterior humeral line is drawn down the anterior cortex of the humerus on the lateral x-ray of the elbow. The anterior humeral line should pass through the center of the ossification center of the capitellum.

Complications

1. Nerve injury occurs in 7% of supracondylar fractures. The median nerve and the radial nerve are most often injured.
2. The anterior interosseous nerve can also be injured. When this occurs the "OK sign" is positive. There is loss of strength of the thumb interphalangeal joint in flexion as well as the index distal interphalangeal joint in flexion. This injury renders the patient unable to perform the "OK sign," with the thumb and index finger apposed against resistance.
3. Brachial artery compromise can lead to Volkmann's contracture (compartment syndrome of the forearm) which will lead to muscle and nerve fibrosis and drastic loss of function.

Consultation

Orthopedics needs to hear about all of these fractures with the patient in the ED. The urgency of consultation in the ED depends on the degree of displacement, the reliability of outpatient observation, and the availability of urgent follow-up.

Emergency Department Treatment and Disposition

1. Nondisplaced fractures can be securely splinted and discharged from the ED, *if and only if* at-home neurovascular observation *and* early orthopedic referral is possible.
2. Displaced fractures need to be admitted for early reduction.

BOX 19-26. CLINICAL PEARLS: SUPRACONDYLAR FRACTURE

- Most common occult elbow fracture in children
- Ninety-five percent of supracondylar fractures have posterior displacement.
- An anterior fat pad is a normal finding, while the posterior fat pad is seated in the olecranon fossa and normally not visualized in a normal x-ray of the elbow.
- A posterior fat pad on a lateral view suggests a hemarthrosis secondary to intra-articular injury and should be treated like a fracture even in absence of a visible fracture line.
- Need close neurovascular observation at home
- Conservative approach is to admit

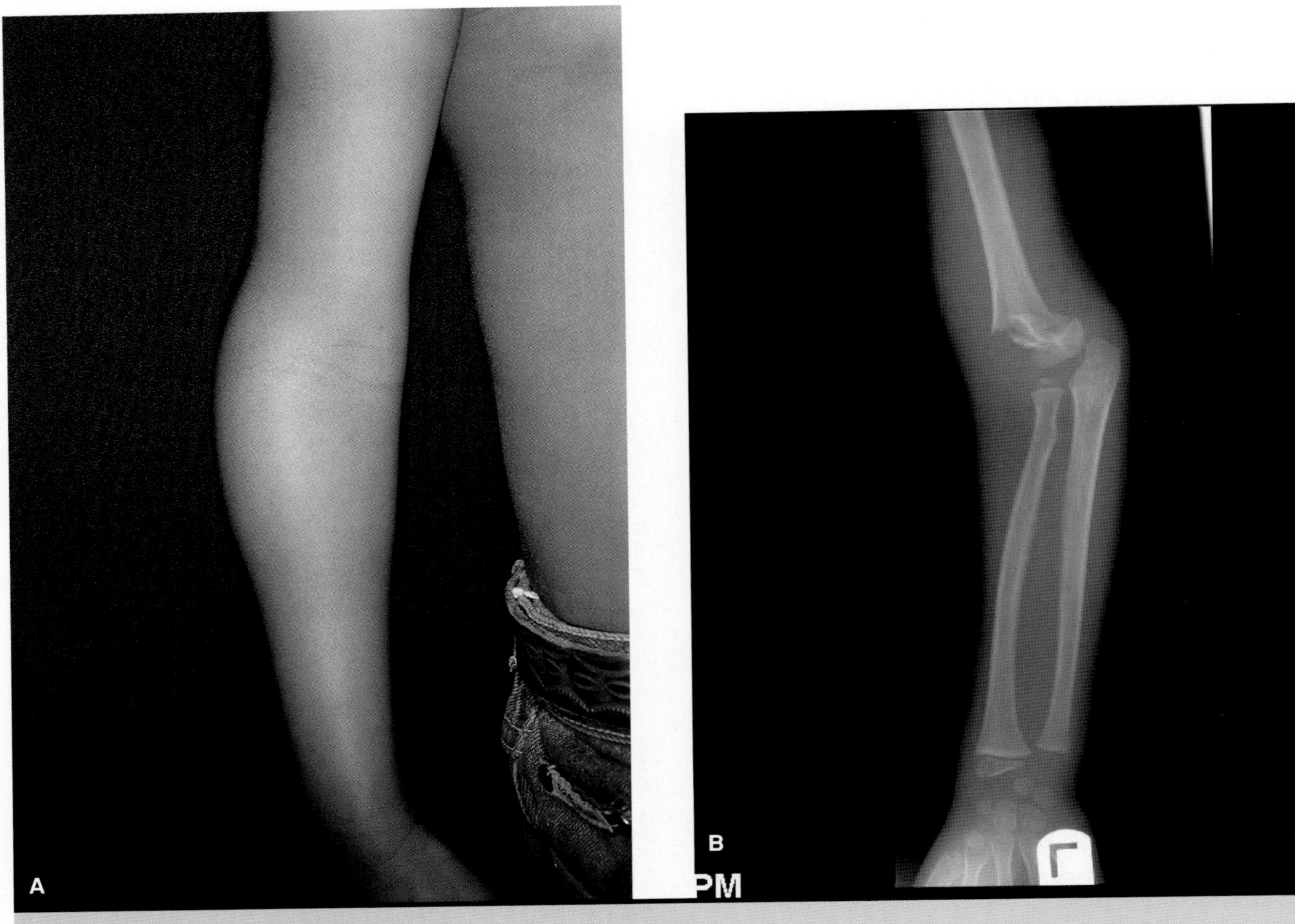

Figure 19-39. Supracondylar Fractures

A. Clinical picture of a supracondylar fracture with marked soft tissue swelling in a child with a history of falling on an outstretched arm. *B*. and *C*. AP and lateral views of the elbow, demonstrating a distal humerus fracture with posterior displacement of the medial and lateral condyles.

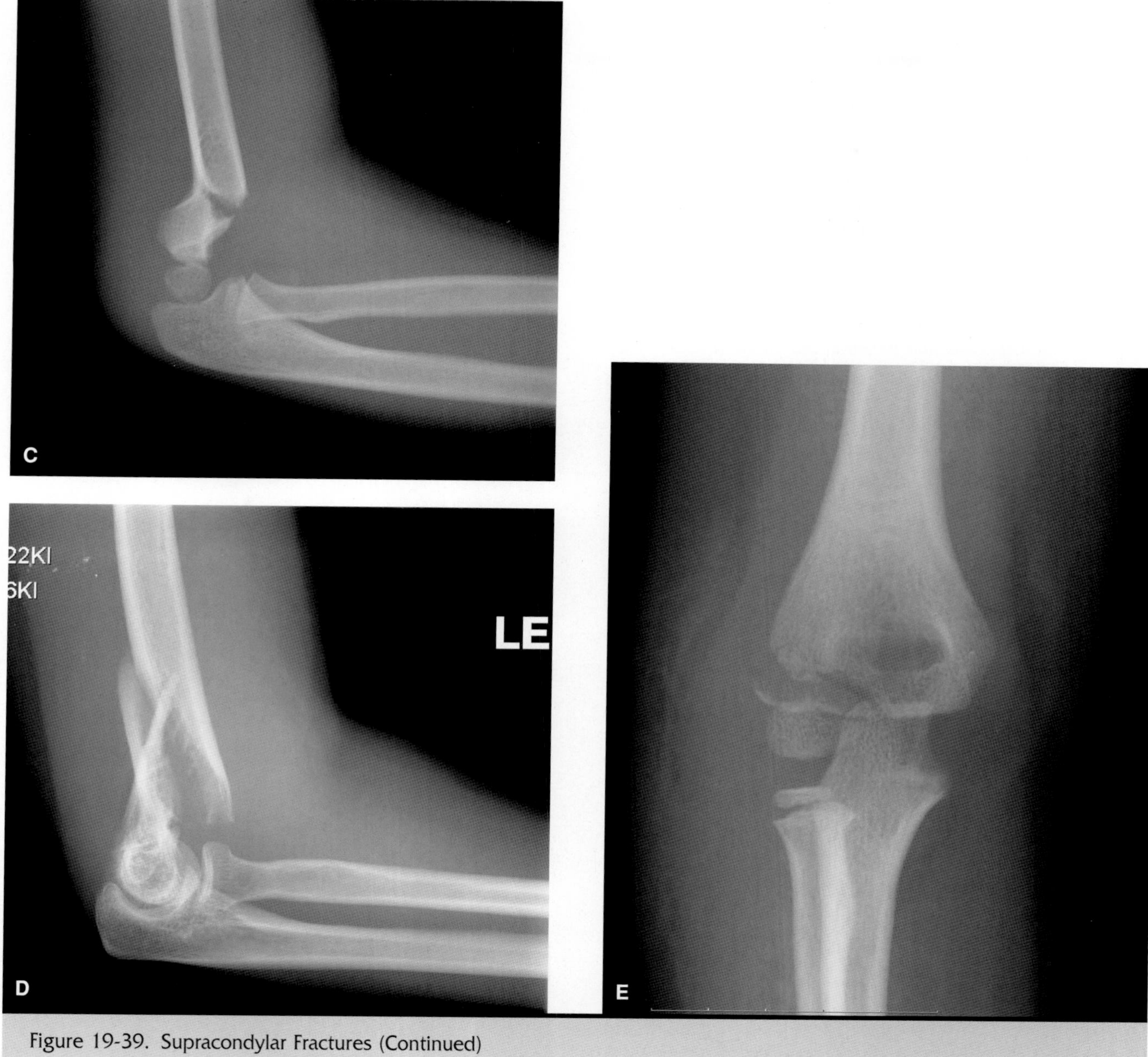

Figure 19-39. Supracondylar Fractures (Continued)

D. In a different patient, this is a lateral view of a comminuted displaced supracondylar fracture. *E*. An AP view of a more subtle, mildly displaced supracondylar fracture in a different patient.

Nursemaid's Elbow

Mechanism of Injury

Sudden traction of the hand or the forearm as occurs in young children when a caretaker pulls a child by the arm to prevent a fall; this results in the annular ligament being pulled over the radial head and becoming displaced between the radial head and the capitellum. Radial head subluxation is also known as "temper-tantrum elbow" or "pulled elbow."

Clinical Features

1. The child usually refuses to move the arm; it is held in pronation at the side and flexed at the elbow (Fig. 19-40).
2. There is pain elicited with supination.
3. Occasionally there is a deformity seen with prominence and displacement of the radial head.

Radiology

1. Radiographs are often unnecessary and may not be helpful, as the radial head and lateral humeral condyle may not be ossified in a young child.
2. When radiographs are obtained, the child often returns with normal arm movement, as these injuries will be often reduced by the radiology technician who will supinate and flex the elbow to 90 degrees (the procedure used for reduction of the subluxation) to obtain a proper lateral x-ray of the elbow.
3. Indications for radiography include either:
   a. Unsuccessful attempts at reduction
   b. The presence of swelling or significant tenderness, suggesting another diagnosis (e.g., fracture or bone infections such as septic arthritis or osteomyelitis)
   c. When there is question or doubt about the mechanism of injury

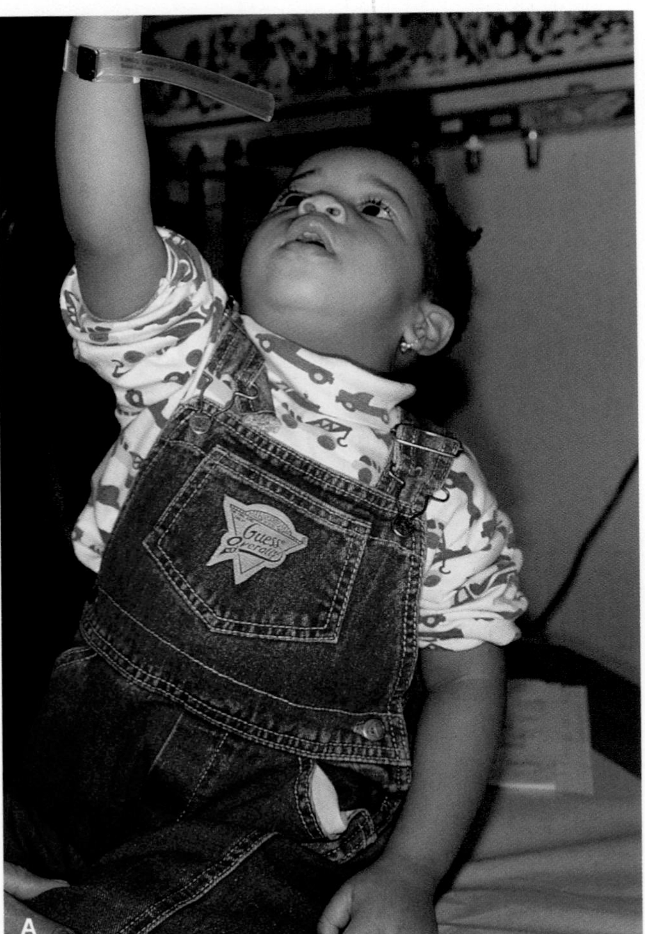

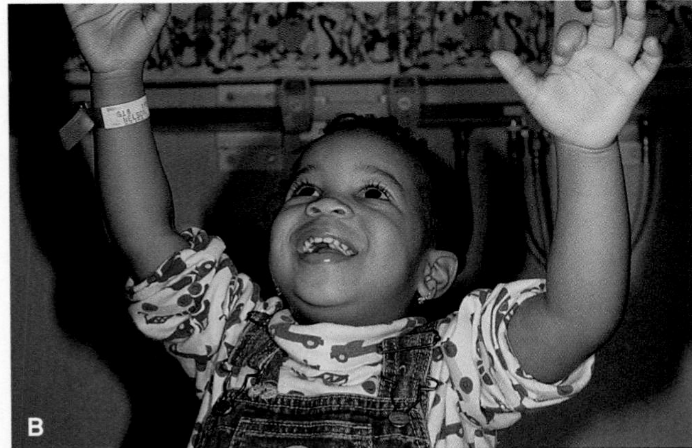

Figure 19-40. Nursemaid's Elbow (Radial Head Subluxation)

A. Image of a child with nursemaid's elbow on the left side, which is the more common side because the adult who pulled on the arm is more likely to be right handed. The child refuses to use the left arm. *B*. Within 15 minutes after reduction the child freely uses the arm.

Complications

Complications are extremely rare with simple subluxation of the radial head or its reduction procedure.

Consultation

Orthopedic consultation is not necessary with simple subluxation of the radial head and successful reduction in the ED.

Emergency Department Treatment and Disposition

1. Reduction in the ED is the definitive treatment.
2. Contraindications for reduction include:
   a. External signs of trauma (e.g., swelling, extreme tenderness, ecchymosis)
   b. Suspicion of elbow or forearm fracture or dislocation
   c. Known mechanism of injury unlikely to result in radial head subluxation
3. Two techniques are used with success for close reduction:
   a. Supination and flexion (traditional reduction technique) *or*
   b. Hyperpronation technique (pronation and flexion); in comparative studies, hyperpronation technique required fewer attempts at reduction compared with supination, was successful more often than supination, and was often successful when supination failed
4. For either of the above mentioned techniques:
   a. Let the child sit comfortably in the caregiver's lap.
   b. Gentle examination of the uninvolved arm first may make the examination of the injured arm easier.
   c. Exclude any point tenderness by palpating the involved arm along the entire length from shoulder to wrist. In the absence of any tenderness, proceed with the reduction.
   d. *Supination and flexion technique:*
      1) The palm of the involved hand is grasped as if to shake it, and the elbow is encircled with the other hand with the thumb placed over the radial head.
      2) In one quick deliberate motion while applying gentle longitudinal traction, the forearm is fully supinated, and in a continuous motion the elbow is flexed to the shoulder.
      3) Successful reduction with the first attempt is seen in 69 to 77% of cases.
   e. *Hyperpronation technique:*
      1) While applying gentle longitudinal traction, the forearm is placed in hyperpronation by a slight counterclockwise motion, then the elbow is flexed.
      2) Successful reduction with the first attempt is seen in 80 to 95% of cases.
5. In 80 to 90% of maneuvers (with either of the above-mentioned techniques), an audible or palpable pop or click is usually felt by the thumb that lies over the radial head as the annular ligament is freed from the joint. This signals successful reduction.
6. Crying and pain are usually seen during the maneuver, but they subside quickly after the reduction and with consolation.
7. With successful reduction, the child usually starts using the arm within 5 to 15 minutes. If the subluxation has been present for several hours it may take longer for normal arm movements to return.
8. A fearful child may not use the arm, even after successful reduction. Removing the child from the examination room and asking the caregiver to distract the child (e.g., with a toy) will help demonstrate the return of normal function to the child.
9. In the absence of a pop or click (with an unsuccessful reduction):
   a. Another attempt is made after 15 minutes.
   b. Some physicians try an alternate maneuver.
10. After a successful reduction, no treatment, radiographs, or immobilization is required.
11. The caretaker should be educated to lift the child using the axilla or upper arm and not the hand or wrist, to prevent recurrences.
12. With recurrent subluxations, immobilization for a few weeks in a posterior splint with the elbow flexed to 90 degrees and the forearm in supination should be done.

BOX 19-27. CLINICAL PEARLS: NURSEMAID'S ELBOW

- Most common injury occurring in children between 2 and 5 years old
- It represents almost 30% of all elbow injuries in young children.
- In actuality, it is a subluxation of the radial head.
- Normal function (i.e., grasping for desirable objects) should take place within 20 to 30 minutes after reduction of nursemaid's elbow.
- Consider an alternative diagnosis with unsuccessful reduction after two to three attempts.
- Recurrence rate for subsequent subluxation is between 24 and 39%. Children 24 months old or younger are at greatest risk. If the child is young (<2 years of age), he or she should be allowed to rest the arm.
- The strength of the annular ligament and the size of the radial head increase with age, making this subluxation uncommon after the age of 5 years.

Elbow Dislocation

Mechanism of Injury

Most commonly associated with a fall on an extended, abducted arm

Clinical Features

The elbow is usually held in flexion and the olecranon process may be palpated posteriorly.

Radiology

Lateral x-ray of the elbow is essential and usually diagnostic (Fig. 19-41).

Complications

1. Medial epicondyle fractures are often associated with elbow dislocations, at a rate that may be as high as 30 to 40%.
2. Ulnar nerve injuries have an association with elbow dislocation.
3. Brachial artery injuries have an association with elbow dislocation.

Consultation

1. All elbow dislocations need to be referred to orthopedics.
2. If the dislocation is associated with a fracture or the reduction is not successful as demonstrated on the lateral elbow x-ray, orthopedics should see the patient in the ED.

Emergency Department Treatment and Disposition

Immediate reduction in the ED is essential.

BOX 19-28. CLINICAL PEARLS: ELBOW DISLOCATION

- Ninety percent of dislocations are posterior.
- Immediate reduction has been associated with a reduction in the complication rate.

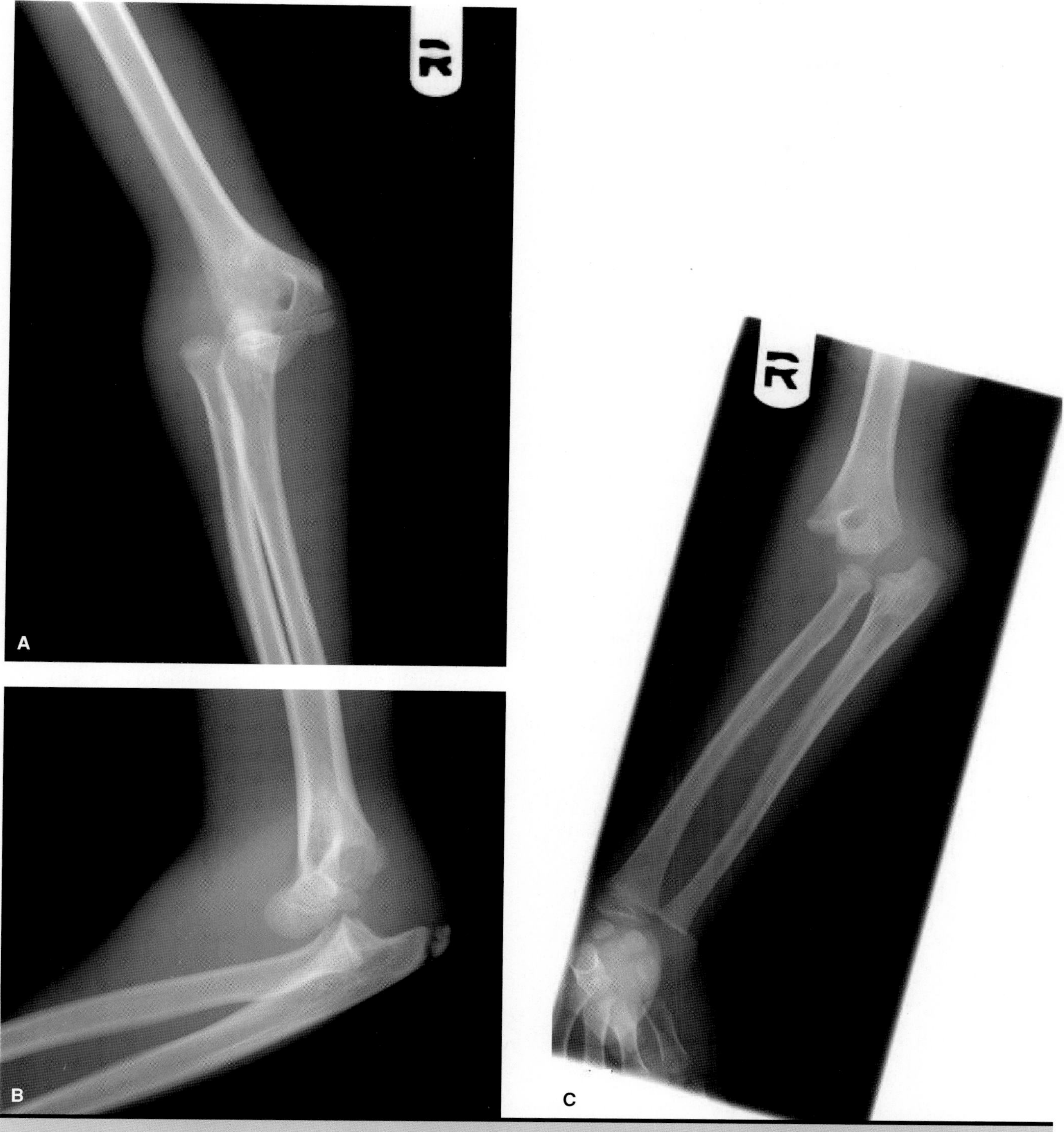

Figure 19-41. Elbow Dislocation and Dislocation of Olecranon and Radial Head

A. AP view of elbow with a posterolateral dislocation of the ulna/radius relative to the distal humerus. *B*. Lateral view of a posterior dislocation of the ulna/radius relative to the distal humerus. *C*. X-ray demonstrating a fracture of the lateral epicondyle of the humerus and a dislocation of the olecranon and radius.

Humerus Fracture

Mechanism of Injury

Humerus fracture can be due to a fall, although a direct blow is also very possible, which should alert the clinician to the possibility of abuse.

Clinical Features

1. Decreased movement of the extremity
2. Localized swelling

Radiology

Perpendicular AP and lateral views of the entire humerus are essential (Fig. 19-42).

Complications

1. *Proximal humerus fractures*
   a. Adhesive capsulitis (frozen shoulder) can occur in children, although it is much more common in adults. When it occurs in children, the possibility of neglect should be investigated.
   b. Brachial plexus injuries and axillary nerve and axillary artery injuries are also associated.
   c. Avascular necrosis is more common in adults, but can occur in children with medical conditions that cause decreased perfusion, such as sickle cell anemia, or circulatory compromise.
2. *Humeral shaft fractures*
   a. Typically involve the middle third
   b. Radial nerve injury is present in 10 to 20%.
   c. The brachial artery can also be injured.
   d. Myositis ossificans of the elbow, which can be avoided by using active routine exercise and not simple passive stretching in the recuperatory phase, sometimes develops (Fig. 19-43).

Consultation

Orthopedic consultation should be obtained for anything greater than one-part fractures or fractures with significant displacement.

Emergency Department Treatment and Disposition

For the majority of fractures, shoulder immobilization and urgent orthopedic referral is adequate. This is particularly true for one-part fractures without significant displacement.

BOX 19-29. CLINICAL PEARLS: HUMERUS FRACTURES

- Young children with open epiphyses usually suffer epiphyseal separation rather than fractures.
- Adolescents with ossified epiphyses have very strong bones and thus have a tendency to develop dislocations sometimes accompanied by fractures.
- More commonly seen in the elderly than in children
- Significant displacement is considered to be separation of >1 cm or angulation of >45 degrees.
- There is extensive muscular attachment to the humeral shaft and may result in distraction of the fragments after the fracture has occurred.

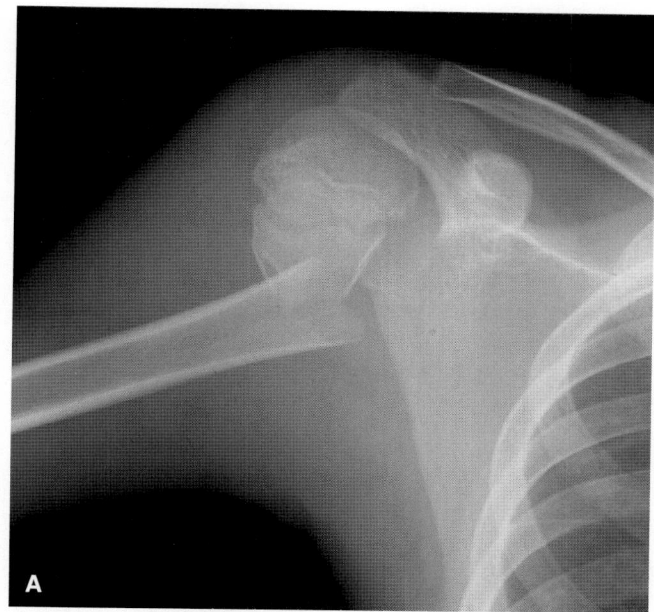

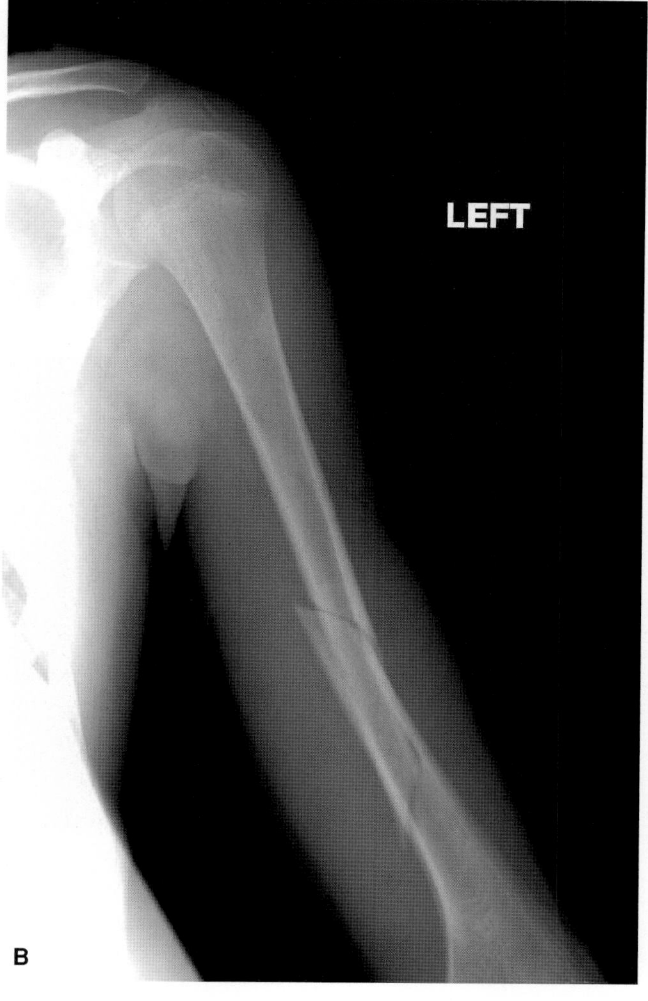

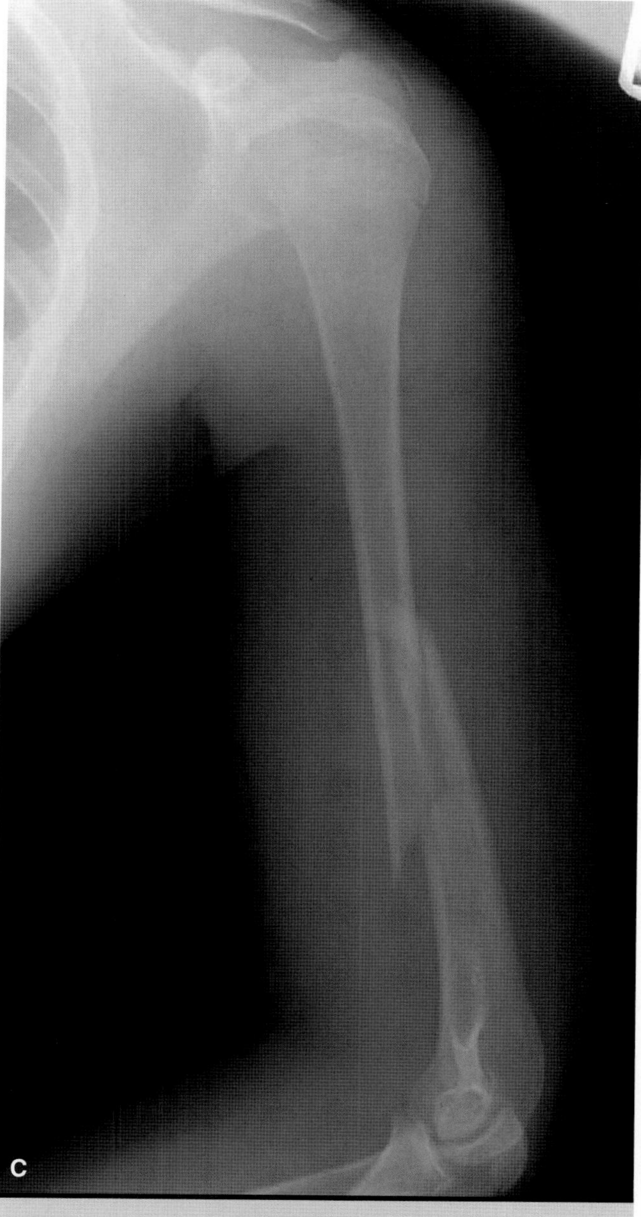

Figure 19-42. Humeral Shaft Fractures

A. Displaced transverse fracture of the proximal humerus. *B* and *C*. AP and lateral views of comminuted midshaft humeral fracture.

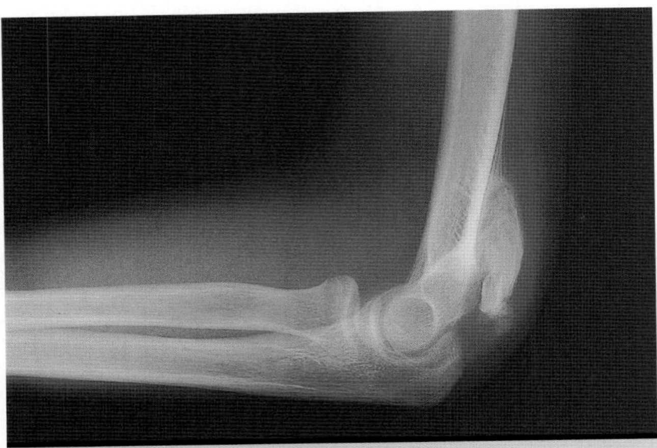

Figure 19-43. Myositis Ossificans

Lateral view of the elbow demonstrates a dense calcification/ossification of the posterior aspect of the elbow joint extending from the distal humeral shaft to the olecranon process. The post-traumatic myositis ossificans was related to a subperiosteal hematoma sustained from a stab wound, which occurred 3 months previously. This 16-year-old presented with a frozen elbow after months of immobilization.

Anterior and Posterior Glenohumeral Joint Dislocations

Mechanism of Injury

Abduction with external rotation of the arm

Clinical Features

1. The arm is held in abduction (Fig. 19-44).
2. Loss of normal contour of the shoulder

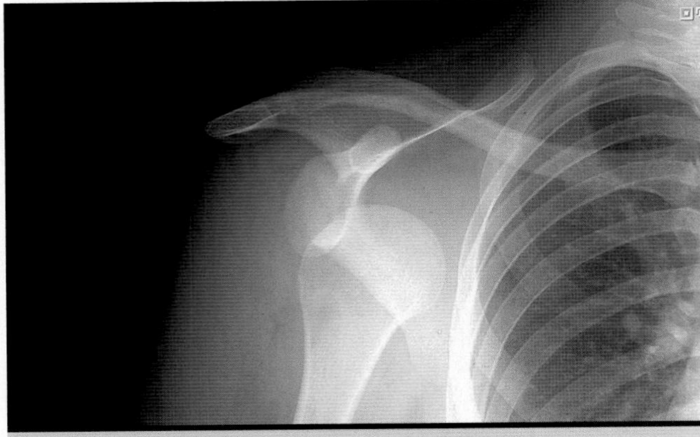

Figure 19-44. Anterior Glenohumeral Joint Dislocation

Anterior dislocation of the right shoulder is seen. The humeral head is displaced anteriorly and inferiorly in relation to the glenoid fossa. There is no evidence of fracture.

3. Pain on any type of movement of the shoulder

Mechanism of Injury

A fall, a seizure, or an electric shock

Clinical Features

1. The arm is held in adduction with internal rotation (Fig. 19-45).
2. Patient cannot abduct or externally rotate to even a minimal extent

Radiology

Standard "trauma series" x-rays should be obtained. These include AP, lateral, and axillary views (Fig. 19-46).

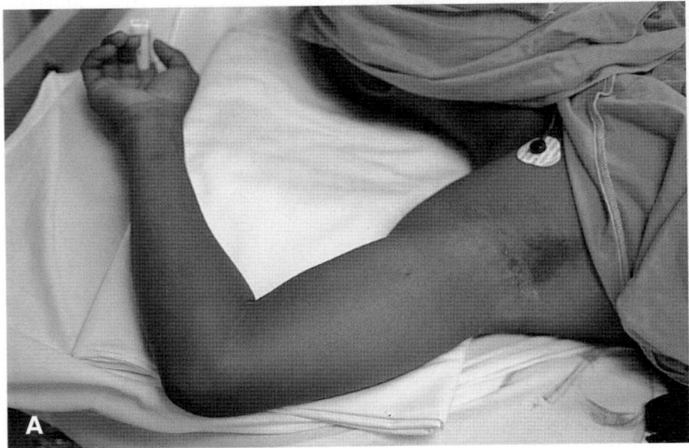

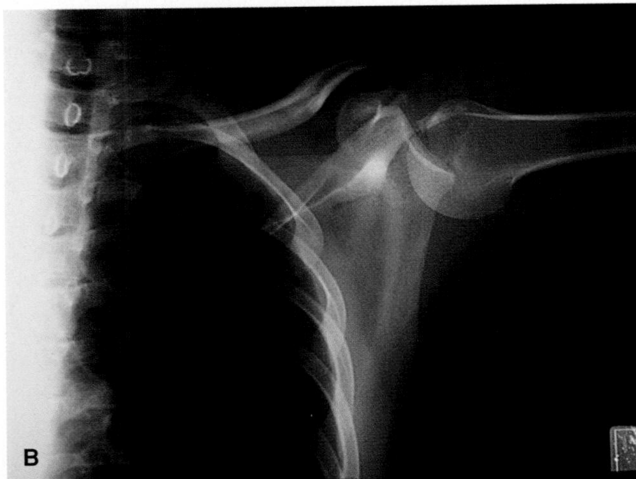

Figure 19-45. Posterior Glenohumeral Joint Dislocation

A. Image of a young boy with a posterior shoulder dislocation postseizure, lying on the stretcher in the position of maximum comfort, as he was unable to adduct the arm. *B*. This AP x-ray of the shoulder, which alone is not diagnostic, suggests dislocation. Note that the humeral head is not inferior to the glenoid fossa, as is usually the case in an anterior dislocation.

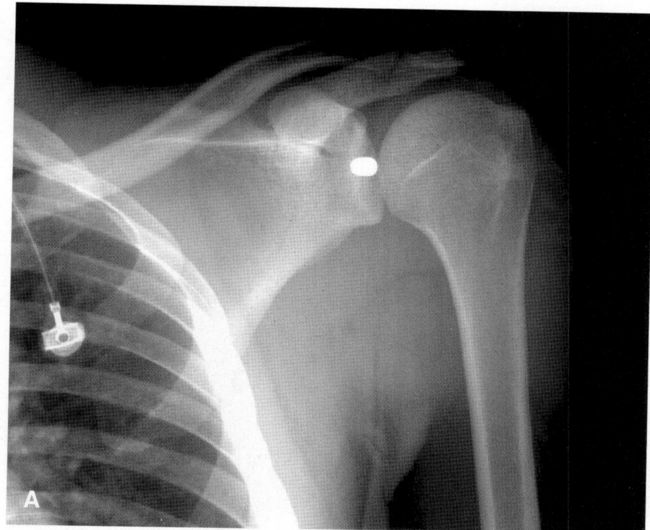

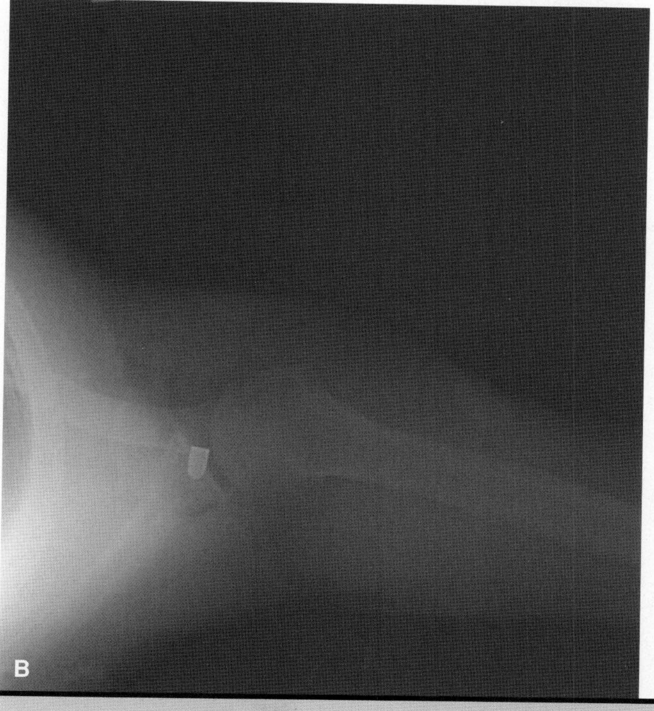

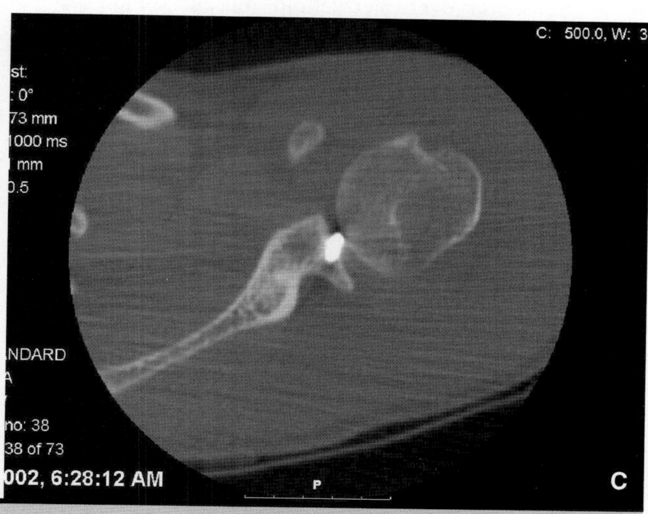

Figure 19-46. Intra-Articular Foreign Body (Bullet)

AP (*A*) and lateral (*B*) views of the glenohumeral joint with an intra-articular bullet lodged within the glenoid fossa, as seen on CT scan (*C*). There is no fracture or dislocation. The bullet required urgent removal in the operating room.

Complications

1. Axillary nerve injury approximately 12% of the time
2. Hill-Sachs lesion (compression fracture of the posterolateral humeral head)
3. Bankart lesion (fracture of the glenoid rim)
4. Detachment or tear of the rotator cuff

Consultation

1. Dislocations that are successfully reduced by the emergency medicine physician should be referred to orthopedics sometime in the next few days.

2. Dislocations that cannot be reduced in the ED need to be evaluated emergently by orthopedics.

Emergency Department Treatment and Disposition

1. Various reduction techniques:
   a. External rotation technique
   b. Scapular manipulation technique
   c. Stimson technique
   d. The traction-countertraction method, in particular axial traction, is best for posterior dislocation. This technique is the most frequently used.
2. After reduction the shoulder should be immobilized with a sling and swathe.

BOX 19-30. CLINICAL PEARLS: SHOULDER DISLOCATIONS

- Anterior shoulder dislocations account for over 95% of the total. Most commonly the humeral head is in the subcoracoid position.
- Sensation over the deltoid muscle should be checked to test the function of the axillary nerve.
- Hill-Sachs lesion occurs when the humeral head impacts on the inferior glenoid rim, and occurs most commonly with inferior dislocations.
- The axillary view, which is difficult to obtain in a patient with a posterior dislocation, is diagnostic for dislocation, in particular for differentiating between anterior and posterior dislocations.
- Posterior dislocations are rare (<5%), and are commonly missed.
- An isolated fracture of the lesser tuberosity of the humerus should lead the physician to investigate for a posterior dislocation that may not be immediately radiologically apparent.

Clavicular Fractures

Mechanism of Injury

A direct blow or fall on the shoulder

Clinical Features

1. Pain on palpation of the clavicle
2. Swelling is usually minor and usually occurs directly over the fracture.

Radiology

Standard x-rays of the clavicle including AP and oblique (Fig. 19-47)

Complications

Injury to the subclavicular artery or vein does occur, but not without significant distraction of the clavicle.

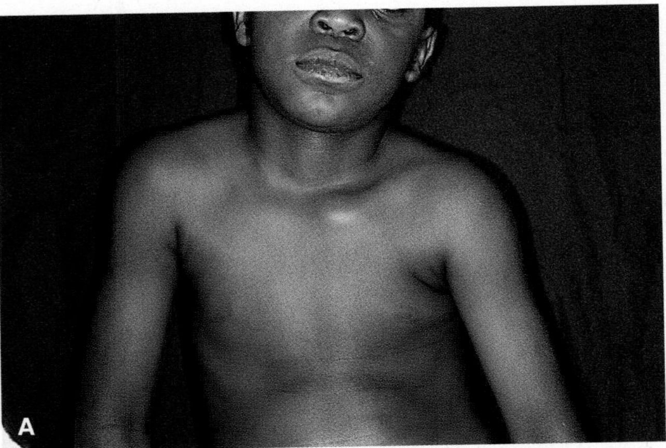

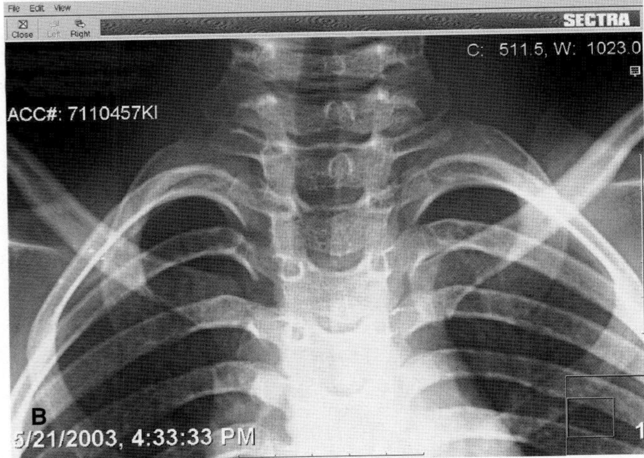

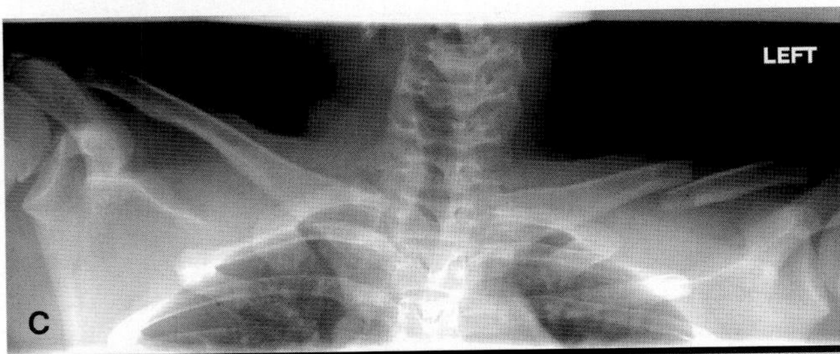

Figure 19-47. Clavicular Fracture/Dislocation

A. A picture of a 9-year-old male who suffered a fall, sustaining a clavicular dislocation. *B*. The x-ray demonstrates that the left clavicle is superiorly displaced at the manubrium, but not fractured. *C*. X-ray of a transverse fracture of the mid–left clavicle with bone overriding by 1.5 cm. The distal fragment is under the proximal fragment. This injury occurred in a 15-year-old who was playing football and fell on his shoulder.

Consultation

Orthopedic consultation is rarely necessary unless there is suspicion of vascular injury.

Emergency Department Treatment and Disposition

A sling has been shown to be as effective as the traditional sling and swathe.

BOX 19-31. CLINICAL PEARLS: CLAVICULAR FRACTURES

- Clavicular fractures are the most common fractures in children.
- Eighty percent involve the middle third of the clavicle.
- Educate parents that fractures heal with the formation of a lump that may take several months to resolve.

Acromioclavicular Injuries

Mechanism of Injury

1. A direct blow to the lateral arm or a blow to the acromion itself
2. These injuries are common in hockey players, who often hit the boards with their shoulders.

Definitions of Acromioclavicular (AC) Injuries

1. First-degree injury
   a. There is an incomplete tear of the AC ligament.
   b. There is no subluxation.
   c. X-rays including stress views are negative.
2. Second-degree injury
   a. There is subluxation of the AC joint.
   b. Routine x-rays are usually normal, although subluxation with stress views is often present.
   c. By definition, the separation of the distal clavicle is less than one-half its diameter in relation to the acromion.
3. Third-degree injury: separation of the distal clavicle by more than one-half its diameter in relation to the acromion

Clinical Features

1. The appearance is usually normal.
2. Pain with gravity traction of the arm

Radiology

Acromioclavicular x-rays including weight-bearing views

Complications

1. Future contact sport activity is limited.
2. Neurovascular complications are extremely rare.

Consultation

1. First- and second-degree injuries need referral to orthopedics after sling and swathe immobilization in the ED.
2. Third-degree separations (obvious dislocation of the AC joint with separation of the distal clavicle by more than one-half its diameter) need to be evaluated by orthopedics in the ED.

Emergency Department Treatment and Disposition

1. First-degree and second-degree injuries are treated with a sling and swathe for 4 to 6 weeks.
2. It remains controversial whether third-degree injuries necessitate operative repair. What is certain is that all third-degree injuries should have verbal orthopedic evaluation with the patient in the ED and definitive follow-up in the next several days (Fig. 19-48).

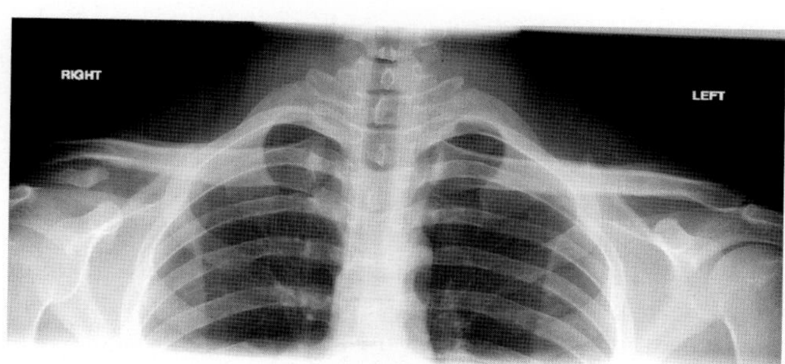

Figure 19-48. Acromioclavicular Separation

Third-degree AC separation of the right shoulder. Note the complete overlap of the acromion process with the clavicle.

BOX 19-32. CLINICAL PEARLS: ACROMIOCLAVICULAR INJURIES

- Fairly common injury among athletes in contact sports
- Acromioclavicular joint pain can occur after an old injury.
- The acromioclavicular stress test is performed by bringing the arm across the body, approximating the elbow with the contralateral shoulder. A positive test produces pain in the area.

Scapular Fractures

Mechanism of Injury

Usually due to a direct blow to the scapular area

Clinical Features

1. Local pain and swelling
2. A decrease in abduction due to pain

Radiology

Scapular x-rays (Fig. 19-49)

Complications

Due to the great force necessary to produce a scapular fracture, complications are always related to associated injuries.

Consultation

Isolated scapular fractures without associated injuries are rare. If the mechanism of injury is localized and other injuries have been ruled out, consultation in the ED is not necessary.

Emergency Department Treatment and Disposition

If no other injuries are identified, a sling with shoulder immobilization can be applied in the ED and limited exercise begun after 2 weeks.

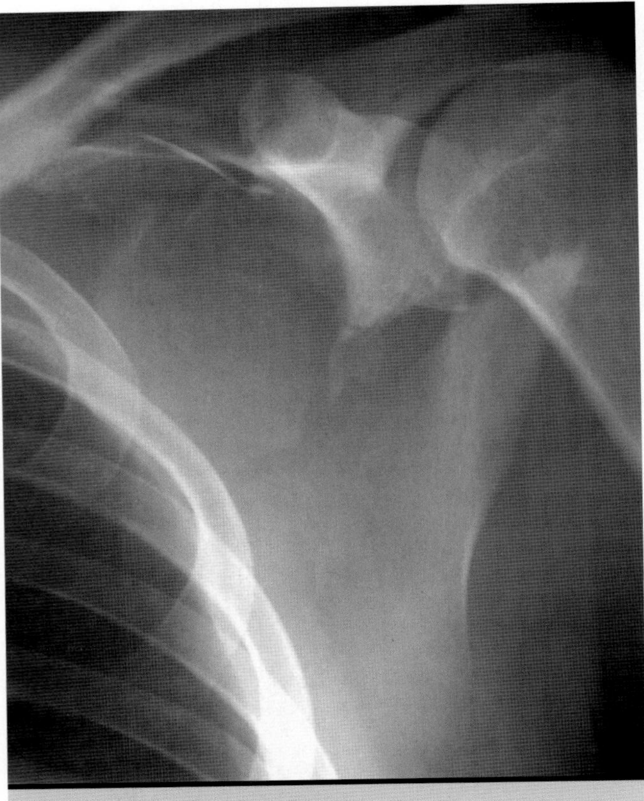

Figure 19-49. Scapular Fracture

This is a scapular x-ray of a youth who was beaten with a golf club. The x-ray demonstrates a variety of scapular fractures. Note the fracture through the glenoid fossa, which will be the most problematic for the orthopedic surgeon.

BOX 19-33. CLINICAL PEARLS: SCAPULAR FRACTURES

- Scapular fractures are rare in childhood.
- Scapular fractures necessitate investigation for other injuries (rib fractures, pneumothoraces, and vertebral fractures).

DIAGNOSIS LOWER EXTREMITY INJURIES

Hip Dislocation

Mechanism of Injury

1. Posterior dislocations result from a direct blow along the axis of the femur. It often occurs with a front end motor vehicle accident in which the patient is thrown forward and the knee strikes the dashboard.
2. Anterior dislocations result from forced abduction, as is the case with external blunt trauma as occurs when a pedestrian is struck by an automobile.

Clinical Features

1. Posterior dislocations: the leg is adducted, flexed, and internally rotated
2. Anterior dislocations: the leg is abducted, flexed, and externally rotated at the hip

Radiology

Routine hip and pelvic x-rays are required.

Complications

1. Frequently associated with acetabular fractures
2. Twenty-five percent are associated with knee injuries and almost 5% are associated with ipsilateral femur fractures.
3. Avascular necrosis of the femoral head
4. Sciatic nerve injury may occur with posterior dislocations.

Consultation

All hip dislocations should have emergent orthopedic consultation in the ED.

Emergency Department Treatment and Disposition

1. Closed reduction in the ED should take place as soon as possible and only after adequate sedation and analgesia.
2. Posterior dislocations
    a. With the patient supine, one caretaker applies steady pressure on both superior iliac crests to stabilize the pelvis.
    b. The person performing the reduction straddles the patient and with the knee flexed to 90 degrees pulls the leg toward the ceiling (Fig. 19-50).
3. Anterior dislocations
    a. Best managed with early closed reduction under spinal or general anesthesia
    b. With the patient supine, the hip is flexed, which converts the anterior dislocation to a posterior dislocation. The posterior dislocation is then reduced as described above.
4. Even with successful reduction in the ED, admission to orthopedics is required.

BOX 19-34. CLINICAL PEARLS: HIP DISLOCATION

- Posterior dislocations account for 90% of hip dislocations.
- All hip dislocations need emergent consultation by orthopedics.
- The neurovascular status of the involved extremity must be evaluated and documented upon arrival, prior to and after any reduction attempts.

Slipped Capital Femoral Epiphysis

Definition

Loss of alignment of the femoral epiphysis

Clinical Features

1. Symptoms are often reported as fatigue when doing strenuous activities, increasing to pain in the hip or the knee with even mild exertion.
2. If undiagnosed, the classic limp becomes apparent.

Etiology

Due to the rapid bone growth and activity level in prepubescent children, there is displacement of the femoral epiphysis.

Radiology

1. Anteroposterior views of both hips as well as a lateral view in the frog-leg position with the hip flexed 90 degrees and abducted 45 degrees
2. There is widening and displacement of the capital epiphysis, which is also displaced posteriorly and inferiorly (Fig. 19-51).

Complications

1. Avascular necrosis

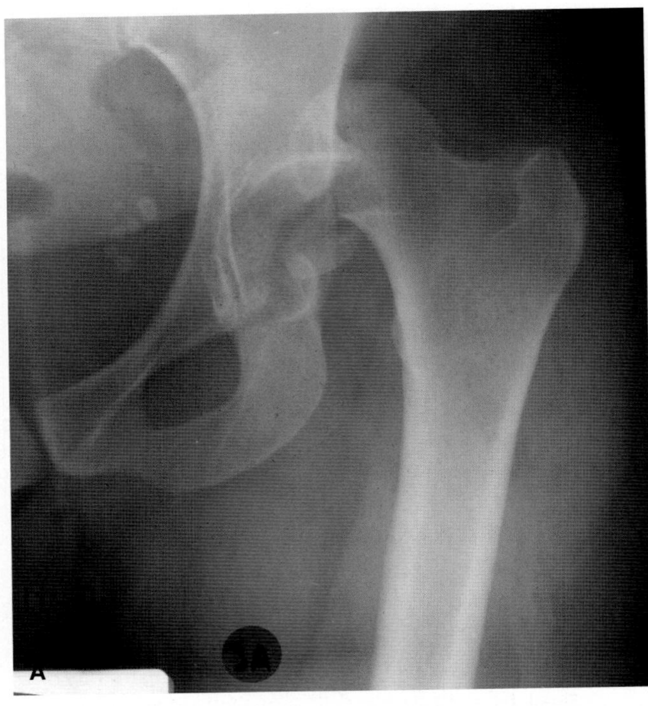

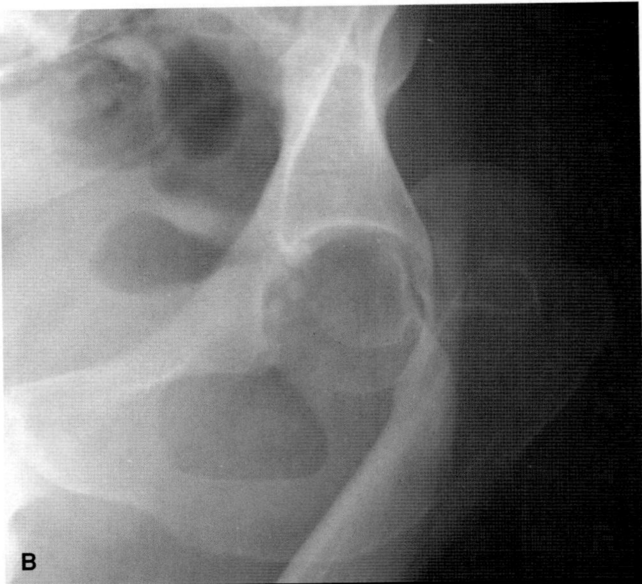

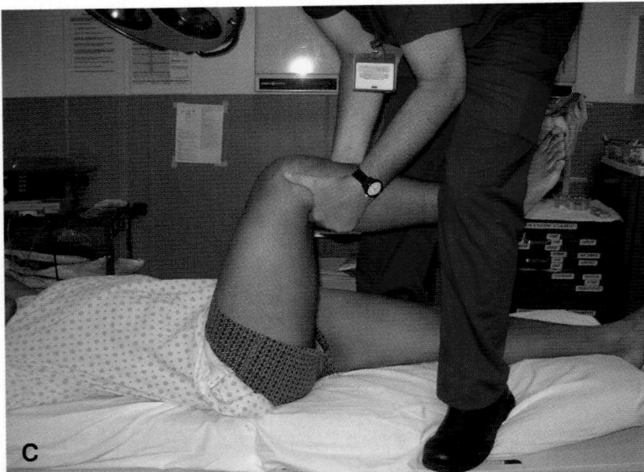

Figure 19-50. Hip Dislocation

A. An AP radiograph of the hip, demonstrating a hip dislocation. The x-ray is suggestive of, but not pathognomonic for, a posterior dislocation. *B*. An anterior oblique x-ray of the same hip confirms the diagnosis of a posterior dislocation. *C*. Image of the proper technique for reduction of a posterior hip dislocation. With the patient lying on the back and the hip and knee flexed to 90 degrees, reduction is performed by applying traction perpendicular to the bed, towards the ceiling.

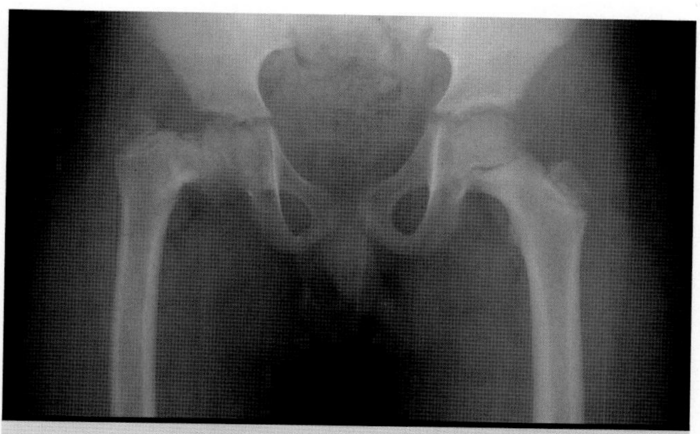

Figure 19-51. Slipped Capital Femoral Epiphysis

This x-ray shows an AP view of the pelvis with a slipped capital femoral epiphysis on the right. Note the obliteration of the epiphyseal plate and the more superior position of the femoral neck and greater trochanter (there is nearly a 90-degree angle formed by the femoral neck and the femoral shaft) in relationship to the left.

BOX 19-36. CLINICAL PEARLS: SLIPPED CAPITAL FEMORAL EPIPHYSIS

- It occurs in children from ages 10 to 16 years, the years of rapid bone growth.
- There is a higher association with children who are overweight.
- Boys predominate over girls.
- In 25% of cases both hips are involved.
- There is a peak incidence in the summer months, when there is increased outdoor physical activity.
- The history may include minor trauma, but it usually has an insidious onset of symptoms.

2. Chondrolysis
3. Further slippage
4. Degenerative arthritis of the hip

Consultation

All patients with slipped capital femoral epiphysis should have emergent orthopedic consultation in the ED.

Emergency Department Treatment and Disposition

Depending upon the degree of slippage, treatment may be conservative or may require internal fixation with application of screws.

BOX 19-35. DIFFERENTIAL DIAGNOSIS OF SLIPPED CAPITAL FEMORAL EPIPHYSIS

- Transient synovitis of the hip
- Septic arthritis
- Degenerative arthritis
- Bursitis

Femur Fracture

Mechanism of Injury

Most commonly associated with motor vehicle accidents and falls from significant heights. In toddlers, child abuse should always be suspected.

Clinical Features

1. Swelling and tenderness on palpitation
2. Deformity may or may not be present.

Radiology

1. X-rays include AP and internal and external rotation views (Fig. 19-52).
2. Hip and knee views may be desired due to the high incidence of associated injuries.

Complications

1. Hemorrhage is the most serious complication. Large adolescents can extravasate 1.5 liters of blood into the thigh after a femur fracture.
2. Neurovascular injury
3. Avascular necrosis of the femoral head

Consultation

All femur fractures should have emergent orthopedic consultation in the ED.

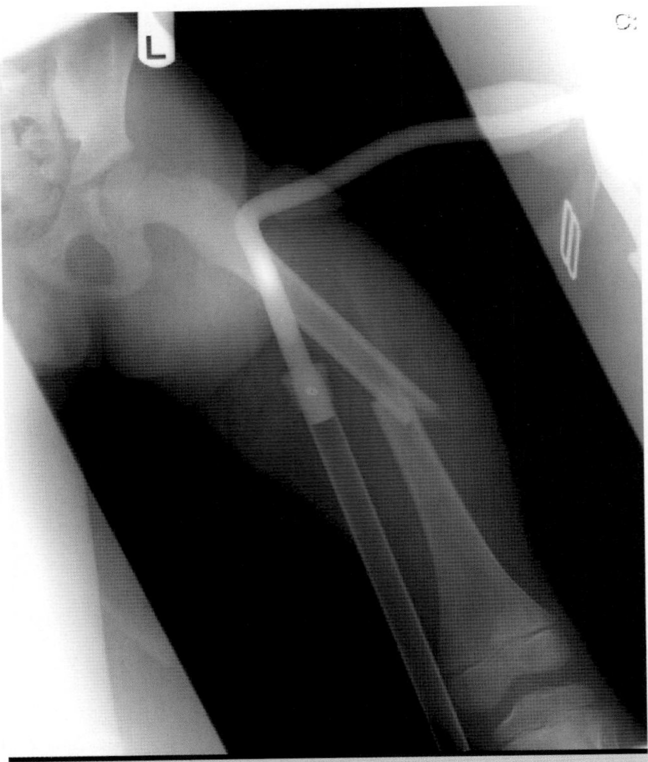

Figure 19-52. Femur Fracture

An x-ray of an 8-year-old pedestrian who was struck by an auto, which demonstrates a complete oblique fracture of the femur mid-shaft with posterior displacement and foreshortening. A splint is also seen.

Emergency Department Treatment and Disposition

1. Immobilization, neurovascular evaluation and documentation, analgesics, and admission.
2. The ultimate treatment of femoral fractures in children less than 6 years of age is more complex than in older children.
3. Depending upon the fracture, definitive treatment may be with various types of external splinting or open reduction internal fixation.

BOX 19-37. DIFFERENTIAL DIAGNOSIS OF FEMUR FRACTURE

- Thigh contusions

BOX 19-38. CLINICAL PEARLS: FEMUR FRACTURE

- More common in males than females
- There is a vascular ring around the base of the femoral neck. Fractures in that area have a higher association with avascular necrosis.
- Mid-shaft femur fractures, especially spiral fractures, should alert the clinician to the possibility of child abuse.

Legg-Calvé-Perthes Disease

Definition

Not secondary to injury, avascular necrosis of the femoral head results from an ill-defined etiology (Fig. 19-53). It is also known as osteochondrosis of the femoral head.

Clinical Features

1. The onset is usually insidious and may progress from months to years.
2. The child will usually present with a limp and a vague complaint of pain in the groin, inner thigh, or hip.
3. Limited abduction of the hip and internal rotation on flexion or extension
4. Symptoms are exaggerated during times of excessive activity or exertion.

Radiology

X-rays (a pelvic view) early on may demonstrate only joint-space widening. Later findings will demonstrate a flattening of the femoral head known as coxa plana.

Complications

1. With its subclinical presentation, there are not many acute complications.
2. Long-term complications include arthritis and limited mobility.

Consultation

Orthopedic consultation is not necessary in the ED.

Emergency Department Treatment and Disposition

Definitive referral to orthopedics

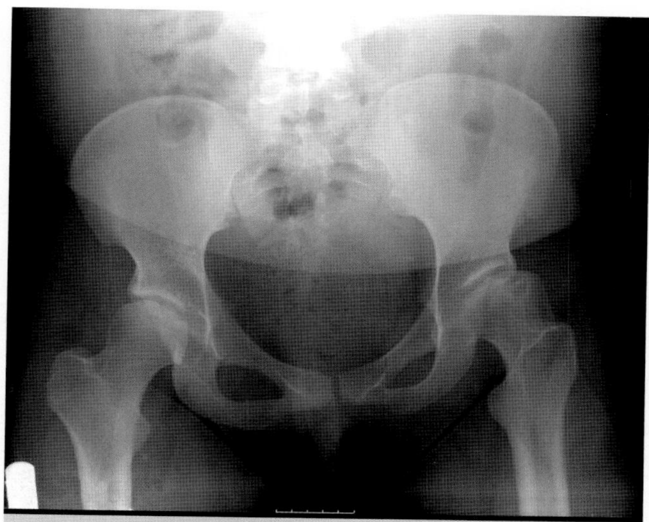

Figure 19-53. Legg-Calvé-Perthes Disease

Chronic and significant deformity of the left femoral head is apparent. Subcortical cysts are also present. The joint space is normal.

BOX 19-39. DIFFERENTIAL DIAGNOSIS OF LEGG-CALVÉ-PERTHES DISEASE

- Contusion
- Myofascial strain
- Avascular necrosis of the femoral head

BOX 19-40. CLINICAL PEARLS: LEGG-CALVÉ-PERTHES DISEASE

- Usually self-limiting disorder
- It affects boys three to five times more often than girls.
- Most commonly seen in children 5 to 7 years of age
- Unilateral in the vast majority of cases (80 to 90%)
- Fairly rare in African-Americans

Patella Fractures

Mechanism of Injury

Usually a direct blow to the patella or a fall directly on the anterior knee

Clinical Features

1. Tender swollen prepatellar area
2. With complete transverse fracture there will be inability to maintain the leg extended against gravity.

Radiology

Patella x-rays including a sunrise view (Fig. 19-54)

Complication

Nonunion of the patella, especially in displaced fractures

Consultation

1. All patients with a patella fracture need orthopedic referral.
2. Displaced/transverse fractures need emergent consultation in the ED.

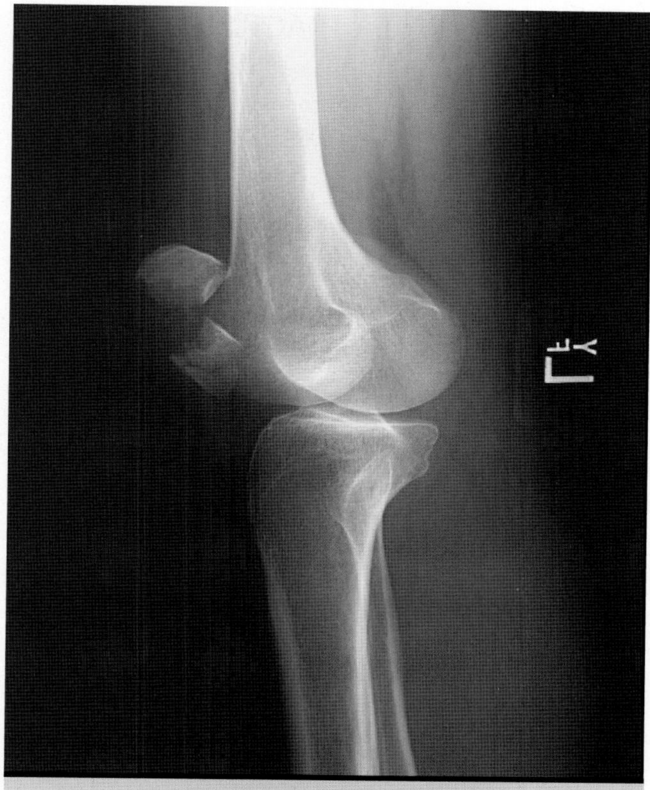

Figure 19-54. Patella Fracture

Lateral x-ray of the knee demonstrates a comminuted patella fracture.

Emergency Department Treatment and Disposition

1. Nontransverse/complete fractures can be treated with immobilization.
2. Transverse or displaced fractures require emergent orthopedic evaluation in the ED.

BOX 19-41. DIFFERENTIAL DIAGNOSIS OF PATELLA FRACTURE

- Contusion
- Tendon rupture
- Strain
- Patellar tendon rupture
- Quadriceps tendon rupture

BOX 19-42. CLINICAL PEARL: PATELLA FRACTURE

- Complete transverse fractures, especially if displaced, need surgical open reduction internal fixation.

Knee Dislocation

Mechanism of Injury

A direct blow to the knee as in a motor vehicle accident or significant fall

Clinical Features

1. Dislocations are classified according to the tibial displacement relative to the femur.
2. Anterior and posterior dislocations are the most common. Others include medial, lateral, and rotary.
3. Obvious deformity is common.
4. Tenderness on palpation
5. Distal pulses may be diminished.

Radiology

Standard x-rays of the knee including AP and lateral of the knee and sunrise view of the patella

Complications

1. Complications are very common.
2. Popliteal artery injury occurs (up to 40%), especially with anterior dislocations.
3. Peroneal nerve injury in 25 to 35%

Consultation

Orthopedic consultation is emergent for all knee dislocations or unstable knees that are highly suspicious for spontaneously reduced dislocations.

Emergency Department Treatment and Disposition

1. Due to the high incidence of neurovascular injury, reduction should take place emergently and in the ED.
2. Hospitalization is recommended for all patients with popliteal artery injuries (Fig. 19-55).

BOX 19-43. DIFFERENTIAL DIAGNOSIS OF KNEE DISLOCATION

- Anterior cruciate ligament tear
- Other ligamentous tear
- Patella fracture
- Contusion or sprain

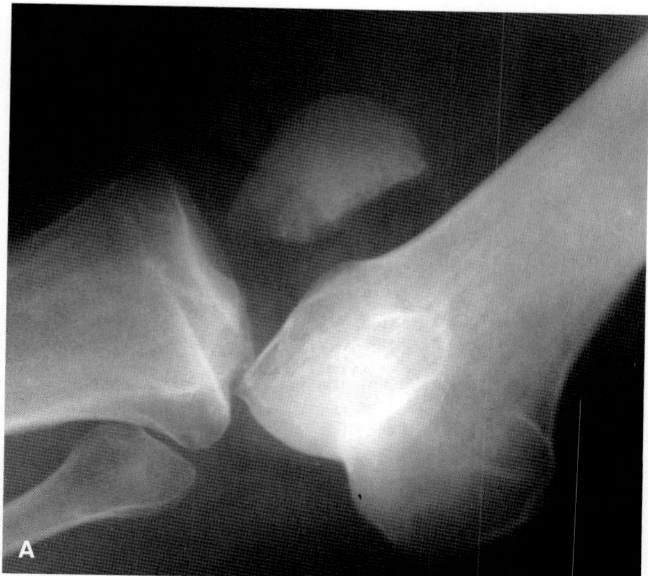

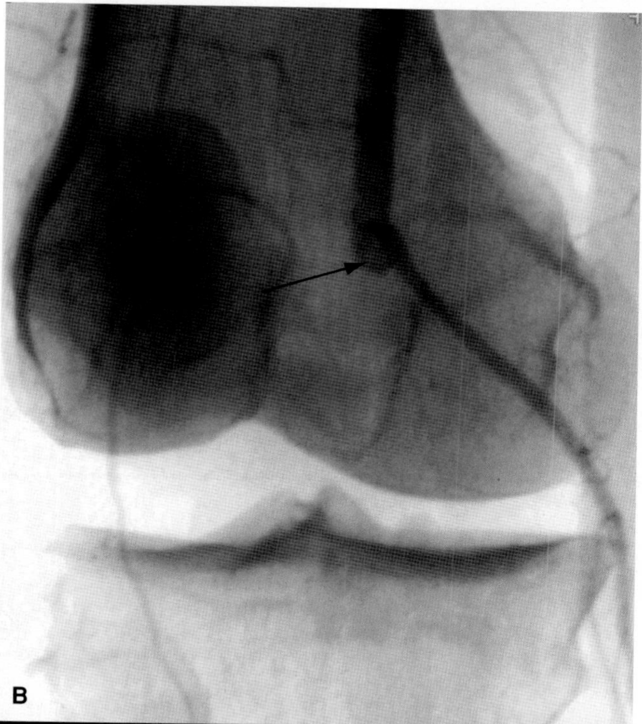

Figure 19-55. Knee Dislocation (Tibiofemoral Dislocation)

A. The tibia is displaced far anterior to the femoral condyles. Besides the transitional component to this dislocation, there is also a rotational component. This is the most common form of knee dislocation and results from forceful hyperextension. There is a great risk of popliteal artery injury. *B*. Despite immediate reduction of the dislocation, the popliteal artery was torn and completely thrombosed (*arrow*). For this reason, all knee dislocations need to undergo angiography to evaluate the popliteal artery.

BOX 19-44. CLINICAL PEARLS: KNEE DISLOCATION

- Peroneal nerve injury will produce paresthesias over the dorsum of the foot, diminished dorsiflexion of the foot, and/or decreased sensation between the first and second toes.
- If orthopedic consultation is not immediately available, the emergency medicine physician should perform the reduction with longitudinal traction and pressure towards the normal knee position.
- Any unstable knee joint should be *treated and evaluated* like a spontaneously reduced dislocation.
- All knee dislocations need to undergo angiography.

Patella Dislocation

Mechanism of Injury

Twisting injury to an extended knee

Clinical Features

1. Obvious deformity is common.
2. Limited movement of the knee secondary to pain
3. Tenderness on palpitation

Radiology

Standard x-rays including AP and lateral of the knee and sunrise view of the patella (Fig. 19-56)

Complications

Few complications are associated with a patella dislocation.

Consultation

Orthopedic consultation is rarely emergent and can be made in several days to a week, only after successful reduction.

Emergency Department Treatment and Disposition

1. Dislocations are easily reduced in the extended knee. Mild pressure is applied toward the normal position.
2. Reduction is usually noneventful and sedation analgesia should be reserved for initial failed attempts.
3. After successful reduction the knee should be immobilized in a dynamic splint and referred for orthopedic consultation.

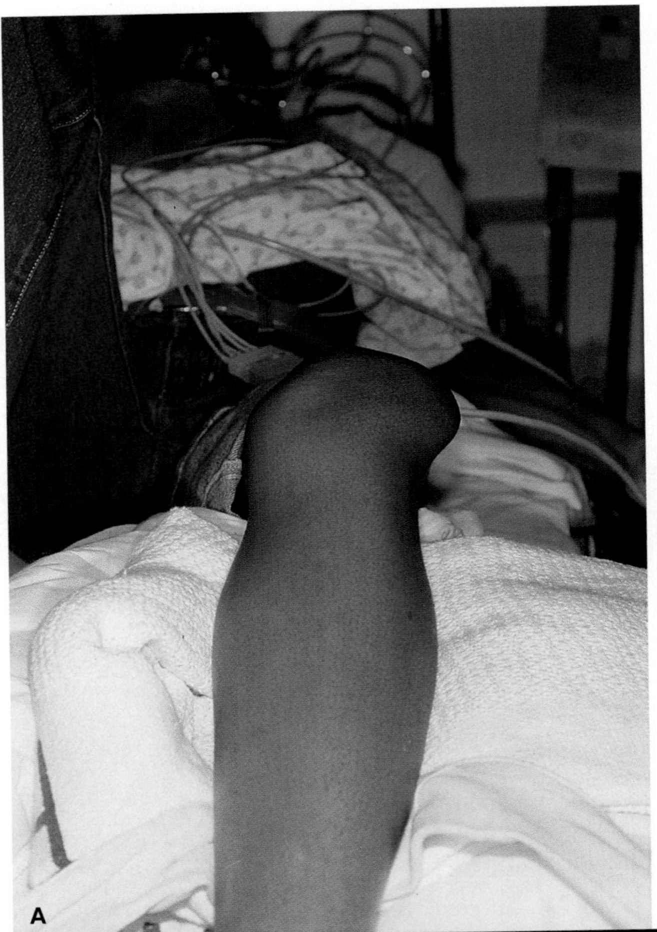

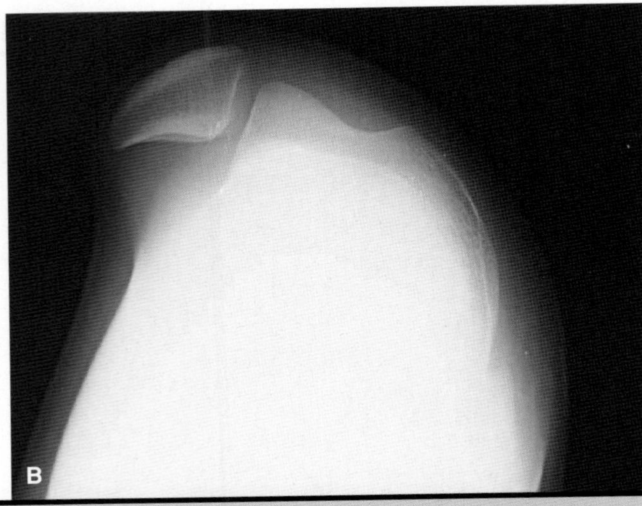

Figure 19-56. Patella Dislocation

A. Image of a 12-year-old girl after a fall, with blunt trauma to the knee and obvious deformity. *B*. Sunrise view x-ray of the patella demonstrating a patella dislocation.

BOX 19-45. DIFFERENTIAL DIAGNOSIS OF PATELLA DISLOCATION

- Anterior cruciate tear
- Other ligamentous tear
- Patella fracture
- Contusion or sprain

BOX 19-46. CLINICAL PEARL: PATELLA DISLOCATION

- Over 90% of patella dislocations are lateral.

Maisonneuve Fracture

Definition

Proximal fibular fracture with disruption of the tibiofibular syndesmosis

Mechanism of Injury

External rotation of the ankle

Clinical Features

1. Usually an obvious ankle fracture
2. Ankle may appear to be without deformity.
3. Pain on palpitation of the proximal calf

Radiology

1. Ankle studies may be negative, but may also show a widened mortise.
2. When x-rays include the proximal fibula, fractures are usually obvious (Fig. 19-57).

Complications

1. Significant arthritic changes and future difficulty in ambulation if left untreated
2. Nonunion of the tibiofibular syndesmosis

Consultation

Orthopedic consultation in the ED

Emergency Department Treatment and Disposition

1. Immobilization, elevation
2. Although most patients with these injuries can eventually be discharged from the ED, they should not do so without orthopedic consultation.

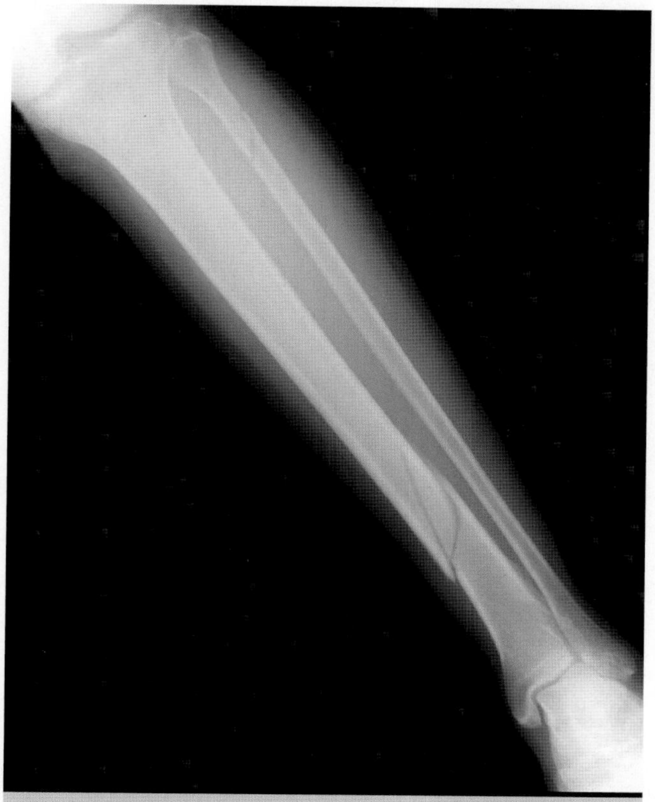

Figure 19-57. Maisonneuve Fracture

X-ray of the lower leg demonstrating a maisonneuve fracture through the proximal fibula and diathesis of the tibiofibular ligament. In this view the mortise appears intact, but there is an obviously comminuted fracture of the distal tibia.

BOX 19-47. DIFFERENTIAL DIAGNOSIS OF MAISONNEUVE FRACTURE

- Tibial plateau fracture
- Ankle fracture
- Ankle sprain
- Knee sprain or ligamentous injury
- Calf compartment syndrome

BOX 19-48. CLINICAL PEARLS: MAISONNEUVE FRACTURE

- When evaluating an injured ankle, always squeeze the calf and anterior lower extremity and look for tenderness.
- Usually associated with deltoid ligament rupture and ankle fractures; evaluate the proximal lower leg when these are diagnosed.

Ankle Sprains and Fractures

Mechanism of Injury

Inversion of the ankle

Clinical Features

1. Swelling, most pronounced over the lateral malleolus
2. Joint instability due to a third-degree sprain can usually be seen with laxity on manipulation, as with the drawer sign.

Radiology

1. X-rays are usually negative.
2. Soft tissue swelling is the most common finding (Fig. 19-58).
3. Avulsion off the distal fibula in anterior talofibular tears is occasionally seen.

Complications

1. Arthritis
2. Undiagnosed proximal metatarsal fractures may produce chronic pain.

Consultation

1. Without documented fracture or neurovascular deficit, consultation in the ED is not indicated.
2. Nonfractures with clinical ligamentous injury need telephone orthopedic consultation and urgent orthopedic follow-up (within 1 week).

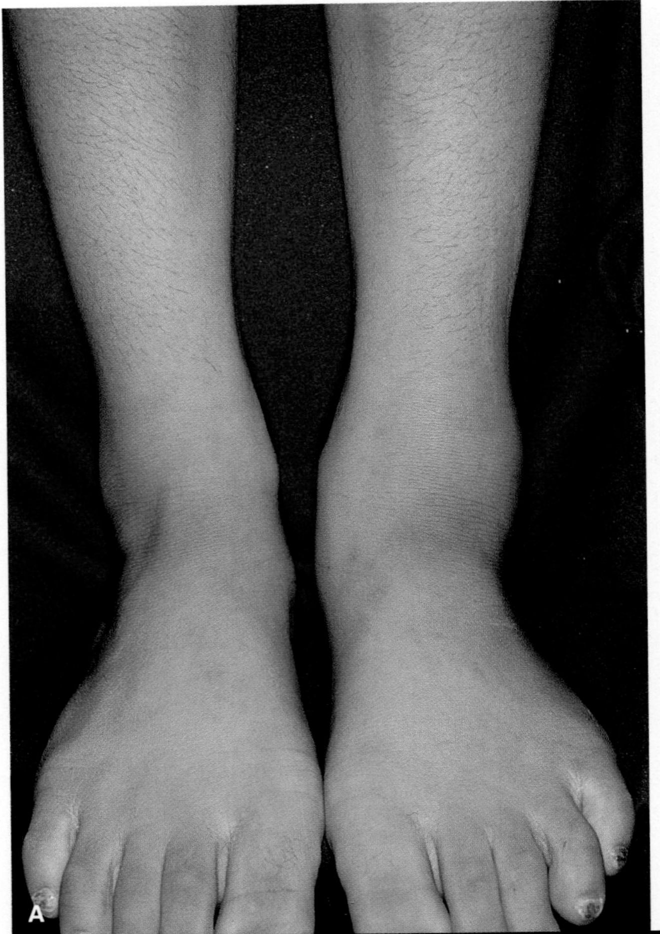

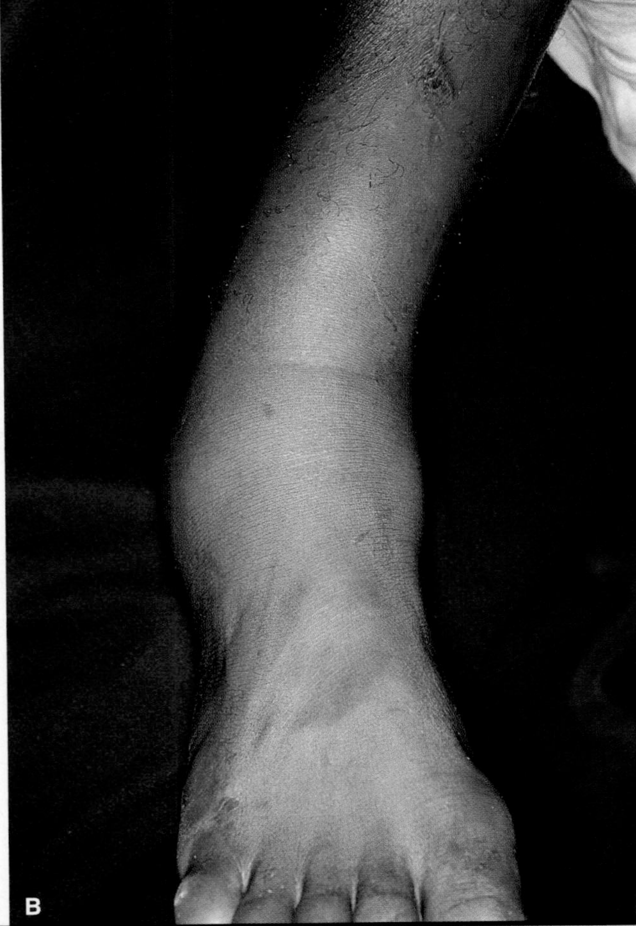

Figure 19-58. Ankle Sprains and Fractures

A. Image of a left ankle sprain with soft tissue swelling in a child who presented after an inversion injury. *B*. Image of a grossly deformed ankle with surrounding soft tissue swelling.

3. Gross ligamentous deformities (laxity on examination), or any neurovascular deficits, need emergent orthopedic consultation in the ED.

Emergency Department Treatment and Disposition

1. For those that do not involve joint instability, ice, elevation, and splinting are appropriate.
2. Sprains in which ligamentous injury is indeterminate should be referred to orthopedic follow-up within 1 to 2 weeks.
3. Obvious ligamentous injuries need to be adequately immobilized until expeditious follow-up (within 1 week) with orthopedics.

BOX 19-49. DIFFERENTIAL DIAGNOSIS OF ANKLE SPRAINS AND FRACTURES

- Ankle fracture
- Maisonneuve fracture
- Proximal metatarsal fracture

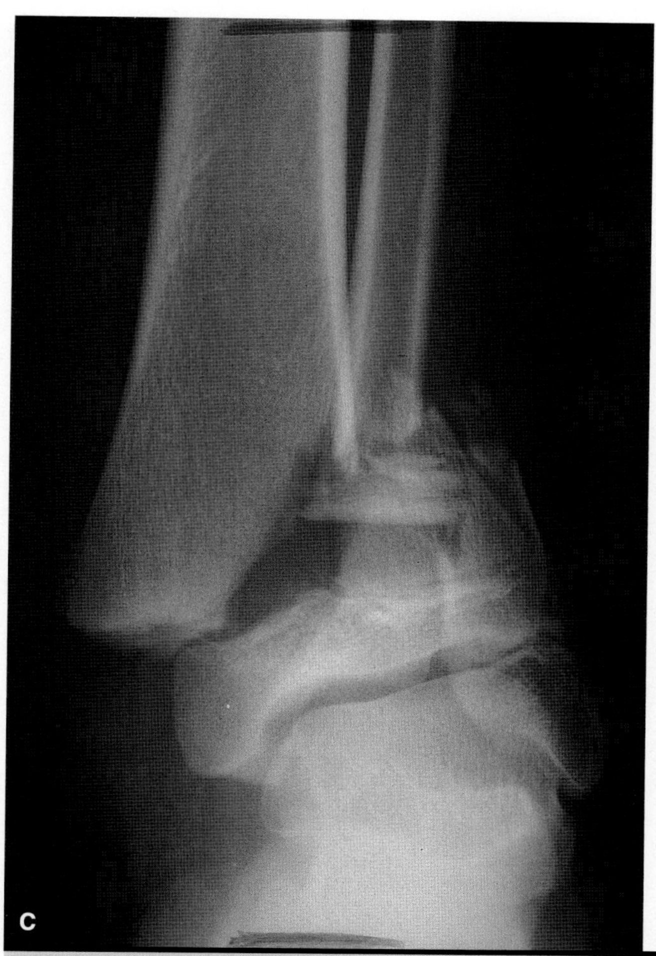

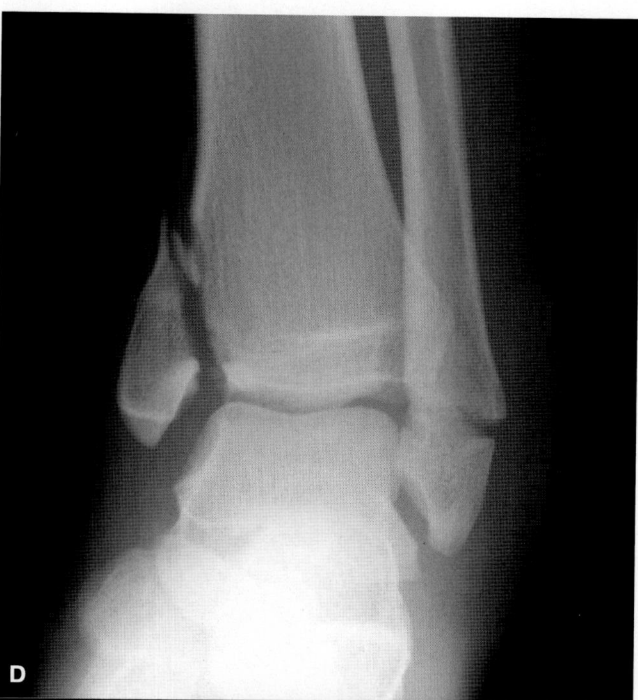

Figure 19-58. Ankle Sprains and Fractures (Continued)

C. X-ray of the patient in figure B showing a comminuted fracture of the distal fibula and a Salter-Harris type II fracture of the distal tibia with lateral displacement of the distal fragment. The ankle mortise appears to be intact. *D*. In a different patient, the radiograph demonstrates a bimalleolar fracture with a comminuted fracture of the medial malleolus and a distal fibular fracture.

BOX 19-50. CLINICAL PEARLS: ANKLE SPRAINS AND FRACTURES

- Ninety percent involve the lateral ligaments.
- Ligamentous injuries occur in the following order of frequency:
  (1) Anterior talofibular
  (2) Calcaneofibular
  (3) Posterior talofibular

Ankle Dislocation

Mechanism of Injury

1. Forced inversion or eversion
2. Direct external force

Clinical Features

1. Obvious deformity is usually present.
2. Types include anterior, posterior (common), superior (diastasis), and lateral (most common).
3. With lateral dislocation, the foot is usually obviously displaced laterally and the skin on the medial side will be tense.

Radiology

Standard three-view look at the ankle, including the AP, lateral, and mortise views (Fig. 19-59)

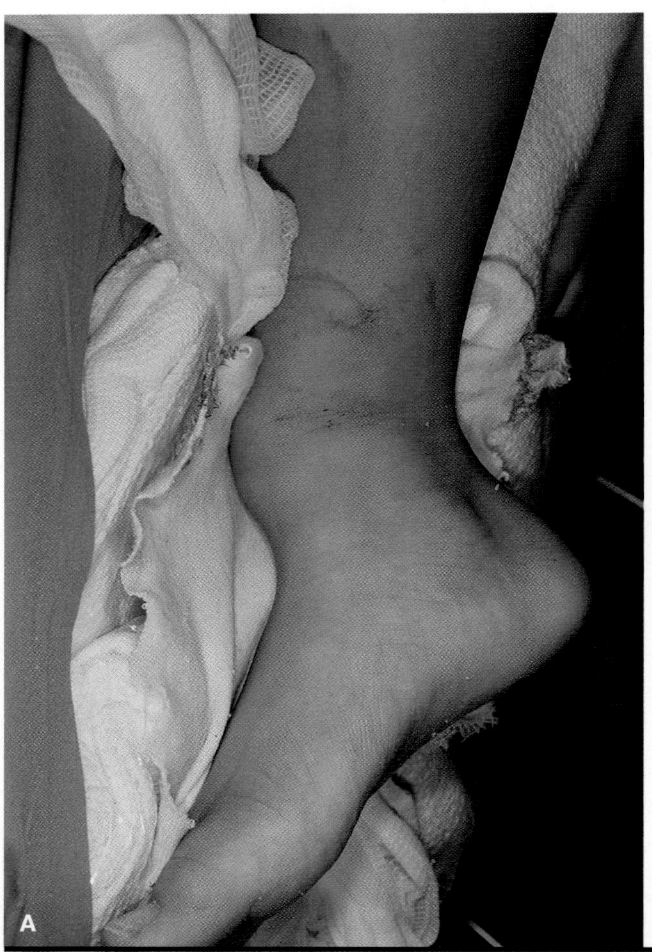

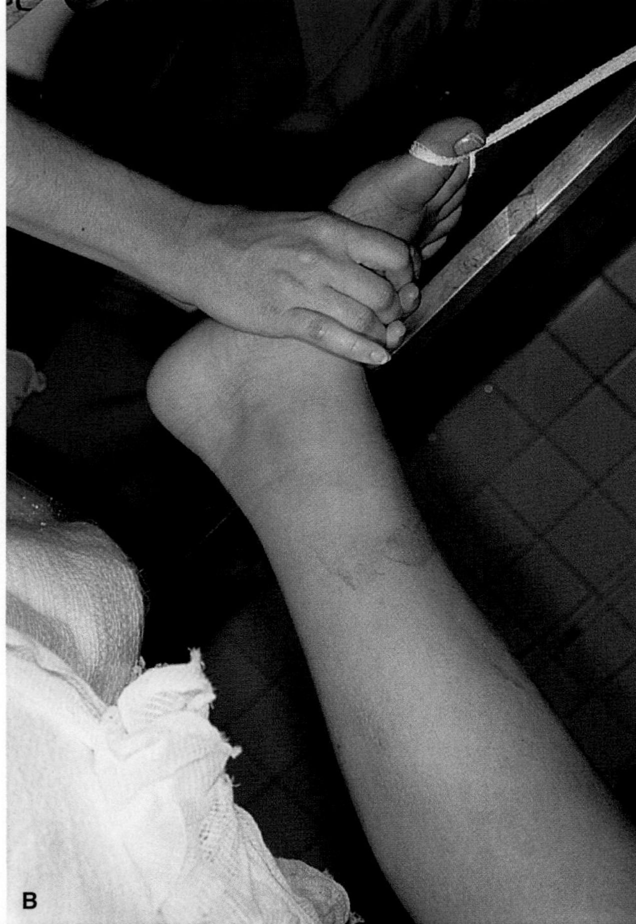

Figure 19-59. Ankle Fracture/Dislocation

A. and *B.* Image of ankle fracture/dislocation prior to reduction.

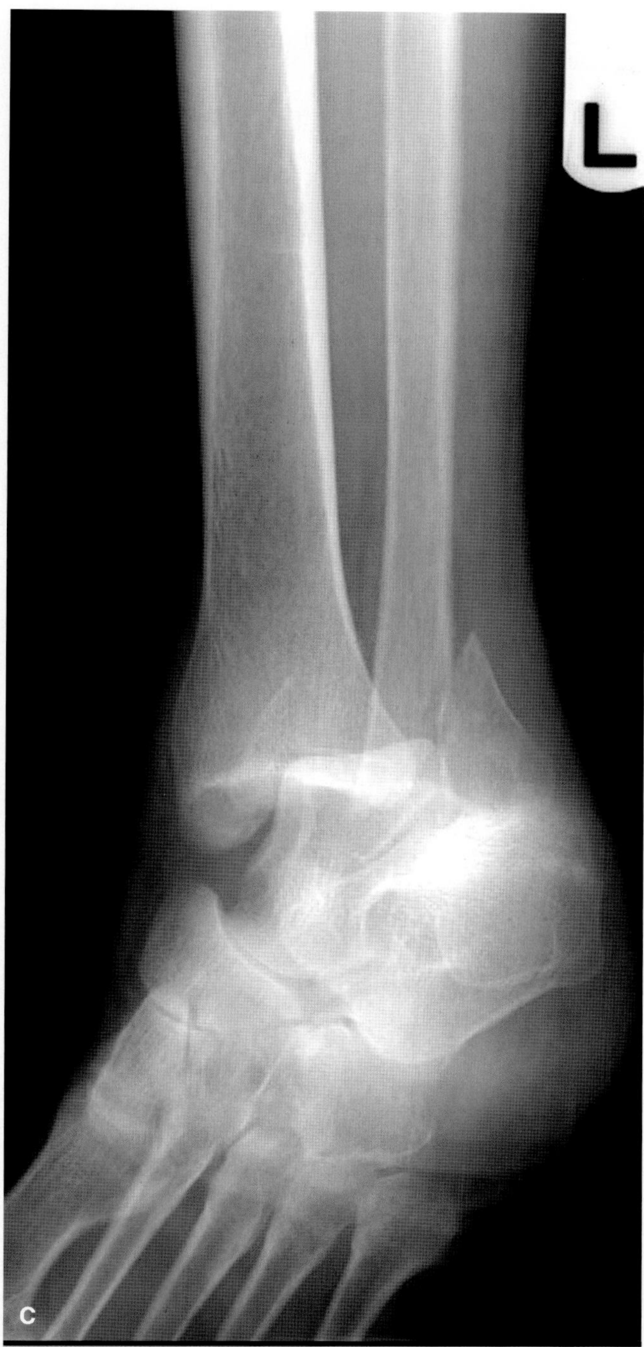

Figure 19-59. Ankle Fracture/Dislocation (Continued)

C. Posteriorly displaced oblique fracture of the distal fibula. Anterior dislocation of the tibia on the talus is also noted.

Complications

1. Avascular necrosis
2. Reflex sympathetic dystrophy

Consultation

All dislocations need emergent orthopedic consultation.

Emergency Department Treatment and Disposition

1. If consultation is not immediately available, reduction should be performed with inline traction by grasping the calcaneus and the forefoot.
2. Vascular integrity should always be checked prior to reduction.
3. Lack of pulses will necessitate reduction prior to x-ray evaluation.
4. Open ankle dislocations require urgent surgery.

BOX 19-51. DIFFERENTIAL DIAGNOSIS OF ANKLE DISLOCATION

- Ankle fracture
- Ankle sprain
- Subtalar dislocation

BOX 19-52. CLINICAL PEARLS: ANKLE DISLOCATION

- Fifty percent are open dislocations.
- Often associated with malleolar fractures
- Lack of pulses necessitates reduction prior to x-ray evaluation; otherwise x-rays should always be taken before emergent reduction.
- Lateral dislocations are almost always associated with fractures of the malleolus or distal fibula.

Calcaneal Fractures

Mechanism of Injury

Compression, usually resulting from a fall from a height

Clinical Features

1. Bohler's angle (normally 20 to 40 degrees) may be decreased.
2. Bohler's angle is formed by the intersection of the two lines between the superior margin of the posterior tuberosity of the calcaneus, through the superior tip of the posterior facet and the superior margin of the posterior tuberosity through the superior tip of the anterior process.

Radiology

1. Standard foot x-rays (PA, lateral, and axial) with the addition of a calcaneal view (Fig. 19-60)
2. CT scan for displaced fractures

Complications

1. Acutely, compartment syndrome
2. Disruption of the subtalar joint
3. Chronic arthritis
4. Heel spurs
5. Plantar fasciitis

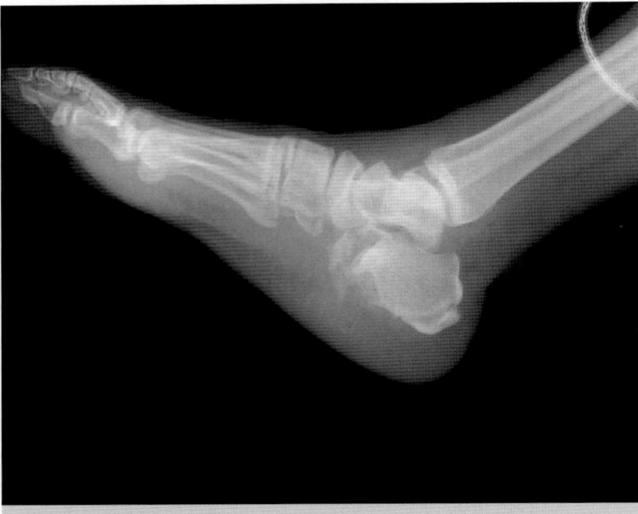

Figure 19-60. Calcaneal Fracture

X-ray of a young girl who fell from a height and sustained a comminuted calcaneal fracture. There is also a linear navicular fracture. The left lateral malleolus also shows a nondisplaced fracture. She also had comminuted right calcaneal fracture.

Consultation

1. Urgent orthopedic or podiatric referral (within several days)
2. Emergent orthopedic or podiatric consult for displaced fractures that may require open reduction

Emergency Department Treatment and Disposition

Immobilization in a compression dressing, ice, elevation, and avoidance of weight bearing

BOX 19-53. DIFFERENTIAL DIAGNOSIS OF CALCANEAL FRACTURES

- Foot contusion
- Plantar myofascial sprain
- Ankle sprain

BOX 19-54. CLINICAL PEARLS: CALCANEAL FRACTURES

- Most commonly, the tarsal bone is also fractured.
- Injury of the calcaneus should warrant evaluation of the lumbar sacral spine, which has a high rate of associated injury.
- Ten percent are associated with calcaneal fractures of the other foot.

Jones Fracture

Mechanism of Injury

Forceful load placed on the ball of the foot or forced oblique lateral plantar flexion

Clinical Features

Mild swelling and point tenderness over the base of the fifth metatarsal

Radiology

Standard x-rays of the foot (Fig. 19-61)

Complications

Uncommonly, chronic pain

Consultation

1. Orthopedic or podiatric consultation for true Jones fractures with minimal pain can be made urgently within several days.
2. Orthopedic or podiatric consultation for fractures with severe pain or proximal shaft transverse fractures should be done emergently for placement of a cylindrical cast.

Emergency Department Treatment and Disposition

1. Bulky dressing
2. Analgesics and weight bearing as tolerated
3. Patients with severe pain will benefit from a walking cast for 3 weeks.

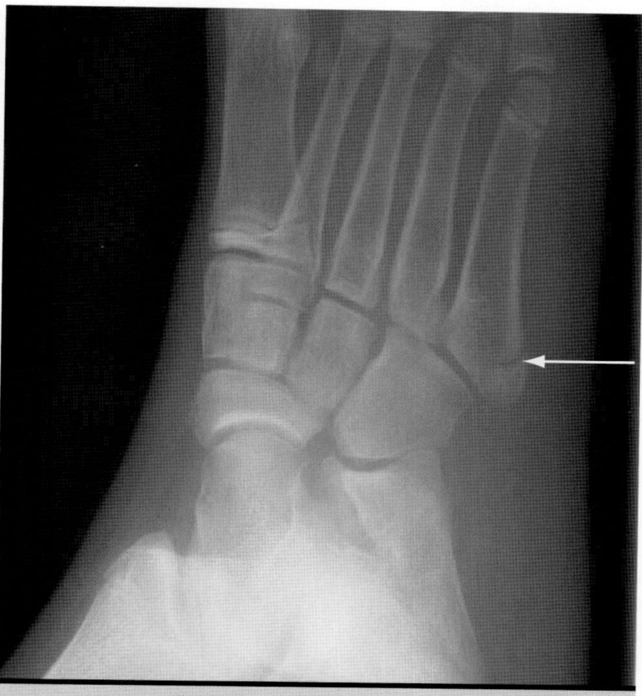

Figure 19-61. Jones Fracture

Classic x-ray appearance of a Jones fracture (fracture of the base of the fifth metatarsal) sustained by forced dorsiflexion of the foot.

BOX 19-55. DIFFERENTIAL DIAGNOSIS OF JONES FRACTURE

- Foot contusion
- Fifth digit fracture
- Proximal shaft fifth metatarsal fracture

BOX 19-56. CLINICAL PEARLS: JONES FRACTURE

- Transverse proximal fifth metatarsal fractures:
  (1) Have a completely different prognosis
  (2) Require urgent/emergent or orthopedic or podiatric consultation
  (3) Have a high incidence of delayed union or nonunion

Lisfranc's Fracture

Definition

Tarsometatarsal dislocation or fracture

Mechanism of Injury

1. Most commonly seen with strong blunt or compressional force, as in a motor vehicle accident
2. Severe rotational stress may also produce this type of dislocation.

Clinical Features

1. Significant midfoot swelling and tenderness
2. Inability to bear weight

Radiology

1. AP, lateral, and oblique views of the foot (Fig. 19-62)
2. CT scan is useful in occult injuries.

Complications

1. Degenerative arthritis
2. Decreased circulation to the distal foot

Consultation

Orthopedic consultation should be done emergently, as these cases most commonly require open reduction and internal fixation.

Emergency Department Treatment and Disposition

1. Ice, immobilization, elevation, analgesics
2. Most commonly admitted for open reduction and internal fixation

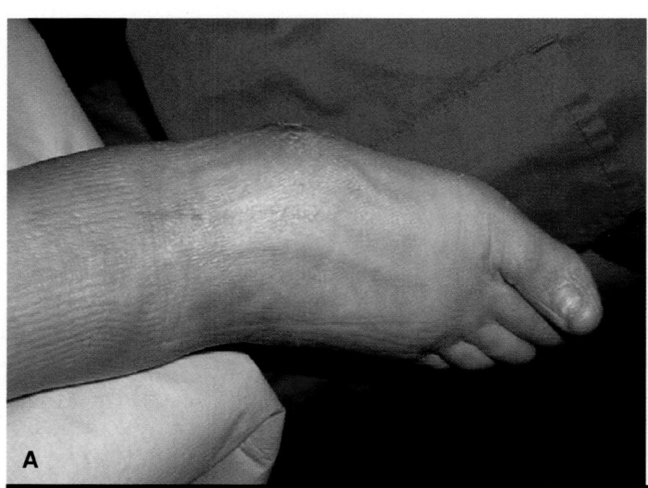

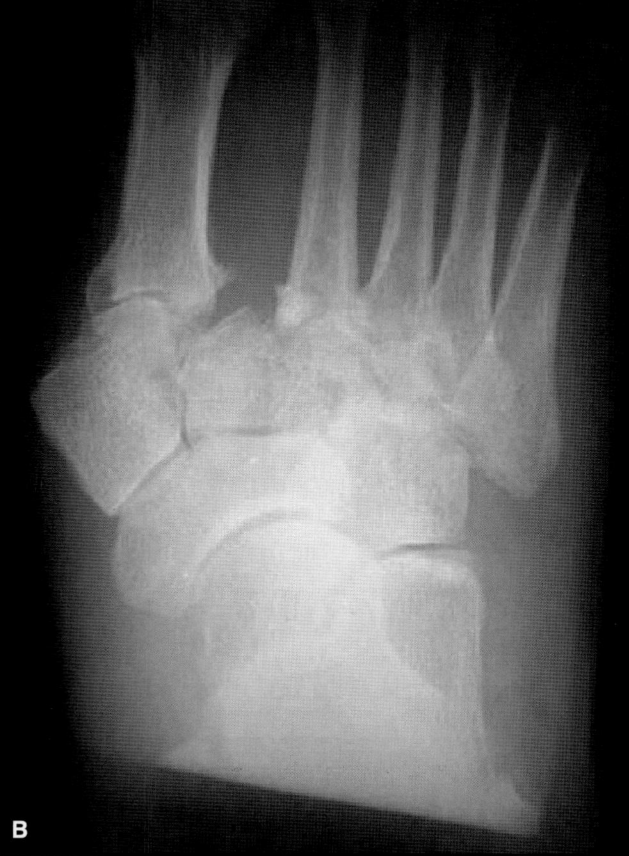

Figure 19-62. Lisfranc's Fracture

A. Picture of a developmentally delayed adolescent whose foot was caught in a metal door, resulting in tenderness and deformity of the midfoot. *B*. X-ray reveals fractures of the base of the second and third metatarsals with lateral dislocations of the second through fifth metatarsals. Note the greatly widened space between the first and second metatarsals.

BOX 19-57. DIFFERENTIAL DIAGNOSIS OF LISFRANC'S FRACTURE

- Metatarsal shaft fracture
- Subtalar fracture/dislocation
- Tarsal fracture

BOX 19-58. CLINICAL PEARLS: LISFRANC'S FRACTURE

- Most common midfoot fracture
- Fracture of the base (proximal) of the second metatarsal is nearly pathognomonic.
- Dislocations may involve one or several tarsometatarsal joints.
- Separation of the base of the first and second metatarsals is highly suggestive.

Osgood-Schlatter Disease

Mechanism of Injury

Microtrauma to the tibial tubercle tuberosity apophysis; this occurs during a normal or slightly advanced activity level for normal adolescents; there is usually no direct injury associated with the pain.

Clinical Features

1. Tender swollen tibial tuberosity (Fig. 19-63)
2. Erythema over the tibial tuberosity may be present.

Laboratory Tests

Since this is not an acute infectious/inflammatory process, there are no laboratory values that contribute to the diagnosis.

Complications

1. The only complication is a lack of participation in the routine activities of an adolescent.
2. There are no significant long-term complications of diagnosed Osgood-Schlatter disease.

Consultation

Not necessary unless the patient is a high-functioning individual; when the diagnosis is made, only rarely is there a reason for a consultant to see the patient in the ED

Emergency Department Treatment and Disposition

Rest and nonsteroidal anti-inflammatory drugs

BOX 19-59. DIFFERENTIAL DIAGNOSIS OF OSGOOD-SCHLATTER DISEASE

- Contusion
- Cellulitis
- Sprain

BOX 19-60. CLINICAL PEARLS: OSGOOD-SCHLATTER DISEASE

- Extremely common
- The activity level of the patient and point tenderness are the keys to diagnosis.
- If systemic signs or symptoms are present, another diagnosis is likely.

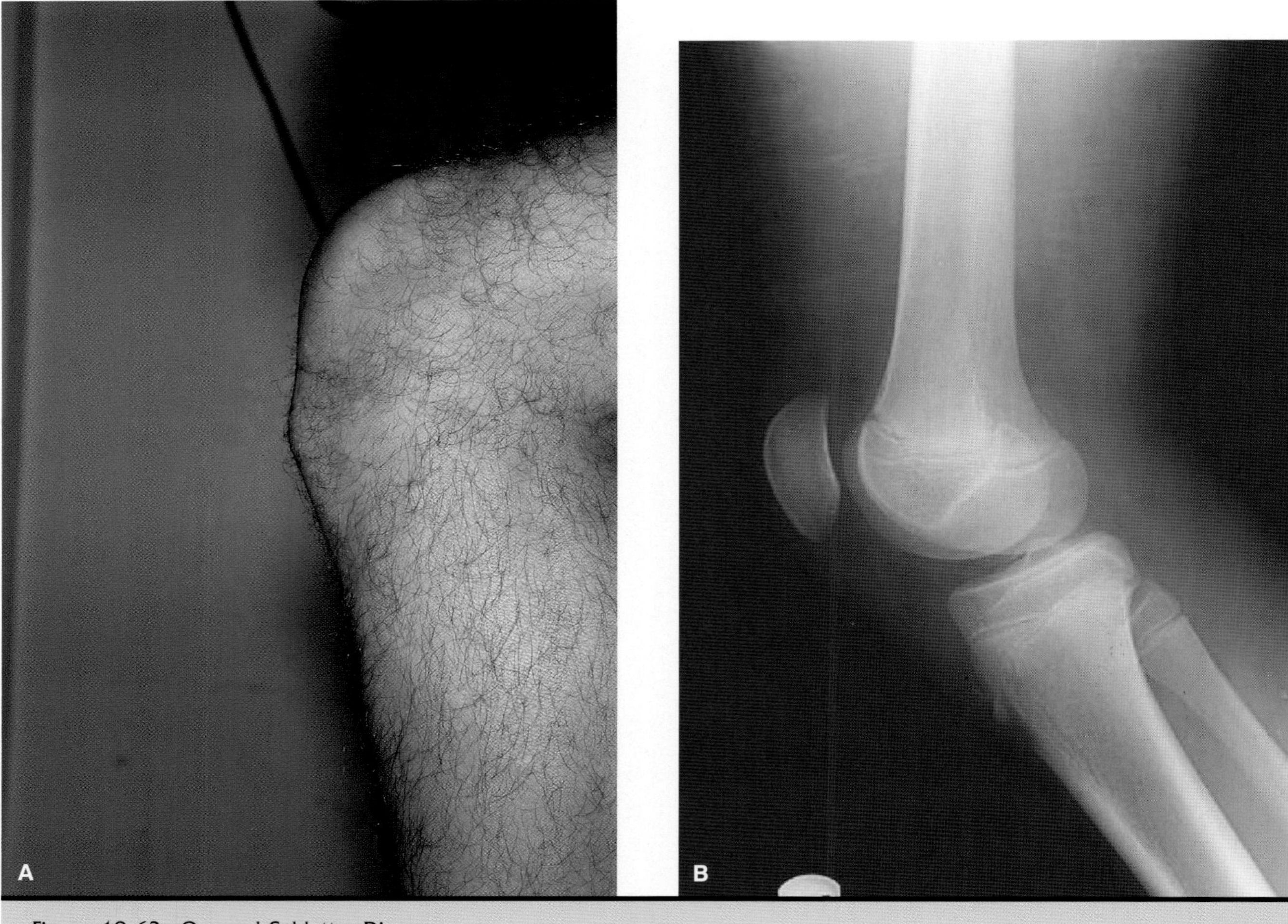

Figure 19-63. Osgood-Schlatter Disease

A. A lateral picture of the knee demonstrating a tender protuberance over the tibial tuberosity in this young basketball player. *B*. A lateral knee x-ray showing fragmentation and calcification over the tibial tuberosity.

Achilles Tendon Rupture

Mechanism of Injury

Forced dorsiflexion of the ankle, usually related to strenuous athletic activity; direct trauma to a taut tendon is a secondary cause

Clinical Features

1. Tender distal calf
2. A palpable defect in the tendon occurs 1½ to 2 inches (narrowest point) proximal to the calcaneus.
3. Thompson's test (no plantar flexion when the calf is squeezed) is positive (Fig. 19-64).

Radiology

Tibia/fibula and ankle films are usually negative.

Complications

1. Complete tears are rarely undiagnosed but lead to a difficult surgical repair.
2. Partial tears that are undiagnosed could lead to complete tears.

Consultation

1. In closed injuries, it is not necessary for orthopedics to see the patient in the ED. Contact should be made with orthopedics with definitive urgent follow-up.
2. Suspicion of a partial tear should also have orthopedic referral for extended immobilization.

Emergency Department Treatment and Disposition

1. A posterior splint should be applied and weight bearing avoided with crutches.
2. All complete Achilles tendon tears need surgical repair.

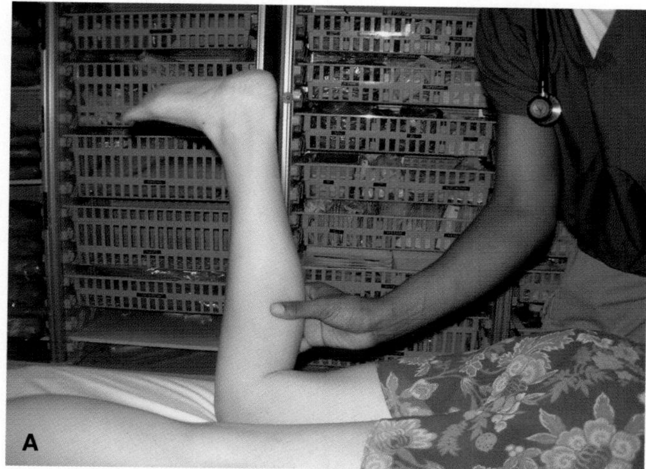

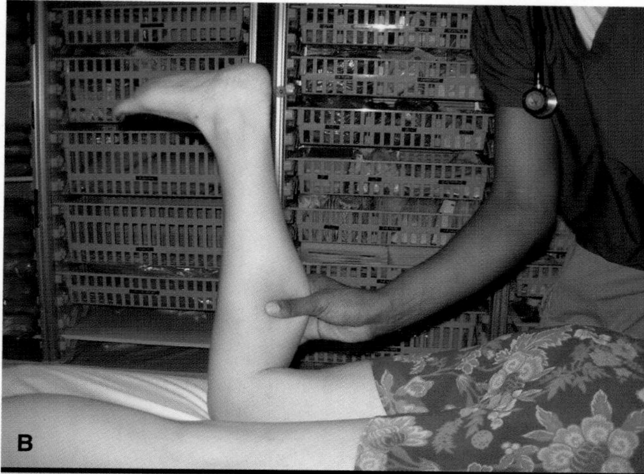

Figure 19-64. Positive Thompson's Test Seen in Achilles Tendon Rupture

A. Image of a patient in the proper position for a Thompson's test prior to squeezing the calf. *B*. Image of a positive Thompson's Test, demonstrating no plantar flexion of the foot after the calf is squeezed. This test is positive with complete tears of the Achilles tendon.

BOX 19-61. DIFFERENTIAL DIAGNOSIS OF ACHILLES TENDON RUPTURE

- Myofascial strain
- Calcaneal fracture
- Posterior malleolar fracture

BOX 19-62. CLINICAL PEARLS: ACHILLES TENDON RUPTURE

- Most common in middle aged men
- Most common in the adolescent athlete in the pediatric population
- Normally the posterior splints are applied with the ankle at 90 degrees, but in this case the ankle should be splinted in gravity equinus position, in which the ankle lies in when the leg is hanging off the examination table.
- The Achilles tendon is able to regenerate when partially sectioned, and heals well with immobilization.
- Partial tears can be missed in 25% of cases.

Anterior Cruciate Ligament Tear

Mechanism of Injury

Direct force to the knee, most commonly in contact sports

Clinical Features

1. A swollen, diffusely tender knee within 1 hour of injury
2. The anterior drawer sign and positive Lachman test are fairly sensitive.

Radiology

Standard x-rays including AP and lateral films of the knee usually demonstrate joint effusion and soft tissue swelling but no bony abnormalities (Fig. 19-65).

Complications

1. Arthritis
2. Chronic pain
3. Limited range of motion

Consultation

Stable knee joints without fracture or dislocation on x-ray can have outpatient orthopedic follow-up.

Emergency Department Treatment and Disposition

1. Immobilization, crutches, and avoidance of weight bearing
2. Orthopedic consultation within 48 hours
3. Definitive treatment is surgical by orthopedics.

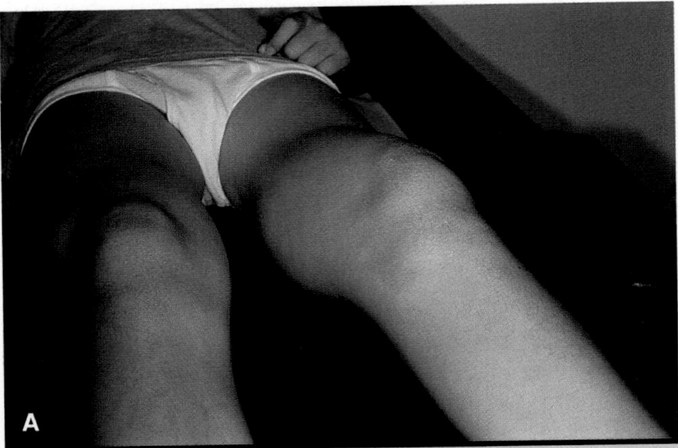

Figure 19-65. Anterior Cruciate Ligament Tear

Image of a 10-year-old male who sustained an anterior cruciate ligament tear while playing football. Note the marked diffuse swelling of the left knee in comparison to the normal right knee.

BOX 19-63. DIFFERENTIAL DIAGNOSIS OF ANTERIOR CRUCIATE LIGAMENT TEAR

- Other ligamentous tear
- Meniscal injury
- Contusion and sprain

BOX 19-64. CLINICAL PEARLS: ANTERIOR CRUCIATE LIGAMENT TEAR

- The most common serious ligament injury of the knee
- Seventy-five percent of anterior cruciate ligament tears will present with hemarthrosis.
- A tense hemarthrosis may decrease the sensitivity of the anterior drawer sign and Lachman test.
- All tender, swollen knees should be immobilized and weight bearing avoided until orthopedic follow-up.

DIAGNOSIS OTHER BONE AND JOINT DISORDERS

Septic Arthritis

Definition

Inflammation of the synovium of the joint by the direct presence of bacterial microorganisms

Clinical Features

1. The skin overlying the joint is usually warm, erythematous, and tender to palpation.
2. The joint is tender to both active and passive range of motion.
3. Systemic signs and symptoms such as fevers and malaise may or may not be present, but when present strengthen the diagnosis.

Pathogenesis

1. The most common cause is an osteomyelitis in close proximity to the joint or a direct inoculation into the joint space.
2. Penetrating (puncture) injuries in proximity to a joint should always be scrutinized.

Etiology

1. *Staphylococcus aureus* (most common)
2. Group A streptococci (second most common)
3. *Streptococcus pneumoniae*
4. *Haemophilus influenzae* type b (unvaccinated patients)
5. Gram-negative bacteria (e.g., Enterobacteriaceae, *Salmonella*)
6. Group B beta-hemolytic streptococci (neonates) (Fig. 49-66)
7. *Neisseria gonorrhoeae* (sexually active adolescents)

Complications

1. Untreated septic arthritis will always result in subsequent degenerative joint disease.
2. Osteomyelitis
3. Avascular necrosis, especially in the hip, where intra-articular pressure is increased due to increased intracapsular pressure.
4. Sepsis

Emergency Department Treatment and Disposition

1. If there is any suspicion of septic arthritis, the patient should be admitted to the hospital for parenteral antibiotics.
    a. In infants and children <5 years of age, provide coverage for *H. influenzae,* particularly those who have not been immunized adequately.
    b. Penicillinase-resistant coverage (e.g., oxacillin for *S. aureus* and other gram-positive bacteria) and a cephalosporin (e.g., cefotaxime)
    c. Cefuroxime alone is another alternative. It covers gram-positive bacteria including *S. aureus* and *H. influenzae.*
    d. Neonates or adolescents: provide coverage for gonococci
    e. Duration of antimicrobial therapy
        1) *S. aureus* septic arthritis: usually 4 to 6 weeks
        2) Uncomplicated group A streptococci, *S. pneumoniae*, or *H. influenzae* septic arthritis: usually 14 to 21 days
        3) Gonococcal arthritis: usually 7 to 10 days
        4) Longer duration of antibiotic therapy is needed if there is concomitant osteomyelitis.
2. Outpatient oral antibiotic therapy is not an acceptable treatment for septic arthritis.

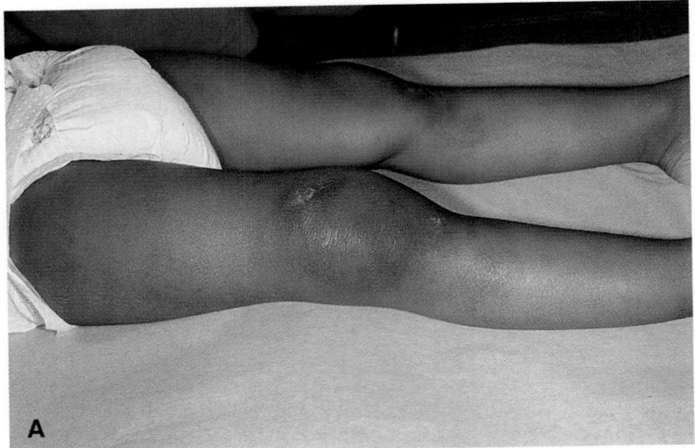

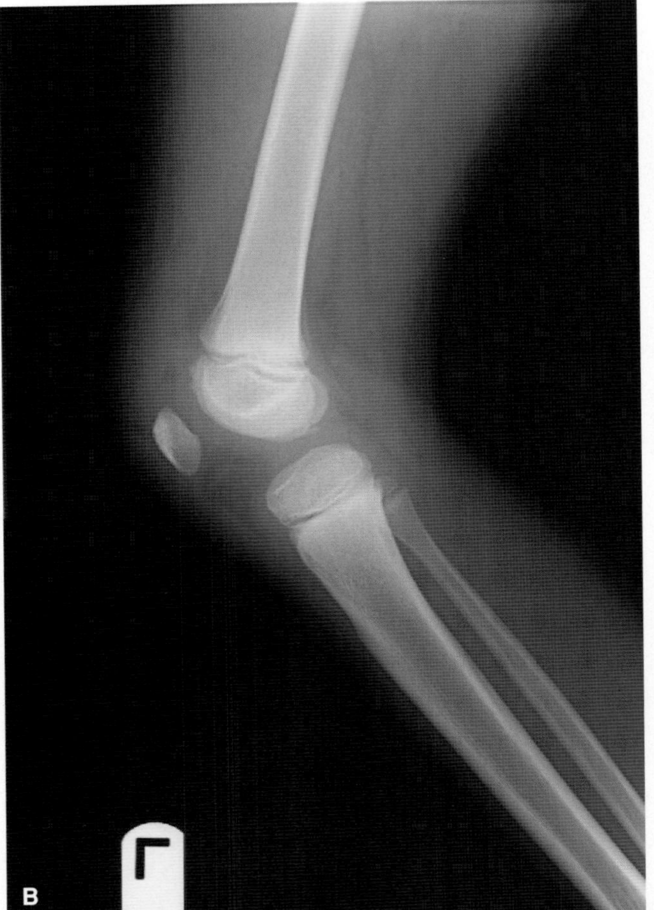

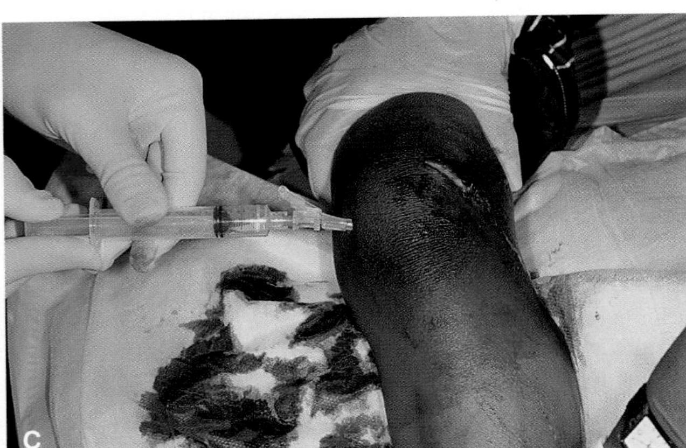

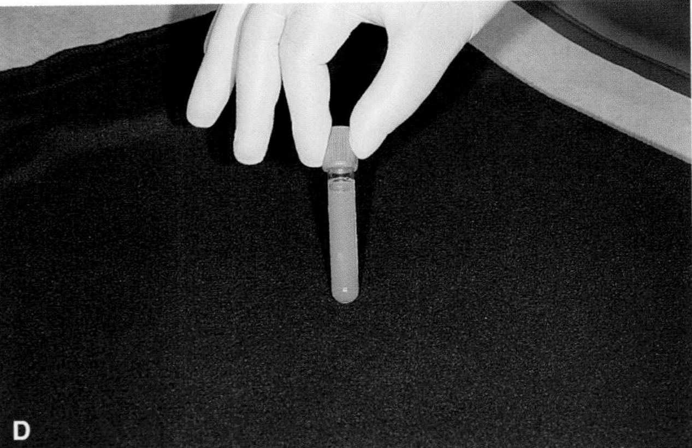

Figure 19-66. Septic Arthritis

A. A picture of a young child with septic arthritis of the right knee. *B*. The x-ray demonstrates an opacification of the suprapatellar bursa indicative of a joint effusion. *C*. An older child who underwent a laceration repair 1 week previously who presented with septic arthritis. He underwent a diagnostic arthrocentesis in the ED. Interestingly enough his ESR was elevated to 80, but his WBC count was only 8.5. *D*. The arthrocentesis yielded 15 mL of purulent straw-colored fluid, which on analysis had a WBC count of 110,000 WBCs/high-power field. Subsequently it grew group A beta-hemolytic streptococci.

BOX 19-65. DIAGNOSIS OF SEPTIC ARTHRITIS

- Diagnosis is made by a positive culture from a synovial aspirate or direct visualization of bacteria on Gram's stain.
- WBC count of the synovial fluid is the test which is essential in the ED.
- The following WBC counts assist in the diagnosis:

  Under 50,000/high-power field (HPF): likely inflammatory

  50,000 to 75,000/HPF: possibly infectious; differential of the WBC should be done; the presence of immature neutrophils (bands) suggest infection

  75,000 to 100,000/HPF: likely infectious; strongly consider septic arthritis if the differential shows any immature neutrophils (bands)

  >100,000/HPF: makes the diagnosis of septic arthritis until proven otherwise by repeated negative cultures

BOX 19-66. DIFFERENTIAL DIAGNOSIS OF SEPTIC ARTHRITIS

- Contusion
- Cellulitis
- Sprain
- Chondromalacia patella (differential diagnosis of septic arthritis of knee)
- Sepsis

BOX 19-67. CLINICAL PEARLS: SEPTIC ARTHRITIS

- There may be a vague history of previous trauma.
- Previously injured joints are the most common sites, followed by the knee, shoulder, and hip.
- WBC count of the synovial fluid is only suggestive; the overall appearance and presence of toxic features in the patient need to be considered.
- Septic arthritis of the hip, in which increased intra-articular pressure can lead to avascular necrosis, is a surgical emergency.

Osteomyelitis

Definition and Pathogenesis

Osteomyelitis is an infection of the bone. It is seen at the junction of the metaphysis and the epiphysis, and is due to deposition of pathogens during bacteremia (hematogenous spread). Infection of the bone can also occur as a result of direct inoculation of pathogens, as in penetrating injury or extension from local infection.

Etiology

1. *Staphylococcus aureus* (most common)
2. Group A streptococci (second most common)
3. *Streptococcus pneumoniae*
4. Gram-negative organisms (*e.g., Haemophilus influenzae* type B [unvaccinated patients], *Pseudomonas aeruginosa, Salmonella* spp., *Escherichia coli, Klebsiella* spp.)

Clinical Features

1. Fevers that may be low-grade
2. Refusal to use the limb or walk
3. Tenderness on palpation over the metaphysis, which is commonly infected
4. Joint swelling
5. Fever and irritability in neonates

Laboratory Tests

1. The first x-ray finding is periosteal elevation (detection of bone destruction and repair is not seen until 7 to 10 days after onset) (Fig. 19-67).
2. Bone demineralization and lytic lesions are a late finding.
3. An elevated WBC count is often seen.
4. Elevated ESR
5. Blood cultures are positive in 60% of cases.
6. Bone scans are positive in 90% of cases.
7. MRI is also sensitive.

Complications

1. Loss of bony architecture
2. Local spread with septic arthritis
3. Avascular necrosis
4. Sepsis

Consultation

1. Emergent consultation is required for all suspected cases of osteomyelitis.
2. All noninfectious bony tenderness should be urgently referred to orthopedics for evaluation of potential mitotic processes.

Emergency Department Treatment and Disposition

1. Antibiotics should be initiated in the ED after cultures.
2. Oxacillin is a good initial antibiotic in suspected cases of osteomyelitis.
3. For patients allergic to penicillin, clindamycin or vancomycin can be substituted.
4. All patients with confirmed or suspected osteomyelitis require admission to the hospital.

BOX 19-68. DIFFERENTIAL DIAGNOSIS OF OSTEOMYELITIS

- Septic arthritis
- Bony tumors (e.g., osteogenic or Ewing's sarcoma)
- Metastatic bony lesions (e.g., leukemia, lymphoma, neuroblastoma)
- Cellulitis
- Hemoglobinopathies (bone infarction)
- Fracture

BOX 19-69. CLINICAL PEARLS: OSTEOMYELITIS

- Consider osteomyelitis in any infant or child with unexplained irritability, fever, or asymmetrical use of an extremity.
- The femur and the tibia are the bones most commonly infected.
- Osteomyelitis may be associated with septic arthritis in young children.
- X-ray abnormalities may take 7 to 10 days to become apparent.
- CT scan is not helpful in making the diagnosis.
- *Staphylococcus aureus* is the most common pathogen involved in hematogenous spread.
- In children with sickle cell disease, there is an increased incidence of *Salmonella*.
- Infections in the foot after plantar puncture wounds are often caused by *Pseudomonas aeruginosa*, which requires extensive evaluation and treatment.

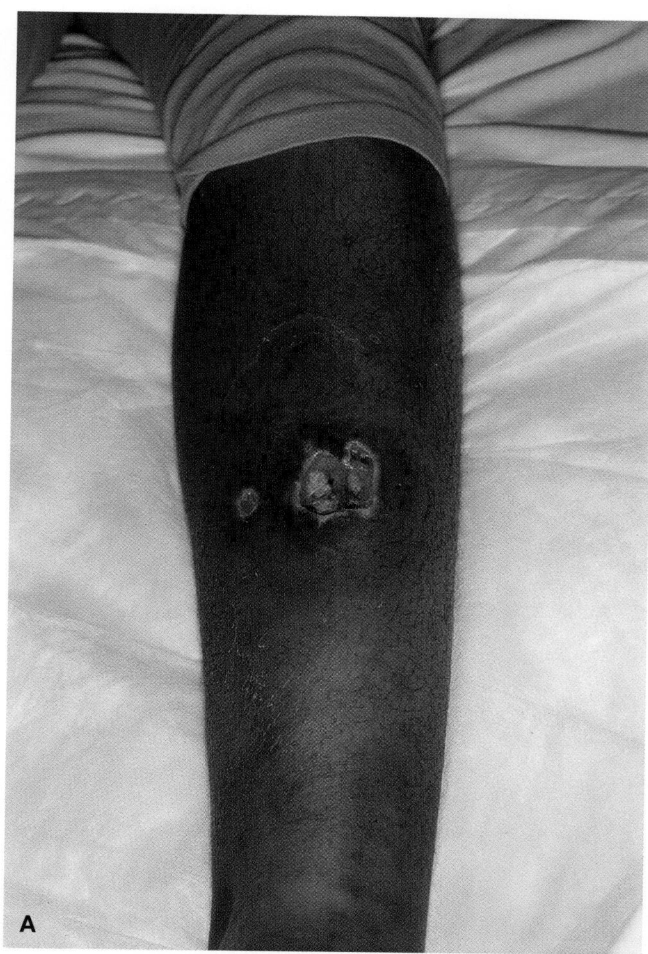

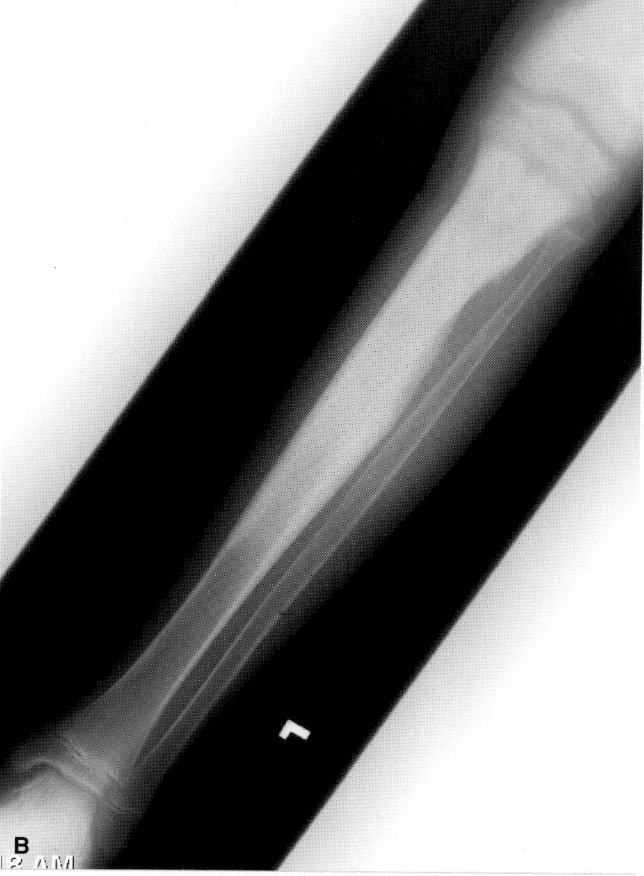

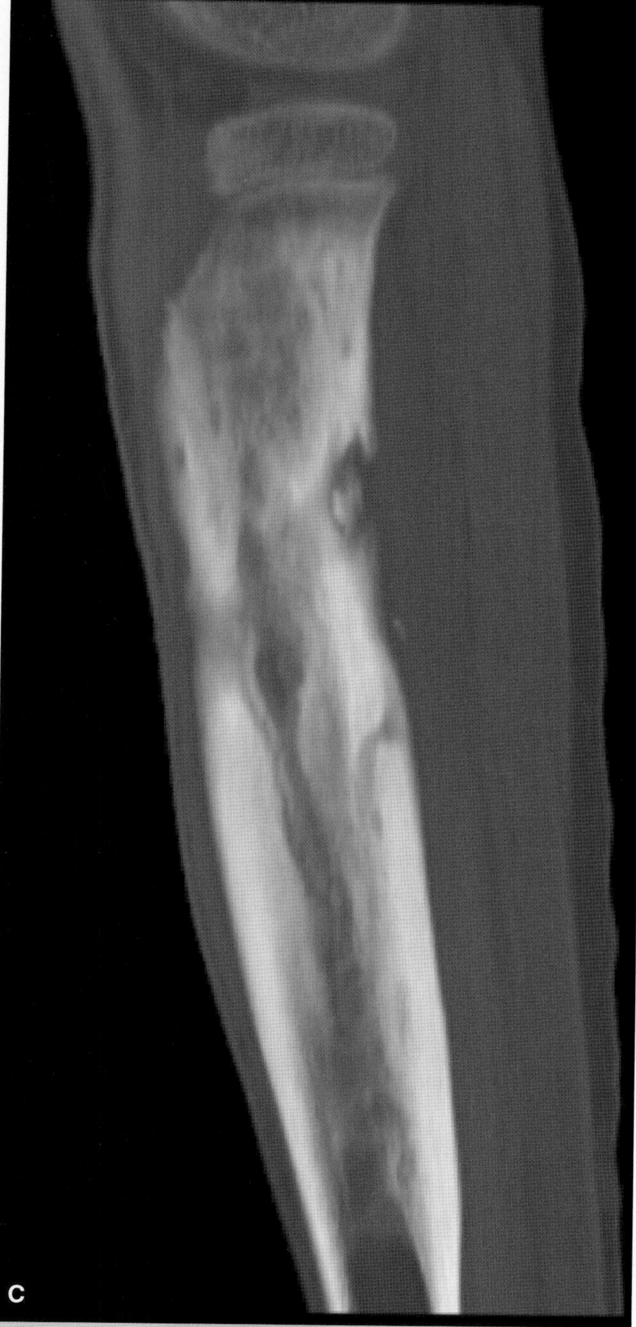

Figure 19-67. Osteomyelitis

A. Image of an 11-year-old girl who recently arrived in the United States from Ghana and presented with a nonhealing ulcer over her lower leg after injuring herself while playing soccer 1 month previously. *B*. X-ray of the tibia demonstrates a heterogenous sclerosis involving the proximal and mid-tibial diaphysis. There is also an area of lucency involving the lateral aspect of the proximal tibial metaphysis. The findings are highly suggestive of osteomyelitis. *C*. MRI of the leg demonstrates a large bony sequestrum and draining sinus tract with Brodie's abscesses and soft tissue enhancement, confirming the diagnosis of osteomyelitis. The patient was subsequently taken to the operating room for débridement and *Staphylococcus aureus* grew in the cultures.

Osteogenesis Imperfecta

Definition

1. Also known as brittle bone disease, osteogenesis imperfecta (OI) is a genetic disorder caused by a quantitative defect in type I collagen.
2. The spectrum of the disease is very broad, with the most severe cases being lethal in the perinatal period, and a much milder form in which the diagnosis may not be made, even in adulthood.

Clinical Features

1. The classic triad consists of fragile bones, blue sclera, and early deafness.
2. In all but the mildest cases there is limitation of early activity with frequent fractures and bowed legs.
3. Even in the mild form, fractures result from only minimal trauma, but fortunately usually these decrease after puberty.

Etiology

An autosomal dominant disorder which causes a defect in the amount of type I collagen, an essential component of the matrix of skin and bone

Laboratory and Radiography

1. The diagnosis is made by using collagen biochemical studies from fibroblasts cultured from skin biopsy.
2. Besides the obvious fractures as a result of the brittle bones, other abnormalities seen on x-ray include a beaded appearance of the ribs on chest x-ray, bowed legs, rib cage flaring at the bases, scoliosis, vertebral compressions, and a popcorn-like appearance of the metaphyses of bones due to disorganization of the bone matrix (Fig. 19-68).

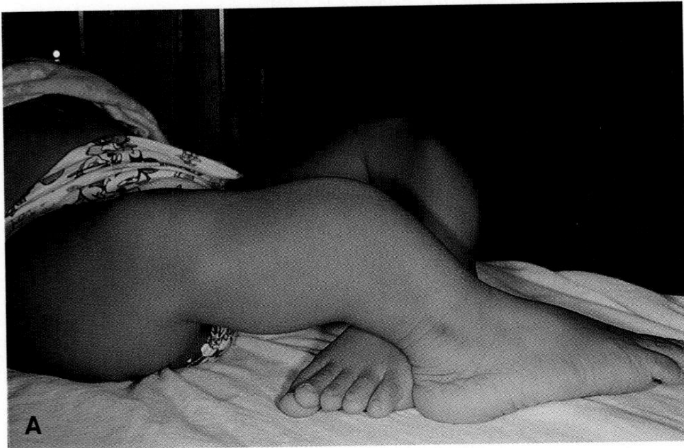

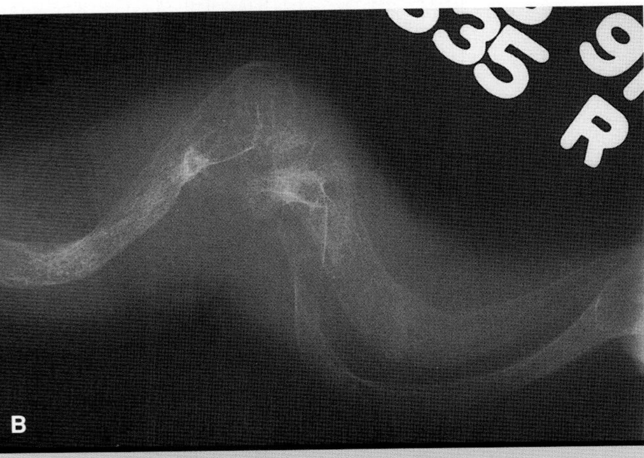

Figure 19-68. Osteogenesis Imperfecta

A. Image of an 8-year-old girl with osteogenesis imperfecta. *B*. X-rays of the lower extremities demonstrate the demineralized and contorted bone.

Complications

1. Multiple fractures, degenerative joint disease, deafness, recurrent pneumonia, cardiac failure, and cor pulmonale
2. There are also multiple neurologic complications, including hydrocephalus, basilar invagination, and brainstem compression.

Emergency Department Treatment and Disposition

1. There is no curative treatment.
2. In milder cases physical rehabilitation may help.
3. For moderate cases, braces, gait aids, and orthopedic management including fracture management and placement of intramedullary rods are indicated.

BOX 19-70. DIFFERENTIAL DIAGNOSIS OF OSTEOGENESIS IMPERFECTA

- Primary bony tumors
- Pathologic fractures
- Bony cysts
- Child abuse

BOX 19-71. CLINICAL PEARLS: OSTEOGENESIS IMPERFECTA

- An inherited autosomal dominant trait
- Most common cause of genetic osteoporosis
- Moderate to severe cases are usually diagnosed in infancy.
- Due to its autosomal dominant nature, there is a strong familial disposition.
- The mildest cases may remain occult, with multiple fractures being the only clue to the diagnosis.

Foreign Bodies and Penetrating Injuries

Mechanism of Injury

1. Most often occur on the plantar aspect of the foot or the palmar surface of the hand.
2. Less commonly it can occur from falling objects or projectiles.

Clinical Features

1. There is always a nearby puncture wound.
2. When on the plantar foot, it may be subtle.
3. Pain will usually be present, but to a much greater extent if there is associated bony involvement.

Radiology

1. X-rays should always be performed with suspicion of any penetrating injury (Fig. 19-69).
2. Foreign bodies of higher density are radiopaque.
3. The ability to see glass on x-ray is dependent on its lead content, with fine crystal having a high content and bottles a lower content.
4. Ultrasound is also useful at detecting subcutaneous foreign bodies.

Complications

1. Cellulitis
2. Osteomyelitis is common after inoculation into the bony matrix.
3. Septic arthritis, either from direct penetration of the joint capsule, or via direct spread from a focus of osteomyelitis
4. Retained foreign body, fibrosis, and pain

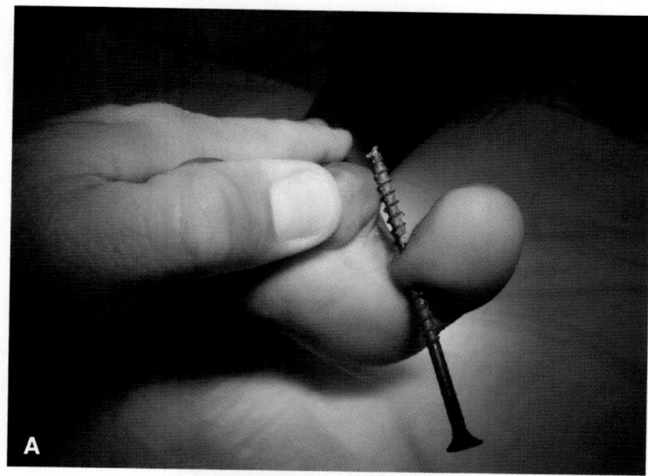

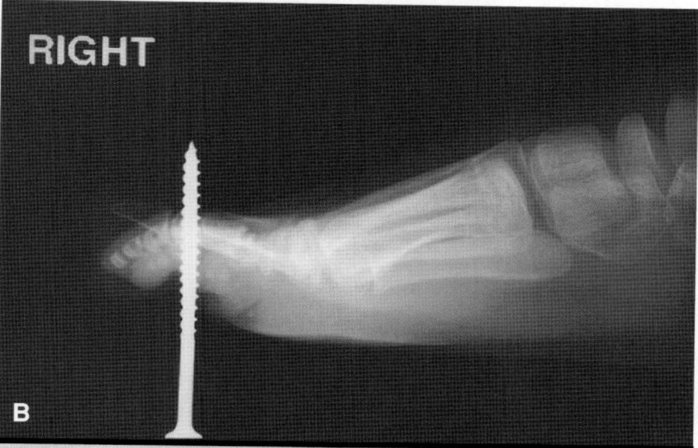

Figure 19-69. Foreign Bodies and Penetrating Injuries

A. Image of a large screw penetrating through the great toe. This 6-year-old child was playing basketball barefoot in a dirt lot. *B*. The x-ray reveals the metallic screw traversing the proximal portion of the great toe.

Consultations

1. All highly suspicious or documented retained foreign body penetrating injuries require consultation in the ED.
2. The service consulted depends on the body site involved and the consultation policy of the institution (extremity injuries usually require orthopedic involvement, torso injuries require trauma/surgery involvement, ocular injuries require ophthalmology involvement, etc).

Emergency Department Treatment and Disposition

1. All suspected foreign bodies should be thoroughly investigated.
2. High suspicion should prompt consultation and parenteral antibiotics in the ED.
3. Penetrating foreign bodies should be admitted to the hospital for definitive removal when indicated, or an initial course of parenteral antibiotics given when removal is not indicated.

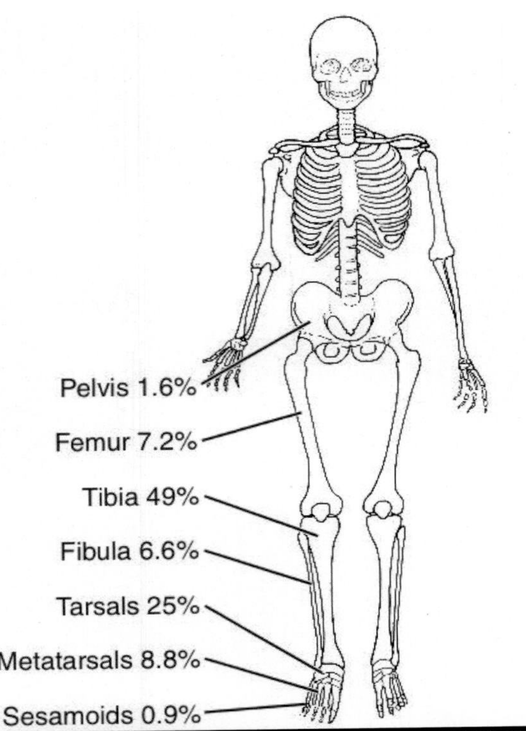

Figure 19-70. The distribution and frequency of stress fractures

Reproduced with permission. Fracture principles. In: Emergency Orthopedics. The Extremities. Simon RR and Koenigsknecht SJ. 2001. McGraw-Hill Co. page 21, 4th ed., New York.

BOX 19-72. DIFFERENTIAL DIAGNOSIS OF FOREIGN BODIES AND PENETRATING INJURIES

- Contusion
- Cellulitis
- Septic arthritis
- Puncture without foreign body retention

BOX 19-73. CLINICAL PEARLS: FOREIGN BODIES AND PENETRATING INJURIES

- Plantar foreign bodies, even when identified on two view x-rays, are extremely difficult to remove in the ED.
- Penetrating injuries through a sneaker may result in *Pseudomonas* osteomyelitis and therefore require aggressive investigation and parenteral antibiotics in the ED, followed by oral antibiotics (covering *Pseudomonas*) and urgent follow-up for wound checks if the patient is discharged home.
- Penetrating injuries resulting in bony fractures require aggressive treatment with expeditious parenteral ED antibiotics, consultation, and admission.

Stress Fractures

Mechanism of Injury

Almost always secondary to overtraining

Clinical Features

1. Pain on ambulation, and in particular exertion
2. Erythema, swelling, or pain on palpation are all rare.

Radiology

1. Stress fractures are mechanical problems and do not cause laboratory abnormalities.
2. Initial x-rays are usually negative.
3. Bone scans may be positive.

Complications

1. Arthritis
2. Chronic pain

Consultation

1. Not necessary in the ED
2. When dealing with an athletic adolescent, referral to an orthopedic sports medicine specialist is always helpful.

Emergency Department Treatment and Disposition

Rest and nonsteroidal anti-inflammatories if necessary

BOX 19-74. DIFFERENTIAL DIAGNOSIS OF STRESS FRACTURE

- Shin splints
- Contusion
- Cellulitis
- Sprain

BOX 19-75. CLINICAL PEARLS: STRESS FRACTURES

- Second most common cause of fractures after metatarsal fractures
- The main differential diagnosis is shin splints, which are usually bilateral; stress fractures are usually unilateral.

Suggested Readings

4th Edition McGraw-Hill Co. Simon RR, Koenigsknecht SJ: *Emergency Orthopedics. The Extremities*. 2001.

Schwartz DT, Reisdorff EJ: *Emergency Radiology*. McGraw-Hill, New York, 2000.

CHAPTER 20

TRAUMA

Karen Santucci / Bonny Baron / Ayman Chritah / Karen L. Stavile / Kevin J. McSherry / David Listman / Binita R. Shah / Eileen C. Quintana / Michael Lucchesi

Edited by Michael Lucchesi

DIAGNOSIS — HEAD TRAUMA

Background

Head trauma is one of the most common childhood injuries. It accounts for 600,000 ED visits, 95,000 hospital admissions, 29,000 permanent disabilities, and 7000 deaths.

Mechanism of Injury

1. The most common cause of head injury in children is falls.
2. Motor vehicle accidents, physical assault including child abuse, and bicycle collisions account for severe head injuries in children (for abusive head injuries, see page 16).
3. Blunt trauma is the most common type of head injury in infants, children, and adolescents (Figs. 20-1, 20-2 and 20-3).
4. Penetrating head injuries are uncommon in children. They occur from gunshot wounds or sharp objects penetrating the skull.

Pathophysiology

1. Acceleration-deceleration injuries
   a. The brain moves within the skull and is injured by impact with it.
   b. Contusions
   c. Subdural hematoma
   d. Alteration in consciousness
2. Compression injuries
   a. The inner table of the skull compresses the dura and brain.
   b. Depressed skull fracture
   c. Epidural hematoma
3. Primary brain injury: injury immediately caused by trauma (blunt, penetrating, or perforating)
4. Secondary brain injury: subsequent insults from hypoxia, hypercarbia, hypotension or hypertension, cerebral edema, expansile lesions, seizures, increased intracranial pressure, electrolyte abnormalities (e.g., hyponatremia, hypoglycemia)

Associated Clinical Features

1. The patient may present with loss of consciousness, vomiting, seizures, depressed mental status, or abnormal neurologic findings.
2. In a recent study of 608 infants (all <2 years of age), 14 of the 30 children with intracranial injury had no loss of consciousness, seizure activity, behavioral change, bulging fontanelle, depressed mental status, or abnormal neurologic findings. Thus, maintain a high index of suspicion for possible intracranial injury in infants, even in the absence of any findings.
3. Glasgow coma scale (GCS) score
   a. Allows quantification of neurologic findings and allows uniformity in description and communication among team members involved in taking care of the patient
   b. Not applicable once the patient is sedated and paralyzed
   c. GCS of 14 to 15 is categorized as mild head injury
   d. GCS of 9 to 13 is categorized as moderate head injury
   e. GCS <3 to 8 is categorized as severe head injury

Consultation

Neurosurgical consultation is warranted when you suspect the possibility of intracranial injury, and for all patients with penetrating injuries and those with abnormal CT findings.

Emergency Department Treatment and Disposition

1. Particular attention must be paid to airway, breathing, and circulation, and protection of the cervical spine in the event that there is concurrent spinal cord injury.

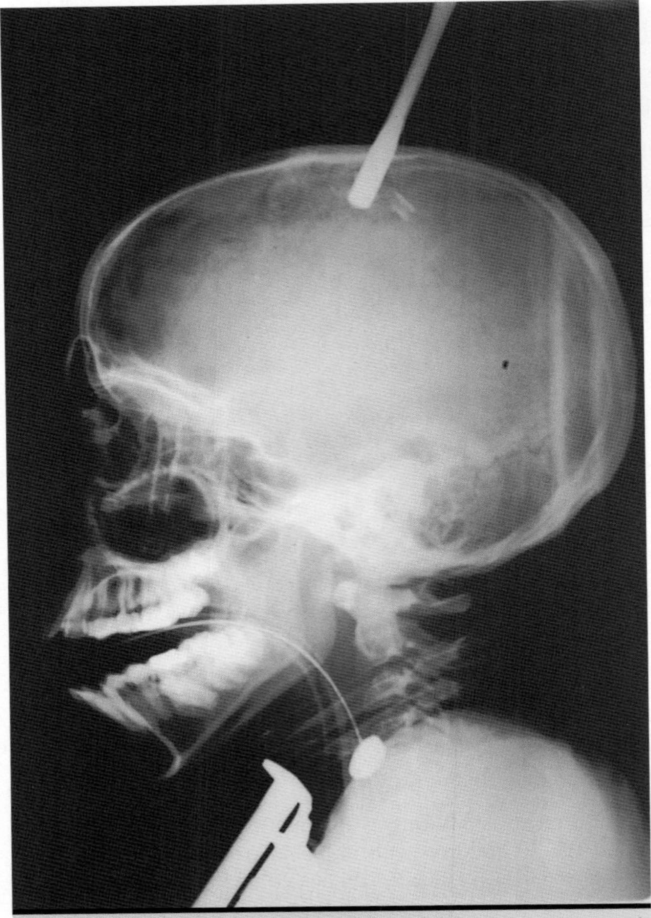

Figure 20-1. Penetrating Head Injury

Lateral skull x-ray of a 16-year-old male who was stabbed in the head with a screwdriver by another youth. The screwdriver, which is approximately 7 mm in diameter, is seen piercing through the top of the skull. The associated fracture and fracture fragments are also seen.

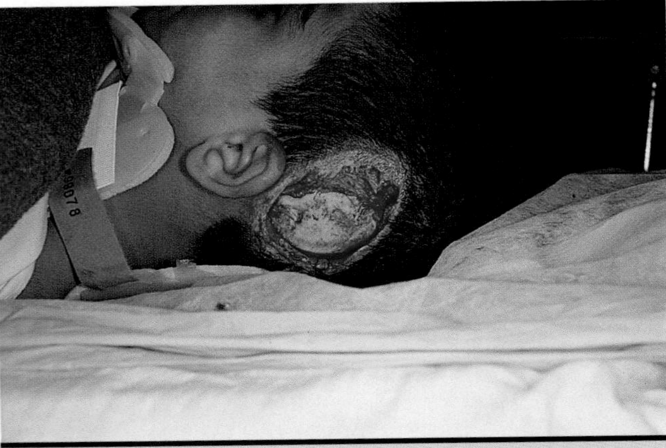

Figure 20-2. Scalp Laceration

A picture of a 6-year-old male who was dragged by a car. He sustained full-thickness scalp avulsions with extensive tissue loss. After initial stabilization and treatment of other injuries, the boy eventually required plastic surgical repair of the wound.

2. For the management of increased intracranial pressure, see page 555.
3. Seizures following head injuries (in either patients actively seizing or for prophylaxis) are usually treated with fosphenytoin.
4. In general, in children with serious head injuries, a complete blood count, type and cross-match, electrolytes, and coagulation studies should be performed. In adolescents, and if there is suspicion of their use, ethanol and toxicologic screens should be drawn.
5. Cervical spine films should be obtained in any alert patient with neck pain or neurologic deficits, and in all unconscious patients (see also C-spine injuries, Figs. 20-16 to 20-20).
6. CT scan of the head (without contrast) is the diagnostic study of choice to exclude intracranial injuries. Some examples of indications for CT scanning include:
   a. Loss of consciousness
   b. GCS <13
   c. Penetrating injury
   d. High-risk mechanism of injury
   e. Clinical signs of basilar or depressed skull fracture
   f. Posttraumatic seizure
   g. Focal neurological findings
   h. Scalp hematoma (especially parietal/temporal)
   i. Prolonged vomiting
   j. Prolonged lethargy
   k. Presence of amnesia
   l. Past history of bleeding diathesis (e.g., hemophilia)
   m. Significant past medical history (e.g., shunts)
   n. Suspected head injury in child abuse
7. All penetrating injuries require emergent neurosurgical evaluation and intervention. No attempt should be made to remove a foreign body penetrating the head in the ED.
8. Hospitalization is recommended for all patients with any of the following:
   a. Abnormal CT scan (abnormality due to acute trauma)
   b. History of loss of consciousness or deteriorating level of consciousness
   c. Penetrating injuries
   d. Focal or abnormal neurological examination
   e. Suspected abusive injuries
   f. Evidence of depressed or basilar skull fracture
   g. Skull fracture
   h. Other significant associated injuries
   i. Patients who are persistently symptomatic even with a normal CT scan (e.g., headache)
   j. Amnesia
   k. Unreliable caretaker at home
9. The American Academy of Pediatrics (AAP) guidelines for minor head injury for patients 2 to 20 years of age include:
   a. Definition of minor injury
      1) Isolated head injury

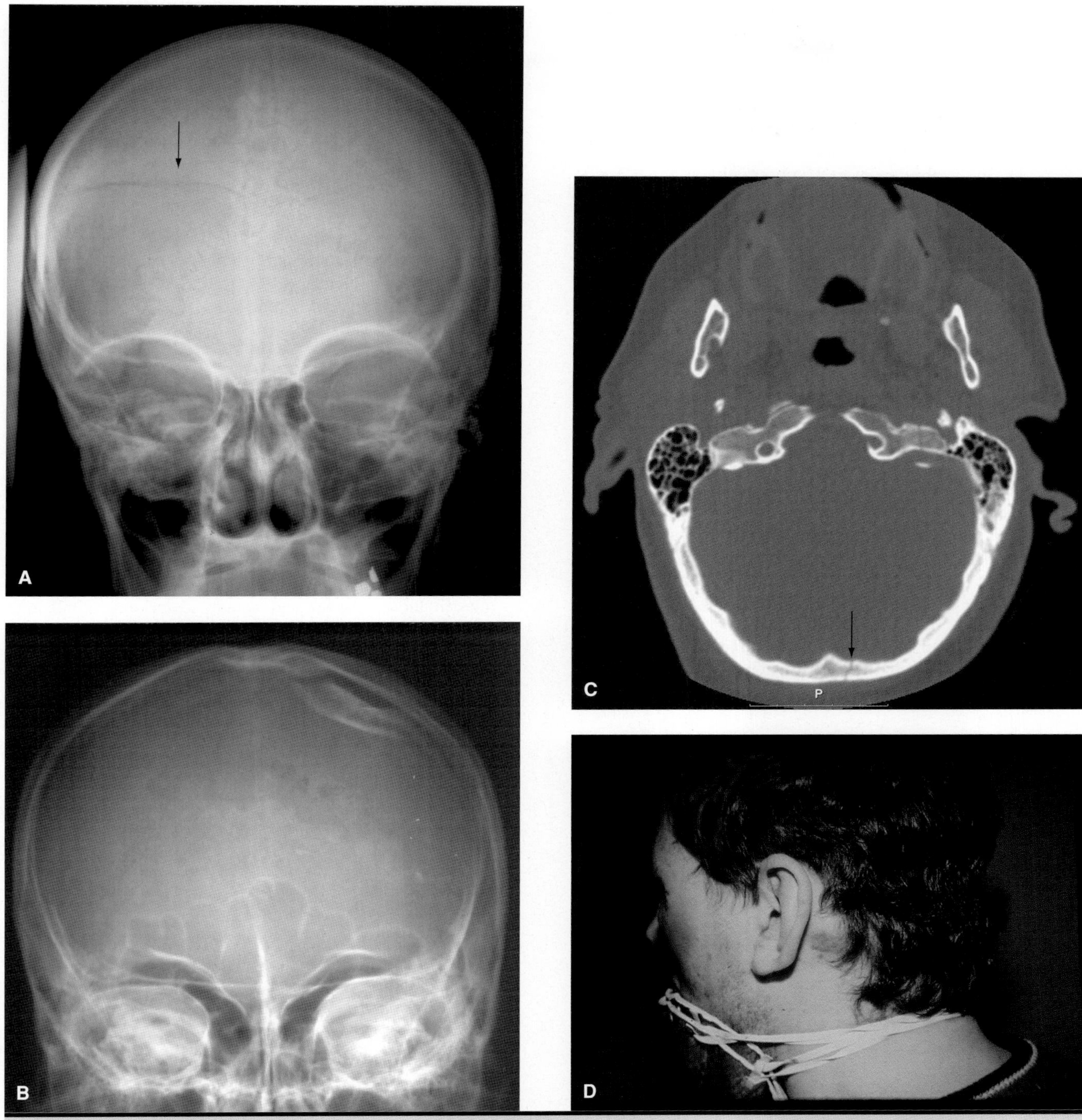

Figure 20-3. Skull Fractures

A. An AP skull x-ray of a young man who was struck on the head during a mugging. Note the linear fracture, which predominantly involves the right parietal bone. Since we rarely get skull films today, you will most frequently encounter skull fractures on the margins of cervical spine films and on facial films. *B*. This is a skull film of a youth who was beaten over the head with a hammer. On the AP view, note the depression of both tables and the diploic space of the left side of the cranium. Depressed skull fractures are more obvious when seen tangentially. *C*. CT scan with bony windows of a basilar skull fractures, including the petrous portion of the left temporal bone and the occipital bone. *D*. An image of a young man who sustained a basilar skull fracture after being beaten by several youths. He actually presented to the emergency department several days later with headaches and dizziness. The ecchymosis over the mastoid process is referred to as Battle's sign. (An image of a 4-year-old male who was involved in a motor vehicle accident and sustained a basilar skull fracture is shown in Fig. 2-13. Note the bilateral periorbital ecchymosis, giving the appearance of raccoon eyes. Also noteworthy is the fact that the child is free of subconjunctival hemorrhages which would likely be present had he sustained facial and ocular trauma).

2) Normal physical and neurological exam (including funduscopy)
3) Normal mental status
4) Loss of consciousness (LOC) <1 minute
5) Normal mental status at initial examination, even if prior emesis, headache, lethargy, or impact seizure

b. Recommendations include:
1) In the absence of LOC: observation in the ED or at home (with a reliable caretaker) and usually no need for head CT
2) In the presence of LOC: head CT
3) Head CT for high-risk patients (e.g., multiple trauma, children with unobserved LOC, patients with suspected C-spine injury, past history of bleeding diathesis, AV malformations or shunts, child abuse, or patients with a language barrier)

10. AAP guidelines for mild head injury for patients <2 years of age include:
a. Head CT for all patients with multiple trauma, bleeding diathesis, penetrating trauma, or suspected abusive head injuries
b. Head CT for those in the high-risk group (e.g., patients with depressed mental status or LOC, focal neurological findings, signs of depressed or basilar skull fracture, acute skull fracture, irritability, bulging fontanelles, seizures, progressively worsening vomiting, or <6 months of age)
c. Head CT for those in the intermediate-risk group (e.g., unwitnessed trauma, vague history, high-impact mechanism, scalp hematoma [especially temporoparietal], falls onto hard surfaces [especially in younger children], vomiting, lethargy or irritability, abnormal behavior, altered behavior for extended period)
d. Observation for those in the low-risk group (e.g., low-impact mechanism with infants >3 months of age)

11. All patients who are discharged home must be given written instructions that are clear to the caretaker, who must understand to return to the ED immediately with any of the following:
a. Excessive sleepiness or difficulty in awakening patient
b. Confusion or abnormal behavior
c. Progressive headache
d. Progressive vomiting or nausea
e. Abnormal gait
f. Ataxia
g. Unequal pupils, double vision, or any visual disturbance
h. Convulsions
i. Bleeding or watery drainage from the nose or ear

Clinical Pearls: Head Trauma

1. Diffuse brain injury (concussion or diffuse axonal injury) is the most common type of head injury.

2. Patients with epidural hematoma may present with the classic lucid interval and acutely deteriorate ("talk and die").

3. Prevent secondary brain injury in patients presenting with head trauma or multiple trauma (Fig. 20-4).

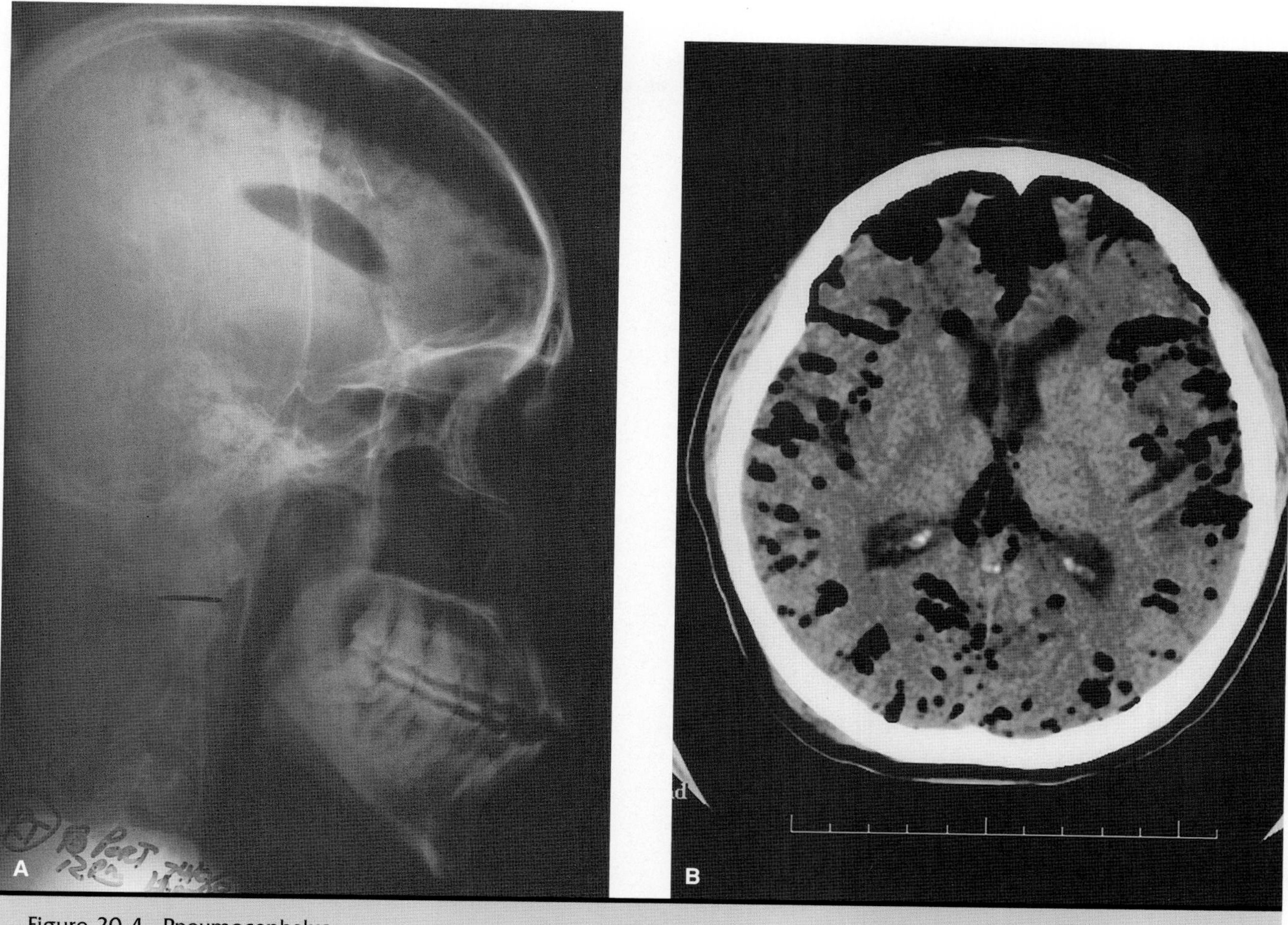

Figure 20-4. Pneumocephalus

A. Lateral skull film of a 19-year-old male who sustained multiple stab wounds to the head, demonstrating extensive pneumocephalus. The bony matrix could not be conclusively evaluated due to the pneumocephalus. *B*. A CT scan of the head of the same patient demonstrates numerous pockets of air in the sulci with marked subarachnoid pneumocephalus.

BOX 20-1. SCALP INJURIES

- Tend to bleed extensively secondary to the rich vascularization
- Subgaleal hematoma presents with extensive soft tissue swelling hours or days after the traumatic event.
- A subgaleal hematoma may persist for days or weeks.
- May require surgical (e.g., plastic surgeon) consultation
- Immediately control bleeding and fully evaluate the patient.

Clinical pearls

- Open scalp wounds should be carefully explored for foreign bodies, skull integrity, and evidence of a step-off or a depressed skull fracture.
- Relatively small scalp wounds may lead to hemodynamically significant blood loss.

BOX 20-2. CEREBRAL CONCUSSION

- A concussion is defined as a transient loss of responsiveness following head trauma.
- Presenting signs may include focal neurologic findings and seizures.
- Head CT scan may be used in addition to observation in the initial evaluation/management of children with minor closed head injury with LOC
- Concussion may be further classified as:

A. *Mild concussion*

(1) Consciousness is preserved.
(2) Associated with temporary neurologic dysfunction
(3) Patients may appear confused and disoriented.
(4) Either associated with no loss of memory (mild cases) or associated with lack of memory for events before (retrograde amnesia) or after (antegrade amnesia) the injury.
(5) Complete recovery is expected.

B. *Classic cerebral concussion*

(1) Associated with loss of consciousness
(2) Associated with post-traumatic amnesia

Clinical pearls

- Severity of injury correlates with duration of amnesia

BOX 20-3. CENTRAL NERVOUS SYSTEM INJURIES

- *Cerebral contusions (intracerebral hematomas)*
  (1) Cerebral contusions occur as the brain moves about within the skull.
  (2) A classic coup injury will occur at the site of impact, and a contrecoup injury will occur at a site remote to the impact site (Fig. 20-5).
  (3) Diagnosis by CT scan
  (4) A majority of contusions are seen in the frontal and temporal lobes (but they can occur anywhere in the brain).
  (5) Characterized by brain parenchymal swelling, tears of brain tissue, and small areas of hemorrhage
  (6) Often associated with subdural hematoma
  (7) Variable signs and symptoms
  (8) Neurosurgical consultation and admission required
- *Diffuse axonal injuries*
  (1) Prolonged posttraumatic coma that is not due to a mass lesion or ischemic insult
  (2) Patients remain comatose for prolonged periods.
  (3) Seen with acceleration-deceleration injuries
  (4) Diffuse brain swelling on CT scan
  (5) Shearing of axons with edema and punctate hemorrhages
  (6) Patients may show evidence of decortication or decerebration.
  (7) Significant morbidity with survival

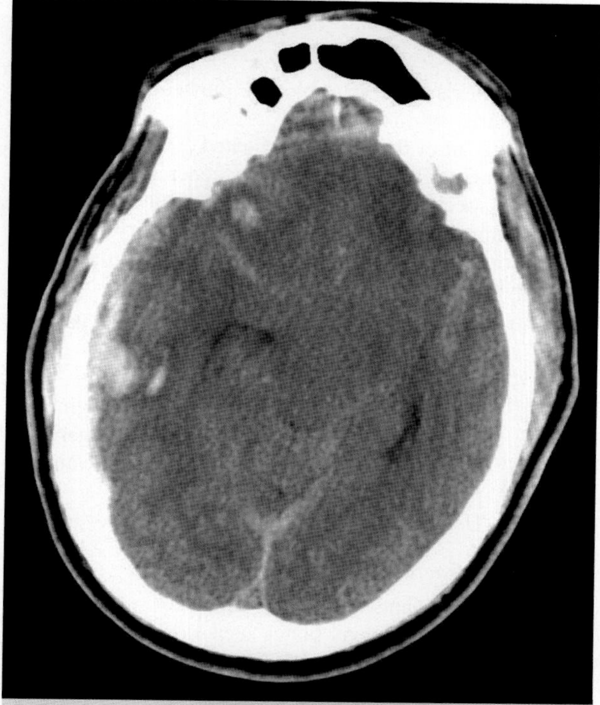

Figure 20-5. Coup and Contrecoup Injury

The head CT scan of a young male who after becoming intoxicated fell to the ground, striking the left side of his head. Note the large left-sided scalp contusion. Also note the right-sided cerebral contusion (contrecoup injury).

BOX 20-4. SKULL FRACTURES

(See also child abuse, Box 1-11)

A. *Linear nondepressed skull fractures*

- Implies a significant blow to the head (but not necessarily brain injury)
- CT scan of the head is indicated.
- Neurosurgical consultation is generally warranted.
- No specific treatment is required but management is directed to the underlying brain injury.
- Complication: growing fractures (leptomeningeal cyst)
  - (1) Unique to infants/young children (<2 years of age) after a skull fracture
  - (2) Associated with dural tears
  - (3) A leptomeningeal cyst may form (evagination of the dura matter, arachnoid membranes, and CSF into the fracture margins) in the postinjury period, and mandates follow-up.
  - (4) Usually seen 3 to 6 months after a linear fracture

B. *Diastatic fracture*

- Seen in infants and young children
- Separation of bony plates seen along suture lines

C. *Depressed fracture*

- Direct impact injury (e.g., hammer or baseball bat) (Figs. 20-3 and 20-6)
- Palpable bony depression or step-off unless presence of large hematoma
- Most common location occipital or temporal region
- Depressed portion can penetrate tissue and dura
- As a general guideline, fragments that are depressed more than the thickness of the skull require neurosurgical elevation.

D. *Open or compound fracture*

- Scalp laceration overlying the fracture (direct communication between scalp laceration and cerebral surface due to torn dura)
- Emergent neurosurgical consultation and early operative intervention (débridement of the brain and closure of the dura)
- Parenteral antibiotics

Clinical pearls

- Suture lines may be mistaken for skull fractures.
- Multiple fractures suggest child abuse.
- It takes considerable force to fracture the skull, and the significance of skull fracture should not be underestimated.
- Skull fractures are a better predictor of intracranial injury (ICI); however, ICI may occur in absence of skull fracture.
- Skull fractures increase the risk of ICI 20-fold.
- Skull fractures are often associated with scalp hematomas (particularly subgaleal).
- A boggy hematoma is a more sensitive predictor of intracranial injury than any other clinical sign.

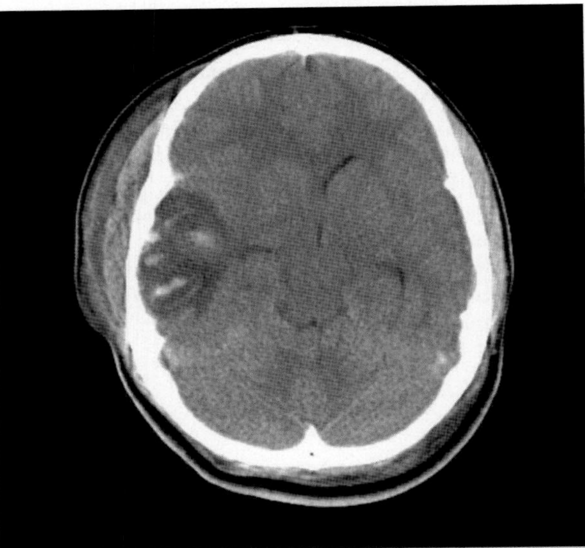

Figure 20-6. Cerebral Contusion with a Depressed Skill Fracture

Seen here is the head CT scan of a 15-year-old female involved in a motor vehicle accident that demonstrates a depressed skull fracture of the right frontoparietal bone with a large overlying scalp hematoma; also seen is a large right temporal and frontoparietal hemorrhagic contusion. There is also a mass effect with a slight shift in the midline toward the left.

BOX 20-5. BASILAR SKULL FRACTURE

- A basilar skull fracture is a fracture that occurs along the base of the skull.
- Typically occurs at the petrous portion of the temporal bone; however, it can occur anywhere along the base of the skull
- Clinical signs that suggest a basilar skull fracture include:
  (1) Hemotympanum
  (2) Cerebrospinal fluid (CSF) otorrhea
  (3) CSF rhinorrhea (double-ring test useful)
  (4) Raccoon eyes (see Fig. 2-13)
    a. Periorbital ecchymosis due to intraorbital bleeding from orbital roof fractures
    b. Absence of conjunctival injection or irritation
  (5) Battle's sign (postauricular ecchymosis suggesting a mastoid fracture)
  (6) Cranial nerve palsies
    a. Cranial nerves I, VII, VIII, and X may be involved.
    b. May be seen immediately or a few days after the injury
- Neurosurgical consultation is required.
- Radiologic investigation should include head CT, including imaging of the temporal bone.
- About 40% fractures are missed by CT.
- Admit the patient for observation of head injury.
- CSF leaks usually resolve in 1 week.
- Prophylactic antibiotics are usually not given (unless otherwise indicated).

Clinical pearls

- Usually results from considerable force; always rule out brain injury
- Must avoid nasogastric tube (may lead to inadvertent passage through an injured cribriform plate)
- Always suspect coincidental cervical spine injury.

BOX 20-6. EPIDURAL HEMATOMA

- Epidural hematoma (EDH) is a collection of blood between the skull and dura, causing compression of the underlying gyri and sulci (Fig. 20-7).
- The hemorrhage may be of arterial or venous origin.
- EDH is most often located in the temporal or temporoparietal area.
- A temporal EDH is often secondary to injury to the middle meningeal artery (about 80% of EDH) or injury to the middle meningeal vein and dura sinus.
- Diagnosis is confirmed by CT scan of the head.
- Typically seen as lenticular or biconvex areas of increased density
- EDH is usually unilateral and localized.
- About 60 to 80% are associated with fractures.
- EDH may cause shift of underlying ventricles across the midline.
- EDH can occur after seemingly trivial injuries (e.g., short falls) or in asymptomatic patients.
- A patient with EDH may present with an asymptomatic period (lucid period), followed by headache, vomiting, and altered mental status that may progress to signs and symptoms of uncal herniation.
- Signs of uncal herniation
  (1) Papillary changes (fixed or dilated pupil on the same side as EDH)
  (2) Hemiparesis on the opposite side
- About 30% present with a classic lucid interval, 30% with altered mental status, and 30% with seizures.
- Neurosurgical consultation is required
  (1) If EDH is small and patient is asymptomatic, close observation in a critical care unit with serial head CT scans are appropriate.
  (2) Operative intervention is warranted if EDH is large, expanding, or symptomatic.
- If treated early, the prognosis is usually excellent.

Clinical pearls

- Patients may occasionally develop an EDH after only minor head trauma. Their only symptoms may be headache or persistent vomiting. One must have a high index of suspicion, as rapid deterioration can ensue.
- Patients with EDH may present with the classic lucid interval followed by a sudden deterioration (so-called "talk and die").

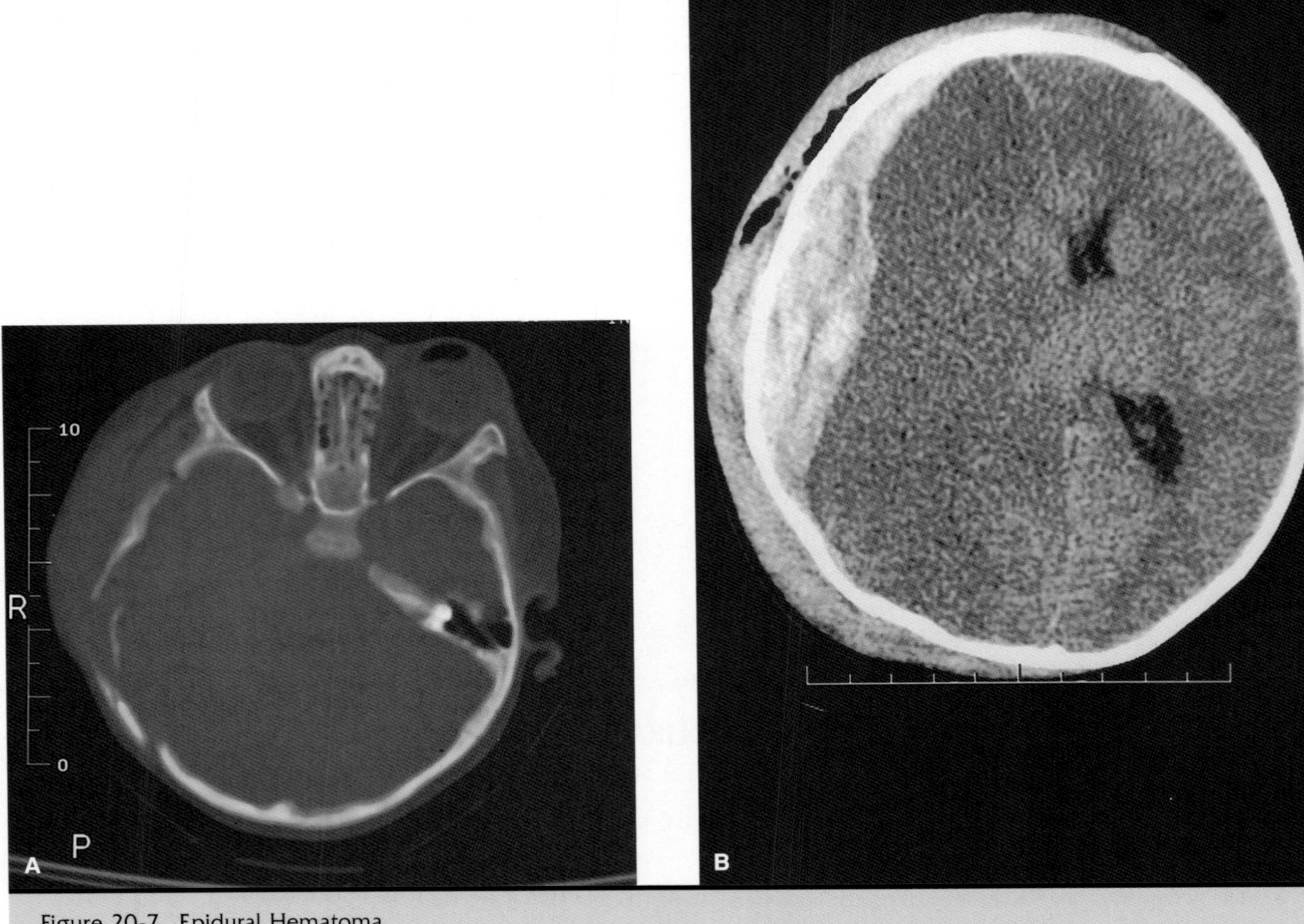

Figure 20-7. Epidural Hematoma

The head CT scan of a 12-month-old male who had a 27-inch television fall from a desktop onto his head as he lay on the floor below. *A*. This bony window demonstrates multiple skull fractures of the right frontal, temporal, and occipital bones. *B*. There is a large area of hyperdensity extending from the right frontal to the right parietal region, representing a large epidural hematoma. There is also extensive hypodensity involving the right cerebral hemisphere and left frontal lobe, with a significant mass effect compressing the right lateral ventricles and causing a midline shift to the left. Diffuse soft tissue swelling overlying the right side of the skull is also seen.

BOX 20-7. ACUTE SUBDURAL HEMATOMA

- Subdural hematoma (SDH) is venous bleeding from bridging veins between the dura and arachnoid membranes that cover the brain parenchyma (Fig. 20-8).
- SDHs are associated with significant mechanisms of injury and are often associated with underlying brain injury (e.g., intracerebral hematomas or contusions).
- About 30% have associated fractures.
- Typically seen as areas of increased density that appear concave or crescent-shaped, covering and compressing the gyri and sulci over an entire hemisphere.
- SDH may be bilateral.
- SDH occurs more commonly than epidural hematoma.
- SDH may cause a shift of underlying ventricles across the midline.
- Symptoms commonly include irritability, vomiting, lethargy (or fluctuations in level of consciousness), seizures, focal neurologic signs, and headache.
- Consultation with neurosurgery is required.
- Clinical triad of shaken impact syndrome (see child abuse, Figs. 1-17 through 1-19).
  (1) Intracranial injury (most often SDH), retinal hemorrhages, and skeletal fractures
  (2) Examine all patients with SDH closely for any other evidence of abuse (e.g., retinal hemorrhages, bony fractures, contusions, or bite marks).
- Keep a low threshold for consulting child protective services and social services in patients with SDH.

Clinical pearls

- Acute SDH occurs four times more commonly in adults than in children.
- SDH may result from direct trauma or from shaking injuries (tearing of the cortical bridging veins or bleeding from the cortex).
- The mechanism of injury for SDH is believed to be acceleration-deceleration; thus, SDH tends to be associated with more diffuse brain injury.

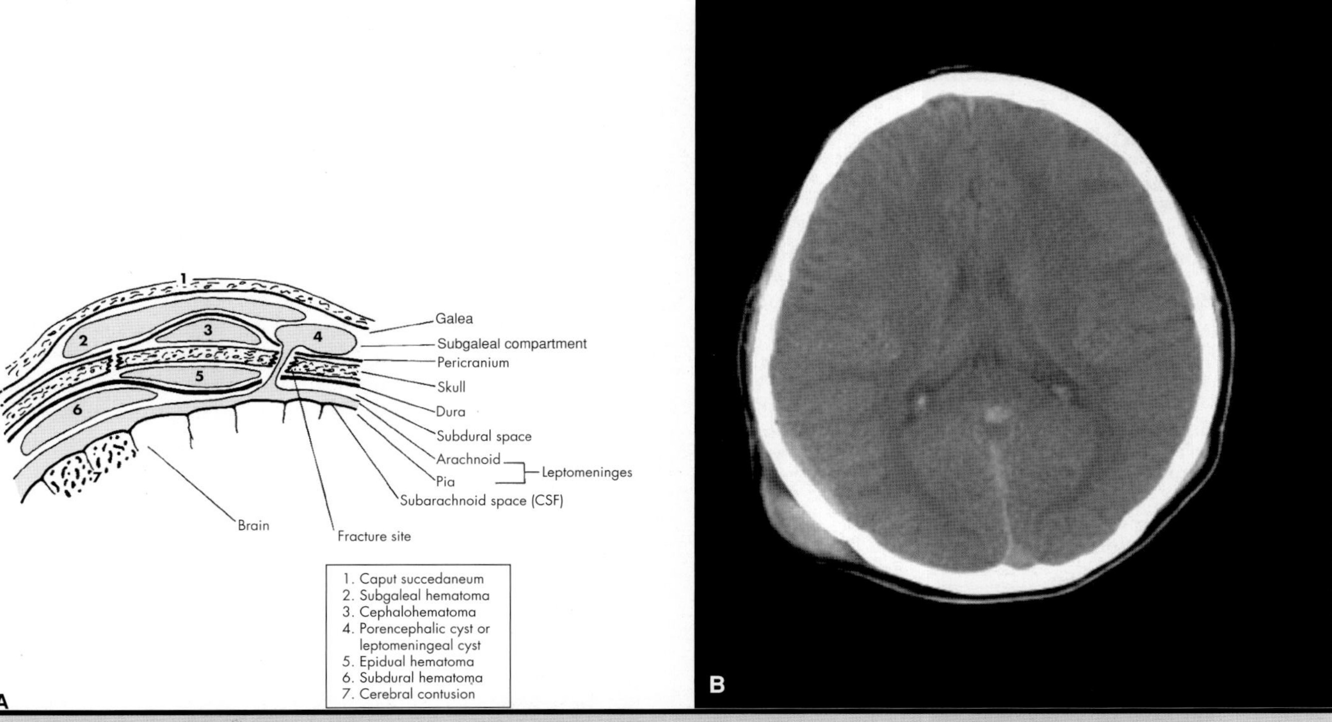

Figure 20-8. Subdural Hematoma

A. Traumatic head injuries. A schematic diagram demonstrating the different levels of the cranium and possible areas of bleeding. (Reproduced with permission from: Barkin RM, Rosen P: *Emergency Pediatrics*, 3rd ed. St. Louis, Mosby-Year Book, 1990, p. 59.) *B*. A CT scan showing a small subdural hematoma in the right posterior parietal area. There is also an overlying soft tissue contusion.

DIAGNOSIS MAXILLOFACIAL TRAUMA

Mechanism of Injury

1. The distribution of maxillofacial injuries in children is different from that in adults.
   a. Children have a preponderance of soft tissue injuries and a low incidence of facial fractures. This injury pattern occurs because infants and children have large craniums and foreheads, underdeveloped paranasal sinuses, prominent buccal fat pads, and elastic facial bones. Because of these anatomic differences, infants and young children most often sustain trauma to the frontal bone and rarely to the midface.
   b. By adolescence, injuries in children more closely parallel those of adults. The fracture pattern shifts to the midface and lower face.
2. The causes of facial trauma vary with age and activity level.
   a. Infants and young children are vulnerable to injury from birth trauma, falls, toys, motor vehicle crashes (MVCs), animal bites, and child abuse.
   b. Older children sustain injury from MVCs (passenger or pedestrian), bicycle crashes, falls, sports, or assaults.
   c. Children injured in MVCs most often are front-seat passengers or are inappropriately restrained for age and size.
3. Facial injuries from gunshot or stab wounds are uncommon in children. The incidence of these penetrating injuries increases in the adolescent population.

Associated Clinical Features

1. Soft tissue injury may result in abrasions, ecchymoses, hematomas, lacerations (Fig. 20-9), or edema.
2. Foreign bodies may be embedded in open wounds.
3. Blood or secretions inside the mouth should prompt a thorough evaluation for intraoral lacerations and dental injuries.
4. Numbness and sensory or motor deficits occur with nerve injury or entrapment.
5. Facial asymmetry or deformities, tenderness, step-offs, and crepitus are suggestive of fractures (Fig. 20-10).
6. Sublingual hematomas, malocclusion, and trismus are seen with mandible fractures.
7. Epistaxis can occur with midfacial fractures or nasal contusions.
8. Diplopia, changes in vision, restriction of extraocular movements, eye pain, photophobia, scleral injection, and abnormal papillary responses are indicative of globe injury or orbital fracture.
9. Altered mental status or neurological deficits suggest an associated head injury.

Laboratory Tests and Diagnostic Radiology

1. The timing and sequence of diagnostic imaging studies will depend on the patient's hemodynamic status and associated injuries. The diagnosis and treatment of life-threatening injuries always take precedence over imaging of facial fractures.
2. Plain radiography is readily available and can be used as the initial diagnostic study for evaluating facial fractures.
   a. Screening radiographs should consist of three views: Waters', posteroanterior (PA), and lateral. These views will identify most fractures. However, the value of plain radiography for diagnosing facial fractures in children is limited, because plain films may fail to clearly define an injury.
   b. Additional views may be helpful for specific injuries:
      1) Submental vertex view: ideal for diagnosing zygomatic arch fractures
      2) Towne's view: images the condyles of the mandible
      3) Right and left lateral oblique: demonstrates the body and ramus of the mandible
   c. Mandible fractures
      1) Plain radiographs are generally acceptable to diagnose mandible fractures.
      2) CT is not routinely used to assess these fractures.
      3) The typical mandible series includes a PA, Towne's, and right and left lateral oblique views.
      4) The panoramic radiograph is most informative and remains the gold standard for identifying mandible fractures.
3. CT scanning is generally superior to plain films for delineating facial fractures.
   a. Noncontrast CT scanning can be performed as the initial diagnostic imaging study, or it may be used selectively to further define injuries seen on plain films.
   b. In addition, a high percentage of patients with facial injury will require diagnostic imaging to evaluate an associated head injury. In stable patients, the head, neck, and face can all be scanned in a matter of minutes.
   c. If there is clinical suspicion of an orbital fracture, axial and coronal cuts in 2- to 3-mm sections through the orbits should be requested.

Complications

1. Airway compromise may occur from blood, secretions, or mechanical obstruction of the tongue.
2. Concomitant head injury may result in altered mental status or neurological deficits.
3. Infection may complicate facial injuries, particularly those with oral or sinus communication, wounds with devitalized tissue, and open fractures.
4. Bleeding from facial injuries may be profuse.

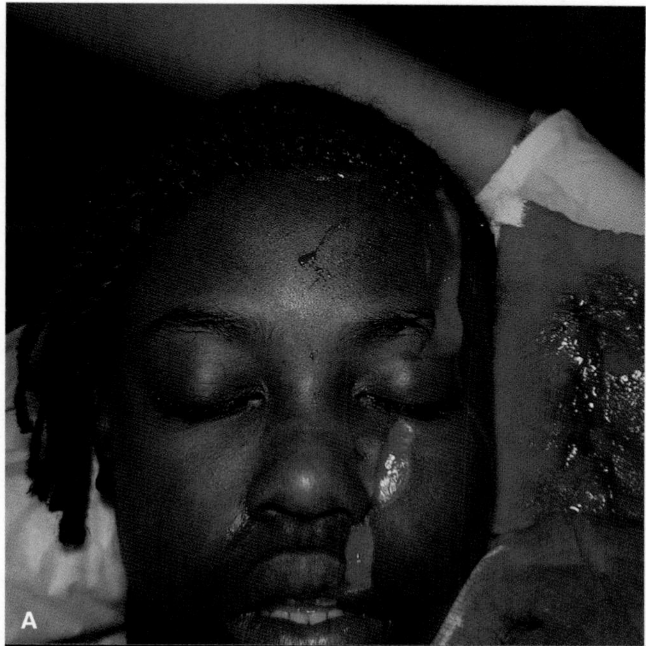

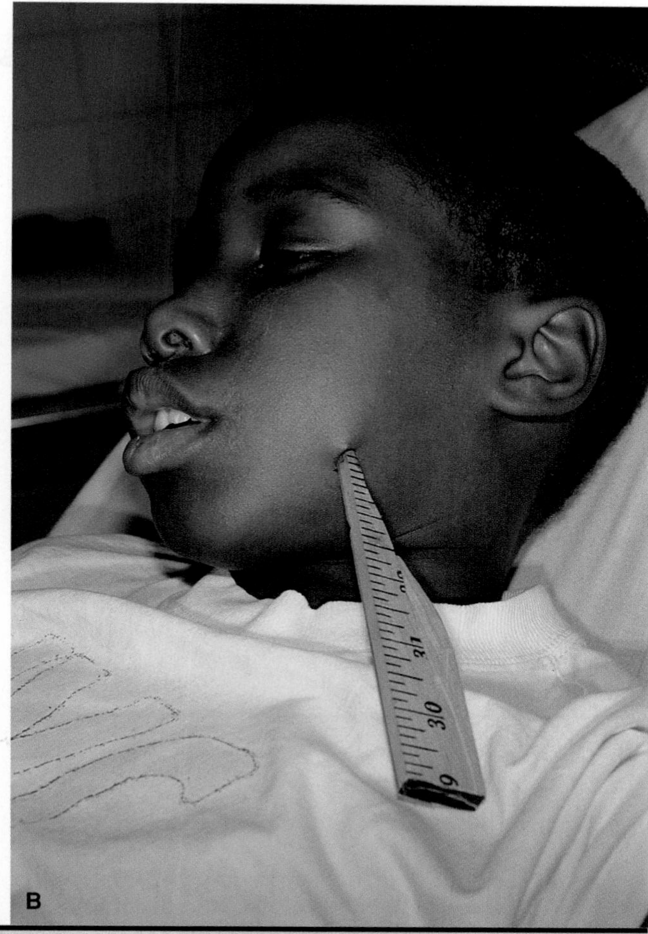

Figure 20-9. Facial Lacerations

A. An image of an 11-year-old female who sustained a slash to the face involving the forehead, upper eyelid, cheek, and upper lip. The eye was not involved, but the lip laceration went through the vermilion border. Extensive lacerations such as this one should always be repaired with specialist consultation, preferably in the operating room. *B*. Picture of a 7-year-old boy who fell while running with a wooden ruler in his hand. The ruler broke and the sharp end pierced his cheek and became embedded in his gingival-buccal fold. The wooden piece was removed and the oral lesions were repaired. After thorough irrigation, the cheek laceration was repaired.

5. Facial lacerations can result in transection of the lacrimal apparatus or parotid duct. The facial and trigeminal nerves are also at risk for injury.
6. Fractures in childhood heal quickly. Diagnostic delay in recognition and treatment of fractures may require later revisional procedures. This can result in cosmetic deformities.
7. There may be long-term developmental complications due to abnormal growth of injured pediatric facial bones.
8. Scarring of the face may cause long-term psychological problems.

Consultation

Generally, children with maxillofacial injuries have sustained major trauma and have multiple associated injuries. Early involvement of subspecialists and a coordinated team approach will ensure optimal care from initial stabilization through definitive treatment of specific injuries. Management of facial trauma may require the expertise of multiple specialists, including oral and maxillofacial surgeons; ear, nose, and throat specialists; plastic surgeons; and ophthalmologists.

Emergency Department Treatment and Disposition

1. Most children with facial trauma have significant associated injuries. They are particularly vulnerable to skull fractures and intracranial injuries. Initial management should be directed at stabilization of life-threatening injuries.
   a. Establishing a patent airway is the primary concern. Blood or secretions may obstruct the airway. Loss of

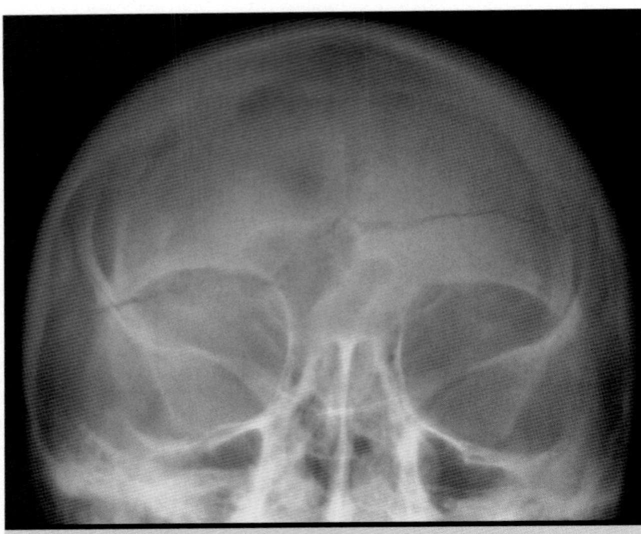

Figure 20-10. Frontal Bone Fracture

This is an x-ray of a youth who sustained a blow to the forehead. The fracture through the frontal bone communicates with the frontal sinus. Communication of a fracture with an air-containing structure necessitates treatment as an open fracture.

tongue support and airway obstruction can occur in patients with mandible fractures. In addition, an altered mental status can further compromise the airway. Oropharyngeal suctioning and an oral airway may relieve the obstruction. Endotracheal intubation establishes a definitive airway and should be performed in any unstable patient.

   b. Intravenous access should be established. Active bleeding should be controlled with digital pressure. Intraoral bleeding may require repair with absorbable sutures for hemostasis.
   c. There is a risk of associated cervical spine injuries. Cervical spine immobilization should be maintained.

2. Once the patient is stabilized, the maxillofacial region can then be evaluated. A thorough history should be elicited. Details of the mechanism of injury and any signs or symptoms of injury should be documented. Physical examination should be performed in an organized manner so that subtle injuries are not missed. In particular, attention should be directed at examination of the eyes, soft tissues, nerves, facial bones, and dentition.

3. The globe and orbits should be the initial focus of examination. Acute intervention may be required to repair injuries that could permanently impair sight. In addition, progressive lid and periorbital edema may make delayed examination of the globe difficult or impossible.
   a. Test visual acuity (as appropriate for age).
   b. Inspect eyelids for lacerations, edema, ptosis, and possible lacrimal injury.
   c. Assess extraocular movements.
   d. Perform a complete examination of the globe, including a funduscopic and slit lamp exam if suspicion of injury
   e. If suspicion of ruptured globe, place a protective eye shield and request immediate ophthalmology consultation
   f. Palpate the orbital rim for tenderness, step-offs, crepitus, and subcutaneous emphysema.

4. Visually inspect the face for asymmetry, edema, ecchymosis, and lacerations.
   a. Lacerations may be in proximity to bony injuries.
   b. If suspicion of fracture, treat as open fracture with intravenous antibiotics, tetanus update, and subspecialty consultation

5. Palpate facial bones for evidence of mobility and fractures.

6. Examine the nose both externally and internally.
   a. Control persistent epistaxis with nasal packing.
   b. Drain septal hematomas.

7. Examine the ears for bleeding, otorrhea, lacerations, avulsions, and auricular hematomas. Auricular hematomas require drainage, compressive dressings, and antibiotics.

8. The mandible should be evaluated for tenderness, displacement, and malocclusion.

9. The alveolar ridge should be examined for stability and tenderness. Loose or avulsed teeth should be noted. Be aware of possible aspiration of avulsed teeth.

10. A full motor and sensory exam should be performed to evaluate nerve injury.

11. Assess possible parotid gland or duct injuries in patients with penetrating trauma.

12. Antibiotics may be beneficial for intraoral lacerations or wounds with significant devitalized tissue.

13. Check status of tetanus prophylaxis in patients with penetrating injuries.

14. Children may be difficult to evaluate because they are frightened, confused, or in pain.
    a. Analgesia must be given promptly.
    b. Sedation may be required to ensure cooperation during diagnostic evaluation and repair of injuries.

15. Following complete clinical evaluation, radiographic studies are performed to assess facial fractures.

16. Children with maxillofacial injuries who have concomitant intracranial or multiple organ system injuries should be admitted to a pediatric intensive care unit.

17. Complex facial fractures, severe ocular injuries, or extensive facial lacerations may require hospitalization for surgical repair.

18. Simple soft tissue or bony injuries can generally be treated in the emergency department, with subspecialty consultation as needed. If specialty expertise is unavailable, patients with significant maxillofacial trauma should be stabilized and transferred to a regional trauma center.

Clinical Pearls: Maxillofacial Trauma

1. Airway compromise is a potential complication of facial trauma. Maintaining airway patency is always the primary concern.
2. Facial injuries in children are often part of a compendium of injuries. Care must initially be directed at treatment of life-threatening injuries. Once stabilization is achieved, focus can then turn to evaluation and treatment of facial injuries.
3. Children may be uncooperative and therefore difficult to evaluate and treat. The consequences of delayed recognition and treatment of injuries can be devastating. Adequate analgesia and sedation will expedite patient care.
4. Nasal trauma with subsequent bleeding into the nasal septum can result in a septal hematoma (Fig. 20-11). The hematoma must be evacuated immediately. Complications of an untreated septal hematoma include septal necrosis, infection, perforation, and collapse (saddle-nose deformity).
5. Knowledge of the anatomical relationships between various facial structures will aid in identification of specific injuries.
6. Early involvement of subspecialists will ensure optimal patient care.

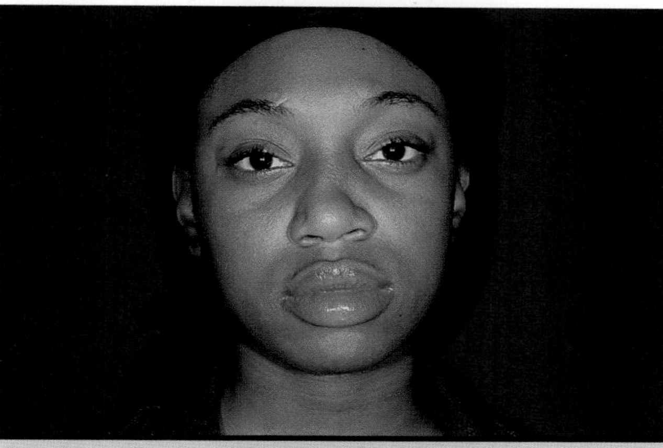

Figure 20-11. Nasal Fracture

This is an image of a 17-year-old female who fell against a chair. There is obvious deviation of the bridge of the nose. In the ED bleeding was controlled with local pressure. The patient was referred for ENT consultation. There was no nasal septal hematoma upon inspection of either nostril.

BOX 20-8. FACIAL FRACTURES

- *Frontal bone fractures*
  (1) Occur frequently in young children because of their prominent foreheads
  (2) These fractures should raise concern of an underlying intracranial injury.
  (3) Linear fractures are managed conservatively.
  (4) Significant bony depression or an underlying hematoma of the brain warrant surgical intervention.
- *Nasal fractures*
  (1) May be diagnosed clinically by deviation, gross deformity, crepitus, step-off, or mobility of nasal bones. Edema of the nose may mask these signs of fracture.
  (2) Always examine the nose with an internal speculum to identify a septal hematoma.
  (3) The nasal septum plays an important role in midfacial growth and aesthetics. Thus, the presence of a hematoma, if not emergently drained, may lead to necrosis and damage to the cartilaginous septum.
  (4) Persistent epistaxis should be controlled with nasal packing. When packing is placed, prophylactic antibiotics are indicated to prevent toxic shock syndrome.
  (5) Simple nasal fractures require no acute intervention beyond control of epistaxis, ice, and analgesics.
  (6) Rapid healing of nasal bones in children necessitates closed reduction of significantly displaced fractures within 5 to 7 days.
- *Naso-orbital-ethmoid (NOE) fractures*
  (1) Fracture involves the bone to which the medial canthal tendon is attached.
  (2) NOE structures are driven back into the intraorbital space.
  (3) Classic findings are a flattened nasal dorsum and telecanthus (widening of the interpalpebral distance).
  (4) Injuries to the lacrimal apparatus and orbital structures are common.
  (5) Examine for CSF rhinorrhea
  (6) Adequate fracture reduction by subspecialists will prevent significant deformity.
- *Zygomaticomaxillary complex fractures (tripod fractures)*
  (1) Involve separation of all three major attachments of the zygoma to the face
  (2) Fracture lines are at the zygomaticotemporal suture, zygomaticofrontal suture, and infraorbital rim.
  (3) Clinical signs may include flatness of the cheek, paresthesia (due to infraorbital nerve impingement), trismus, epistaxis, step deformities, or diplopia (secondary to edema, hematoma, or entrapment of extraocular muscles).
  (4) Associated with a large amount of facial edema that may mask facial deformities
  (5) The patient needs ophthalmologic evaluation for any suspected ocular injury.
  (6) *Key point: Isolated zygomatic arch fractures are uncommon in children.*
- *Maxillary fractures*
  (1) Rare in young children
  (2) Incidence increases in older children as paranasal sinuses develop
  (3) Often secondary to high-speed MVCs
  (4) *Le Fort I (transmaxillary fracture):* separation of the maxilla from the midface; a mobile maxilla and open bite are present
  (5) *Le Fort II (pyramidal fracture):* involves the maxilla, nasal bones, and medial aspect of the orbits; both the nose and maxilla are mobile
  (6) *Le Fort III (craniofacial dysjunction):* complete separation of the midface from the base of the skull; patients have a dish-shaped facial appearance with mobility at the nasofrontal and zygomaticofrontal sutures
  (7) LeFort II and III: bilateral periorbital ecchymosis (raccoon eyes) may be present; epistaxis is common; if CSF rhinorrhea is present, treat as an open skull fracture
  (8) *Key point:* Pure Le Fort injuries are rarely seen; patients can have a combination of any of these fractures.
- *Mandible fractures* (Fig. 20-12)
  (1) Risk of airway compromise, especially if bilateral fractures
  (2) May present with malocclusion, trismus, hematoma, ecchymosis, or inability to close the jaw due to severe displacement
  (3) Paresthesia of the lower lip and chin are present if the inferior alveolar nerve is injured.
  (4) A single fracture necessitates a thorough search for a second fracture on the contralateral side of the mandible.
  (5) Potential complications include injury to permanent teeth, growth disturbances with subsequent facial asymmetry, and ankylosis of the mandibular condyle.
  (6) Most fractures are managed with closed reduction and intermaxillary fixation.

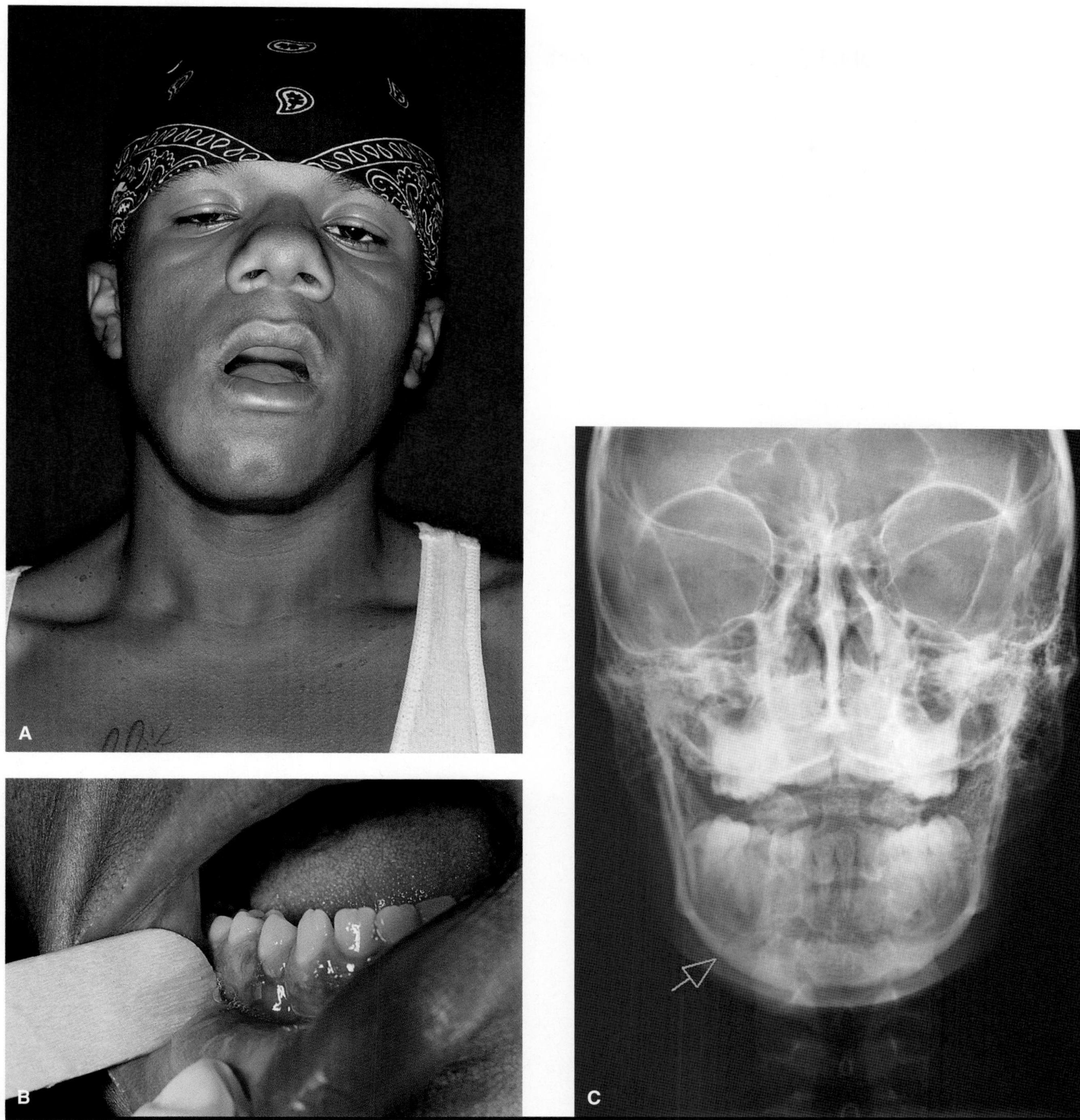

Figure 20-12. Mandible Fracture

A. Picture of a 17-year-old male who was hit in the jaw with a bat, sustaining a mandible fracture on the right side. The fracture line went through the body of the mandible and caused malalignment of the teeth on that side. The malalignment and pain caused an inability to fully open the mouth. *B*. Examination of the oral cavity demonstrated that the fracture line had extended up through the gingiva and into the oral cavity. Apart from the ultimate fixation of the fracture, the patient required admission for parenteral antibiotics, which were started in the ED. *C*. An x-ray of the frontal view of the mandible, demonstrating the fracture on the right (*arrow*).

BOX 20-9. SOFT TISSUE FACIAL INJURIES ASSOCIATED WITH FACIAL FRACTURES

- *Parotid duct injury*
  (1) The location of the parotid duct is approximated by drawing a line from the tragus of the ear to the middle of the upper lip. The duct usually enters the mouth at the level of the second maxillary molar.
  (2) Intraoral blood at the orifice of the duct signifies injury.
  (3) The transverse facial artery and buccal branches of the facial nerve are located superiorly to the duct. Buccal branch palsy is suggestive of duct transection.
  (4) If suspicion of parotid duct injury, cannulate the distal duct intraorally, irrigate with saline, and watch the wound for effluent
  (5) The most commonly injured portion of the duct is superficial to the masseter muscle. Immediate operative repair is advised for duct injuries at this location.
  (6) Parotid fistulas or sialoceles (periductal accumulation of saliva) are complications of unrecognized injury.
- *Facial nerve injury*
  (1) Evaluate facial nerve integrity prior to administration of local anesthetic for laceration repair.
  (2) The buccal branch of the facial nerve is superficial to the parotid duct. Presume facial nerve damage if the parotid duct is injured.
  (3) Immediately explore and operatively repair branches of the facial nerve posterior to a line perpendicular to the lateral canthus of the eye. Anterior to this line, repair is usually not warranted due to spontaneous reinnervation of smaller branches.
- *Trigeminal nerve injury*
  (1) If injury occurs to the trigeminal nerve, suspect an associated facial fracture.
  (2) The inferior alveolar (mandibular fracture) and infraorbital (zygomaticomaxillary complex fractures) are the most commonly injured nerve branches.
  (3) Treat by reducing fractures. If symptoms persist in 6 to 12 weeks, consider nerve exploration.
- *Injury to the lacrimal outflow system*
  (1) Increased frequency with naso-orbital-ethmoid fractures and damage to the medial canthal ligament
  (2) Suspect in eyelid lacerations located in the medial third
  (3) Can test patency of the duct by injecting fluorescein into the conjunctival sac and observing dye in the nose (Jones I test)
  (4) Primary repair by specialists recommended within 48 hours of injury
- *Eyelid injuries*
  (1) Always check for underlying globe injury.
  (2) Improper repair of lid margin lacerations may lead to deformity (entropion, ectropion). Optimal repair is performed in the operating room.
  (3) Horizontal lacerations of the upper lid may sever the levator palpebrae muscle. Careful approximation is necessary to prevent ptosis and loss of levator function.
- *Auricular hematomas (cauliflower ear)*
  (1) Occur as a result of shearing forces to the auricle that cause hematoma formation between the perichondrium and the underlying cartilage
  (2) As the perichondrial blood supply is cut off by the expanding hematoma, cartilage dies and is replaced by fibrocartilaginous scar tissue, resulting in cauliflower ear.
  (3) Treat with incision and drainage of the hematoma, compression (to prevent recurrence), and antibiotics.
- *Lip lacerations involving the vermilion border*
  (1) Careful alignment is required in order to ensure good cosmetic results.
  (3) Mark the wound with methylene blue prior to repair, as local anesthesia may cause distortion of the border.
- *Through-and-through lacerations involving the oral mucosa and skin*
  (1) Layered closure is required: first, irrigate and repair the inner mucosa with absorbable sutures. Next, irrigate and repair the muscularis, subcutaneous tissue, and skin.
  (2) Failure to perform a careful, layered closure may result in a buccal hematoma or infection.
  (3) Antibiotics with anaerobic coverage are recommended.

BOX 20-10. ORBITAL FRACTURES

- *Medial wall fractures*
  (1) The medial wall of the orbit is formed primarily by the thin lamina papyracea of the ethmoid bone; thus, the anatomic weakness makes it susceptible to fracture.
  (2) Orbital emphysema may be present.
  (3) Entrapment of the medial rectus muscle can lead to limited abduction.
  (4) Evaluate possible lacrimal injury.
  (5) Treatment is supportive.
  (6) Follow-up eye examinations are recommended.
  (7) Surgery is indicated if persistent symptoms of enophthalmos or diplopia are present.
- *Orbital blowout fractures* (Fig. 20-13)
  (1) Caused by a sudden increase in intraorbital pressure when an object larger than the size of the orbit (e.g., baseball, fist) impacts the orbit
  (2) The thin orbital floor fractures easily.
  (3) Intraorbital soft tissue contents herniate into the maxillary sinus.
  (4) Entrapment of extraocular muscles may occur.
  (5) Clinical signs include periorbital edema/ ecchymosis, enophthalmos, and numbness along the infraorbital nerve distribution.
  (6) Diplopia and restricted extraocular movements are signs of muscle entrapment.
  (7) Always evaluate possible globe injury.
  (8) Immediate ophthalmologic consultation for globe injury or muscle entrapment

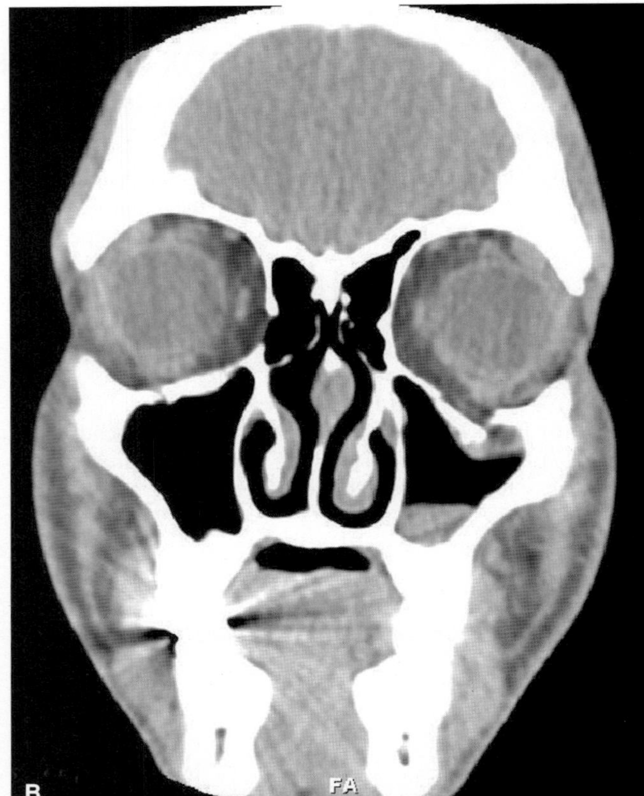

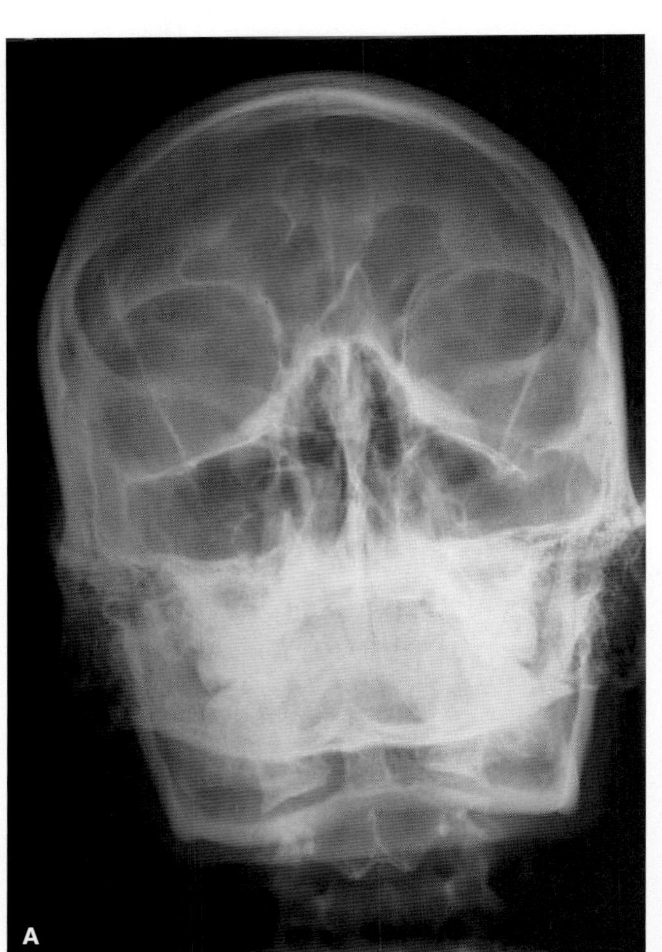

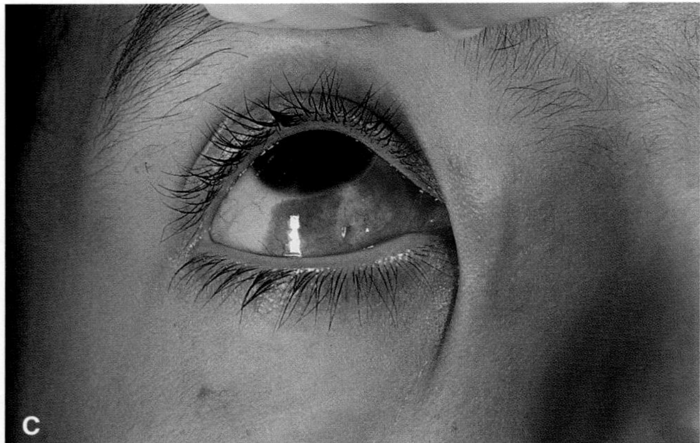

Figure 20-13. Orbital Fracture and Subconjunctival Hemorrhage

A. A facial film of a 16-year-old male who sustained a punch to the face. There is an orbital floor fracture on the left with a fluid level in the left maxillary sinus, most likely caused by blood. *B*. A CT scan of the orbits of the same patient as in part *A*. Here, the blowout fracture of the left orbital floor is clearly displayed, as is the blood in the left maxillary sinus. No evidence of inferior rectus muscle entrapment is noted. *C*. An image of a 6-year-old girl who sustained a subconjunctival hemorrhage as a result of an air bag deployment in a low-speed motor vehicle accident. This was an isolated finding and there was no other ocular injury. When not associated with other ocular injuries, subconjunctival hemorrhages are purely cosmetic, but they are often of great concern to the patient's family. With direct ocular trauma, the cornea, anterior chamber, and visual acuity should be scrutinized. In this case, slit-lamp evaluation should be performed. Occasionally subconjunctival hemorrhages can be caused by rubbing the eye with a conjunctival foreign body or even by a forceful sneeze or cough. It is rare for these mechanisms to have associated ocular injuries. Subconjunctival hemorrhages fade to green and yellow and resolve spontaneously in several weeks.

DIAGNOSIS PEDIATRIC CERVICAL SPINE TRAUMA

Mechanism of Injury

1. Cervical spine injuries (CSI) in infants and children are caused by motor vehicle crashes (MVCs), falls from heights, sports injuries (e.g., diving, football), child abuse, and rarely birth trauma.

2. Gunshot and stab wounds occur infrequently in young children. The incidence of CSI from penetrating trauma increases during adolescence.

3. Spinal injuries are rare in children, accounting for 1 to 10% of all spinal injuries reported. Despite this lower incidence, mortality is higher among spine-injured children than adults. Serious neurologic sequelae occur in less than 1% of all children hospitalized with a history of spinal injury.

4. Spinal cord injury in children <8 years of age occurs mainly in the upper cervical vertebrae and is associated with a high risk of neurologic sequelae. This is due to the relative ligamentous and joint capsule laxity, relative muscle weakness, large head-to-body ratio, incomplete ossification of cartilaginous elements, and horizontal orientation of shallow facet joints. After 8 years of age, the fulcrum of cervical spinal movement changes to the adult pattern of C5 to C6.

5. Multilevel spinal injuries occur more frequently in children. Sixteen percent occur at noncontiguous levels.

Associated Clinical Features

1. Clinical signs and symptoms associated with CSI include:
   a. Paresis, paralysis, flaccidity, ataxia, spasticity and loss of rectal tone
   b. Pain, sensory deficits, temperature instability, paresthesias and loss of anal wink
   c. Altered mental status secondary to concomitant head trauma
   d. Neck pain, torticollis (Fig. 20-14), limitation of motion, and muscle spasm
   e. Abnormal or absent reflexes
   f. Clonus without rigidity
   g. Diaphragmatic breathing without retractions
   h. Neurogenic shock (hypotension with bradycardia)
   i. Blood pressure variability with flushing and sweating
   j. Fluctuating body temperature
   k. Priapism and decreased bladder function
   l. Fecal retention and unexplained ileus
   m. Autonomic hyperreflexia

2. There may be associated injuries. These include head and facial trauma, soft tissue injury, and abdominal, chest, and extremity trauma.

3. There is an increased risk of cervical spine (C-spine) trauma associated with various congenital anomalies. These include aplasia, hypoplasia of the odontoid, block vertebrae, Klippel-Feil syndrome, Down syndrome, skeletal dysplasia (e.g., Morquio's syndrome and diastrophic dwarfism), juvenile chronic arthritis, pharyngeal infection, and os odontoideum. The latter abnormality refers to an oval or round ossicle with a smooth cortical border located in the position of the odontoid process and thought to arise from nonunion of an unrecognized odontoid fracture.

Radiologic Studies

1. For initial assessment of the cervical spine:
   a. The minimum studies required for initial assessment of the cervical spine include a *supine lateral view, an AP view, and an open-mouth odontoid view* (Fig. 20-15).

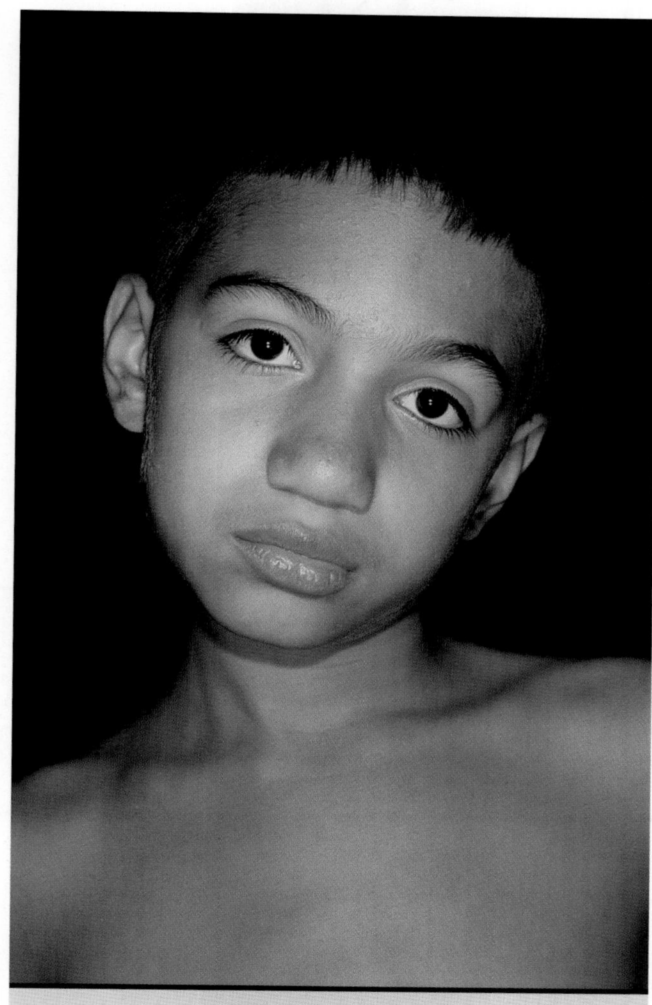

Figure 20-14. Torticollis

An image of an 11-year-old male with an acute onset of atraumatic torticollis. Although torticollis may be a presenting sign of cervical spine injury, it more commonly has an atraumatic cause.

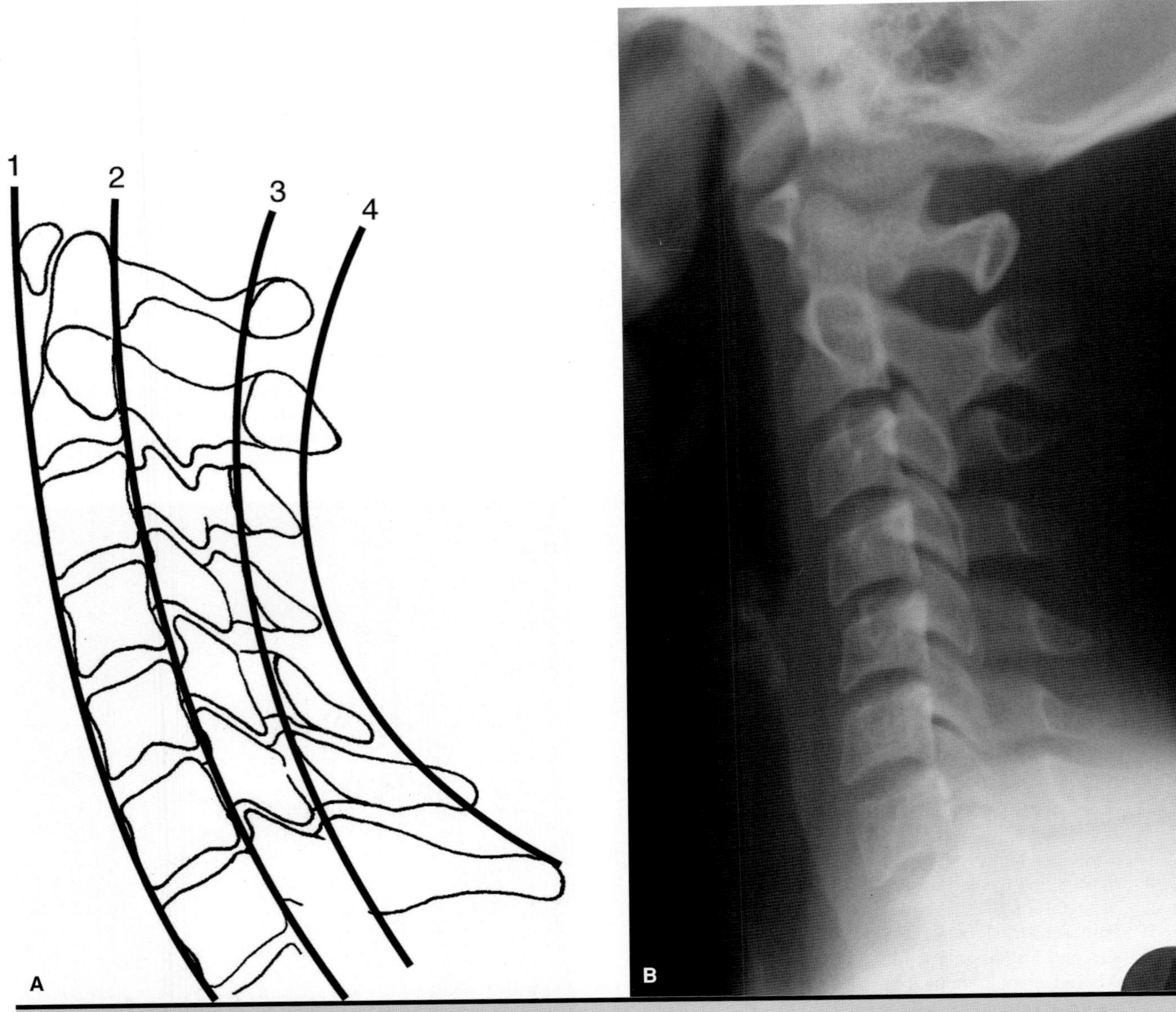

Figure 20-15. Normal Cervical Spine

A. Vertebral alignment of the lateral cervical spine. The four curves of the lateral cervical spine are shown: (1) anterior vertebral body line, (2) posterior vertebral body line, (3) spinolaminar line, and (4) tips of the spinous processes. (Reproduced with permission from: Ruoff B, West OC: The cervical spine. In: Schwartz DT, Reisdorff EJ, (eds). *Emergency Radiology*. McGraw-Hill, New York, 2000, p. 284.) *B*. Normal lateral cervical spine. Note the uniformity without bulging of the prevertebral soft tissue spaces, the normal alignment of the anterior and posterior vertebral margins, the uniformity in height of the disc spaces, and the uniformity of intervals between the spinous processes.

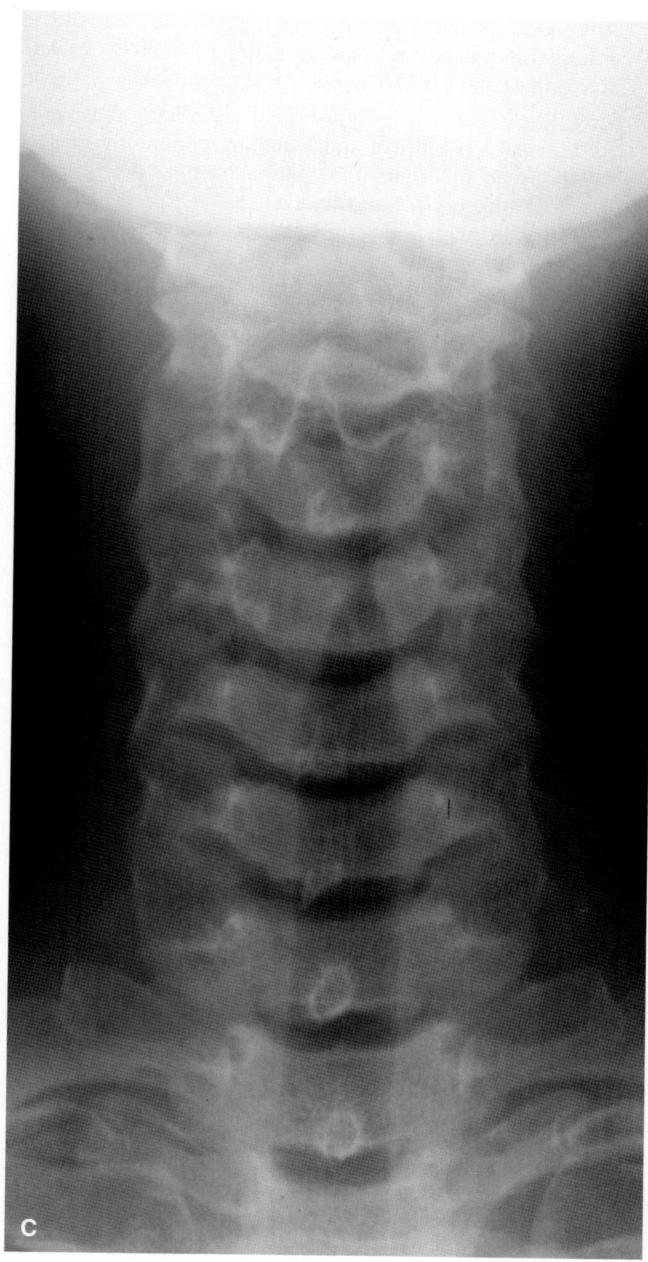

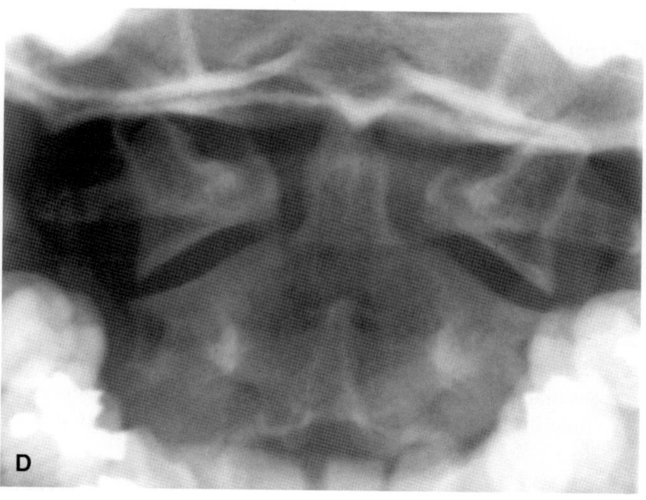

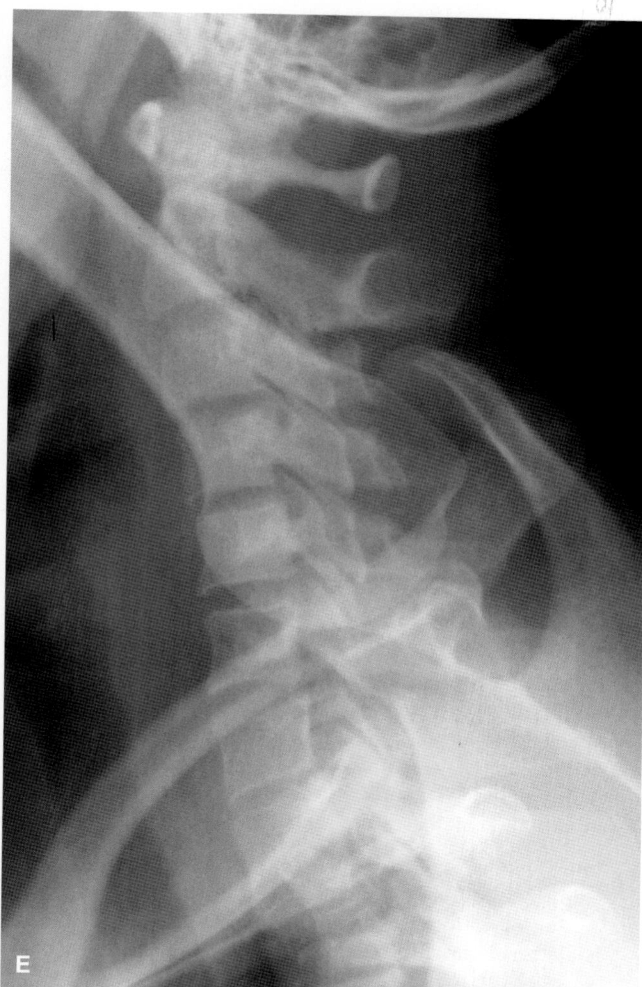

Figure 20-15. Normal Cervical Spine (Continued)

C. Normal anteroposterior view of the cervical spine. The lateral vertebral margins merge with each other creating a wavy line and giving a false impression of a continuous bony column. The vertebral bodies do not demonstrate any vertical fracture line. Such a vertical fracture may not be appreciated on the lateral view. Note that the oval densities of the spinous processes seen on end are also projected in a vertical line. *D*. Normal open-mouth view. The lateral masses of C1 are nicely aligned and flush with the superior facets of C2. Also note the odontoid process of C2 is equidistant between the lateral masses of C1. *E*. A high-quality swimmer's view. Notice that even under the best circumstances the lower cervical vertebral arches are obscured by the shoulder girdle, though C7 is seen normally positioned on T1. This view is difficult and often cumbersome to obtain; thus it is reserved for the patient with very low suspicion of an unstable injury.

b. The lateral spine image must visualize all seven cervical vertebrae and include the cervicothoracic junction.
c. In certain circumstances, either downward traction on the shoulders or a *"swimmer's view"* may help to better visualize the lower cervical spine.
d. Special studies, such as *oblique radiographs,* may show details of the facet joints and pedicles.

2. It is recommended that the entire spine be imaged in any child with evidence of spinal injury. MRI is mandatory for any child with a neurologic deficit.

3. Pseudosubluxation versus acute traumatic subluxation.
   a. The spinolaminar line (Fig. 20-15) is the most important line in children. It joins the bases of the spinous processes and should appear in a smooth arc
   b. The spinous process of C2 may appear to lie posterior to the spinous processes of C1 and C3. This "pseudosubluxation" is a normal variant in 40% of children below the age of 7 years, and in 24% of children up to age 16 years
   c. Pseudosubluxation reduces with extension
   d. This is in contrast to acute traumatic subluxation, which does not reduce with extension because of pain and muscle spasm
   e. The *anterior and posterior spinal lines,* joining the anterior and posterior borders of the cervical spine, respectively, are useful in children over 7 years of age. Pseudosubluxation of C2 on C3 or C3 on C4 is a normal variant that can cause disruption of these lines
   f. The *spinous processes* should form a straight line on AP projection; any offset suggests unilateral facet dislocation. All four of these lines should appear in a smooth and even contour

4. Complaints of significant neck pain (Fig. 20-16), neurologic findings, or a history of high-risk mechanism of injury appear to be the best predictors of CSI. Approximately 14% of all spinal fractures are missed on initial lateral radiographic evaluation. The addition of an AP and open-mouth view increases the sensitivity to 94%.

5. Interspinous distances more than 1.5 times the one above or below on the AP view indicate anterior cervical dislocation. A lack of uniform angulation of the interspaces in flexion is a normal variant in children under 16 years of age.

6. A number of normal variants make the interpretation of cervical spine films in children especially difficult. These variants include:
   a. Absence of normal cervical lordosis
   b. "Pseudospread" of the atlas on the axis up to age 7 years
   c. Pseudosubluxation
   d. Anterior wedging of the vertebral bodies of up to 3 mm
   e. Overriding of the anterior arch of C1 above the odontoid
   f. Lack of uniform angulation at the interspaces in flexion

7. Persistence of synchondrosis at the base of the odontoid, the apical odontoid epiphysis, incomplete ossification of the posterior arch of C1, and secondary ossification centers of the spinous processes may resemble bony fractures in children.

8. Any child with apparent neurologic injury requires radiologic assessment of the entire spine, including CT scan to evaluate bony injury and MRI to assess spinal cord damage.
   a. CT scan is particularly useful at visualizing those portions of the cervical spine that are commonly missed and frequently injured in children, such as the occiput / C1-2 and cervicothoracic levels.
   b. CT scan may detect injuries not readily apparent on plain radiographs.
   c. Thin cut sections (2-3 mm) with sagittal and coronal 3-D reconstruction is recommended and should be tailored to the plain radiographic findings.
   d. CT scan provides detailed anatomical information and allows assessment of impingement of the thecal sac and spinal cord from extradural sources, such as retropulsed bony fragments or hematoma.
   e. Since children are more likely than adults to suffer ligamentous injury, the role of CT scanning in children below age 8 years is less beneficial, unless there is concern of bony abnormality.

9. MRI is mandatory for any child with a neurologic deficit. MRI best assesses spinal cord, disc, and ligamentous disruption. MRI can also detect soft tissue injury, herniated disks, and hematoma not visualized on other imaging modalities.

Complications

1. Neurologic sequelae from spinal cord injury include deformity, vertebral instability, post-traumatic stenosis, paralysis, and paresthesias.

2. Spinal cord transection and major hemorrhage are associated with poor outcome and significant neurologic sequelae in survivors. Minor hemorrhage or edema is associated with moderate-to-good recovery.

3. Neurologic injury from trauma at the C1 to C2 level (atlanto-occipital level; Fig. 20-17) depends on the degree of subluxation sustained. The spinal canal is at its widest at this point and affords some degree of protection.

4. Patients with CSI are at risk for associated head, face, chest, abdominal, and extremity injuries.

5. Death most often occurs as a result of injury to associated organs, particularly the brain.

Consultation

Emergent neurosurgical/orthopedic consultation should be obtained promptly for any child with an obvious neurologic deficit, altered mental status, or documented radiologic evidence of vertebral fracture, dislocation, or spinal cord injury.

Emergency Department Treatment and Disposition

1. The acute management of a patient with a spinal cord injury requires the rapid restoration of airway, breathing, and circulation, with concurrent attention to neutral cervical spine immobilization. A brief neurologic examination with

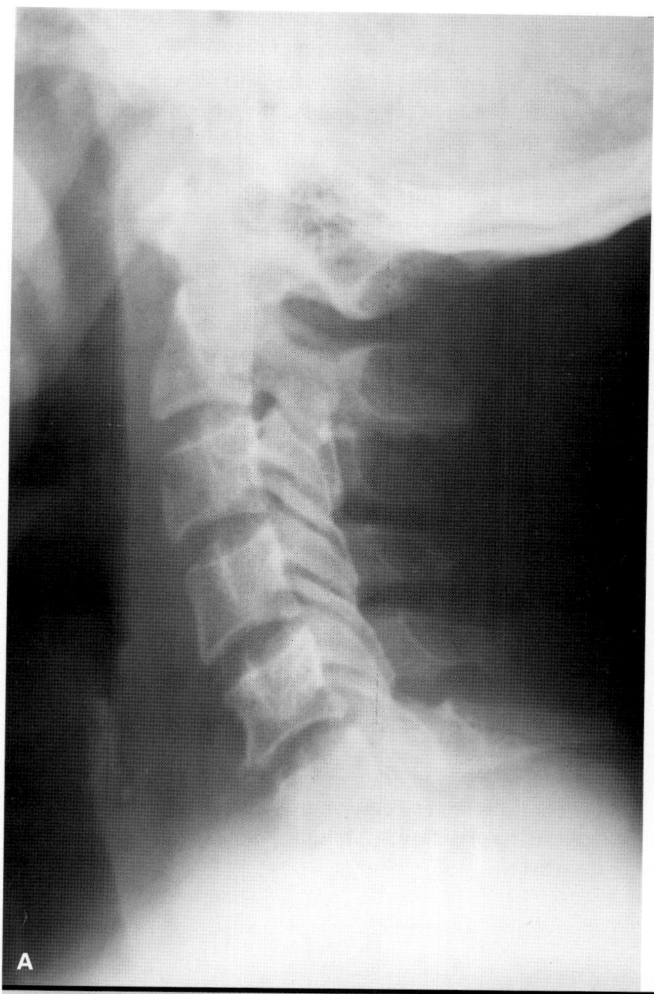

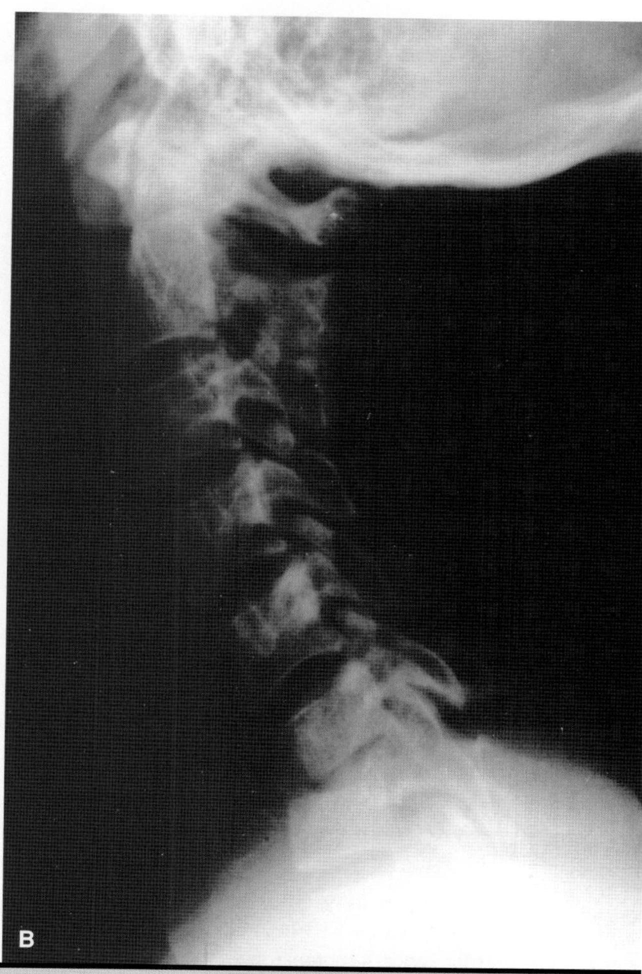

Figure 20-16. Subluxation of Vertebra C6 on C7

A. The general rule in radiology, that you can't diagnose what you can't see, is nowhere more applicable than with a cervicothoracic lateral c-spine film. This is an x-ray of an adolescent inmate who was taken to the ED with complaints of neck pain after striking the back of his head while slipping in the shower. This is an incomplete lateral c-spine x-ray. The bony structures to C5 are normal, but there is a subtle abnormality with a widening of the prevertebral soft tissue space anterior to C6. *B*. Repeat full study taken with traction applied to both arms. While admittedly of poor quality, it demonstrates an unstable subluxation of C6 on C7.

recording of the GCS should be done as part of the primary survey.

2. Indications for cervical spine immobilization after trauma include:
   a. Loss of consciousness
   b. Altered mental status (GCS <13)
   c. A mechanism of injury consistent with spinal cord injury
   d. Neck pain or guarding of the neck
   e. Associated head or facial trauma
   f. Distracting injury
3. The entire spine should be inspected using a log-rolling technique with in-line cervical immobilization. Examination of the spine begins with inspection and palpation for abnormalities, including sites of tenderness, deformity, ecchymoses, contusions, abrasions, head tilt, and penetrating wounds. A high index of suspicion for occult CSI should be maintained in a child who has sustained multiple trauma.
4. Cervical spine immobilization must be maintained until complete clinical and radiologic assessment is made. Trauma series radiographs should include a lateral cervical spine radiograph, visualizing all seven cervical vertebrae from the occiput to the cervicothoracic junction, and supine chest and pelvic radiographs.
5. Maintenance infusion of IV fluids without glucose should be given, with boluses as needed. Appropriate cardiorespiratory monitoring should be instituted and serial neurologic examinations conducted.

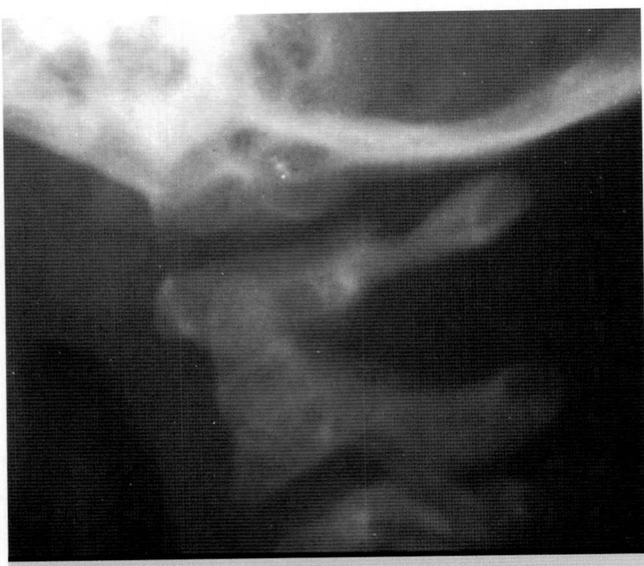

Figure 20-17. Atlanto-Occipital Dislocation

An x-ray of a young child brought in on a long board in a cervical collar after a motor vehicle collision. Note the alarming space between the base of the cranium and the cervical spine. This is a lateral cervical spine view that shows findings consistent with atlanto-occipital dislocation. An x-ray such as this mandates an emergent CT scan or MRI, which in this case was normal. This normal variant can be seen in young children due to the laxity of the cervical spine ligaments, in combination with an oversized cervical collar, resulting in slight axial traction.

6. Neurogenic shock manifests as a loss of descending sympathetic tone, which will be evident by a combination of bradycardia and hypotension. Early recognition is essential because fluid resuscitation alone may not be effective and vasopressors may be required to restore adequate perfusion.
7. There is a great deal of controversy surrounding the effectiveness of steroids in spinal cord injury.
   a. The current recommendation is to administer IV high-dose steroids for 24 hours, if started within 3 hours of spinal cord injury, and to administer steroids for 48 hours if started between 3 and 8 hours after injury.
   b. The initial bolus of methylprednisolone is 30 mg/kg, followed by an infusion of 5.4 mg/kg per hour.
8. Children with documented CSI, neurologic deficit, or history of a high-risk mechanism of injury (e.g., head injury, MVC, fall from a height greater than body height, diving accidents, vehicular ejection, distracting injuries, and altered mental status) should be hospitalized for observation in a PICU. If specialty expertise is unavailable, patients with significant CSI should be stabilized and transferred to a regional trauma center.

Clinical Pearls

1. A high clinical index of suspicion for CSI should be anticipated in the presence of midline cervical tenderness, altered level of consciousness, neurologic injury, and distracting injury.
2. There is an increased risk of cervical spine trauma associated with various congenital anomalies. These include aplasia, hypoplasia of the odontoid, os odontoideum, block vertebrae, Klippel-Feri syndrome. Down syndrome, and skeletal dysplasias (e.g. Morquio's syndrome and diastrophic dwarfism).

BOX 20-11. CERVICAL SPINE INJURIES

- *Atlanto-occipital dislocation*
  (1) Is a rare occurrence following MVC, falls, and forceps delivery
  (2) It is usually fatal and most survivors suffer severe neurologic damage.
  (3) Young children are particularly at risk
  (4) Cardiorespiratory arrest is common and frequently results in anoxic brain injury.
- *Axial compression fractures*
  (1) Resulting in a Jefferson burst fracture (Fig. 20-18) of C1 are rare in children, but are typically seen in teenagers following MVCs and diving accidents
  (2) This injury was originally described by Jefferson as a burst injury of C1 secondary to a blow on the vertex of the skull
  (3) The ring of C1 is crushed between the bulky base of the cranium and the C2 vertebra
- *Odontoid fractures* (Fig. 20-19)
  (1) Among the most common CSIs in children
  (2) Fractures must not be confused with normal anatomic variations in the odontoid due to synchondrosis between the body of the axis and the odontoid, which may be seen in children up to age 7 years.
  (3) Eighty percent of odontoid fractures are displaced in the sagittal plane and can be seen on the lateral view
  (4) These fractures may be completely absent or may be more easily seen on the open-mouth or submental views (these additional views may not be easily obtained, especially in an unstable patient)
- *Fractures of the body and neural arch of the axis (C2)*
  (1) Less common than fractures of the odontoid process and the atlas
  (2) The usual mechanism involves hyperextension resulting in a "hangman's fracture" (the second most common injury of the axis; Fig. 20-20), with bilateral fracture of the pars interarticularis of the axis, horizontal tearing of the C2/C3 disk, and anterior subluxation of C2 on C3
  (3) The name comes from the autopsy findings seen in some hanging victims
  (4) In clinical practice, this fracture is much more often seen with hyperextension of the neck due to hitting one's face on a windshield in a MVC
  (5) Neurologic damage occurs if the fracture extends to the vertebral foramina with injury to the vertebral artery
  (6) It is considered an unstable fracture
- *Injuries to the middle and lower cervical spine*
  (1) More closely follow the adult-type pattern
  (2) Facet disruption without associated fractures may occur in children due to ligamentous laxity
- Pure ligamentous injuries
  (1) May result in delayed instability, even when initial radiographs appear normal
  (2) Children present clinically with persistent neck pain, stiffness, or muscle spasm. Prevertebral swelling, loss of lordosis, widening of interspinous distances, and occasional dimple fracture of a vertebral body are clues to the diagnosis.

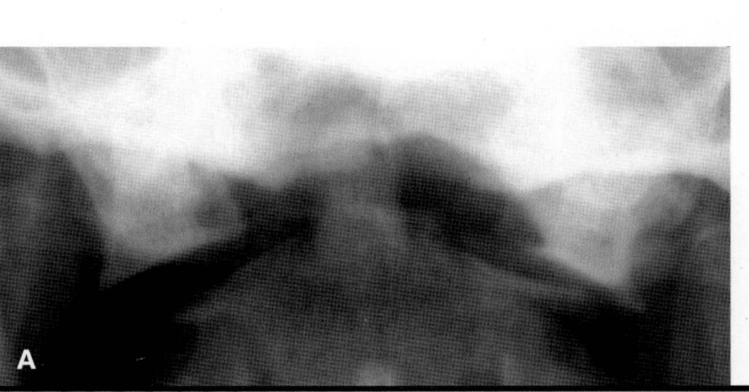

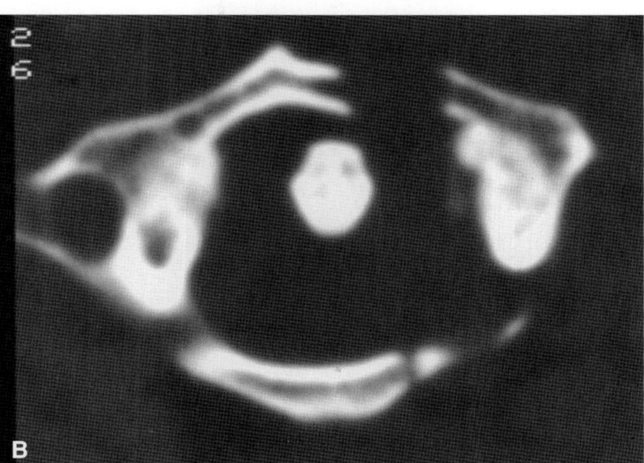

Figure 20-18. Jefferson's Burst Fracture

A. The open-mouth view of a young man who was struck on top of the head with a baseball bat. Note the lateral displacement of the C1 lateral masses on the C2 superior facets. Although a fracture line is not seen, this abnormality should prompt one to get a CT scan of the area. The subsequent CT scan (*B*) demonstrates both an anterior and a posterior arch fracture. In children, differential growth rates of portions of the cervicocranium can give rise to alarming but totally benign lateral displacement of the C1 lateral masses, a normal variant called *pseudospread*. A CT scan of pseudospread would be normal.

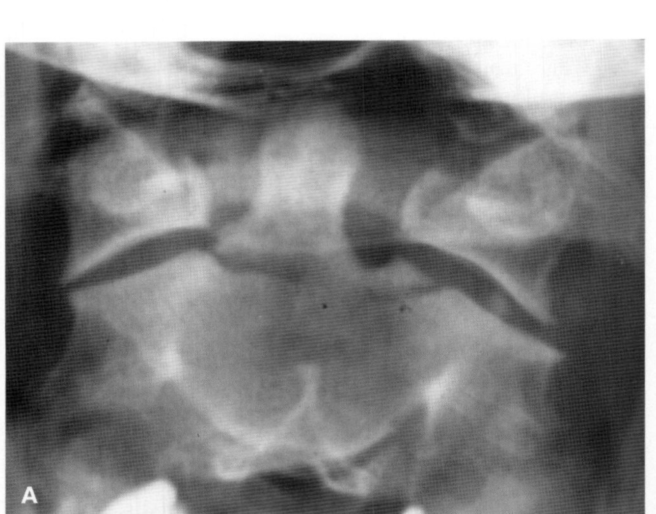

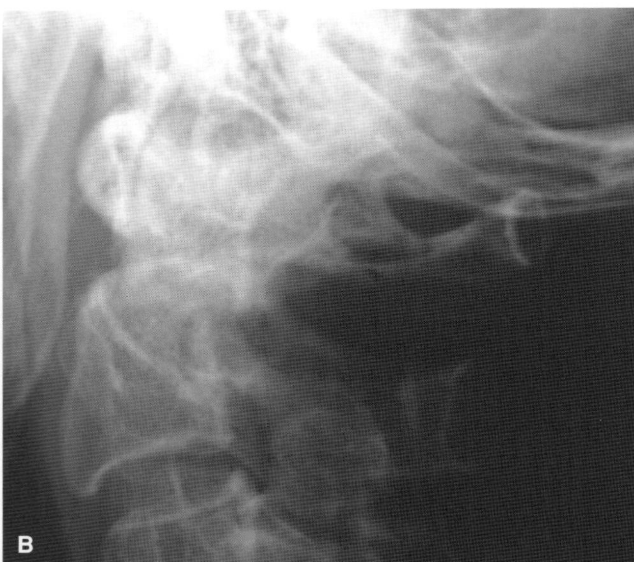

Figure 20-19. Odontoid Fracture

A. This is an open-mouth view of the odontoid of a young man who was hit by a car while riding his bicycle. There was significant impact and he was thrown onto the hood. Despite this, he refused assistance at the scene and continued to ride his bicycle home. Later that evening while eating dinner he complained of shoulder pain. The open-mouth view demonstrates an obvious low dens fracture. Note also the asymmetry in the spaces of the odontoid and the lateral masses of C1. *B*. In a different patient who sustained a blow to the face, the odontoid fracture can be clearly seen on the lateral cervical spine view. Note the posterior displacement of the upper portion of the odontoid, which can be easily seen if one follows the vertical line created by the pre-dens space and the vertical line created by the anterior cortex of the lower portion of the odontoid.

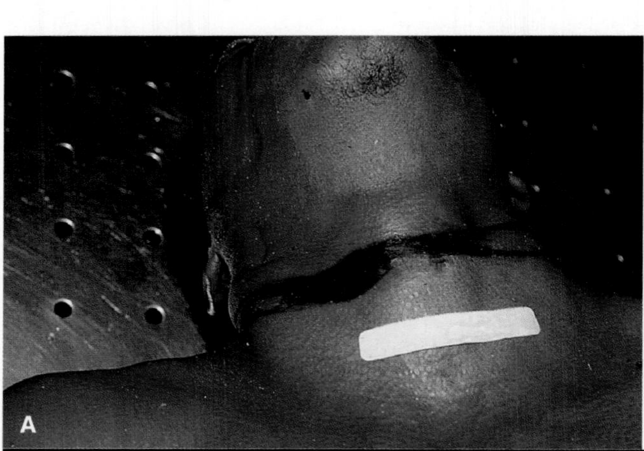

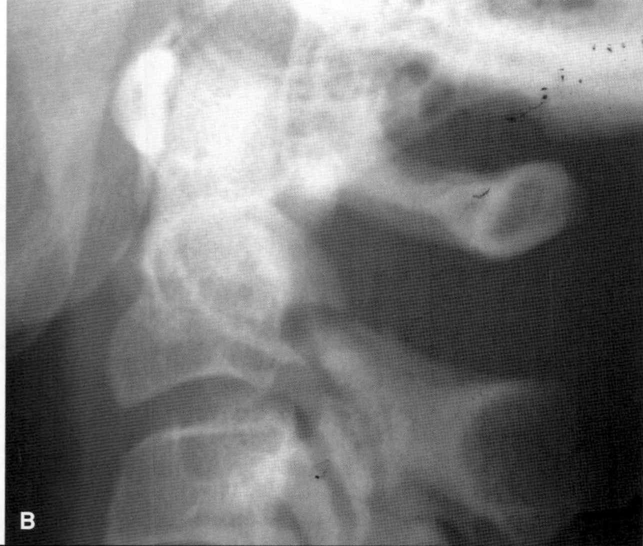

Figure 20-20. Hangman's Fracture

A. An image of a young man who committed suicide by hanging. Note the rope burn on the neck. What is not seen in this picture are the petechial hemorrhages of the face and the subconjunctival hemorrhages of both eyes due to venous engorgement. *B*. An x-ray of a different patient who sustained a horizontally-oriented hangman's fracture.

BOX 20-12. DIFFERENTIAL DIAGNOSIS OF CERVICAL SPINE INJURIES

- *SCIWORA*
  (1) Refers to *s*pinal *c*ord *i*njury *w*ith*o*ut *r*adiographic *a*bnormality.
  (2) It is more common in younger children and occurs most frequently with CSI.
  (3) MRI has shown significant pathology in many of these patients.
  (4) One theory about the pathophysiology of SCIWORA in children is that developmental characteristics of the immature spine allow for *transient excessive movement* during trauma with resulting cord distraction or compression.
  (5) *Cord ischemia* due to direct vessel injury or hypoperfusion is another postulated cause.
  (6) Delayed onset of neurologic damage is usually apparent within 48 hours.
  (7) Numbness, paresthesias or shock-like sensations in the extremities are suggestive of SCIWORA.
  (8) These patients should be evaluated thoroughly for evidence of spinal cord injury.
  (9) MRI is indicated to differentiate cord edema from hemorrhage, as well as to assess ligamentous injury.
- *Atlanto-axial rotatory fixation (AARF)*
  (1) It is a rare condition.
  (2) It can arise spontaneously from minor trauma or in association with congenital cervical spine abnormalities.
- *Transient quadriparesis*
  (1) It is seen relatively frequently in children.
  (2) It is more often seen in young boys following sports-related injuries.
  (3) Clinically, there is a period of paralysis lasting from seconds to minutes, with complete recovery over a period of less than 24 hours.
  (4) No radiologic abnormalities are found.
  (5) The etiology is thought to be a concussion of the spinal cord.
- *Shaken impact syndrome or child abuse*
  (1) Suspect when there is a discrepancy between the history and the degree of physical injury or there has been a delay in seeking treatment.
  (2) Suspect with a history of repeated injuries, or when informants appear to be inconsistent in their reports of injuries.
- *Acquired torticollis*
  (1) (Spasm of the sternocleidomastoid muscle or "wry neck") occurs far more commonly than CSI.
  (2) The contracted sternocleidomastoid muscle is on the side opposite the direction of head rotation.
  (3) Torticollis can be treated conservatively with analgesia.
- *Cervicothoracic junction injury* is rarely reported in children less than 10 years of age.

BOX 20-13. KEY POINTS OF CERVICAL SPINE INJURY

- Knowledge of the anatomy and physiology of the pediatric spine and its relationship to the mechanism of injury is essential in the assessment of the spine-injured child.
- Children present unique problems in evaluation and management because of fear and anxiety as well as their inability to localize or describe pain or to cooperate with the examination.
- Appropriate initial management combined with a thorough clinical and radiologic assessment is imperative in any child presenting with a potential spinal cord injury.
- Normal variants in the pediatric cervical spine may present difficulties in interpretation. Variations in alignment may appear as vertebral displacement; variations in curvature may resemble muscle spasm or ligamentous injury; and growth centers may be confused with fractures.
- Long-term neurologic sequelae from significant spinal cord injury will have a major impact on the quality of life of a child. Because spinal cord injuries are permanent and devastating, injury prevention remains paramount.

DIAGNOSIS DENTAL TRAUMA

Mechanisms of Injury

1. Falls (e.g., inside the home) for primary dentition
2. Altercations, motor vehicle accidents, or sports-related injuries for permanent dentition
3. Dental injuries may also occur due to child abuse.

Associated Clinical Features

1. The peak age for dental injuries is 2 to 4 years (range, 8 to 10 years).
2. Injuries to periodontal structures can lead to disruption of the periodontal ligament. This may lead to pulpal necrosis (can happen even with minor injuries).

Consultation

Dental consult for significant injuries of the teeth

Emergency Department Treatment and Disposition

1. When there is significant injury to the teeth, dental x-rays are indicated to identify alveolar fractures.
2. General principles of management of specific dental injuries are detailed in Boxes 20-14, 20-15, and 20-16.

Clinical Pearls: Dental Trauma

1. Make every attempt to locate the dislodged tooth following any dental trauma; it may be aspirated, fractured, or intruded. As indicated, radiographs are obtained to exclude impediment of the airway or esophagus.
2. Differentiate primary teeth from permanent teeth when evaluating dental injuries.
3. Do not re-implant primary teeth.

BOX 20-14. INJURIES TO PERIODONTAL STRUCTURES

- *Concussion*
  (1) A minor traumatic injury to the supporting structures and tooth
  (2) No evidence of loosening or displacement of the tooth
  (3) May cause increased sensitivity to percussion
  (4) Management is the same for primary teeth and permanent teeth.
  (5) Nonemergent dental consultation
  (6) Advise the patient to avoid exposure to extremes of temperature.
- *Subluxation* (Fig. 20-21)
  (1) Subluxation is due to more severe injury to the supportive structures than concussion, causing abnormal loosening of the tooth but without displacement of the tooth.
  (2) Manifested by slight mobility of the tooth (but the tooth remains in place)
  (3) Presence of discomfort to percussion
  (4) The risk of pulpal necrosis is low if there is <2 mm of mobility.
  (5) Management depends on the degree of mobility.
  (6) Management is the same for both primary and permanent teeth.
  (7) Consult a dentist if there is >2 mm of mobility.
  (8) Follow-up and observation for <2 mm of mobility
  (9) Splinting is recommended for >2 mm of mobility.
- *Luxation*
  (1) Increased mobility of the tooth in the lateral plane
  (2) May have an associated fracture of the tooth socket
  (3) There is an increased risk of pulpal necrosis.
  (4) Dental consult in the ED
  (5) Need to reposition and stabilize by bracing
- *Intrusion*
  (1) Traumatic impaction of the tooth into the socket by an axial force
  (2) May have an associated fracture of the root system
  (3) Clinically apparent shortening of the intruded tooth
  (4) Dental consultation and follow-up are indicated.
  (5) If damage to the developing permanent tooth, extraction of the intruded tooth is more likely to be indicated
  (6) The re-erupted tooth may need endodontic treatment or root canal.
- *Extrusion*
  (1) An outward displacement of the tooth
  (2) Evaluate the integrity of the structures supporting the tooth.
  (3) Severely extruded primary teeth may be extracted to reduce the risk of foreign body aspiration.
  (4) Repositioning and splinting of the extruded tooth, especially a permanent tooth
  (5) Dental consultation and follow-up are imperative.

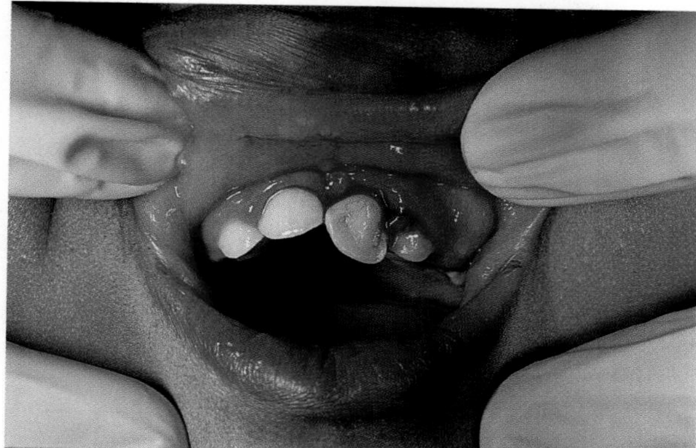

Figure 20-21. Tooth Subluxation

An image of a 2-year-old male who was running and fell, sustaining a subluxation of an upper anterior primary tooth. The injury was managed conservatively with frequent mouth rinsing and oral antibiotics. Had the tooth been completely avulsed, it would not have been reimplanted, as primary teeth are never reimplanted.

BOX 20-15. TOOTH AVULSION

- Avulsion is a complete displacement of the tooth out of its socket (Fig. 20-22).
- Damage to the periodontal ligament
- Determine whether the tooth is primary or permanent.
- Do not replant a primary tooth (due to potential for pulp necrosis with subsequent inflammation and damage to the underlying permanent tooth bud).
- Management of the avulsed permanent tooth:
  (1) If the tooth cannot be reimplanted immediately, the tooth must be kept moist.
  (2) Transport to the ED in a balanced salt solution: Hank's balanced salt solution (3M Save-a-Tooth kit), cold milk, saliva, or water (storing the tooth under the patient's or parent's tongue or in the buccal fold may be considered during patient transport to the ED; however, there is a risk of aspiration)
  (3) Hold the tooth by the crown and not the root.
  (4) The tooth can be rinsed gently to remove debris.
  (5) *Do not scrub, scrape, or brush the tooth (especially the root).*
  (6) Reimplant as soon as possible (ideally within 30 minutes) by using a gentle rotating motion.
  (7) Maintain firm pressure, then ask the patient to bite down firmly on a piece of folded gauze.
  (8) Consult an oral surgeon emergently for stabilization of the newly reimplanted tooth (bracing).
  (9) Dental consultation and follow-up are necessary.
  (10) Root canal is generally necessary.

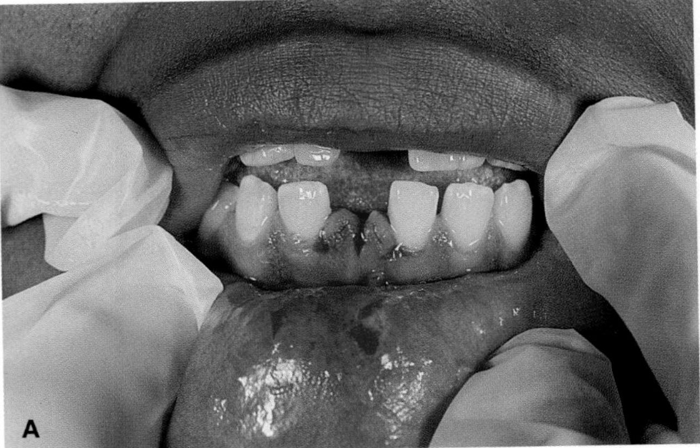

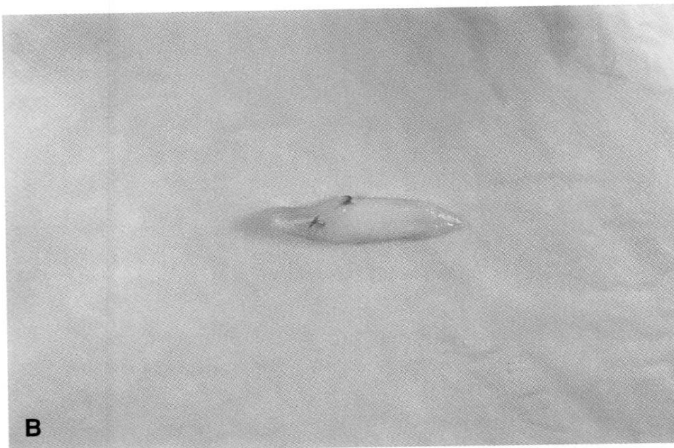

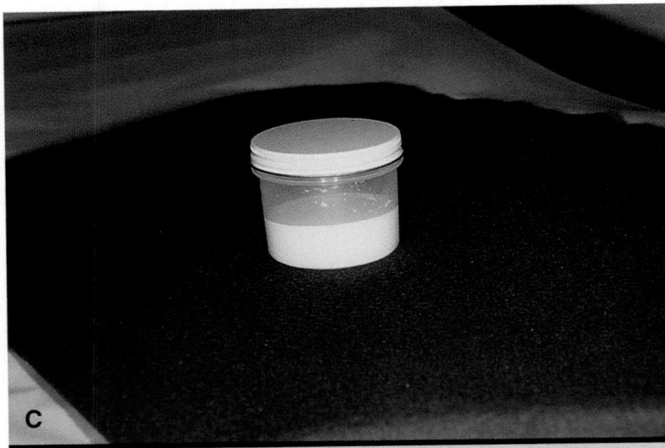

Figure 20-22. Tooth Avulsion

A. An image of a 16-year-old who was punched in the mouth and suffered an avulsion of her lower anterior incisor (#26). The blow also caused subluxation of #23, #24, and #25. The ideal scenario would have been for a family member to rinse the tooth with tap water and place it back into its socket, and getting to the ED as soon as possible. Other less desirable but acceptable first aid measures include placing the tooth in Hank's solution, having the child place the tooth under her tongue, or placing it in a small container of milk. Unfortunately the avulsed tooth (*B*) was left out to dry for over 2 hours before being placed in a container of milk (*C*). The patient arrived in the ED within 30 minutes, but the tooth in the container of milk did not arrive for over 3 hours, and the tooth could not be replaced.

BOX 20-16. DENTAL INJURIES: THE ELLIS CLASSIFICATION OF DENTAL FRACTURES

- The Ellis classification of dental fractures for permanent teeth and their management:
  a. *Class I Ellis fracture*
     (1) Fracture through enamel only
     (2) May leave a jagged edge
     (3) Emergent dental consult unnecessary
     (4) Follow-up with dentist
     (5) Filing of jagged edges or cosmetic repair is sometimes needed.
  b. *Class II Ellis fracture*
     (1) Fracture through both enamel and dentin
     (2) Site on the tooth may be sensitive
     (3) Dental consult should be requested emergently (within hours)
     (4) Temporary coating to decrease sensitivity and risk of infection
     (5) Consider antibiotic therapy, as the exposed dentin may be a portal of entry for infection of the underlying pulp.
     (6) Eventual cosmetic repair as indicated
  c. *Class III Ellis fracture* (Fig. 20-23)
     (1) Fracture through enamel and dentin with pulp exposure
     (2) May be associated bleeding
     (3) The tooth may be sensitive to touch and temperature.
     (4) There is an increased risk of infection with this type of fracture.
     (5) Emergent dental consultation is warranted.
     (6) Management includes temporary coating and antibiotics.
     (7) Early root canal and eventual cosmetic repair are required.

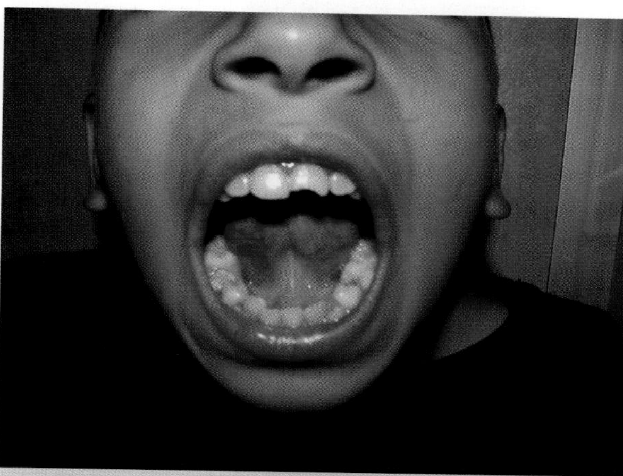

Figure 20-23. Ellis II Fracture and Tongue Laceration

An image of a 9-year-old male who fell and bit his tongue. There is an Ellis type II fracture of the left upper incisor (#8), and also a tongue laceration. The laceration line approximated well and did not involve the edge of the tongue. It was treated conservatively with frequent mouth rinsing and oral antibiotics. Most tongue lacerations are small and are caused when the tongue is caught between the upper and lower incisors. These do not usually require repair. Larger through-and-through lacerations (approaching 1 cm), those that don't approximate well, or lacerations extending through the edge of the tongue require repair in the ED or operating room.

DIAGNOSIS DENTAL CARIES AND DENTOALVEOLAR ABSCESS

Definitions

1. Dental caries: Bacterial disease of teeth characterized by demineralization of tooth enamel and dentine by acid produced during the fermentation of dietary carbohydrates by oral bacteria
2. A dentoalveolar abscess: An acute infection characterized by localization of pus in the structures surrounding the teeth (Fig. 20-24)

Pathogenesis

1. Dental decay presents as opaque areas of enamel with grayish hues. More advanced decay appears as brownish cavitations. Dental caries, while initially asymptomatic, become painful when the decay impinges upon the pulp (inflammation develops). Destruction of enamel and dentin by caries results in bacterial invasion of the pulp to produce pulpitis.
2. Dentoalveolar abscess consists of one of the following processes:
   a. Periapical abscess: Infection originates in the dental pulp due to dental caries. This is the most common type of dental abscess in children. As mentioned earlier, dental caries erodes enamel and dentin and allows bacteria to invade the pulp, producing pulpitis. Pulpitis can progress to necrosis, with bacterial invasion of the alveolar bone, causing an abscess.
   b. A periodontal abscess: This involves the supporting structures of the teeth (periodontal ligaments, alveolar bone). This is the most common type of dental abscess seen in adults. It may occur in children with impaction of a foreign body in the gingiva.

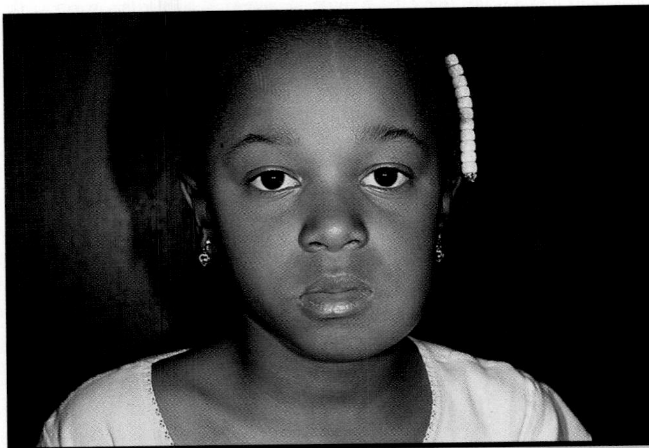

Figure 20-24. Dental Abscess

An image of a 6-year-old female who complained of pain in her mouth for 2 days. The child had a dental filling placed 1 week previously. She was brought to the ED when her mother noted facial swelling. In the ED she was found to have left mandibular vestibular swelling with fluctuance. An maxillofacial surgeon was called and the abscess was drained in the ED under conscious sedation. A Penrose drain was placed and the child was discharged with saline mouth rinses and oral antibiotics with follow-up the next day.

Etiology

1. Odontogenic infections are caused by normal oral flora that comprise the bacteria found on mucosal surfaces, bacteria of the plaque, and bacteria that are found in gingival sulcus.
2. Bacterial pathogens primarily include aerobic gram-positive cocci, anaerobic gram-positive cocci, and anaerobic gram-negative rods (e.g., *Bacteroides*, *Fusobacterium*, *Peptococcus*, *Peptostreptococcus* spp., and viridans streptococci).

Associated Clinical Features

1. Ludwig's angina is unusual in children.
   a. Abscesses of the second and third mandibular molars may perforate the mandible and spread into the submandibular and submental spaces.
   b. Ludwig's angina is manifested by swelling of the floor of the mouth and elevation and posterior displacement of the tongue.
   c. The infection usually begins unilaterally but quickly spreads to include the entire neck and may produce a brawny edema of the suprahyoid region of the neck.
   d. The most common presenting symptoms are oral, neck, and dental pain, and neck swelling, odynophagia, dysphagia, dysphonia, trismus, and tongue swelling.
   e. It may compromise airway patency.
2. No laboratory studies or imaging studies are required for uncomplicated dentoalveolar abscess.
3. A panoramic radiograph may identify carious or impacted or broken tooth and radiolucent changes within the bone.

Complications

1. Facial cellulitis
2. Intracranial complications (e.g., cavernous sinus thrombosis [due to the close approximation of the apex of the maxillary canine root to the infraorbital fissure], brain abscess)
3. Airway obstruction (infection tracking through the submandibular or sublingual space [Ludwig's angina] or through the lateral pharyngeal or retropharyngeal space)
4. Maxillary sinusitis secondary to decompression of an abscess (roots of premolars and molars are in close approximation to the floor of the maxillary sinus)

5. Maxillary odontogenic infections may spread superiorly to cause secondary periorbital or orbital cellulitis.
6. Septicemia

Consultation

Oral-maxillofacial surgeon (complicated dentoalveolar abscess) or a dentist (uncomplicated abscess)

Emergency Department Management and Disposition

1. Incision and drainage of a fluctuant mass or establishing drainage by creating an opening into the offending tooth and extraction of the tooth, if necessary
2. Hospitalization is recommended for any of the following:
   a. Patients who are not able to take fluids orally or those unable to handle secretions
   b. Patients with complications (e.g., facial or mandibular cellulitis with potential airway compromise)
   c. Patients with systemic signs of infection
   d. Failure of outpatient therapy
3. Antibiotic therapy usually includes either penicillin or clindamycin (either covers all likely pathogens that are involved in the polymicrobial etiologies of dentoalveolar abscess).
4. Analgesic therapy for pain management is given as indicated.

Clinical Pearls: Dental Caries and Dentoalveolar Abscess

1. The most common type of dental abscess in children is periapical abscess.
2. An infection of a primary tooth must be treated aggressively; if left untreated, it can damage the developing un-erupted permanent tooth bud.
3. Odontogenic infections are polymicrobial in nature and are caused by normal oral flora. These primarily include aerobic gram-positive cocci, anaerobic gram-positive cocci, and anaerobic gram-negative rods.

BOX 20-17. VARIOUS STAGES OF DENTAL CARIES

- *Reversible pulpitis*
  (1) Mild inflammation of the tooth pulp caused by caries encroaching on the tooth pulp
  (2) Pain is triggered by hot, cold, and sweet stimuli, and is usually transient and resolves spontaneously.
  (3) Dental consultation is necessary for removal of the carious tissue and placement of dental restoration or filling.
  (4) Generally, pain control and referral
- *Irreversible pulpitis*
  (1) Severe inflammation of the pulp
  (2) Pain becomes severe, spontaneous, and more persistent (often poorly localized).
  (3) Dental consultation/referral is warranted.
  (4) A definitive way to relieve discomfort is via root canal (removal of the pulp chamber and canal), or in advanced disease, extraction of the tooth.
  (5) Pain management (until definitive care can be performed) includes nonsteroidal anti-inflammatory drugs, acetaminophen, or a weak opioid (codeine).
- *Apical periodontitis*
  (1) Severely inflamed pulp eventually necroses and inflammation around the apex of the tooth ensues.
  (2) Pain is severe, spontaneous, and persistent and localizes to the affected tooth.
  (3) Tooth is sensitive to percussion.
  (4) Regional lymphadenopathy may be apparent.
  (5) Dental referral necessary for definitive care (root canal or extraction)
  (6) Appropriate pain management
  (7) Antibiotics are generally not necessary.
- *Apical abscess*
  (1) Localized, purulent form of apical periodontitis
  (2) Fluctuant buccal or palatal swelling (may or may not have a draining fistula)
  (3) Regional adenopathy is often present.
  (4) Dental referral necessary for definitive care (root canal or extraction).
  (5) Appropriate pain management
  (6) Antibiotics generally are not necessary unless concurrent cellulitis present.

BOX 20-18. CLINICAL FEATURES OF DENTOALVEOLAR ABSCESS

- Pain (severe, often stimulated by chewing pressure and heat)
- Percussion tenderness (extreme pain to percussion of the involved tooth)
- Increased mobility of the tooth owing to resorption of root and supporting bone
- Signs of inflammation (edema, erythema, and tenderness of soft tissue surrounding the tooth) may be present.
- Purulent discharge (gentle probing of swollen, fluctuant area may disclose pus)
- Systemic signs and symptoms (fever, malaise) may be present.
- Cervical lymphadenopathy may be present.
- The tooth may become extruded because of pressure or fluid in the periradicular space.
- Infections of the lower jaw
  - (1) Pain
  - (2) Swelling (submandibular or intraoral sublingual)
  - (3) Trismus (spread of infection into the spaces around the muscles of mastication)

BOX 20-19. FACIAL CELLULITIS AS A COMPLICATION OF ODONTOGENIC INFECTIONS

- May follow apical periodontitis
- Infection may spread to major fascial spaces of the head and neck, and airway compromise is a potential complication.
- Facial space swelling may involve any of the following areas:
  - (1) Submandibular swelling
    - a. Dental abscesses from the second or third molars
    - b. An ill-defined but often impressive swelling below the mandible
    - c. The inferior border and angle of the mandible are often difficult to palpate.
  - (2) Buccal swelling
    - a. Results from infection of maxillary or mandibular molars
    - b. A large area of involvement (often extends from the philtrum to the parotid border and up to the periorbital area)
    - c. Tender swelling of the cheek without trismus
    - d. Maxillary infection may seed the periorbital area (complications include loss of vision, cavernous sinus thrombosis, central nervous system involvement)
  - (3) Sublingual swelling
    - a. Abscess involving any of the lower teeth whose apex is above the mylohyoid muscle attachment (e.g., incisors, canines, premolars)
    - b. Usually unilateral elevation of floor of the mouth near the offending tooth (infection can spread across the midline)
    - c. Common presenting complaints include pain and dysphagia
    - d. Risk of airway compromise (due to elevation of the base of the tongue)
  - (4) Other less frequently involved facial space areas include submental, masticator, lateral pharyngeal, and retropharyngeal areas.
- Other clinical features of facial cellulitis:
  - (1) Diffuse, painful swelling of the affected tissue
  - (2) Fever may be present.
  - (3) Regional adenopathy common

Management

- Patients with localized (contained) infection:
  - (1) Treat with antistreptococcal oral antibiotics (e.g., penicillin)
  - (2) If penicillin allergy, consider erythromycin or clindamycin
  - (3) Needs evaluation by a dentist within 1 to 2 days (but return earlier if pain or swelling progresses)
  - (4) Definitive therapy is root canal or extraction.
- With infection extending regionally into deep spaces of the head and neck:
  - (1) Hospitalization and surgical and infectious disease consultation
  - (2) CT imaging is mandatory.
  - (3) If an abscess is identified it must be drained.
  - (4) Intravenous antibiotics (to include anaerobic coverage) should be started immediately.

BOX 20-20. DIFFERENTIAL DIAGNOSIS OF DENTOALVEOLAR ABSCESS

- Gingivostomatitis (various etiologies)
- Parotiditis (other etiologies [e.g., mumps, coxsackie virus])
- Facial cellulitis (infection from other etiologies [e.g., arthropod bite])
- Buccal cellulitis (e.g., infection from *Streptococcus pneumoniae*)
- Periorbital cellulitis (infection from other etiologies [e.g., sinusitis, trauma, arthropod bite])
- Neoplasms

DIAGNOSIS THORACIC TRAUMA

Mechanism of Injury

1. Blunt thoracic trauma may occur as a result of motor vehicle, motorcycle, or bicycle crashes; pedestrians collision with motor vehicles; falls; and assaults. In addition, the increased popularity of high-risk sports, such as snowboarding and moto-cross, has led to an increase in sports-related blunt chest injuries. Injuries occur by direct trauma, compression, or acceleration/deceleration forces.
2. Penetrating thoracic injuries in children are much less common than those caused by blunt mechanisms. The incidence of penetrating injuries increases dramatically, however, in the adolescent population.
   a. Penetrating injuries result from gunshot, stab, or shotgun wounds.
   b. Stab wounds refer to direct injury to structures caused by a thrust of a sharp instrument.
   c. Injuries from firearms are due to both direct trauma from bullet and bone fragments and that from blast effect (permanent and temporary tissue cavities are created by a projectile).

Associated Clinical Features

1. External signs of injury may be present. These include abrasions, ecchymoses, lacerations, crepitus, and tenderness; however, the lack of these findings does not exclude significant injury.
2. Tachypnea may be the earliest sign of pulmonary compromise or hypoxia. Cyanosis is a late finding.
3. Tachycardia and peripheral vasoconstriction are indicators of significant blood loss. Hypotension occurs just prior to circulatory collapse.
4. Decreased breath sounds and changes in percussion are associated with pulmonary parenchymal injury or air or blood in the pleural space.
5. Tracheal deviation may be seen with a tension pneumothorax. As air is forced into the thoracic cavity, the mediastinum and trachea are displaced to the opposite side.
6. Jugular venous distention may signify cardiac tamponade or a tension pneumothorax (Fig. 20-25).
7. Paradoxical chest wall motion occurs when the structural integrity of the chest wall is compromised (flail chest).

Laboratory Tests and Radiology

1. During the initial resuscitation, blood should be sent for baseline hematologic and metabolic studies as well as type and cross-match. Serial hemoglobin and hematocrit levels should be monitored in order to gauge blood loss.
2. Pulse oximetry provides a rapid initial indication of oxygen saturation. Arterial blood gas (ABG) analysis should subsequently be performed on all patients with significant thoracic trauma or abnormal pulse oximetry. ABG provides

additional information about the adequacy of ventilation and oxygenation. Respiratory abnormalities could be detected by obtaining an alveolar-arterial oxygen difference.

3. Chest radiographs are the initial imaging modality to rapidly screen patients with blunt chest trauma.
   a. Portable chest radiography should be done during the primary trauma survey.
   b. If patient immobilization is unnecessary, an upright chest x-ray aids in diagnosing small pneumo- and hemothoraces. If immobilization is required, a supine chest x-ray will suffice.
   c. Initial chest x-rays may not reveal the extent of pulmonary injuries. Delayed chest x-rays should be performed if there is clinical suspicion of pulmonary contusions or parenchymal injury.
4. Spiral computed tomography (CT) is more sensitive and specific than chest radiographs for diagnosing thoracic pathology.
   a. CT is useful for the evaluation of aortic, airway, pulmonary, skeletal, and diaphragmatic injuries.
   b. In addition, since thoracic injury in children is an indicator of multisystem trauma, CT scans can be used to further identify abdominal and pelvic injuries.

Complications

1. Airway
   a. A child's smaller airway diameter collapses and occludes more easily than that of an adult. This results in hypoxia and respiratory failure.
   b. High metabolic demand and anatomic differences (large tongue, small mandible, soft epiglottis) make children more susceptible to airway compromise than adults. Early airway management is imperative.
   c. Laryngeal or upper tracheal injury may accompany major thoracic trauma. Lethal consequences generally occur early after the injury; however, long-term sequelae

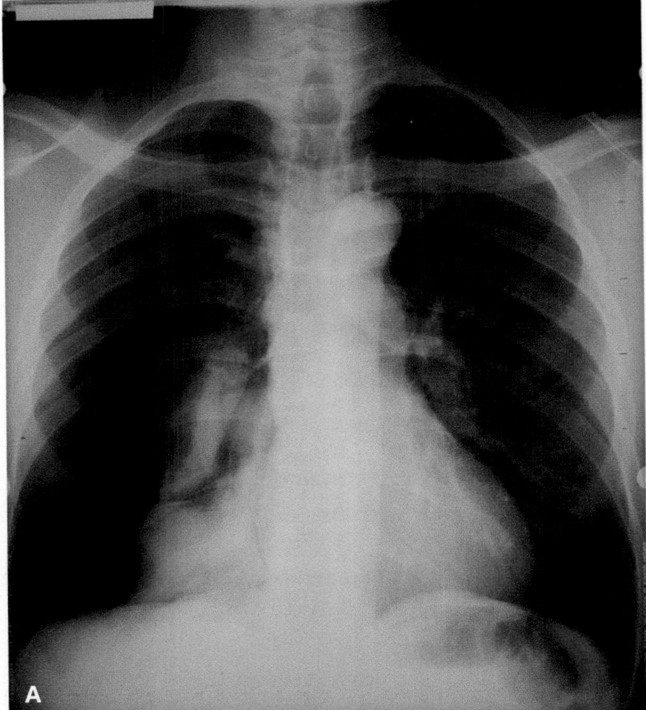

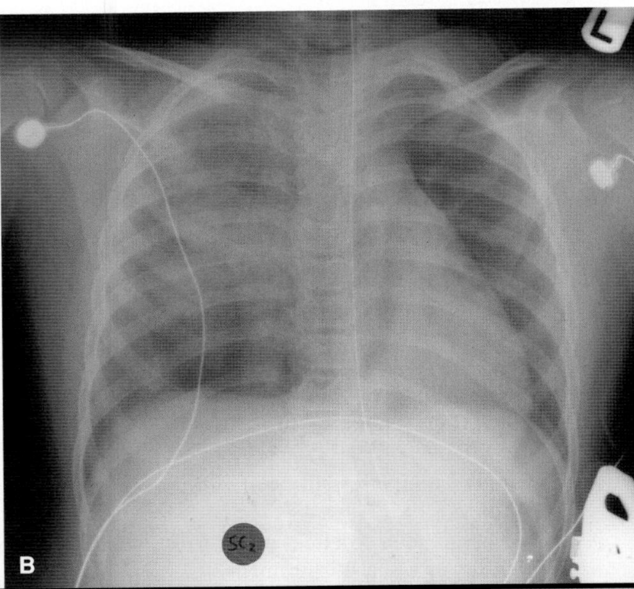

Figure 20-25. Pneumothorax and Pneumomediastinum

A. An x-ray of an adolescent male who sustained a stab wound to the chest resulting in a 100% pneumothorax on the right side. *B*. An x-ray of another young male who also sustained a stab wound to the right chest. Shortly after this chest radiograph was taken, the patient had deterioration in his clinical status necessitating needle decompression of the chest and placement of a chest tube. Both were performed prior to the development of the x-ray.

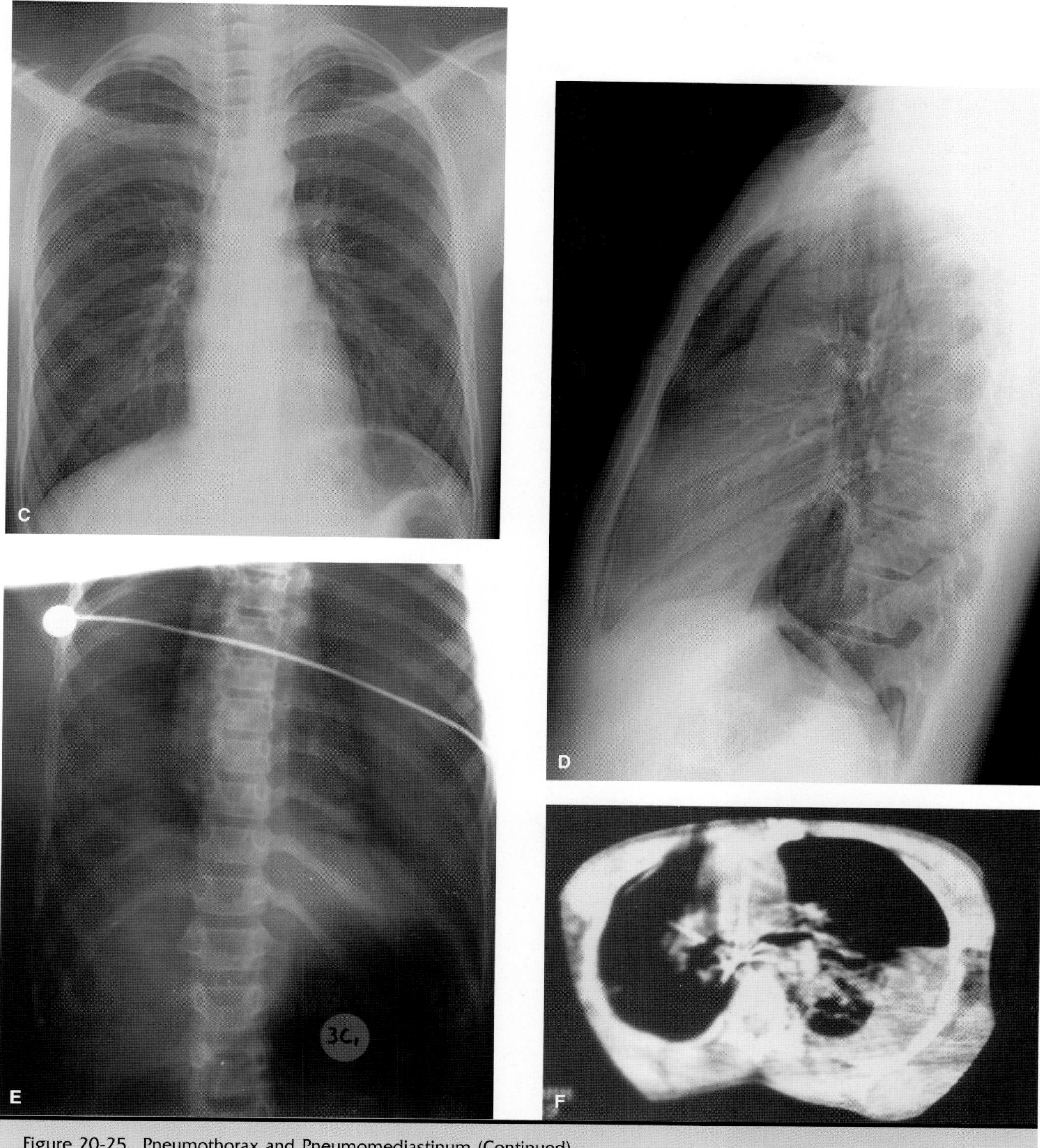

Figure 20-25. Pneumothorax and Pneumomediastinum (Continued)

C. AP chest radiograph of an adolescent male who sustained a parasternal stab wound with an ice pick. The youth was relatively asymptomatic and initial portable chest x-ray was normal. Even this AP view taken in the radiology suite is normal. *D.* The lateral chest radiograph, demonstrating the vertical streaking lucencies related to the ascending aorta and root of the great vessels, as well as the retrosternal space. This example demonstrates that it is easier to identify a pneumomediastinum on a lateral chest x-ray than on the frontal view. *E.* A chest x-ray of a 12-year-old boy who was struck by a car. This hastily done, poor-quality film was taken when the child's mental status began to deteriorate. Note the left costophrenic angle which is surprisingly deep. This is an example of a deep sulcus sign seen in an anterior pneumothorax. *F.* The chest CT scan of the same patient clearly demonstrates the anterior pneumothorax.

include airway stenosis, atelectasis, pneumonia, and loss of distal functional lung parenchyma.

2. Breathing
   a. Due to the lack of cartilaginous ossification, the ligamentous attachments of the ribs allow significant damage without any radiographic evidence.
   b. Rib fractures or flail chest require early, aggressive respiratory supportive care. High priorities are early maintenance of adequate oxygenation, prevention of atelectasis and pneumonia, and adequate pain management (Fig. 20-26).
   c. Behavioral immaturity of children compromises their ability to communicate early complaints of respiratory difficulties.
   d. Pneumonia is a common complication that often develops within hours of the initial pulmonary injury.
   e. Pulmonary injuries, such as contusions, may not initially be clinically apparent. Early chest radiographs often appear normal. Over time hypoxia and respiratory distress develop. Severe cases may result in acute respiratory distress syndrome (ARDS). This occurs less frequently in children than in adults. It is associated with high mortality.

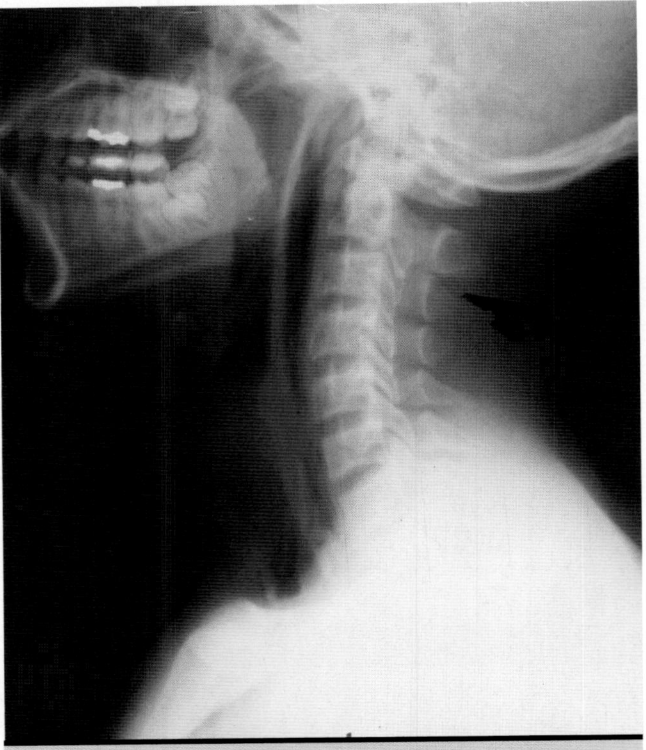

Figure 20-26. Traumatic Airway Obstruction

Soft tissue neck x-ray of an adolescent who sustained a laryngeal fracture resulting in subcutaneous emphysema of the neck. Note the obvious soft tissue air tracking along the fascial planes.

3. Circulation
   a. Vital signs may underestimate the degree of metabolic derangement. Children have tremendous cardiovascular reserve and may maintain normal vital signs up until the point of circulatory collapse. Tachycardia and peripheral vasoconstriction indicate significant blood loss.
   b. Precordial blunt chest trauma can result in myocardial contusions. Dysrhythmias and hypotension may occur. Additionally, sudden death can occur after chest wall impact (commotio cordis). This disorder has been most commonly described in athletes who were injured during sporting events. Ventricular fibrillation is the most commonly described dysrhythmia in commotio cordis.
   c. Pericardial tamponade is more commonly caused by penetrating than by blunt trauma. If unrecognized in the early stages of clinical evaluation, it results in rapid circulatory collapse.
   d. Laxity of mediastinal fixation allows significant organ shifts and may result in aortic injury. If not identified and treated early, aortic injuries result in high mortality.
   e. Massive blood loss with multiple blood transfusions may lead to hypothermia, acid-base disorders, electrolyte abnormalities, thrombocytopenia, and coagulopathies.

4. Disability
   a. Thoracolumbar spinal injuries may occur with severe chest trauma.
   b. Thoracic pediatric trauma victims can present with spinal cord injury without radiologic abnormality (mnemonic: SCIWORA).
   c. Clinical suspicion of spinal cord injuries warrants immobilization and further diagnostic evaluation.

Consultation

Children who have sustained significant thoracic trauma are at high risk for multisystem injuries. Care of these patients should always involve a team approach. Pediatric emergency personnel must work in conjunction with surgical specialists during initial stabilization and throughout diagnostic evaluation. Additional subspecialists may be consulted as complex injuries are identified.

Emergency Department Treatment and Disposition

1. Methodical evaluation of airway, breathing, and circulation is of prime importance in patients with thoracic trauma.
   a. Provide high-flow oxygen and suction any secretions or blood that may obstruct the airway.
   b. Establish and secure a patent airway.
   c. Indications for emergent intubation:
      1) Upper respiratory obstruction
      2) Inability to control secretions
      3) Respiratory fatigue, hypoxia, apnea, loss of protective airway reflexes
      4) Airway protection in patients with neurologic dysfunction

2. Monitor vital signs with a cardiac monitor, pulse oximetry, and frequent blood pressure measurements.
3. Maintain cervical immobilization for blunt injuries and penetrating injuries with a cervical trajectory.
4. Inspection and auscultation of the chest will provide information about the ventilatory status and associated injuries.
   a. If decreased breath sounds, deviated trachea, and hypoxia are present, immediate needle decompression, followed by chest thoracostomy, are indicated for treatment of a tension pneumothorax. Chest radiographs should not delay this intervention.
   b. A chest tube should also be placed for a hemothorax, simple pneumothorax, or hemopneumothorax (Fig. 20-27).
5. Intravenous access with simultaneous collection of blood samples should be obtained.
6. Initial fluid resuscitation with a bolus of normal saline or lactated Ringer's (20 mL/kg) should be performed. After three boluses of 20 mL/kg of crystalloid, blood products are used.
   a. Packed RBCs in a type-specific bolus of 10 mL/kg or whole blood in a type-specific bolus of 20 mL/kg
   b. Blood that is not cross-matched (type O) can be used if immediate blood replacement is necessary or if there is a delay in obtaining type-specific blood.
   c. Indications for blood transfusions include:
      1) Massive or continuous blood loss
      2) Need for additional fluid resuscitation beyond crystalloid
      3) Hypotension secondary to blood loss
      4) Resuscitation during laparotomy or thoracotomy
7. Open thoracotomy is indicated in patients with penetrating precordial wounds if there is clinical suspicion of cardiac tamponade. Outcome in these pediatric trauma patients is dismal.
8. Children with documented thoracic injuries, respiratory compromise, or multiple organ system injuries should be admitted to a pediatric ICU. Any child with a significant mechanism of injury should be hospitalized for observation. If specialty expertise is unavailable, patients with significant thoracic trauma should be stabilized and transferred to a regional trauma center.

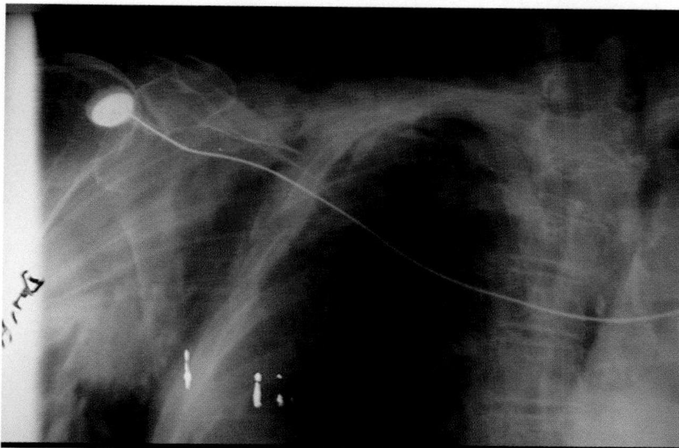

Figure 20-27. Subcutaneous Emphysema

An x-ray of a young man who was struck by a car and sustained multiple rib fractures. The patient had easily palpable subcutaneous emphysema. Note the lucency in the axilla and the entire right upper thorax caused by the subcutaneous air.

Clinical Pearls: Thoracic Trauma

1. Airway, breathing, and circulation may all be adversely affected. Rapid evaluation and treatment must be undertaken during the primary trauma survey.
2. Significant injuries to the pulmonary parenchyma may be present without any signs of external trauma or skeletal injuries. This occurs because the child's compliant cartilaginous ribs allow transmission of forces upon the thoracic skeleton directly to the lungs.
3. Children have tremendous cardiovascular reserve. They may exhibit only subtle changes in heart rate or respirations despite severe cardiothoracic injury.
4. If a clear history of severe trauma is lacking, young children who present with rib fractures should be considered possible victims of child abuse.
5. Thoracic trauma in children is an indicator of multisystem injury. A thorough examination must be performed in order to avoid missed injuries.

BOX 20-21. IMMEDIATELY LIFE-THREATENING THORACIC INJURIES

Derangements of airway, breathing, or circulation that must be identified and treated during the primary trauma survey:

- Airway obstruction
  (1) Laryngeal or upper tracheal injury may accompany major thoracic trauma.
  (2) Blood or secretions
  (3) Change in voice quality, gurgling, snoring, stridor
- Tension pneumothorax
  (1) Air under pressure in the pleural cavity causes a shift of the mediastinum and compression of the great vessels and contralateral lung.
  (2) Respiratory distress
  (3) Tachycardia and hypotension
  (4) Ipsilateral decreased breath sounds and hyperresonance to percussion
  (5) Jugular venous distention (JVD may be absent if concomitant hypovolemia present)
  (6) Tracheal deviation to the opposite side
- Open pneumothorax (sucking chest wound)
  (1) Air preferentially enters through a large defect in the chest wall.
  (2) Normal lung expansion becomes impossible.
  (3) Paradoxical breathing
  (4) Hypoxia and hypercarbia
- Flail chest (Fig. 20-28)
  (1) Two or more adjacent ribs fractured in two or more places cause disruption of normal chest wall movement.
  (2) Associated with underlying lung contusion and hypoxia
  (3) Paradoxical chest wall movements
  (4) Tenderness and crepitus at fracture sites
  (5) Rare in children because of their compliant chest walls, but when present, flail chest is a marker of severe underlying pulmonary injury
- Massive hemothorax (Fig. 20-29)
  (1) Massive bleeding from lung parenchyma or intercostal vessels
  (2) Respiratory distress
  (3) Tachycardia, followed by hypotension, with progressive hemorrhagic shock
  (4) Absent breath sounds and dullness to percussion on affected side
  (5) Indications for operative intervention: initial blood loss of 10 to 15 mL/kg of body weight or persistent blood loss of 2 to 4 mL/kg per hour
- Cardiac tamponade (Fig. 20-30)
  (1) Blood fills the pericardial sac, venous return is compromised, ventricular filling is limited, and stroke volume is reduced.
  (2) Most commonly caused by stab wounds; the presence of a precordial wound suggests the diagnosis.
  (3) Tachycardia and increased total peripheral resistance are initial compensatory mechanisms. If untreated, progression to hypotension and cardiac arrest may occur.
  (4) Classic diagnostic description of Beck's triad (rising venous pressure, falling arterial pressure, and muffled heart sounds) may be absent or incomplete.

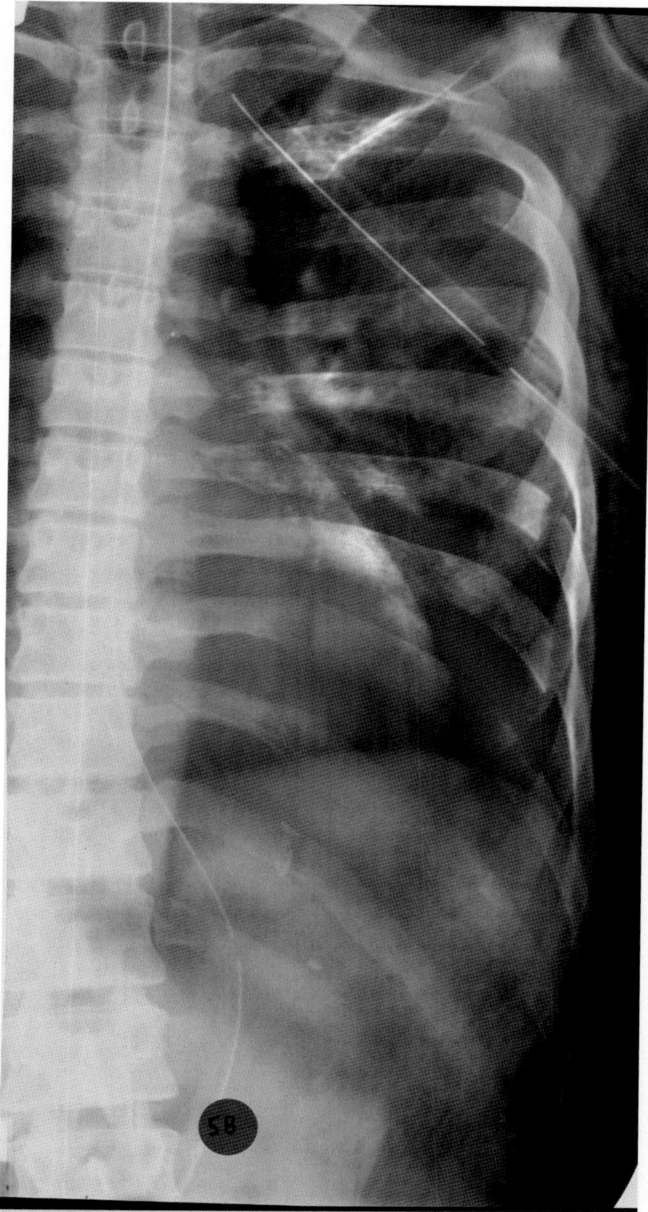

Figure 20-28. Flail Chest

This is the x-ray of an adolescent who sustained significant blunt chest trauma. Note the fractures of ribs 4 through 10 seen medially that are indicative of posterior rib fractures, and the more peripheral fractures seen in ribs 4 through 8. This patient presented with paradoxical movement of the chest with breathing, crepitus of subcutaneous emphysema, and a pneumothorax that required placement of the chest tube (also seen on the x-ray).

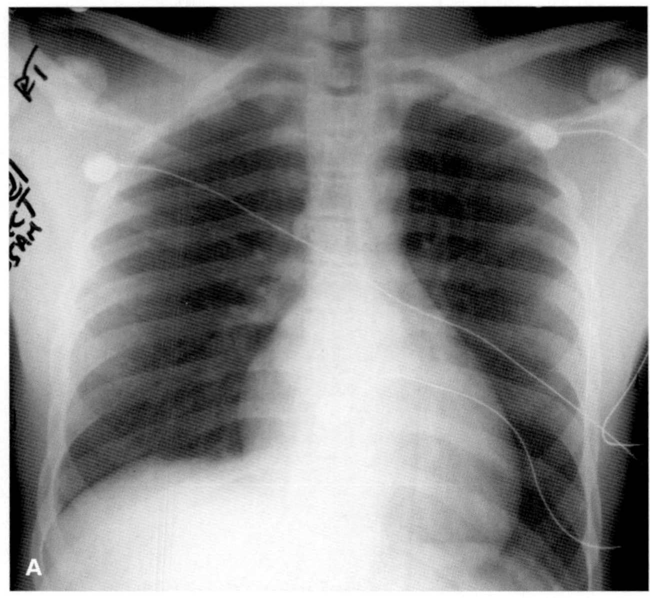

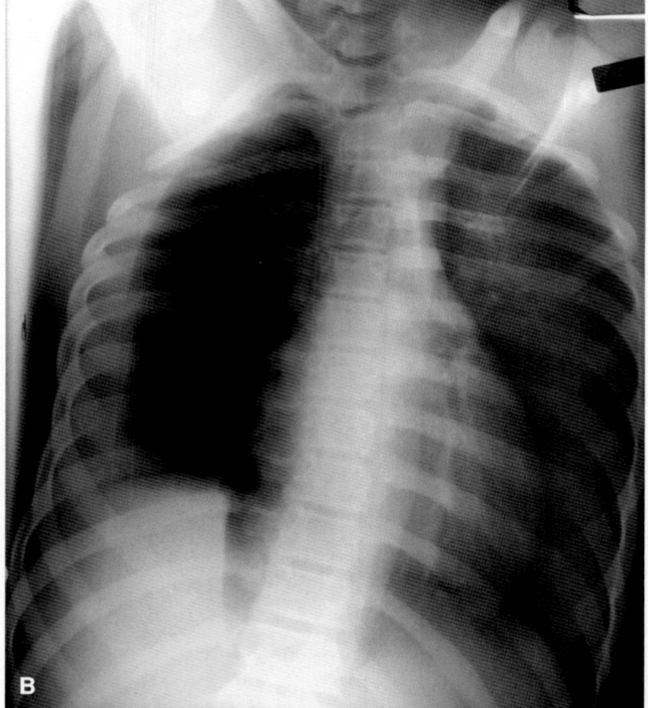

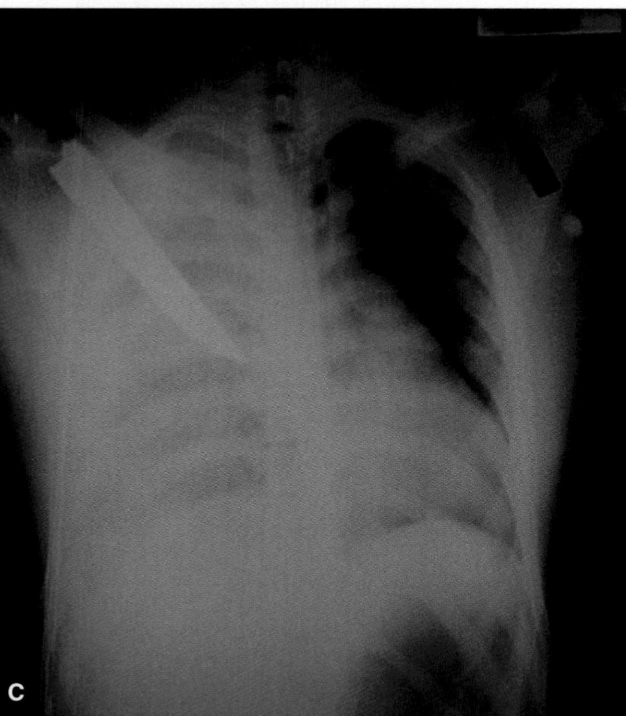

Figure 20-29. Hemothorax

A. An AP radiograph of a 14-year-old boy who was hit by a car. While there are no pathognomonic findings indicative of a hemothorax, in this clinical context the caretakers were concerned about the elevation of the right hemidiaphragm. In particular the lateral position of the right hemidiaphragm apex makes the possibility of subpulmonic fluid even more likely. *B*. The subsequent right lateral decubitus film, also done as a portable, demonstrates a significant hemothorax. *C*. An x-ray of an 18-year-old male who presented with a knife in his right chest. The portable x-ray demonstrates a massive right-sided hemothorax. The patient was intubated and resuscitated, had chest tube placement in the ED and was quickly taken to the operating room where the knife was removed.

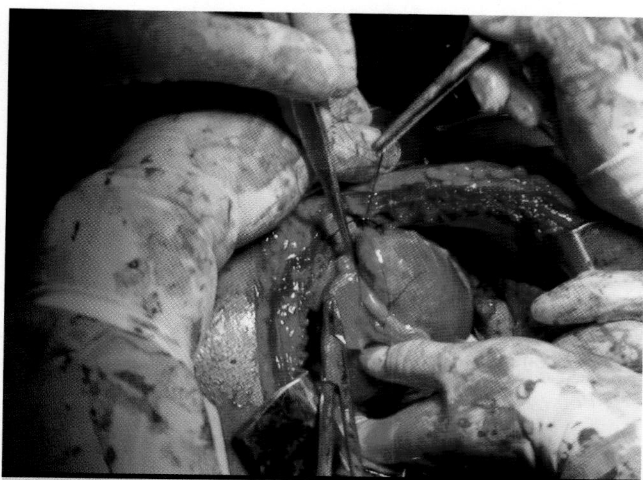

Figure 20-30. Cardiac Tamponade

The clinical picture of an ED thoracotomy performed on a 16-year-old male who sustained a stab wound to the chest. The patient developed pulseless electrical activity upon arrival. His pulse and blood pressure returned after relief of a cardiac tamponade. The image demonstrates the suture closure of a 1-cm right ventricular injury. Luckily for the patient, this was his only injury and he went on to a full recovery, leaving the hospital in approximately 2 weeks.

BOX 20-22. ADDITIONAL THORACIC INJURIES

- *Pulmonary contusion* (Fig. 20-31)
  (1) One of the most common thoracic injuries in children
  (2) External signs of injury are often absent.
  (3) Initial clinical signs and chest x-ray findings may be normal.
  (4) Ventilation/perfusion ($\dot{V}/\dot{Q}$) mismatch and respiratory failure develop later.
- *Rib fractures*
  (1) Uncommon in young children due to their incompletely calcified, pliable ribs; adolescents may present with rib fractures
  (2) Identification of a rib fracture suggests a high-energy force. This is often associated with severe underlying organ injury.
  (3) *If trauma history is inconsistent with injury, particularly if there are multiple rib fractures in various stages of healing, child abuse must be suspected*
- *Simple pneumothorax, hemothorax, or hemopneuomthorax*
  (1) Air or blood in the pleural space
  (2) Decreased breath sounds on the affected side
  (3) $\dot{V}/\dot{Q}$ mismatch and hypoxia occur.
  (4) Upright, expiratory chest x-ray aids in diagnosis of pneumothorax
  (5) Treatment is tube thoracostomy.
- *Tracheobronchial tree injury* (Fig. 20-32)
  (1) Rare in children, but high mortality rate
  (2) Associated with crush injury to the chest
  (3) Presents with hemoptysis, subcutaneous emphysema, tension pneumothorax, or persistent air leak with inability to re-expand the lung after tube thoracostomy
  (4) Bronchoscopy confirms the diagnosis.
- *Blunt cardiac injury (myocardial contusion)*
  (1) Direct blunt trauma to the anterior chest; chest pain and anterior chest wall tenderness
  (2) Tachycardia most common; significant dysrhythmias and hypotension may occur
  (3) May result in sudden death (commotio cordis)
- *Aortic disruption* (Fig. 20-33)
  (1) Associated with rapid deceleration mechanism of injury
  (2) May present with chest or back pain, hypotension, or cardiovascular collapse
  (3) Requires immediate surgical repair
  (4) High morbidity and mortality rate
- *Traumatic diaphragmatic injury* (Fig. 20-34)
  (1) Most frequently caused by blunt force injury; often associated with lap belts
  (2) Presents with abdominal pain or significant respiratory distress
  (3) Majority of the injuries are left-sided
  (4) Early recognition and airway management are key.

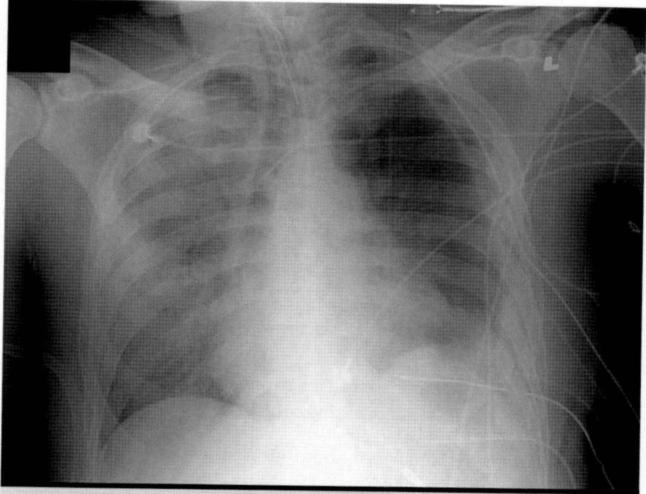

Figure 20-31. Pulmonary Contusion

An x-ray of a young man who fell from a roof and sustained significant blunt chest trauma. His initial chest x-ray was relatively normal. During the course of his work-up he became progressively more hypoxic, necessitating endotracheal intubation. This subsequent chest x-ray, taken several hours after presentation, demonstrates a large right-sided pulmonary contusion.

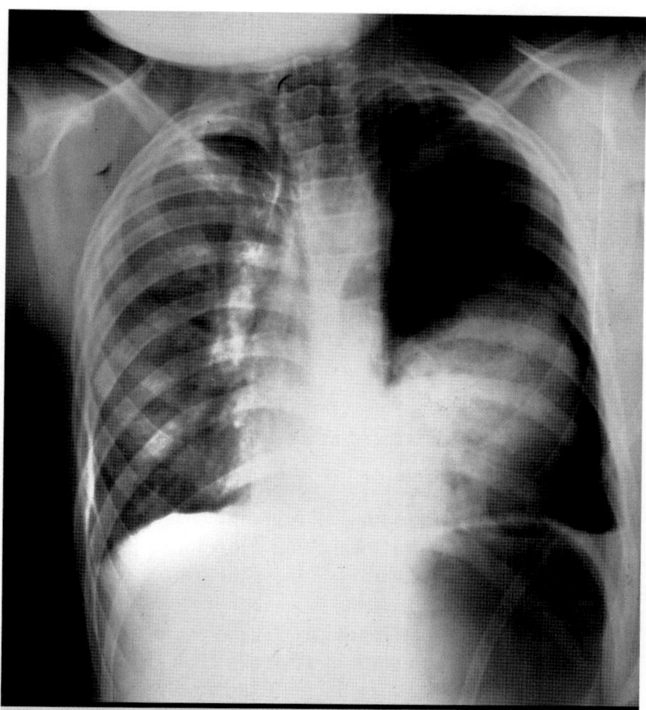

Figure 20-32. Tracheobronchial Tree Injury

This 13-year-old child was hit by a car. The AP chest x-ray demonstrates an obvious left-sided pneumothorax, but the position of the left lung is peculiar. Rather than collapsing toward the hilum, the lung seems to have fallen to the dependent portion of the thorax. This is called the "fallen-lung sign." This is an extremely rare finding on x-ray, but when present, the abnormal position of the lung, together with the left-sided pneumothorax, are highly suggestive of rupture of the tracheobronchial tree. This was confirmed on a subsequent CT scan.

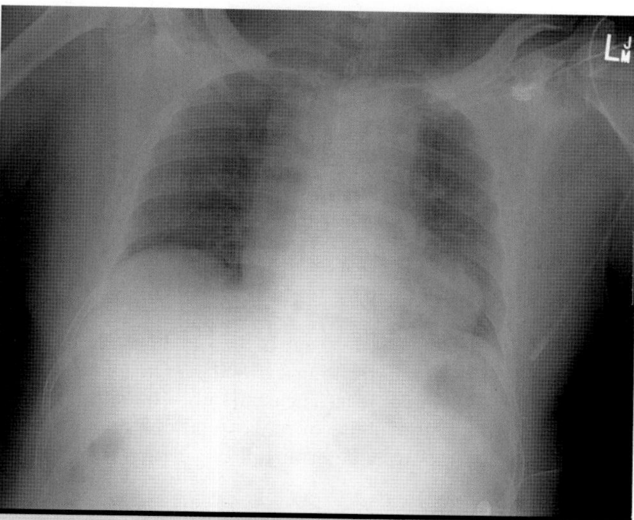

Figure 20-33. Aortic Disruption

This is an AP chest x-ray of a young man who had been struck by a minibus. He had sustained pelvic fractures as well as long-bone extremity fractures. This AP view clearly demonstrates a widened mediastinum. A subsequent CT scan confirmed that the widened mediastinum was due to a hematoma from an aortic injury.

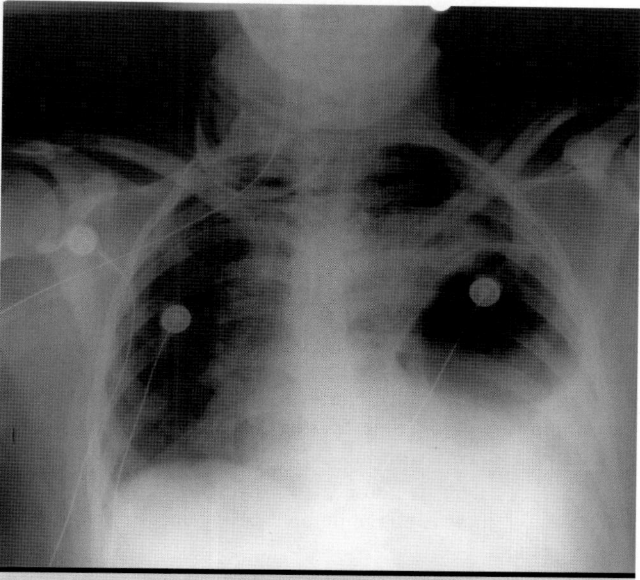

Figure 20-34. Traumatic Diaphragmatic Injury

A portable chest x-ray of a young man who sustained massive blunt abdominal trauma. There is no clear diaphragmatic contour on the left and the bowel has apparently been pushed up into the chest. An NG tube could not be passed and had doubled back on itself in the distal esophagus. Many cases of traumatic diaphragmatic rupture are far more subtle and may be difficult to diagnose, even with the aid of CT. In these less obvious cases, simple elevation of the diaphragm or blurring of its contour could be a soft sign of injury. Where the diagnosis is missed, the patient is at risk for developing herniation of bowel through the defect weeks, months, or even years after the injury.

DIAGNOSIS ABDOMINAL TRAUMA

Background

1. Trauma is the leading cause of morbidity and mortality in children more than 1 year of age in the United States. Trauma accounts for 1.5 million injuries, 500,000 hospitalizations, and 20,000 deaths per year. The availability, quality, training, and timeliness of response of prehospital care resources are a potentially important determinant of outcome in pediatric trauma.
2. Abdominal trauma is the leading cause of initially unrecognized fatal injury in children. Among the various causes of death in children suffering trauma, abdominal injuries account for about 22% of the cases.
3. Up to 20% of children who present with a normal blood pressure and a Glasgow Coma Scale score ≤10 have associated intra-abdominal injuries.

Mechanism of Injury

1. Most common causes of abdominal trauma are:
   a. Automobile occupant–related
   b. Pedestrian struck by a vehicle
   c. Falls account for a small number of abdominal injuries in children. Falls typically occur in younger children (<1 to 2 years of age), and these children more frequently sustain head and extremity injuries.
   d. Accidents involving recreational vehicles (e.g., about 25% injuries sustained by all-terrain vehicles [ATVs] are abdominal in nature)
   e. Penetrating trauma
2. Blunt trauma from motor vehicle crashes (MVCs) is the most common cause of abdominal trauma in children. Additionally, children have multisystem injuries more frequently than adults.
3. Several factors place children at increased risk of morbidity and mortality when they sustain abdominal trauma.
   a. The smaller body size of a child leads to traumatic forces that are often distributed over a smaller body mass, increasing the number of systems injured during trauma.
   b. Solid abdominal organs are proportionately larger in children than in adults. There is an increased risk of direct injury to them in blunt and penetrating injury.
   c. Young children have less well developed abdominal muscles and a more protuberant abdomen with less insulating fat.
   d. The urinary bladder is an abdominal organ in young children.

Associated Clinical Features

1. Pediatric victims of blunt trauma sustain head injury more frequently than do adults, so a history of abdominal trauma might be difficult to obtain. The younger the patient, the more difficult and less reliable the physical exam.
2. Many children swallow large amounts of air from excessive crying after trauma and develop abdominal distension, making the physical exam less reliable.
3. Most children with blunt abdominal trauma caused by MVCs also have associated nonabdominal trauma. Data from the National Pediatric Trauma Registry (NPTR) confirm that associated head injury accounts for >50% of trauma-related deaths, and thoracic injuries for 20% of deaths.
4. Hematuria is an important marker for serious renal and nonrenal trauma in children.
   a. In the presence of gross hematuria, 22% of the time there is renal trauma, but 17% of the time there is splenic injury, and in 8% hepatic injury.
   b. Hematuria alone can occur without gross renal injury (due to capillary disruption).
   c. Hematuria may be absent in up to 50% of patients with renal pedicle injuries and isolated ureteral injuries.
5. Children who are resuscitated with multiple units of blood are at risk for transfusion-related coagulopathies.
6. Mortality in children with isolated liver, spleen, kidney, or pancreatic trauma has been reported to be less than 10%. This percentage increases to 20% if the GI tract is involved, and may be as high as 50% if any major blood vessels are injured.

Emergency Department Management and Disposition

1. Details regarding the exact mechanism of injury will assist in making an early and correct diagnosis.
2. Laboratory tests:
   a. Ancillary laboratory testing rarely identifies unsuspected injuries in awake and cooperative patients. One must recognize the usefulness and limitations of individual laboratory tests.
   b. In the recent past, trauma victims were assessed with CBC, platelet counts, electrolytes, liver (LFT) and renal function tests, ABG, PT/PTT, amylase, urinalysis, and a type and cross-match. This management has recently been scrutinized. A report of a review of 3939 laboratory screening tests in 285 consecutive children with minimal to moderate injury and 91 patients with proven abdominal injury found that a thorough abdominal exam combined with a urinalysis could detect 98% of all injuries.
   c. A reasonable diagnostic approach in hemodynamically stable children with blunt abdominal trauma would be to obtain baseline hemoglobin (Hgb), serum amylase, urinalysis, and a type and screen or cross-match.

d. LFTs may be very useful in assessing the severity of blunt abdominal trauma. If aspartate aminotransferase is >450 units/L and the alanine aminotransferase is >250, there is 100% sensitivity and 92% specificity for detecting hepatic trauma.

e. Serum amylase and lipase values are commonly elevated in patients with blunt abdominal trauma. The sensitivity of these tests in proving pancreatic injury increases with serial values. Amylase and lipase have little utility in differentiating between pancreatic and nonpancreatic insult.

3. Plain abdominal radiographs:
   a. Serve a major role in penetrating trauma (identification of foreign bodies and detection of pneumoperitoneum)
   b. Plain radiographs are often normal (>95%) in cases of blunt abdominal trauma.

4. FAST (Focused abdominal sonography for trauma; Fig. 20-35)
   a. Abdominal ultrasound can be used to rule in intraabdominal fluid or organ damage in children.
   b. Negative us does not rule out intraabdominal injury and if clinical suspicion persists, abdominal computed tomography (CT) scanning should be performed.

5. The radiologic procedure of choice for evaluating stable trauma patients is CT scanning.
   a Indications for abdominal and pelvic CT scan include:
      1) Suspected blunt abdominal trauma
      2) Significant fluid resuscitation (without obvious foci of blood loss)
      3) Multisystem trauma
      4) A Hgb of <10 g/dL without obvious blood loss and/or hematuria
   b. All solid organ injuries and about 96% of hollow viscus injuries are identified by CT scan.
   c. CT scan will identify most significant solid viscus injury, including hepatic, splenic, adrenal, and renal (and assist with grading such injuries).
   d. CT scanning may miss some mesenteric injuries, but peritoneal lavage is useful for discriminating between mesenteric injury and bowel perforation (immediate clinical symptoms of mesenteric injuries include hypotension secondary to hemorrhage, abdominal distention, pain, and tenderness).

6. Once hemoglobin and hematocrit (Hct) values have been obtained and are being followed serially, the goal is to maintain the Hct values above 30% (some experts allow the hemoglobin to fall to 7 g/dL before blood transfusion, only if the patient remains hemodynamically stable).

7. Laparotomy is indicated if 40 to 50% of the patient's blood volume has been replaced in the first 24 hours.

8. There is still debate regarding the management of microscopic hematuria. Renal imaging is indicated only in children with abdominal trauma if they have another indication for the CT (e.g., severe pain or more than 50 RBCs/high power field [hpf]).

9. Children with documented abdominal injuries or multiple organ system injuries should be admitted to a pediatric ICU. Any child with a significant mechanism of injury should be hospitalized for observation. Many experts believe that the optimal location for the treatment of children with acute trauma is a designated pediatric center. If specialty expertise is unavailable, patients with significant trauma should be stabilized and transferred to a regional trauma center.

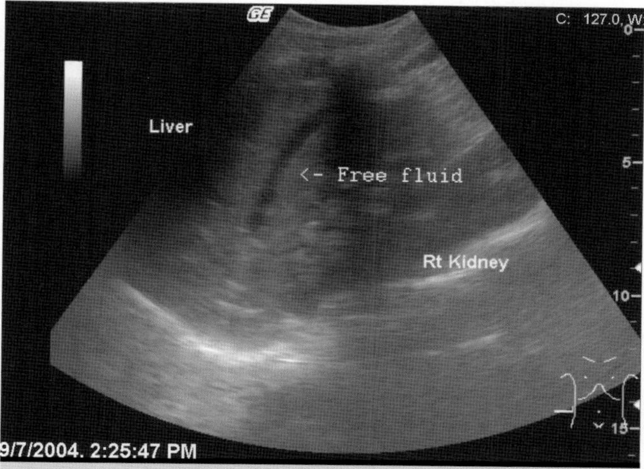

Figure 20-35. Positive FAST Examination

A FAST (*f*ocused *a*bdominal *s*onography for *t*rauma) exam of a 15-year-old male who was brought to the ED after being struck by a car. This study was performed in the ED. The lucent line between the kidney and liver is indicative of free fluid, in this case blood. The patient was successfully resuscitated and maintained perfusion, and further work-up failed to reveal any additional life-threatening injuries. His liver laceration was successfully embolized in the angiography suite and he did not require laparotomy.

Clinical Pearls: Abdominal Trauma

1. The spleen and the liver are the most frequently injured organs in blunt trauma (followed by the kidney, the stomach, and the intestines).
2. Children may maintain a normal blood pressure even with a significant amount of blood loss (25%). Persistent tachycardia in a trauma patient can be due to blood loss or a variety of other factors (e.g., age, pain, temperature, or stress).
3. Initial Hgb and Hct values might be normal despite significant bleeding and blood loss. Serial Hgb and Hct values are extremely useful.
4. While electrolyte abnormalities are exceedingly rare in acute trauma, a metabolic acidosis is to be expected in children in hypovolemic shock. The base deficit has proven to be a useful marker for the presence of abdominal trauma requiring surgery.
5. Hematuria is an important marker for serious renal and nonrenal trauma in children.

BOX 20-23. SPLENIC INJURY

- The spleen is the most commonly injured abdominal organ related to blunt abdominal trauma (Fig. 20-36).
- Patients who have splenic injuries may present with either diffuse abdominal pain or localized tenderness.
- Hallmarks of splenic injury:
  (1) Upper abdominal pain
  (2) Kehr's sign (left shoulder pain secondary to diaphragmatic irritation)
  (3) Left upper quadrant pain

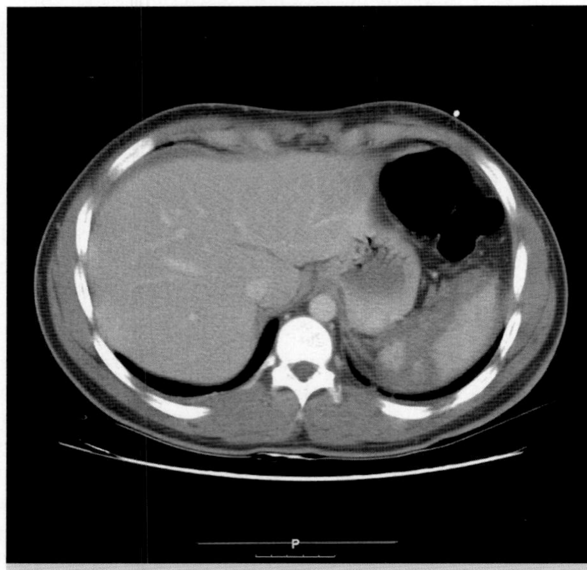

Figure 20-36. Splenic Laceration

An abdominal CT scan of a 19-year-old male who was a restrained passenger involved in a motor vehicle crash. The scan revealed a shattered spleen with hemorrhage contained within the splenic capsule.

- Abdominal radiographs occasionally reveal a medially displaced gastric bubble.
- Abdominal CT is proven accurate at identifying and grading the severity of splenic injury.
- Radionuclide splenic scan will also identify the extent of injury.
- More than 90% of splenic injuries are managed nonoperatively.
- Risk factors for predicting the need for surgery include older age, lower initial hematocrit, injury secondary to MVC, and multiple associated injuries.
- The usual indications for laparotomy include:
  (1) Child presenting with hypotension that is unresponsive to fluids and blood replacement
  (2) Child requiring >40 mL/kg of blood transfused over <24 hours
  (3) Other associated intra-abdominal injuries
- If a child has a splenic injury but does not undergo laparotomy, he or she should be admitted for close observation and serial Hct measurements.

Clinical pearls: Splenic injury

- Suspect splenic injury when children present with altered mental status, aberration of vital signs, anemia, left lower rib fractures, or persistent abdominal pain and/or grunting after abdominal trauma.
- Nonoperative management of splenic injuries has widely replaced the traditional treatment (splenectomy or splenorrhaphy).
- The decision for operative intervention is predominantly based on the child's hemodynamic stability and blood requirement, far more so than the grade of the anatomic injury.

BOX 20-24. LIVER INJURY

- The liver is the second most common solid organ to be injured in blunt trauma (Fig. 20-37).
- The liver is the most common organ to be injured in penetrating trauma.
- Liver injury is the most common lethal abdominal injury in blunt trauma.
- Suspect liver injury with right upper quadrant pain and/or tenderness.
- CT scan is still considered the gold standard for the detection and management of hepatic injury.
- The higher the grade of injury, the more likely the probability of surgery
- Usual indications for surgery include:
  - (1) Unresponsive hypotension
  - (2) Other associated injuries
  - (3) Need for a transfusion of >40 mL/kg
- Other risk factors for surgery include:
  - (1) Lower pediatric trauma score
  - (2) More than 25% lobar disruption
  - (3) Juxtahepatic venous injury
  - (4) Hepatic avulsion
  - (5) Necessity of transfusion within 2 hours of presentation
  - (6) Major hepatic vein trauma

Clinical pearls: Liver injuries

- Liver injuries are generally more severe than splenic injuries.
- Liver injuries are also more likely to rebleed.
- Some unique complications of nonoperative management include bile leaks, delayed bleeding, and hemobilia.

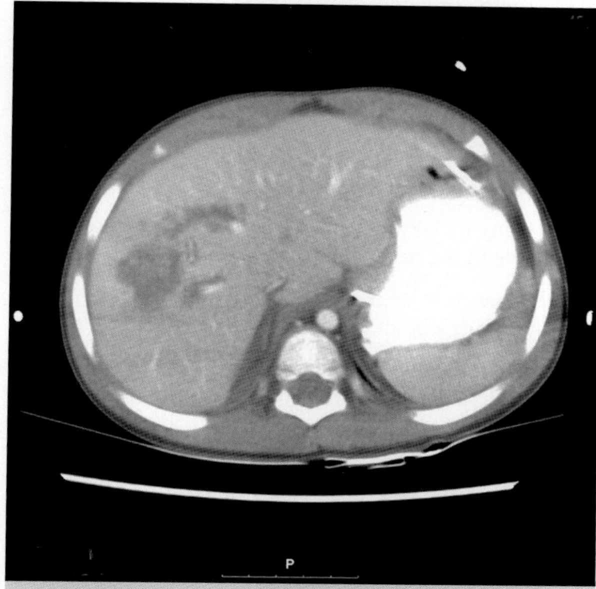

Figure 20-37 Liver Laceration

An abdominal CT scan of a 4-year-old male who was a pedestrian struck by a motor vehicle. The scan revealed a large complex laceration involving the right lobe of the liver. The laceration is seen centrally and does not reach the capsular surface. There is no active extravasation of contrast or blood. If this had been his only life-threatening injury, he would likely have done well, but unfortunately he also sustained a pelvic fracture, a femur fracture, and intracranial hemorrhage. He was successfully resuscitated but ultimately succumbed to his intracranial injuries.

BOX 20-25. RENAL TRAUMA

- Kidneys are the third most common solid organs injured via blunt force trauma (Figs. 20-38 and 20-39).
- The most commonly reported mechanism for renal trauma is related to MVCs.
- The usual mechanism of insult is direct flank impact or rapid deceleration injury.
- As many as 80% of renal injuries will have associated injuries to the head, chest, liver, and spleen.
- Less than 10% of renal injuries after blunt trauma will require surgical intervention.
- Urologists often attempt conservative management unless hypotension, urinary extravasation, or ongoing hemorrhage are present.

Clinical pearls: Renal trauma

- In the past, a cutoff of ≥20 RBCs/HPF on urinalysis generally indicated the necessity for imaging to assess potential renal injury in clinically stable patients.
- A significant number of children with posttraumatic microscopic hematuria have underlying congenital renal anomalies or minor renal injuries.
- Delayed complications of renal injury include hypertension, nephrectomy, and infection.

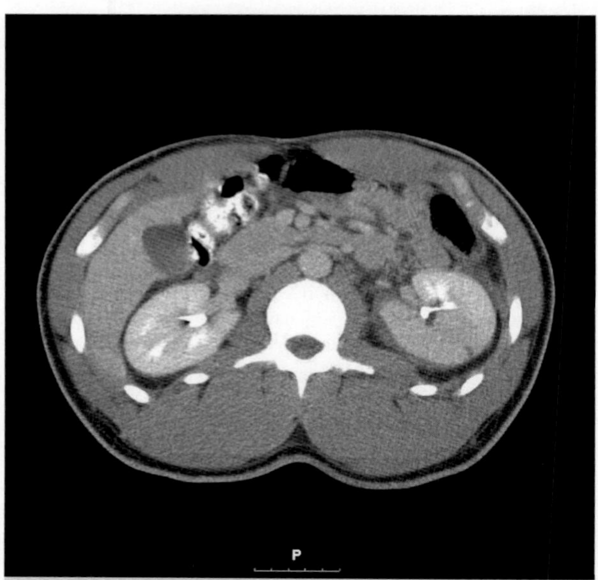

Figure 20-38. Kidney Laceration without Extravasation

An abdominal CT scan of an adolescent male who was riding on the back of a motorcycle that was involved in an crash with a car. The scan demonstrates an abnormal wedge-shaped area involving the entire posterior part of the left kidney, with a small linear low-density lesion extending to the lateral renal cortex. This region does not show contrast concentration and is suggestive of a renal laceration. There is no evidence of contrast extravasation; however, a collection is noted in the left perinephric space.

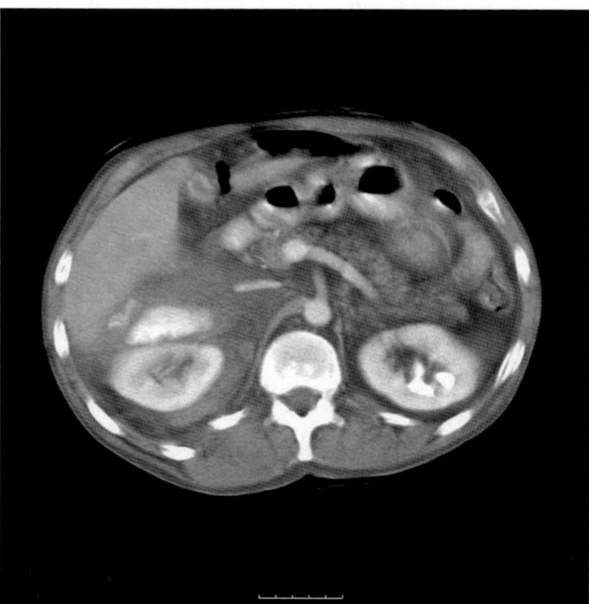

Figure 20-39. Kidney Laceration with Extravasation

An abdominal CT scan of a young male struck by a car. There is evidence of a fracture seen through the anterosuperior portion of the upper pole of the right kidney. The fracture line extends from the renal hilum to the lateral cortex. Significant extravasation of intravenous contrast is seen around the fractured fragment. A large perinephric hematoma is also seen. On delayed sections not shown here, contrast was seen to opacify only one of two calyces on the right, and there was delayed excretion by the right kidney, which suggested a renal pedicle injury.

BOX 20-26. GASTROINTESTINAL INJURIES

- The most common mechanisms associated with GI injuries include direct trauma, seat belt–related injuries, handlebar injuries, and penetrating trauma.
- The jejunum is most commonly injured, followed by the duodenum, ileum, and cecum.
- Initial signs and symptoms of GI perforation may be so mild that there may be a clinical delay of 12 to 18 hours before the diagnosis is made.
- Peritoneal signs are initially present in only 30 to 38% of patients with bowel injury (far fewer have evidence of pneumoperitoneum).
- Physical exam findings in children with GI injuries are often very benign; however, all children with bowel perforation will eventually develop peritonitis, fever, and tachycardia over a 12- to 24-hour period.
- Free air may only be present 30 to 47% of the time.
- Consider other nonspecific findings of bowel injury, including free intraperitoneal fluid, bowel wall thickening or enhancement, bowel dilation, or mesenteric infiltration.
- Pediatric surgery must be consulted when there is clinical or radiologic evidence of bowel injury.
- If an immediate diagnostic peritoneal lavage is performed, an elevated RBC count ($>$100,000 RBCs/mm^3) or evidence of bile, particulate matter, elevated lavage amylase, or alkaline phosphatase is suggestive of bowel injury.

Clinical pearls: Gastrointestinal injuries

- The presence of abdominal ecchymosis in a child after a seat belt–related injury signifies a 50% or greater chance of harboring an intra-abdominal injury.
- CT scan cannot reliably exclude bowel injury.
- Only careful repeated examinations will allow for early detection of all bowel injuries.
- All children who are at risk for bowel injury (e.g., seat belt and handlebar injuries) require surgical admission, close observation, and serial exams, in addition to diagnostic imaging.

BOX 20-27. LAP SEAT BELT INJURY

- A constellation of symptoms ("lap belt complex") can occur in children who have a seat belt applied inappropriately (Fig. 20-40).
- It generally occurs in young children (4 to 9 years of age) who are wearing seat belts that have been improperly positioned over their immature iliac crests.
- When there is rapid deceleration of the vehicle, the lap belt can migrate onto the abdomen.
- Typical injuries include:
  (1) Small bowel contusions and lacerations
  (2) Lumbar flexion-distraction injuries
  (3) Lumbar spine fractures
  (4) Chance fracture (lumbar spine flexion injuries with distraction of the posterior elements)

Clinical pearl: Lap belt injury

- Abdominal ecchymosis due to lap belt use signifies a high risk of intra-abdominal injury, but the absence of it does not exclude it.
- The most common site of intestinal injury is the jejunum, followed by the duodenum, ileum, and cecum.
- Other injuries may include mesenteric hematomas, bladder disruption, diaphragm rupture, renal trauma, pelvic fractures, and pulmonary contusions.

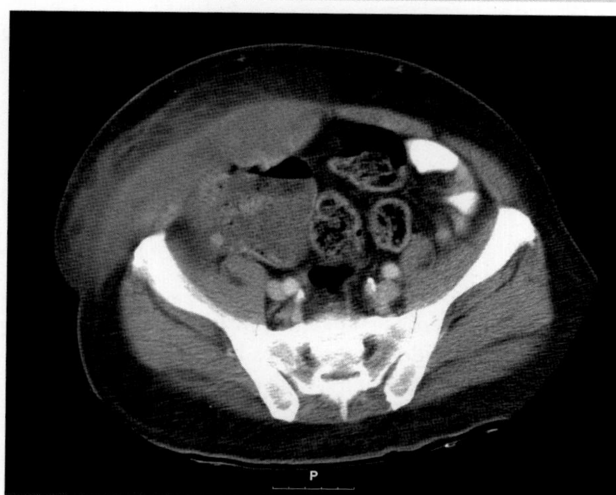

Figure 20-40. Rectus Muscle Hematoma

An abdominal CT scan of a 16-year-old male who was the back seat passenger in a car involved in an MVC. He was only wearing the lap portion of the restraint and presented to the ED complaining of right-sided abdominal pain. As he was hemodynamically stable without a base deficit he was sent for a CT scan, which demonstrated a large rectus muscle hematoma. Fortunately, he did not sustain a spinal injury, which is more commonly associated with this type of mechanism.

BOX 20-28. BICYCLE-RELATED INJURIES

- Bicycle-related injuries mainly occur when a child loses control of the bicycle or when he or she is struck by a car while riding.
- The most frequently incurred injuries are extremity fractures and trauma to the head and neck.
- A common mechanism of injury is a child falling forward and striking the abdomen against the handlebars.
- If a child presents with symptoms consistent with a significant handlebar injury, the child should have a CT scan and be admitted for observation.

Clinical pearls: Bicycle-related injuries

- Handlebar injuries are often interpreted as trivial by evaluating physicians when they initially examine the child (prior to the onset of severe pain and vomiting).
- The average reported delay to diagnosis of intra-abdominal injury is about 23 hours.
- The most common abdominal injuries are traumatic pancreatitis, renal and splenic trauma, duodenal hematoma, bowel perforation, and hepatic trauma.

BOX 20-29. PEDESTRIAN INJURIES

- These are the second most common cause of abdominal trauma in children.
- The most common associated injuries include those to the extremities (44%) and head (32%).
- A child's mortality is related to the extent of multisystem trauma (80% of deaths result from head trauma).

Clinical pearls: Pedestrian injuries

- Patient age is a very important determinant of location and type of injury.
- Children <5 years of age are more likely to sustain crush injuries to the head and trunk (because of their short stature and site of impact).
- Children >5 years of age are more likely to sustain impact-related injuries.
- Waddel's triad is a classic example of the constellation of injuries associated with an impact injury. It consists of left-sided abdominal trauma (spleen), extremity trauma (femur fracture), and closed head injury.

BOX 20-30. PENETRATING TRAUMA

- Penetrating injuries (stab and gunshot wounds) account for far fewer abdominal injuries in children (only 1.5% of all trauma admissions) than other means.
- It is estimated that gunshot wounds occur twice as often as stabbings.
- The GI tract and liver are the most commonly injured sites (Fig. 20-41).
- Any penetrating injury that occurs below the nipples anteriorly and the scapula posteriorly can potentially involve the peritoneal cavity.
- It has been reported that 30 to 40% of thoracic gunshot wounds have associated abdominal injuries.
- Absolute indications for laparotomy include any of the following: abdominal tenderness away from the location of the stab wound, hypotension, evisceration, or ongoing blood loss.
- Pneumoperitoneum, unexplained fever, and leukocytosis are considered relative indications for laparotomy.

Clinical pearls: Penetrating trauma

- Gunshot wounds to the abdomen generally require surgery.

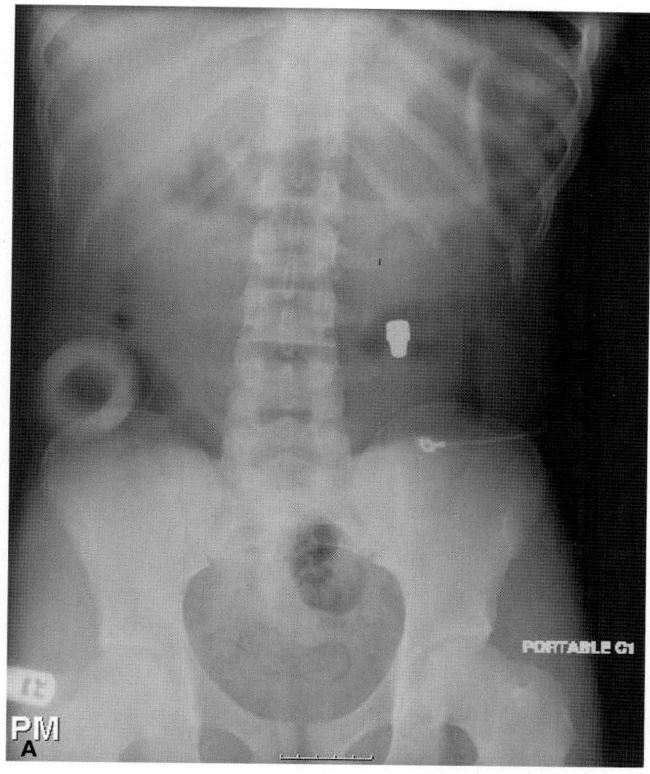

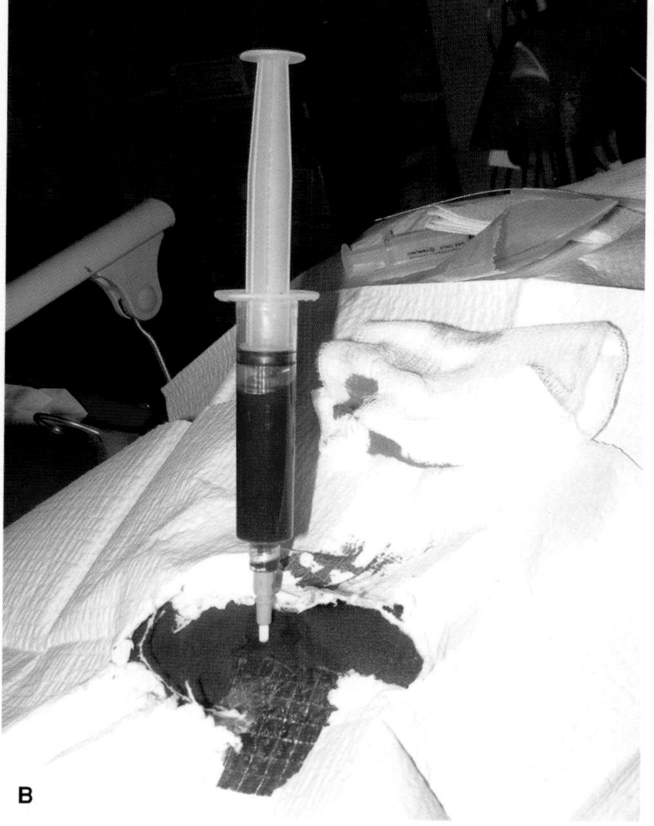

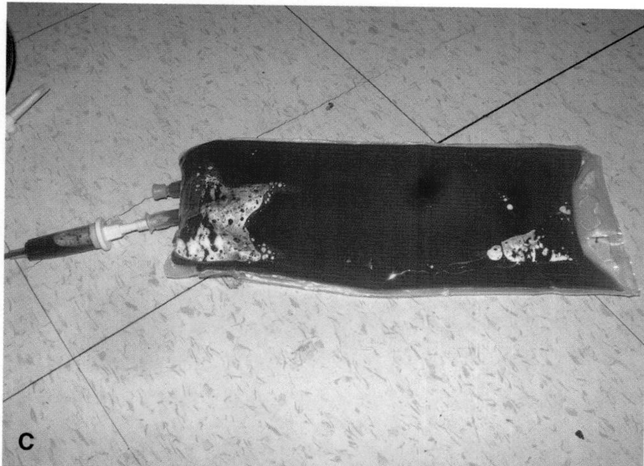

Figure 20-41. Gunshot Wound to the Abdomen with Diagnostic Peritoneal Lavage

A. An abdominal flat plate of a 16-year-old female who was caught in a cross-fire and sustained a gunshot wound to the abdomen. This x-ray was obtained because she was hemodynamically stable without a base deficit or peritoneal signs. The surface wound was tangential and could have been mistaken for a graze. The radiograph demonstrates the intra-abdominal metallic foreign body, which turned out to be the bullet. The decision to perform a diagnostic peritoneal lavage was made, and to the surprise of the ED team, the tap was positive (*B*). She was subsequently rushed to the operating room. *C*. A different patient who sustained blunt abdominal trauma in an MVC also underwent an diagnostic peritoneal lavage. The tap was negative, but as one can see in the image, the lavage fluid on the floor of the resuscitation room appears to be positive for blood. Indeed, analysis of the fluid demonstrated a RBC count of $>100{,}000/\text{mm}^3$. Exploratory laparotomy identified a liver laceration, which was successfully repaired. With the advent of ED ultrasound, the role of diagnostic peritoneal lavage is becoming increasingly limited.

BOX 20-31. PANCREATIC INJURIES

- The most common mechanisms for pancreatic injuries include bicycle handlebar injury, MVCs, and direct blows to the abdomen.
- The classic triad of epigastric pain, a palpable abdominal mass, and hyperamylasemia are detected only rarely in children, and furthermore may develop very slowly.
- Abdominal ultrasound and contrast CT are used to make the diagnosis.
- Simple pancreatitis is treated with bowel rest and nasogastric decompression.
- A transection of the pancreas requires surgical repair.

Clinical pearls: Pancreatic injuries

- Traumatic pancreatitis is notoriously difficult to diagnose, as both CT scan and laboratory tests may be normal in early injury. Over time an elevated amylase will ensue.
- An elevated serum amylase should suggest the possibility of pancreatic injury, but the absolute value does not directly correlate with the severity of injury.
- Pancreatic pseudocysts occur fairly commonly (in 38 to 78% of cases and approximately 3 to 7 days after the injury).

BOX 20-32. ABDOMINAL TRAUMA DUE TO CHILD ABUSE

- Many factors make the diagnosis of abuse and its underlying injuries difficult.
- Male caretakers are the usual offenders and most caregivers presenting to the ED may be reluctant to provide an accurate and detailed history.
- Mortality is extremely high (45 to 50%) secondary to delays in presentation and the extent of injury.
- In order of decreasing frequency, inflicted abdominal injuries include ruptured liver or spleen, intestinal perforation, duodenal hematoma, pancreatic injury, and kidney trauma.
- In most cases of child abuse with intra-abdominal injuries, there are also other associated traumatic injuries (soft tissue injuries such as bruises in 95%, head trauma in 45%, fractures in 27%, and skull fractures estimated to be in 18% of the cases).
- Consultations should include pediatric surgery, child protective services, social workers, primary care providers, and law enforcement personnel.

Clinical pearls: Abdominal trauma due to child abuse

- Liver and spleen injuries are the most common types of intra-abdominal injury seen in child abuse.
- Other injuries include duodenojejunal rupture, duodenal rupture, and pancreatic and vena cava trauma.
- The most common presentation is shock, but massive intra-abdominal bleeding and peritonitis may also occur after hollow viscus rupture, and a clinical picture of an obstructive pattern may also ensue with bilious emesis.
- Suspect abusive abdominal trauma in any child with unexplained peritonitis or shock (especially in the presence of bilious vomiting and/or anemia).

DIAGNOSIS PELVIC TRAUMA

Definition

1. Type I: single fracture of the pelvic bone without a fracture of the pelvic ring
2. Type II: single fracture of the pelvic ring without displacement
3. Type III: double fracture of the pelvic ring with a free floating segment. Examples:
   a. Malgaigne fracture
   b. Straddle fracture
4. Type IV: acetabular fracture

Mechanism of Injury

Usually results from a strong external force applied to the pelvis, as in a fall from a significant height, high-impact MVC, or a pedestrian struck by a motor vehicle

Associated Clinical Features

1. Ecchymosis over the pubis, iliac wings, scrotum, or labia may suggest pelvic fractures.
2. Injuries to intraperitoneal and retroperitoneal visceral and vascular structures are commonly associated with pelvic fractures.
3. Assessment of peripheral pulses can identify vascular injuries associated with pelvic fractures.

Laboratory Tests

1. An anteroposterior radiograph in the ED is the initial diagnostic test of choice (Fig. 20-42).
2. Subtle fractures may be picked up on oblique, lateral, inlet, or 35° AP views.
3. CT scanning is more sensitive for acetabular and sacral fractures.
4. CT scanning is also very helpful in evaluating the posterior pelvis and determining hematoma size.
5. A retrograde urethrogram to evaluate the lower genitourinary tract is essential with anterior pelvic fractures, and in males with blood at the penile meatus, a movable high-riding prostate, or scrotal hematoma (Fig. 20-43).

Complications

1. Hemorrhagic shock
2. Neurologic injuries, especially with sacral fractures
3. Urologic injury
4. Pulmonary and fat emboli

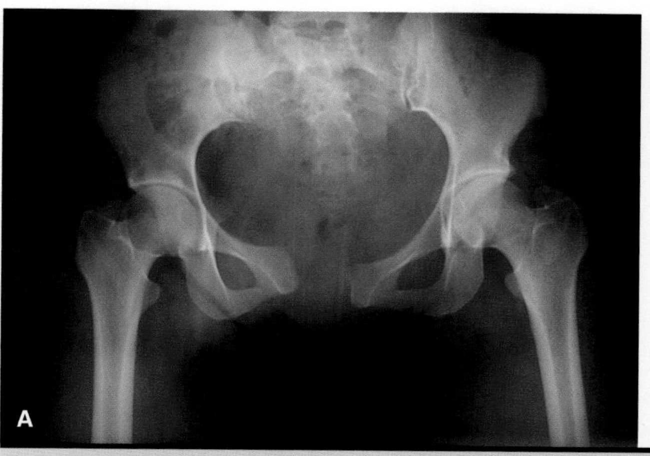

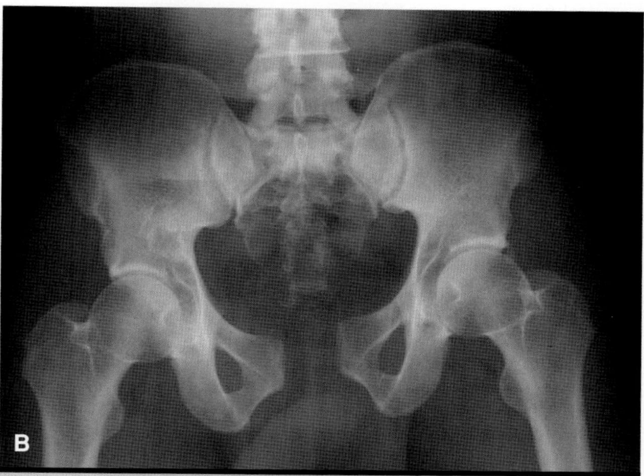

Figure 20-42. Pelvic Fractures

A. Pelvic radiograph of an adolescent who was struck by a car and sustained injury due to an AP compression mechanism. The AP force caused a rupture of the anterior pelvis (symphysis pubis) and disruption of the right sacroiliac joint. Note the compression and loss of joint space of the right sacroiliac joint, in comparison to the left sacroiliac joint. In this type of fracture, in addition to the disruption of the ligament holding together the symphysis pubis, the anterior sacroiliac, sacrotuberous, and sacrospinous ligaments on the affected side would have also been disrupted. *B*. Pelvic radiograph of another youth who was also struck by a car. Again there is widening of the symphysis pubis due to the AP compression forces. In addition, in this x-ray the right sacroiliac joint is markedly widened, and this is commonly known as an "open-book pelvis." In addition to the more anterior ligamentous structures disrupted seen in the patient in *A*, this patient also had disruption of the posterior sacroiliac ligaments. Posterior involvement increases the risk for excessive bleeding, and indeed this patient required fluid and blood resuscitation, as well as an emergent trip to the angiography suite for embolization of the bleeding vessels.

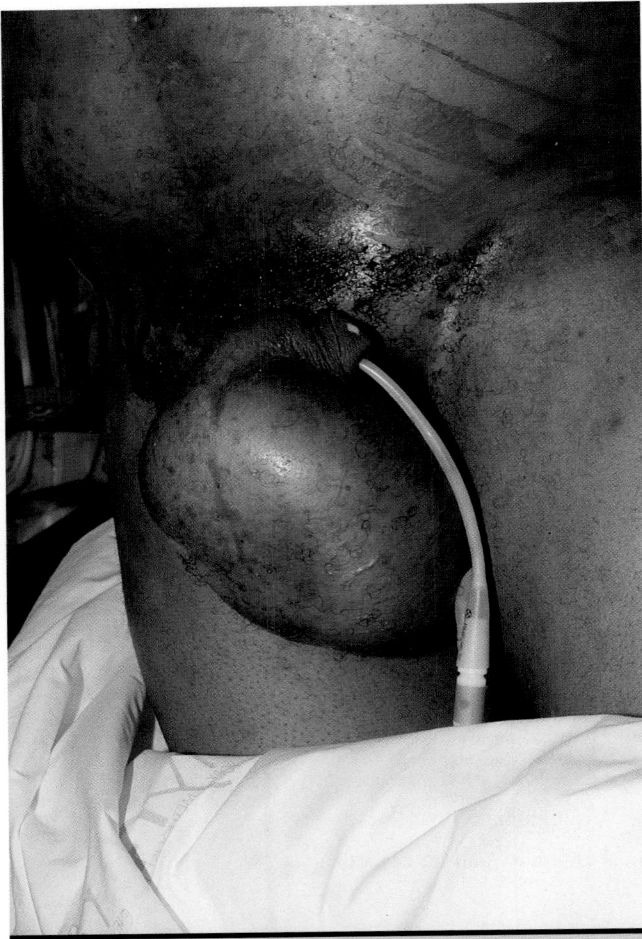

Figure 20-43. Scrotal Hematoma

An image of the same patient shown in Fig. 20-42a, who was a pedestrian struck by an automobile. This image demonstrates his large scrotal hematoma, which was subtle upon presentation, but increased dramatically during his short stay in the ED. After his "open-book pelvic fracture" was demonstrated on x-ray and his scrotal hematoma was discovered on physical examination, a retrograde urethrogram was performed, which showed no injury to the urethra. Only then was the Foley catheter seen in this image placed.

Consultation

Emergent orthopedic and trauma consultation is necessary for all pelvic fractures.

Emergency Department Treatment and Disposition

1. Type I and II fractures are stable fractures.
2. Type III and IV fractures are unstable fractures.
3. IV resuscitation with two large-bore lines should be placed in all patients with pelvic fractures before there is any evidence of hemorrhagic shock.
4. Since children who do not respond to fluid resuscitation have the highest mortality, resuscitation with blood should be instituted for those with worsening base deficits.
5. There should be emergent immobilization by orthopedics for any unstable fractures.

Clinical Pearls: Pelvic Fractures

1. There is a high incidence of concomitant injuries including head, intra-abdominal, and long bone injuries.
2. The pelvis is shaped like a pretzel, so it is extremely rare for there to be a disruption of the ring in one location, without a second ring disruption in a different location.
3. There is often an associated hip dislocation.
4. There is a high association of genitourinary injury in males. A high-riding prostate, blood at the penile meatus, or a scrotal hematoma mandates a retrograde urethrogram.
5. As increased level of suspicion, due either to the mechanism of injury or peroneal tenderness, should also trigger an investigation. In fact, all pelvic fractures are assumed to have accompanying urologic injury until proven otherwise.
6. When pain is elicited on manipulation of the iliac wings or when a pelvic ring fracture is diagnosed, further distraction or manipulation of the ring can cause increased bleeding and should be strictly avoided.
7. Hemorrhagic shock is the leading cause of death in pelvic fractures.
8. Children who do not respond to transfusions equal to the estimated total blood volume (TBV = 88 mL/kg times the child's weight in kilograms) are likely to have major vascular injuries and are likely to require embolization.
9. Posterior involvement, especially sacroiliac fractures, are associated with the most significant bleeding.
10. Seemingly hemodynamically stable patients can deteriorate very quickly.
11. Base deficits should be obtained upon arrival and repeated, as it is an early indicator of shock.

BOX 20-33. CLINICAL FEATURES OF PELVIC FRACTURES

- Physical examination in unconscious patients or patients with distracting injuries is unreliable.
- Patients may present in hemorrhagic shock due to retroperitoneal blood loss.
- Direct, gentle palpation of the symphysis pubis, sacroiliac joints, and sacrum may elicit pain in the nonimpaired, alert patient.
- Medial or posterior pressure on each iliac wing will elicit pain.

BOX 20-34. DIFFERENTIAL DIAGNOSIS OF PELVIC FRACTURES

- Hip fracture
- Lumbar-sacral fracture
- Bony contusion
- Buttock or rectal injury
- Bladder rupture
- Genital injury

Suggested Readings

Amsterdam JT: Dental emergencies: Part I—Pain and trauma. *Emerg Med* 1994;26:21.

Bliss D, Silen M: Pediatric thoracic trauma. *Crit Care Med* 2002;30(11 Suppl):S409.

Brown RL, Brunn MA, Garcia VF: Cervical spine injuries in children: a review of 103 patients treated consecutively at a level 1 pediatric trauma center. *J Pediatr Surg* 2001;36:1107.

Cantor RM, Leaming JM: Evaluation and management of pediatric major trauma. *Contemp Issues Trauma* 1998;16:229.

Centers for Disease Control and Prevention: Childhood injuries in the United States. Division of Injury Control. Center for Environmental Health and Injury Control, Centers for Disease Control and Prevention. *Am J Dis Child* 1990;144:627.

Cooper A, Foltin GL: Thoracic trauma. In: Barkin R (ed.) *Pediatric Emergency Medicine: Concepts and Clinical Practice*, 2nd ed. Mosby, Philadelphia,1997, p. 318.

Dormans JP: Evaluation of children with suspected cervical spine injury. *J Bone Joint Surg Am* 2002;84-A:124.

Furnival RA: Controversies in pediatric thoracic and abdominal trauma. *Clin Pediatr Emerg Med* 2001;2:48.

Gaines BA, Ford HR: Abdominal and pelvic trauma in children. *Crit Care Med* 2002;30(11 Suppl):S416.

Garcia VF, Gotschall CS, Eichelberger MR, Bowman LM: Rib fractures in children: a marker of severe trauma. *J Trauma* 1990;30:695.

Gassner R, Tuli T, Hächl O, Moreira R, Ulmer H: Craniomaxillofacial trauma in children: a review of 3385 cases with 6060 injuries in 10 years. *J Oral Maxillofacial Surg* 2004;62:399.

Greenes DS, Schutzman SA: Clinical indicators of intracranial injury in head-injured infants. *Pediatrics* 1999;104:861.

Greenes DS, Schutzman SA: Isolated skull fractures in infants: what are their clinical characteristics, and do they require hospitalization? *Ann Emerg Med* 1997;30:253.

Haug RH, Foss J: Maxillofacial injuries in the pediatric patient. *Oral Surg Oral Med Oral Pathol Oral Radiol Endodontics* 2000;90:126.

Holland AJ, Broome C, Steinberg A, Cass DT: Facial fractures in children. *Pediatr Emerg Care* 2001;17:157.

Holmes JF, Sokolove PE, Brant WE, Kuppermann N: A clinical decision rule for identifying children with thoracic injuries after blunt torso trauma. *Ann Emerg Med* 2002;39:537.

Kadish H: Thoracic trauma. In: Fleisher G, Ludwig S (eds.) *Textbook of Pediatric Emergency Medicine*, 4th ed. Baltimore, Lippincott Williams & Wilkins, 2000, p. 1341.

Klauber MR, Marshall LF, Luerssen TG, et al: Determinants of head injury mortality: importance of the low risk patient. *Neurosurgery* 1989;24:31.

Koltai PJ, Rabkin D: Management of facial trauma in children. *Pediatr Clin North Am* 1996;43:1253.

Krasner P: Modern treatment of avulsed teeth by emergency physicians. *Am J Emerg Med* 1994;12:241.

Kureishi A, Chow AW: The tender tooth: Dentoalveolar, pericoronal and periodontal infections. *Infect Dis Clin North Am* 1988; 2:163.

Proctor M: Spinal cord injury. *Crit Care Med* 2002;30(Suppl):S489.

Reynolds R: Pediatric spinal injury. *Curr Opin Pediatr* 2000;12:67.

Roche C, Carty HL: Spinal trauma in children. *Pediatr Radiol* 2001;31:677.

Rothrock SG, Green SM, Morgan R: Abdominal trauma in infants and children: Prompt identification and early management of serious and life-threatening injuries. Part I: Injury patterns and initial assessment. *Pediatr Emerg Care* 2000;16:106. Part II: Specific injuries and ED management. *Pediatr Emerg Care* 2000;16:189.

Schafermeyer RW: Pediatric trauma. *Emerg Med Clin North Am* 1993;11:187.

Schneider K, Segal G: Dental abscess. *EMedicine J* 2002;3(4).

Shusterman S: Pediatric dental update. *Pediatr Rev* 1994;15:311.

Towbin JA, Gajarski RJ: Cardiac troponin I: A new diagnostic gold standard of cardiac injury in children? *J Pediatr* 1997;130:853.

Viccellio P, Simon H, Pressman B, et al: A prospective multicenter study of cervical spine injury in children. *Pediatrics* 2001;108:E20.

INDEX

Note: Page numbers followed by *f* indicate figures; page numbers followed by *b* indicate boxes